NEONATAL DERMATOLOGY

Renewing Items

Commissioning Editor: Karen Bowler
Development Editor: Nani Clansey
Project Manager: Kathryn Mason
Design Manager: Judith Wright
Designer: Charles Gray
Illustration Manager: Merlyn Harvey
Illustrator: Danny Pyne
Marketing Manager(s) (UK/USA): Clara Toombs/Kathy Neely

NEONATAL DERMATOLOGY
Second Edition

Lawrence F. Eichenfield MD
Professor of Pediatrics and Medicine (Dermatology)
University of California, San Diego School of Medicine
Chief, Division of Pediatric and Adolescent Dermatology
Rady Children's Hospital, San Diego
San Diego, California
USA

Ilona J. Frieden MD
Professor of Dermatology and Pediatrics
Chief, Division of Pediatric Dermatology
University of California, San Francisco School of Medicine
San Francisco, California
USA

Nancy B. Esterly MD
Professor Emerita of Dermatology and Pediatrics
Medical College of Wisconsin
Milwaukee, Wisconsin
USA

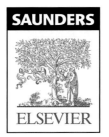
SAUNDERS
ELSEVIER

SAUNDERS
ELSEVIER

Mosby is an affiliate of Elsevier Inc.

First edition 2001
© 2008, Elsevier Inc. All rights reserved.

978-1-4160-3432-2

British Library Cataloguing in Publication Data
A catalogue record for this book is available from the British Library

Library of Congress Cataloging in Publication Data
A catalog record for this book is available from the Library of Congress

Notice
Medical knowledge is constantly changing. Standard safety precautions must be followed, but as new research and clinical experience broaden our knowledge, changes in treatment and drug therapy may become necessary or appropriate. Readers are advised to check the most current product information provided by the manufacturer of each drug to be administered to verify the recommended dose, the method and duration of administration, and contraindications. It is the responsibility of the practitioner, relying on experience and knowledge of the patient, to determine dosages and the best treatment for each individual patient. Neither the Publisher nor the author assume any liability for any injury and/or damage to persons or property arising from this publication.
The Publisher

Printed in China
Last digit is the print number: 9   8   7   6   5   4   3   2   1

Contents

Foreword

In the 33 years since Larry Solomon and Nancy Esterly first wrote a monograph devoted to describing skin diseases of the newborn, the field of neonatology has changed from a descriptive one (without a physiological or biochemical basis to recommend treatment), to one in which the molecular pathogenesis for many disorders is now known. Although many of these disorders are quite rare, clinicians are now able to identify them with great precision, tailor therapies, and offer families genetic counseling and prognostic information that, until recently, were unknowns. The skin offers extraordinary opportunities for gene transfer, not only to treat rare metabolic disorders, but also to deliver immunomodulatory agents (e.g., IL-12) and/or growth factors to aid healing. With its unique capacity to heal without scar formation, the skin of the young fetus can teach us much about wound repair.

Over the last 30 years, the increased survival rate of extremely low birth weight (ELBW) infants has posed the greatest challenge in the neonatal ICU. Neonatologists have long recognized that the skin of the premature newborn infant is unusual, but until recently did not appreciate the magnitude of the physiological, biochemical and structural differences, nor conceived of potential interventions to lessen morbidities. For example, the vernix caseosa has been shown to contain a significant number of antimicrobial substances, including the defensins, lactoferrin, lysozyme, bactericidal/permeability-increasing protein, calprotectin, secretory leukocyte protease inhibitor and a cathelicidin [LL-37]. Beta defensins and LL-37 protect epithelial surfaces. On dry epithelia, they function as 'preservatives.' On mucosal surfaces, they can be secreted into the biofilm that covers the epithelial surface, creating a milieu that is antibacterial. The presence of vernix in fetal life may help prevent infections from microorganisms colonizing the amniotic fluid. Vernix caseosa may also enhance wound healing and has been suggested as a possible treatment for burn patients. The loss of the vernix caseosa with washing and handling not only increases the magnitude of insensible water losses, but also alters the types of skin bacteria, and may increase susceptibility to nosocomial infection. Hospital-acquired infections are a major problem worldwide; they increase mortality, prolong hospitalization and are associated with adverse neurodevelopmental outcomes. Breaches in skin integrity (through the use of central lines and venous/capillary sampling) are likely a major contributor to this increased risk of infection in hospitalized newborn infants. The application of topical emollients (e.g., sunflower seed oil) can improve skin integrity (thereby decreasing insensible water losses) and may also be a useful strategy to decrease the risk of nosocomial infections in selected high-risk populations.

The first edition of *Neonatal Dermatology* was a remarkable achievement and brought the subspecialty of neonatal dermatology into the modern era. The second edition comprehensively addresses the questions of practicing neonatologists and pediatricians as well as pediatric subspecialists. For example, the addition of algorithms to aid in differential diagnosis and new chapters on topics such as *Diaper Dermatitis* will certainly be of great interest to practitioners, while the additional basic science information and new chapters on *Erythrodermas, Immunodeficiency, and Metabolic Disorders* will be welcomed by pediatric-subspecialists (geneticists, neurologists, hematologists, oncologists and dermatologists). The extensive number of detailed photographs has been increased by thirty percent. Furthermore, the up-to-date references and the clarity of prose that characterized the last edition have been retained. This textbook represents an extraordinary accomplishment for Drs Eichenfield, Frieden and Esterly, and they should be congratulated.

By Richard A. Polin MD
Professor of Pediatrics
Columbia-Babies & Childrens Hospital
New York
USA

Preface

Seven years have passed since the publication of the first edition of this textbook. For Nan, this book reflects a lifelong interest in the newborn skin and the joys and challenges of teaching. For Larry and Ilona it was a tremendous opportunity to work with our co-editor Nancy Esterly. We thank her for her inspiration in helping us create this book, and for holding the bar for academic rigor high in pediatric dermatology, a field which she helped to create as the 'mother of pediatric dermatology' and editor *par excellence*.

While no book is perfect, we have been gratified by the success of the first edition, both in its brisk sales and, more importantly, in its use as an authoritative reference. In our own busy clinical practices we have turned to the textbook again and again as we try to diagnose or think about management of infants and newborns with skin diseases. For us, the first edition truly passed the 'use test,' as attested to by the frayed copies in our offices and clinics.

For this second edition, we faced an important question: how could we make it better, and even more useful? The first and most obvious way was to add more high-quality photographs of both common and uncommon conditions. We have increased our photo number by 212. We have also added several new chapters. 'Diaper Area Eruptions' highlights, with both illustrations and text, the multitude of conditions which can present in this anatomic area. A chapter on 'Epidermolysis Bullosa' emphasizes the diagnosis and management of this group of genetic diseases, which pose tremendous management challenges in affected newborns. All chapters in the book have been updated and several chapters, including 'Vascular Birthmarks' and 'Selected Genetic Disorders,' have been extensively revised, since these are subjects where knowledge is rapidly changing.

Although the text title is *Neonatal Dermatology*, this scope of the book's content goes beyond the neonatal period well into infancy. As a direct result of our commitment to this, we have devoted an entire chapter to 'Eczematous Disorders', with a particular emphasis on atopic dermatitis, which can begin in the neonatal period but becomes increasingly common and significant soon afterwards.

As in the first edition, we were blessed to have had help from many generous colleagues from all over the world, who contributed their time and expertise to make this second edition even better than the first. We thank them for their great efforts in helping this book live up to its potential as a day-to-day resource for evaluating infants and newborns. We also thank the tremendously supportive colleagues, medical staff and administrative support teams in our workplaces, and our patients who continue to inspire us.

LFE
IJF
NBE

List of Contributors

Richard J. Antaya MD
Associate Professor of Dermatology
and Pediatrics
Director, Pediatric Dermatology
Yale University School of Medicine
New Haven, CT
USA

Eulalia Baselga MD
Pediatric Dermatologist
Hospital de la Santa Creu i. Saint Pau
Barcelona, Spain
Consultant Pediatric Dermatologist
Department of Dermatology
Institut Universitari Dexeus
Barcelona, Spain

Laurie A. Bernard MD
Assistant Clinical Professor of Pediatrics,
UCSD School of Medicine
Pediatric Hospitalist, Rady Children's
Hospital San Diego
Department of Pediatrics
San Diego, CA
USA

John S. Bradley MD
Director, Division of Infectious Disease
Rady Children's Hospital, San Diego
San Diego, CA
USA

Alanna F. Bree MD
Assistant Professor of Dermatology and
Pediatrics
Department of Dermatology and Pediatrics
Baylor College of Medicine
Texas Children's Hospital
Houston, TX
USA

Anna L. Bruckner MD
Assistant Professor of Dermatology and
Pediatrics
Stanford University School of Medicine
Director, Pediatric Dermatology
Lucile Packard Children's Hospital
Stanford, CA
USA

Craig N. Burkhart MD
Pediatric Dermatology Fellow
Department of Pediatric Dermatology
Children's Memorial Hospital
Chicago, IL
USA

K. Robin Carder MD
Clinical Assistant Professor of Dermatology
University of Texas, Southwestern Medical
Center at Dallas
Pediatric Dermatology of Dallas
Dallas, TX
USA

Yuin-Chew Chan MD
Consultant Dermatologist and Chief
Paediatric Dermatology Unit
National Skin Centre
Singapore

David H. Chu MD PhD
Howard Hughes Medical Institute
The Rockefeller University;
The Ronald O. Perelman Department of
Dermatology
New York University School of Medicine
New York, NY
USA

Bernard A. Cohen MD
Professor of Pediatrics and Dermatology
Division of Pediatric Dermatology
Johns Hopkins University School of Medicine
Baltimore, MD
USA

Bari B. Cunningham MD
Director, Dermatologic Surgery
Pediatric & Adolescent Dermatology
Rady Children's Hospital, San Diego
Associate Professor of Pediatrics & Medicine
(Dermatology), University of California, San
Diego School of Medicine
San Diego, CA
USA

James G.H. Dinulos MD
Associate Professor of Medicine and
Pediatrics (Dermatology)
Section of Dermatology
Dartmouth-Hitchcock Medical Center
Lebanon, NH
USA

Beth A. Drolet MD
Professor of Dermatology and Pediatrics
Medical College of Wisconsin
Medical Director of Dermatology and
Birthmarks and Vascular Anormales
Children's Hospital of Wisconsin
Milwaukee, WI
USA

Odile Enjolras MD
Director, Consultation des Angiomes
Hôpital d'enfants Armand Trousseau
Paris
France

Sheila Fallon Friedlander MD
Director, Fellowship Training Program
Pediatric & Adolescent Dermatology
Rady Children's Hospital, San Diego
Professor of Pediatrics & Medicine
(Dermatology)
University of California, San Diego School
of Medicine
San Diego, CA
USA

Sheila S. Galbraith MD
Assistant Professor of Dermatology
Department of Dermatology
Medical College of Wisconsin
Milwaukee, WI
USA

Maria C. Garzon MD
Associate Professor of Clinical Dermatology
and Clinical Pediatrics, Columbia
University, NY
Director, Pediatric Dermatology,
Morgan Stanley Children's Hospital of
NY Presbyterian
New York, NY
USA

Neil F. Gibbs MD
Assistant Clinical Professor of Pediatrics and
Medicine (Dermatology)
University of California, San Diego School of
Medicine;
Assistant Clinical Professor
Department of Dermatology
Uniformed Services University of the Health
Sciences School of Medicine
Bethesda, MD;
San Diego, CA
USA

Amy E. Gilliam MD
Assistant Clinical Professor of Dermatology
and Pediatrics
Department of Dermatology and Pediatrics
University of California, San Francisco
San Francisco, CA
USA

Adelaide A. Hebert MD
Professor of Dermatology and Pediatrics
Department of Dermatology
University of Texas Medical School
Houston, TX
USA

Paul J. Honig MD
Attending Physician, Pediatric Dermatology
Professor Emeritus, Pediatrics and
Dermatology
Children's Hospital of Philadelphia
University of Pennsylvania School of
Medicine
Philadelphia, PA
USA

Renee J. Howard MD
Assistant Clinical Professor of Dermatology
University of California, San Francisco
San Francisco, CA
USA

Alan D. Irvine MD FRCPI MRCP
Associate Professor Department of Clinical
Medicine Trinity College Dublin;
Consultant Paediatric Dermatologist
Our Lady's Hospital for Sick Children
Crumlin
Dublin
Ireland

Ho Jin Kim MD
Dermatologist and Pediatric Dermatologist
McLean, VA
USA

Liborka Kos, MD
Assistant Clinical Professor of Dermatology
Department of Dermatology
Medical College of Wisconsin
Milwaukee, WI
USA

Tamara Koss MD
Instructor in Clinical Dermatology
Department of Dermatology
Columbia University
New York, NY
USA

Bernice R. Krafchik MBChB FRCPC
Professor Emeritus
Departments of Pediatrics and Medicine
University of Toronto
Toronto, ON
Canada

Alfons L. Krol MD FRCPC
Professor of Dermatology and Pediatrics
Department of Dermatology
Oregon Health and Science University
Director, Pediatric Dermatology, Doernbecher
Children's Hospital
Portland, OR
USA

Leslie P. Lawley MD
Assistant Professor of Pediatrics and
Dermatology
Emory University School of Medicine
Atlanta, GA
USA

Moise L. Levy MD
Professor, Departments of Pediatrics and
Dermatology
Baylor College of Medicine
Dermatology, Chief of Service
Texas Children's Hospital
Houston, TX
USA

Cynthia A. Loomis MD PhD
Assistant Professor of Pathology and
Dermatology
NYU School of Medicine
New York, NY
USA

Anne W. Lucky MD
Acting Director
Division of Pediatric Dermatology
The Cincinnati Children's Hospital
Volunteer Professor of Dermatology and
Pediatrics
The University of Cincinnati College of
Medicine
Cincinnati, Ohio
Dermatology Research Associates, Inc.
Cincinnati, OH
USA

Hanspaul S. Makkar MD FRCP(C)
Assistant Professor of Dermatology,
Pediatrics and Surgery
University of Connecticut School of Medicine
Farmington, CT
USA

Anthony J. Mancini, MD
Associate Professor of Pediatrics &
Dermatology
Northwestern University Feinberg School of
Medicine
Head, Division of Pediatric Dermatology
Children's Memorial Hospital
Chicago, IL
USA

Denise W. Metry MD
Associate Professor Dermatology and
Pediatrics
Texas Children's Hospital
Baylor College of Medicine
Houston, TX
USA

Brandie J. Metz MD
Assistant Professor of Dermatology and
Pediatrics
Departments of Dermatology and Pediatrics
University of California, Irvine
Irvine, CA
USA

Dean S. Morrell MD
Associate Professor
Director of Pediatric and Adolescent
Dermatology
UNC Department of Dermatology
Chapel Hill, NC
USA

Nicole C. Pace MD
Instructor of Medicine and Pediatrics
(Dermatology)
Section of Dermatology
Dartmouth-Hitchcock Medical Center
Lebanon, NH
USA

Amy S. Paller MD
Professor and Chair, Department of
Dermatology
Professor, Department of Pediatrics
Northwestern University
Chicago, IL
USA

Julie S. Prendiville MB MRCPI FRCPC
Clinical Professor
Department of Pediatrics
University of British Columbia
Head, Division of Pediatric Dermatology
British Columbia's Children's Hospital
Vancouver, BC
Canada

Neil S. Prose MD
Professor of Dermatology and Pediatrics
Duke University Medical Center
Durham, NC
USA

Maureen Rogers MBBS FACD
Emeritus Consultant Dermatologist
Department of Dermatology
The Children's Hospital at Westmead
Sydney
Australia

Dawn Siegel MD
Assistant Professor of Dermatology and
Pediatrics
Oregon Health and Sciences University
Portland, OR
USA

Elaine C. Siegfried MD
Professor of Pediatrics and Dermatology
Department of Pediatrics
Saint Louis University Medical School
St. Louis, MO
USA

Robert A. Silverman MD
Clinical Associate Professor of Pediatrics
Georgetown University, Washington, DC;
INOVA Fairfax Hospital for Children
University of Virginia, Charlottesville
Fairfax, VA
USA

Yong-Kwang Tay MD
Head and Senior Consultant Dermatologist
Department of Dermatology
Changi General Hospital
Singapore

Antonio Torrelo MD
Pediatric Dermatologist
Director, Department of Dermatology
Hospital Infantil del Niño Jesús
Madrid
Spain

Annette M. Wagner MD
Assistant Professor of Pediatrics and
Dermatology
Northwestern University Medical School
Specialist in Pediatric Dermatologic Surgery
and Lasers
Children's Memorial Hospital
Chicago, IL
USA

Mary L. Williams MD
Adjunct Professor of Dermatology and
Pediatrics
Department of Dermatology
University of California, San Francisco
San Francisco, CA
USA

Li-Chuen Wong MD
Consultant Dermatologist
Department of Dermatology
The Children's Hospital at Westmead
Sydney
Australia

Albert C. Yan MD
Section Chief, Pediatric Dermatology
Assistant Professor, Pediatrics and
Dermatology
Children's Hospital of Philadelphia
University of Pennsylvania School of
Medicine
Philadelphia, PA
USA

Dedication

To
Lori, Matthew, Julia and to my parents, Frances and Stuart Eichenfield
LFE

To Mark, Mike, and Sarai and to the rest of the 'Four Friedens': Bonnie, Karl, and Sarajo
IJF

To my four-legged friends
NBE

Fetal Skin Development

Cynthia A. Loomis, Tamara Koss, David Chu

Skin is a complex tissue made up of many different cell types, derived from both embryonic mesoderm and ectoderm. Skin cells originating from embryonic mesoderm include fibroblasts, vascular cells, and adipocytes, as well as the bone marrow-derived Langerhans' cells, which reside in the epidermis. Skin cells originating from embryonic ectoderm include epidermal keratinocytes and the neural crest-derived melanocytes. Development, growth, and regional patterning of the skin are regulated by sequential and tightly regulated inductive interactions between these various cell types within the skin, as well as between skin and adjacent nonskin tissues. Genetic or teratogenic disruptions in these regulatory interactions result in serious congenital anomalies that can directly affect the care of the infant. Moreover, premature birth before full maturation of the skin can lead to impaired thermoregulation and defective barrier function in the neonate.

A timeline highlighting several important morphologic events that occur during skin morphogenesis is illustrated in Figure 1-1. In this figure, and throughout the text, two distinct dating systems are indicated. We use the term estimated gestational age (EGA), as it is used in basic embryology texts and by researchers, to refer to the age of the fetus.[1] In this system, fertilization occurs on day 1. However, the dating system used by obstetricians and most other clinicians as a reliable and convenient method for staging the pregnancy defines day 1 as the first day of the last menstrual period (LMP) and is synonymous with menstrual age.[2] In this dating system, fertilization occurs on approximately day 14. Thus a woman who is 14 weeks pregnant (LMP) is carrying a 12-week-old fetus (EGA).

From a functional point of view, fetal skin development can be divided into three temporally overlapping stages – organogenesis, histogenesis, and maturation[3] – that correspond roughly to the embryonic period (0–60-plus days), the early fetal period (60 days to 5 months), and the late fetal period (5–9 months) of development. The first stage, organogenesis, involves the specification of ectoderm lateral to the neural plate to become epidermis and the allocation of subsets of mesenchymal and neural crest cells to become dermis. During this stage, embryonic ectoderm and mesoderm become physically apposed, and they initiate the signaling cross-talk necessary for basement membrane and subsequent skin appendage (hair, nail, and sweat gland) formation. The second stage, histogenesis, is characterized by dramatic morphologic changes in the presumptive skin, including epidermal stratification, epidermal appendage involution and differentiation, mesenchymal subdivision of the dermis and hypodermis, and vascular neogenesis. The third stage, maturation, entails the functional evolution of these skin components so that they provide adequate thermoregulatory capacity, surface tensile strength, and barrier function for postnatal survival in the harsh, arid environment outside the uterus.

EPIDERMIS

Overview

The epidermis is a self-renewing stratified epithelium that covers the entire surface of an individual. The predominant cell within this epithelium is the keratinocyte. In its mature form, the epidermis consists of four histologically distinct keratinocyte layers, described from deep to superficial: the basal layer, the spinous layers, the granular layer, and the stratum corneum. The proliferative basal keratinocytes are anchored to the basement membrane, an extracellular meshwork separating the epidermis from the underlying dermis. As the daughter cells produced by this layer differentiate, they down-regulate the synthesis of matrix adhesion proteins, detach from the basement membrane, and move outward into the spinous layers. In this zone, the keratinocytes expend much of their energy in the production of keratin intermediate filaments. These rigid rods insert into the numerous desmosomal adhesion junctions and through these interconnections provide tensile strength and mechanical integrity for the epidermis.[4] On further differentiation, keratinocytes accumulate large protein and lipid granules, structures that define the most superficial viable layer, the granular layer. As the cells undergo terminal differentiation, moving from the granular layer into the stratum corneum, several biochemical events occur simultaneously, including (1) cell enucleation, (2) the aggregation of keratin filaments by the protein filaggrin, (3) transglutaminase-mediated protein cross-linking to form an insoluble cornified envelope, and (4) lamellar granule extrusion of lipid sheets to form the water-impermeable mortar surrounding the cornified envelopes.

Keratinocytes are not the only cells present within the epidermis, however. Melanocytes are pigment-producing cells interspersed among the basal keratinocytes.[5] Transport of their pigment-containing melanosomes to nearby keratinocytes provides protection from the mutagenic effects of ultraviolet irradiation. Langerhans' cells are antigen-presenting cells located primarily within the suprabasal epidermal layers, and they act as immunologic sentinels responding to the invasion of skin pathogens. Merkel cells are specialized neuroendocrine cells that are important in mechanoreception. Both Langerhans' cells and melanocytes migrate into the epidermis

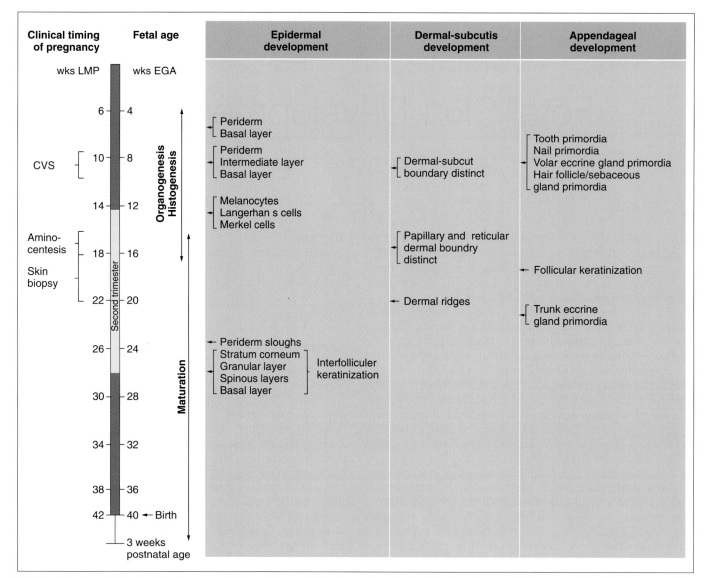

FIG. 1-1 Critical events in the development of skin and its specialized structures, indicating their times of initiation as defined by fetal age (EGA) and duration of pregnancy (LMP). Unless otherwise stated, times refer to the skin of the back.

during embryonic development, whereas Merkel cells appear to be derived from a pluripotent keratinocyte.

Embryonic Development

During the third week after fertilization the human embryo undergoes gastrulation, a complex process of involution and cell redistribution that generates the three primary embryonic germ layers: endoderm, mesoderm, and ectoderm.[1] Shortly after gastrulation, the ectoderm is further subdivided into neuroectoderm, a medial strip parallel to the long axis of the developing embryo, and presumptive epidermis on either side of this strip. The early presumptive epidermis is a loosely associated single cell layer.[6,7] By 6 weeks' EGA (8 weeks LMP), the earliest point in time that human embryos are generally available for study, the surface ectoderm covering most regions of the body already consists of basal cells and more superficial periderm cells (Fig. 1-2), which are not attached to basement

membrane.[8–10] The periderm layer is a transient embryonic layer that does not participate in the production of definitive epidermal progenitors, and the presumptive epidermis at these early stages is not considered a true stratified epithelium.

The basal cells of the embryonic epidermis display morphologic and biochemical features similar – but not identical – to basal cells of later developmental stages. Embryonic basal cells are slightly more columnar than later fetal basal cells and lack the morphologically distinct matrix adhesion structures called hemidesmosomes.[11,12] Matrix adhesion of the early embryonic epidermis is probably mediated largely by the actin-associated $\alpha6\beta4$ integrin, as suggested by expression and genetic studies in mice and humans.[12–15]

Intercellular attachment between individual basal cells at this stage appears to be mediated by classic cadherin adhesion molecules, such as E- and P-cadherin, as well as by a few desmosomal junctions. E- and P-cadherin have both been detected on basal cell membranes as early as 6 weeks' EGA, whereas

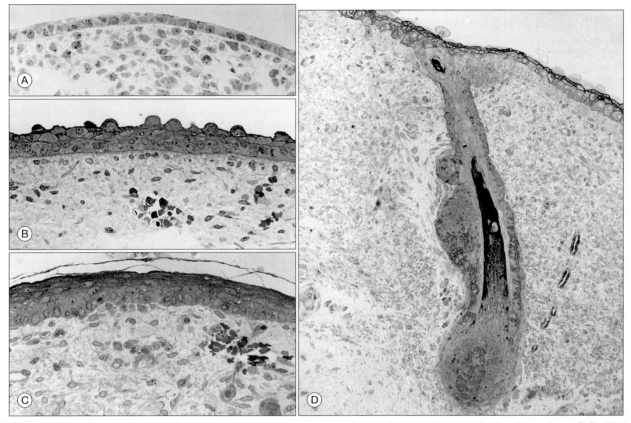

FIG. 1-2 Epidermal morphogenesis. **A** At 36 days the epidermis consists only of a basal layer and a superficial periderm layer. **B** By 72 days a well-formed intermediate layer is present between the basal and periderm layers. By the end of the second trimester, there are several intermediate cell layers and the stratified epidermis begins to keratinize. **C** In neonatal skin, a distinct granular layer and stratum corneum are present. Hair follicles first begin to bud down in the dermis between 75 and 80 days. **D** An early bulbous hair peg-stage follicle from a mid-second trimester fetus. (Photomicrographs courtesy Dr Karen Holbrook.)

E-cadherin alone is expressed on the early periderm.[16] Cytoplasmic filaments in the basal cells include both actin microfilaments and the less abundant keratin intermediate filaments, which even at these early stages are composed of K5 and K14 keratins, proteins generally restricted to definitive stratified epithelia.[17-19]

Periderm cells of the embryonic epidermis are larger and flatter than the underlying basal cells. As such, periderm cells have been termed a pavement epithelium.[8,20] Apical surfaces in contact with the amniotic fluid are studded with microvilli. Their lateral surfaces in contact with adjacent peridermal cells are sealed with tight junctions, possibly precluding passive – but not active – diffusion of fluids across this outer layer of the embryo.[10] Periderm cells, like the embryonic basal cells, express the stratified epithelial keratins K5 and K14, but also express simple epithelial keratins K8, K18, and K19.[21-24] Towards the end of the second trimester these superficial cells are eventually sloughed and become a component of the vernix caseosa covering the newborn.[25] At this stage of fetal development, the maturing epidermis begins to form its own barrier to the external environment.[26]

Early Fetal Development

By the end of 8 weeks' gestation (10 weeks LMP), the basic components of most organ systems have been laid down and hemopoietic production has shifted to the bone marrow. This marks the classic division between embryonic and fetal development, and it corresponds to the timing of definitive epidermal stratification and the formation of the third 'intermediate' layer between the two pre-existing cell layers (Fig. 1-2). Mouse studies indicate that p63, a protein closely related to the tumor suppressor gene p53, plays a critical role in directing the simple-to-stratified epithelial transition.[27] Cells in the intermediate layer of the early fetal epidermis express the K1/10 skin differentiation-type keratin markers, as well as the desmosomal protein desmoglein 3, which is also known as the pemphigus vulgaris antigen.[28,29] Moreover, intermediate filaments and desmosomal junctions are more abundant in this layer than in the basal or periderm layers. In contrast to the spinous cells of the mature nonwounded epidermis, cells within the intermediate layer remain highly proliferative.[30,31] Over the next several weeks more layers are gradually added to this intermediate zone of the developing epidermis, such that by 22–24 weeks' EGA the epidermis contains four to five layers in addition to the degenerating periderm.

After the onset of stratification, the basal layer also displays characteristic morphologic and biochemical changes. Basal cells become more cuboidal and begin to synthesize other keratin peptides, including K6, K8, K19, and the K6/K16 hyperproliferative pair.[25,26] This latter keratin pair is not normally expressed in mature interfollicular epidermis but is upregulated in response to wounding and hyperproliferative conditions.[32] During early fetal development, the basal cell layer also begins to express the hemidesmosomal proteins BPA1 and BPA2, and to secrete collagen types V and VII, the latter being the major component of the anchoring fibrils of the dermis.[28,33–35] DNA-labeling studies indicate that by 80–90 days' EGA a distinct subset of slow-cycling cells exists within the basal cell population, suggesting that an epidermal stem cell population has already been set aside at these early stages.[30]

Late Fetal Development

Maturation of the epidermis during late fetal development is characterized by the generation of granular and stratum corneal layers, the formation of a water-impermeable barrier, and the sloughing of the periderm. Keratinization, which is the type of terminal differentiation mediated by granular layer and stratum corneum formation, is initiated first in the skin appendages between 11 and 15 weeks' EGA, and only begins to involve the interfollicular epidermis from about 22–24 weeks' EGA.[25] Initiation of keratinization is characterized morphologically by the marked increase in cytoplasmic density of the superficial keratinocytes and the precursor of the keratin-aggregating protein filaggrin. The early granular layer continues to mature with the formation of more granules. More superficial layers arise that undergo incomplete terminal differentiation, resulting in the formation of transglutaminase-mediated cross-linked envelopes that still encase remnant organelles. At slightly later stages the terminal differentiation is more complete, resulting in the complete absence of organelles in keratinized cells of the stratum corneum. During the third trimester the cornified cell layers increase in number, aiding in the formation of a barrier. Although the third-trimester stratum corneum is structurally similar to that of the adult, functional studies indicate that it is much less effective at preventing water loss and is less permeable to exogenous compounds.[36–40]

Clinical Relevance

Gross defects in early epidermal specification and organogenesis are rarely observed in the neonate, probably because they are incompatible with fetal survival. Using mice as an animal model system, researchers demonstrated that obliteration of p63 gene function precludes the formation of most multilayered epithelia in the body, leading to perinatal lethality due to loss of skin barrier function (Table 1-1). Humans who have been found to carry mutations in this gene still retain some functionality and therefore display less severe alterations in their epidermis and appendages (see below).

Unlike defects in early epidermal organogenesis, congenital defects in epidermal maturation are not uncommon as they do not usually impinge on in utero survival. Lamellar ichthyosis is usually inherited in an autosomal recessive manner and in 30% of patients is caused by mutations in the gene encoding epidermal transglutaminase,[41–44] the enzyme that cross-links submembranous proteins to form the insoluble cornified envelope of the stratum corneum. In its absence, large dark polygonal scales form over the entire body, and at birth the infant may be transiently wrapped in a waxy, collodion-like membrane.[45] A similar clinical presentation can be seen in patients homozygous for mutations in the ABCA12 gene, which encodes an ATP-binding cassette thought to be important for lipid trafficking across keratinocyte membranes. Infants with the more severe 'harlequin ichthyosis' are born encased in armor-like plates of thickened, adherent stratum corneum,[46–49] and this extreme variant also appears to be due to mutations in the ABCA12 gene. Additional disorders associated with impaired epidermal maturation and the relevant genes are listed in Table 1-2.

In contrast to the permanent manifestations of genetic defects, the inadequate epidermal keratinization and maturation of the premature epidermis are transient. Immaturity of the stratum corneum, especially in infants born before 28 weeks' EGA (30 weeks LMP), places these neonates at increased risk for dehydration, excessive penetration of topical drugs or

TABLE 1-1 Specification/patterning/morphogenesis

EPIDERMIS		DERMIS	
Protein/GENE	Disorder	Protein/GENE	Disorder
p63	AEC	Lmx1b	Nail-Patella syn
	Appendages	LaminA, SMPSTE24	Restrictive Dermopathy
Protein/GENE	Disorder	LaminA	Lipodystrophy, partial, 2
Lmx1b	Nail Patella syn	PPARG	Lipodystrophy, partial 3
EDA	X-linked hypohidrotic ED	AcetylcholineR (fetal subunit)	Multiple pterygium syn's
EDAR	Autosomal hypohidrotic ED, Ty3	PTPN11, KRAS, NF1	Noonan syn
Connexin 30	Autosomal hydrotic ED, Ty2	GNAS1	Progressive osseus heteroplasia
p63	Hay-Wells, AEC, EEC syn's	GNAS1	Albright hereditary osteodystrophy
Msx1	Wtkop syn		
Dlx3	Tichodento-osseous syn		

ED, ectodermal dysplasia; syn, syndrome

TABLE 1-2 Differentiation

EPIDERMIS		DERMIS		Appendages	
Protein/GENE	Disorder	Protein/GENE	Disorder	Protein/GENE	Disorder
Structural proteins		Structural proteins		Structural proteins	
K1, K10	BCIE	Collagen VII	Dystrophic EB	Plakoglobin	Naxos Dz
K1, K9	Vorner, Unna-Thost, Greither keratinopathies	Col1a1 or 1a2	Osteogenesis imperfecta, I, II, IV	Plakophilin	Skin fargility syndrome
K5, K14	EB simplex	Col5A1, Col5A2	Ehlers-Danlos, I	Desmoplakin	skin fragility–woolly hair syndrome
ATP2A2 (Ca-ATPase)	Darier White Dz	Col5A1, Col5A2, Col1A2	Ehlers-Danlos, II	Claudin 1	Ichthyosis-Sclerosing cholangitis (alopecia) syn
ATP2C1 (Ca-ATPase)	Hailey-Hailey Dz	Col3A1, tenascin-XB	Ehlers-Danlos, III	K6a, K16	Pachyonychia congenita, Type I
Connexin 26 GJB2	KID syn	Col3A1	Ehlers-Danlos, IV	K6b, K17	Pachyonychia congenita, Type II
Claudin 1	Ichthyosis-Sclerosing cholangitis syn	FBN1 (fibrillin)	Marfan syn	K6b, K18	Steatocystoma multiplex
Loricrin	NBCIE, Vohwinkel syn's	FBLN5, FBLN4	Cutis laxa, AR Type I	KRTHB1, B3, B6	Monilethrix
Plectin	EB with MD	ELN (Elastin)	Cutis laxa	RMRP mitochondrial RNA cartilage-hair hypoplasia	
BPAG2	GABEB				
a6B4 integrin	Junctional EB with PA				
Laminin5	Junctional EB				
Processing proteins		Processing or regulatory proteins		Regulatory proteins	
LEKTI	Netherton syn	lysyl hydroxylase	Ehlers-Danlos, VI	Hairless	Papular atrichia
Transglutaminase 1	Lamellar ichthyosis 1; NCIE	ADAMTS2	Ehlers-Danlos, VII	WHN	T-cell immunodeficiency alopecia, nail dystrophy
ATP-binding casette A12	Lamellar ichthyosis 2	Cu-transporting ATPase, apha pep	Ehlers-Danlos, IX (Cutix laxa, X-linked)		
NAD(P)H steroid dehydrogenase-like protein, NSDHL	CHILD syn	sterol isomerase emopamil-binding protein (EBP)	Chondrodysplassia punctata, X2		
Fatty aldehyde dehydrogenase	Sjogren-Larsson	HRAS	Costello syn		
Steroidsulfatase/ arylsufatase C	X-linked ichthyosis	MRP6	PXE		
Transglutaminase 5	Acral peeling skin syndrome	GNAS1	Osseous Heteroplasia, progressive		
spremidine/spermine N(1)-acetyltransferase	Keratosis follicularis spinulosa decalvans	Col1A1fused to PDGFB	DFSP		
Phytanoyl CoA hydroxylase	Refsum				
Irf6 (transcription factor)	Polpoteal pterygium syn; Wan der Woude syn				

other chemicals, and infection from organisms newly colonizing the skin[36–40,50] (see Chapters 4 and 5). In general, even full-term newborns display a somewhat reduced barrier function, and continued maturation occurs over the first few weeks of life, such that by 3 weeks of age, the newborn's stratum corneum is structurally and functionally equivalent to that of the adult; maturation is accelerated in the premature infant, although the duration may be longer in extremely premature infants.[38,51]

Specialized Cells Within the Epidermis

Two major immigrant cells – melanocytes and Langerhans' cells – populate the epidermis during early embryonic development. Melanocytes are derived from a subset of neuroectoderm cells, the neural crest, which forms along the dorsal neural tube and gives rise to a variety of cell types, including many tissues of the face and peripheral autonomic neurons.[52] Neural crest cells destined to become melanocytes migrate away from the neural tube within the mesenchyme subjacent to the presumptive epidermis. They migrate as semicoherent clones laterally and then ventrally around the trunk to the thoracoabdominal midline, anteriorly over the scalp and face, and distally along the extremities. Postnatally, the embryonic paths taken by these partially coherent clones can be readily visualized in patients with banded pigmentary dyscrasias following Blaschko's lines, such as the disorders classified as hypomelanosis of Ito, and linear and whorled hypermelanosis (see Chapters 21 and 22).[53,54]

The melanocytes can be first detected within the epidermis of the human embryo at approximately 50 days' EGA, based on their dendritic morphology and their specific immunoreactivity.[55] Even at these early developmental time points the density of melanocytes is quite high (1000 cells/mm^2).[56] The density increases further around the time of epidermal stratification (80–90 days' EGA) and initiation of appendageal development. Between 3 and 4 months EGA, depending on body site and the race of the fetus, melanin (visible pigment) production becomes detectable, and by 5 months melanocytes begin transferring melanosomes to the keratinocytes, a process that will continue after birth.[57–59] Although all melanocytes are in place at birth and melanogenesis is well under way, the skin of the newborn infant is not fully pigmented and will continue to darken over the first several months. This is most apparent in individuals with darker skin tones.

Langerhans' cells, the other major immigrant population, are detectable within the epidermis by 40 days' EGA.[60] Similar to melanocytes, the early embryonic Langerhans' cells do not yet possess the specialized organelles characteristic of mature cells, but can be distinguished from other epidermal cells by their dendritic morphology, immunopositive reaction for the HLA-DR surface antigen, and high levels of ATPase activity. After the transition from embryo to fetus they begin to express the CD1 antigen on their surface and to produce characteristic granules of mature Langerhans' cells.[60,61] Although the extent of dendritic processes from individual Langerhans' cells increases during the second trimester, the total number of cells remains low and only increases to typical adult numbers in the third trimester.[62,63]

Another distinct subset of cells within the basal cell layer are Merkel cells, which are highly innervated neuroendocrine cells involved in mechanoreception. Merkel cells can be round or dendritic, and are found at particularly high densities in volar skin. They are frequently associated with epidermal appendageal structures and are occasionally detected within the dermis. Their distinguishing morphologic and immunohistochemical features are cytoplasmic dense-core granules, keratin 18, and neuropeptide expression, which can be detected as early as 8–12 weeks' EGA in palmoplantar epidermis and at slightly later times in interfollicular skin.[17,64] Recent keratin expression data, as well as transplant studies, suggest that Merkel cells are derived from pluripotent keratinocytes, rather than neural progenitors such as neural crest, but the results are not conclusive.[64–67]

Clinical Relevance

Many clinical defects are known to affect normal pigmentation within an individual (Table 1-3). Defects in melanoblast migration, proliferation, and/or survival occur in several clinical syndromes, and many of the genetic mutations responsible for these defects have been identified. Failure of an adequate number of melanoblasts to completely supply distal points on their embryonic migration path occurs in the different types of Waardenburg syndrome, as well as in piebaldism, resulting in depigmented patches on the central forehead, central abdomen, and extremities. These defects are associated with mutations in several different genes, including genes encoding transcription factors, such as Pax3 and MITF, as well as membrane receptors and their ligands, such as endothelin 3, endothelin-receptor B, and c-kit.[68–78] In albinism, on the other hand, melanocyte development is normal, but production of pigment or melanin is inadequate. The most severe form of oculocutaneous albinism results from null mutations in the gene encoding tyrosinase, the rate-limiting enzyme in the production of melanin. Less severe forms of albinism are caused by mutations in tyrosinase alleles, which lead to partial loss of function, as well as by mutations in other genes encoding proteins important in melanin assembly in melanosomes or transport.[5]

DERMIS AND SUBCUTIS

Overview

The mature dermis is characterized by complex interwoven collagen and elastic fibers enmeshed in a proteoglycan matrix. Fibroblasts, mast cells, and macrophages are scattered throughout this mesh, and nerve fibers and vascular networks course through it, dividing it into distinct domains. In contrast, the embryonic dermis is quite cellular and amorphous, lacking organized extracellular fibers. Embryonic mesenchymal cells capable of differentiating into a wide variety of cell types are embedded in a highly hydrated gel, rich in hyaluronic acid. Moreover, only a few nerve fibers have reached this peripheral location, and vessels have not evolved into their mature patterns. During the course of fetal development, this so-called cellular dermis, which is conducive to cell migration and tissue remodeling, is transformed into the fibrillar dermis of the adult, which provides increased strength, resilience, and structural support.[79]

Embryonic Dermal Development

The specification and allocation of dermal mesenchymal cells are rather complex and not well understood. The cell of origin

TABLE 1-3 Development and tumor overlaps

Dermis		Epidermis/Appendages	
Protein/GENE	Disorder	Protein/GENE	Disorder
PTEN	Proteus S	PTEN	Cowden syn
Fumarate hydratase	Hereditary Mult leiomyoma	MSH2, MLH1 (mismatch repr)	Muir-Torre syndrome (sebaceous tumors)
B-catenin/APC	desmoid tumors	B-catenin (Wnt?)	pilomatricomas
GNAS	McCune Albright syndrome	APC	Adenomatous polyposis of the colon
PKA reg subunit-1-alpha	Carney; Name, LAMB	Ptch/Shh	Gorlin syn (palmar pits/BCCs)
TSC1, 2, 3, 4	Tuberous sclerosis		
Merlin/Neurofibromin 2/NF2	Neurofibromatosis I	STK11 (ser-thr kinase)	Peutz-Jeghers syndrome
NF2 (merlin)	Neurofibromatosis II	FLCN (folliculin)	Birt-Hogg-Dube syndrome
glomulin	Glomuvenous Malformations		
Col1A1fused to PDGFB	DFSP		

for the presumptive dermis depends on its anatomic location. The dermis of the face is derived from neural crest cells; that of the dorsal trunk is derived from the dermatomyotome portion of the differentiated somite; and the dermis of the limbs is derived from the lateral plate (somatic) mesoderm.[79–81] Regional patterning of the skin and differences in the type and quality of the epidermal appendages produced in the older fetus might in part reflect these early differences in dermal cell precursors. In addition, signaling from adjacent tissues plays a critical role.[82,83]

By 6–8 weeks' EGA the presumptive dermal cells already underlie the epidermis. However, there is as yet no sharp demarcation between cells giving rise to skin dermis and those giving rise to musculoskeletal elements. Electron microscopic (EM) studies of the presumptive dermis at these stages demonstrate fine filaments, but rarely fibers.[84] Although most protein components of collagen fibers and some microfibrillar components of elastin fibers (fibrillin) are synthesized by the embryonic dermal cells, the proteins are not yet assembled into large, rigid fibers.[3,35] Moreover, the ratio of collagen III to collagen I is 3:1, the reverse of what it is in the adult.[35,85,86]

Fetal Dermal Development

After embryonic–fetal transition at 60 days, the presumptive dermis is distinguishable from the underlying skeletal condensations. Moreover, within the dermis there is a progressive change in matrix organization and cell morphology, such that by 12–15 weeks the fine interwoven mesh of the papillary dermis adjacent to the epidermis can be distinguished from the deeper, more fibrillar reticular dermis.[3,35] Large collagen fibers accumulate in the reticular dermis during the second and third trimesters. Definitive elastin fibers first become detectable by EM studies around 22–24 weeks' EGA,[87] although both the microfibrillar protein fibrillin and the microfibrillar structures, which are morphologically similar to elastin-

associated microfibrils of the adult, can be detected at earlier stages.[3] By the end of gestation the dermis is thick and well organized, but is still much thinner than in the adult and has a higher water content, reminiscent of the fetal dermis. Maturation of the dermis is marked by increasing tensile strength and the transition from a nonscarring to a scarring response after wounding. Thus fetal skin biopsies tend to heal with little evidence of the surgical event. This has obvious clinical implications, and the molecular controls critical for nonscarring fetal wound healing are an area of active research by many groups.[88–90]

Clinical Relevance

Congenital defects in the specification and development of the dermis are probably incompatible with survival to term, although there are a few exceptions (see Tables 1-1 and 1-2). Infants with restrictive dermopathy disorder, which is characterized by a thin, flat dermis, lack of elastic tissue fibers, and shortened appendageal structures, do survive to birth but then die in the neonatal period, partly because of insufficient elaboration of the dermis.[91–93] This disorder is caused by mutations in either the LaminA gene or the gene encoding the LaminA processing enzyme. Another syndrome characterized by inadequate dermal development is Goltz syndrome (focal dermal hypoplasia).[45,94] This is an X-linked dominant condition in which males who inherit the mutation on their single X chromosome die in utero. In contrast, females are functional mosaics as a result of random X-inactivation early in embryogenesis, and those with Goltz syndrome display areas of dermal hypoplasia where the mutant X is active. These bands of dermal hypoplasia follow Blaschko's lines and alternate with bands of normal dermal development where the normal X is active.[54,95] Another disorder that displays patchy dermal hypoplasia and in many cases probably reflects mosaicism for an autosomal dominant mutation is Proteus syndrome, although some affected individuals appear to carry mutations in the *PTEN* gene.[96]

Specialized Components of the Dermis

The structure and organization of the cutaneous nerves and vessels begin early in gestation but do not develop into those of the adult until a few months after birth. And although the pattern of the vasculature varies among regions of the body, vessels of the endoderm–mesoderm interface form through the in situ differentiation of endothelial cells (vasculogenesis).[97,98] Originally, they form horizontal plexuses within the subpapillary and deep reticular dermis, which are interconnected by groups of vertical vessels. This vascular framework has been elegantly reconstructed by the use of computer graphics to illustrate the complexity that already exists by 45–50 days' EGA.[99] Such structure does not remain constant even throughout fetal life, but varies depending on the body region and gestational age, as well as on the presence of hair follicles and glands that may require an increased blood supply. Furthermore, vascular emergence and development correlate directly with the particular tissue, determined specifically by the influences of pressure and function.

Regional variation also depends on gestational age. Blood vessels have been identified in fetal skin as early as 9 weeks' EGA. At this stage, they help delineate the dermal–hypodermal junction. By 3 months, the distinct horizontal and vertical networks have formed. And by the fifth month vasculogenesis has largely ceased and the formation of the complex vascular plexus is initiated by angiogenesis, the budding and migration of endothelium from pre-existing vessels. With increasing gestational age the superficial architecture becomes more organized, culminating at birth in an extensive capillary network responsible for the skin redness often observed in the newborn. Within the first few postnatal months the complexity decreases as skin surface area increases, lanugo hairs are lost, and sebaceous gland activity decreases. It is during this time that the rate of skin growth is greatest. By approximately 3 months of age, the vascular patterns most closely resemble those of the (mature) adult.

Development of the cutaneous innervation closely parallels that of the vascular system in terms of its pattern, rate of maturation, and organization. Nerves of the skin consist of somatic sensory and sympathetic autonomic fibers, which are predominantly small and unmyelinated. The development of these nerve fibers consists of myelination with a concomitant decrease in the number of axons, and is far from complete at birth. It may in fact continue until puberty.

Clinical Relevance

Not only do the number and caliber of the blood vessels change over time, so too does the direction of blood flow. Considering the dynamic nature of this circulatory system, it is not surprising that, of the congenital malformations seen in newborns, vascular defects are the most common (Table 1-4). The Klippel–Trenaunay and Sturge–Weber syndromes are examples of these. In the former, unilateral cutaneous vascular malformations, usually involving an extremity, are seen in association with venous varicosities and hypertrophy of the associated soft tissue and/or bone. In the latter, cutaneous capillary malformations are also often unilateral and may involve the lips, tongue, and nasal and buccal mucosae. Studies

TABLE 1-4 Skin development

Vascular regulators	
CMG2	Fibromatosis, Juvenile Hyaline
TIE2	Inherited venous malformations
Endoglin, activin receptor-like kinase 1	HHT/Osler-Weber Rendu
VEGF-3	Hereditary lymphedema, Type I
Foxc2	Hereditary lymphedema, Type II (Lymphedema w/distichiasis)
Foxc2	Lymphedema and yellow nail Syndrome
SOX18	Hypotrichosis-Lymphedema-Telangiectasia Syndrome
VG5Q translocation	Some cases of Klippel-Trenaunay syndrome

of families with heritable vascular anomalies have begun to provide insights into the pathways critical for normal fetal vascular development and subsequent postnatal remodeling. Specifically, increased activity of the TIE2 receptor tyrosine kinase, one of the vascular endothelial cell-specific receptor tyrosine kinases that have been characterized, has been described in some families with inherited venous malformations.[100,101] In addition, aberrant activities of TGF-β binding proteins, endoglin and activin receptor-like kinase 1, have been reported in patients with hereditary hemorrhagic telangiectasia (Osler–Weber–Rendu syndrome), resulting in remodeling of the apparent abnormal capillary bed.[102,103] The importance of early fetal innervation to normal skin morphogenesis is the recent demonstration that lack of the fetus-specific component of the acetylcholine receptor produces the extensive dermal webbing seen in multiple pterygium syndrome.

Development of the Hypodermis

A distinct region that is the hypodermis can be delineated by 50–60 days' EGA.[3] It is separated from the overlying cellular dermis by a plane of thin-walled vessels. Toward the end of the first trimester the sparse matrix of the hypodermis can be distinguished morphologically from the slightly denser, more fibrous matrix of the dermis.[79,104] In the second trimester, mesenchymally derived preadipocytes begin to differentiate and accumulate lipids,[105] and by the third trimester the more mature adipocytes are aggregated into large lobules of fat divided by fibrous septa. Although the molecular pathways that direct mesenchyme cells to commit to the adipocyte pathway are not well understood, many regulators involved in the subsequent preadipocyte differentiation have been identified.[106,107] An example is the gene that encodes leptin, whose abnormal regulation has been implicated in the pathogenesis of obesity.[108–110]

COMBINED DERMOEPIDERMAL STRUCTURES

Dermoepidermal Junction

The dermoepidermal junction (DEJ) is the region where the epidermis and dermis abut. In the broadest definition, it includes the specialized extracellular matrix on which the basal keratinocytes sit, known as the basement membrane, as well as the basal-most portion of the basal cells and the superficial-most portion of the dermis. Importantly, both dermal and epidermal compartments contribute to the molecular synthesis, assembly, and integration of this region.

A simple basement membrane, separating the dermis and epidermis, can be discerned as early as 8 weeks' EGA. The basic protein constituents common to all basement membranes can already be detected immunohistochemically at this stage.[12,34,111] These include collagen IV, laminin, and heparin sulfate and proteoglycans.

Specialized components of the DEJ do not appear until after the embryonic–fetal transition, around the time of initial epidermal stratification.[12,34,111] With a few exceptions, all basement membrane antigens are in place by the end of the first trimester.[3] As discussed, the α6 and β4 integrin subunits are expressed quite early by embryonic basal cells.[12] However, they do not become localized to the basal surface until after 9.5 weeks, which is coincident with the time when bullous pemphigoid antigens are first detected immunohistochemically and hemidesmosomes are recognized ultrastructurally.[11,12,34,112] Similarly, anchoring filaments and anchoring fibrils, the basement membrane components that mediate basal cell attachment to extracellular matrix, are recognizable by 9 weeks' EGA.[3,11] Collagen VII, the anchoring fibril protein, is detected slightly earlier, at 8 weeks.[11]

Recent experimental data have delineated many of the molecular interactions crucial for connecting the cytoskeletal networks of the basal cells with the extracellular filamentous networks important in matrix adhesion (Fig. 1-3). On the outer surface of the basal cell α6β4, the hemidesmosome integrin binds laminin-5, the major constituent of anchoring filaments.[113] Laminin-5 in turn binds collagen VII, the major component of anchoring fibrils, thus indirectly connecting the hemidesmosome to the anchoring fibrils.[114] On the inner side of the basal cell membrane, the cytoplasmic tail of β4 interacts with the submembranous plaque protein plectin, which then binds with keratin intermediate filament proteins.[115] In addition, the cytoplasmic tail of BPA2 binds the hemidesmosomal plaque protein BPA1, which in turn appears to bind the keratin intermediate filaments.[116]

Clinical Applications

Several congenital disorders characterized by severe blistering of the skin occur as a result of mutations in genes encoding DEJ components[117] (see Chapter 10). The severity of the disorder, the exact plane of tissue separation, and the involvement of nonskin tissues depend in part on which proteins are affected by the genetic mutations (see Table 1-2). Because these blistering disorders are associated with a high postnatal morbidity and mortality they are frequent candidates for prenatal testing, and when the responsible genetic mutation is one that has been identified, this can be accomplished by chorionic villus sampling (CVS) or amniocentesis (see section on Prenatal Diagnosis of Severe Congenital Skin Disorders).

Development of Appendages

Skin appendages (hair, nails, sweat and mammary glands in mammals, and feathers and scales in birds and reptiles) all

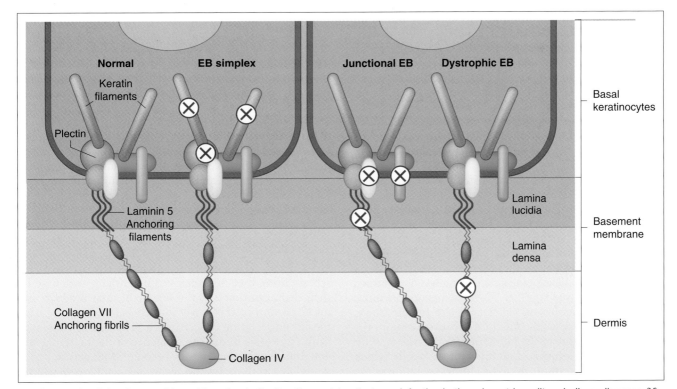

FIG. 1-3 Schematic of the dermoepidermal junction indicating the proteins that are defective in the relevant hereditary bullous diseases (X). Mutations in genes encoding keratin 5 or keratin 14 cause epidermolysis bullosa (EB simplex). Plectin function is disrupted in EB associated with muscular dystrophy. One of the subunits of laminin-5 is defective in most forms of junctional EB. However, the β4 subunit of α6β4 integrin is altered in the form associated with pyloric atresia, and bullous pemphigoid antigen 2 (BPA2) is mutated in generalized atrophic benign EB. Collagen VII is defective in all forms of dystrophic EB published to date.

consist of two distinct components: an epidermal component that elaborates the differentiated end-product, such as the hair or nail, and the dermal component that regulates specification and differentiation of the appendage. Fetal development of these structures depends on rigidly choreographed, collaborative interactions between early epidermis and dermis.[79,118,119] Defects in dermal induction or specification of the overlying ectoderm, or in the ectoderm's responses to these instructions, result in aberrant development, as has been demonstrated in genetic studies and transplant experiments in animal model systems.[79,118–120] Moreover, the recent demonstration that defects in human homologs of mouse hairless, LMX1B, and tabby genes result in clinically significant developmental abnormalities in humans confirms the relevance of such animal studies to our understanding of human skin appendage development.[121–125]

Hair Follicle and Sebaceous Gland Development

Hair follicle formation begins on the head and then spreads caudally and ventrally in waves, resulting in regularly spaced rows and whorls of follicles.[126,127] The first morphologic evidence of follicle formation in humans is the focal crowding of small groups of basal keratinocytes at regularly spaced intervals, starting between 75 and 80 days on the face and scalp.[126,128–130] This ectodermal structure is called the placode of the pregerm-stage follicle. Slightly later in development, mesenchymal cell clusters are observed beneath these ectodermal placodes. Although morphologically similar to other dermal fibroblasts, these clustered mesenchymal cells are biochemically distinguishable based on their continued expression of certain molecular markers, such as nerve growth factor receptor (NGFR).[3] On the trunk at approximately 80 days' EGA, a cluster of basal epidermal cells thickens and begins to bud downward into the dermis, forming the early hair germs.[130,131] Transplant studies in other species indicate that ectodermal budding requires an induction signal from the underlying mesenchymal cells. The cells of the early ectodermal bud or placode then respond with their own signal, which elicits a second mesenchymal signal. This second signal directs the species-specific type of mesenchymal appendage that will ultimately develop.[79,119]

The next stage of hair development involves further proliferation and resulting downward elongation of the ectodermal bud, forming the so-called hair peg.[126] At 12–14 weeks' EGA the hair peg develops a widened bulb at its base that flattens and then invaginates, engulfing the subjacent clustered mesenchymal cells, which become the follicular dermal papilla. In addition to the widened bulb at the base, two other bulges form along the length of the developing follicle, which is now termed the bulbous hair peg (see Fig. 1-2).[126,132] The uppermost bulge is the presumptive sebaceous gland, and the middle bulge, which forms at approximately one-third the distance from the follicular base, is the site of the future insertion of the arrector pili muscle and is the location of multipotent stem cells, which give rise to all the progenitors necessary for regeneration of the lower portion of follicle during postnatal follicular cycling, as well as to cells capable of replenishing the overlying epidermal covering in the event of extensive surface wounds or burns. Recent lineage studies indicate that progeny of the follicular stem cells do not take up permanent residence in the epidermis, but function transiently until resident epidermal stem cells can functionally replace them.[133,134]

Maturation of the hair peg into a definitive follicle is a complex process involving the formation of a patent hair canal and the elaboration of at least six distinct concentric rings of cells.[135] The most peripheral ring of ectodermal cells makes up the outer root sheath, whose upper portion is continuous with the interfollicular epidermis and undergoes a similar process of keratinization. The lower portion of the outer root sheath, in contrast, does not form a granular layer or classic stratum corneum. The inner root sheath forms just internal to the outer root sheath. The cells in this sheath do form a granular layer through the keratin proteins, and keratin-aggregating products produced here differ from those produced by the normal epidermis. Cells in this inner root sheath arise from self-renewing progenitor cells at the base of the follicle, which differentiate as they move upward toward the skin surface surrounding the hair shaft. Likewise, the three internal concentric layers of the hair shaft – cuticle, cortex, and medulla (from outer to inner) – arise from the matrix cells at the base of the follicle. These deep matrix cells sit on the basement membrane 'mat,' along the concavity of the hair follicle invagination, and as such are in close proximity to the dermal papillae mesenchymal cells.

By 19–21 weeks' EGA, the hair canal has fully formed and the scalp hairs are visible just above the surface of the fetal epidermis.[127,136,137] They continue to lengthen until 24–28 weeks, when they shift from the active growing phase (anagen) to the short-lived degenerative phase (catagen) and then to the resting phase (telogen).[3,138] They then re-enter the active growing stage (second anagen), and the first wave of hairs is shed into the amniotic fluid as the new hairs grow out. Cycling through active and inactive phases continues for all hairs throughout the life of an individual,[139] although cycles for individual hairs become asynchronous postnatally. The maintenance of a tight anatomic relationship between dermal papilla cells and the cycling ectodermal portion of the hair follicle is critical for follicular self-renewal, and the inability to maintain this relationship results in a form of inherited alopecia in which hair neogenesis is normal but, after the first resting phase, cycling is aberrant.[122]

Perinatally the second wave of fine lanugo hairs is shed. With subsequent cycles, hairs increase in diameter and coarseness, forming first vellus and then adult-type terminal hair shafts on the scalp and brow.[138] During adolescence, vellus hairs of androgen-sensitive areas undergo a similar transition to terminal-type hair follicles.

Sebaceous gland maturation occurs in parallel with that of the follicle proper and begins between 13 and 16 weeks' EGA.[140] Lipogenic cells produced by the outer proliferative layer of the sebaceous gland progressively accumulate lipid/sebum until they terminally differentiate, which results in their disintegration and the release of their products into the upper portion of the newly formed hair canal.[141,142] The synthesis and secretion of sebum is accelerated in the second and third trimesters under the influence of the maternal steroids, and the glands themselves become hyperplastic.[143,144] This stimulated activity by the sebaceous glands is believed to be responsible for the common condition known as neonatal acne. In the absence of exogenous maternal hormones, these glands become quiescent during the first few months of life and again increase in activity during the hormonal changes of adolescence.[143]

Nail Development

The first evidence of nail formation is delineation of the flat surface of the future nail bed on the dorsal digit tip at 8–10 weeks (Fig. 1-4),[10,145] slightly earlier than the initiation of hair follicle development. Along the proximal boundary of the early nail field a wedge of ectoderm buds inward at an oblique angle to the surface, forming the proximal nail fold. The presumptive nail matrix cells, which will give rise to the differentiated nail plate, reside on the ventral (deeper) side of the proximal invagination. At around 11 weeks, the dorsal surface of the nail bed begins to keratinize, a process similar to subsequent keratinization of the embryonic epidermis.[146–149] In the fourth month, the definitive nail plate grows out distally from the proximal fold, replacing the embryonic cornified layers, and completely covers the nail bed by the fifth month. Keratinization of the nail resembles that of the epidermis except that nail terminal differentiation, like hair shaft differentiation,

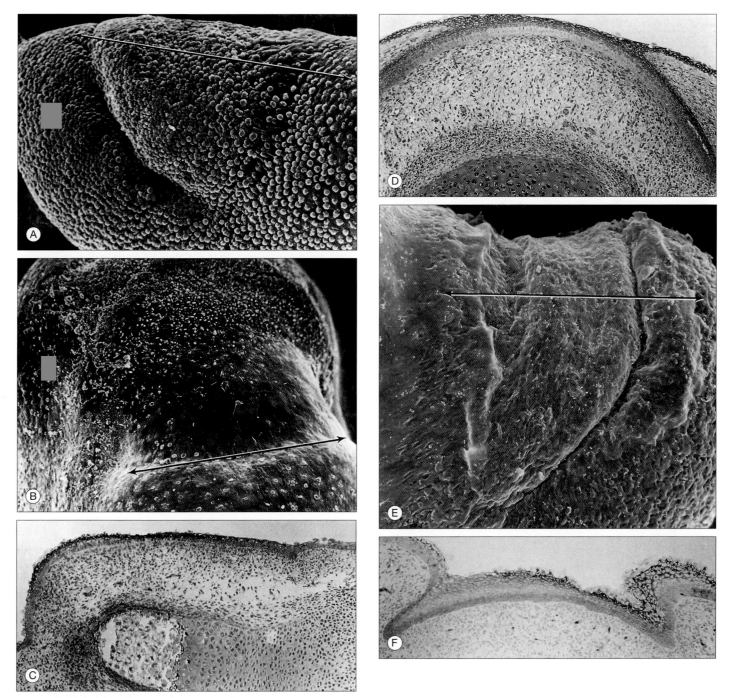

FIG. 1-4 Nail development. The developing nail from 65 to 85 days' EGA, by scanning electron and light microscopy. The nail field boundaries are marked by folds seen clearly in **A, B** and **E**. The lines delimited by arrows indicate the plane of the section taken for the accompanying histologic sections. **C, D** and **F** show the increasing thickness and differentiation of the epidermis forming the presumptive nail plate. Reproduced with permission from Schachner LA, Hansen RC (eds) Pediatric dermatology, 2nd edn. Edinburgh: Churchill Livingstone, 1995.

involves the synthesis of distinct keratins and keratin-aggregating proteins normally not expressed in epidermis.[150–152] The keratins found in hairs and nails provide greater structural stability and rigidity than those in epidermis.

Eccrine and Apocrine Sweat Gland Development

The first morphologic indicators of palmoplantar eccrine gland development are the formation of large mesenchymal bulges or pads on the volar surfaces of the hands and feet between 55 and 65 days' EGA, and the induction of parallel ectodermal ridges overlying these bulges between 12 and 14 weeks (Fig. 1-5).[153,154] The curves and whorls that these ridges adopt are intimately related to the size and shape of the embryonic volar pads and result in the characteristic dermatoglyphic patterns, or 'fingerprints,' which can be visualized on the surface of the digit tips in the fifth month.[154,155] In contrast to those of most other animal species, the volar mesenchymal pads in humans regress by the third trimester.

Individual eccrine gland primordia bud at regularly spaced intervals along the ectodermal ridges, elongating as cords of cells into the pad mesenchyme. By 16 weeks, the glandular regions at the terminal portion of this downgrowth have formed, and the secretory and myoepithelial components become discernible. Canalization of the dermal components of the glands occurs by loss of desmosome adhesion along the innermost ectodermal surfaces with maintenance of lateral adhesion between cells of the duct and gland walls. This process is complete by 16 weeks, whereas the opening of the epidermal portion of the duct by vesicular fusion and autolysis and keratinization of the wall are not complete until 22 weeks' EGA.[156,157] Although the primary ectodermal ridges are established quite early in embryonic development, secondary ridges form at later stages and the complexity of the undulating DEJ increases further at late fetal stages and postnatally with the formation of dermal papillae protruding into the overlying epidermis.

In contrast to volar eccrine glands, interfollicular eccrine glands and apocrine glands do not begin budding until the fifth month of gestation.[136,158] Apocrine sweat glands, like sebaceous glands, usually bud from the upper portion of a hair follicle, whereas eccrine sweat glands arise independently. Over the next several weeks, the glandular cords of cells elongate. By 7 months EGA the clear cells and mucin-secreting

dark cells characteristic of apocrine glands are distinguishable. At birth, the secretory portions of nonvolar sweat glands remain high in the dermis but postnatally extend progressively down to the subcutis. The apocrine gland functions transiently in the third trimester and then becomes quiescent in the neonate,[144,159] whereas the eccrine gland does not appear to function in utero but progressively reaches functional maturity postnatally.[160–164]

Ectodermal Appendages: Clinical Relevance

Genetic studies in mice have suggested that mutations in the genes that direct early regional patterning of the mammalian embryo can have a profound impact on later skin appendage specification and differentiation.[82,83,165,166]

One such gene, *LMX1B*, which encodes a homeobox-containing transcription factor, acts several stages before the initiation of appendageal downgrowths and is important in distal limb patterning.[166] Experimental ablation of *LMX1B* function in mice results in the transformation of dorsal limb musculoskeletal elements and dermal structures to a more ventral (volar side) phenotype. Viewed from the side, *Lmx1b* mutant mouse limbs appear perfectly symmetrical, with the paw pads present on both the ventral and dorsal aspects. Mutations in *LMX1B* have been observed in at least some people with the autosomal dominant disease nail–patella syndrome.[121] These patients display a much less dramatic limb phenotype, characterized by aberrant or absent development of the nails and patellae (elbows). This milder effect on dorsal limb structures reflects the fact that individuals with nail–patella syndrome are heterozygotes. Thus they carry a single defective copy of *LMX1B*, together with a wild-type copy, resulting in only partial loss of gene function.

Several other genes have been identified that appear to regulate skin appendage formation. Positional cloning strategies have been used to identify genes affected in several different types of ectodermal dysplasias, a heterogeneous group of disorders defined by their involvement of hair, nails, glands, and/or teeth (see Tables 1-1 and 1-2). The most common type of ectodermal dysplasia, anhidrotic (hypohidrotic) ectodermal dysplasia, is caused by mutations in the *EDA* or *EDAR* genes, which encode a ligand/receptor pair related to TNF signaling components.[125] The gene encoding MSX1, another homeobox-containing transcription factor, has been shown to be mutated in familial tooth agenesis, which affects not only tooth development but also the formation of nails and hair.[167,168]

Studies in mice suggest that other classic embryonic patterning genes play a direct role in epidermal appendage development, including genes encoding components of the Notched, Wnt, and Sonic hedgehog signaling pathways.[118,169] The importance of such genes in human skin homeostasis has already been demonstrated by the finding that *PATCHED* is the tumor suppressor gene mutated in nevoid basal cell carcinoma (Gorlin) syndrome, and that it and other genes of the pathway are frequently mutated in spontaneous basal cell carcinomas.[170–174] Indeed, several genes involved in tumor formation are critical regulators during embryonic development (Table 1-5). Finally, it is important to consider potential teratogenic effects on normal skin appendage development. Dilantin, for example, can cause broadening of the nail associated with distortions in the underlying distal phalange.

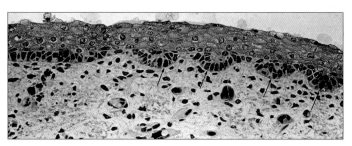

FIG. 1-5 Sweat gland development. Plantar epidermis from the digit of a late first-trimester human fetus showing a multilayered epidermis and the primary epidermal ridges (arrows) that will develop into sweat glands and ducts. Reproduced with permission from Schachner LA, Hansen RC (eds) Pediatric dermatology, 2nd edn. Edinburgh: Churchill Livingstone, 1995.

TABLE 1-5 Skin development

Melanocytic regulators		
KIT	growth factor	Piebaldism
PAX3	transcription factor	Waardenburg syndrome 1,3
MITF	transcription factor	Waardenburg syndrome 2A
SNA12	transcriptional repressor (zn finger, Snail homolog, Neural crest)	Waardenburg syndrome 2D
SOX10, Endothelin-3, EDNRB	transcription factor; G-protein coupled receptor & ligand	Waardenburg syndrome 4
PTPN11 (SHP2)	tyrosine phophotase 2C	LEOPARD syndrome
MYO5	organelle movement	Griscelli syndrome
LYST	lysosomal trafficing	Chediak-Higashi
TYR	tyrosinase	Oculocutaneous albinism, 1A & 1B
TYRP1	tyrosinase-related protein	Oculocutaneous albinism, 3
MATP	Memb asso transporter prot	Oculocutaneous albinism, 4
AP3B1	prot trafficking to lysosomes	Hermansky Pudlak 2
DTNBP1	biogenesis of lysosomes	Hermansky Pudlak 7
BLOC1S3	biogenesis of lysosomes	Hermansky Pudlak 8

PRENATAL DIAGNOSIS OF SEVERE CONGENITAL SKIN DISORDERS

A number of inherited skin disorders are compatible with in utero survival but are life-threatening or result in severe morbidity after birth. Often these disorders can be diagnosed during the first or second trimesters of pregnancy. Candidates for prenatal testing include those fetuses with an affected sibling or other family member. Importantly, the need for prenatal testing depends on the familial relationship, the mode of inheritance of the disorder in question, and in some cases the sex of the fetus. DNA from parents and from both affected and unaffected siblings should be analyzed before conception to determine the exact mutational event responsible for the disorder in the relevant pedigree, and the likelihood that the fetus will in fact inherit the disease.[175] With this in mind, prenatal and genetic counseling should be a critical component of early interventional care of infants affected with severe genodermatoses.

Until recently, prenatal diagnosis of inherited disorders has relied on fetal skin biopsies performed between 19 and 22 weeks' EGA.[176,177] The procedure is carried out under ultrasound guidance, and multiple biopsies must be taken, although the number of biopsies and the sites from which they are taken depend on the disorder for which the fetus is at risk. In some disorders, such as those in which keratinization of the interfollicular dermis is not yet complete, analysis of the developing appendageal structures is required for accurate diagnosis.[177] Fortunately, because of the identification of the genetic mutations responsible for many of these disorders, diagnosis can be made using cells obtained from CVS at 8–10 weeks' EGA, or amniocentesis at 16–18 weeks' EGA.[9] The obvious advantages of these procedures is that they can be performed early in the pregnancy with minimal risk to the mother and fetus.

Fundamental knowledge of those skin disorders whose etiologies are genetic is crucial for the practicing pediatric dermatologist. Awareness of the resources available for both diagnosis and treatment of those fetuses suspected of having an inherited disorder is equally as important and must frequently be reviewed as our understanding of the molecular bases for genetic abnormalities evolves. Data on genetic test availability, provided by both commercial and research laboratories, are provided by GeneTest (http://www.genetests.org), a database for healthcare providers. Information regarding the identity of genes critical for specific disorders, as well as whether laboratories exist that conduct relevant testing, can also be accessed through the website for Online Mendelian Inheritance in Man (*http://www.ncbi.nlm.nih.gov/entrez/query.fcgi?db=OMIM&i tool=toolbar*).[178] It is only through physicians' awareness of the different genodermatoses, as well as their understanding of normal fetal skin development, that the need for evaluation can be recognized, the necessary therapies and supports provided, and the patients best served.

ACKNOWLEDGMENTS

The authors are grateful to Angela Christiano, Karen Holbrook, and William Larsen for their thought-provoking discussions and insights into human genetics and embryology.

REFERENCES

1. Larsen WL. Human Embryology. New York: Churchill Livingstone, 1997.
2. Cunningham FG, MacDonald PC, Gant NF, et al. Williams' obstetrics. Stanford: Appleton & Lange, 1997.
3. Holbrook KA. Structural and biochemical organogenesis of skin and cutaneous appendages in the fetus and newborn. In: Polin RA, Fox WW, eds. Fetal and neonatal physiology. Philadelphia: WB Saunders, 1998; 729–752.
4. Fuchs E. The cytoskeleton and disease: genetic disorders of intermediate filaments. Ann Rev Genet 1996; 30: 197–231.
5. Barsch GS. The genetics of pigmentation: from fancy genes to complex traits. Trends Genet 1996; 12: 99–305.
6. Matsunaka M, Mishima Y. Electron microscopy of embryonic human epidermis at seven and ten weeks. Acta Dermatol Venereol 1969; 49: 241–250.
7. Breathnach AS, Robins J. Ultrastructural features of epidermis of a 14 mm (6 weeks) human embryo. Br J Dermatol 1969; 81: 504–516.
8. Holbrook KA, Odland GF. The fine structure of developing human epidermis: light, scanning, and transmission electron microscopy of the periderm. J Invest Dermatol 1975; 65: 16–38.
9. Holbrook KA, Odland GF. Regional development of the human epidermis in the first trimester embryo and the second trimester fetus (ages related to the timing of amniocentesis and fetal biopsy). J Invest Dermatol 1980; 74: 161–168.
10. Holbrook KA. Structure and function of the developing human skin. In: Goldsmith LA, ed. Physiology, biochemistry, and molecular biology of the skin. New York: Oxford Press, 1991: 63–110.
11. Smith LT, Sakai LY, Burgeson RE, et al. Ontogeny of structural components at the dermal–epidermal junction in human embryonic and fetal skin: the appearance of anchoring fibrils and type VII collagen. J Invest Dermatol 1988; 90: 480–485.
12. Hertle MD, Adams JC, Watt FM. Integrin expression during human epidermal development in vivo and in vitro. Development 1991; 112: 193–206.
13. Thorsteinsdottir S, Roelen BA, Freund E, et al. Expression patterns of laminin receptor splice variants alpha 6A beta 1 and alpha 6B beta 1 suggest different roles in mouse development. Dev Dyn 1995; 204: 240–258.
14. Hodivala-Dilke KM, DiPersio CM, Kreidberg JA, et al. Novel roles for alpha3beta1 integrin as a regulator of cytoskeletal assembly and as a trans-dominant inhibitor of integrin receptor function in mouse keratinocytes. J Cell Biol 1998; 142: 1357–1369.
15. DiPersio CM, Hodivala-Dilke KM, Jaenisch R, et al. alpha3 beta1 Integrin is required for normal development of the epidermal basement membrane. J Cell Biol 1997; 137: 729–742.
16. Furukawa F, Fujii K, Horiguchi Y, et al. Roles of E- and P-cadherin in the human skin. Microsc Res Tech 1997; 38: 343–352.
17. Moll R, Moll I, Franke WW. Identification of Merkel cells in human skin by specific cytokeratin antibodies: changes of cell density and distribution in fetal and adult plantar epidermis. Differentiation 1984; 28: 136–154.
18. Sun TT, Eichner R, Nelson WG, et al. Keratin classes: molecular markers for different types of epithelial differentiation. J Invest Dermatol 1983; 81: 109s–115s.
19. Moll R, Franke WW, Schiller DL, et al. The catalog of human cytokeratins: patterns of expression in normal epithelia, tumors and cultured cells. Cell 1982; 31: 11–24.
20. Hoyes AD. Electron microscopy of the surface layer periderm of human foetal skin. J Anat 1968; 103: 321–336.
21. Lehtonen E, Lehto VP, Vartio T, et al. Expression of cytokeratin polypeptides in mouse oocytes and preimplantation embryos. Dev Biol 1983; 100: 158–165.
22. Jackson BW, Grund C, Winter S, et al. Formation of cytoskeletal elements during mouse embryogenesis. II. Epithelial differentiation and intermediate-sized filaments in early postimplantation embryos. Differentiation 1981; 20: 203–216.
23. Dale BA, Holbrook KA, Kimball JR, et al. Expression of epidermal keratins and filaggrin during human fetal skin development. J Cell Biol 1985; 101: 1257–1269.
24. Moll R, Moll I, Wiest W. Changes in the pattern of cytokeratin polypeptides in epidermis and hair follicles during skin development in human fetuses. Differentiation 1982; 23: 170–178.
25. Nieland ML, Parmley TH, Woodruff JD. Ultrastructural observations on amniotic fluid cells. Am J Obstet Gynecol 1970; 108: 1030–1042.
26. Benzie RJ, Doran TA, Harkins JL, et al. Composition of the amniotic fluid and maternal serum in pregnancy. Am J Obstet Gynecol 1974; 119: 798–810.
27. Boon LM, Mulliken JB, Vikkula M. RASAI variable phenotype with capillary and arteriovenous malformations. Curr Opin Genet Dev 2005 Jun; 15(3): 265–269
28. Lane AT, Helm KF, Goldsmith LA. Identification of bullous pemphigoid, pemphigus, laminin, and anchoring fibril antigens in human fetal skin. J Invest Dermatol 1985; 84: 27–30.
29. Woodcock-Mitchell J, Eichner R, Nelson WG, et al. Immunolocalization of keratin polypeptides in human epidermis using monoclonal antibodies. J Cell Biol 1982; 95: 580–588.
30. Bickenbach JR, Holbrook KA. Label-retaining cells in human embryonic and fetal epidermis. J Invest Dermatol 1987; 88: 42–46.
31. Bickenbach JR, Holbrook KA. Proliferation of human embryonic and fetal epidermal cells in organ culture. Am J Anat 1986; 177: 97–106.
32. Weiss RA, Eichner R, Sun TT. Monoclonal antibody analysis of keratin expression in epidermal diseases: a 48- and 56-kdalton keratin as molecular markers for hyperproliferative keratinocytes. J Cell Biol 1984; 98: 1397–1406.
33. Muller HK, Kalnins R, Sutherland RC. Ontogeny of pemphigus and bullous pemphigoid antigens in human skin. Br J Dermatol 1973; 88: 443–446.
34. Fine JD, Smith LT, Holbrook KA, et al. The appearance of four basement membrane zone antigens in developing human fetal skin. J Invest Dermatol 1984; 83: 66–69.
35. Smith LT, Holbrook KA, Madri JA. Collagen types I, III, and V in human embryonic and fetal skin. Am J Anat 1986; 175: 507–521.
36. West DP, Halket JM, Harvey DR, et al. Percutaneous absorption in preterm infants. Pediatr Dermatol 1987; 4: 234–237.
37. Evans NJ, Rutter N. Percutaneous respiration in the newborn infant. J Pediatr 1986; 108: 282–286.
38. Evans NJ, Rutter N. Development of the epidermis in the newborn. Biol Neonate 1986; 49: 74–80.
39. Harpin VA, Rutter N. Barrier properties of the newborn infant's skin. J Pediatr 1983; 102: 419–425.
40. Nachman RL, Esterly NB. Increased skin permeability in preterm infants. J Pediatr 1971; 79: 628–632.
41. Laiho E, Ignatius J, Mikkola H, et al. Transglutaminase 1 mutations in autosomal recessive congenital ichthyosis: private and recurrent mutations in an isolated population. Am J Hum Genet 1997; 61: 529–538.
42. Epstein EH Jr. The genetics of human skin diseases. Curr Opin Genet Dev 1996; 6: 295–300.
43. Huber M, Rettler I, Bernasconi K, et al. Mutations of keratinocyte transglutaminase in lamellar ichthyosis. Science 1995; 267: 525–528.
44. Russell LJ, DiGiovanna JJ, Rogers GR, et al. Mutations in the gene for transglutaminase 1 in autosomal recessive lamellar ichthyosis. Nature Genet 1995; 9: 279–283.

45. Novice FM, Collison DW, Burgdorf WHC, et al. Handbook of genetic skin disorders. Philadelphia: WB Saunders, 1994.

46. Akiyama M, Kim DK, Main DM, et al. Characteristic morphologic abnormality of harlequin ichthyosis detected in amniotic fluid cells. J Invest Dermatol 1994; 102: 210–213.

47. Akiyama M, Dale BA, Smith LT, et al. Regional difference in expression of characteristic abnormality of harlequin ichthyosis in affected fetuses. Prenat Diagn 1998; 18: 425–436.

48. Dale BA, Holbrook KA, Fleckman P, et al. Heterogeneity in harlequin ichthyosis, an inborn error of epidermal keratinization: variable morphology and structural protein expression and a defect in lamellar granules. J Invest Dermatol 1990; 94: 6–18.

49. Milner ME, O'Guin WM, Holbrook KA, et al. Abnormal lamellar granules in harlequin ichthyosis. J Invest Dermatol 1992; 99: 824–829.

50. Lane AT. Development and care of the premature infant's skin. Pediatr Dermatol 1987; 4: 1–5.

51. Kalia YN, Nonato LB, Lund CH, et al. Development of skin barrier function in premature infants. J Invest Dermatol 1998; 111: 320–326.

52. Anderson DJ. Stem cells and transcription factors in the development of the mammalian neural crest. FASEB J 1994; 8: 707–713.

53. Loomis CA. Linear hypopigmentation and hyperpigmentation, including mosaicism. Semin Cutan Med Surg 1997; 16: 44–53.

54. Loomis CA, Orlow SJ. Cutaneous findings in mosaicism and chimerism. Curr Probl Dermatol 1996; 3: 87–92.

55. Gown AM, Vogel AM, Hoak D, et al. Monoclonal antibodies specific for melanocytic tumors distinguish subpopulations of melanocytes. Am J Pathol 1986; 123: 195–203.

56. Holbrook KA, Underwood RA, Vogel AM, et al. The appearance, density and distribution of melanocytes in human embryonic and fetal skin revealed by the anti-melanoma monoclonal antibody, HMB-45. Anat Embryol 1989; 180: 443–455.

57. Zimmerman AA, Cornbleet T. The development of epidermal pigmentation in the Negro fetus. J Invest Dermatol 1948; 11: 383–395.

58. Mishima Y, Widlan S. Embryonic development of melanocytes in human hair and epidermis. J Invest Dermatol 1996; 46: 263–277.

59. Breathnach AS, Wyllie LM. Electron microscopy of melanocytes and Langerhans' cells in human fetal epidermis at 14 weeks. J Invest Dermatol 1965; 44: 51–60.

60. Foster CA, Holbrook KA, Farr AG. Ontogeny of Langerhans' cells in human embryonic and fetal skin: expression of HLA-DR and OKT-6

determinants. J Invest Dermatol 1986; 86: 240–243.

61. Berman B, Chen VL, France DS, et al. Anatomical mapping of epidermal Langerhans' cell densities in adults. Br J Dermatol 1983; 109: 553–558.

62. Drijkoningen M, De Wolf-Peeters C, Van der Steen K, et al. Epidermal Langerhans' cells and dermal dendritic cells in human fetal and neonatal skin: an immunohistochemical study. Pediatr Dermatol 1987; 4: 11–17.

63. Foster CA, Holbrook KA. Ontogeny of Langerhans' cells in human embryonic and fetal skin: cell densities and phenotypic expression relative to epidermal growth. Am J Anat 1989; 184: 157–164.

64. Moll I, Lane AT, Franke WW, et al. Intraepidermal formation of Merkel cells in xenografts of human fetal skin. J Invest Dermatol 1990; 94: 359–364.

65. Moll I, Kuhn C, Moll R. Cytokeratin 20 is a general marker of cutaneous Merkel cells while certain neuronal proteins are absent. J Invest Dermatol 1995; 104: 910–915.

66. Moll I, Moll R. Early development of human Merkel cells. Exp Dermatol 1992; 1: 180–184.

67. Moll I, Paus R, Moll R. Merkel cells in mouse skin: intermediate filament pattern, localization, and hair cycle-dependent density. J Invest Dermatol 1996; 106: 281–286.

68. Nobukuni Y, Watanabe A, Takeda K, et al. Analyses of loss-of-function mutations of the MITF gene suggest that haploinsufficiency is a cause of Waardenburg syndrome type 2A. Am J Hum Genet 1996; 59: 76–83.

69. Hofstra RM, Osinga J, Tan-Sindhunata G, et al. A homozygous mutation in the endothelin-3 gene associated with a combined Waardenburg type 2 and Hirschsprung phenotype (Shah–Waardenburg syndrome). Nature Genet 1996; 12: 445–457.

70. Edery P, Attie T, Amiel J, et al. Mutation of the endothelin-3 gene in the Waardenburg-Hirschsprung disease (Shah–Waardenburg syndrome). Nature Genet 1996; 12: 442–444.

71. Attie T, Till M, Pelet A, et al. Mutation of the endothelin-receptor B gene in Waardenburg–Hirschsprung disease. Hum Molec Genet 1995; 4: 2407–2409.

72. Ezoe K, Holmes SA, Ho L, et al. Novel mutations and deletions of the KIT steel factor receptor gene in human piebaldism. Am J Hum Genet 1995; 56: 58–66.

73. Tassabehji M, Newton VE, Read AP. Waardenburg syndrome type 2 caused by mutations in the human microphthalmia MITF gene. Nature Genet 1994; 8: 251–255.

74. Puffenberger EG, Hosoda K, Washington SS, et al. A missense mutation of the endothelin-B receptor gene in multigenic Hirschsprung's disease. Cell 1994; 79: 1257–1266.

75. Spritz RA, Droetto S, Fukushima Y. Deletion of the KIT and PDGFRA genes in a patient with piebaldism. Am J Med Genet 1992; 44: 492–495.

76. Tassabehji M, Read AP, Newton VE, et al. Waardenburg's syndrome patients have mutations in the human homologue of the Pax-3 paired box gene. Nature 1992; 355: 635–636.

77. Fleischman RA, Saltman DL, Stastny V, et al. Deletion of the c-kit protooncogene in the human developmental defect piebald trait. Proc Natl Acad Sci USA 1991; 88: 10885–10889.

78. Giebel LB, Spritz RA. Mutation of the KIT mast/stem cell growth factor receptor protooncogene in human piebaldism. Proc Natl Acad Sci USA 1991; 88: 696–699.

79. Sengal P. Morphogenesis of the skin. Cambridge: Cambridge University Press, 1976.

80. Christ B, Jacob HJ, Jacob M. Differentiating abilities of avian somatopleural mesoderm. Experientia 1979; 35: 1376–1378.

81. Noden DM. Vertebrate craniofacial development: novel approaches and new dilemmas. Curr Opin Genet Dev 1992; 2: 576–581.

82. Loomis CA, Harris E, Michaud J, et al. The mouse Engrailed-1 gene and ventral limb patterning. Nature 1996; 382: 360–363.

83. Parr BA, McMahon AP. Dorsalizing signal Wnt-7a required for normal polarity of D-V and A-P axes of mouse limb. Nature 1995; 374: 350–353.

84. Smith LT, Holbrook KA. Development of dermal connective tissue in human embryonic and fetal skin. Scanning Electron Microsc 1982; 1745–1751.

85. Sykes B, Puddle B, Francis M, et al. The estimation of two collagens from human dermis by interrupted gel electrophoresis. Biochem Biophys Res Commun 1976; 72: 1472–1480.

86. Epstein EH Jr. α[3]3 human skin collagen. Release by pepsin digestion and preponderance in fetal life. J Biol Chem 1974; 249: 3225–3231.

87. Deutsch TA, Esterly NB. Elastic fibers in fetal dermis. J Invest Dermatol 1975; 65: 320–323.

88. Martin P. Wound healing – aiming for the perfect skin regeneration. Science 1998; 276: 75–81.

89. Cass DL, Bullard KM, Sylvester KG, et al. Wound size and gestational age modulate scar formation in fetal wound repair. J Pediatr Surg 1997; 32: 411–415.

90. Stelnicki EJ, Bullard KM, Harrison MR, et al. A new in vivo model for the study of fetal wound healing. Ann Plast Surg 1997; 39: 374–380.

91. Smitt JH, van Asperen CJ, Niessen CM, et al. Restrictive dermopathy. Report of 12 cases. Dutch Task Force on Genodermatology. Arch Dermatol 1998; 134: 577–579.

92. Mau U, Kendziorra H, Kaiser P, et al. Restrictive dermopathy: report and review. Am J Med Genet 1997; 71: 179–185.

93. Holbrook KA, Dale BA, Witt DR, et al. Arrested epidermal morphogenesis in three newborn infants with a fatal genetic disorder (restrictive dermopathy). J Invest Dermatol 1987; 88: 330–339.

94. Mucke J, Happle R, Theile H. MIDAS syndrome respectively MLS syndrome: a separate entity rather than a particular lyonization pattern of the gene causing Goltz syndrome. Am J Med Genet 1995; 57: 117–118.

95. Happle R. Lyonization and the lines of Blaschko. [Review]. Hum Genet 1985; 70: 200–206.

96. Happle R, Steijlen PM, Theile U, et al. Patchy dermal hypoplasia as a characteristic feature of Proteus syndrome. Arch Dermatol 1997; 133: 77–80.

97. Risau W, Lemmon V. Changes in the vascular extracellular matrix during embryonic vasculogenesis and angiogenesis. Dev Biol 1988; 125: 441–450.

98. Noden DM. Embryonic origins and assembly of blood vessels. Am Rev Respir Dis 1989; 140: 1097–1103.

99. Johnson CL, Holbrook KA. Development of human embryonic and fetal dermal vasculature. J Invest Dermatol 1989; 93: 10S–17S.

100. Sato TN, Tozawa Y, Deutsch U, et al. Distinct roles of the receptor tyrosine kinases Tie-1 and Tie-2 in blood vessel formation. Nature 1995; 376: 70–74.

101. Vikkula M, Boon LM, Carraway KLR, et al. Vascular dysmorphogenesis caused by an activating mutation in the receptor tyrosine kinase TIE2. Cell 1996; 87: 1181–1190.

102. Johnson DW, Berg JN, Baldwin MA, et al. Mutations in the activin receptor-like kinase 1 gene in hereditary haemorrhagic telangiectasia type 2. Nature Genet 1996; 13: 189–195.

103. McAllister KA, Grogg KM, Johnson DW, et al. Endoglin, a TGF-beta binding protein of endothelial cells, is the gene for hereditary haemorrhagic telangiectasia type 1. Nature Genet 1994; 8: 345–351.

104. Smith LT, Holbrook KA, Byers PH. Structure of the dermal matrix during development and in the adult. J Invest Dermat 1982; 79: 93s–104s.

105. Fujita H, Asagami C, Oda Y, et al. Electron microscopic studies of the differentiation of fat cells in human fetal skin. J Invest Dermatol 1969; 53: 122–139.

106. Fajas L, Fruchart JC, Auwerx J. Transcriptional control of adipogenesis. Curr Opin Cell Biol 1998; 10: 165–173.

107. Klaus S. Functional differentiation of white and brown adipocytes. Bioessays 1997; 19: 215–223.

108. Skolnik EY, Marcusohn J. Inhibition of insulin receptor signaling by TNF: potential role in obesity and non-insulin-dependent diabetes mellitus. Cytokine Growth Factor Rev 1996; 7: 161–173.

109. Digby JE, Montague CT, Sewter CP, et al. Thiazolidinedione exposure increases the expression of uncoupling protein 1 in cultured human preadipocytes. Diabetes 1998; 47: 138–141.

110. Ioffe E, Moon B, Connolly E, et al. Abnormal regulation of the leptin gene in the pathogenesis of obesity. Proc Natl Acad Sci USA 1992; 95: 11852–11857.

111. Lane AT. Human fetal skin development. Pediatr Dermatol 1986; 3: 487–491.

112. Riddle CV. Focal tight junctions between mesenchymal cells of fetal dermis. Anat Rec 1986; 214: 113–117.

113. Giancotti FG. Integrin signaling: specificity and control of cell survival and cell cycle progression. Curr Opin Cell Biol 1997; 9: 691–700.

114. Rousselle P, Keene DR, Ruggiero F, et al. Laminin 5 binds the NC-1 domain of type VII collagen. J Cell Biol 1997; 138: 719–728.

115. Rezniczek GA, de Pereda JM, Reipert S, et al. Linking integrin alpha6beta4-based cell adhesion to the intermediate filament cytoskeleton: direct interaction between the beta4 subunit and plectin at multiple molecular sites. J Cell Biol 1998; 141: 209–225.

116. Guo L, Degenstein L, Dowling J, et al. Gene targeting of BPAG1: abnormalities in mechanical strength and cell migration in stratified epithelia and neurologic degeneration. Cell 1995; 81: 233–243.

117. Christiano AM, Uitto J. Molecular complexity of the cutaneous basement membrane zone. Revelations from the paradigms of epidermolysis bullosa. Exp Dermatol 1996; 5: 1–11.

118. Oro AE, Scott MP. Splitting hairs: dissecting roles of signaling systems in epidermal development. Cell 1998; 95: 575–578.

119. Hardy MH. The secret life of the hair follicle. Trends Genet 1992; 8: 55–61.

120. Sundberg JP. Handbook of mouse mutations with skin and hair abnormalities: Animal models and biomedical tools. Boca Raton: CRC Press, 1994.

121. Dreyer SD, Shou G, Antonio B, et al. Mutations in LMX1B cause abnormal skeletal patterning and renal dysplasia in nail patella syndrome. Nature Genet 1998; 19: 47–50.

122. Ahmad W, Faiyaz ul Haque M, Brancolini V, et al. Alopecia universalis associated with a mutation in the human hairless gene. Science 1998; 279: 20–24.

123. Ferguson BM, Brockdorff N, Formstone E, et al. Cloning of Tabby, the murine homolog of the human EDA gene: evidence for a membrane-associated protein with a short collagenous domain. Hum Molec Genet 1997; 6: 1589–1594.

124. Srivastava AK, Pispa J, Hartung AJ, et al. The Tabby phenotype is caused by mutation in a mouse homologue of the EDA gene that reveals novel mouse and human exons and encodes a protein ectodysplasin-A with collagenous domains. Proc Natl Acad Sci USA 1997; 94: 13069–13074.

125. Kere J, Srivastava AK, Montonen O, et al. X-linked anhidrotic (hypohidrotic) ectodermal dysplasia is caused by mutation in a novel transmembrane protein. Nature Genet 1996; 13: 409–416.

126. Pinkus H. Embryology of hair. In: Montagna W, Ellis RA, eds. The biology of hair growth. New York: Academic Press, 1958: 1–32.

127. Holbrook KA, Odland GF. Structure of the human fetal hair canal and initial hair eruption. J Invest Dermatol 1978; 71: 385–390.

128. Carlsen RA. Human fetal hair follicles: the mesenchymal component. J Invest Dermatol 1974; 63: 206–211.

129. Wessells HK, Roessner KD. Nonproliferation in dermal condensation of mouse vibrissae and pelage hairs. Dev Biol 1965; 12: 419–433.

130. Hashimoto K. The ultrastructure of the skin of human embryos V. The hair germ and perifollicular mesenchymal cells. Br J Dermatol 1970; 83: 167–176.

131. Breathnach AS, Smith J. Fine structure of the early hair germ and dermal papilla in the human foetus. J Anat 1968; 102: 511–526.

132. Robins EJ, Breathnach AS. Fine structure of the human foetal hair follicle at hair-peg and early bulbous-peg stages of development. J Anat 1969; 104: 553–569.

133. Cotsarelis G, Sun TT, Lavker RM. Label-retaining cells reside in the bulge area of pilosebaceous unit: implications for follicular stem cells, hair cycle, and skin carcinogenesis. Cell 1990; 61: 1329–1337.

134. Lavker RM, Sun TT. Hair follicle stem cells: present concepts. J Invest Dermatol 1995; 104: 8S–39S.

135. Montagna W, Van Scott E. The anatomy of the hair follicle. In: Montagna W, Ellis RA, eds. The biology of hair growth. New York: Academic Press, 1958: 39–64.

136. Serri F, Montagna W, Mescon H. Studies of the skin of the fetus and the child. J Invest Dermatol 1962; 39: 99–217.

137. Smith DW, Gong BT. Scalp-hair patterning: its origin and significance relative to early brain and upper facial development. Teratology 1974; 9: 7–34.

138. Barth JH. Normal hair growth in children. Pediatr Dermatol 1987; 4: 173–184.

139. Paus R. Control of the hair cycle and hair diseases as cycling disorders. Curr Opin Dermatol 1996; 3: 248–258.

140. Serri F, Huber MW. The development of sebaceous glands in man. In: Montagna W, Ellis RA, Silver AF, eds. Advances in biology of skin. The sebaceous glands. Oxford: Pergamon Press, 1963: 1–18.

141. Fujita H. Ultrastructural study of embryonic sebaceous cells, especially of their droplet formation. Acta Dermatol Venerol 1972; 52: 99–155.

142. Williams ML, Hincenbergs M, Holbrook KA. Skin lipid content during early fetal development. J Invest Dermatol 1988; 91: 263–268.

143. Pochi PE, Strauss JS, Downing DT. Age-related changes in sebaceous gland activity. J Invest Dermatol 1979; 73: 108–111.

144. Solomon LM, Esterly NB. Neonatal dermatology. I. The newborn skin. J Pediatr 1970; 77: 888–894.

145. Holbrook KA. Structural abnormalities of the epidermally derived appendages in skin from patients with ectodermal dysplasias: Possible insight into developmental errors. In: Salinas C, ed. The ectodermal dysplasias, birth defects: original article series. New York: Liss, 1988: 15–44.

146. Zaias N. Embryology of the human nail. Arch Dermatol 1963; 87: 37–53.

147. Zaias N, Alvarez J. The formation of the primate nail plate. An autoradiographic study in squirrel monkey. J Invest Dermatol 1968; 51: 120–136.

148. Lewis BL. Microscopic studies, fetal and mature nail and surrounding soft tissue. Arch Dermatol 1954; 70: 732–747.

149. Hashimoto K, Gross BG, Nelson R, et al. The ultrastructure of the skin of human embryos. 3. The formation of the nail in 16–18 weeks old embryos. J Invest Dermatol 1966; 47: 205–217.

150. Lynch MH, O'Guin WM, Hardy C, et al. Acidic and basic hair/nail 'hard' keratins: their colocalization in upper cortical and cuticle cells of the human hair follicle and their relationship to 'soft' keratins. J Cell Biol 1986; 103: 2593–2606.

151. O'Guin WM, Galvin S, Schermer A, et al. Patterns of keratin expression define distinct pathways of epithelial development and differentiation. Curr Topics Dev Biol 1987; 22: 97–125.

152. O'Guin WM, Sun TT, Manabe M. Interaction of trichohyalin with intermediate filaments: three immunologically defined stages of trichohyalin maturation. J Invest Dermatol 1992; 98: 24–32.

153. Mulvihill JJ, Smith DW. The genesis of dermatoglyphics. J Pediatr 1969; 75: 579–589.

154. Hirsch W, Schweichel JU. Morphological evidence concerning the problem of skin ridge formation. J Mental Defic Res 1973; 17: 58–72.

155. Okajima M. Development of dermal ridges in the fetus. J Med Genet 1975; 12: 243–250.

156. Hashimoto K, Gross BG, Lever WF. The ultrastructure of the skin of human embryos. I. The intraepidermal eccrine sweat duct. J Invest Dermatol 1965; 45: 139–151.

157. Hashimoto K, Gross BG, Lever WF. The ultrastructure of human embryo skin. II. The formation of intradermal portion of the eccrine sweat duct and of the secretory segment during the first half of embryonic life. J Invest Dermatol 1966; 46: 205–217.

158. Hashimoto K. The ultrastructure of the skin of human embryos. VII. Formation of the apocrine gland. Acta Dermatol Venereol 1970; 50: 241–251.

159. Montagna W, Parakkal PF. Apocrine glands. In: Montagna W, Parakkal PF, eds. The structure and function of skin. New York: Academic Press, 1974: 332–365.

160. Foster KG, Hey EN, Katz G. The response of the sweat glands of the newborn baby to thermal stimuli and to intradermal acetylcholine. J Physiol 1969; 203: 13–29.

161. Green M, Behrendt H. Sweating capacity of neonates. Nicotine-induced axon reflex sweating and the histamine flare. Am J Dis Children 1969; 118: 725–732.

162. Bagnara JT, Ferris W, Turner WA Jr, et al. Melanophore differentiation in leaf legs. Dev Biol 1978; 64: 149–164.

163. Behrendt H, Green M. Nature of the sweating deficit of prematurely born neonates. Observations on babies with the heroin withdrawal syndrome. N Engl J Med 1972; 286: 1376–1379.

164. Sinclair JD. Thermal control in premature infants. Annu Rev Med 1972; 23: 129–148.

165. Loomis CA, Kimmel RA, Tong CX, et al. Analysis of the genetic pathway leading to formation of ectopic apical ectodermal ridges in mouse Engrailed-1 mutant limbs. Development 1998; 125: 1137–1148.

166. Chen H, Lun Y, D, O, et al. Limb and kidney defects in Lmx1b mutant mice suggest an involvement of LMX1B in human nail patella syndrome. Nature Genet 1988; 19: 51–55.

167. Lyngstadaas SP, Nordbo H, Gedde-Dahl T Jr, et al. On the genetics of hypodontia and microdontia: synergism or allelism of major genes in a family with six affected members. J Med Genet 1996; 33: 37–42.

168. Vastardis H, Karimbux N, Guthua SW, et al. A human MSX1 homeodomain missense mutation causes selective tooth agenesis. Nature Genet 1996; 13: 417–421.

169. Cheng-Ming C. Molecular basis of epithelial appendage morphogenesis. Austin, TX: RG Landes, 1998.

170. Aszterbaum M, Rothman A, Johnson RL, et al. Identification of mutations in the human PATCHED gene in sporadic basal cell carcinomas and in patients with the basal cell nevus syndrome. J Invest Dermatol 1998; 110: 885–888.

171. Gailani MR, Stahle-Backdahl M, Leffell DJ, et al. The role of the human homologue of *Drosophila* patched in sporadic basal cell carcinomas. Nature Genet 1996; 14: 78–81.

172. Hahn H, Wicking C, Zaphiropoulous PG, et al. Mutations of the human homolog of *Drosophila* patched in the nevoid basal cell carcinoma syndrome. Cell 1996; 85: 841–851.

173. Johnson RL, Rothman AL, Xie J, et al. Human homolog of patched, a candidate gene for the basal cell nevus syndrome. Science 1996: 272: 668–671.

174. Xie J, Murone M, Luoh SM, et al. Activating smoothened mutations in sporadic basal-cell carcinoma. Nature 1998; 391: 90–92.

175. Sybert VP, Holbrook KA. Prenatal diagnosis and screening. Dermatol Clin 1987; 5: 17–41.

176. Blanchet-Bardon C, Dumez Y. Prenatal diagnosis of a harlequin fetus. Semin Dermatol 1984; 3: 225–228.

177. Holbrook KA. The biology of human fetal skin at ages related to prenatal diagnosis. Pediatric Dermatol 1983; 1: 97–111.

178. Online Mendelian Inheritance in Man, OMIM (TM). McKusick-Nathans Institute for Genetic Medicine, Johns Hopkins University (Baltimore, MD) and National Center for Biotechnology Information, National Library of Medicine (Bethesda, MD), {date of download}. World Wide Web URL: http://www.ncbi.nlm.nih.gov/omim/

Structure and Function of Newborn Skin

Anthony J. Mancini and Leslie P. Lawley

The skin of the newborn serves a pivotal role in the transition from the aqueous intrauterine environment to extrauterine terrestrial life and is integral to the vital functions of mechanical protection, thermoregulation, cutaneous immunosurveillance, and maintenance of a barrier that prevents insensible loss of body fluids. The anatomy and function of skin are most easily understood by dissecting the individual compartments (stratum corneum, epidermis, dermoepidermal junction (DEJ), dermis and subcutaneous tissue) and their component cell types. Specialized structures found within these compartments, such as pilosebaceous units, sweat glands, nerves, and vascular networks, play an essential role both anatomically and functionally in cutaneous homeostasis in the neonate. The anatomy of these compartments and structures of the skin, and the physiologic processes involved in their functions, are the focus of this chapter.

Human skin consists of three layers: epidermis, dermis, and subcutaneous fat (Fig. 2-1). All elements of skin are derived from either ectoderm or mesoderm, the former giving rise to the epidermis and other cutaneous epithelial components.[1] A brief description of fetal skin development is helpful in understanding the structure and function of newborn skin, and is incorporated into some of the following discussions of the various compartments and structures. A more thorough review of cutaneous embryology is the focus of Chapter 1.

STRATUM CORNEUM AND EPIDERMIS

The most obvious clinical difference between the skin of the term newborn and that of an adult is the presence of the moist, greasy, yellow-white substance called vernix caseosa, which is a coating comprising a combination of sebaceous gland secretions, desquamated skin cells, and shed lanugo hairs.[2,3] The vernix caseosa has an important role in maintaining hydration and pH balance, and preventing infection during the first few days of life.[4,5] Certain components of the innate immune system, termed antimicrobial polypeptides (see later this chapter, Cutaneous Immunosurveillance, Langerhans' Cells, and Cytokines), have been isolated in the vernix and probably play an important role in surface defense in the newborn.[4,6,7] This coating persists for the first several days of postnatal life, eventually disappearing completely to reveal the more typical, moderately dry newborn skin.

The structure of term newborn skin is histologically similar to that of older individuals, whereas premature infant skin reveals several unique features that have increased our understanding of fetal skin development. The outermost compartment of the skin, the epidermis, arises from surface ectoderm and at about the third week of fetal life consists of a single layer of undifferentiated cells that becomes two-layered by around 4 weeks.[8] The outer layer of cells, the periderm, is found only in developing skin and is transiently present, eventually undergoing a series of apoptotic cellular events as the epidermis becomes multilayered and the stratum corneum, the outermost layer of flattened, nonnucleated skin cells, is forming.[9] By 24 weeks of gestation the periderm is largely absent,[8,9] and the epidermis shows considerable progressive maturation, which is largely complete by 34 weeks.[10] A thin, hydrophobic layer of the periderm may persist for several days postnatally and may participate in protective and thermoregulatory functions.[11]

The epidermis is a stratified epithelium, the number of cell layers varying between different body regions. The various layers, from the dermal side toward the skin surface, are termed the stratum basale, stratum spinosum, stratum granulosum, and stratum corneum. In areas of thicker skin, such as the palms and soles, the stratum lucidum is interposed between the granular and corneal layers. These epidermal layers are shown in Figure 2-2.

Individual cells within the epidermis are referred to as keratinocytes, so named for the intermediate-sized filament proteins (keratins) that are synthesized within them. Keratins are the major structural proteins of the epidermis and its appendages, constituting up to 85% of the total protein of fully differentiated epidermal keratinocytes.[12] They have been divided into types I and II based on their acidic or basic nature, respectively, and are frequently configured in specific pairs of a type I and a type II protein as obligatory heteropolymers.[13] Terminal differentiation of the epidermis involves the sequential expression of different proteins, including the keratins, in the basal and spinal layers.[14] An important function of the keratins is imparting mechanical integrity to epithelial cells. Mutations in the genes encoding these proteins have been confirmed as the basis of several inherited skin defects, such as the simplex form of the mechanobullous disease epidermolysis bullosa.[12]

The stratum basale consists of a single layer of cells, the basal portions of which are in contact with the dermis and contribute to the DEJ. The cells of the basal layer are cuboidal to columnar in shape and are anchored to the underlying

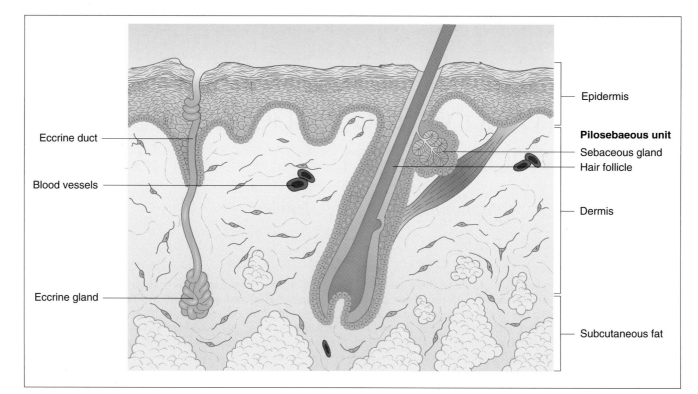

FIG. 2-1 Basic anatomy of the skin, which is composed of three major divisions: epidermis, dermis, and subcutaneous fat. Adnexal structures include pilosebaceous units and eccrine ducts and glands (shown), and apocrine glands (not shown). (Courtesy of Randall Hayes.)

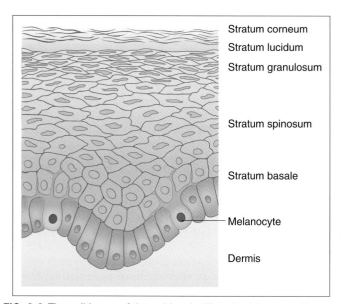

FIG. 2-2 The cell layers of the epidermis. Note the interspersed distribution of melanocytes in the basal cell layer. (Courtesy of Randall Hayes.)

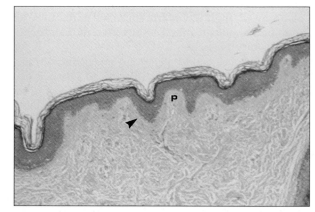

FIG. 2-3 Histologic appearance of normal skin. The basal portion of the epidermis has an undulating surface, resulting in rete ridges (arrowhead) interposed between dermal papillae (p).

dermis by cytoplasmic processes. The stratum basale has an undulating surface inferiorly, forming projections called rete ridges, which lie interposed between the dermal papillae of the superficial (papillary) dermis (Fig. 2-3). The basal cell layer contains cells that eventually replace those continually lost from the epidermis through terminal differentiation, maturation and desquamation. Interspersed among the cells in the basal cell layer are the dendritic, pigment (or melanin)-producing cells (melanocytes), which are discussed in more detail below, under Melanocytes and Pigmentation of the Skin.

The stratum spinosum consists of the cells between the stratum basale and the stratum granulosum and forms the bulk of mammalian epidermis. The keratinocytes in this layer are polyhedral in shape and have numerous tiny, spiny projections spanning the intercellular space between contiguous cells.[15] These projections are composed ultrastructurally of desmosomes, which form communication junctions between the cells. Keratinocytes of the spinous layer become larger, flatter, and more desiccated as they progress from the basal layer toward the skin surface. Also present in this layer are

Langerhans' cells, bone marrow-derived cells that are involved in cutaneous immunosurveillance through antigen processing and presentation (see Cutaneous Immunosurveillance, Langerhans' Cells and Cytokines).

The stratum granulosum comprises a thin layer of darkly stained keratinocytes at the outermost surface of the stratum spinosum. The dark appearance of these cells is due to the presence of keratohyalin granules, which are composed of an electron-dense protein (profilaggrin) and keratin intermediate filaments.[16] Profilaggrin is subsequently converted to filaggrin, a protein involved in the aggregation and disulfide bonding of keratin filaments,[17,18] and it has been suggested that keratohyalin serves to form a matrix that provides structural support by linking keratin filaments to one another.[15] The granular cell layer is also where lamellar bodies (Odland bodies, membrane-coating granules) are produced.[19] These intracellular organelles participate in the formation of the epidermal permeability barrier through the production and discharge of lipid substances into the intercellular corridors of the stratum corneum.

In areas of thicker skin, such as the palms and soles, the stratum lucidum is present as a layer with a clear hyaline appearance. At this level one can visualize transitional cells that exhibit marked degeneration of the nucleus and other organelles and, ultramicroscopically, keratin filaments and keratohyalin granules, which are abundant but not yet as compact as in the stratum corneum.[15]

The stratum corneum, or cornified layer, is composed of several layers of flattened, nonnucleated keratinized cells (corneocytes) arranged in an overlapping fashion. The thickness of this layer varies by body region, being thinnest on the face (especially over the eyelids) and genitalia, and thickest on the palms and soles. It is now widely accepted that the epidermal permeability barrier resides in the stratum corneum and serves the vital functions of preventing excessive transepidermal water loss (TEWL) and preventing penetration of a variety of substances.[20–24]

The formation of the epidermal barrier is accomplished through the lipid secretions of lamellar bodies, which include free fatty acids, ceramides, and cholesterol. These lipids are deposited in the intercellular interstices within the stratum corneum. This arrangement has been likened to 'bricks and mortar,' where the corneocytes represent the bricks and the intercellular lipids represent the mortar.[25] Although these lipids represent only about 10% of the dry weight of the stratum corneum[26] their location and composition are vital, and cutaneous barrier function is dependent on both the generation of sufficient quantities of these lipids and their strategic secretion and organization into lamellar bilayer unit structures.[24,25,27–29] In fact, the epidermis is equipped with the necessary machinery to autonomously regulate its lipid-synthesis apparatus in response to specific barrier requirements.[30–32] The development of a functional barrier has been shown to be closely correlated with normal ontogenesis and does not appear to be disrupted by somatic growth retardation.[33] Hence, more mature infants, even those who are small for gestational age, have a competent epidermal barrier.[34]

The epidermis and stratum corneum in the full-term infant are well developed, and the barrier properties are excellent.[35] Conversely, premature infants have greater skin permeability and a more poorly functioning barrier. Histologically, the term infant has a well-developed epidermis, which is several layers thick, and a well-formed stratum corneum.[2,10] This maturity is lacking in preterm infants.[35–39] An acceleration of skin maturation may occur postnatally in preterm infants, although in extremely low-birthweight infants (23–25 weeks' gestational age) complete development of a fully functional barrier may require up to 8 weeks.[36,37,40] Recent studies support the long-held notion that the shift from an aqueous to an air environment, and hence water flux, may be an important factor in this acceleration of barrier formation.[41] Nonetheless, during the period of postnatal maturation large transepidermal water losses contribute to the morbidity of the preterm infant, and therefore a major focus of past studies has been the development of a therapeutic strategy to accelerate epidermal barrier maturation or augment its function, including the use of semipermeable membranes[42–45] or topical emollients.[46,47] Premature infant skin and barrier maturation are discussed in more detail in Chapter 4.

In addition to the prevention of insensible water losses across the skin by the epidermal barrier, the epidermis and stratum corneum of the newborn provide important protection against toxicity from exposure to ultraviolet rays (UVR), and this protective effect may be greater for UVB than for UVA radiation.[48] As previously noted, melanin is primarily responsible for UVR protection, although the 'protein barrier' of the stratum corneum may augment this cutaneous function.[49] Epidermal lipids may also play a role in protection from UVR. Another function of the superficial skin layers is protection against microorganisms, which are blocked from invasion across the skin by an intact stratum corneum. In addition to such physical factors, the antimicrobial qualities of skin may be related to the relative dryness of the stratum corneum, the presence of skin surface lipids, and the degree of epidermal cellular differentiation.[49–52] Skin is also a vital participant in the process of neonatal thermoregulation (discussed in more detail later) through regulation of cutaneous blood flow and evaporative water loss.

Percutaneous absorption of substances across neonatal skin requires passage through the stratum corneum and epidermis, diffusion into the dermis, and eventual transfer into the systemic circulation. Transfer across the stratum corneum and epidermis may be through the intercellular corridors (favoring nonpolar or hydrophobic compounds) or via a transcellular route (which favors polar or hydrophilic substances).[53] Hair follicles and eccrine sweat ducts may serve as diffusion shunts for certain substances (i.e. ions, polar compounds, very large molecules), which would otherwise traverse the stratum corneum slowly (because of their large molecular weight).[54] The rate-limiting step of percutaneous absorption seems to be diffusion through the stratum corneum,[54] and hence the effectiveness of the epidermal permeability barrier correlates inversely with percutaneous absorption. Percutaneous absorption, although continuously being explored in terms of its therapeutic applications, may contribute to systemic absorption and potential toxicity after topical application of some substances to newborn skin, especially in preterm infants or those with cutaneous damage.[36] Importantly, although the barrier function of intact skin in the term infant is usually normal, the surface area-to-weight ratio is greater than in older children and adults. Caution should therefore be exercised in the use of topical agents in any newborn, with extra caution and a thorough risk–benefit analysis being employed in the case of premature infants or any neonate with a compromised skin barrier. Percutaneous absorption is discussed in more detail in Chapter 5.

DERMOEPIDERMAL JUNCTION

The dermoepidermal junction (DEJ) is an important site of attachment in skin, occurring at the interface between the basal epidermis and the papillary dermis. It appears that the various components of the DEJ are expressed in term newborn skin in a manner similar to that in adults, without apparent differences in their quantity or associations.[2] For reasons that are poorly understood, however, skin appears to be more fragile during the newborn period, even in term infants, as evidenced by blisters or erosions developing in situations that do not cause blisters later in life (e.g. erosions due to diapering, sucking blisters on fingers and hands, and disease states such as bullous syphilis).

Specialized structures called hemidesmosomes assist in anchoring the basal keratinocytes to the underlying plasma membrane. Ultrastructurally the DEJ can be broken down into several planes, including (from the epidermal side to the dermal side) the inferior portion of the basal keratinocyte; an empty-appearing, electron-lucent clear plane known as the lamina lucida; a thin, dark, electron-dense layer known as the lamina densa; and the sublamina densa fibrillar region[16,55] (Fig. 2-4). Each of these layers contains individual components that function harmoniously in concert to create cohesion between the epidermis and the underlying dermis. Defects in, or antibodies directed against, some of these components have been etiologically linked to cutaneous disease.

Major constituents of the DEJ include bullous pemphigoid (BP) antigens, α6β4 integrin, laminin-5, type IV collagen, and type VII collagen. The BP antigens are large glycoproteins with both intracellular (BP antigen 1) and transmembrane (BP antigen 2) components. BP antigen 2, also known as collagen type XVII, extends from the basal keratinocyte across the lamina lucida into the lamina densa,[56] and autoantibodies directed against it have been found in the sera of patients with BP, pemphigoid gestationis, mucous membrane pemphigoid, linear IgA disease, lichen planus pemphigoides, and recently, pemphigoid nodularis.[57,58] Reduced or absent expression of BP antigen 2 is found in patients with a hereditary junctional form of epidermolysis bullosa (EB) termed generalized atrophic benign EB, and has recently been described in a rare variant of EB simplex.[58-62]

α6β4 integrin is a membrane glycoprotein component of the hemidesmosome, and defects in this integrin have been identified in a subset of patients with junctional EB in combination with pyloric atresia.[63-66] Laminin-5 is a glycoprotein localized mainly to the lamina densa and lower lamina lucida,[67] and is also associated predominantly with hemidesmosomes.[68] Mutations in the genes encoding various chains of laminin-5 have been identified in patients with the lethal (Herlitz) junctional type of EB.[69-72]

Type IV collagen predominates in the lamina densa region, whereas type VII collagen, which is also known as the epidermolysis bullosa acquisita (EBA) antigen, is situated in the zone beneath the lamina densa. EBA antigen was so named because it was first defined by circulating autoantibodies in the sera of patients with EBA, an acquired autoimmune blistering disease.[73] The dystrophic forms of inherited EB have been shown to be a result of defects in the gene encoding type VII collagen.[74]

DERMIS AND SUBCUTANEOUS FAT

The dermis of human skin consists primarily of connective tissues, including proteins (collagen and elastic tissue) and ground substance. This compartment lies between the epidermis superiorly and the subcutaneous fat inferiorly and forms a resilient and flexible layer that envelops the entire organism. It is divided into superficial (papillary) and deep (reticular) components, which are anatomically divided by a thin plexus of blood vessels. Although differentiation between these dermal compartments can be ascertained on the basis of the size of the collagen fiber bundles in adult skin, this criterion is less helpful in newborn skin, where there is a more gradual transition in fiber bundle size.[2] Structures found within the dermis, which are discussed in different sections of this chapter, include the cutaneous appendages (pilosebaceous units, eccrine and apocrine sweat glands), as well as nerves, blood vessels, and lymphatics.

Collagen is the major constituent of mammalian dermis and accounts for approximately 75% of the dry weight of the skin.[16] The collagens are a family of related, yet individually distinct, structural proteins, and in the skin they provide tensile strength and elasticity. Types I and III collagen are the major collagens found in human dermis, and smaller amounts of types IV (a primary component of the basement membrane as noted above), V, VI, and VII are also present.[75] Eighty to 90% of dermal collagen is type I. Type III collagen was initially termed fetal collagen because of its predominance in fetal tissues, where it accounts for over half of total skin collagen. However, synthesis of type I collagen accelerates during the postnatal period, and eventually the ratio of type I to type III collagen increases, such that in adult skin it is around 5:1–6:1.[76] Abnormalities in collagen synthesis or posttranslational processing may result in clinical disease, including osteogenesis imperfecta and the Ehlers–Danlos syndromes.

Elastic fibers play an important role in the structure and function of skin, providing elasticity and resilience. They consist of two components: elastin, which is a connective tissue protein, and elastic fiber-associated microfibrillar component, a complex of glycoproteins.[75] Elastic fibers are distrib-

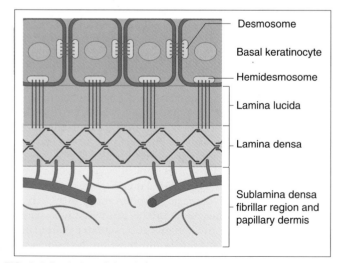

FIG. 2-4 Depiction of the ultrastructure of the dermoepidermal junction (DEJ). Hemidesmosomes assist in anchoring the basal keratinocyte to the underlying plasma membrane. Planes of division within the DEJ include the lamina lucida, lamina densa, and sublamina densa fibrillar region. (Courtesy of Randall Hayes.)

Desmosome

Basal keratinocyte

Hemidesmosome

Lamina lucida

Lamina densa

Sublamina densa fibrillar region and papillary dermis

uted in the papillary and reticular dermis. Fibers in the papillary dermis have been subdivided into elaunin fibers, which are oriented parallel to the DEJ, and oxytalan fibers, which connect the elaunin fibers to the DEJ.[1] It has been demonstrated that elastic fibers are distributed in the term newborn dermis in a manner similar to that of the adult, albeit with a decreased elastin content in the papillary dermal bundles, and with a finer fiber diameter in the reticular dermis.[2] The most widely recognized disease related to abnormalities in elastin production is cutis laxa, a heterogeneous group of disorders featuring lax skin and occasional systemic involvement in the form of hoarseness, emphysema, hernias, and diverticulae.[77]

The ground substance of the dermis is an amorphous material that surrounds and embeds the fibrous and cellular components found in this compartment. Glycosaminoglycans (GAGs), which are long chains of aminated sugars, and proteoglycans (PGs), which are large molecules consisting of a core polypeptide linked to GAGs, are major constituents of ground substance.[1,16] Major GAGs and PGs in the dermis are chondroitin sulfate, dermatan sulfate, heparin/heparin sulfate, chondroitin 6-sulfate, and hyaluronic acid (hyaluronan).[1,16,78] These components are capable of retaining large amounts of water and may also play a role in binding growth factors and providing structural support, anticoagulation, and adhesion.[1,79,80] Hyaluronic acid has been demonstrated in large amounts in fetal dermis and amniotic fluid and is thought by some to be associated with the rapid wound healing without scarring that has been observed to occur in fetal wounds.[81] These observations have been applied to the study of diabetic ulcers, where hyaluronic acid levels have been shown to be decreased, leading to the hypothesis that application of this substance may induce healing.[82] Fibronectin is a large glycoprotein also found in the dermis and is associated with a variety of putative functions, including organization of the extracellular matrix, wound healing, attachment, and chemotaxis.[1,16]

The subcutaneous fat is an important layer, playing a role in shock absorption, energy storage, and maintenance of body heat. The individual cells in the subcutaneous fat – adipocytes – form lobules that are separated by fibrous septa. The fibrous septa contain neural and vascular elements and connect deeper with the fascia of underlying skeletal muscle. In contrast, brown fat is a distinct type of adipose tissue present only in newborns that plays a vital role in neonatal thermoregulation (discussed in more detail later) through the oxidation of fatty acids.[83] Brown fat makes up 2–6% of the neonate's total body weight and is found primarily in the scapular region, the mediastinum, around the kidneys and adrenal glands, and in the axilla.[84] The nonshivering thermogenesis that occurs in this tissue appears to be regulated by the enzyme-uncoupling protein thermogenin, which serves as a protonophore through the mitochondrial membrane, enabling high rates of cellular respiration and proton conductivity.[85] Brown fat is depleted over time and is virtually absent in adults.

PILOSEBACEOUS UNITS, APOCRINE GLANDS, AND NAILS

Hair Follicles

The earliest hair follicles begin to form at 9–12 weeks' gestation[86] primarily in a facial location, and the bulk of the remaining hairs start developing around 16–20 weeks, progressing in a cephalocaudad fashion.[86,87] In some full-term infants, and especially in premature infants, the skin surface is covered with lanugo hairs, which are soft, fine hairs with limited growth potential.[2] These hairs are usually shed by term, or shortly thereafter, and are replaced by vellus hairs, which are eventually replaced on the scalp by coarse terminal hairs. The majority of hairs present at birth are synchronized in their growth phase,[3,88] although this synchrony of growth is disrupted within a few months and may result in a period of temporary alopecia.[88] The growth of a hair follicle is cyclic, the stages being divided into anagen (active growth), catagen (transitional involution), and telogen (resting) phases. The typical length of each of these phases is 2–5 years, 3 days, and 3 months, respectively.[87] No new hair follicles are formed after birth.

The hair follicle is organized into a series of concentric cellular compartments, the details of which are beyond the scope of this chapter. The structure of a pilosebaceous unit is depicted in Figure 2-5. Longitudinally, the hair follicle can be divided into three zones: the infundibulum, extending from the opening of the follicle to the entrance of the sebaceous duct; the isthmus, extending from the entrance of the sebaceous duct to the insertion of the arrector pili muscle; and the inferior segment, which forms the remainder of the follicle from the insertion of the pili muscle to the base. A subpopulation of hair follicle keratinocytes has been identified in the upper follicle near the insertion site of the arrector pili.[89,90] This area has been termed the bulge, and these cells may be involved not only in the regeneration of the anagen hair follicle, but also in the long-term maintenance of the epidermis.[91] Within the specialized environment of the bulge are multipotent stem cells, Merkel cells, and melanocytes which are thought to interact, leading to the differentiation of stem cells into the components of the hair follicle, sebaceous gland and epidermis.[92–96] The exact signaling and control of these stem cells is not known, but adhesion molecules, epidermal growth factor, nerve growth factor, and platelet-derived growth factor are all felt to play a role.[94] The integrity of the hair shaft is related to its protein constituents, including the intermediate filament

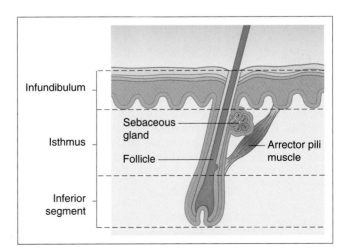

FIG. 2-5 The pilosebaceous unit, divided into three zones: the infundibulum, extending from the opening of the follicle to the entrance of the sebaceous duct; the isthmus, extending from the entrance of the sebaceous duct to the insertion of the arrector pili muscle; and the inferior segment, extending from the insertion of the arrector pili muscle to the base. (Courtesy of Randall Hayes.)

hair keratins and high-sulfur proteins, and to the strong disulfide bonding between these proteins.[87] In neonates, hair may be a source of valuable clinical information, the utility of neonatal hair shaft analysis as a marker for intrauterine exposure to drugs of abuse having emerged as a valuable tool over the last decade.[91-100]

Sebaceous Glands

Sebaceous glands begin to develop between 13 and 15 weeks of fetal life.[101] They are nearly always associated with hair follicles and are found diffusely in the skin, except on the palms, soles, and dorsal feet.[102] The locations of the most prominent glands are the face and scalp, and in term neonates may be quite evident over the nose, forehead, and cheeks. Modified glands are found in the skin of the nipples and areolae (Montgomery's tubercles), on the labia minora and prepuce (Tyson's glands), on the vermilion border of the lips (Fordyce's condition), and in the eyelids (meibomian glands). Sebaceous glands are well formed at birth and are quite active during the neonatal period, when they are stimulated by transplacentally derived steroid hormones and possibly by endogenous steroid production.[3] This sebaceous activity in the newborn is reflected by the common finding of neonatal acne. Sebum, the substance produced by the holocrine sebaceous glands, is a composite of triglycerides, wax esters, squalene, cholesterol, and cholesterol esters and serves a role in lubrication of the follicle and epidermal surface.[1] Sebum levels sharply decline over the first year of life,[103] putatively in response to diminished levels of circulating hormones. The glands then remain relatively quiescent, producing only small amounts of sebum, until puberty.[2]

Apocrine Glands

The apocrine glands are limited in distribution and are found primarily in the axillae, areolae, mons pubis, labia minora, scrotum, perianal area, external ear canal, and eyelids (Moll's glands).[102] Their function in humans is unclear, although they may serve as scent glands. Apocrine glands remain small until puberty, when they enlarge and begin the process of secreting a milky white fluid. Body odor in postadolescent individuals is related to bacterial action on these secretions.

The Nail

The nail acts as a hard, protective covering over the distal end of the digit and may have served a function in evolution to assist in grasping small objects. The nail unit is depicted in Figure 2-6. The nail plate consists of cornified cells with a high protein (primarily keratin) content and is produced by the matrix, a cellular zone situated underneath the proximal nail fold at the base of the nail. The nail plate is situated on top of the nail bed, a highly vascular zone. The lateral nail folds consist of skin that envelops the lateral borders of the nail plate. The average growth rate of the human fingernail is 0.10–0.12 mm/day and appears to be greatest during the second decade of life.[104] Toenails, which grow at a slower rate, may appear to be abnormal or 'ingrown' in newborns as a result of relative nail plate hypoplasia with a bulbous distal phalanx.[105] Despite their abnormal appearance, these nails eventually grow out and take on a more normal appearance.

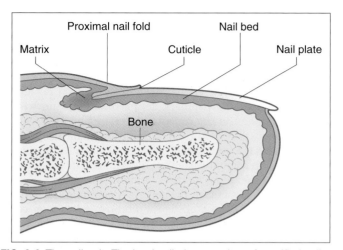

FIG. 2-6 The nail unit. The hard nail plate consists of cornified cells and is produced by the mitotically active cells of the nail matrix, which is situated underneath the proximal nail fold. (Courtesy of Randall Hayes.)

ECCRINE GLANDS AND NEONATAL SWEATING

Eccrine sweating is a physiologic response to increased body temperature and is the most effective means by which humans regulate their body temperature through evaporative heat loss.[106] Gestational age, postnatal age, and body site are all important variables with regard to eccrine glands, and much of what is known about the process of neonatal sweating has been learned from studies of the normal physiologic eccrine gland responses of term and preterm neonates to various sweat-inducing stimuli.

Eccrine sweat glands first appear during fetal development at 14 weeks and are initially limited to the volar surface of the hands and feet.[107] They then appear in the axillae and eventually in a generalized distribution, with a full complement of anatomically normal glands present by the 28th week of gestation, although functionally the glands are immature until 36 weeks of gestation.[108] The total number of eccrine sweat glands is formed before birth[97] and is estimated to be between 2 and 4 million.[107]

The eccrine sweat gland consists of two segments: a secretory coil and a duct. The secretory coil is composed of secretory cells and myoepithelial cells, the latter being contractile cells with smooth muscle-like characteristics.[107] The duct is composed of two cell layers, the basal and luminal ductal cells, which are involved in secretion and reabsorption of solutes. Components of eccrine sweat include water, sodium, chloride, potassium, urea, lactate, and ammonia.[107] Although newly formed sweat is isotonic, reabsorption of water and solutes occurs in the duct such that the expelled product is hypotonic. Evaporation of sweat from the surface of skin removes 0.58 calorie of heat for each gram of water that evaporates.[109]

Eccrine sweat glands are innervated anatomically by fibers of the sympathetic nervous system, although functionally they are under cholinergic influence, and acetylcholine is the major neurotransmitter released from the periglandular nerve endings.[107] Circulating catecholamines can also have a stimulatory effect on eccrine sweat production,[109] as can a variety of other peptides or neurotransmitters.

Sweating can be induced by pharmacologic stimulation and by emotional or thermal stress, and all mechanisms appear to be developed to some extent at birth in term infants. Levels of sweat production in response to the intradermal injection of pharmacologic agents have been demonstrated to bear a direct relation to gestational age,[110–113] as well as to birthweight.[110] Thermal stress-induced sweating, although present in infants, appears to require a greater thermal stimulus in neonates than in adults, and this response also appears to be less developed in premature infants,[113–117] increasing with increasing postnatal age.[115] However, the thermal stimulus of sweating is an important contributor to increased insensible water loss in certain infants at risk, such as those treated with phototherapy for hyperbilirubinemia[118] and those under radiant warmers.[119,120] The core temperature at which sweating begins in full-term newborns has been estimated at around 37.2°C.[121]

'Emotional sweating' also appears to be well developed at birth in full-term but not premature neonates.[108] In one study, skin conductance after heel prick for routine blood testing rose sharply, and to a greater extent, in infants of more advanced gestational ages,[122] supporting the role of postconceptual age in maturation of the sweating response to emotional stress. Another study using auditory stimuli revealed that the sympathetic nervous system innervating the eccrine glands developed over the first 10 weeks of life.[123]

The process of neonatal sweating, therefore, appears to develop early anatomically in fetal life and functionally at later stages, and the sweating response appears to be well developed at birth in term but not preterm infants. Hypotheses on the potential mechanisms for progressive postnatal maturity of the sweating response include anatomic development of the sweat gland, functional development of the gland, or nervous system maturation.[115]

NERVES, VASCULAR NETWORKS, AND THERMOREGULATION

The cutaneous neural and vascular networks both develop early in the fetus, and their architecture becomes organized into adult patterns with increasing postnatal age.[2] Nerve networks in the skin contain both somatic sensory and sympathetic autonomic fibers and function as innervation for arrector pili muscles, cutaneous blood vessels, and sweat glands, as well as serving as receptors for touch, pain, temperature, itch, and mechanical stimuli. Large myelinated fibers, which are cutaneous branches of musculoskeletal nerves, innervate the skin in a pattern similar to that of vascular supply, whereas sensory nerves follow segmental dermatomes, which often show some overlap. Although cutaneous nerve fibers in the neonate are similar in structure and distribution to those in the adult, ultramicroscopic examination has revealed a higher percentage of unmyelinated fibers with bundling of axons, suggesting cytoarchitectural immaturity or incomplete growth.[124]

Sensory cutaneous nerves may end freely or in encapsulated terminals. Free nerve endings in skin represent the most important of sensory receptors and include penicillate fibers found in a subepidermal location in hairy skin,[125] multiple types of free endings in digital (nonhairy) skin,[126] and papillary nerve endings found at the orifice of hair follicles.[16] Free nerve endings may also be associated with Merkel cells, neurosecretory cells of uncertain biologic significance that are of epithelial derivation and which become scarce in human skin after

fetal development.[2,127,128] Studies suggest that Merkel cells may actually be trophic for developing nerves and therefore play an inductive role in the development of the human cutaneous nerve plexus.[129] Specialized sensory receptors are present to varying degrees at birth, including Pacinian corpuscles, which are well developed and abundant in palm and sole skin, and Meissner's corpuscles, which are not fully formed and undergo continued morphologic changes with age.[2]

The vasculature of human dermis comprises two plexuses that parallel the skin surface: one in the lower dermis (deep plexus) and one just beneath the papillary dermis (superficial plexus).[102] These two systems are connected by intercommunicating vessels, and vertical vessel arcades project superiorly from the superficial plexus toward the epidermis to form papillary loops (Fig. 2-7). This subpapillary plexus also gives rise to vessels that infuse the periadnexal structures.[102] The cutaneous vascular system also contains arteriovenous shunts, or glomi, which are specialized anastomoses that assist in the regulation of skin blood flow and thermoregulatory shunting.[3,114] The cutaneous capillary network is fairly disordered at birth and assumes a more orderly network pattern by the second week of life,[130] with continued development until around 3 months.[131]

Vasomotor tone is under the control of a complex series of neurogenic, myogenic, and pharmacologic mechanisms,[3] and the ability to control skin blood flow is now known to be well developed in neonates.[132] It was previously suggested that skin blood flow and total peripheral blood flow both correlate inversely (and decrease) with increasing birthweight, gestational maturity, and postnatal age, along with the development of increasing peripheral vascular resistance.[133] However, studies of capillary blood cell velocity (CBV) in full-term infants have demonstrated a correlation between CBV and postnatal age, making the significance of previous microvascular findings in the neonate unclear.[134]

Thermoregulation, which maintains an equilibrium between heat production and heat loss, is a crucial requirement in the neonate for maintenance of optimal core body temperature. It is a complex physiologic process under the control of the nervous (most importantly the hypothalamus) and endocrine

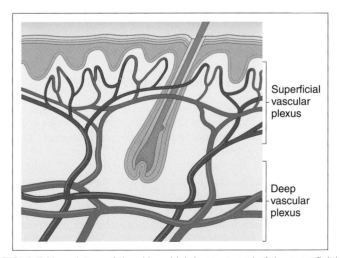

FIG. 2-7 Vasculature of the skin, which is composed of the superficial plexus and the deep plexus with intercommunicating vessels. The superficial plexus gives rise to vertical vessel arcades that project superiorly into the dermal papillae and form papillary loops. (Courtesy of Randall Hayes.)

systems. Although the thermoregulatory response is present in both term and preterm neonates, it is more pronounced in term infants.[135] The primary contributors to thermogenesis are muscles (voluntary and involuntary, or 'shivering' thermogenesis), sweat glands, blood vessels, and adipose tissue.[136] Heat loss, or thermolysis, is accomplished by flow of heat from the center of the body to the surface and, subsequently, flow of heat from the body surface to the environment.[136] Heat transfer to the surroundings can be accomplished through conduction (thermal exchange between the body surface and objects with which it is in contact), convection (heat loss from mass flow of moving air over the body surface), or radiation (electromagnetic heat loss to cool surfaces within the environment). Water evaporation, the fourth mechanism of heat loss, is discussed in the section on neonatal sweating.

Thermal stimuli providing information to the hypothalamus are transmitted from skin thermal receptors, as well as from deeper receptors present in the abdominal cavity and central nervous system.[136,137] In general, increased environmental temperature results in cutaneous arteriolar vasodilatation and heat dissipation, whereas cold stress leads to vasoconstriction, with resultant decreased skin blood flow and reduced heat loss from the body core. Heat production in the neonate is accomplished primarily through nonshivering thermogenesis, which utilizes the increased number of mitochondria, increased glycogen stores, and abundant blood supply of brown fat.[137] The primary mechanism utilized by the overheated neonate to dissipate heat is evaporative water loss through sweating.

Although temperature regulation is developed to some extent in most infants, they are susceptible to both cold and heat stress. Transition out of the stable thermal environment of the uterus, as well as birth trauma, malformations, drugs, and respiratory deficiency, may predispose the newborn to hypothermia, whereas birth trauma and exogenous sources of heat may lead to hyperthermia.[136] Studies of both full-term and preterm infants reveal a decreased ability to vasoconstrict blood vessels in the extremities following exposure to cool temperatures, further predisposing infants to hypothermia.[121,138] Thermoregulation is a multifaceted process, which at times may be inadequate in the maintenance of the homeothermic state in the neonate. An understanding of these processes is therefore vital for providing appropriate thermal support to such infants.

MELANOCYTES AND PIGMENTATION OF THE SKIN

As mentioned, interspersed among the basal layer cells are the dendritic, melanin-producing cells called melanocytes. These cells first appear between a gestational age of 40 and 50 days and migrate to the skin from the neural crest.[139] Whereas melanocytes are found in both basal and suprabasal locations during embryogenesis, neonatal skin reveals a more limited distribution restricted to the basal epidermal layer.[140,141] Melanin is manufactured within organelles called melanosomes, which are formed in melanocytes and transferred to neighboring keratinocytes via dendritic connections. Each melanocyte is in contact with roughly 36 keratinocytes, an association that is referred to as the epidermal melanin unit. The transfer of melanin from the melanocyte to the keratinocytes within this unit results in pigment being distributed in the basal layer, as well as more superficially, where melanin serves a protective role by absorbing and scattering ultraviolet radiation (UVR).[16]

Two forms of melanin are present in human skin: eumelanin, which is brown, and pheomelanins, which are red and yellow.[115,142] Differences in native skin pigmentation among individuals are related to the concentration, as well as the distribution and retention, of melanin in the basal cell layer, rather than to the absolute number of melanocytes.[1,143,144] Although melanocytes in newborn skin are quantitatively comparable to those in older individuals, melanin production, and hence skin pigmentation, is relatively decreased during the neonatal period,[2,3] with gradual darkening over several months following birth. Several disorders of either increased or decreased pigmentation, as well as proliferation of melanocytes, are seen in the newborn period. These include disorders such as albinism, piebaldism, café au lait macules, congenital nevi, and others. Disorders of pigmentation and melanocytes are discussed in Chapters 21 and 22.

CUTANEOUS IMMUNOSURVEILLANCE, LANGERHANS' CELLS, AND CYTOKINES

Cutaneous Immunosurveillance

While participating in the important roles of physical protection, barrier function, and thermoregulation, the skin also occupies a niche in the immunologic system of the host as a peripheral immune organ. Various models and terms have been used to describe the immunologic capacities of the skin, including skin-associated lymphoid tissues (SALT), skin immune system (SIS), dermal microvascular unit (DMU), and dermal immune system (DIS).[145,146] SALT are composed of epidermal Langerhans' cells and keratinocytes, as well as dermal endothelial cells and the skin-draining lymph nodes, and are an important system in the induction of immunity and tolerance.[146] The broader terminology of the SIS refers to the entire complex interplay of immune response-related systems in the skin, including cellular components and humoral factors,[146,147] and both dermal and epidermal components.

These immunologic systems in the skin provide cutaneous immunosurveillance, which functions in the prevention of the development of cutaneous neoplasms and mediates against persistent infections with intracellular pathogens.[148] Cellular components include keratinocytes, antigen-presenting cells (APCs), monocytes and macrophages, granulocytes, mast cells, lymphocytes, and endothelial cells, whereas humoral constituents include antimicrobial peptides, complement proteins, immunoglobulins, cytokines, and prostaglandins.[146] Antimicrobial peptides and proteins are an important innate cutaneous defense mechanism against microbial intruders. They have a broad-spectrum killing activity, and their presence in both amniotic fluid and vernix caseosa has been well documented, suggesting that effective innate immune protection begins during fetal and early neonatal life.[4,6,149,150] Human antimicrobial peptides include the cathelicidin and β-defensin families.

Characterization of lymphocyte populations within normal human skin has revealed that they are predominantly T cells, with 90% of cells clustered around postcapillary venules or adjacent to cutaneous appendages.[147,151] Intraepidermal localization of T lymphocytes accounts for less than 2% of skin lymphocytes normally present. B lymphocytes are not present in normal human skin, but may be found in mucosal locations.

Langerhans' Cells

The cell that sets the SIS apart from others is the Langerhans' cell (LC). This APC resides in the epidermis and is involved in skin allograft rejection, delayed hypersensitivity reactions, and specific T-cell responses.[152] LCs are derived from the bone marrow and migrate via a hematogenous route to the skin. They are present in the fetus as early as 16 weeks' gestation, with early restriction to the basal layer and eventual distribution among suprabasal cells.[153]

The function of the LC was unclear until the 1970s, when surface Fc receptors, major histocompatibility complex (MHC) class II molecules, and C3 receptors were described on its surface,[148] suggesting an immunologic role. It is now well accepted that the epidermal LC is involved in antigen processing and presentation in a variety of skin-induced immune responses against a variety of antigens, including contact allergens, alloantigens, tumor antigens, and microorganisms.[154] These cells have been found to have positive staining for other characteristic surface markers, including CD1a and S100 proteins and membrane-bound adenosine triphosphatase (ATPase).[154] Although the exact function of the CD1a glycoprotein remains unclear, relatively weak expression of the antigen on LCs from neonatal skin has been demonstrated[155] and may partially explain why neonatal donor skin demonstrates extended survival compared to adult donor skin after transplantation in animal models.[156–158] Ultrastructurally, LCs are found to contain Birbeck granules, distinctive cytoplasmic organelles with central striations and a characteristic 'tennis racket' appearance on thin sections.[152] Although the exact function of these granules is unknown, it has been suggested that they may be involved in receptor–ligand interactions and surface antigen trafficking.[159]

LCs are a member of the dendritic family of cells, which are stellate cells with cytoplasmic extensions, or dendrites. Other dendritic APCs are present in human skin, including dermal dendritic cells, which also contribute to the surveillance function of the immune system and initiation of the primary immune response. These cells were also shown to express high levels of MHC class II molecules, as well as factor XIIIa, and are isolated primarily from the dermis.[160] Some dermal dendritic cells may acquire the ultrastructural characteristics of LCs and therefore may be precursors of these epidermal APCs.[160]

Cytokines

In addition to the role of such cellular components in cutaneous immunity, a complex interplay with several humoral factors is also present, including the biologic proteins known as cytokines. These autocrine, paracrine, endocrine, exocrine, and intracrine proteins include the interleukins (ILs), interferons (IFNs), colony-stimulating factors (CSFs), tumor necrosis factors (TNFs), and growth factors (GFs).[147,154] They are produced by various cell types, including keratinocytes, which have been demonstrated to be capable of secreting several types of cytokine.[147]

Cytokines have multiple biologic functions and act on target cells by binding to specific receptors. The result of such binding is signal transduction to the cell interior followed by activation of various second-messenger pathways and eventual altered gene expression and cell function.[154] For instance, on exposure to contact allergens LCs may show enhanced migration after induction of local IL-1β production, ultimately resulting in activation and expansion of allergen-specific T-cell populations,[146] whereas IL-10 inhibits the ability of LCs to stimulate T cells.[152] Cytokines are involved in many cutaneous processes, both physiologic and pathologic, the details of which are beyond the scope of this chapter. Although not clearly elucidated, the secretion, activity, and effector functions of cytokines in neonates may differ from those in adults. An example is the hypothalamic response to IL-1, also known as endogenous pyrogen, in newborns. The synthesis of prostaglandins in response to this protein normally shifts the thermoregulatory set-point, resulting in fever, but this responsiveness is decreased in the neonate, which may account for the attenuated fever response in the setting of infection.[142]

REFERENCES

1. White CR, Bigby M, Sangueza OP. What is normal skin? In: Arndt KA, LeBoit PE, Robinson JK, Wintroub BU, eds. Cutaneous medicine and surgery. an integrated program in dermatology. Philadelphia: WB Saunders, 1996; 3–45.
2. Holbrook KA. A histological comparison of infant and adult skin. In: Maibach HI, Boisits EK, eds. Neonatal skin, structure and function. New York: Dekker, 1982; 3–31.
3. Solomon LM, Esterly NB. Neonatal dermatology. I. The newborn skin. J Pediatr 1970; 77: 888–894.
4. Marchini G, Lindow S, Brismar H, et al. The newborn infant is protected by an innate antimicrobial barrier: peptide antibiotics are present in the skin and vernix caseosa. Br J Dermatol 2002; 147: 1127–1134.
5. Visscher MO, Narendran V, Pickens WL, et al. Vernix caseosa in neonatal adaptation. J Perinatol 2005; 25: 440–446.
6. Yoshio H, Tollin M, Gudmundsson GH, et al. Antimicrobial polypeptides of human vernix caseosa and amniotic fluid: implications for newborn innate defense. Pediatr Res 2003; 53: 211–216.
7. Yoshio H, Lagercrantz H, Gudmundsson GH, et al. First line of defense in early human life. Semin Perinatol 2004; 28: 304–311.
8. Serri F, Montagna W. The structure and function of the epidermis. Pediatr Clin North Am 1961; 8: 917–941.
9. Holbrook KA, Sybert VP. Basic science. In: Schachner LA, Hansen RC, eds. Pediatric dermatology, 2nd edn. New York: Churchill Livingstone, 1995; 1–70.
10. Evans NJ, Rutter N. Development of the epidermis in the newborn. Biol Neonate 1986; 49: 74–80.
11. Wickett RR, Mutschelknaus JL, Hoath SB. Ontogeny of water sorption–desorption in the perinatal rat. J Invest Dermatol 1993; 100: 407–411.
12. Fuchs E. Keratins: Mechanical integrators in the epidermis and hair and their role in disease. Prog Dermatol 1996; 30: 1–12.
13. Fuchs E, Weber K. Intermediate filaments: Structure, dynamics, function, and disease. Annu Rev Biochem 1994; 63: 345–382.
14. Byrne C, Tainsky M, Fuchs E. Programming gene expression in developing epidermis. Development 1994; 120: 2369–2383.

15. Bressler RS, Bressler CH. Functional anatomy of the skin. Clin Podiatr Med Surg 1989; 6: 229–246.

16. Haake AR, Holbrook KA. The structure and development of skin. In: Freedberg IM, Eisen AZ, Wolff K, et al. (eds) Dermatology in general medicine, 5th edn. New York: McGraw-Hill, 1999; 70–114.

17. Dale BA, Holbrook KA, Steinert PM. Assembly of stratum corneum basic protein and keratin filaments in macrofibrils. Nature 1978; 276: 729–731.

18. Manabe M, Sanchez M, Sun TT, et al. Interaction of filaggrin with keratin filaments during advanced stages of normal human epidermal differentiation and in ichthyosis vulgaris. Differentiation 1991; 48: 43–50.

19. Odland GF, Holbrook K. The lamellar granules of epidermis. Curr Probl Dermatol 1981; 9: 29–49.

20. Elias PM. Lipids and the epidermal permeability barrier. Arch Dermatol Res 1981; 270: 95–117.

21. Elias PM. Epidermal lipids, barrier function and desquamation. J Invest Dermatol 1983; 80(Suppl): 44S–49S.

22. Proksch E, Holleran WM, Menon GK, et al. Barrier function regulates epidermal lipid and DNA synthesis. Br J Dermatol 1993; 128: 473–482.

23. Elias PM, Feingold KR. Lipids and the epidermal water barrier: metabolism, regulation, and pathophysiology. Semin Dermatol 1992; 11: 176–182.

24. Grubauer G, Feingold KR, Harris RM, et al. Lipid content and lipid type as determinants of the epidermal permeability barrier. J Lipid Res 1989; 30: 89–96.

25. Elias PM. Dynamics of the epidermal barrier: New implications for percutaneous drug delivery, topical therapeutics and disease pathogenesis. Prog Dermatol 1992; 26: 1–8.

26. Friberg SE. Micelles, microemulsions, liquid crystals, and the structure of stratum corneum lipids. J Soc Cosmet Chem 1990; 41: 155–171.

27. Elias PM, Goerke J, Friend DS. Mammalian epidermal barrier layer lipids: Composition and influence on structure. J Invest Dermatol 1977; 69: 535–546.

28. Elias PM, Friend DS. The permeability barrier in mammalian epidermis. J Cell Biol 1975; 65: 180–191.

29. Aszterbaum M, Menon GK, Feingold KR, et al. Ontogeny of the epidermal barrier to water loss in the rat: Correlation of function with stratum corneum structure and lipid content. Pediatr Res 1992; 31: 308–317.

30. Menon GK, Feingold KR, Moser AH, et al. De novo sterologenesis in the skin. II. Regulation by cutaneous barrier requirements. J Lipid Res 1985; 26: 418–427.

31. Grubauer G, Feingold KR, Elias PM. Relationship of epidermal lipogenesis to cutaneous barrier function. J Lipid Res 1987; 28: 746–752.

32. Monger DJ, Williams ML, Feingold KR, et al. Localization of sites of lipid biosynthesis in mammalian epidermis. J Lipid Res 1988; 29: 603–611.

33. Williams ML, Aszterbaum M, Menon GK, et al. Preservation of permeability barrier ontogenesis in the intrauterine growth-retarded fetal rat. Pediatr Res 1993; 33: 418–424.

34. Hammarlund K, Sedin G, Stromberg B. Transepidermal water loss in newborn infants. VIII. Relation to gestational age and post-natal age in appropriate and small for gestational age infants. Acta Paediatr Scand 1983; 72: 721–728.

35. Barker N, Hadgraft J, Phil D, et al. Skin permeability in the newborn. J Invest Dermatol 1987; 88: 409–411.

36. Harpin VA, Rutter N. Barrier properties of the newborn infant's skin. J Pediatr 1983; 102: 419–424.

37. Evans NJ, Rutter N. Percutaneous respiration in the newborn infant. J Pediatr 1986; 108: 282–286.

38. Rutter N. The immature skin. Br Med Bull 1988; 44: 957–970.

39. Hammarlund K, Sedin G. Transepidermal water loss in newborn infants. III. Relation to gestational age. Acta Paediatr Scand 1979; 68: 795–801.

40. Kalia YN, Nonato LB, Lund CH, Guy RH. Development of skin barrier function in premature infants. J Invest Dermatol 1998; 111: 320–326.

41. Hanley K, Jiang Y, Elias PM, et al. Acceleration of barrier ontogenesis in vitro through air exposure. Pediatr Res 1997; 41: 293–299.

42. Bustamante SA, Steslow J. Use of a transparent adhesive dressing in very low birthweight infants. J Perinatol 1989; 9: 165–169.

43. Knauth AK, Gordin M, McNelis W, et al. Semipermeable polyurethane membrane as an artificial skin for the premature neonate. Pediatrics 1989; 83: 945–950.

44. Vernon HJ, Lane AT, Wischerath LJ, et al. Semipermeable dressing and transepidermal water loss in premature infants. Pediatrics 1990; 86: 835–847.

45. Mancini AJ, Sookdeo-Drost S, Madison KC, et al. Semipermeable dressings improve epidermal barrier function in premature infants. Pediatr Res 1994; 36: 306–314.

46. Lane AT, Drost SS. Effects of repeated application of emollient cream to premature neonates' skin. Pediatrics 1993; 92: 415–419.

47. Nopper AJ, Horii KA, Sookdeo-Drost S, et al. Topical ointment therapy benefits premature infants. J Pediatr 1996; 128: 660–669.

48. Corsini E, Sangha N, Feldman SR. Epidermal stratification reduces the effects of UVB (but not UVA) on keratinocyte cytokine production and cytotoxicity. Photodermatol Photoimmunol Photomed 1997; 13: 147–152.

49. Jackson SM, Elias PM. Skin as an organ of protection. In: Fitzpatrick TB, Eisen AZ, Wolff K, et al. (eds) Dermatology in general medicine, 4th edn. New York: McGraw-Hill, 1993; 241–253.

50. Wyatt JE, Poston SM, Noble WC. Adherence of Staphylococcus aureus to cell monolayers. J Appl Bacteriol 1990; 69: 834–844.

51. Romero-Steiner S, Witek T, Balish E. Adherence of skin bacteria to human epithelial cells. J Clin Microbiol 1990; 28: 27–31.

52. Darmstadt GL, Fleckman P, Jonas M, et al. Differentiation of cultured keratinocytes promotes the adherence of Streptococcus pyogenes. J Clin Invest 1998; 101: 128–136.

53. Ebling FJG. Functions of the skin. In: Champion RH, Burton JL, Ebling FJG, eds. Textbook of dermatology, 5th edn. Oxford: Blackwell Scientific, 1992; 125–155.

54. Hurley HJ. Permeability of the skin. In: Moschella SL, Hurley HJ, eds. Dermatology, 3rd edn. Philadelphia: WB Saunders, 1992; 101–106.

55. Woodley D, Sauder D, Talley MJ, et al. Localization of basement membrane components after dermal–epidermal junction separation. J Invest Dermatol 1983; 81: 149–153.

56. Pulkkinen L, Uitto J. Hemidesmosomal variants of epidermolysis bullosa. Mutations in the Greek α6β4 integrin and the 180-kDa bullous pemphigoid antigen/type XVII collagen genes. Exp Dermatol 1998; 7: 46–64.

57. Zone JJ, Taylor TB, Meyer LJ, et al. The 97 kDa linear IgA bullous disease antigen is identical to a portion of the extracellular domain of the 180 kDa bullous pemphigoid antigen, BPAg2. J Invest Dermatol 1998; 110: 207–210.

58. Powell AM, Sakuma-Oyama N, Oyama N, et al. Collagen XVII/BP180: a collagenous transmembrane protein and component of the dermoepidermal anchoring complex. Clin Exp Dermatol 2005; 30: 682–687.

59. Jonkman MF, deJong MC, Heeres K, et al. 180-kD bullous pemphigoid antigen (BP180) is deficient in generalized atrophic benign epidermolysis bullosa. J Clin Invest 1995; 95: 1345–1352.

60. Pohla-Gubo G, Lazarova Z, Giudice GJ, et al. Diminished expression of the extracellular domain of bullous pemphigoid antigen 2 (BPAG2) in the epidermal basement membrane of patients with generalized atrophic benign epidermolysis bullosa. Exp Dermatol 1995; 4: 199–206.

61. Gatalica B, Pulkkinen L, Li K, et al. Cloning of the human type XVII collagen gene (COL17A1), and detection of novel mutations in generalized atrophic benign

epidermolysis bullosa. Am J Hum Genet 1997; 60: 352–365.

62. Huber M, Floeth M, Borradori L, et al. Deletion of the cytoplasmic domain of BP180/collagen XVII causes a phenotype with predominant features of epidermolysis bullosa simplex. J Invest Dermatol 2002; 118: 185–192.

63. Vidal F, Aberdam D, Miquel C, et al. Integrin beta 4 mutations associated with junctional epidermolysis bullosa with pyloric atresia. Nature Genet 1995; 10: 229–234.

64. Pulkkinen L, Bruckner-Tuderman L, et al. Compound heterozygosity for missense (L156P) and nonsense (R554X) mutations in the beta4 integrin gene (ITGB4) underlies mild, nonlethal phenotype of epidermolysis bullosa with pyloric atresia. Am J Pathol 1998; 152: 935–941.

65. Ruzzi L, Gagnoux-Palacios L, Pinola M, et al. A homozygous mutation in the integrin alpha6 gene in junctional epidermolysis bullosa with pyloric atresia. J Clin Invest 1997; 99: 2826–2831.

66. Brown TA, Gil SG, Sybert VP, et al. Defective integrin alpha 6 beta 4 expression in the skin of patients with junctional epidermolysis bullosa and pyloric atresia. J Invest Dermatol 1996; 107: 384–391.

67. Stanley JR, Woodley DT, Katz SI, et al. Structure and function of basement membrane. J Invest Dermatol 1982; 79: 69S–72S.

68. Masunaga T, Shimizu H, Ishiko A, et al. Localization of laminin-5 in the epidermal basement membrane. J Histochem Cytochem 1996; 44: 1223–1230.

69. Uitto J, Pulkkinen L, Christiano AM. Molecular basis of the dystrophic and junctional forms of epidermolysis bullosa: mutations in the type VII collagen and kalinin (laminin 5) genes. J Invest Dermatol 1994; 103: 39S–46S.

70. Pulkkinen L, McGrath J, Airenne T, et al. Detection of novel LAMC2 mutations in Herlitz junctional epidermolysis bullosa. Mol Med 1997; 3: 124–135.

71. Kivirikko S, McGrath JA, Pulkkinen L, et al. Mutational hotspots in the LAMB3 gene in the lethal (Herlitz) type of junctional epidermolysis bullosa. Hum Mol Genet 1996; 5: 231–237.

72. Kivirikko S, McGrath JA, Baudoin C, et al. A homozygous nonsense mutation in the alpha 3 chain gene of laminin 5 (LAMA3) in lethal (Herlitz) junctional epidermolysis bullosa. Hum Mol Genet 1995; 4: 959–962.

73. Woodley DR. Importance of the dermal–epidermal junction and recent advances. Dermatologica 1987; 174: 1–10.

74. Hovnanian A, Rochat A, Bodemer C, et al. Characterization of 18 new mutations in COL7A1 in recessive dystrophic epidermolysis bullosa provides evidence for distinct molecular mechanisms underlying defective anchoring fibril formation. Am J Hum Genet 1997; 61: 599–610.

75. Uitto J, Olsen DR, Fazio MJ. Extracellular matrix of the skin: 50 years of progress. J Invest Dermatol 1989; 92: 61S–77S.

76. Uitto J, Perejda AJ, Abergel RP, et al. Altered steady-state ratio of type I/III procollagen mRNAs correlates with selectively increased type I procollagen biosynthesis in cultured keloid fibroblasts. Proc Natl Acad Sci USA 1985; 82: 5935–5939.

77. Micali G, Bene-Bain MA, Guitart J, et al. Genodermatoses. In: Schachner LA, Hansen RC, eds. Pediatric dermatology, 2nd edn. New York: Churchill Livingstone, 1995; 347–411.

78. Couchman JR, Caterson B, Christner JE, et al. Mapping by monoclonal antibody detection of glycosaminoglycans in connective tissues. Nature 1984; 307: 650–652.

79. Hardingham TE, Fosang AJ. Proteoglycans: many forms and many functions. FASEB J 1992; 6: 861–870.

80. Scott JE. Proteoglycan: collagen interactions and subfibrillar structure in collagen fibrils. Implications in the development and ageing of connective tissues. J Anat 1990; 169: 23–35.

81. Longaker MT, Adzick NS, Hall JL, et al. Studies in fetal wound healing. VII. Fetal wound healing may be modulated by hyaluronic acid stimulating activity in amniotic fluid. J Pediatr Surg 1990; 25: 430–433.

82. Colwell AS, Longaker MT, Lorenz HP. Fetal wound healing. Front Biosci 2003; 8: s1240–1248.

83. West DP, Worobec S, Solomon LM. Pharmacology and toxicology of infant skin. J Invest Dermatol 1981; 76: 147–150.

84. Buczkowski-Bickmann MK. Thermoregulation in the neonate and the consequences of hypothermia. Clin Forum Nurse Anesth 1992; 3: 77–82.

85. Nedergaard J, Cannon B. Brown adipose tissue: Development and function. In: Polin RA, Fox WW, eds. Fetal and neonatal physiology, 2nd edn. Philadelphia: WB Saunders, 1998; 478–489.

86. Muller M, Jasmin JR, Monteil RA, et al. Embryology of the hair follicle. Early Hum Dev 1991; 26: 159–166.

87. Bertolino AP, Klein LM, Freedberg IM. Biology of hair follicles. In: Fitzpatrick TB, Eisen AZ, Wolff K, et al. (eds) Dermatology in general medicine, 4th edn. New York: McGraw-Hill, 1993; 289–293.

88. Barman JM, Pecoraro V, Astore I, et al. The first stage in the natural history of the human scalp hair cycle. J Invest Dermatol 1967; 48: 138–142.

89. Cotsarelis G, Sun TT, Lavker RM. Label-retaining cells reside in the bulge area of pilosebaceous unit: implications for follicular stem cells, hair cycle and skin carcinogenesis. Cell 1990; 61: 1329–1337.

90. Sun TT, Cotsarelis G, Lavker RM. Hair follicular stem cells: The bulge-activation hypothesis. J Invest Dermatol 1991; 96: 77S–78S.

91. Yang JS, Lavker RM, Sun TT. Upper human hair follicle contains a subpopulation of keratinocytes with superior in vitro proliferative potential. J Invest Dermatol 1993; 101: 652–659.

92. Blanpain C, Lowry WE, Geoghegan A, et al. Self-renewal, multipotency, and the existence of two cell populations within an epithelial stem cell niche. Cell 2004; 118: 530–532.

93. Christiano AM. Epithelial stem cells: stepping out of their niche. Cell 2004; 118: 530–532.

94. Lavker RM, Sun TT, Oshima H, et al. Hair follicle stem cells. J Invest Dermatol Symp Proc 2003; 8: 28–38.

95. Narisawa Y, Hashimoto K, Kohda H. Merkel cells participate in the induction and alignment of epidermal ends of arrector pili muscles of human fetal skin. Br J Dermatol 1996; 134: 494–498.

96. Kim DK, Holbrook KA. The appearance, density, and distribution of Merkel cells in human embryonic and fetal skin: their relation to sweat gland and hair follicle development. J Invest Dermatol 1995; 104: 411–416.

97. Klein J, Forman R, Eliopoulos C, et al. A method for simultaneous measurement of cocaine and nicotine in neonatal hair. Ther Drug Monit 1994; 16: 67–70.

98. Koren G. Measurement of drugs in neonatal hair: a window to fetal exposure. Forensic Sci Int 1995; 70: 77–82.

99. Kintz P, Mangin P. Determination of gestational opiate, nicotine, benzodiazepine, cocaine and amphetamine exposure by hair analysis. J Forensic Sci Soc 1993; 33: 139–142.

100. Eliopoulos C, Klein J, Chitayat D, et al. Nicotine and cotinine in maternal and neonatal hair as markers of gestational smoking. Clin Invest Med 1996; 19: 231–242.

101. Pochi PE, Strauss JS, Downing DT. Age-related changes in sebaceous gland activity. J Invest Dermatol 1979; 73: 108–111.

102. Stal S, Spira M, Hamilton S. Skin morphology and function. Clin Plast Surg 1987; 14: 201–208.

103. Agache P, Blanc D, Barrand C, et al. Sebum levels during the first year of life. Br J Dermatol 1980; 103: 643–649.

104. Baden HP, Kvedar JC. Biology of nails. In: Fitzpatrick TB, Eisen AZ, Wolff K, et al. (eds) Dermatology in general medicine, 4th edn. New York: McGraw-Hill, 1993; 294–297.

105. Wagner AM, Hansen RC. Neonatal skin and skin disorders. In: Schachner LA, Hansen RC, eds. Pediatric

dermatology, 2nd edn. New York: Churchill Livingstone, 1995; 263–346.

106. Mancini AJ, Lane AT. Sweating in the neonate. In: Polin RA, Fox WW, eds. Fetal and neonatal physiology, 2nd edn. Philadelphia: WB Saunders, 1998; 767–770.

107. Sato K. Biology of the eccrine sweat gland. In: Fitzpatrick TB, Eisen AZ, Wolff K, et al. (eds) Dermatology in general medicine, 4th edn. New York: McGraw-Hill, 1993; 221–231.

108. Atherton DJ. The neonate. In: Champion RH, Burton JL, Ebling FJG, eds. Textbook of dermatology, 5th edn. Oxford: Blackwell Scientific, 1992; 382–383.

109. Guyton AC. Textbook of medical physiology, 8th edn. Philadelphia: WB Saunders, 1991; 799–801.

110. Green M, Behrendt H. Sweating capacity of neonates. Nicotine-induced axon reflex sweating and the histamine flare. Am J Dis Child 1969; 118: 725–732.

111. Behrendt H, Green M. Drug-induced localized sweating in full-size and low-birth-weight neonates. Am J Dis Child 1969; 117: 299–306.

112. Green M, Behrendt H. Drug-induced localized sweating in neonates. Am J Dis Child 1970; 120: 434–438.

113. Foster KG, Hey EN, Katz G. The response of the sweat glands of the newborn baby to thermal stimuli and to intradermal acetylcholine. J Physiol 1969; 203: 13–29.

114. Green M. Comparison of adult and neonatal skin eccrine sweating. In: Maibach HI, Boisits EK, eds. Neonatal skin, structure and function. New York: Dekker, 1982; 35–66.

115. Harpin VA, Rutter N. Sweating in preterm babies. J Pediatr 1982; 100: 614–618.

116. Green M, Behrendt H. Sweating responses of neonates to local thermal stimulation. Am J Dis Child 1973; 125: 20–25.

117. Hey EN, Katz G. Evaporative water loss in the newborn baby. J Physiol 1969; 200: 605–619.

118. Oh W, Karecki H. Phototherapy and insensible water loss in the newborn infant. Am J Dis Child 1972; 124: 230–232.

119. Jones RWA, Rochefort MJ, Baum JD. Increased insensible water loss in newborn infants nursed under radiant heaters. Br Med J 1976; 2: 1347–1350.

120. Williams PR, Oh W. Effects of radiant warmer on insensible water loss in newborn infants. Am J Dis Child 1974; 128: 511–514.

121. Karlsson H, Hanel SE, Nilsson K, et al. Measurement of skin temperature and heat flow from skin in term newborn babies. Acta Paediatr 1995; 84: 605–612.

122. Gladman G, Chiswick ML. Skin conductance and arousal in the newborn. Arch Dis Child 1990; 65: 1063–1066.

123. Hernes KG, Morkrid L, Fremming A, et al. Skin conductance changes during the first year of life in full-term infants. Pediatr Res 2002; 52: 837–843.

124. Sato S, Ogihara Y, Hiraga K, et al. Fine structure of unmyelinated nerves in neonatal skin. J Cutan Pathol 1977; 4: 1–8.

125. Cauna N. The free penicillate nerve endings of the human hairy skin. J Anat 1973; 115: 277–288.

126. Cauna N. Fine morphological characteristics and microtopography of the free nerve endings of the human digital skin. Anat Rec 1980; 198: 643–656.

127. Moll R, Moll I, Franke WW. Identification of Merkel cells in human skin by specific cytokeratin antibodies: changes of cell density and distribution in fetal and adult plantar epidermis. Differentiation 1984; 28: 136–154.

128. Moll I, Moll R, Franke WW. Formation of epidermal and dermal Merkel cells during human fetal skin development. J Invest Dermatol 1986; 87: 779–787.

129. Narisawa Y, Hashimoto K, Nihei Y, et al. Biological significance of dermal Merkel cells in development of cutaneous nerves in human fetal skin. J Histochem Cytochem 1992; 40: 65–71.

130. Perera P, Kurban AK, Ryan TJ. The development of the cutaneous microvascular system in the newborn. Br J Dermatol 1970; 82: 86–91.

131. Mayer KM. Observations on the capillaries of the normal infant. Am J Dis Child 1921; 22: 381–387.

132. Beinder E, Trojan A, Bucher HU, et al. Control of skin blood flow in pre- and full-term infants. Biol Neonate 1994; 65: 7–15.

133. Wu PYK, Wong WH, Guerra G, et al. Peripheral blood flow in the neonate. 1. Changes in total, skin, and muscle blood flow with gestational and postnatal age. Pediatr Res 1980; 14: 1374–1378.

134. Norman M, Herin P, Fagrell B, et al. Capillary blood cell velocity in full-term infants as determined in skin by videophotometric microscopy. Pediatr Res 1988; 23: 585–588.

135. Jahnukainen T, van Ravenswaaij-Arts C, Jalonen J, et al. Dynamics of vasomotor thermoregulation of the skin in term and preterm neonates. Early Hum Dev 1993; 33: 133–143.

136. Risbourg B, Vural M, Kremp O, et al. Neonatal thermoregulation. Turk J Pediatr 1991; 33: 121–134.

137. Thomas K. Thermoregulation in neonates. Neon Network 1994; 13: 15–22.

138. Karlsson H, Olegard R, Nilsson K. Regional skin temperature, heat flow and conductance in preterm neonates nursed in low and in neutral environmental temperature. Acta Pediatr 1996; 85: 81–7.

139. Holbrook KA, Underwood RA, Vogel AM, et al. The appearance, density and distribution of melanocytes in human embryonic and fetal skin revealed by the anti-melanoma monoclonal antibody, HMB-45. Anat Embryol 1989; 180: 443–455.

140. Haake AR, Scott GA. Physiologic distribution and differentiation of melanocytes in human fetal and neonatal skin equivalents. J Invest Dermatol 1991; 96: 71–77.

141. Scott GA, Haake AR. Keratinocytes regulate melanocyte number in human fetal and neonatal skin equivalents. J Invest Dermatol 1991; 97: 776–781.

142. Jimbow K, Quevedo WC, Prota G, et al. Biology of melanocytes. In: Freedberg IM, Eisen AZ, Wolff K, et al. (eds) Dermatology in general medicine, 5th edn. New York: McGraw-Hill, 1999; 192–220.

143. Boissy RE. The melanocyte. Its structure, function, and subpopulations in skin, eyes, and hair. Dermatol Clin 1988; 6: 161–173.

144. Szabo G, Gerald A, Pathak MA. Racial differences in the fate of melanosomes in human epidermis. Nature 1969; 222: 1081–1082.

145. Bos JD. The skin immune system: lupus erythematosus as a paradigm. Arch Dermatol Res 1994; 287: 23–27.

146. Bos JD. The skin as an organ of immunity. Clin Exp Immunol 1997; 107: 3–5.

147. Bos JD, Kapsenberg ML. The skin immune system: progress in cutaneous biology. Immun Today 1993; 14: 75–78.

148. Streilein JW, Bergstresser PR. Langerhans cells: antigen presenting cells of the epidermis. Immunobiol 1984; 168: 285–300.

149. Dorschner RA, Lin KH, Murakami M, et al. Neonatal skin in mice and humans expresses increased levels of antimicrobial peptides: innate immunity during development of the adaptive response. Pediatr Res 2003; 53: 566–572.

150. Braff MH, Hawkins MA, DiNardo A, et al. Structure-function relationships among human cathelicidin peptides: dissociation of antimicrobial properties from host immunostimulatory activities. J Immunol 2005; 174: 4271–4278.

151. Bos JD, Zonneveld I, Das PK, et al. The skin immune system (SIS): distribution and immunophenotype of lymphocyte subpopulations in normal human skin. J Invest Dermatol 1987; 88: 569–573.

152. Hogan AD, Burks AW. Epidermal Langerhans' cells and their function in the skin immune system. Ann Allergy Asthma Immunol 1995; 75: 5–12.

153. Drijkoningen M, de Wolf-Peters C, Van Der Steen K, et al. Epidermal Langerhans' cells and dermal dendritic cells in human fetal and neonatal skin: an immunohistochemical study. Pediatr Dermatol 1987; 4: 11–17.

154. Stingl G, Hauser C, Wolff K. The epidermis: an immunologic microenvironment. In: Fitzpatrick TB, Eisen AZ, Wolff K, et al. (eds) Dermatology in general medicine, 4th edn. New York: McGraw-Hill, 1993; 172–197.

155. Kowolenko M, Carlo J, Gozzo JJ. Histologic identification of cellular differences that may contribute to the reduced immunogenicity of transplanted neonatal versus adult skin tissue. Int Arch Allergy Appl Immunol 1986; 80: 274–277.

156. Silvers WK. Studies on the induction of tolerance of the H-Y antigen in mice with neonatal skin grafts. J Exp Med 1968; 128: 69–83.

157. Silvers WK, Collins NH. The behavior of H-Y-incompatible neonatal skin grafts in rats. Transplantation 1979; 28: 57–59.

158. Kowolenko M, Gozzo JJ. Comparative study of neonatal and adult skin transplants in mice. Transplantation 1984; 38: 84–86.

159. Hanau D, Fabre M, Schmitt DA, et al. Appearance of Birbeck granule-like structures in anti-T6 antibody-treated human epidermal Langerhans cells. J Invest Dermatol 1988; 90: 298–304.

160. Nestle FO, Nickoloff BJ. Dermal dendritic cells are important members of the skin immune system. Adv Exp Med Biol 1995; 378: 111–116.

3

Lesional Morphology and Assessment

Albert C. Yan, Paul J. Honig, Ho Jin Kim

The skin of the newborn infant can exhibit a vast spectrum of conditions. Neonatal cutaneous findings may indicate transitory, benign processes such as erythema toxicum neonatorum, or may represent important harbingers of internal disease or genetic alteration, as might be observed in patients with herpes simplex virus infection or incontinentia pigmenti. Fortunately, dermatologic manifestations are readily visible to the clinician, and it is often more efficient to first assess lesional morphology and then focus history-taking on the basis of the observed clinical findings. The timely identification and accurate diagnosis of skin findings in the newborn infant therefore relies on obtaining a comprehensive history and a meticulous physical examination, as well as on a proper understanding of physiologic differences between neonatal, pediatric, and adult skin that will influence both the diagnosis and the management of skin conditions appropriate to the neonate. This chapter reviews the salient aspects of the prenatal and perinatal history, as well as the principles of morphologic assessment in the term and preterm infant.

A COMPREHENSIVE HISTORY AND ITS IMPACT

The comprehensive history is a vital part of any neonatal skin evaluation. In the newborn setting this includes not only prenatal and perinatal histories but also maternal, paternal, and family medical histories (Box 3-1).

Prenatal History

Prenatal history should focus on questions about possible antenatal exposures to medications, drugs, or infections. Questions should examine the use of prescription and non-prescription medications, as well as controlled and uncontrolled substances such as tobacco, alcohol, cocaine and other illicit drugs. Certain drugs, for example phenytoin, valproic acid, coumadin, diethylstilbestrol, systemic retinoids, tetracycline derivatives, and penicillamine, are known teratogens. As substance abuse among mothers has become more prevalent, our knowledge of their effects on the fetus is expanding. Specific cutaneous features may be observed with specific substances, as noted in fetal alcohol syndrome, where patients may manifest with short palpebral fissures, a broad flat nasal bridge, and a long upper lip with an absent or ill-defined philtrum.[1] Other cutaneous findings of substance abuse are less specific and

defined, but have been linked with premature birth and fetal growth retardation and its inherent cutaneous susceptibilities.[2] Additional factors important in the prenatal history include maternal infections, especially within the first trimester when organogenesis occurs. The TORCH constellation of infections (toxoplasmosis, syphilis, rubella, cytomegalovirus, herpes), human papilloma virus, and human immunodeficiency virus (HIV) may have significant systemic and cutaneous effects on the infant, as addressed specifically in later chapters.

Maternal History

Maternal history should include age, medical history, and outcomes of prior pregnancies. Certain genetic disorders have been linked to advanced maternal age during pregnancy, particularly chromosomal abnormalities, the most frequent being Down syndrome.[3] Maternal disease may have a significant impact on the developing fetus. Systemic lupus erythematosus and related collagen vascular disorders highlight neonatal diseases that occur as a result of transplacental transmission of pathogenic antibodies – in this case anti-Ro/SSA, anti-La/SSB, or U1RNP antibody may result in an infant with neonatal lupus erythematosus.[4] Other autoimmune disorders (such as bullous disorders), as well as chronic medical conditions requiring systemic medications, are also important in assessing the newborn. Medical conditions acquired during pregnancy, such as gestational diabetes, will also affect fetal development. Previous pregnancies that resulted in spontaneous abortions may suggest X-linked dominant conditions or autosomal recessive conditions that are fatal in utero. Failure to initiate or poor progression of labor may be the first clue to X-linked ichthyosis in the infant.[5] Polyhydramnios has been associated with trisomies, and junctional epidermolysis bullosa with associated pyloric atresia.[6,7] Paternal history, although less significant, may be useful. Increased paternal age has been linked to chromosomal abnormalities, in particular Down syndrome, Apert's syndrome, achondroplasia, and neurofibromatosis.[8–13] Finally, a detailed family history may help identify possible congenital anomalies or genetic disorders. The pattern of affected family members may indicate a specific mode of inheritance. A history of consanguinity should be sought if recessive genetic disorders are suspected.

The history of labor and delivery should include approximate gestational dates. Premature, term, and postdate infants

bility can be subtle early signs of sepsis. Cutaneous findings of infection may include a full or bulging fontanelle, generalized erythema, petechiae, purpura, and vasomotor instability, with poor peripheral circulation (i.e. mottling and cyanosis of the acral areas).[14] The umbilical area, as well as central venous or arterial catheterization sites, should be evaluated closely as potential portals of entry. Prolonged labor, abnormal presentation, and artificial extraction measures may account for petechiae, ecchymoses, and hematomas which may herald the onset of hyperbilirubinemia. In certain disorders, such as congenital malignancies (e.g. melanoma) or congenital infections (e.g. chorioamnionitis), examination of the placenta may be helpful.

CUTANEOUS EXAMINATION AND EVALUATION

Although historical evidence is important, the cornerstone of dermatology remains a careful, detailed cutaneous examination. This requires both visual and tactile assessment of the skin. Special precautions must be followed in the newborn nursery, especially in the intensive care unit setting. Careful handwashing or the use of newer topical broad-spectrum antimicrobial hand preparations, with removal of jewelry, must be performed to reduce the risk of nosocomial infections.[15,16] Some infants may require incubators to maintain their temperature and fluid balance. During examination, prolonged exposure outside of the isolette can result in hypothermia. Open radiant warmers are helpful, but prolonged exposure should be avoided because open warmers will increase transepidermal water loss. When examining an infant, good lighting and adequate exposure are essential. Although natural lighting is best, this is rarely available. Fluorescent lights and bilirubin lights may mask some of the subtle contours and colors of individual lesions. Where practical, the infant should routinely have all clothing removed, including diapers, so that the entire skin surface can be examined.

A great deal of similarity may occur between pathologic processes. Although some diagnoses are obvious, there is only a finite number of ways that skin can express disease. An organized approach to evaluating and describing lesions is of paramount importance.

Examination of the skin surface should proceed systematically from inspection to palpation, separating the body into segments to ensure complete evaluation. Inspection of the lesions should characterize the primary and secondary lesions; the colors involved; the borders; the configuration; and the distribution of relevant cutaneous findings. Relevant primary and secondary lesions should first be identified (Box 3-2). An understanding of the significance of these primary and secondary lesions will not only help generate an appropriate differential diagnosis but also allow for concise communication of pertinent data to colleagues. We have attempted to use the most commonly used definitions for primary and secondary lesions. Unfortunately, a review of the core dermatologic textbooks and literature reveals a great deal of inconsistency among these definitions.[17–21] Subsequently, the color, borders, configuration, and distribution of lesions are assessed (Box 3-3). When evaluating color, one should take into account the variations in different ethnic groups because background color will alter the overall color of lesions. The border should be examined for distinct or indistinct margins. Next,

present with different cutaneous examinations, and are differentially susceptible to cutaneous disease. For instance, premature infants have a higher incidence of hemangiomas; term infants are more likely to develop erythema toxicum neonatorum; and postdate infants undergo significant desquamation shortly after birth. Identification of congenital cutaneous candidiasis in a preterm infant at high risk for systemic infection will warrant a different approach from term infants, for whom the disease poses significantly less of a risk. An excessively prolonged labor may indicate X-linked ichthyosis. Premature rupture of membranes, prolonged labor, and evidence of fetal distress due to hypoxia or meconium aspiration, may predispose an infant to cutaneous infection and subsequent sepsis. Low-birthweight infants must be watched with particular vigilance for signs of septicemia. Other risk factors for sepsis include male gender and prematurity, the risk being inversely proportional to gestational age. Apnea, bradycardia, irritability, feeding intolerance, temperature instability, abdominal distension, increased respiratory effort, hypotonia, and glucose insta-

configuration should be assessed. Are the lesions linear, annular, nummular, targetoid, grouped, or retiform? Finally, the last step is the evaluation of distribution. Is the lesion single or multiple, localized or generalized, symmetric or asymmetric, extensor or flexural, acral, or inverse? This is then followed by palpation of the lesion, with particular attention to the border. Lesions may be soft, firm, fluctuant, indurated, or tender.

Mucous membranes, teeth, hair, and nails should be included in a full cutaneous examination. Teeth, hair, and nails are ectodermal structures like the skin, and can be intimately linked to cutaneous pathologic processes. Teeth are normally absent at birth, but natal teeth, which represent prematurely erupted primary incisors, can be seen. Delayed onset of eruption, absent or abnormal teeth, or enamel dysplasia can be seen in the ichthyoses, ectodermal dysplasias, and other genodermatoses such as incontinentia pigmenti and tuberous sclerosis. Sparse to abundant hairs can be seen as a variation of normal. Synchronous loss of hair followed by regrowth is a normal finding until the development of an adult hair distribution, usually during the first year of life. Subtle changes in hair texture with a matted, lusterless, brittle, or unruly appearance should prompt closer evaluation by light microscopy for hair shaft abnormalities, which can be elucidated with scanning electron microscopy. Diffuse hypotrichosis can be seen in hidrotic and anhidrotic ectodermal dysplasia, ichthyoses, and incontinentia pigmenti. Diffuse hypertrichosis can be seen in mucopolysaccharidosis, Cornelia de Lange syndrome, and hypertrichosis lanuginosa. Nail abnormalities, in particular aplasia, hypoplasia, and dysplasia, have been associated with chromosomal disorders, ectodermal dysplasias, and epidermolysis bullosa. Absent nails or triangular lunulae have been associated with nail–patella syndrome. Finally, to complete the cutaneous examination, the lymph nodes, liver, and spleen should be palpated, particularly when infectious or neoplastic diagnoses are suspected.

CONSIDERATIONS UNIQUE TO THE NEONATAL PERIOD

Cutaneous reaction patterns in newborns can differ significantly from those seen in children and adults, because of the immaturity of the skin and its components. Although the precise mechanisms have not been fully elucidated, there are numerous clinical examples of such differences. Although all the known dermoepidermal junction antigens are made by the middle of the second trimester, the lack of a developed rete ridge pattern and well-developed collagen fibrils within the papillary dermis may explain the greater propensity for vesicle formation in the newborn.[22] The epidermis, particularly in immature infants, has a relatively thin stratum corneum, which results in increased transepidermal water loss, making infants more susceptible to xerosis. Furthermore, the immature epidermis is quite fragile and prone to trauma at sites of maceration and friction, such as the neck, axillae, and groin. Even mild adhesive can strip the epidermis, causing significant damage.[23] The loss of this barrier function increases susceptibility to cutaneous infection with both bacteria and *Candida* species. The composition of neonatal subcutaneous fat, with its greater proportion of saturated fatty acids, makes it more prone to hypoxic trauma, leading to subcutaneous fat necrosis.[24] The immaturity of the cutaneous vasculature, with its exaggerated vasomotor tone in response to hypothermia, contributes to the prevalence of cutis marmorata in infancy.[25]

REACTION PATTERNS

An understanding of the specialized reaction patterns is outlined in Boxes 3-2 and 3-3, and in conjunction with a comprehensive history and assessment of cutaneous morphology will aid the clinician in making the proper dermatologic diagnosis.

Box 3-2 Primary and secondary lesions

Primary Lesions

Primary lesions are defined as lesions that arise de novo and are therefore most characteristic of the disease process. The graphic representations are intended to demonstrate three-dimensional and topographic relationships and not necessarily the histology of the example shown.

Macule
A circumscribed, flat lesion with color change, up to 1 cm in size, although the term is often used for lesions larger than 1 cm. By definition, they are not palpable

Examples
Ash leaf macules, café au lait macules, capillary malformations

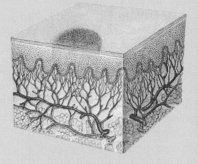

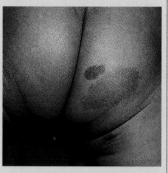

Café au lait macules

Patch
A circumscribed, flat lesion with color change, greater than 1 cm in size

Examples
Nevus depigmentosus, mongolian spots, nevus simplex

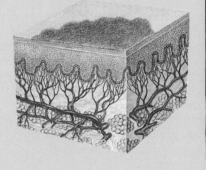

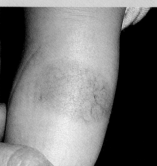

Hemangioma precursor

Papule
A circumscribed, elevated, solid lesion, up to 1 cm in size. Elevation may be accentuated with oblique lighting

Examples
Verrucae, milia, and juvenile xanthogranuloma.

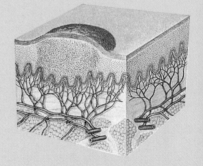

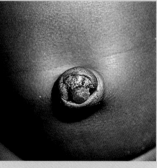

Umbilical granuloma

Plaque
A circumscribed, elevated, plateau-like, solid lesion, greater than 1 cm in size

Examples
Mastocytoma, nevus sebaceous

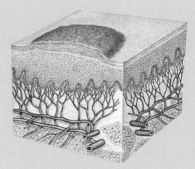

Nevus sebaceous

Continued

Box 3-2 Primary and secondary lesions—cont'd

Nodule
A circumscribed, elevated, solid lesion with depth, up to 2 cm in size.

Examples
Dermoid cysts, neuroblastoma

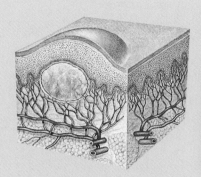

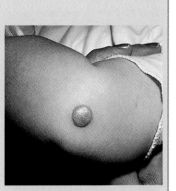

Juvenile xanthogranuloma

Tumor
A circumscribed, elevated, solid lesion with depth, greater than 2 cm in size

Examples
Hemangioma, lipoma, rhabdomyosarcoma

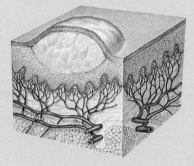

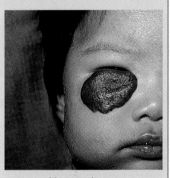

Hemangioma

Vesicle
A circumscribed, elevated, fluid-filled lesion up to 1 cm in size

Examples
Herpes simplex, varicella, miliaria crystallina

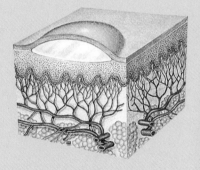

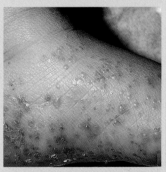

Acropustulosis of infancy

Bulla
A circumscribed, elevated, fluid-filled lesion greater than 1 cm in size

Examples
Sucking blisters, epidermolysis bullosa, bullous impetigo

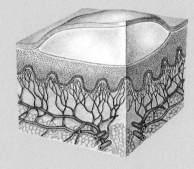

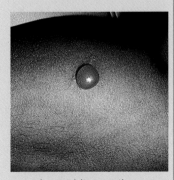

Insect bite reaction

Box 3-2 Primary and secondary lesions—cont'd

Wheal
A circumscribed, elevated, edematous, often evanescent lesion, caused by accumulation of fluid within the dermis

Examples
Urticaria, bite reactions, drug eruptions

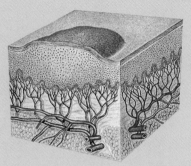
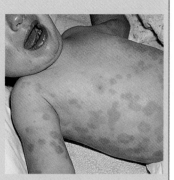

Drug eruption

Pustule
A circumscribed, elevated lesion filled with purulent fluid, less than 1 cm in size

Examples
Transient neonatal pustular melanosis, erythema toxicum neonatorum, infantile acropustulosis

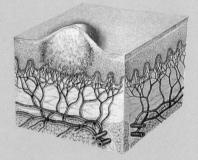
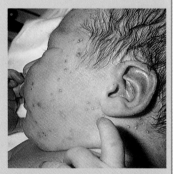

Transient neonatal pustular melanosis

Abscess
A circumscribed, elevated lesion filled with purulent fluid, greater than 1 cm in size

Example
Pyodermas

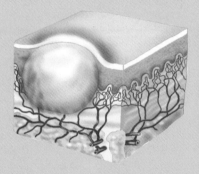
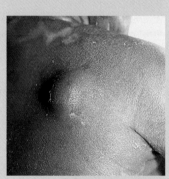

Abscess

Secondary Lesions
Secondary lesions are characteristically brought about by modification of primary lesions, either by the individual or through the natural evolution of the lesion in the environment. The graphic representations are intended to demonstrate three-dimensional and topographic relationships and not necessarily the histology of the example shown.

Crust
Results from dried exudate overlying an impaired epidermis. Can be composed of serum, blood, or pus

Examples
Epidermolysis bullosa, impetigo

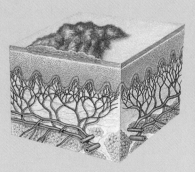
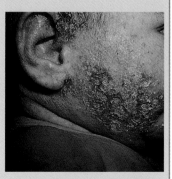

Infected atopic dermatitis

Continued

Box 3-2 Primary and secondary lesions—cont'd

Scale
Results from increased shedding or accumulation of stratum corneum as a result of abnormal keratinization and exfoliation. Can be subdivided further into pityriasiform (branny, delicate), psoriasiform (thick, white, and adherent), and ichthyosiform (fish scale-like)

Examples
Ichthyoses, postmaturity desquamation, seborrheic dermatitis

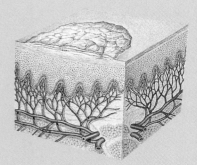

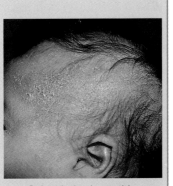

Seborrheic dermatitis

Erosion
Intraepithelial loss of epidermis. Heals without scarring

Examples
Herpes simplex, certain types of epidermolysis bullosa

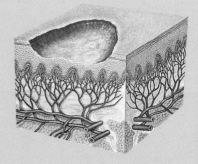

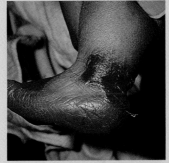

Epidermolysis bullosa

Ulcer
Full-thickness loss of the epidermis, with damage into the dermis. Will heal with scarring

Examples
Ulcerated hemangiomas, aplasia cutis congenita

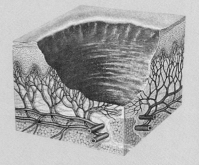

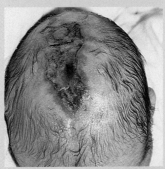

Aplasia cutis congenita

Fissure
Linear, often painful break within the skin surface, as a result of excessive xerosis.

Examples
Inherited keratodermas, hand and foot eczema

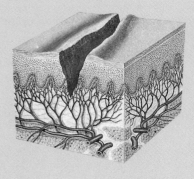

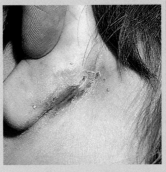

Atopic dermatitis

Box 3-2 Primary and secondary lesions—cont'd

Lichenification
Thickening of the epidermis with exaggeration of normal skin markings caused by chronic scratching or rubbing

Examples
Sucking callus, atopic dermatitis

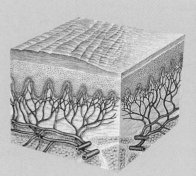
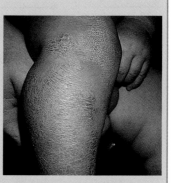
Atopic dermatitis

Atrophy
Localized diminution of skin. Epidermal atrophy results in a translucent epidermis with increased wrinkling, whereas dermal atrophy results in depression of the skin with retained skin markings. Use of topical steroids can result in epidermal atrophy, whereas intralesional steroids may result in dermal atrophy. Dyschromia and telangiectasia may also be present in the context of steroid-induced atrophy

Examples
Aplasia cutis congenita, intrauterine scarring, and focal dermal hypoplasia

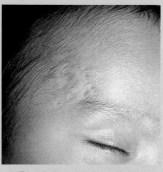
Focal dermal hypoplasia

Scar
Permanent fibrotic skin changes that develop as a consequence of tissue injury. In utero scarring can occur as a result of certain infections or amniocentesis or postnatally from a variety of external factors

Examples
Congenital varicella, aplasia cutis congenita

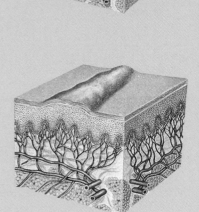
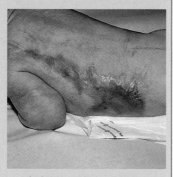
Aplasia cutis congenita

Box 3-3 Color, borders, configuration, and distribution of lesions

Color: To the untrained eye, the appreciation of subtle variations in color is often the most difficult concept to grasp. Fortunately, this assessment does not carry the diagnostic weight of the primary or secondary lesions. When evaluating the color, one must take into account the background pigmentation of the patient. In infants with darker skin type, subtle erythema or jaundice may be difficult to appreciate. Likewise, pigment dilution is more difficult to evaluate in lighter skin. The most prominent colors seen in cutaneous pathologic processes are described.

Red	Red color can be the result of vasodilation or hyperemia caused by inflammation. Deeper red or purple hues suggest extravasation of red blood cells. Diascopy is a diagnostic maneuver to help differentiate these possibilities. By applying pressure to the lesion, one can whether the lesion blanches, which suggests rubor due to vasodilation or inflammation. Conversely, nonblanching lesions suggest vascular damage, with consequent extravasation of blood into the dermis.
White	White color can be the result of loss of pigment within the epidermis or the accumulation of white material such as purulent exudate or keratinous material. One should not use the term white to describe skin-colored lesions.
Yellow	Yellow coloration can be seen in lipid-containing lesions such as xanthomas, or as a result of bile accumulation, as in jaundice.
Brown/blue/grey/black	Variations in color are related to increased melanin or hemosiderin in the skin. The more superficial the pigmentation, the darker the color. Melanin in the deep dermis appears blue to gray, owing to the Tyndall effect. Evaluation of hyperpigmentation and hypopigmentation must take into account the infant's genetic and racial background. Diffuse hyperpigmentation is rare and may signify systemic disease, such as congenital Addison's disease and other endocrinopathies, nutritional disorders, and hepatic disease. Likewise, diffuse hypopigmentation can be seen in systemic diseases such as albinism and phenylketonuria.

Box 3-3 Color, borders, configuration, and distribution of lesions—cont'd

Border

The border of a cutaneous lesion may also help in the differential diagnosis. Some lesions, such as acrodermatitis enteropathica, ichthyosis linearis circumflexa, and erysipelas, have distinct borders.

Examples of lesions with indistinct borders include cellulitis and atopic dermatitis. The borders of the lesion may be raised and indurated, as in granuloma annulare and neonatal lupus.

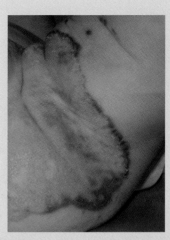

Border Acrodermatitis enteropathica Note the characteristically well-demarcated border in these lesions of acrodermatitis enteropathica.

Configuration

Linear

Several lesions follow a linear pattern. If they are found to be discordant with normal lines of demarcation, one should search for an external insult. Linear lesions can be subdivided (see below).

Blaschko (Linear)

These linear V- and S-shaped lines are believed to represent patterns of neuroectodermal migration, and skin lesions in this distribution indicate areas of cutaneous mosaicism. They do not follow any known vascular, nervous, or lymphatic pattern.

Examples

Linear epidermal nevus, incontinentia pigmenti

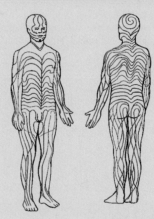

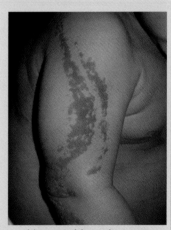

Linear epidermal nevus

Dermatomal/Zosteriform (Linear)

Lines demarcating a dermatome supplied by one dorsal root ganglia.

Example

Herpes zoster

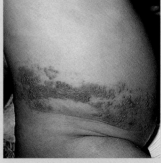

Herpes zoster

Segmental Patterns

The configuration of segmental lesions is thought to be determined by the location of embryonic placodes or other embryonic territories, as can be seen in PHACE(S) syndrome.

Examples

Infantile hemangioma
Nevus of Ota

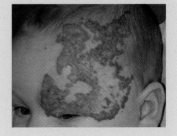

Box 3-3 Color, borders, configuration, and distribution of lesions—cont'd

Koebnerization (Linear)
Certain skin conditions tend to recapitulate at sites of skin injury, which may give them a linear configuration. Classic examples include: psoriasis, lichen planus, and lichen nitidus.

Examples
Lichen nitidus, psoriasis

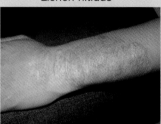

Koebnerization (Linear)
Lichen nitidus

Anatomic Lesions (Linear)
Skin lesions that occur in a linear configuration may indicate underlying involvement of a vascular structure, as might be encountered with infiltration of an intravenous cannulation site. Infectious organisms, such as *Aspergillus*, *Rhizopus*, or mycobacteria, may also spread along a vascular or 'sporotrichoid' distribution.

Examples
Sporotrichosis, atypical mycobacterial infection

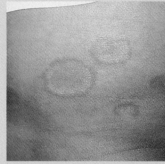

Anatomic Pattern (Linear): Iatrogenic calcinosis cutis resulting from extravasation of calcium from an intravenous catheter

Annular
A round, ring-shaped lesion, where the periphery is distinct from the center.

Examples
Tinea corporis, neonatal lupus, syphilis, annular erythema of infancy

Annular lesions of neonatal lupus

Nummular
A coin-shaped lesion, with homogenous character throughout.

Examples
Nummular eczema, discoid lesions neonatal lupus

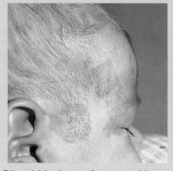

Discoid lesions of neonatal lupus

Gyrate/Polycyclic/Arciform/Serpiginous
Variations in the spectrum of annular lesions.

Examples
Neonatal lupus erythematosus, urticaria.

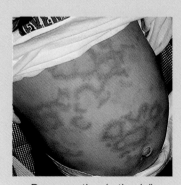

Drug eruption (urticarial)

Continued

Box 3-3 Color, borders, configuration, and distribution of lesions—cont'd

Targetoid/Iris
Concentric ringed lesions, often with a dusky or bullous center. This is characteristic of erythema multiforme.

Example
Erythema multiforme

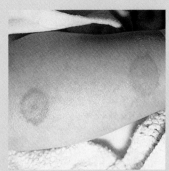

Early lesions of erythema multiforme

Herpetiform
An example is herpes simplex.

Example
Herpes simplex.

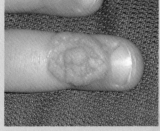

Herpes simplex infection

Corymbiform
Defined as a central cluster of lesions surrounded by scattered individual lesions.

Example
Verrucae.

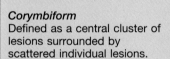

Retiform/Reticulate
A netlike pattern of lesions.

Examples
Cutis marmorata, cutis marmorata telangiectatica congenita.

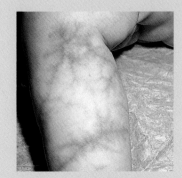

Cutis marmorata telangiectatica congenita

REFERENCES

1. Clarren SK, Smith DW. The fetal alcohol syndrome. N Engl J Med 1978; 298: 1063–1067.
2. Buchi KF. The drug-exposed infant in the well-baby nursery. Clin Perinatol 1998; 25: 335–350.
3. Hansen JP. Older maternal age and pregnancy outcome: a review of the literature. Obstet Gynecol Surv 1986; 41: 726–742.
4. McCauliffe DP. Neonatal lupus erythematosus: a transplacentally acquired autoimmune disorder. Semin Dermatol 1995; 14: 47–53.
5. Bradshaw KD, Carr BR. Placental sulfatase deficiency: maternal and fetal expression of steroid sulfatase deficiency and X-linked ichthyosis. Obstetr Gynecol Survey 1986; 41: 401–413.
6. Carlson DE, Platt LD, Medearis AL. The ultrasound triad of fetal hydramnios, abnormal hand posturing, and any other anomaly predicts autosomal trisomy. Obstet Gynecol 1992; 79: 731–734.
7. Lin AN. Management of patients with epidermolysis bullosa. Dermatol Clin 1996; 14: 381–387.
8. McIntosh GC, Olshan AF, Baird PA. Paternal age and the risk of birth defects in offspring. Epidemiol 1995; 6: 282–288.
9. Moloney DM, Slaney SF, Oldridge M, et al. Exclusive paternal origin of new mutations in Apert syndrome. Nature Genet 1996; 13: 48–53.
10. Zhu JL, Madsen KM, Vestergaard M, et al. Paternal age and congenital malformations. Hum Reprod. 2005; 20: 3173–3177.
11. Wilkin DJ, Szabo JK, Cameron R, et al. Mutations in fibroblast growth-factor receptor 3 in sporadic cases of achondroplasia occur exclusively on the paternally derived chromosome. Am J Hum Genet. 1998; 63: 711–716.
12. McIntosh GC, Olshan AF, Baird PA. Paternal age and the risk of birth defects in offspring. Epidemiology. 25; 6: 282–288.
13. Riccardi VM, Dobson CE 2nd, Chakraborty R, et al. The pathophysiology of neurofibromatosis: IX. Paternal age as a factor in the origin of new mutations. Am J Med Genet. 1984; 18: 169–76.
14. Fanaroff AA, Korones SB, Wright LL, et al. Incidence, presenting features, risk factors and significance of late onset septicemia in very low birth weight infants. Pediatr Infect Dis J 1998; 17: 593–598.
15. Baltimore RS. Neonatal nosocomial infections. Semin Perinatol 1998; 22: 25–32.
16. Gaynes RP, Edwards JR, Jarvis WR, et al. Nosocomial infections among neonates in high-risk nurseries in the United States. Pediatrics 1996; 98: 357–361.
17. Fitzpatrick TB, Bernhard JD. Dermatologic diagnosis by recognition of clinical morphologic patterns. In: Fitzpatrick TB, Eisen AZ, Wolff K, et al. (eds) Dermatology in general medicine, 4th edn. Vol 1. New York: McGraw Hill, 1993; 55.
18. Hurwitz S. An overview of dermatologic diagnosis. In: Hurwitz S. Clinical pediatric dermatology, 2nd edn. Philadelphia: WB Saunders, 1993; 1.
19. Jackson R. Definitions in dermatology. A dissertation on some of the terms used to describe the living gross pathology of the human skin. Clin Exp Dermatol 1978; 3: 241–247.
20. Lewis EJ, Dahl MV. On standard definitions: 33 years hence. Arch Dermatol 1997; 133: 1169.
21. Ashton RE. Standard definitions in dermatology: the need for further discussion. Arch Dermatol 1998; 134: 637–638.
22. Solomon LM, Esterly NB. Neonatal dermatology. I. The newborn skin. J Pediatr 1970; 77: 888–894.
23. Harpin VA, Rutter N. Barrier properties of the newborn infant's skin. J Pediatr 1983; 102: 419–425.
24. Hicks MJ, Levy ML, Alexander J, et al. Subcutaneous fat necrosis of the newborn and hypercalcemia: case report and review of the literature. Pediatr Dermatol 1993; 10: 271–276.
25. Smales OR, Kime R. Thermoregulation in babies immediately after birth. Arch Dis Child 1978; 53: 58–61.

4

Skin of the Premature Infant

Amy E. Gilliam, Mary L. Williams

The premature infant assumes the challenge of independent life despite the immaturity of essential functions. Skin functions are primarily protective, and immaturity of these functions contributes to the vulnerability of the preterm infant. The main function of the skin is to provide a permeability barrier that both protects the aqueous interior of the infant from desiccation in the xeric atmosphere and prevents massive influx of water when immersed in hypotonic solutions.[1] Other important functions of skin include barriers to percutaneous absorption of exogenous xenobiotics, to injury from mechanical trauma, to colonization and penetration by microorganisms, and to injury from ultraviolet light. In addition to its barrier functions, skin also participates in the thermoregulatory, neurosensory, and immunologic systems.

The consequences of skin immaturity for the premature infant depend on the infant's position on the maturational timetable for each cutaneous function, which is in turn dependent on the infant's gestational and postnatal ages. All skin layers (i.e. epidermis, dermis, and subcutaneous fat) are thinner in the preterm infant than at term.[2,3] Because the outermost layers of the epidermis (i.e. the stratum corneum) are the primary effector of most of the barrier properties of skin, the timetable for maturation of the stratum corneum predicts the competence of many skin functions. Stratum corneum begins to form around hair follicles at about 14 weeks' gestational age and spreads to include the epidermis between hair follicles by 22–24 weeks' gestational age.[2] During the ensuing weeks the thickness of the stratum corneum increases from only a few to several cell layers,[3] such that by term it is actually thicker than adult stratum corneum. The 'excess,' outermost layers of stratum corneum are then shed during the first days of life; this process of physiologic desquamation is accentuated in postmature babies.

These histological features underlie the clinical characteristics of skin maturation embodied in the Ballad scale, widely used for assessing gestational age[4] (Fig. 4-1). In the extremely premature infant (<24 weeks) the skin is sticky, friable, and transparent; lanugo hairs are absent. As gestation progresses, the skin becomes less transparent and peeling and surface cracking are increasingly seen, indicative of a thickening stratum corneum, and lanugo hair density peaks and then regresses. Despite definition of these milestones of gross and microscopic skin development, with the exception of the permeability barrier little is known about the competency or developmental timetable of most skin functions in premature infants.

THE PERMEABILITY BARRIER IN THE PRETERM INFANT

The permeability barrier resides in the stratum corneum through its provision of a hydrophobic lipid shield over the underlying nucleated cell layers.[1] Because of their plasma and intracellular membranes, most cells are hydrophobic relative to the vascular and extracellular compartments; however, in stratum corneum this pattern is reversed. Instead, the extracellular compartment of stratum corneum is filled with a highly organized series of hydrophobic lipid membranes in the extracellular spaces, whereas the anucleate corneocytes form an aqueous compartment as a result of loss of their plasma and organelle membranes. This interposition of hydrophobic lipid membranes in the extracellular compartment retards the movement of water inward or outward across the stratum corneum. The stacking of multiple layers of cornified cells surrounded by extracellular lipid bilayers further enhances this barrier to water movement through the generation of a tortuous intercellular pathway for water movement.

As a multilayered stratum corneum develops in the third trimester,[2,3] the barrier to transepidermal water loss (TEWL) also matures, such that by 34 weeks' gestation TEWL rates approximate adult values.[5–7] The immaturity of permeability barrier function in infants less than 34 weeks' gestational age can be demonstrated either by measuring TEWL rates directly using one of several noninvasive instruments that measure water vapor pressure at the skin surface, or by assessing the degree of vasoconstriction after application of topical phenylephrine (i.e. with a competent barrier this small hydrophilic molecule is not absorbed, and hence no skin blanching occurs).[6–8] Other, indirect methods of assessing permeability barrier maturity during stratum corneum formation measure electrical properties of the skin, for example capacitance[9] or electrical resistance,[10,11] as influenced by stratum corneum water and lipid content. By all of these measures, the extent of permeability barrier immaturity parallels the degree of prematurity. In addition to increasing stratum corneum thickness, the development of a competent permeability barrier in fetal rat skin is accompanied by (1) deposition of neutral lipid in the intercellular domains of stratum corneum; (2) increasing stratum corneum cholesterol and ceramide content; and (3) the organization of these lipids into mature lamellar membrane structures, as viewed by electron microscopy.[12,13] Whether these same lipid biochemical and ultrastructural changes also underlie barrier formation during human skin development has not yet been determined, but a large body of

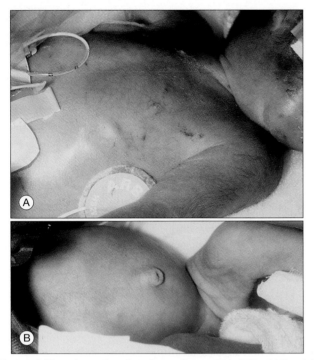

FIG. 4-1 **A** Note the moist glistening surface of this 900 g birthweight, 29 weeks' gestational age infant on day 2 of life, reflecting an impaired barrier to TEWL. Note also the multiple abrasions, demonstrating the fragility of the newborn preterm infants' skin to trauma. **B** This 700 g birthweight, 27 weeks' gestational age infant at 28 days of age exhibits the dull skin surface reflectance of a mature barrier to TEWL, illustrating the acceleration of skin maturation after birth.

evidence from other sources predicts that this will be the case.

Permeability barrier maturation accelerates after birth, such that by 2–3 weeks' postnatal age most premature infants, regardless of gestational age, have competent barriers[6]. Thus, maturation that may require approximately 10 weeks to complete in utero is accelerated following premature delivery. However, as the limits of viability have been lowered to include survivors of 25 weeks' (<750 g) to even 22 weeks' gestational age, barrier function may take as long as 8 weeks following birth to mature.[14,15] The gestational ages of these very immature infants directly abut the timetable for stratum corneum formation (see the previous discussion). It may not be surprising, therefore, that extremely premature infants do not respond as rapidly to maturational signals initiated by birth. In fetal rat skin, it is air exposure with evaporation of water from the skin surface that stimulates accelerated barrier formation, because this acceleration can be prevented by covering the skin surface with a vapor-impermeable membrane.[16] This may also occur if preterm human skin is covered with occlusive materials.[17]

Permeability barrier ontogenesis is developmentally regulated; hence, small-for-dates infants exhibit a barrier function that is appropriate for their gestational age.[18] In fetal rats, barrier maturation is regulated by glucocorticoids[19], thyroid hormone, and sex hormones, as well as by activators and ligands of the PPARα and LXR nuclear hormone receptors[13] (Table 4-1). Some of these agents also regulate lung development; and glucocorticoids often are administered prepartum to mothers to accelerate fetal lung maturation when premature

delivery is imminent.[20] Whether barrier maturation is also stimulated by these interventions in humans has not been determined. One group demonstrated that preterm infants of mothers treated with glucocorticoids have reduced insensible water losses and lower serum sodium concentrations in the first 4 days of life, consistent with a maturational effect on the skin barrier.[20a] In contrast, Jain et al.[21] reported that epidermal maturation and barrier function, which was measured directly to determine TEWL using an Evaporimeter, did not appear to be influenced by antenatal steroids.

Another aspect of the permeability barrier that undergoes postnatal maturation is the 'acid mantle,' which refers to the development of an acidic pH within the stratum corneum that is required for normal permeability barrier homeostasis and stratum corneum integrity as well as cohesion. At birth, human stratum corneum has a near-neutral surface pH. This pH declines over the ensuing days to weeks to become acidic, comparable to that of adults. As has been demonstrated in the neonatal rat, this postnatal decline in stratum corneum pH can be accelerated by the application of liver X receptor (LXR) activators, which are members of the nuclear hormone receptor superfamily. The accelerated formation of the acid mantle results in correction of abnormalities in permeability barrier homeostasis and improved stratum corneum integrity and cohesion, demonstrating the importance of the development of the acid mantle for skin barrier function.[22] In very low-birthweight and premature infants, this pattern of postnatal change in skin pH has been shown to be similar to that described in term infants.[23]

CONSEQUENCES OF PERMEABILITY BARRIER IMMATURITY

Fluid and Electrolyte Imbalance and Evaporative Energy Loss

The primary consequences of permeability barrier immaturity are (1) increased evaporative loss of free water from the skin surface, placing the infant at risk for volume depletion, particularly hypernatremic dehydration; and (2) energy loss through heat of evaporation; that is, 0.58 kilocalories (kcal) are expended for each milliliter of water that evaporates.[7] Therefore, optimal care of the premature infant requires both accurate compensation for cutaneous water losses to preserve fluid and electrolyte balance and maintenance of the infant in a thermally neutral environment, such that caloric intake can be directed toward growth and not heat production.[7,24,25] Although concurrent cutaneous water losses can be measured directly (i.e. by measuring TEWL), this procedure is not standard practice in most nurseries. Instead, cutaneous water losses and respiratory fluid losses are together considered insensible (i.e. not directly measured).[24] In term infants, TEWL accounts for approximately two-thirds of insensible losses; but cutaneous water losses are much higher in preterm infants, whereas respiratory fluid losses remain relatively constant.[26,27] Neonatal fluid requirements are estimated using complex formulas that take into account the following:

- Measured losses in urine and feces
- Estimates of insensible losses
- Requirements to support growth (increasing with postgestational age).

TABLE 4-1 Regulatory signals for skin barrier formation in fetal rats

Activator	Effect	Nuclear receptor	Class
Dexamethasone	Accelerate	Glucocorticoid	I
Thyroid hormone	Accelerate	Thyroid hormone	II
Diethylstilbestrol	Accelerate	Estrogen	I
Testosterone	Retard	Androgen	I
Linoleic acid	Accelerate	PPARα	II
Clofibric acid	Accelerate	PPARα	II
Farnesol	Accelerate	?FXR or PPARα	II
25-hydroxycholesterol	Accelerate	LXR	II
Ciglitazone Prostaglandin J_2	No effect	PPARγ	II
GW-1514 (free fatty acids)	Accelerate	PPAR-β/Δ	II

Class I: Steroid hormone receptors. Ligand binds in cytosol, translocates to nucleus after ligand binding; regulates gene transcription as homodimer.

Class II: RXR-interacting subfamily of receptors. Ligand binds to receptor in nucleus; regulates gene transcription as heterodimer with the RXR receptor and its ligand, 9-cis retinoic acid (e.g. RXR-T3R; RXR-Vitamin D3R).

TABLE 4-2 Factors modifying cutaneous water losses in preterm infants

Factor	Effect on TEWL
Decreasing gestational age	Increased TEWL; rates proportional to degree of prematurity
Increasing postnatal age	TEWL decreases towards mature rates: >1000 g, mature by 2–3 weeks; <1000 g, mature by 4–8 weeks
Increasing ambient temperature	Increased TEWL; proportional to increase in temperature
Increasing ambient humidity	Decreased TEWL; proportional to increased humidity
Radiant warmer	Increased TEWL (by 40–100%)
Radiant warmer with heat shield	Increased TEWL (by 20–40%)
Phototherapy	Increased by (up to 50%)
Skin diseases (absent or abnormal stratum corneum)	Increased; depends on percent body surface involved and severity of defect

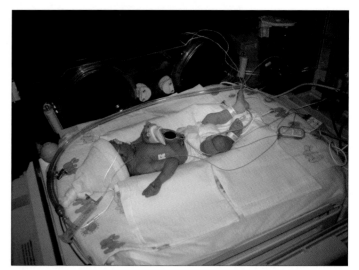

FIG. 4-2 Former 33-week premature infant at 4 days of age in a humidified incubator (opened for purposes of photograph). Photograph courtesy of Eric S. Patrick, MD.

ity. It is the vapor pressure of water at the skin surface that determines the rate of evaporation.[18]

A humidified incubator (Fig. 4-2) can provide a thermally neutral environment with low rates of evaporative water loss, because at a relative humidity of 80% or more, skin surface evaporation effectively ceases.[28–30] Scrupulous antisepsis, however, is required to prevent bacterial colonization of this environment, particularly with water-loving organisms such as *Pseudomonas* spp. Moreover, these devices obstruct access to extremely ill or unstable infants. Therefore, these infants are commonly cared for on an open bed, where a radiant warmer provides a thermally neutral environment at the expense of greatly increased rates of TEWL.[29–32] Infants requiring care under radiant warmers are typically the youngest and most premature: that is, the population with the poorest skin barriers. Use of a plastic cover or plastic bubble blanket may increase the humidity and mitigate to some extent the adverse effects of the radiant heating on TEWL.[33–35] Although these plastic shields are widely employed, standards for thermal stability and transmission have not been established.[36] Phototherapy, required in many preterm infants to treat hyperbilirubinemia, also increases TEWL[37] and fluid requirements, particularly when white light systems are used.[38–40] Many skin disorders also adversely affect the competence of the permeability barrier (see below and Table 4-2).

There is considerable variability in TEWL among infants of the same gestational and postgestational ages. The timetable for maturation of barrier function varies between infants of the same gestational age, and maturation is often quite precipitous.[7,8,14] Hence, formulas that estimate 'insensible' cutaneous losses are inherently inaccurate. Moreover, such formulas rely heavily on retrospective adjustments and inevitably result in 'chasing' fluids. It should not be forgotten that cutaneous losses are not inherently insensible (i.e. unmeasurable). Indeed, it has been shown that measurement of TEWL using rapid and noninvasive instrumentation from as few as three body sites permits accurate estimation of total cutaneous losses in preterm infants.[41] Despite this, measurement of TEWL has not been adopted widely by intensive care nurseries in the approach to fluid management. Clinical studies that

Neonatal fluid requirements must be modified by postnatal age to compensate for fluid redistribution (i.e. requirements on the first extrauterine day are decreased as a result of contraction of the extracellular compartment) and adjusted, retrospectively, to compensate for excessive weight loss or gain and/or serologic parameters of fluid or electrolyte imbalance.[24]

In addition, fluid replacements must adjust for a number of environmental conditions (Table 4-2), because cutaneous losses are not merely a function of stratum corneum maturity: they are also modified by the ambient temperature and humid-

compare outcomes using methods that incorporate direct measurement of skin losses versus traditional methods of estimating 'insensible' losses are needed to determine the clinical value of more accurate, prospective determination of cutaneous losses.

Other strategies to reduce TEWL in the preterm infant include the use of protective skin dressings or ointments. Semipermeable dressings (e.g. Bioclusive, Omniderm, Opsite, Tegaderm) that permit some passage of water vapor and other gases, but are impervious to water and microorganisms, can reduce TEWL rates and also are protective against the trauma caused by adhesives from monitors.[42–46] Moreover, barrier maturation is not inhibited by these dressings, and neither have increased rates of infection nor colonization by microorganisms been observed. Nonetheless, increased bacterial colonization under such dressings is observed in other clinical settings[47] and remains a serious consideration with their use on preterm infants. In addition, many of these dressings contain adhesive materials, and even those without adhesives can cling to the moist skin surface of the preterm newborn and injure the epidermis, unless they are either removed carefully or allowed to detach spontaneously. Furthermore, partial body applications (i.e. trunk and abdomen) to very immature infants (<1000 g), may not be sufficient to reduce total fluid requirements.[42] These limitations hinder the widespread adoption of artificial dressings in routine skin care. It should also be remembered that the benefits of these agents have only been shown in studies with small numbers of subjects. Confirmation of these findings in larger cohorts is required before their routine use can be generally recommended.

Topical ointments, such as petrolatum[48,49] or Aquaphor[50] also reduce TEWL, although the effect from a single application lasts only 4–8 hours.[50–52] Less-frequent applications do not decrease fluid requirements, but they appear to improve the overall condition of the skin and protect against skin trauma.[50] Although largely composed of nonphysiologic lipids (e.g. long-chain hydrocarbons and wax esters), these emollients have a long history of dermatologic use without associated toxicity or evidence of significant percutaneous absorption. Nonetheless, internal hydrocarbon accumulations (paraffinomas) are reported, albeit rarely,[53,54] and gastrointestinal absorption of hydrocarbons is documented.[55a] Hence, the possibility remains that these lipids may not be entirely innocuous when applied to the skin of very premature infants, whose absorptive characteristics may more closely approximate those of gastrointestinal mucosa than mature skin. (See also discussion on 'Control of Transcutaneous Water Loss' in Chapter 5). In a recent systematic review of randomized controlled trials comparing prophylactic application of topical ointment in preterm infants to routine skin care, Conner et al.[56] reported that daily application of topical ointment increases the risk for coagulase-negative staphylococcal and nosocomial infections in these patients. Therefore, routine application of topical ointment is no longer recommended for premature infants. However, increased rates of infection described with the use of topical ointments should not be extrapolated to developing countries, where natural oils are commonly used to enhance skin barrier function. Circumstances may be very different in these settings: survival is much lower, care practices differ, and the range of agents that cause infection is divergent. Moreover, these oils supply essential fatty acids and nutrients that may be particularly critical in the setting of maternal nutritional deficiency. Thus, topical treatment with sunflower seed oil was shown to reduce the incidence of nosocomial infections in very low-birthweight infants in both Bangladesh[57] and Egypt,[58] whereas the application of Aquaphor did not significantly increase or reduce the risk of infection.[57]

An alternate approach to barrier fortification in these infants would be use of mixtures of lipids physiologic to the skin. The extracellular membranes of the stratum corneum that provide the barrier to TEWL comprise an approximately equimolar mixture of ceramides, long-chain free fatty acids, and cholesterol.[55] The effect of various mixtures of these physiologic lipids on permeability barrier function has been examined in mature skin in experimental systems, in which the barrier is initially perturbed (e.g. by solvent wipes to extract native stratum corneum lipids), the test lipids are applied, and the rate of barrier recovery (i.e. normalization of TEWL) determined.[52,59] Whereas applications of any one or two of the physiologic lipids (i.e. incomplete mixtures) aggravate barrier homeostasis in mature epidermis, equimolar mixtures allow normal barrier recovery. Moreover, optimized ratios of the three key physiologic lipid classes can actually accelerate barrier recovery following insult[60] and in aged skin.[61] Yet despite the theoretic advantages of employing physiologic lipid mixtures, these have not been examined for efficacy in treating the barrier immaturity of the preterm infant.

Increased Percutaneous Absorption of Xenobiotics

Another direct consequence of skin barrier immaturity is the increased absorption of topically applied substances (Table 4-3), sometimes with tragic consequences (see Chapter 5).[36,62–65] This vulnerability was first recognized historically when preterm infants developed methemoglobinemia through the absorption of aniline dyes in the laundry marks placed on diapers.[64] Subsequently, the demonstration of neurotoxicity due to percutaneous absorption of hexachlorophene, commonly in use in nurseries as an antibacterial cleanser,[62] led to wider recognition of the vulnerability of the preterm infant to toxicity from topically applied agents.

The same factors that determine the movement of water from inside out also regulate the movement of low molecular weight substances from outside in.[65] Small (<800 Da) hydrophilic molecules are effectively excluded by the extracellular membrane system from penetration across a mature stratum corneum, whereas small hydrophobic molecules or those with amphipathic properties (containing both hydrophilic and hydrophobic parts) are able to penetrate through the tortuous intercellular, lipid bilayer pathway.[1,66,67] In the preterm infant, the thinner stratum corneum results in a reduction in the length (tortuosity) of the intercellular pathway, which would enhance percutaneous absorption of hydrophilic molecules. Whether there are also qualitative changes in the lipid composition and structural integrity of the lipid bilayers of immature stratum corneum that alter its permeability function is unknown.

In addition to immaturity of the permeability barrier, several other factors in premature infants may contribute to toxicity from topical xenobiotics.[62,64] First, the surface area/volume ratio is increased in all infants, but even more so in premature infants; this effectively increases the absorptive surface while reducing the volume of distribution for the absorbed drug. Once absorbed, reduced levels of serum-binding proteins, such as albumin, may increase the proportion of free drug. Simi-

TABLE 4-3 Hazardous or potentially hazardous compounds that may be absorbed across the skin of preterm infants[†] (see also Chapter 5)

Compound	Toxicity	Sources
Alcohol (methylated spirits)	Skin necrosis; neurotoxic	Topical antiseptic
Aluminum*	Neurotoxicity	Metal containers for topical ointments
Aniline dyes	Methemoglobinemia	Laundry marks
Boric acid, borax	Shock, renal failure	Antifungals, talc powders
Benzocaine	Methemoglobinemia	Topical analgesics; teething products
Benzethonium chloride*	Carcinogen	Antiseptic soap
Benzoyl benzoate*	Neurotoxicity	Scabicide
Bicarbonate	Metabolic alkalosis	Baking soda for diaper dermatitis
Camphor*	Gastrointestinal toxin, neurotoxicity	Topical antipruritic; camphorated oils (Vaporub; Campho-Phenique)
Coal tars*	Carcinogen	Topical anti-inflammatory products
Corticosteroid	Adrenal suppression; hyperadrenocorticism	Topical corticosteroids
Diphenhydramine	Neurotoxicity	Topical analgesics (Caladryl)
Epinephrine	High output failure	Topical vasoconstriction
Glycerin*	Hyperosmolarity	Emollients; cleansers (Aquanil)
Hexachlorophene	Neurotoxicity	Antiseptic soaps (pHisoHex)
Iodochlorhydroxyquine	Optic neuritis	Topical antibiotic (Vioform)
Isopropyl alcohol	Skin necrosis; neurotoxicity	Topical antiseptics
Lactic acid*	Metabolic acidosis	Topical keratolytics (Lac-Hydrin)
Lindane	Neurotoxicity	Scabicide (Kwell)
Mercury	Neurotoxicity; acrodynia; nephrotic syndrome	Disinfectants; teething powder (historical)
Methylene blue	Methemoglobinemia	Vital stain
Neomycin	Ototoxicity	Topical antibiotic (Neosporin)
Nystatin*	Nephrotoxicity	Topical antifungal (Mycostatin)
Phenol	Cardiac and neurotoxicity	Disinfectants (e.g. commercial laundries); local anesthetic/antimicrobials (e.g. Castellani's paint)
Propylene glycol*	Hyperosmolarity; neurotoxicity	Topical vehicles; emollients, cleansers (Cetaphil)
Povidone–iodine	Skin necrosis; hypothyroidism	Topical antiseptic (Betadine)
Prilocaine	Methemoglobinemia	Topical anesthetic (EMLA)
Resorcinol	Methemoglobinemia	Topical antiseptic
Salicylic acid	Salicylism	Topical keratolytics
Silver sulfadiazine	Kernicterus; argyria	Topical antibiotic (Silvadene)
Sulfur*	Paralysis; death	Scabicide ointment
Triclosan*	Neurotoxicity	Topical antiseptic
Urea	Elevated BUN	Topical keratolytics/emollients

*Potentially hazardous compounds.
[†]References 62–72, 149–160.

larly, deficiency of an adipose reservoir to buffer against the redistribution of fat-soluble drugs, such as lindane, to lipid-enriched neural tissues, may make the premature infant particularly vulnerable to central nervous system (CNS) toxicity from such agents. Immaturity of detoxification mechanisms, such as hepatic conjugation, and of renal function, also alter drug pharmacodynamics and can increase toxicity.

The increased permeability of premature skin to small hydrophilic molecules has also been exploited to enhance the percutaneous delivery of medications such as theophylline.[64,68] Transdermal drug delivery offers the theoretic advantages of (1) the avoidance of first-pass hepatic metabolism; (2) a slow and continual reservoir of release, minimizing peaks and valleys; (3) the ability to easily remove the drug source (in the case of patch delivery systems), if needed; and (4) a painless method of drug delivery with easy access.[64] A confounding factor in developing these systems for the premature infant is the variability of barrier competence, both between infants of the same gestational ages and as the dynamics of barrier competence change as the infants mature.

In the care of the preterm infant, it is safest to assume that any medication applied to the skin may be absorbed systemically. As a corollary, the ideal topical medications for preterm infants are those with low systemic toxicity. It is also necessary to consider the composition and potential toxicity of vehicles used for topical drug delivery, because components of these may also be absorbed across the immature skin barrier (see Chapter 5).[36] In addition, the provision of a safe antiseptic for use on premature infant skin is particularly problematic, especially in the most immature infants, who have not only the most immature but also the most unstable barriers, and are therefore exposed to repeated applications of antiseptics for intravenous access.[69] In recent years, topical iodine-containing antiseptics (10% povidone–iodine) have been largely replaced by chlorhexidine-containing antiseptics (0.5% chlorhexidine gluconate solution in 70% isopropanol) in the neonatal intensive care nursery because of the potential risk for transient hypothyroxinemia and hypothyroidism due to systemic iodine absorption from the use of topical iodine-containing antiseptics.[70,71] Even the use of alcohol poses a risk for percutaneous absorption in the premature neonate, especially when used under occlusion, and has led to complications such as hemorrhagic skin necrosis.[72]

Impact of Permeability Barrier Immaturity on other Organ Systems

Excluding congenital malformations and genetic diseases, the major causes of morbidity and mortality in premature infants are respiratory distress syndrome, patent ductus arteriosus (PDA), necrotizing enterocolitis (NEC), periventricular/intraventricular hemorrhage (IVH), and overwhelming infection. Maintenance of normal blood pressure and 'optimal' blood volume protects against these major causes of morbidity and mortality in the preterm infant. Cutaneous fluid losses are perhaps the most important destabilizing factor in fluid homeostasis of the premature infant, and this influence is likely to be even more pronounced in the extremely premature. For example, overhydration contributes to the development of symptomatic PDA,[73] as larger blood volumes increase shunting through the ductus arteriosus. Conversely, systemic hypotension may increase the likelihood of an intracranial hemorrhage. Alterations in cerebral blood pressure induce hemorrhage into the periventricular germinal matrix, a gelatinous and highly vascular fetal structure which is present up to 34 weeks' gestational age.[74] The preterm infant may be unable to maintain cerebral blood flow in the presence of systemic hypotension. The period of greatest risk for IVH is in the first week of life, particularly the first 2 days, which coincides not only with the time of greatest permeability barrier incompetence but also with the time when tissue fluids undergo redistribution with contraction of the extracellular fluid compartment.[75] Thus, to the extent that IVH is precipitated by fluctuations in systemic blood pressure, overcompensated or uncompensated cutaneous water losses may be an exacerbating factor.

The pathogenesis of NEC is attributed to a triad of ischemia, oral feeding, and infection;[76,77] each of these pathogenic factors may be exacerbated by skin immaturity. As in PDA and IVH, fluid imbalance resulting from skin immaturity could be a cofactor, as both overcorrection of fluids[78] and

hypotensive ischemia–reperfusion injury[79] are implicated in NEC. Early initiation of oral feeds[80] is undertaken to reverse a negative energy balance in the preterm infant. Caloric losses caused by increased evaporative water loss from the skin surface contribute to this caloric drain. *Staphylococcus epidermidis* has also been implicated in the pathogenesis of NEC.[81-83] An impaired cutaneous barrier to this normal skin resident could be a factor not only in the development of *S. epidermidis* septicemia (see following discussion) but also in abnormal gastrointestinal colonization by this organism,[84] although a connection between these two phenomena is not obvious.

It seems likely, therefore, that efforts to closely monitor cutaneous losses through direct measurements of TEWL, with the goal of tight control of replacement fluids, would decrease the incidence and severity of these major complications of prematurity and improve the outcome of these infants.[85]

IMMATURITY OF OTHER SKIN BARRIERS

Cutaneous Barrier to Mechanical Injury

The skin of the premature infant is much more vulnerable to mechanical injury than that of term infants, as a consequence of several factors. In addition to a thinner stratum corneum, the epidermal–dermal interface is smooth, lacking interdigitations (i.e. rete ridges or dermal papillary projections) until the middle of the third trimester.[2] Both of these factors result in decreased resistance to shear forces. Moreover, the dermis is also thinner, less collagenized, and more gelatinous. Although the major structural proteins that underlie the mechanical strength of skin are expressed before the onset of keratinization, they may not be as abundant or organized into functionally mature units as in adult or even term infants' skin.[2] Whatever its basis, skin fragility is a major problem in the neonatal care of the preterm infant.[51] It is particularly vulnerable to abrasions and deeper wounds from adhesive tapes used to secure monitors, airways, and intravenous lines. Similarly, the threshold for irritant contact dermatitis from fecal contact (diaper dermatitis), for chemical burns from prolonged contact with antiseptics,[86] or for thermal burns is much reduced. Gentle handling, minimal use of adhesives, and use of hydrophilic gel[87] or pectin barrier[88] adhesives only when required can minimize these injuries. A regimen of emollient lubrication or use of nonadherent, semipermeable dressings may also protect against mechanical injuries (see previous discussion).

Cutaneous Barrier to Infection

Although mature skin is colonized by a variety of bacteria and other microorganisms, these organisms are effectively excluded from the interior. The basis for the barrier to transcutaneous infection is not entirely understood, but includes both the mechanical shield of the stratum corneum against invading microorganisms and specific components, such as certain lipids[89,90] and antimicrobial peptides (defensins and cathelicidins), that may both inhibit the growth of microorganisms and modulate immune responses.[91,92] The thinner, easily abraded stratum corneum of the preterm infant constitutes an impaired mechanical shield against the ingress of microorganisms. In addition, it is possible that specific biochemical components of the cutaneous barrier to infection are also immature in preterm infants, although this has not been determined. Preterm infants' skin is colonized soon after birth with coagulase-negative staphylococci, predominantly *S. epidermidis*. Colonization with *Malassezia* and *Proprionobacteria* occurs later, that is, after 3 weeks,[84] coincident with maturation of the permeability barrier. *S. epidermidis* has become the most frequent cause of postnatally acquired systemic infections in these infants.[93–98] *Malassezia furfur*, a common colonizing yeast on human skin, and *M. pachydermatitis*, a colonizer of canine skin, as well as the opportunistic fungi *Aspergillus*, *Candida*, and *Rhizopus*, are also systemic pathogens in this group.[99–103] Direct invasion across the immature epidermis by fungi of low pathogenicity in very preterm infants has been documented,[104] demonstrating that the stratum corneum barrier to infection is incompetent in these neonates. Exploitation of a portal of entry, such as site of skin injury or along transcutaneous catheter lines, may be a more common means of entry than direct invasion of the stratum corneum. Regardless of the route of transcutaneous entry, the immaturity of the immune system, particularly opsonic mechanisms, then permits organisms of low pathogenic potential to mature hosts to establish disease in the preterm infant.[105] The use of intravenous lipid supplements also favors the establishment of a nidus of infection once entry into the circulation has been obtained.[94]

Cutaneous Barrier to Light Injury

Energy absorbed from ultraviolet (UV) light passing through the skin may damage critical cellular functions through the generation of free radicals, principally singlet oxygen, as well as through inflammatory responses initiated by cytokine release and the generation of eicosanoids.[106,107] For example, free radical damage to deoxyribonucleic acid (DNA) may either result in cell death or initiate carcinogenic mutations. Although shorter wavelengths are more energetic and hence more damaging, they do not penetrate as deeply. In mature skin, ultraviolet B (UVB) (290–320 nm) does not penetrate into the dermis, but ultraviolet A (UVA) (320–400 nm) does, and visible wavelengths (400–800 nm) reach even deeper levels.[108] Hence, in considering the effects of light on the skin, one must consider not only the cumulative energy of the light absorbed but also the depth of penetration. Cutaneous defenses against UV light injury include:

- Mechanisms that absorb or reflect light (e.g. stratum corneum, melanin)
- Enzymatic (e.g. superoxide dismutase, catalase, glutathione peroxidase) and nonenzymatic (e.g. ascorbate, β-carotene) systems that absorb singlet oxygen or interrupt free radical cascades initiated by superoxide and hydroxyl radicals
- Mechanisms to repair cellular and DNA damage.

In mature skin, the stratum corneum is the first line of defense, filtering out approximately 80% of incident UVB light.[108] Therefore, the much thinner stratum corneum of the premature infant is one factor that must result in increased vulnerability to UV injury. In addition, rules about depth of penetration of different wavelengths based on studies of mature skin may not hold for premature skin. Melanocytes are present in the basal epidermis by the end of the first trimester, and melanin granules are synthesized and begin to be transferred to keratinocytes by mid-gestation.[2] However, inherent skin color is lighter in neonates, and melanin granule formation is not fully mature, even at term.[109] Moreover, the ability of melanocytes in the skin of preterm infants to increase melanin synthesis in response to UV stress has not been examined. Although maturation of other antioxidant defenses in the epidermis has not been studied either, these antioxidant systems are immature in the lungs of preterm infants.[110] Hence, the same may also be true for skin. Taken together, it is apparent that the premature infant is particularly vulnerable to UV injury.

UVB is filtered out by window glass, but UVA is not. Therefore the preterm infant in the nursery may be exposed to solar UVA, as well as longer wavelengths from artificial light sources. UVA is implicated in certain phototoxic and photoallergic responses.[111] Although its role in carcinogenesis is still controversial, a role in the causation of melanoma has not been excluded.[112,113] It should be assumed that the cutaneous barrier to UV light is immature in the preterm infant, hence they should be physically shielded from exposure to sunlight from exterior windows and other sources of ultraviolet light.

Portions of the visible light spectrum (420–500 nm) induce isomerization of bilirubin to compounds that can be excreted without hepatic conjugation. Hence, phototherapy with a variety of light sources is standard therapy for neonatal unconjugated hyperbilirubinemia. Because the commonly used fluorescent daylight bulbs emit UVA, the interposition of a Plexiglas shield is essential to avoid burns in preterm infants.[114] No deleterious long-term effects of visible light phototherapy on skin are documented.[115,116] However, as more extremely premature infants are exposed to these modalities, the possibility that they may be unusually vulnerable should be considered. For example, severe phototoxicity occurred in a preterm infant following use of intravenous fluorescein and prolonged dye retention as a result of renal immaturity.[117] Moreover, even internal organs are potentially affected by phototherapy, because light may penetrate more deeply through the skin of the preterm infant. For example, phototherapy has been linked to an increased incidence of symptomatic PDA in preterm infants.[118,119] Because merely shielding the chest wall overlying the heart can mitigate this complication, a direct photo effect on ductal tissue is likely.[120,121] Limitation on the intensity of ambient nursery lighting is recommended, largely out of concern for a contribution to the retinopathy of prematurity.[122,123] It would also seem prudent to consider the potential deleterious cutaneous and transcutaneous effects of nursery lighting on the vulnerable premature infant.

Cutaneous Contribution to Immaturity of Thermal Homeostasis

Body heat may escape through a number of mechanisms, as listed below:

- Evaporative heat loss
- Conduction: that is, direct gain or loss of heat to objects in direct contact with the infant's body
- Convection: that is, loss of body heat to the atmosphere, a function both of ambient air temperature and airflow (increased heat transfer with increased flow)
- Radiation (i.e. infrared energy exchanged between objects not in contact that absorb and remit radiant energy).[25]

Maintenance of a thermally neutral environment, minimizing unwanted heat loss or heat gain, is a major challenge to those who care for premature infants. The skin participates in thermal homeostasis through several mechanisms. Evaporation of water from the skin's surface results in caloric loss (0.58 kcal/mL). Water loss occurs both through passage of water across the stratum corneum as a function of barrier competency (see the previous discussion) and from secreted water delivered to the skin surface by ducts (eccrine sweating) in response to neural and other stimuli.[123] Caloric losses caused by an immature skin barrier are a major contributor to the preterm infant's heat loss, particularly in the first week of life.[124] Conversely, because eccrine function is immature, the premature infant is unable to compensate for heat stress by sweating.[125] Even in term infants, sweating is not functionally mature because the term infant's set point is higher than in mature individuals. Sweating in preterm infants matures rapidly following birth; however, the efficiency remains poor, with fewer body sites sweating in response to thermal stimuli and maintenance of a high set point.[125] Vasomotor control of cutaneous blood flow is a third component of the skin's contribution to thermal homeostasis. Both vasoconstriction and vasodilation in response to thermal stimuli are attenuated in the skin of preterm infants, although these responses appear to mature within 2–3 weeks.[126] Finally, the subcutaneous adipose reservoir is deficient in preterm infants, reducing both their insulation against heat loss and their energy reserves for thermal conversion.

Neurocutaneous Development in the Premature Infant

Responsiveness to touch is present at a very early age: that is, by the end of the first trimester the fetus withdraws in response to skin stroking.[127] In the preterm infant, neurocutaneous responses may be immature and 'globalized.' Thus, in the unstable premature infant handling is minimized to avoid adverse effects of skin stimulation, such as changes in heart rate, hypoxia, and apneic episodes.[128,129] However, older and more stable preterm infants may benefit from skin contact.[130] Originally, skin-to-skin contact was explored as a mechanism to facilitate maternal bonding with the term infant.[131] A modification of this principle, designated 'kangaroo mother care,' has been advocated for preterm infants in developing countries as a safe and effective mode of care for stable premature infants.[132,133] Kangaroo mother care is based on the marsupial model of transition to independent life, in which the infant is continually housed against the mother's skin and permitted ad libitum breastfeeding. In economies that cannot provide routine nursery equipment such as incubators, the adoption of kangaroo mother care can reduce both morbidity and mortality from inadequate thermal protection and infections associated with overcrowding in nurseries and formula feedings.[132] Briefer periods of maternal skin-to-skin contact during neonatal nursery residence have also been advocated in the care of the preterm infant in developed economies as a means to enhance maternal confidence and to humanize the nursery experience.[131–135] When infants are carefully selected to avoid the inclusion of unstable ones, the practice does not appear to be deleterious to the babies and may be beneficial (e.g. reduce periods of 'purposeless' activity). Long-term benefits to mother and child of skin-to-skin contact are difficult to distinguish from the benefits of more conventional mother–child contact, but may include prolonged maternal lactation and less infant crying.[132] Although it may seem intuitively obvious that both parents and infants would benefit psychologically from the humanizing effects of skin-to-skin contact, the neurocutane-

ous pathways that are likely to underlie these responses are only beginning to be delineated in mature skin.[136] It will be important as this work proceeds, to examine the maturation of these pathways in the preterm infant, so as both to better understand the capacity of the maturing infant to respond to these external stimuli and to develop systems of care that are both rational and 'humanistic.'

SKIN DISEASES IN THE PREMATURE INFANT

Barrier Function of Abnormal Skin

The consequences of barrier immaturity in premature infants may be compounded if the infant also has a primary skin disorder. Infants with severe genetic skin disorders are often born prematurely.[137] Skin diseases that result in hyperkeratosis (scaling) or a thickened stratum corneum, such as the ichthyoses, are commonly associated with impaired barrier function:[137,138] that is, a thick stratum corneum is not necessarily a competent one. These infants are at risk for hypernatremia as a result of increased evaporative loss of free water from the skin surface.[139,140] Similarly, infants with widespread blistering diseases, whether resulting from underlying infection, as in staphylococcal scalded skin syndrome, or from one of the genetic mechanobullous diseases, e.g. epidermolysis bullosa, have increased fluid requirements as a result of loss of barrier integrity. Skin disease also increases the risk of systemic absorption of topical medications, both because of a further compromise in barrier competence and because of increased exposure to topical medications. Instances of this include prolonged use of topical steroids to dermatitic skin, resulting in adrenal suppression and other signs of hypercorticism,[141,142] and use of salicylate-containing ointments to remove excessive scale, resulting in salicylism.[143]

Scars of Prematurity

A number of nursery procedures may lead to scars; the number of scars nursery graduates bear is correlated with their degree of prematurity and the duration of intensive care[144] (see also Chapter 8). Although most of these scars are not of great concern, more severe scarring sequelae can occur, particularly those resulting from wounds from chest tubes, skin strippings from adhesive tapes, and extravasated intravenous fluids. In addition, very premature infants (<29 weeks) may develop atrophic scars or so-called 'anetoderma of prematurity.'[145] Although the term 'anetoderma' implies a loss of elastic tissue and clinically manifests as an 'outpouching' of the skin, scars of prematurity can also be flat. These scars are often apparently absent in the early neonatal period, becoming evident at a few weeks to months of life. They often develop at sites of previous application of monitors and adhesives. The exact source of injury may be obvious if the pattern and location correspond to a known intervention (such as a cardiac monitor lead), but scars can also develop in areas not corresponding to known areas of injury (Fig. 4-3).

Hemangiomas

Hemangiomas of infancy are more common in preterm infants and their frequency is related to the degree of prematurity.[146] Premature infants also have higher risk of having multiple hemangiomas, but the exact basis for this increase is not

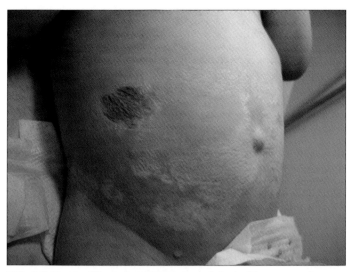

FIG. 4-3 Former 25-week gestational age infant with scars on the abdomen. Such scarring is not rare in very premature infants but may not be noted until several months of age. (Courtesy of Linda Beets-Shay, MD).

known (Fig. 4-4). Hypotheses include the presence of angioblasts which have not yet differentiated toward to more a mature phenotype, and an imbalance of growth and inhibitory angiogenic control mechanisms as a result of being born prematurely, thus removing a developing fetus from maternal and placental influences.[147,148]

SUMMARY

Because skin reliably performs its life-enabling functions throughout life, it and its diseases have often been trivialized. Only in rare instances of skin failure, such as in extensive burns, drug-induced toxic epidermal necrolysis, or severe autoimmune pemphigus vulgaris, is the importance of the skin barrier readily apparent. Yet, neonatologists have long been cognizant of the importance of fluid balance and thermal homeostasis in the care of the premature infant. Now, through advances in the care of fragile premature infants, and particularly through the advent of surfactant replacement therapy, neonates of ever-greater prematurity survive, relentlessly pushing backward the age of viability. In this context, the consequences of skin barrier immaturity emerge as a critical frontier in their management. Barrier failure contributes to the morbidity and mortality of the preterm neonate through fluid and electrolyte instability and the effects of fluid imbalance on blood volume and blood pressure, as well as an increased susceptibility to transcutaneous infections and toxicity from transcutaneous absorption of xenobiotics. As a result of the interlocking interdependence of organ systems, all of which are immature, the magnitude of the skin's contribution to neonatal morbidity cannot currently be estimated. Further study is needed to determine whether direct measurement of skin fluid losses would result in more precise, prospective fluid management and improved nursery outcomes. Insights from studies of barrier ontogenesis in experimental animals also suggest promising areas for clinical evaluation.

At present, it is only possible to outline broad principles for the care of the premature infant's skin.[34,47] Most of these are self-evident, such as the need to avoid exposure to topical agents of potential systemic toxicity, or for gentle handling to

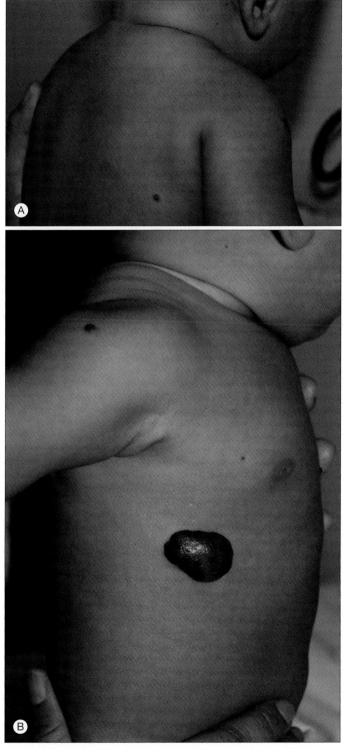

FIG. 4-4 A Former 34-week premature infant at 5 months of age with small hemangiomas of infancy on trunk and extremities. **B** The same infant with a larger hemangioma of infancy in addition to the small ones. He had approximately 30 lesions in total.

prevent abrogation of the skin's integrity. However, the optimal application of these principles in practice is often less evident. For example, all ingredients in topical medicaments, emollients, or cleansers need to be identified and their potential for toxicity considered, yet this information may not be easily obtained.[36] Moreover, preferred products, such as an aqueous solution of chlorhexidine for skin antisepsis, may not be commercially available.[36] In most instances skin care practices have not been systematically studied to determine optimal regimens. Just as the term infant's skin is more resilient and protective than the skin of a premature infant of 30 weeks' gestation, procedures that may not be hazardous to an infant of this gestational age may be toxic to the extremely immature 'micropreemie.' Therefore, in designing future studies, it will be important to consider the differences in skin function in babies of varying gestational and postnatal ages. Greater awareness of skin functions and their physiologic bases, as well as the infant's position on the maturational timetable of these functions, will be needed for the development of rational regimens of skin care in the future.

ACKNOWLEDGMENTS

The authors are indebted to Dr Khanh-Van Le-Bucklin for assistance with the literature review and to Dr Peter M. Elias for critical review of the manuscript.

REFERENCES

1. Elias PM, Menon GK. Structural and lipid biochemical correlates of the epidermal permeability barrier. Adv Lipid Res 1991; 21: 1–26.
2. Holbrook KA. Structural and biochemical organogenesis of skin and cutaneous appendages in the fetus and newborn. In: Polin RA, Fox WW, eds. Fetal and neonatal physiology, 2nd edn. Vol I. Phildelphia: WB Saunders, 1998; 729.
3. Evans NJ, Rutter N. Development of the epidermis in the newborn. Biol Neonate 1986; 49: 74–80.
4. Ballard JL, Khoury JC, Wedig K, et al. New Ballard score, expanded to include extremely premature infants. J Pediatr 1991; 119: 417–423.
5. Hammarlund K, Sedin G. TEWL in newborn infants. III. Relation to gestational age. Acta Pediatr Scand 1979; 68: 795–801.
6. Harpin VA, Rutter N. Barrier properties of the newborn infant's skin. J Pediatr 1983; 102: 419–425.
7. Cartlidge PHT, Rutter N. Skin barrier function. In: Polin RA, Fox WW, eds. Fetal and neonatal physiology, 2nd edn. Vol I. Phildelphia: WB Saunders, 1998; 771.
8. Nachman RL, Esterly NB. Increased skin permeability in preterm infants. J Pediatr 1971; 79: 628–632.
9. Okah FA, Wickett RR, Pickens WL, et al. Surface electrical capacitance as a noninvasive bedside measure of epidermal barrier maturation in the newborn infant. Pediatrics 1995; 96: 688–692.
10. Muramatsu K, Hirose S, Yukitake K, et al. Relationship between maturation of the skin and electrical skin resistance. Pediatr Res 1987; 21: 21–24.
11. Emery MM, Hebert AA, Aguirre V-C, et al. The relationship between skin maturation and electrical skin impedance. J Dermatol Sci 1991; 2: 336–340.
12. Aszterbaum M, Feingold KR, Menon GK, et al. Ontogeny of the epidermal barrier to water loss in the rat: Correlation of function with stratum corneum structure and lipid content. Pediatr Res 1992; 31: 308–317.
13. Williams ML, Hanley K, Elias PM, et al. Ontogenesis of the epidermal permeability barrier. J Invest Dermatol (Symposium Proceedings) 1998; 3: 75–79.
14. Kalia YN, Nonato LB, Lund CH, et al. Development of skin barrier function in premature infants. J Invest Dermatol 1998; 111: 320–326.
15. Ågren J, Sjörs G, Sedin G. Transepidermal water loss in infants born at 24 and 25 weeks of gestation. Acta Paediatr 1998; 87: 1185–1190.
16. Hanley K, Jiang Y, Elias PM, et al. Acceleration of barrier ontogenesis in vitro through air exposure. Pediatr Res 1997; 41: 293–299.
17. Williams ML, Feingold KR. Barrier function of neonatal skin [letter]. J Pediatr 1998; 133: 467–468.
18. Hammarlund K, Sedin G. Transepidermal water loss in newborn infants. IV. Small for gestational age infants. Acta Paediatr Scand 1980; 69: 377–383.
19. Aszterbaum M, Feingold KR, Menon GK, et al. Glucocorticoids accelerate fetal maturation of the epidermal permeability barrier in the rat. J Clin Invest 1993; 91: 2703–2708.
20. NIH Consensus Conference. Effect of corticosteroids for fetal maturation on perinatal outcome. JAMA 1995; 273: 413–418.
20a. Omar SA, DeCristofaro JD, Agarwal BI, LaGamma EF. Effects of prenatal steroids on water and sodium homeostasis in extremely low birth weight neonates. Pediatrics 1999; 104: 482.
21. Jain A, Rutter N, Cartlidge PH. Influence of antenatal steroids and sex on maturation of the epidermal barrier in the preterm infant. Arch Dis Child Fetal Neonatal Ed. 2000; 83: F112–116.
22. Fluhr JW, Crumrine D, Mao-Qiang M, et al. Topical liver X receptor activators (LXR) accelerate post-natal acidification of stratum corneum and improve function in the neonate. J Invest Dermatol (in press).
23. Fox C, Nelson D, Wareham J. The timing of skin acidification in very low birth weight infants. J Perinatol 1998; 18: 272–275.
24. Oh W. Fluid and electrolyte management. In: Fanaroff AA, Martin RJ, eds. Neonatal–perinatal medicine: Diseases of the fetus and infant, 6th edn. Vol I. St Louis: Mosby, 1997; 622.
25. Perlstein PH. Physical environment. In: Fanaroff AA, Martin RJ, eds. Neonatal–perinatal medicine: Diseases of the fetus and infant, 6th edn. Vol I. St Louis: Mosby, 1997; 481.
26. Fanaroff AA, Rand MB, Wald M, et al. Insensible water loss in low birth weight infants. Pediatrics 1972; 50: 236–245.
27. Wu PYK, Hodgman JE. Insensible water loss in preterm infants: Changes with postnatal development and non-ionizing radiant energy. Pediatrics 1974; 54: 704–712.
28. Harpin VA, Rutter N. Humidification of incubators. Arch Dis Child 1985; 60: 219–224.
29. Bell EF. Infant incubators and radiant warmers. Early Hum Dev 1983; 8: 351–375.
30. Williams PR, Oh W. Effects of radiant warmer on insensible water loss in newborn infants. Am J Dis Child 1974; 128: 511–514.
31. Bell EF, Neidich GA, Cashore WJ, et al. Combined effect of radiant warmer and phototherapy on insensible water loss in low-birth-weight infants. J Pediatr 1979; 94: 810–813.
32. Kjartansson S, Arsan S, Hammarlund K, et al. Water loss from the skin of term and preterm infants nursed under a radiant heater. Ped Res 1995; 37: 233–238.
33. Marks KH, Friedman Z, Maisels MJ. A simple device for reducing insensible water loss in low-birth-weight infants. Pediatrics 1977; 60: 223–226.
34. Baumgart S. Reduction of oxygen consumption, insensible water loss, and radiant heat demand with use of a plastic blanket for low-birth-weight infants under radiant warmers. Pediatrics 1984; 74: 1022–1028.
35. Cramer K, Wiebe N, Hartling L, et al. Heat loss prevention: a systematic review of occlusive skin wrap for premature neonates. J Perinatol 2005; 25: 763–769.
36. Siegfried EC. Neonatal skin and care. Dermatol Clin 1998; 16: 437–446.
37. Maayan-Metzger A, Yosipovitch G, Hadad E, et al. Transepidermal water loss and skin hydration in preterm

infants during phototherapy. Am J Perinatol. 2001; 18: 393–396.

38. Oh W, Karecki H. Phototherapy and insensible water loss in the newborn infant. Am J Dis Child 1972; 124: 230–232.

39. Wu PYK, Hodgman JE. Insensible water loss in preterm infants: Changes with postnatal development and non-ionizing radiant energy. Pediatrics 1974; 54: 704–712.

40. Kjartansson S, Hammarlund K, Sedin G. Insensible water loss from the skin during phototherapy in term and preterm infants. Acta Paediatr 1992; 81: 764–768.

41. Hammarlund K, Nilsson GE, Oberg PA, et al. TEWL in newborn infants. I. Relation to ambient humidity and site of measurement and estimation of total transepidermal water loss. Acta Pediatr Scand 1977; 66: 553–562.

42. Knauth A, Gordin M, McNelis W, et al. Semipermeable polyurethane membrane as an artificial skin for the premature neonate. Pediatrics 1989; 83: 945–950.

43. Barak M, Hershkowitz S, Rod R, et al. The use of a synthetic skin covering as a protective layer in the daily care of low birth weight infants. Eur J Pediatr 1989; 148: 665–666.

44. Vernon HJ, Lane AT, Wischerath LJ, et al. Semipermeable dressing and transepidermal water loss in premature infants. Pediatrics 1990; 86: 357–362.

45. Donahue ML, Phelps DL, Richter SE, et al. A semipermeable skin dressing for extremely low birth weight infants. J Perinatol 1996; 16: 20–26.

46. Mancini AJ, Sookdeo-Drost S, Madison KC, et al. Semipermeable dressings improve epidermal barrier function in premature infants. Pediatr Res 1994; 36: 306–314.

47. Katz S, McGinley K, Leyden JJ. Semipermeable occlusive dressings: Effects on growth of pathogenic bacteria and re-epithelialization of superficial wounds. Arch Dermatol 1986; 122: 58–62.

48. Lane AT. Development and care of the premature infant's skin. Pediatr Dermatol 1987; 4: 1–5.

49. Rutter N, Hull D. Reduction of skin water loss in the newborn. I. Effect of applying topical agents. Arch Dis Child 1981; 56: 669–672.

50. Nopper AJ, Horii KA, Sookdeo-Drost S, et al. Topical ointment therapy benefits premature infants. J Pediatr 1996; 128: 660–669.

51. Ghadially R, Halkier-Sorenson L, Elias P. Effects of petrolatum on stratum corneum structure and function. J Am Acad Dermatol 1992; 26: 387–396.

52. Mao-Qiang M, Brown BE, Wu-Pong S, et al. Exogenous nonphysiologic vs. physiologic lipids: Divergent mechanisms for correction of permeability barrier dysfunction. Arch Dermatol 1995; 131: 809–816.

53. Brown BE, Diembeck W, Hoppe U, et al. Fate of topical hydrocarbons in the skin. J Soc Cosmet Chem 1995; 46: 1.

54. Lester DE. Normal paraffins in living matter: Occurrence, metabolism, and pathology. Prog Food Nutr Sci 1979; 3: 1.

55. Mao-Qiang M, Feingold KR, Elias PM. Exogenous lipids influence permeability barrier recovery in acetone treated murine skin. Arch Dermatol 1993; 129: 728–738.

55a. Cockayne SE, Lee JA, Herrington CI. Oleogranulomatous response in lymph nodes associated with emollient use in Netherton's syndrome. Br J Dermatol 1999; 141: 562.

56. Conner JM, Soll RF, Edwards WH. Topical ointment for preventing infection in preterm infants. Cochrane Database Syst Rev. 2004; 1: CD001150.

57. Darmstadt GL, Saha SK, Ahmed AS, et al. Effect of topical treatment with skin barrier-enhancing emollients on nosocomial infections in preterm infants in Bangladesh: a randomised controlled trial. Lancet. 2005; 365: 1039–1045.

58. Darmstadt GL, Badrawi N, Law PA, et al. Topically applied sunflower seed oil prevents invasive bacterial infections in preterm infants in Egypt: a randomized, controlled clinical trial. Pediatr Infect Dis J. 2004; 23: 719–725.

59. Yang L, Mao-Qiang M, Taljebini M. Topical stratum corneum lipids accelerate barrier repair after tape stripping, solvent treatment and some but not all types of detergent treatment. Br J Dermatol 1995; 133: 679–685.

60. Mao-Qiang M, Feingold KR, Thornfelt CR, et al. Optimization of physiological lipid mixtures for barrier repair. J Invest Dermatol 1996; 106: 1096–1101.

61. Zettersten EM, Ghadially G, Feingold KR, et al. Optimal ratios of topical stratum corneum lipids improve barrier recovery in chronologically aged skin. J Am Acad Dermatol 1997; 37: 403–408.

62. West DP, Worobec S, Soloman LM. Pharmacology and toxicology of infant skin. J Invest Dermatol 1981; 76: 147–150.

63. West DP, Halket JM, Harvey DR, et al. Percutaneous absorption in preterm infants. Pediatr Dermatol 1987; 4: 234–237.

64. Rutter N. Percutaneous drug absorption in the newborn: Hazards and uses. Clin Perinatol 1987; 14: 911–930.

65. Scheuplein RJ, Blank LH. Permeability of skin. Physiol Rev 1971; 51: 702–747.

66. Potts RO, Franceur ML. The influence of stratum corneum morphology on water permeability. J Invest Dermatol 1991; 96: 495–499.

67. Menon GK, Elias PM. Morphologic basis for a pore-pathway in mammalian stratum corneum. Skin Pharmacol 1997; 10: 235–246.

68. Barrett DA, Rutter N. Transdermal delivery and the premature newborn. Crit Rev Ther Drug Carrier Syst 1994; 11: 1–30.

69. Froman RD, Owen SV, Murphy C. Isopropyl pad use in neonatal intensive care units. J Perinatol 1998; 18: 216–220.

70. Linder N, Davidovitch N, Reichman B, et al. Topical iodine-containing antiseptics and subclinical hypothyroidism in preterm infants. J Pediatr 1997; 131: 434–439.

71. Smerdely P, Lim A, Boyages SC, et al. Topical iodine-containing antiseptics and neonatal hypothyroidism in very-low-birthweight infants. Lancet 1989; 16: 661–664.

72. Harpin V, Rutter N. Percutaneous alcohol absorption and skin necrosis in a preterm infant. Arch Dis Child 1982; 57: 477–479.

73. Bell EF, Warburton D, Stonestreet BS, et al. Effect of fluid administration on the development of symptomatic patent ductus arteriosus and congestive heart failure in premature infants. N Engl J Med 1980; 302: 598–604.

74. Papile L. Intracranial hemorrhage. In: Fanaroff AA, Martin RJ, eds. Neonatal–perinatal medicine: Diseases of the fetus and infant, 6th edn. Vol I. St Louis: Mosby, 1997; 891.

75. Bauer K, Versmold H. Postnatal weight loss in preterm neonates 1500 g is due to isotonic dehydration of the extracellular volume. Acta Paediatr Scand 1989; 360(Suppl): 37–42.

76. Musemeche CA, Kosloske AM, Bartow SA, et al. Comparative effects of ischemia, bacteria, and substrate on the pathogenesis of intestinal necrosis. J Pediatr Surg 1986; 21: 536–538.

77. Willoughby RE, Pickering LK. Necrotizing enterocolitis and infection. Clin Perinatol 1994; 21: 307–315.

78. Bell EF, Warburton D, Stonestreet BS, et al. High volume fluid intake predisposes premature infants to necrotizing enterocolitis. [Letter] Lancet 1979; 2: 90.

79. Nowicki PT, Nankervis CA. The role of the circulation in the pathogenesis of necrotizing enterocolitis. Clin Perinatol 1994; 21: 219–234.

80. Crissinger KD, Granger DN. Mucosal injury induced by ischemia and reperfusion in the piglet intestine: Influences of age and feeding. Gastroenterol 1989; 97: 920–926.

81. Gruskay JA, Abbasi S, Anday E, et al. Staphylococcus epidermidis-associated enterocolitis. J Pediatr 1986; 109: 520–524.

82. Scheifele DW, Bjornson GL, Dyer RA, et al. Delta-like toxin produced by coagulase-negative staphylococci is associated with neonatal necrotizing

enterocolitis. Infect Immun 1987; 55: 2268–2273.

83. Mollit DL, Tepas JJ, Talbert JL. The role of coagulase-negative staphylococcus in neonatal necrotizing enterocolitis. J Pediatr Surg 1988; 23: 60–63.

84. Eastick K, Leeming JP, Bennett D, et al. Reservoirs of coagulase negative staphylococci in preterm infants. Arch Dis Child 1996; 74: F99–104.

85. Williams ML, Le KVT. The permeability barrier in the preterm infant: Review of the clinical consequences of barrier immaturity and of insights derived from an animal model of barrier ontogenesis, with a call for further studies. Eur J Pediatr Dermatol 1998; 8: 101.

86. Watkins AMC, Keogh EJ. Alcohol burns in the neonate. J Pediatr 1992; 28: 306–308.

87. Lund CH, Nonato LB, Kuller JM, et al. Disruption of barrier function in neonatal skin associated with adhesive removal. J Pediatr 1997; 131: 367–372.

88. Dollison EJ, Beckstrand J. Adhesive tape vs. pectin-based barrier use in preterm infants. Neonatal Network 1995; 14: 35–39.

89. Miller SJ, Aly R, Shinefeld HR, et al. In vitro and in vivo antistaphylococcal activity of human stratum corneum lipids. Arch Dermatol 1988; 124: 209–215.

90. Bibel DJ, Aly R, Shinefeld HR. Topical sphingolipids in antisepsis and antifungal therapy. Clin Exp Dermatol 1995; 20: 395–400.

91. Gallo RL, Huttner KM. Antimicrobial peptides: an emerging concept in cutaneous biology. J Invest Dermatol 1998; 111: 739–743.

92. Braff MH, Bardan A, Nizet V, et al. Cutaneous defense mechanisms by antimicrobial peptides. J Invest Dermatol 2005; 125: 9–13.

93. Patrick CC, Kaplan SL, Baker CJ, et al. Persistent bacteremia due to coagulase-negative staphylococci in low birth weight neonates. Pediatrics 1989; 84: 977–985.

94. Freeman J, Goldman DA, Smith NE, et al. Association of intravenous lipid emulsion and coagulase-negative staphylococcal bacteremia in neonatal intensive care units. N Engl J Med 1990; 323: 301–308.

95. Klein JO. From harmless commensal to invasive pathogen. [Editorial] N Engl J Med 1990; 323: 339–340.

96. Freeman J, Epstein MF, Smith NE, et al. Extra hospital stay and antibiotic usage with nosocomial coagulase-negative staphylococcal bacteremia in two neonatal intensive care populations. Am J Dis Child 1990; 144: 324–329.

97. St Geme JW, Bell LM, Baumgart S, et al. Distinguishing sepsis from blood culture contamination in young infants with blood cultures growing coagulase-negative staphylococci. Pediatrics 1990; 86: 157–162.

98. Nataro JP, Corcoran L, Zirin S, et al. Prospective analysis of coagulase-negative staphylococcal infection in hospitalized infants. J Pediatr 1994; 125: 798–804.

99. Aschner JL, Punsalang A, Maniscalco WM, et al. Percutaneous central venous catheter colonization with *Malassezia furfur*: Incidence and clinical significance. Pediatrics 1987; 80: 535–539.

100. Stuart SM, Lane AT. *Candida* and *Malassezia* as nursery pathogens. Semin Dermatol 1992; 11: 19–23.

101. Chang HJ, Miller HL, Watkins N, et al. An epidemic of *Malassezia pachydermatis* in an intensive care nursery associated with colonization of health care worker's pet dogs. N Engl J Med 1998; 338: 706–711.

102. Rowen JL, Correa AG, Sokol DM, et al. Invasive aspergillosis in neonates: Report of five cases and literature review. Pediatr Infect Dis J 1992; 11: 576–582.

103. Linder N, Keller N, Huri C, et al. Primary cutaneous mucormycosis in a premature infant: Case report and review of the literature. Am J Perinatol 1998; 15: 35–38.

104. Rowen JL, Atkins JT, Levy ML, et al. Invasive fungal dermatitis in the 1000-gram neonate. Pediatrics 1995; 95: 682–687.

105. Yoder MC, Polin RA. Developmental immunology. In: Fanaroff AA, Martin RJ, eds. Neonatal–perinatal medicine: Diseases of the fetus and infant, 6th edn. Vol I. St Louis: Mosby, 1997; 685.

106. Granstein RD. Photoimmunology. In: Fitzpatrick TB, Eisen AZ, Wolff K, et al., eds. Dermatology in general medicine, 4th edn. Vol I. New York: McGraw Hill, 1993; 1638.

107. Norris G, Gange RW, Hawk JLM. Acute effects of ultraviolet radiation on the skin. In: Fitzpatrick TB, Eisen AZ, Wolff K, et al., eds. Dermatology in general medicine, 4th edn. Vol I. New York: McGraw Hill, 1993; 1651.

108. Kohevar IE, Pathak MA, Parrish JA. Photophysics, photochemistry, and photobiology. In: Fitzpatrick TB, Eisen AZ, Wolff K, et al., eds. Dermatology in general medicine, 4th edn. Vol I. New York: McGraw Hill, 1993; 1627.

109. Holbrook KA, Sybert V. Basic Science, embryogenesis of the skin. In: Schachner LA, Hanson RC, eds. Pediatric dermatology. Vol I. New York: Churchill Livingstone, 1988; 3.

110. Frank L, Sosenko IRS. Development of the lung antioxidant system in late gestation: Possible implications for the prematurely born infant. J Pediatr 1987; 110: 9–14.

111. Hawk JLM, Norris PG. Abnormal responses to ultraviolet radiation: Idiopathic. In: Fitzpatrick TB, Eisen AZ, Wolff K, et al., eds. Dermatology in general medicine, 4th edn. Vol I. New York: McGraw Hill, 1993;1661.

112. Koh HK, Kligler BE, Lew RA. Sunlight and cutaneous malignant melanoma: Evidence for and against causation. Photchem Photobiol 1990; 51: 765–779.

113. Setlow RB, Woodhead AD. Temporal changes in the incidence of malignant melanoma: Explanation from action spectra. Mutat Res 1994; 307: 365–374.

114. Siegfried EC, Stone MS, Madison KC. Ultraviolet light burn: a cutaneous complication of visible light phototherapy of neonatal jaundice. Pediatr Dermatol 1992; 9: 278–282.

115. Halmek LP, Stevenson DK. Neonatal jaundice and liver disease. In: Fanaroff AA, Martin RJ, eds. Neonatal–perinatal medicine: Diseases of the fetus and infant, 6th edn. Vol I. St Louis: Mosby, 1997; 1345.

116. Berg P, Lindelof B. Is phototherapy in neonates a risk factor for malignant melanoma development? Arch Pediatr Adolesc Med 1997; 151: 1185–1187.

117. Kearns GL, Williams BJ, Timmons OD. Fluorescein phototoxicity in a premature infant. J Pediatr 1985; 107: 796–798.

118. Barefield ES, Dwyer MD, Cassady G. Association of patent ductus arteriosus and phototherapy in infants weighing less than 1000 grams. J Perinatol 1993; 13: 376–380.

119. Rosenfeld W, Sadhev S, Brunot V, et al. Phototherapy effect on the incidence of patent ductus arteriosus in premature infants: prevention with chest shielding. Pediatrics 1986; 78: 10–14.

120. Clyman RI, Rudolph AM. Patent ductus arteriosus: a new light on an old problem. Pediatr Res 1978; 12: 92–94.

121. Ancott SW, Walsh-Sukys MC. Recommendations for newborn care. In: Fanaroff AA, Martin RJ, eds. Neonatal–perinatal medicine: Diseases of the fetus and infant, 6th edn. Vol I. St Louis: Mosby, 1997; 408.

122. Glass P, Avery GB, Subramanian KN, et al. Effect of bright light in the hospital nursery on the incidence of retinopathy of prematurity. N Engl J Med 1985; 313: 401–404.

123. Mancini AJ, Lane AT. Sweating in the neonate. In: Polin RA, Fox WW, eds. Fetal and neonatal physiology, 2nd edn. Vol I. Phildelphia: WB Saunders, 1998; 767.

124. Hammarlund K, Stromberg B, Sedin G. Heat loss from the skin of preterm and fullterm newborn infants during the first weeks after birth. Biol Neonate 1986; 50: 1–10.

125. Harpin VA, Rutter N. Sweating in preterm infants. J Pediatr 1982; 100: 614–619.

126. Jahnukainen T, van Ravenswaaij-Arts, Jalonen J, et al. Dynamics of vasomotor thermoregulation of the skin in term and preterm neonates. Early Hum Dev 1993; 33: 133–143.

127. Hogg ID. Sensory nerves and associated structures in the skin of human fetuses of 8 to 14 weeks of menstrual age correlate with functional capability. J Comp Neurol 1941: 75: 371.

128. Long JG, Philip AG, Lucey JF. Excessive handling as a cause of hypoxemia. Pediatr 1980; 65: 203–207.

129. Lynch ME. Iatrogenic hazards, adverse occurrences, and complications involving NICU nursing practice. J Perinatal Neonatal Nurs 1991; 5: 78–86.

130. Field TM, Schanberg SM, Scafidi F, et al. Tactile/kinesthetic stimulation effects on preterm neonates. Pediatrics 1986; 77: 654–658.

131. Klaus MH, Kennell JH. Care of the mother, father and infant. In: Fanaroff AA, Martin RJ, eds. Neonatal–perinatal medicine: Diseases of the fetus and infant, 6th edn. Vol I. St Louis: Mosby, 1997; 548.

132. Cattaneo A, Davanzo R, Uxa F, et al. Recommendations for the implementation of kangaroo mother care for low birthweight infants. Acta Paediatr 1998; 87: 440–445.

133. Tessier R, Cristo M, Velez S, et al. Kangaroo mother care and the bonding hypothesis. Pediatrics 1998; 102: e17.

134. Whitelaw A, Heisterkamp G, Sleath K, et al. Skin to skin contact for very low birthweight infants and their mothers. Arch Dis Child 1988; 63: 1377–1381.

135. Ludington-Hoe SM, Thompson C, Swinth J, et al. Kangaroo care: Research results and practice implications and guidelines. Neonatal Network 1994; 13: 19–27.

136. O'Sullivan RL, Lipper G, Lerner EA. The neuro-immuno-cutaneous–endocrine network: Relationship of mind and skin. Arch Dermatol 1998; 134: 1431–1435.

137. Williams ML, LeBoit PE. The ichthyoses: disorders of cornification. In: Arndt KA, Leboit PE, Robinson JK, Wintroub BU, eds. Cutaneous medicine and surgery: An integrated program in dermatology. Vol II. Philadelphia: WB Saunders, 1996; 1681.

138. Buyse L, Graves C, Marks R, et al. Collodion baby dehydration: the danger of high transepidermal water loss. Br J Dermatol 1993; 129: 86–88.

139. Garty BB, Metzker A, Nitzan M. Hypernatremia in congenital lamellar ichthyosis. J Pediatr 1979; 95: 814.

140. Jones SK, Thomason LM, Surbrugg SK, et al. Neonatal hypernatraemia in two siblings with Netherton's syndrome. Br J Dermatol 1986; 114: 741–743.

141. Turpeinen M. Influence of age and severity of dermatitis on the percutaneous absorption of hydrocortisone in children. Br J Dermatol 1988; 118: 517–522.

142. Feinblatt BI, Aceto T, Beckhorn G, et al. Percutaneous absorption of hydrocortisone in children. Am J Dis Child 1966; 112: 218–224.

143. Chiaretti A, Schembri Wismayer D, Tortorolo L, et al. Salicylate intoxication using a skin ointment. Acta Pediatr 1997; 86: 330–331.

144. Cartlidge PH, Fox PE, Rutter N. The scars of newborn intensive care. Early Hum Dev 1990; 21: 1–10.

145. Prizant TL, Lucky AW, Frieden IJ, et al. Spontaneous atrophic patches in extremely premature infants. Arch Dermatol 1996; 132: 671–674.

146. Amir J, Metzker A, Krikler R, et al. Strawberry hemangioma in preterm infants. Pediatr Dermatol 1986; 3: 331–332.

147. Bree AF, Siegfried E, Sotelo-Avila C, et al. Infantile hemangiomas: speculation on placental trophoblastic origin. Arch Dermatol 2001 May; 137: 573–577.

148. Garzon MC, Drolet BA, Haggstrom A, Frieden IJ. Incidence and clinical associations of multiple haemangiomas of infancy. [Abstract] Proceedings of the 15 ISSVA Congress, Wellington, New Zealand, 2004.

149. Rogers SCF, Burrows D, Neill D. Percutaneous absorption of phenol and methyl alcohol in Magenta Paint BPC. Br J Dermatol 1978; 98: 559–560.

150. Segal S, Cohen SN, Freeman J, et al. Camphor: Who needs it? Pediatrics 1978; 62: 404–406.

151. Benda GI, Hiller JL, Reynolds JW. Benzyl alcohol toxicity: Impact on neurologic handicaps among surviving very low birth weight infants. Pediatrics 1986; 77: 507–512.

152. Bamford MFM, Jones LF. Deafness and biochemical imbalance after burns treatment with topical antibiotics in young children. Arch Dis Child 1978; 53: 326–329.

153. Stohs SJ, Ezzedeen FW, Anderson AK, et al. Pecutaneous absorption of iodochlorhydroxyquin in humans. J Invest Dermatol 1984; 82: 195–198.

154. McDonald MG, Getson PR, Glasgow AM, et al. Propylene glycol: Increased incidence of seizures in low birth weight infants. Pediatrics 1987; 79: 622–625.

155. Bishop NJ, Morley R, Day JP, et al. Aluminum neurotoxicity in preterm infants receiving intravenous feeding solutions. N Eng J Med 1997; 336: 1557–1561.

156. Barker N, Hadgraft J, Rutter N. Skin permeability in the newborn. J Invest Dermatol 1987; 88: 409–411.

157. Armstrong RW, Eichener ER, Klein DE, et al. Pentachlorophenol poisoning in a nursery for newborn infants. II. Epidemiologic and toxicologic studies. J Pediatr 1969; 75: 317–325.

158. Pramanik AK, Hansen RC. Transcutaneous gamma benzene hexachloride absorption and toxicity in infants and children. Arch Dermatol 1979; 115: 1224–1225.

159. L'Allemand D, Gruters A, Beyer P, et al. Iodine in contrast agents and skin disinfectants is the major cause for hypothyroidism in premature infants during intensive care. Horm Res 1987; 28: 42–49.

160. Parravicini E, Fontana C, Paterlini GL, et al. Iodine, thyroid function, and very low birth weight infants. Pediatrics 1996; 98: 730–734.

5

Neonatal Skin Care and Toxicology

Alanna F. Bree, Elaine C. Siegfried

BACKGROUND

The skin of the neonate is distinctive in many ways, including its immature anatomy and physiology. An understanding of the principles of human skin development and a more uniform approach to skin care in the neonatal nursery can minimize risks to this special population of patients. Well-defined and standardized guidelines for skin care of premature infants have recently been published.[1-4]

STRUCTURE AND FUNCTION OF NEONATAL SKIN

As discussed in Chapters 1, 2 and 4, there are structural and developmental differences in the skin of adults, full-term infants and premature neonates. The skin of a full-term newborn is structurally and functionally more ready to adapt to an air environment. In contrast, the skin of a premature infant is in homeostasis with a fluid environment. After abrupt exposure to the xeric, postnatal world, premature skin matures rapidly over 2–8 weeks, taking significantly longer for the most premature and lowest-birthweight neonates.[5] Despite this rapid maturation, skin barrier function is inadequate, with associated morbidity and mortality.

Infants less than 24 weeks' gestation have minimally protective stratum corneum at birth.[5,6] In addition, their ratio of body surface area to weight is up to five times that of an adult.[7,8] These differences make premature infants much more susceptible to transepidermal water loss (TEWL), which is 10 times greater in a 24-week than in a full-term newborn.[9] Increased TEWL is accompanied by fluid/electrolyte disturbances, percutaneous absorption of topically applied agents, and percutaneous infection, and may be exacerbated by iatrogenic exposure to infrared radiant warming and blue light phototherapy.

At the dermoepidermal junction, anchoring fibrils, anchoring filaments and hemidesmosomes are fewer and smaller in premature infants,[6] with resultant skin fragility and risk of inadvertent cutaneous injury. Healing is compromised by increased metabolic demands and suboptimal nutrient stores in these infants. The dermis is composed of smaller collagen fibrils in both premature and full-term infants. Elastic fibers in the premature infant are tiny, immature and sparse, whereas those in the full-term newborn are also small but similar in distribution to an adult.[6] This dermal immaturity allows for increased dependant and postinflammatory edema, with resultant risk of ischemic injury. Premature infants also have an attenuated layer of subcutaneous fat and nonfunctional eccrine glands at birth, leading to compromised thermoregulatory capabilities.[10]

The antimicrobial defenses of neonatal skin are also immature, which leads to a greater risk of infectious complications.[10] An acidic skin surface pH, historically known as the 'acid mantle,' coincides with normal postnatal bacterial colonization. A full-term newborn is born with an alkaline pH that rapidly becomes acidic over the first few days of life. In preterm infants this process can take a few weeks. Additionally, the skin's antimicrobial lipids and peptides may not be fully functional at birth, thus failing to provide important innate immunity.[11]

PERCUTANEOUS ABSORPTION AND TOXICITY

An infant's immature skin barrier, coupled with a high ratio of body surface area to weight, significantly increases the risk of percutaneous absorption. Facile percutaneous absorption can be utilized with therapeutic advantage to neonates. For example, a side effect of phenylephrine eye drops was classically described as 'raccoon facies,' a visible periorbital ring of pallor due to cutaneous vasoconstriction.[12] This finding has since been quantified and is directly proportional to measurements of transepidermal water loss. Both methods have been established as useful markers of stratum corneum integrity in infants.[12,13] Transdermal delivery has also been utilized for the administration for theophylline[12,14] and diamorphine[15] in premature infants. Even supplemental oxygen has been administered percutaneously to very small preterm infants with poor pulmonary function.[16,17]

Numerous reports have documented percutaneous poisoning from agents applied to the skin of infants and children (Table 5-1). Further compounding this risk are the developmentally distinct aspects of pediatric pharmacokinetics: absorption, tissue distribution, metabolism and detoxification.[18,19] In addition, toxicologic data are lacking for most of these topically applied agents, especially for infants and children, a group known as therapeutic orphans.[10,20] Revered clinicians have historically overlooked the potential for percutaneous

TABLE 5-1 Reported hazards of percutaneous absorption in infants and children

Compound	Product	Toxicity
Alcohols[124,125]	Skin antiseptic	Cutaneous hemorrhagic necrosis, elevated blood alcohol levels
Aniline[16]	Dye used as a laundry marker	Methemoglobinemia, death
Adhesive remover solvents[129]	Skin preparations to aid in adhesive removal	Epidermal injury, hemorrhage and necrosis
Benzocaine[154]	Mucosal anesthetic (teething products)	Methemoglobinemia
Boric acid[24]	Baby powder, diaper paste	Vomiting, diarrhea, erythroderma, seizures, death
Calcipotriol[155]	Topical vitamin D_3 analogue	Hypercalcemia, hypercalcemic crisis
Chlorhexidine[120]	Topical antiseptic	Systemic absorption but no toxic effects
Corticosteroids[156]	Topical anti-inflammatory	Skin atrophy, striae, adrenal suppression
Diphenhydramine[157]	Topical anti-pruritic	Central anticholinergic syndrome
Lidocaine[85]	Topical anesthetic	Petechiae, seizures
Lindane[158]	Scabicide	Neurotoxicity
Mercuric chloride[159]	Diaper rinses, teething powders	Acrodynia, hypotonia
Methylene blue[160]	Amniotic fluid leak	Methemoglobinemia
N,N-dimethyl-m-toluamide (DEET)[113]	Insect repellant	Neurotoxicity
Neomycin[108]	Topical antibiotic	Neural deafness
Phenolic compounds (pentachlorophenol, hexachlorophene, resorcinol)[19]	Laundry disinfectant, topical antiseptic	Neurotoxicity, tachycardia, metabolic acidosis, methemoglobinemia, death
Phenylephrine[13]	Ophthalmic drops	Vasoconstriction, periorbital pallor
Povidone–iodine[122]	Topical antiseptic	Hypothyroidism
Prilocaine[86]	Topical anesthetic	Methemoglobinemia
Salicylic acid[161]	Keratolytic emollient	Metabolic acidosis, salicylism
Silver sulfadiazine[137,139]	Topical antibiotic	Kernicterus (sulfa component), agranulocytosis, argyria (silver component)
Tacrolimus[162]	Topical immunomodulator	Elevated blood levels of immunosuppressive medication
Triple dye (brilliant green, gentian violet, proflavine hemisulfate)[71]	Topical antiseptic for umbilical cord	Ulceration of mucous membranes, skin necrosis, vomiting, diarrhea
Urea[163]	Keratolytic emollient	Uremia

poisoning in designing therapy for infants. This was evidenced by an epidemic of neonatal cyanosis in London in the late 1800s. At that time, cloth diapers were labeled with aniline dye stamps. The imprint of the stamp on the perineum and buttock of one of the affected infants was a clue to the diagnosis. Despite this discovery, diapers labeled with aniline were used for decades, resulting in at least six infant deaths.[12] Another example is Cooke's 1926 review of diaper dermatitis. Here, he recommended a rapid and permanent 'cure' for 'ammoniacal' dermatitis by rinsing diapers in either dilute mercuric chloride or saturated boric acid solution.[21] Over the last 70 years, published accounts have served to document only the most severe toxicities – in some cases manifesting as nursery epidemics of obvious clinical illness or deaths.

With regards to topical therapy in infants, both active ingredients and vehicles are important to consider. The vehicle affects the absorption of the active medication. Hydrophilic agents are able to penetrate the lipid bilayer better than water-soluble compounds. Topically applied lipids also enhance epidermal hydration, widening intracellular bonds and facilitating enhanced absorption.[22] Preservatives are bacteriostatic compounds required for any product that contains an aqueous component. Emulsifiers are required to enable the mixing of aqueous and oil components in a product and help make the product easier to apply to the skin. Fragrances may be added to enhance product appeal. Preservatives are often classified as emulsifiers or fragrances by manufacturers to allow for marketing as a 'preservative-free' product.[23] A variety of other additives, including vitamins and plant extracts, may be added to enhance marketing allure. Any of these inactive ingredients can be an occult cause of irritation, allergic contact sensitization, and toxicity. Table 5-2 reviews products that should be used with caution in newborns based on potential toxicity and side effects. The best approach is to use topical products with simple vehicles, and to be aware of the quantity applied as well as the duration of skin contact.

SKIN CARE GUIDELINES

In 1999, the skin care practices in neonatal nurseries were often based in tradition,[24] with wide variability and no consistency noted in multiple surveys.[25–27] An evidence-based

TABLE 5-2 Topical agents that should be used with caution in the newborn

Compound	Product	Concern
Ammonium lactate	Keratolytic emollient	Possible lactic acidosis
Benzethonium chloride	Skin cleansers	Poisoning by ingestion, carcinogenesis
Coal tar	Shampoos, anti-inflammatory ointments	Excessive use of polycyclic aromatic hydrocarbons are associated with an increased risk of cancer
Glycerin	Emollients, cleansing agents	Hyperosmolality, seizures
Propylene glycol	Emollients, cleansing agents	Excessive enteral and parenteral administration has caused hyperosmolality and seizures
Triclosan	Deodorant and antibacterial soaps	Toxicities seen with other phenolic products

As published in Siegfried EC. Neonatal skin and skin care. Dermatol Clin 1998; 16: 437–448.[25]

TABLE 5-3 Neonatal Skin Condition Scale. Based on the Association of Women's Health, Obstetric and Neonatal Nurses Evidence-based clinical practice guideline for neonatal skin care[3]

	Dryness	Erythema	Breakdown
1	Normal, no signs of dryness	No evidence of erythema	None
2	Dry skin, visible scaling	Visible erythema <50% body surface	Small localized area
3	Very dry skin, cracking/fissures	Visible erythema >50% body surface	Extensive

comprehensive practice guideline was published in 2001.[1,2] This landmark reference includes a validated 9-point scale that rates dryness, erythema, and skin breakdown, which is helpful in monitoring neonates who are at exceptionally high risk for skin problems (Table 5-3).[28]

Although established guidelines have improved skin care for infants in the neonatal intensive care unit (NICU), there is still a paucity of literature on the optimal skin care of healthy, full-term newborns.[29–31] Anticipatory guidance for new parents should include information about safe skin-care techniques and dispel misconceptions regarding some baby care products.[32] In the first month of life newborns are exposed to an average of eight skin-care products with a minimum of 48 ingredients.[33] New parents often receive sample products provided by manufacturers and distributed in the hospital at the time of delivery. This can be misinterpreted as an endorsement for a particular product. Some companies further utilize this relationship to market their products as the 'choice of hospitals.'

The principles of product selection and use are similar for infants of any gestational age: avoiding exposure to unnecessary products and ingredients while seeking products that have been tested in newborns. Product manufacturers can be asked for available data that support marketing claims.

SKIN CARE PRACTICES

Skin Cleansing

For both children and adults, bathing is often a hygienic necessity. However, frequent bathing of infants is more of a cultural and aesthetic practice that allows for tactile interaction with the caregiver. Benefits must be carefully balanced with the detrimental effects that can occur with bathing, especially in premature infants.[34,35]

For neonates, bathing can lead to hypothermia, increased oxygen consumption, respiratory distress, and destabilized vital signs.[36] Therefore, the first bath should be delayed until after vital signs and temperature have remained stable for at least 2–4 hours.[1,2] Immersion bathing, when feasible, may be beneficial from a developmental perspective. It is more soothing, and can promote enhanced sleep,[37,38] and in studies was not associated with significant differences in oxygen saturation, respiratory rate, or heart rate in premature infants less than 32 weeks' gestation.[39] The water level should be high enough to cover the infant's entire body to aid temperature control and decrease evaporative heat loss. The optimal temperature of bath water is 100.4°F, which should always be accurately measured. Second-degree burns have been reported after immersion into overly hot bath water tested only by touch.[40] Sponge bathing with a moistened cotton ball or cloth is an acceptable alternative. Immediately after bathing, the infant's skin should be gently towel dried and a head covering applied.[2]

Vernix caseosa, composed of sebaceous gland secretions, desquamated skin cells, and shed lanugo hairs,[41] is negligible in preterm infants. Vernix need not be removed,[34] as this layer may aid in thermoregulation, hydration, bacterial protection, and wound healing.[41–44]

There is scant medical literature addressing the claims of the mildness of 'baby' soaps.[45] The most common problem associated with cleansing products is irritation. Liquid cleansers and superfatted soaps are less irritating than traditional soap product derived from lye. The safest products for term neonates are mild, neutral pH cleansers without added dyes or fragrances.[2] Cleansing products should be used sparingly and rinsed off well.

The first bath should be given respecting universal precautions to limit contact with transmissible pathogens. There have been no studies to support the routine use of antiseptics. The once-conventional use of antimicrobial cleansers for routine infant bathing diminished following recognition of the toxicity risks. Hexachlorophene was widely used prior to 1975, and subsequently associated with serious adverse reactions in infants, including fatal neurotoxicity. There has been only one subsequent report of an infectious complication possibly linked to a change in bathing with nonantiseptic cleanser.[46] However, in an era of increasing antibiotic-resistant colonization and infection with *Staphylococcus aureus*, the use of antimicrobial cleansers may be reconsidered. One economical, safe and effective option is dilute sodium hypochlorite. Household bleach sold for use in laundering clothes is 3–6% sodium hypochlorite. A 0.025% solution can be made by adding 2 mL bleach per gallon of water.[47] It should be noted that mild skin irritation from contact with dilute solution may occur, and that more concentrated or prolonged contact can cause skin necrosis.[48] Sensitization dermatitis is rare. In premature infants <26 weeks' gestation the safest option is to bathe with sterile water alone to minimize the risks of irritation, chemical absorption, and potential toxicity.[2]

Care of the infant scalp and hair follows the same principles as skin care. The same or similar gentle liquid cleansers may be used.[49] 'Baby' shampoos are distinguished by a low ocular irritation index and a pH and saline concentration similar to those of tears.[34] Allergic contact dermatitis from cleansing products, including shampoos, is rare[50] as they have very brief contact with the skin before being rinsed off. Fragrance and preservatives in moisturizers that are left on the skin are more common causes of allergic contact dermatitis and pruritis. However, cocamidopropyl betaine, a gentle surfactant very commonly used in shampoos and cleansers marketed for infants, is substantive, and is a well-recognized allergen to avoid.

Mouth and Nail Care

Little attention has been directed towards oral care in the neonate.[51] Some NICU protocols include recommendations for mouth care, such as wiping the lips with a water-soaked gauze or cloth every 3–4 hours. This is important for patients with oral devices in place, who are prone to mucosal drying. There is no data or theoretical basis to support the use of medicated mouth rinses in infants, as has been advocated for adults.[52]

Minimal nail care is needed in the neonatal period. Fingernails should be trimmed to limit self-inflicted excoriation, avoiding close trimming that can cause bleeding and lead to infection.[32] Of note, artificial and long natural fingernails in healthcare workers have been associated with an outbreak of *Pseudomonas aeruginosa* in a neonatal intensive care unit[53] and linked to a case report of an infant infection and resultant death.[54]

Emollients

In full-term infants moisturizers enhance epidermal hydration and may increase the absorption of topically applied medications. Ointments provide a more effective moisture barrier than creams or lotions. In addition, oil-and water emulsions utilize several potentially irritating, sensitizing, or toxic ingredients. White petrolatum is a safe, inexpensive, and highly effective emollient. Wool alcohols, along with methylchloroisothiazolinone/methylisothiazolinone (CMI/MI, a common preservative), thimerosal, nickel, fragrances, and neomycin, rank among the most common causes of allergic contact dermatitis in children.[55] (Eucerin Creme (Beiersdorf AG, Hamburg, Germany) is a popular product that has been studied for use in the nursery. It contains water, petrolatum, mineral oil, ceresin, lanolin alcohol, and methylchloroisothiazolinone/methylisothiazolinone (CMI/MI, also known as Kathon CG). Although the susceptibility of premature infants to allergic contact sensitization is unknown, CMI/MI has been associated with allergic contact sensitization in up to 10% of exposed adults and is the third most common sensitizer in children with chronic dermatitis[55a]). Aquaphor ointment (Beiersdorf AG, Hamburg, Germany), a petroleum wax-based emollient, contains white petrolatum, mineral oil, ceresin, lanolin alcohol (a wool alcohol), panthenol, glycerin, and bisabolol.)

Infant Massage

Infant massage, a tradition in some cultures, has recently been popularized, along with manufacture and marketing of related products. These products are usually formulated with fragrance, preservatives, and other agents not previously studied in this population. Because these products are liberally applied to the skin of infants, there is a risk of toxicity and sensitization.

Infant massage has many reported and theoretical benefits, including increased interaction and bonding opportunities between infants and parents, improved parental understanding of the infant's behavior, and reduced parental stress.[56] Variables studied in hospitalized premature infants include decreased motor variability and distress, and enhanced weight gain and development, leading to reduced length of stay.[57] However, an evidence-based review did not recommend this practice,[58] calling into question the methodological quality of the studies.

Interestingly, several studies have suggested that weight gain associated with infant massage may be due primarily to percutaneous absorption of essential fatty acids from the massage oil. Animal studies first documented a reversal of fatty acid deficiency in rats treated with cutaneous application of essential fatty acid (EFA)-rich safflower oil.[59] This was not reproduced in neonates treated with sunflower seed oil,[60] but subsequent studies in premature and full-term infants have shown positive effects of oil massage. Weight and length gain velocity were statistically increased in newborns receiving oil massage four times a day for the first 31 days of life, coconut oil being superior to mineral oil in these parameters.[61] Infants massaged with safflower oil had significant rises in serum essential fatty acids, including linolenic acid and arachidonic acid, whereas infants massaged with coconut oil had increases in saturated fats.[62]

Circumcision Care

Topical anesthetics that contain lidocaine or lidocaine/prilocaine mixtures are effective when used prior to circumcision,[63] and are safe if used appropriately, although systemic absorption and toxicity have been reported.[64,65] Preoperatively, the skin may be cleansed with an antiseptic (see section on Skin

Cleansing, above). Following the procedure, the antiseptic should be gently removed from the skin using a water-dampened gauze, special attention being paid to the leg creases, low back, and buttocks.[2] Bland emollients should be applied liberally to the area, either alone or in combination with a semiocclusive dressing. Antibiotic ointments, which may increase the risk of sensitization, have not been shown to be beneficial over white petrolatum in preventing infection.[66] Postoperative wound care is recommended for 3–4 days after the procedure, with gentle debridement using a water-dampened cotton swab, followed by the application of petroleum jelly or zinc oxide ointment.[67]

Diapering and Diaper Care Products

The first disposable diapers marketed in 1963, had an absorbent core of cellulose fluff. In the mid-1980s, a superabsorbent core material containing a cross-linked sodium polyacrylate was developed. This material, contained in all superabsorbent disposable diapers, transforms and holds fluid within a gel and has the capacity to absorb many times its own weight. As a result of this, pseudoanuria has been reported in an infant, because of the inability to feel moisture on a superabsorbent diaper.[68] Urine output, monitored by weighing diapers, can also be erroneous if diapers are allowed to remain open under a radiant warmer.[69]

Irritant diaper dermatitis is rare in the immediate neonatal period, but increases in incidence over the first month,[70] with overall prevalence between 4% and 15%.[71] There is a complex interplay in the occlusive diaper environment, with many components contributing to the pathogenesis of diaper dermatitis. Excessive hydration leads to maceration and increased skin permeability. Now prone to injury, the addition of alkaline urine changes the normal protective acidic pH of the skin[72] and permits the growth of microorganisms, including *Candida albicans*, *S. aureus*, and *Streptococcus*.[73] This pH also activates fecal lipases, proteases, and bile salts, which can lead to further injury.[74] Additives contained in the myriad products marketed for diaper area cleansing and rash compound the problem.

Superabsorbent diapers are clearly superior to cloth ones in preventing irritant diaper dermatitis.[75] Disposable diapers effectively reduce maceration, help create a favorable pH, decrease exposure to urine and feces, and better contain enteric pathogens.[76,77] Other contactants in the diaper area may not have such a favorable profile and can worsen the factors that lead to diaper dermatitis. Topically applied medications in the diaper area are also more readily absorbed and can lead to irritation, sensitization, and percutaneous toxicity.

The use of commercial diaper wipes and rash balms is ubiquitous in the neonatal nursery, but product selection is extremely variable and is affected more by marketing than by medicine.[25] Diaper wipes are typically used several times a day for the first 1–2 years of life, but there are only limited published reports in the medical literature evaluating tolerance of these products.[76,78,79] The conclusions of these limited studies indicate no demonstrable differences in skin condition and integrity with use of these products. One study even advocated disposable baby wipes as the 'gold standard,' as they were found to be more mild than a cotton washcloth and water.[80] In a company-sponsored trial no irritation was demonstrated in chamber scarification tests in adults using the lotion contained in high-quality wipes.[79] Most are alcohol free with the

addition of emollients, but all are laden with preservatives and fragrance that can lead to contact sensitization. Of note, there was one report of 'baby-wipe dermatitis' which was reported in nine adults who suffered from hand eczema due to preservatives in diaper wipes.[81]

Many emollients and diaper care products contain similar ingredients. Of these, a few have documented percutaneous toxicity, especially under diaper occlusion. Even now only the more infamous compounds listed in Table 5-1 are scarce in topical products. Some of these ingredients may have underappreciated toxicities, as listed in Table 5-2. Because there are no regulations that require disclosure of all inactive ingredients in over-the-counter products, only a painstaking mission can obtain this proprietary information. Regardless, it is always important to review the label and consider the toxicities of both active and inactive ingredients before applying them to the skin of an infant.

Routine care of the diaper area begins with prompt changing after soiling. Disposable diaper wipes may be used for routine cleansing. Compromised skin should be cleansed with lukewarm water and a soft cloth or mineral oil on cotton squares. The area should be patted dry. A hairdryer should not be used for this purpose as thermal burns from their use have occurred.[82] A barrier paste is recommended for prophylaxis or treatment of dermatitis. Generic, preservative-free 20% zinc oxide ointment is a safe and inexpensive agent. Powders are not recommended because of the risk of aspiration.[83] Supine diaper changes can impair heart rate and oxygen saturation in premature infants. These adverse effects can be minimized by decreasing the lifting angle to less than 30°.[84]

Ultraviolet Protection, Phototherapy, and Thermal Injury

The overall density of melanocytes in skin is greater in children than in adults, but melanin production is limited and melanocytes in children may be more susceptible to ultraviolet (UV)-induced damage.[85] In addition, infants and children have not had the gradual UV exposure that stimulates facultative pigmentation. For these reasons, pediatric patients are more susceptible to the damaging effects of excessive exposure to sunlight.

More than 500 000 new cases of skin cancer are diagnosed in the United States every year, with an increased incidence of all types of skin cancers, including melanoma. A child born in 1935 had a 1:1500 chance of developing melanoma, while a newborn now has a projected risk of 1 : 71. To help with this risk, sun protection measures are more important than ever.

A sunscreen is a compound that absorbs, reflects, or scatters the harmful spectrum of UV light (290–400 nm). An increasingly wide variety of sunscreen products are available. Ingredients that reflect and scatter a large portion of the solar spectrum, including UVB, UVA, and visible light, are zinc oxide and titanium dioxide.

The selection of an appropriate vehicle is just as important as the active ingredient. Variables include degree of water resistance, ease of application, emollient versus drying properties, and the number of potentially irritating or sensitizing additives. Adverse reactions, seen in 19% of patients, include subjective irritation, irritant contact dermatitis, allergic contact dermatitis, contact urticaria, and photosensitivity and acne formation.[86,87]

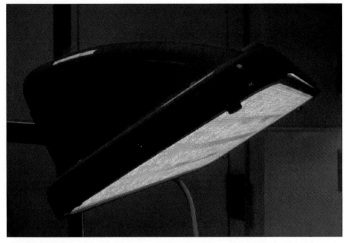

FIG. 5-1 Phototherapy light source, which can be wheeled to the bedside for treatment of infants with hyperbilirubinemia.

The safety of topically applied sunscreens has not been established for infants under 6 months of age, but the theoretical risk of toxicity is low. Concerns have focused on neonatal metabolism of p-aminobenzoic acid (PABA), a folic acid analog with structural similarities to those of the sulfonamides. The safest first-line strategy for sun protection in infants is sun avoidance, followed by the use of appropriate clothing and zinc oxide-containing sunscreens to areas which cannot be adequately covered with clothing such as the face and hands.

Phototherapy is the standard therapy for hyperbilirubinemia. Light sources vary, including fluorescent bulbs (320–700 nm, including UVA and visible light spectrum), light emission diodes (blue visible light spectrum) (Fig. 5-1), and fiberoptic halogen light sources (green visible light spectrum). Burns can occur in infants treated with phototherapy, especially if protective Plexiglas covers are not used appropriately.[88] The units should be positioned the correct distance from the infant and monitored to ensure the correct emission wavelength, so as to limit complications. The use of emollients does not increase the risk of burns during therapy,[89] although phototherapy can increase TEWL;[90] appropriate measures should therefore be taken.

Thermal burns can also occur with the use of transcutaneous CO_2 monitoring, heat lamps, heating/warming pads, heel warming techniques, and radiant warmers.[10] Caution should always be used with these devices, and the infant closely monitored for any side effects. The use of these devices should be limited or avoided if possible.

Insect Repellants

Parents, especially of infants born in the summer months, are often concerned about insect bites and arthropod-borne illness. N,N,-diethyl-m-toluamide (DEET) is the most effective topical insect repellant available. It appears to be safe in concentrations of up to 30% for use on children over 2 months of age when used according to the directions on the product labels. Concentrations greater than 30% and excessively frequent applications are associated with toxicity, including encephalopathy and seizures.[91] Oral ingestion of DEET can be fatal, therefore DEET-containing products are not recommended for infants and should be avoided.

Formulations with higher concentrations of DEET remain effective for longer periods: 10% DEET is effective for approxi-

mately 2 hours, and 24% DEET provides an average of 5 hours of protection. DEET is effective against mosquitoes, biting flies, fleas, gnats, chiggers, and ticks, but does not protect against stinging insects. DEET should be applied sparingly to exposed skin or clothing, but *not* under clothes. The effectiveness will be decreased when the child sweats or gets wet. Products that combine sunblock with DEET should not be used because sunblock needs repeated applications and DEET should be applied only once a day. DEET should not be used on young children's hands, periorificial areas, compromised skin, or near food. Two other insect repellents Picaridin (KBR 3023) and oil of lemon eucalyptns are commercially available. However, at the time of publication, the American Academy of Pediatrics had not yet commented upon the safety of these repellents in children.

Formulations containing oil of citronella are marketed as insect repellants. Citronella is less effective than DEET, with a duration of action less than 30 minutes, and so requires frequent reapplication.[92] Citronella candles and incense can reduce the number of mosquitoes in the environment. Small studies have demonstrated a mosquito-repellant efficacy comparable to that of DEET in a soybean oil extract, but with a short duration of action that requires frequent reapplication.

Permethrin is an insect repellant and insecticide that is nontoxic to humans and without systemic effects. It is approved for skin application in different concentrations to treat head lice and scabies. Permethrin is deactivated on skin within 20 minutes. It is only effective as a repellant on exterior clothing when it dries and binds to the cloth fiber. It is nonstaining, odorless, and resistant to degradation by sunlight (UV), heat, and water. When applied to clothing it remains active for 2–6 weeks even through weekly launderings.

SPECIAL ISSUES IN THE NICU

Skin Antisepsis

Skin antisepsis practices such as cord care regimens and the use of antimicrobial washes prior to invasive procedures are used to help control nursery epidemics of localized and invasive streptococcal and staphylococcal infections. Prospective, controlled comparative outcome studies on the safety and efficacy of these practices are lacking.

Common cord care practices include nonintervention ('dry cord care')[1] or the use of an antimicrobial agent. The most commonly used antiseptics are isopropyl alcohol, triple dye (brilliant green, gentian violet, and proflavine hemisulfate), povidone–iodine, bacitracin, hexachlorophene, and chlorhexidine. The data regarding control of bacterial colonization and prevention of omphalitis are conflicting.[46,93–96] Although antiseptic cord care may reduce the risk of colonization and subsequent infection, it exposes infants to potentially toxic and sensitizing agents (see Table 5-1) and delays cord separation. Important variables to consider when selecting antiseptic agents for cord care include efficacy against bacterial colonization and the potential for percutaneous toxicity. With regard to bacterial colonization, chlorhexidine has been shown to be superior to 70% ethanol,[97] hexachlorophene,[98] and povidone–iodine[99] in reducing group A streptococcus and S. aureus, but not coagulase-negative staphylococci, group B streptococci, or Gram-negative bacilli. Triple dye has been superior to bacitracin ointment,[100] hexachlorophene,[101] and isopropyl alcohol,[102] but may promote colonization with Gram-negative organisms.[103] The efficacy of any topical antimicrobial agent may diminish with prolonged use. As regards toxicity (Table 5-1), isopropyl alcohol, povidone–iodine, triple dye and hexachlorophene have been shown to have negative effects, but these have not been similarly reported with chlorhexidine.

Chlorhexidine has a broad spectrum of activity against both Gram-positive and Gram-negative bacteria and yeast. It binds strongly to the skin, which may act to reduce its absorption and increase its local efficacy.[10] A 0.5–4% aqueous chlorhexidine-containing product appears to be a safe choice for infants.[104] Several products contain chlorhexidine and isopropyl alcohol at varying concentrations, and cause irritation when impregnated on dressing materials in very low-birthweight infants.[105] Detectable increasing plasma chlorhexidine levels were documented in preterm infants treated with 1% chlorhexidine in an unspecified concentration of ethanol every 4 hours for 5–9 days.[106] Significant absorption could not be documented in a similar group of infants treated with 1% chlorhexidine in a 3% zinc oxide dusting powder, supporting the role of alcohols in facilitating percutaneous absorbtion.[106] Some commercially available formulations also contain the proprietary pluronics, fragrance, and red dye. Pluronics are added solely to enhance lathering and can cause serious corneal damage.

Povidone–iodine is a common topical antiseptic preparation. It is convenient with single-use preparations. Adverse effects of topically applied iodine have been recognized in infants for decades.[107] They include local skin necrosis, and hypothyroidism due to absorption in four infants treated with iodine-containing ointment on open wounds.[108] If povidone–iodine is used, it should be in two consecutive applications with drying for at least 30 seconds to be effective. Any residue should be thoroughly cleansed from the skin after the procedure.[2]

Alcohol is a commonly used topical antiseptic which, because of its volatility, rapidly evaporates before absorption. Generous application followed by occlusion can result in significant absorption, and can also enhance the absorption of other concomitantly applied medications, especially through immature or diseased skin. Hemorrhagic skin necrosis due to alcohol has been reported in preterm infants.[109] Additional potential toxicities include metabolic acidosis, central nervous system dysfunction, and hypoglycemia,[110] with acute intoxication reported in infants where isopropyl alcohol has been used for umbilical cord care.[111] Despite their comfortable familiarity and ready availability in single-use pads, the use of alcohol solutions is not recommended in infants as they are less effective and have more potential side effects.[2,112]

The indiscriminate use of topical antibacterial agents is not recommended.[113] Bland emollients should be used for skin injuries if there is no evidence of infection. Use of topical antimicrobial agents for prophylaxis increases the risks of bacterial resistance and contact sensitization. As they can also disrupt the normal commensal skin flora, their use should be restricted to true cutaneous infections.[114]

Hand hygiene in medical staff is also important in preventing bacterial colonization and infection in hospitalized neonates. Handwashing is a simple, inexpensive method to reduce nosocomial transmission.[10] Chlorhexidine-containing cleansers are effective, as are alcohol-based products. One study[115] showed no significant difference in microbial counts or types of organism with either regimen. In addition, the same study, which was partially supported by the manufacturer, showed that the use of mild soap combined with an alcohol-based rinse improved skin condition over the 4-week trial.[115] The application of an emollient may also improve skin condition and reduce shedding of bacteria from the hands of medical staff.[10]

Fomites can also be the source of bacteria in the NICU. This includes the stethoscopes of the medical staff,[116] which should be routinely cleansed. Toys in the microenvironment can also be a source of bacterial colonization.[117]

The potential for subclinical toxicities must be considered by everyone caring for small neonates. When several topical therapeutic options are available, the one with the greatest antimicrobial efficacy and the least potential for toxicity should be utilized. Poisindex is an extensive, frequently updated, computerized reference source for the identification of potentially toxic compounds.[118]

Adhesives

Adhesives have many applications in the NICU, but there are also underappreciated risks (Fig. 5-2). Adhesives are important for securing monitoring and life-saving equipment. They are also a primary cause of skin breakdown, with up to 90% of stratum corneum being removed after a single tape stripping from neonatal skin.[3] In addition, little is known about the potential for percutaneous toxicity or allergic sensitization from rubber or cyanoacrylate-based products. Despite the routine use of adhesives in the nursery, there are few studies identifying improved products or procedures to minimize

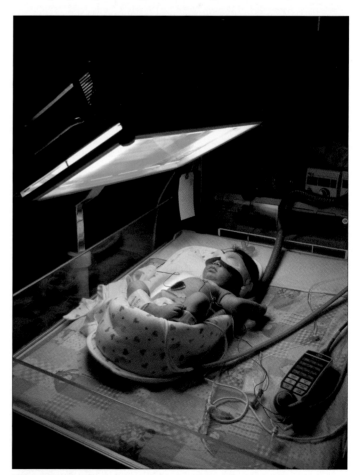

FIG. 5-2 This 27-week gestation premature infant receiving phototherapy demonstrates how many exogenous materials are applied to the skin for standard interventions.

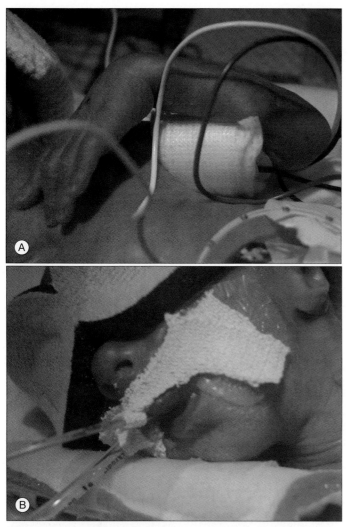

FIG. 5-3 a and b: This preterm infant demonstrates both the translucent, red quality of the skin of a very premature infant as well as some of the techniques used to minimize the effects of adhesives including securing materials with double-backed tape and soft gauze wraps.

oil or emollients are more effective, but limit the ability to reapply tape to the area if necessary. Glue solvents are helpful, but should be avoided in neonates owing to a report of toxic epidermal necrolysis after their use in a premature infant.[119]

Skin Injuries and Extravasations

The potential for skin injury is high in the NICU. Apart from adhesives, friction, heat, and extravasation are the most common causes of injury,[2] but pressure injury is uncommon. Vigilance is important to routinely assess for risk factors, and infants must be handled with great care to limit inadvertent skin trauma. Whereas interval rotation prevents pressure-induced ulceration,[120] minimizing movement can limit friction injury. Pressure injuries are most common on the occiput and ears, especially in infants receiving high-frequency oscillator ventilation or extracorporeal membrane oxygenation.[10] Products to help reduce this pressure in critically ill infants include water, air, gel and sheepskin mattresses. Gel pads for the head are also available for this purpose. Clear transparent dressings can be placed over the elbows and knees in agitated infants, and petrolatum can be applied to intertriginous areas to reduce friction and injury.[2] Tapes and wraps should be applied in a manner that allows for adequate circulation and appropriate visualization, so that the area can be assessed regularly to ensure they are not constrictive and limiting blood flow.[10]

Extravasation injuries from intravenous infusions are common in the NICU, with an incidence of 20–60%.[121] These injuries can lead to significant morbidity, including skin necrosis, infection, scarring, and contracture. Techniques to help limit these complications include prompt discontinuation of the infusion, with elevation of the affected area and removal of any locally constrictive items. The use of warm or cold packs has not been studied. Additional techniques for more severe infiltrations vary according to the clinical situation.

For infants with blanching of skin in the area of an acidic or hyperosmolar solution extravasation, a multiple puncture technique may reduce pressure and prevent necrosis.[122] Under an aseptic technique, multiple skin perforations are made with a blood drawing stylet and the fluid is gently expressed from the area. Saline-soaked gauze is then applied to the area to help encourage drainage.

Alternate techniques include saline flush-outs or liposuction.[123] Liposuction, under local or general anesthesia, utilizes a cannula inserted in the area of extravasation to remove the infiltrated fluid and subcutaneous fat. The saline flush-out technique employs an initial injection of hyaluronidase, which is an enzyme that increases the distribution and absorption of extravasated fluids and has reportedly been used safely in neonates.[121] Four stab wounds are then made at the periphery, and a cannula is used to infiltrate saline in multiple aliquots which is then massaged from the area. These methods, with certain variations, have been found to be highly effective in reducing or eliminating the side effects of intravenous infusion extravasations.

Specific antidotes are also available for certain extravasation injuries. Subcutaneous phentolamine[124] and topical nitroglycerin[125] have both been used in neonates to successfully treat dopamine infiltrations. Close monitoring of vital signs is necessary if these agents are used.

associated side effects.[10] Strategies to limit this trauma are outlined in the AWOHNN guidelines.[2] They include strictly limiting the area of adhesive application and eliminating the use of bonding agents. Attention should be paid to using smaller pieces of tape, backed with cotton or additional tape, and using alternate, nonadhesive-based products such as hydrogel electrodes. These products may, however, be less reliable in securing equipment and should not be used when secure adherence is critical.

Additional strategies to limit adhesive-related trauma include delaying the removal of newly applied adhesives for a minimum of 24 hours, securing probes and other equipment with soft gauze wraps or foam strips (Fig. 5-3), and using semipermeable pectin barriers or hydrocolloid dressings underneath adhesives when possible. Skin protectant wipes are available and coat the skin with plastic polymers to provide a barrier to adhesives, although they are not recommended in this population because of a lack of clinical studies.

Adhesives should be removed with caution. Slow, gentle peeling of the adhesive using parallel force while holding the underlying skin helps limit trauma. Folding the tape onto itself as it is removed from the skin prevents unintended injury. The use of warm water and cotton balls may be helpful. Mineral

Wound Care

Wound cleansing should be gentle and not disrupt the healing process. For superficial erosions, sterile saline can be use to cleanse the area. For deeper injuries involving the dermis, gentle irrigation with half normal saline through a catheter-tipped 20 mL syringe is effective.[2] Hydrogen peroxide and iodine have been shown to delay wound healing and should be avoided.[126]

Optimal hydration is an important parameter for rapid wound healing. Petrolatum-based emollients are semiocclusive and have been shown to facilitate healing.[127] Dressings used to aid in wound healing include transparent polyurethane films, hydrocolloids, hydrogels, foam dressings, and wound stabilizers.

Transparent polyurethane films are adhesive and semipermeable. This type of dressing can be used to secure devices and prevent friction, but should not be frequently removed and reapplied as this can lead to epidermal injury. They are best left in place until they come off on their own, and should not be used over infected wounds.

Hydrocolloid dressings are also widely used. These dressings are typically made from carbohydrate-based materials such as pectin. They are occlusive, nonabsorptive, prevent friction, and mold easily to the skin surface. They are often used in the NICU as a barrier to other more traumatic adhesives. Owing to their occlusive nature, they trap from the wound fluid rich in cytokines, which promote healing, and can be left in place for several days to limit skin stripping.

Hydrogels are also useful in the NICU setting for wound care. They are hydrophilic polymers with a high water or glycerin content. They are nonadherent, soothing, and promote epithelialization. Neonates can lie on sheets, or small pieces can be used for skin tears. The drawbacks with use of hydrogels are secondary maceration of surrounding healthy skin, rapid desiccation when used in the setting of an overhead radiant warmer, and the need for a secondary dressing if secure placement is needed. If applied to large surface areas, they should be warmed appropriately to limit temperature instability in the neonate.[126]

Mepitel (Mölnlycke Health Care Inc., Newtown, PA) is a nonadherent contact layer that acts as a wound stabilizer. It is a transparent, nonabsorptive soft mesh with a hydrophobic silicone layer that is used to protect the wound base and allow for epithelialization. It can be left in place for 7–10 days and allows for concurrent application of ointments. This dressing, and those in the Mölnlycke product line that utilize the Safetac soft silicone technology, are different from most other dressings because of the greatly reduced risk of skin stripping and resultant epidermal injuries with their use.

Foam dressings are sponge-like and nonadherent. They are made of polyurethane or cellulose and can be used to absorb exudates and reduce pressure.

Silver sulfadiazine cream is a popular wound care product, but its topical use is associated with systemic toxicity, including kernicterus and agranulocytosis.[128] More recently a case of acute renal failure was reported in an adult with high serum and urine silver levels following the use of silver sulfadiazine.[129] The cutaneous side effects also include argyria.[130] Ionic silver is known to be an antimicrobial agent with a wide spectrum of activity against Gram-positive bacteria, Gram-negative bacteria, and yeast.[131] Newer dressings using ionic silver, reportedly limit systemic silver absorption. Nevertheless, extreme care should be exercised in the use of this dressing in premature newborns, with the most cautious recommendation for avoidance until appropriate trials can be conducted in this population.

Topical antimicrobial agents, including mupirocin and bacitracin, should not be used prophylactically; instead, their use should be guided by appropriate cultures. Appropriate and limited use helps limit bacterial resistance and secondary contact sensitization.

Transepidermal Water Loss (TEWL)

TEWL is coupled with evaporative heat loss in infants. In premature infants less than 30 weeks' gestation it can be excessive, owing to their limited cutaneous barrier function. Losses range from 40 to 129 mL/kg/day,[132] and this can lead to significant fluid and electrolyte disturbances. The appropriate calculation of replacement fluids can be difficult, as measurable parameters lag behind actual losses.

Several techniques have been reported to minimize heat and water loss in neonates, but three methods have been studied and shown to be effective specifically in limiting TEWL. These include increased ambient humidity, adhesive dressings, and routine use of emollients.

Increased ambient humidity increases water vapor pressure, which inversely decreases evaporative fluid and heat loss.[133] An environment that can provide high ambient water vapor pressure, such as a double-walled incubator or servo-controlled humidification incubator (Fig. 5-4), will decrease TEWL. Lower ambient water pressure under a radiant warmer (Fig. 5-5), not

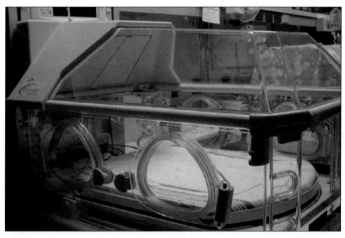

FIG. 5-4 Servo-controlled humidification and double-walled incubators have been shown to decrease TEWL by increasing ambient water vapor pressure.

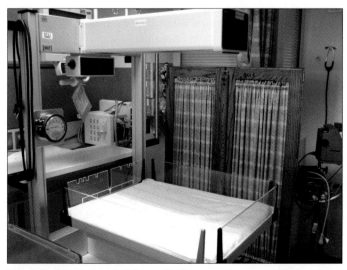

FIG. 5-5 Care in a bed with a radiant warmer increases TEWL owing to decreased ambient water vapor pressure.

irradiation, is the cause of increased TEWL in this setting.[134] Increased ambient humidity also increases the theoretical risk of bacterial contamination;[135] therefore, use of this modality should be limited to no more than 1 week.[2]

Semipermeable, transparent polyurethane dressings have been reported in two studies[136,137] to effectively decrease TEWL with no increased risk of infection, although this was not the case in a study by Donahue et al.[138] One additional study showed reduced fluid and electrolyte disturbances with decreased mortality associated with the use of this type of dressing.[139] It provides an artificial barrier until the cutaneous barrier can develop, and has been shown to reduce TEWL by up to 50%. This type of dressing, once applied, should not be removed if possible, as removal can lead to significant skin injury.[2]

Routine application of emollients has not become standard practice in NICUs owing to conflicting data regarding the associated risks and benefits. In general, bland emollients diminish TEWL, facilitate hydration of the stratum corneum, speed wound healing, and provide barrier protection against percutaneous infection.[10,140] Regular, liberal applications of bland, petrolatum-based ointments to the skin surface have also been shown to decrease TEWL,[141,142] but may also increase the risk of infection.[127,143] The effect on decreasing TEWL is greatest immediately following the application of an emollient, but diminishes over 3–6 hours. Therefore, to be effective, emollients must be applied at a minimum of every 6 hours to limit TEWL.[2]

A series of prospective studies in neonates down to 26 weeks' gestation provided evidence of improved skin integrity, decreased TEWL, and no significant change in cutaneous infections.[141,142,144] Based on these findings, many NICUs instituted topical emollient therapy for premature infants. A subsequent case–control survey documented an increased risk of systemic candidiasis in extremely low-birthweight infants treated with topical petrolatum.[127] The largest prospective, randomized, controlled multisite investigation (Vermont Oxford Network) included 1191 infants <30 weeks' gestation treated with either prophylactic generalized application of ointment twice daily or local application of ointment only to sites of injury.[143] No difference was detected in the combined primary outcome of nosocomial bacterial sepsis or death, but secondary analysis revealed an increase in nosocomial bacterial sepsis, especially with coagulase-negative staphylococcus in the ointment treated group. Therefore an evidence based review did not recommend prophylactic ointment use on a routine basis for premature infants despite improved skin condition.[89] A prospective study[145] evaluated the use of two different topical emollients in preterm Bangladeshi infants <33 weeks' gestation: 159 infants treated with sunflower seed oil and 157 infants treated with Aquaphor were compared to 181 untreated control infants. The sunflower oil group was 41% less likely to develop nosocomial infection than controls, but Aquaphor did not significantly increase or decrease the risk of infection.

Other ceramide-based emollients have recently been developed and are available over the counter. Their use has not been extensively tested in infants and children, and therefore they are not currently recommended in the neonatal population. Based on the products' ingredients, they could theoretically enhance the barrier function of the skin and decrease TEWL with a fairly low toxicity profile.

Several alternatives are used to control water loss and its accompanying thermal and fluid instability in small, prema-ture infants. Enclosed isolettes limit convective heat loss and can maintain high ambient humidity. However, this type of unit impedes easy access to patients (Fig. 5-6). In many high-risk nurseries plastic barriers are placed over infants nursed on open radiant warmers. There are limited data on the safety and efficacy of this practice. Reports have documented that blanketing an infant with a thin, pliable clear plastic wrap reduces insensible water loss.[146] In direct comparison, a plastic blanket is superior to a rigid plastic hood with regard to these parameters.[146] Many adaptations to these reported techniques are currently employed. A wide variety of products and materials are used in diverse ways. The majority of these products are not manufactured or indicated for this purpose, raising several concerns, including inconsistent composition, uncertain shelf-life, the possibility of degradation with prolonged exposure to heat, and the possibility of significant infrared absorption.

The use of transparent polyurethane coverings over radiant warmers (Fig. 5-7) has also been shown to decrease water losses and overall heat demands.[10] The majority of plastic wraps used in hospital nurseries are manufactured for food storage. Their composition varies: For example, Saran Wrap (Dow Brands, Indianapolis, IN) is polyvinylidone chloride sheeting, whereas Anchor Wrap (Anchor Packaging, Senton, MO) is a similar but not identical product of polyvinyl chlo-

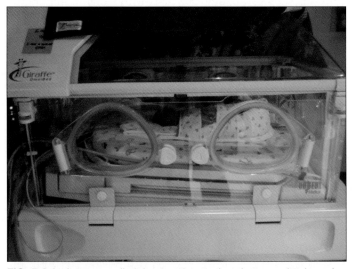

FIG. 5-6 Isolettes may limit heat and water loss but can also impede care.

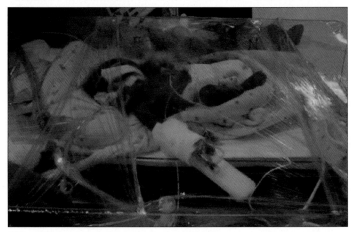

FIG. 5-7 Transparent polyurethane coverings over radiant warmers can limit water and heat loss in premature infants.

Box 5-1 Recommendations for basic skin care of the premature newborn

1. Use adhesives sparingly
- Place protective dressing at sites of frequent taping (endotracheal and nasogastric tube placement)
- Use nonadhesive electrodes and change them only when they become nonfunctional

2. Limit bathing
- Defer initial cleansing until body temperature has stabilized
- Avoid cleansing agents for the first 2 weeks
- Use warm water and moistened cotton pledgets in a humid environment
- Surface cleansing is required no more than twice a week
- If antimicrobial skin preparation is required, use short-contact chlorhexidine (except on the face)

3. Be aware of the composition and quantity of all topically applied agents
- This includes antimicrobial cleansers, diaper wipes, adhesive removers, perineal products
- Dispense from single-use containers, if possible

4. Ensure adequate intake of protein, essential fatty acids, zinc, biotin, and vitamins A, D, and B
- Be aware that erosive periorificial dermatitis is a sign of nutritional deficiency

5. Consider use of ointment emollient for xerosis or minor skin abrasions

6. Guard against excessive thermal and UV exposure
- Use thermally controlled water for bathing
- Avoid surface monitors with metal contacts
- Use Plexiglas shielding over daylight fluorescent phototherapy

7. Protect sites of cutaneous injury with the appropriate occlusive dressing
- Use a film dressing on nonexudative sites
- Use a foam dressing on exudative wounds
- Maintain appropriate hydration at the skin–dressing interface
- Remove necrotic debris with each dressing change

---

ride. The composition of other generic plastic food wraps may vary from box to box. Food wraps are specifically made for use with cold storage and have not been tested for stability after prolonged heating.

In some nurseries plastic 'bubble wrap' is used as a thermal blanket. This practice was introduced in 1971.[147] Two studies have documented its effectiveness when used in the delivery room for infants born at <28 weeks' gestation. This practice has been shown to increase not only heat but also survival.[148,149] Plastic bubble wrap is generically manufactured and distributed as packing material; its composition is variable and difficult to identify reliably. A plastic that is opaque to infrared will acutely block heat transmission when used in the setting of an overhead infrared source. Plastics that retain heat have the potential to burn contacted skin.[150]

Clearly, the use of these techniques to control thermal and fluid losses in small premature infants deserves further study.

There is currently no 'best practice' defined for these parameters, the various methods never having been directly compared to one another to fully assess outcomes.

SUMMARY

Increased understanding of the mechanisms that contribute to skin development may one day provide therapy to accelerate barrier maturation in very premature infants. Prolonged maintenance in a fluid environment would be an alternate approach. Until that time, therapy should be directed towards providing a safe, temporary barrier and minimizing additional skin injury while allowing easy access to and handling of infants (Box 5-1). A well-defined and uniformly accepted standard of care for the skin of premature infants has been established and should be adopted by all hospital personnel.[3,5]

REFERENCES

1. Lund C, Kuller J, Lane A, et al. Neonatal skin care: the scientific basis for practice. J Obstet Gynecol Neonatal Nurs 1999; 28: 241–254.
2. Association of Women's Health, Obstetric and Neonatal Nurses. Evidence-based clinical practice guideline: neonatal skin care. Washington, DC: 2001.
3. Lund CH, Kueller J, Lane AT, et al. Neonatal skin care: evaluation of the AWHONN/NANN research-based practice project on knowledge and skin care practices. J Obstet Gynecol Neonatal Nurs 2001; 30: 30–40.
4. Lund CH, Osborne JW, Kuller J, et al. Neonatal skin care: clinical outcomes of the AWHONN/NANN evidence-based clinical practice guideline. J Obstet Gynecol Neonatal Nurs 2001; 30: 41–51.
5. Kalia YN, Nonato LB, Lund CH, et al. Development of skin barrier function in premature infants. J Invest Dermatol 1998; 111: 320–326.
6. Eady R, Holbrook K. Structure and function: skin development. In: Schachner LA, Hansen RC, eds. Pediatric dermatology, 3rd edn, Philadelphia, PA: 2003;3–13.
7. Holbrook KA. Structure and function of the developing human skin. In: Goldsmith LA, ed. Physiology, biochemistry and molecular biology of the skin. New York: Oxford University Press, 1991; 63–110.
8. Brion L, Fleischman AR, Schwartz GJ. Evaluation of four length–weight formulas for estimating body surface area in newborn infants. J Pediatr 1985; 107: 801–803.
9. Rutter N. The immature skin. Eur J Pediatr 1996; 155: S18–20.
10. Darmstadt GL, Dinulos JG. Neonatal skin care. Pediatr Clinic North Am 2000; 47: 757–782.
11. Fox C, Nelson D, Wareham J. The timing of skin acidification in very low birth weight infants. J Perinatol 1998; 18: 272–275.
12. Rutter N. Percutaneous drug absorption in the newborn: hazards and uses. Clin Perinatol 1987; 14: 911–930.
13. Plantin P, Jouan N, Karangwa A, et al. Variations of the skin permeability in premature newborn infants. Value of the skin vasoconstriction test with neosynephrine. Arch Franç Pédiatr 1992; 49: 623–625.
14. Cartwright RG, Cartlidge PH, Rutter N, et al. Transdermal delivery of theophylline to premature infants using a hydrogel disc system. Br J Clin Pharmacol 1990; 29: 533–539.
15. Barrett DA, Rutter N, Davis SS. An in vitro study of diamorphine permeation through premature human neonatal skin. Pharmacol Res 1993; 10: 583–587.
16. Cartlidge PH, Rutter N. Percutaneous respiration in the newborn infant. Effect of ambient oxygen concentration on pulmonary oxygen uptake. Biol Neonate 1988; 54: 68–72.

17. Cartlidge PH, Rutter N. Percutaneous oxygen delivery to the preterm infant. Lancet 1988; 1: 315–317.

18. Kearns GL, Abdel-Rahman SM, Alander SW, et al. Developmental pharmacology – drug disposition, action and therapy in infants and children. N Engl J Med 2003; 349: 1157–1168.

19. West DP, Worobec S, Solomon LM. Pharmacology and toxicology of infant skin. J Invest Dermatol 1981; 76: 147–150.

20. Blumer JL. The therapeutic orphan – 30 years later. A joint conference of the Pediatric Pharmacology Research Unit Network, the European Society of Developmental Pharmacology, and the National Institute of Child Health and Human Development held in Washington, DC, 2 May 1997. Pediatrics 1997; 104: 581–645.

21. Cooke JV. Dermatitis of the diaper region in infants (Jacquet dermatitis). Arch Dermatol Syphillol 1926; 14: 539–546.

22. Micali G, Lacarrubba F, Bongu A, et al. The skin barrier. In: Freinkel RK, Woodley DT, eds. The biology of the skin. New York: Taylor & Francis, 2001; 219–231.

23. Orchard D, Weston WL. The importance of vehicle in pediatric topical therapy. Pediatr Ann 2001; 30: 208–210.

24. Siegfried EC. Neonatal skin and skin care. Dermatol Clin 1998; 16: 437–446.

25. Siegfried EC, Shah PY. Skin care practices in the neonatal nursery: a clinical survey. J Perinatol 1999; 19: 31–39.

26. Munson KA, Bare DE, Hoath SB, et al. A survey of skin care practices for premature low birth weight infants. Neonatal Netw 1999; 18: 25–31.

27. Baker SF, Smith BJ, Donohue PK, et al. Skin care management practices for premature infants. J Perinatol 1999; 19: 426–431.

28. Lund CH, Osborne JW. Validity and reliability of the neonatal skin condition score. J Obstet Gynecol Neonatal Nurs 2004; 33: 320–327.

29. Walker L, Downe S, Gomez L. Skin care in the well term newborn: two systematic reviews. Birth 2005; 32: 224–228.

30. Anon. Postpartum care of the mother and newborn: a practical guide. Technical Working Group, World Health Organization. Birth 1999; 26: 255–258.

31. Chalmers B, Mangiaterra V, Porter R. WHO principles of perinatal care: the essential antenatal, perinatal, and postpartum care course. Birth 2001; 28: 202–207.

32. Lin RL, Tinkle LL, Janniger CK. Skin care of the healthy newborn. Cutis 2005; 75: 25–30.

33. Cetta F, Lambert GH, Ros SP. Newborn chemical exposure from over-the-counter skin care products. Clin Pediatr 1991; 30: 286–289.

34. Gelmetti C. Skin cleansing in children. Eur Acad Dermatol Venereol 2001; 15(Suppl 1): 12–15.

35. Peters KL. Bathing premature infants: physiological and behavioural consequences. Am J Crit Care 1998; 7: 90–100.

36. Henningsson A, Nystrom B, Tunnel R. Bathing or washing babies after birth? Lancet 1981; 26: 1401–1403.

37. Als H, Lawhon G, Brown E, et al. Individualized behavioural and environmental care for the very low birth weight preterm infant at high risk for bronchopulmonary dysplasia: neonatal intensive care unit and developmental outcomes. Pediatrics 1986; 78: 1123–1132.

38. Kanda K, Tochihara Y, Ohnaka T. Bathing before sleep in the young and in the elderly. Eur J Appl Physiol Occup Physiol 1999; 80: 71–75.

39. Nako Y, Harigaya A, Tomomasa T, et al. Effects of bathing immediately after birth on early neonatal adaptation and morbidity: a prospective randomized comparative study. Pediatr Int 2000; 42: 517–522.

40. Mirowski GW, Frieden IJ, Miller C. Iatrogenic scald burn: a consequence of institutional infection control measures. Pediatrics 1996; 98: 963–965.

41. Joglekar VM. Barrier properties of vernix caseosa. Arch Dis Child 1980; 55: 817–819.

42. Yoshio H, Tollin M, Gudmundsson GH, et al. Antimicrobial polypeptides of human vernix caseosa and amniotic fluid; implications for newborn innate defense. Pediatr Res 2003; 53: 211–216.

43. Hoath SB. The stickiness of newborn skin: bioadhesion and the epidermal barrier. J Pediatr 1997; 131: 338–340.

44. Tollin M, Bergsson G, Kai-Larsen Y, et al. Vernix caseosa as a multi-component defence system based on polypeptides, lipids and their interactions. Cell Mol Life Sci. 2005; 62: 2390–2399.

45. Morelli JC, Weston WL. Soaps and shampoos in pediatric practice. Pediatrics 1987; 80: 634–637.

46. Simon NP, Simon MW. Changes in newborn bathing practices may increase the risk of omphalitis. Clin Pediatr (Phil) 2004; 43: 763–767.

47. Heggers JP, Sazy JA, Stenberg BD, et al. Bactericidal and wound-healing properties of sodium hypochlorite solutions: the 1991 Lindberg Award. J Burn Care Rehab 1991; 12: 420–424.

48. Hostynek JJ, Wilhelm KP, Cua AB, Maibach HI. Irritation factors of sodium hypochlorite solutions in human skin. Contact Dermatitis. 1990; 23: 316–324.

49. Janniger CK, Bryngil JM. Hair in infancy and childhood. Cutis 1993; 51: 336–338.

50. Bree A, Siegfried EC. General principles of skin care in children. In: Schachner LA, Hansen RC, eds. Pediatric dermatology, 3rd edn. Philadelphia, PA: Elsevier Health Sciences, 2003: 93.

51. Jiggins M, Talbot J. Mouth care in PICU. Paediatr Nurs 2000; 11: 23–26.

52. O'Reilly M. Oral care of the critically ill: a review of the literature and guidelines for practice. Aust Crit Care. 2003; 16: 101–110.

53. Moolenaar RL, Crutcher JM, SanJoaquin VH, et al. A prolonged outbreak of Pseudomonas aeruginosa in a neonatal intensive care unit: did staff fingernails play a role in disease transmission? Infect Control Hosp Epidemiol 2000; 21: 80–85.

54. Anonymous. Fingernail bacteria linked to infant infection, death. Rep Med Guidel Outcomes Res 2000; 11: 5.

55. Manzini BM, Ferdani G, Simonetti V, et al. Contact sensitization in children. Pediatr Dermatol 1998; 15: 12–17.

55a. Mancini BM. Contact sensitization in children. Pediatr Dermatol 1998; 15: 12–17.

56. Beyer K, Strauss L. Infant massage programs may assist in decreasing parental perceived stress levels in new parents. Occup Ther 2002; 16: 53–68.

57. Modrcin-Talbott MA, Harrison LL, Groer M, et al. The biobehavioral effects of gentle human touch on preterm infants. Nur Sci Q 2003; 16: 60–67.

58. Vickers A, Ohlsson A, Jacy JB, et al. Massage for promoting growth and development of preterm and/or low birth-weight infants. Cochrane Database Syst Rev 2004; 2: CD000390.

59. Bohles H, Bieber MA, Heird WC. Reversal of experimental essential fatty acid deficiency by cutaneous administration of safflower oil. Am J Clin Nutr 1976; 29: 398–401.

60. Hunt CE, Engel RR, Modler S, et al. Essential fatty acid deficiency in neonates: inability to reverse deficiency by topical applications of EFA-rich oil. J Pediatr 1978; 92: 603–607.

61. Sankaranarayanan K, Mondkar JA, Chauhan MM, et al. Oil massage in neonates: an open randomized controlled study of coconut versus mineral oil. Ind Pediatr 2005; 42: 877–884.

62. Solanki K, Matnani M, Kale M, et al. Transcutaneous absorption of topically massaged oil in neonates. Ind Pediatr 2005; 42: 998–1005.

63. Taddio A. Pain management for neonatal circumcision. Paediatr Drugs 2001; 3: 101–111.

64. Rincon E, Baker RL, Iglesisa AJ, et al. CNS toxicity after topical application of EMLA cream on a toddler with molluscum contagiosum. Pediatr Emerg Care 2000; 16: 252–254.

65. Frayling IM, Addison GM, Chattergee K, et al. Methaemoglobinaemia in children treated with prilocaine–

lignocaine cream. Br Med J 1990; 301: 153–154.

66. Smack DP, Harrington AC, Dunn C, et al. Infection and allergy incidence in ambulatory surgery patients using white petrolatum vs. bacitracin ointment. A randomized controlled trial. JAMA 1996; 276: 972–977.

67. Gelbaum I. Circumcision; refining a traditional surgical technique. J Nurs Midwife 1993; 38: 18S–20S.

68. Barada JH. Pseudoanuria due to superabsorbent diapers. N Engl J Med 1991; 325: 892–893.

69. Hermansen MC, Buches M. Urine output determination from superabsorbent and regular diapers under radiant heat. Pediatrics 1988; 81: 428–431.

70. Visscher MO, Chatterjee R, Muson KA, et al. Development of diaper rash in the newborn. Pediatr Dermatol 2000; 17: 52–57.

71. Kazaks EL, Lane AT. Diaper dermatitis. Pediatr Clin North Am 2000; 47: 909–919.

72. Berg RW, Buckingham KW, Stewart RL. Etiologic factors in diaper dermatitis: the role of urine. Pediatr Dermatol 1986; 3: 102–106.

73. Ferrazzini G, Kaiserr RR, Hirsig Cheng SK, et al. Microbiological aspects of diaper dermatitis. Dermatology 2003; 206: 136–141.

74. Buckingham KE, Berg RW. Etiologic factors in diaper dermatitis: the role of feces. Pediatr Dermatol 1986; 3: 107–112.

75. Lane A, Rehder P, Helm K. Evaluation of diapers containing absorbent gelling material with conventional disposable diapers in newborn infants. Am J Dis Child 1990; 144: 315–318.

76. Odio M, Friedlander ST. Diaper dermatitis and advances in diaper technology. Curr Opin Pediatr 2000; 12: 342–346.

77. Wong DL, Brantley D, Clutter L, et al. Diapering choices: a critical review of the issues. Pediatr Nurs 1992; 18: 41–52.

78. Priestley GC, McVittie E, Aldridge RD. Changes in skin pH after the use of baby wipes. Pediatr Dermatol 1996; 13: 14–17.

79. Ehretsmann C, Schaefer R, Adam R. Cutaneous tolerance of baby wipes by infants with atopic dermatitis, and comparison of the mildness of baby wipe and water on infant skin. J Eur Acad Dermatol Venereol 2001; 15: 16–20.

80. Odio M, Streicher-Scott J, Hansen RC. Disposable baby wipes: efficacy and skin mildness. Dermatol Nurs 2001; 13: 107–112, 117–118, 121.

81. Guin JD, Kincannon J, Church FL. Baby-wipe dermatitis: preservative-induced hand eczema in parents and persons using moist towelettes. Am J Contact Dermatol 2001; 12: 189–192.

82. Deans L, Slater H, Goldfarb IW. Bad advice; bad burn; a new problem in burn prevention. J Burn Care Rehab 1990; 11: 563–564.

83. Silver P, Sagy M, Rubin L. Respiratory failure from corn starch aspiration: a hazard of diaper changing. Pediatr Emerg Care 1996; 12: 108–110.

84. Yung-Weng W, Ying-Ju C. A preliminary study of bottom care effects on premature infants' heart rate and oxygen saturation. J Nurs Res 2004; 12: 161–168.

85. Mancini AJ. Skin. Pediatrics 2004; 113: 1114–1119.

86. Foley P, Nixon R, Marks R, et al. The frequency of reactions to sunscreens: results of a longitudinal population-based study on the regular use of sunscreens in Australia. Br J Dermatol 1993; 128: 512–518.

87. Schauder S, Ippen H. Contact and photocontact sensitivity to sunscreens. Review of a 15-year experience and of the literature. Contact Dermatol 1997; 37: 221–232.

88. Siegfried EC, Stone MS, Madison KC. Ultraviolet light burn: a cutaneous complication of visible light phototherapy of neonatal jaundice. Pediatr Dermatol 1992; 9: 278–282.

89. Conner JM, Soll RF, Edwards WH. Topical ointment for preventing infection in preterm infants. Cochrane Database Systemic Review 2004; 1: CD001150.

90. Maayan-Metzger A, Yosipovitch G, Haded E, et al. Transepidermal water loss and skin hydration in preterm infants during phototherapy. Am J Perinatol 2001; 18: 393–396.

91. Lipscomb J, Kramer J, Leikin J. Seizure following brief exposure to the insect repellent N,N-diethyl-m-toluamide. Ann Emerg Med 1992; 21: 315.

92. Magnon G, Kline D, Roberts L, et al. Repellency of two DEET formulations and Avon Skin-So-Soft against biting midges (Diptera: Ceratopogonide) in Honduras. J Am Mosquito Control Assoc 1991; 7: 80.

93. Janssen PA, Selwood BL, Dobson SR. To dye or not to dye: a randomized, clinical trial of a triple dye/alcohol regime versus dry cord care. Pediatrics. 2003; 111: 15–20.

94. Medves JM, O'Brien BA. Cleaning solutions and bacterial colonization in promoting healing and early separation of the umbilical cord in healthy newborns. Can J Pub Health 1997; 88: 380–382.

95. Dore S, Buchan D, Coulas S, et al. Alcohol versus natural drying for newborn cord care. J Obstet Gynecol Neonatal Nurs 1998; 27: 621–627.

96. Evens K, George J, Angst D, et al. Does umbilical cord care in preterm infants influence cord bacterial colonization or detachment? J Perinatol 2004; 24: 100–104.

97. Belfrage E, Enocksson E, Kalin M, et al. Comparative efficiency of chlorhexidine and ethanol in umbilical cord care. Scand J Infect Dis 1985; 17: 413.

98. Verber IG, Pagan FS. What cord care – if any? Arch Dis Child 1993; 68: 594.

99. Smales O. A comparison of umbilical cord treatment in the control of superficial infection. NZ Med J 1988; 101: 453.

100. Andrich MP, Golden SM. Umbilical cord care: a study of bacitracin ointment vs triple dye. Clin Pediatr 1984; 23: 342–342.

101. Wald ER, Snyder MJ, Gutberlet RL. Group beta-hemolytic streptococcal colonization. Acquisition, persistence and effect of umbilical cord treatment with triple dye. Am J Dis Child 1977; 131: 178.

102. Paes B, Jones CC. An audit of the effect of two cord-care regimens on bacterial colonization in newborn infants. Qual Rev Bull 1987; 13: 109–113.

103. Speck W, Driscoll J, O'Neil J, et al. Effect of antiseptic cord care on bacterial colonization in the newborn infant. Chemother 1980; 26: 372–376.

104. Garland JS, Buck RK, Maloney P, et al. Comparison of 10% povidone–iodine and 0.5% chlorhexidine gluconate for the prevention of peripheral intravenous catheter colonization in neonates: a prospective trial. Pediatr Infect Dis J 1995; 14: 510–516.

105. Garland JS, Alex CP, Mueller CD, et al. Local reactions to a chlorhexidine gluconate-impregnated antimicrobial dressing in very low birth weight infants. Pediatr Infect Dis J 1996; 15: 912–914.

106. Aggett PJ, Cooper LV, Ellis SH, et al. Percutaneous absorption of chlorhexidine in neonatal cord care. Arch Dis Child 1981; 56z: 878–880.

107. Pyati SP, Ramamurthy RS, Krauss MT, et al. Absorption of iodine in the neonate following topical use of povidone iodine. J Pediatr 1977; 91: 825–828.

108. Barakat M, Carson D, Hetherton AM, et al. Hypothyroidism secondary to topical iodine treatment in infants with spina bifida. Acta Paediatr 1994; 83: 741–743.

109. Harpin VA, Rutter N. Percutaneous alcohol absorption and skin necrosis in a preterm infant. Arch Dis Child 1982; 57: 477–479.

110. Howard R. The appropriate use of topical antimicrobials and antiseptics in children. Pediatr Ann 2001; 30: 219–224.

111. Dalt LD, DallAmico R, Laverda AM, et al. Percutaneous ethyl alcohol intoxication in a one-month-old infant. Pediatr Emerg Care 1991; 7: 343–344.

112. Maki DG, Ringer M, Alvarado CJ. Prospective randomised trial of povidone–iodine, alcohol, and chlorhexidine for prevention of infection associated with central venous and arterial catheters. Lancet 1991; 338: 339–343.

113. Light IJ, Sutherland JM. Effect of topical antibacterial agents on the acquisition of bacteria by newborn

infants. Antimicrob Agents Chemother 1968; 8: 274–278.

114. Davies J, Babb JR, Ayliff GA. The effect on the skin flora of bathing with antiseptic solutions. J Antimicrob Chemother 1977; 3: 473–481.

115. Larson E, Silberger M, Jakob K, et al. Assessment of alternative hand hygiene regimens to improved skin health among neonatal intensive care unit nurses. Heart Lung 2000; 29: 136–142.

116. Marinella MA, Pierson C, Chenoweth C. The stethoscope. A potential source of nosocomial infection? Arch Intern Med 1997; 157: 786–790.

117. Hanrahan KS, Lofgren M. Evidence-based practice: examining the risk of toys in the microenvironment of infants in the neonatal intensive care unit. Adv Neonatal Care 2004; 4: 184–201.

118. Poisindex: http://www.micromedex.com/products/poisindex/

119. Ittman PI, Bozynski ME. Toxic epidermal necrolysis in a newborn infant after exposure to adhesive remover. J Perinatol 1993; 13: 476–477.

120. Eichenfield L, Larralde M. Neonatal skin and skin disorders. In: Schachner LA, Hansen RC, eds. Pediatric dermatology, 3rd edn. Philadelphia, PA: 2003; 261–262.

121. Ramasethu J. Prevention and management of extravasation injuries in neonates. NeoReview 2004; 5: e491–497.

122. Chandavasu O, Garrow E, Valda V, et al. A new method for the prevention of skin sloughs and necrosis secondary to intravenous infiltrations. Am J Perinatol 1986; 3: 4–5.

123. Gault DT. Extravasation injuries. Br J Plast Surg 1993; 46: 91–96.

124. Subhani M, Sridhar S, DeCristofaro JD. Phentolamine use in a neonate for the prevention of dermal necrosis caused by dopamine: a case report. J Perinatol 2001; 21: 324–326.

125. Wong AF, McCulloch LMM, Sola A. Treatment of peripheral tissue ischemia with topical nitroglycerin ointment in neonates. J Pediatr 1992; 121: 980–983.

126. Taquino LT. Promoting wound healing in the neonatal setting: process vs. protocol. J Perinat Neonatal Nurs 2000; 14: 104–118.

127. Campbell JR, Zaccaria E, Baker CJ. Systemic candidiasis in extremely low birth weight infants receiving topical petrolatum ointment for skin care: a case–control study. Pediatrics 2000; 105: 1041–1045.

128. Viala J, Simon L, LePommelet C. Agranulocytosis after application of silver sulfadiazine in a 2-month old infant. Arch Pediatr 1997; 4: 1103–1106.

129. Chaby G, Viseux V, Poulain JF, et al. Topical silver sulfadiaxine-induced acute renal failure. Ann Dermatol Venereol 2005; 132: 891–893.

130. Payne CM, Bladin C, Colchester AC, et al. Argyria from excessive use of topical silver sulphadiazine. Lancet 1992; 340: 126.

131. Russel AD, Hugo WB. Antimicrobial activity and action of silver. Prog Med Chem 1994; 31: 351–370.

132. Sedin G, Hammarlund K, Nilsson GE, et al. Measurement of transepidermal water loss in newborn infants. Clin Perinatol 1985; 12: 79–99.

133. Hammarlund K, Nilesson GE, Oberg PA, et al. Transepidermal water loss in newborn infants. Acta Paediatr Scand 1977; 66: 553–562.

134. Kjartansson S, Arsan S, Hammarlund K, et al. Water loss from the skin of term and preterm infants nursed under a radiant warmer. Pediatr Res 1995; 37: 233–238.

135. Harpin VA, Rutter N. Humidification of incubators. Arch Dis Child 1985; 60: 219–224.

136. Knauth A, Gordin M, McNelis W, et al. Semipermeable polyurethane membrane as an artificial skin for the premature neonate. Pediatrics 1989; 83: 945–950.

137. Vernon HJ, Lane AT, Wischerath LJ, et al. Semipermeable dressing and transepidermal water loss in premature infants. Pediatrics 1990; 86: 357–362.

138. Donahue ML, Phelps DL, Richter SE, et al. A semipermeable skin dressing for extremely low birth weight infants. J Perinatol 1996; 16: 20–26.

139. Bhandari V, Brodsky N, Porat R. Improved outcome of extremely low birth weight infants with Tegaderm application to skin. J Perinatol 2005; 25: 276–281.

140. Ghadially R, Halkier-Sorensen L, Elias PM. Effects of petrolatum on stratum corneum structure and function. J Am Acad Dermatol 1992; 26: 387–396.

141. Lane AT, Drost SS. Effects of repeated application of emollient cream to premature neonates' skin. Pediatrics 1993; 92: 415–419.

142. Nopper AJ, Horii KA, Sookdeo-Drost S, et al. Topical ointment therapy benefits premature infants. J Pediatr 1996; 128: 660–669.

143. Edwards WH, Conner JM, Sol RF, for the Vermont Oxford Network Neonatal Skin Care Study Group. The effect of prophylactic ointment therapy on nosocomial sepsis rates and skin integrity in infants with birth weights of 501–1000 g. Pediatrics 2004; 113: 1195–1203.

144. Pabst RC, Starr KP, Qaiyumi S, et al. The effects of application of Aquaphor on skin condition, fluid requirements and bacterial colonization in very low birth weight infants. J Perinatal 1999; 19: 278–283.

145. Darmstadt GL, Saha SK, Nawshad Uddin Ahmed ASM. Effect of topical treatment with skin barrier-enhancing emollients on nosocomial infection in preterm infants in Bangladesh: a randomised controlled trial. Lancet 2005; 365: 1039–1045.

146. Baumgart S. Reduction of oxygen consumption, insensible water loss and radiant heat demand with use of a plastic blanket for low-birth-weight infants under radiant warmers. Pediatrics 1984; 74: 1022–1028.

147. Besch NJ, Perlstein PH, Edwards NK, et al. The transparent baby bag: a shield against heat loss. N Engl J Med 1971; 284: 121–124.

148. Narendran V, Hoath SB. Thermal management of the low birth weight infant: a cornerstone of neonatology. J Pediatr 199; 134: 529–531.

149. Vohra S, Frent G, Campbell V, et al. Effect of polyethylene occlusive skin wrapping on heat loss in very low birth weight infants at delivery: a randomized trial. J Pediatr 1999; 134: 547–551.

150. LeBlanc MH. Thermoregulation: Incubators, radiant warmers, artificial skins, and body hoods. Clin Perinatol 1991; 18: 403–422.

151. Gelman CR, Rumack BH, Hess AJ. Benzocaine. Englewood, CA: Micromedex, 1996.

152. Hoeck HC, Laurberg G, Laurberg P. Hypercalcemic crisis after excessive topical use of a vitamin D derivative. J Intern Med 1994; 235: 281–282.

153. Raimer SS. The safe use of topical corticosteroids in children. Pediatr Ann 2001; 30: 225–229.

154. Reilly JF Jr, Weisse ME. Topically induced diphenhydramine toxicity. J Emerg Med 1990; 8: 59–61.

155. Franz TJ, Lehman PA, Franz SF, et al. Comparative percutaneous absorption of lindane and permethrin. Arch Dermatol 1996; 132: 901–905.

156. Dinehart SM, Dillard R, Raimer SS, et al. Cutaneous manifestations of acrodynia (pink disease). Arch Dermatol 1988; 124: 107–109.

157. Porat R, Gilbert S, Magilner D. Methylene blue-induced phototoxicity: An unrecognized complication. Pediatrics 1996; 97: 717–721.

158. Abidel-Magid EHM, El Awad Ahmed FR. Salicylate intoxication in an infant with ichthyosis transmitted through skin ointment. Pediatrics 1994; 94: 939–940.

159. Allen A, Siegfried E, Silverman R, et al. Significant absorption of topical tacrolimus in 3 patients with Netherton syndrome. Arch Dermatol 2001; 137: 747–750.

160. Anonymous. High plasma urea concentrations in collodion babies. Arch Dis Child 1987; 62: 212.

6

Diagnostic and Therapeutic Procedures

Bari B. Cunningham, Annette M. Wagner

Diagnostic and therapeutic procedures play an important role in the field of neonatal dermatology. Suspected diagnoses can often be rapidly confirmed by simple office-based procedures such as potassium hydroxide (KOH) preparation, Tzanck smears, hair mounts, or scabies preparations. Laboratory tests such as Gram-stained smears, skin cultures, and direct fluorescent antibody testing can identify pathogenic organisms that enable directed therapy. Skin biopsy can provide invaluable information when histopathologic examination is appropriately combined with special stains, immunofluorescence, polymerase chain reactions (PCRs), immunohistochemistry, or electron microscopy.

Performing procedures in neonates can be technically challenging and requires careful attention to pediatric issues such as increased toxicity of anesthetic agents. Special dressings and postoperative wound instructions are often necessary to avert complications following procedures.

Many genetic skin diseases can be diagnosed prenatally with the aid of specific genetic and metabolic tests, such as PCR or fluorescence in situ hybridization (FISH). Specific gene analysis by DNA sequencing may be helpful in the diagnosis of many congenital dermatologic diseases.

This chapter reviews common diagnostic and therapeutic procedures in neonatal dermatology and provides a 'How To' guide for the practitioner. Appropriate use of diagnostic testing and the current status of genetic, metabolic, and prenatal diagnosis are discussed. In anticipation of rapid advances in these areas, referral sources for up-to-date information in these fields are provided.

SPECIFIC DIAGNOSTIC PROCEDURES

Potassium Hydroxide Preparation and Fungal Cultures

Potassium hydroxide (KOH) examination of skin, hair, and nails for suspected fungal infection is one of the most commonly used diagnostic procedures in dermatology. Adequate specimen collection is critical and varies by anatomic site.

Skin scrapings for KOH preparation and fungal culture should be collected from the margins of the lesions because this is the area of active growth of the fungus. Some authors recommend cleansing the skin with alcohol before scraping to reduce bacterial contamination.[1] Unfortunately, this removes much of the scale, making the collection of adequate material difficult. The use of antibacterial agents in the fungal culture medium is preferable for preventing bacterial overgrowth of cultures.

Collection of skin scrapings is accomplished using a #15 scalpel blade, the edge of a glass microscopic slide, or a foman blade.[2] The foman blade, a two-sided, spatula-like instrument, is less likely to inadvertently cut the skin of a moving infant. An adequate specimen should be collected so that if the KOH preparation is equivocal, a fungal culture can be performed without repeating the collection procedure.[3] If blisters are present, use a curved iris scissors to remove the roof of the blister for examination. The KOH preparation technique is outlined in Box 6-1. Hyphae should be differentiated from cell walls, fabric fibers, and small hairs (Fig. 6-1). Cell walls have an irregular linearity; threads appear uniform and lack internal structures. Ink-containing KOH preparations (Swartz–Lamkin) are available to enhance the hyphae and increase the yield of positive examinations.

Scalp scrapings can be obtained in a similar manner. If culture material is needed, a toothbrush, a gynecologic viral collection brush, or a wet cotton-tipped applicator can be rubbed against the scalp surface and placed in the collection

---

Box 6-1 KOH preparation technique

1. Select an area of the lesion – the margin is recommended.
2. Using a #15 blade, the edge of a microscopic slide, or a foman blade, scrape gently across the edge of the scaling skin plaque using the motion of a knife spreading butter on bread.
3. Gently drop the skin scrapings onto a glass slide by tapping the edge of the blade against the glass. Material may be swept into a pile using the blade or cover slip, and a cover slip applied.
4. Apply a few drops of 10–20% KOH to the edge of the cover slip, and apply gentle pressure to the surface to flatten the scales.
5. Rack down the substage condenser and put the light on low.
6. Scan and focus the smear on 4–100× objectives, scanning the material at low power until suspicious areas are identified and then switching to higher power to confirm the diagnosis.

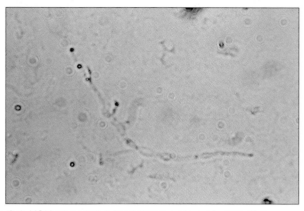

FIG. 6-1 KOH preparation for detection of yeast ×100. Note pseudohyphae.

container or directly on the culture medium.[4] Hair samples from the scalp can be examined directly for the presence of fungus. Often, scraping with the blade is sufficient to retrieve enough hairs for a KOH preparation or culture without the trauma of 'pulling.'

Collection of fungal samples from nails is particularly challenging. A 2 or 3 mm skin curette may be used to scrape out subungual debris, which may be more accessible when the nail is trimmed. Alternatively, a #15 blade can be directed away from the digit toward the underside of the nail to dislodge material. If the suspected infection is on the nail surface, the blade should be used to gently scrape the superficial surface of the nail plate.

Mycosel agar and Mycobiotic agar are commonly used fungal culture media composed of Sabouraud dextrose agar containing chloramphenicol and cyclohexamide to reduce bacterial overgrowth. Dermatophyte test medium (DTM) is a simplified culture system for the detection of dermatophytes. When the culture is positive, dye in the medium turns red. Certain non-dermatophytes, such as *Aspergillus* spp. can also turn the medium red, so colony morphology should also be evaluated. For most fungi, inoculated media can be kept at room temperature. The bottle caps should be kept loose to allow air into the culture bottle. Some diphasic fungi, such as *Cryptococcus* spp., grow poorly at room temperature and should be incubated at 37°C.

For deep fungus, a skin biopsy must be performed. The collected tissue is ground into minute pieces and inoculated onto the culture medium and/or stained for microscopic examination.

The yield of fungal culture is lowest for nails. This can be particularly problematic when distinction between psoriatic and fungal nails is necessary, but is not a major clinical issue in neonates or young infants. Distal nail clippings can be submitted for routine histology and periodic acid–Schiff staining to look for microscopic evidence of fungus.[5] The yield of this procedure has been demonstrated to be superior to KOH preparation and equal to that of fungal culture.

Bacterial Cultures and Stains

Normal skin is colonized with a variety of bacteria. Pathogenic bacteria must be identified and distinguished from 'normal' flora to enable appropriate medical therapy of primary or secondary skin infection. A Gram-stained smear of material from lesions suspected of bacterial infection can allow for prelimi-

nary identification of the infecting organism and provide a guide to appropriate therapy. The presence of polymorphonuclear leukocytes, together with large numbers of bacteria, usually indicates infection.

Cultured skin specimens should be plated on blood agar and inoculated into a thioglycollate (anaerobic) broth. If infection with Gram-negative rods is suspected, MacConkey or EMB agar plates should be inoculated. Suspected meningococcal and gonococcal infections should be plated on Thayer–Martin or chocolate agar plates in a CO_2 atmosphere. Anaerobic cultures for suspected anaerobic streptococcus, *Bacteroides*, and *Clostridium* should be plated on blood agar.

Early identification of infecting organisms is critical in certain rapidly progressive skin infections, such as necrotizing fasciitis. Gram stain and culture of the overlying skin has a low yield; the growth of organisms takes several days, even when cultures are positive. Biopsy of skin for frozen section has improved the rapidity of diagnosis in this disease. The use of a rapid streptococcus test can be helpful in the early identification of streptococcal infection in necrotizing fasciitis.[6]

Tzanck Preparation

Microscopic examination of cells obtained from the base of a vesicle or bulla (Tzanck smear) is used primarily for the diagnosis of viral processes, including herpes simplex and varicella zoster viruses. First introduced in 1947 as a rapid technique for evaluating cutaneous blistering, the Tzanck smear remains widely used[7] despite the development of more sophisticated but costly techniques. This examination can be used for evaluation of other noninfectious causes of vesiculopustules in the neonate. Its use in diseases such as toxic epidermal necrolysis, staphylococcal scalded skin syndrome,[8] pemphigus vulgaris,[9] and Langerhans' cell histiocytosis[10] has been well documented.

The technique for performing Tzanck preparations is described in Box 6-2. The tissue can be air-dried, heat-fixed, or fixed in methanol before staining. Various commercially prepared stains can be used to provide nuclear detail, including Giemsa, crystal violet, toluidine blue, Hemacolor, thiazine–xanthene, and others. Multinucleated giant cells are seen on high, dry power and can be diagnostic of varicella or herpes simplex infection. Examination with the oil immersion objective is often helpful in equivocal cases. Caution must be taken not to over-interpret clumped epithelial or white blood cells as indicative of giant cells. To be positive, epidermal nuclei should be 'molded' together with nuclear membranes that appear to be indenting each other. Homogeneous, ground-glass nucleoplasm is also characteristic of the multinucleated giant cell[11] (Fig. 6-2). Tzanck preparations, along with evaluation of free-floating blister contents by Gram or Wright stain, may display characteristic findings of a variety of diseases, as described in Table 6-1.

Direct Fluorescent Antibody Test for Diagnosis of Herpes Virus Infection

Despite its utility as a screening tool, the Tzanck preparation has limited sensitivity and specificity. The direct fluorescent antibody (DFA) test is a rapid, cost-effective, sensitive, and highly specific[12] method for detecting and distinguishing cutaneous herpes simplex virus (HSV 1 and 2) and varicella zoster virus (VZV) infections. Direct immunofluorescence is most sensitive on vesicles, less sensitive on pustules, and even less

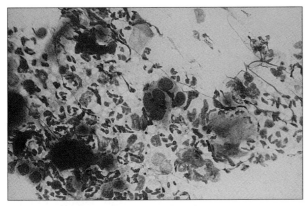

FIG. 6-2 Multinucleated giant cell on Tzanck smear.

TABLE 6-1 Findings on Tzanck smears of blister scrapings and Wright/Gram stains of blister fluid contents of selected neonatal cutaneous conditions

Transient neonatal pustular melanosis	Large numbers of polymorphonuclear leukocytes
Pustular psoriasis	Large numbers of polymorphonuclear leukocytes
Acropustulosis of infancy	Large numbers of polymorphonuclear leukocytes
Incontinenti pigmenti	Large numbers of eosinophils
Erythema toxicum neonatorum	Large numbers of eosinophils
Eosinophilic pustular folliculitis	Large numbers of eosinophils
Toxic epidermal necrolysis	Cuboidal cells with high nuclear to cytoplasmic ratio; inflammatory cells present
Staphylococcal scalded skin syndrome	Broad epidermal cells without inflammation
Histiocytosis	Histiocytes with oval nuclei with longitudinal grooves or 'kidney bean' shape
Varicella or herpes simplex	Multinucleated giant cells

Box 6-2 Tzanck smear technique

1. Select a lesion. The yield for obtaining a positive smear is highest from a fresh vesicle, followed by a pustule, and then a crusted lesion.
2. Wipe the lesion with alcohol and allow it to dry for 1 minute.
3. Using a #15 blade, either remove the crust or unroof the vesicle or pustule.
4. Using a #15 blade at an angle of less than 90°, scrape the lesion base with the edge of the blade.
5. Gently transfer the material from the blade to a glass slide by repeatedly and gently touching the blade to the slide. (Forceful smearing will grind the cells, resulting in crushed nuclei.)
6. Allow the smear to air dry (alternately, tissue may be heat fixed or fixed in methanol).
7. Flood the slide with staining solution for 30–60 seconds. Use either Giemsa, Wright, methylene blue, or toluidine blue stains.
8. Rinse excess stain off of the slide with tap water and allow the slide to air dry.
9. Apply one or two drops of immersion oil or tap water. Then place a cover slip over the slide.
10. Rack up the substage condenser toward the stage and adjust the field diaphragm for optimal illumination and resolution.

so on crusted lesions.[13] DFA testing uses monoclonal antibodies directed against type-specific glycoprotein epitopes of the herpes virus envelope.[14] The base of a blister, erosion, or ulcer is aggressively scraped at the bedside. The material is then smeared on a glass slide and sent to the appropriate laboratory Box 6-3. Clinicians should consult hospital laboratories regarding the requirements for obtaining samples for DFA examination. Some laboratories request commercially prepared, dual-welled glass slides to be inoculated as controls. Slides are prepared with a few drops of fluorescein-conjugated murine monoclonal antibodies against HSV 1 and 2 (prepared as a 1 : 1 mixture) or VZV. After approximately 30 minutes the slides are rinsed and examined by epifluorescence microscopy. Slides emitting bright-green cytoplasmic fluorescence are positive.[15] False-positive DFA results have been reported in rare instances.[16]

Viral Culture

Although Tzanck smears and the DFA technique can provide rapid results in suspected viral infection, the gold standard remains viral culture. After absorbing the fluid of the vesicle with a Dacron-tipped applicator and firmly rubbing the base of the vesicle, the applicator should be placed in a sterile tube containing at least 3 mL of viral transport medium (buffered isotonic balanced salt solution, traditionally containing penicillin and streptomycin or gentamicin to prevent bacterial contamination. Recent studies suggest that less contamination occurs with the addition of vancomycin and amikacin.[17] Specimens should be refrigerated or transported on ice for the best results.

Culture techniques are most useful in suspected herpes virus infection. Herpes simplex virus produces identifiable changes in culture cells in 2–3 days, and culture techniques are quite sensitive. VZV is more difficult to culture and can take 7–14 days, with frequent false-negative results.[18]

Polymerase chain reaction (PCR) is now being more widely used in the diagnosis of many viral infections and in attempts to find the etiology of many common skin disorders of unknown etiology.[19-21] Studies using PCR in the identification of herpes infection in keratoconjuctivitis[22] and in primary genital herpes[23] have found the assay to be superior to viral culture in both sensitivity and ease of collection.

Scabies/Ectoparasite Preparations

The most difficult part of a scabies preparation is finding the appropriate lesion to sample. A linear burrow is an excellent place to scrape but may prove hard to identify. On young infants and children, where mites abound, the palms are a highly fruitful location because the hands and fingers are used for rubbing and scratching. Finger webs, wrists, feet, axillae, vesicles, and untouched pink papules are good sites for scraping.[24] The technique for scabies preparations is described in Box 6-3.

Moving mites are generally easily visible and can be quickly viewed under scanning power. Mites are 0.2–0.4 mm in size, with four pairs of legs (Fig. 6-3). Eggs are oval and one-tenth of the size of the mite. Feces are also oval, but golden brown in color and usually occur in clumps (Fig. 6-4). Air bubbles are the biggest artifacts present in scabies preparations. Gently pressing on the cover slip can dislodge these. In addition, trapped air is round, whereas ova and feces are usually oval.

Epiluminescent microscopy (ELM), utilizing a handheld magnifier through which skin can be viewed through a layer of oil, can also be helpful in the identification of scabies on the skin.[25] Mites appear as dark triangular structures resulting from pigment in the anterior section of the thorax.

Microscopic Hair Examination

Various hair shaft abnormalities can be detected by simple bedside diagnostic examination. Table 6-2 lists the microscopic hair findings in certain syndromes. Hair can be examined with the light microscope, both with and without the use of polarizing lenses (see Fig. 28-31). More detailed information can be obtained from scanning and/or transmission electron microscopic examination of hair. In general, hair obtained for microscopic examination should be snipped rather than pulled. This avoids unnecessary trauma and discomfort for the infant and eliminates artifacts produced by the force of epilation. A few clinical scenarios (e.g. loose anagen syndrome) involve actual abnormalities of the hair bulb, which requires that hair be pulled together with its root for examination. Most hair abnormalities seen in the neonate involve scalp hair. The hair changes of Netherton syndrome, however, are variable and often absent from scalp hair. The diagnosis of Netherton syndrome can be made in these patients by sampling eyebrow or eyelash hair.[26] The reader is referred to Chapter 28 for a detailed discussion of hair disorders in the neonate.

Skin Biopsy

One of the most useful diagnostic tests in dermatology is the skin biopsy. This simple technique allows sampling of skin specimens for diagnostic testing, histopathologic examination, or culture. The type of biopsy performed depends on the size, the suspected depth, and the location on the skin of the lesion to be biopsied.

Box 6-3 Mineral oil scraping for scabies

1. Select a good site, such as the palms, web spaces, wrists, or obvious burrows that are not excoriated.
2. Apply mineral oil to a #15 blade. You may also want to cover the lesion to be sampled with mineral oil to reduce pain and friction.
3. Scrape the lesion vigorously five to six times to remove the stratum corneum. Punctate bleeding will demonstrate that you are at the correct depth.
4. Apply mineral oil to a glass slide.
5. Immerse the #15 blade in the oil and transfer the onto the glass slide.
6. Add a cover slip to the glass slide.
7. View under microscope on low power (4× or 10×). Mites, eggs, or feces are all recognizable (see Figs. 6-3 and 6-4).

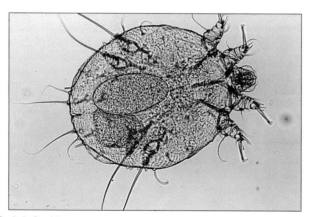

FIG. 6-3 Scabies preparation demonstrating mite *Sarcoptes scabeii*.

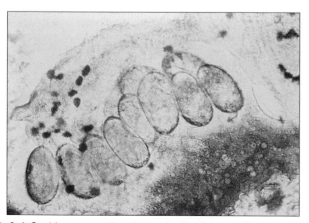

FIG. 6-4 Scabies preparation demonstrating feces and eggs.

TABLE 6-2 Hair examination of selected clinical conditions in the newborn

Condition	Microscopic hair findings
Netherton syndrome	Light microscopy: 'ball and socket' configuration or trichorrhexis invaginata.[27,28] May include golf-tee[29] or tulip-like[26] configurations. May show circumferential strictures (earliest stage of invagination)
Menkes syndrome	Light microscopy: classically reveals pili torti or twisted hair, but monilethrix and trichorrhexis nodosa[30] also reported
Trichothiodystrophy	Light microscopy: wavy, irregular outline with a flattened shaft with folded ribbon configuration. Polarized microscopy: light and dark bands or 'tiger tail' pattern
Chediak–Higashi syndrome	Light microscopy: evenly distributed small, granular melanin aggregates[31]
Griscelli syndrome	Light microscopy: large, unevenly distributed melanin aggregates, primarily located in the medulla

Punch biopsy is the most common method of skin sampling used in dermatology. This approach is excellent for complete removal of small lesions (<6 mm), and for obtaining tissue for diagnostic purposes for routine histology, immunofluorescence, electron microscopy, or culture, but it does have limitations. It may not be the optimal method of sampling if the suspected pathology is located in the subcutaneous fat since this method may be too superficial to include the diseased tissue. For lesions confined to the epidermis and superficial dermis, punch biopsy may not be the best method of sampling, because full-thickness skin is removed and a more prominent scar will result than with a shave biopsy.

Punch biopsies are performed with reusable sterile Keyes skin punches or, more commonly, with inexpensive, extremely sharp, disposable punches. They can be purchased in sizes ranging from 2 to 6 mm. Typically a 3 or 4 mm punch biopsy is performed for diagnostic purposes. When specimens larger than 6 mm are required, or if deeper biopsies containing fat or subcutaneous tissue are optimal for diagnosis or culture, a fusiform or excisional biopsy is indicated (Box 6-4).

Skin Biopsy/Specialized Tests
Special Stains
Routine skin biopsies are usually stained with hematoxylin–eosin (H&E), the standard staining method for tissue. In certain instances, special staining techniques are required to further delineate structures in the skin or pathologic organisms. Many histochemical special stains can be performed on formalin-fixed, paraffin-embedded material.

Electron Microscopy
Electron microscopy (EM) uses thin (1 μm) tissue sections to allow high-resolution images of nuclear membrane abnormalities and organelle changes, which are not routinely seen with light microscopy.[25] It may be very useful in establishing the diagnoses of several diseases, such as Langerhans' cell histiocytosis and epidermolysis bullosa (EB). Specimens for EM may be obtained by punch biopsy and placed in glutaraldehyde fixative. For EB, rotary traction may be applied to the skin just before biopsy in an attempt to elicit a microscopic cleavage plane. This can be achieved by gently pushing and twisting an eraser tip on the skin. The traumatized skin is then locally anesthetized, and a punch biopsy is performed. Transmission EM (TEM) allows for precise localization of the ultrastructural level of cleavage within a given specimen, thereby differentiating simplex, junctional, and dystrophic types of EB.[32] Centers vary widely, however, in their experience with the electron microscopic diagnosis of EB, and referral of the specimen to a major medical center with significant expertise and experience in the ultramicroscopic features of EB should be considered.

Immunofluorescence
Two types of immunofluorescence test can be performed. Direct immunofluorescence tests for immunoreactants localized in the tissues of the patient's skin or mucous membrane, whereas indirect immunofluorescence testing detects circulating antibodies in the patient's serum. Although indirect immunofluorescence is less sensitive than direct, it may at times provide valuable supplementary diagnostic information.

Direct Immunofluorescent Microscopy
Direct immunofluorescent microscopy may be useful for the diagnosis of immune-mediated vesiculobullous diseases, lupus erythematosus, and leukocytoclastic vasculitis. A perilesional biopsy (next to but not including a fresh blister) should be biopsied (Box 6-5). Frozen sections are incubated with fluorescent-linked antibodies to human IgG, IgA, IgM, and C3, as well as other antibodies. Specimens may be frozen until testing or kept in transport medium (Michel's medium: ammonium sulfate, N-ethylmaleimide, and magnesium sulfate in a citrate buffer) for at least 2 weeks without loss of reactivity.[33]

Indirect Immunofluorescent Microscopy
Various dilutions of the patient's serum are incubated on an epithelial substrate, usually primate esophagus. The circulating antibodies are reported as the highest positive dilution, or 'titer.' This diagnostic technique is useful for pemphigus vulgaris, pemphigus foliaceus, bullous pemphigoid, and other autoimmune blistering disorders.

Perhaps the most common neonatal application of these techniques is in the diagnosis of epidermolysis bullosa. In this case, a skin biopsy specimen is submitted for immunofluorescent antigenic mapping. Through this modified indirect immunofluorescence technique, the ultrastructural level of a blister can be determined based on the binding of antibodies having known ultrastructural binding sites.[32] The three most commonly used antibodies are those directed against bullous pemphigoid antigen, laminin, and type IV collagen.[32] Other

---

Box 6-4 Technique for performing a punch biopsy

1. Biopsy the freshest, most recent lesion.
2. Cleanse the skin with alcohol or antiseptic.
3. Anesthetize with 1% lidocaine with epinephrine using a 30-gauge needle.
4. Stretch the skin between the thumb and forefinger. Using firm, downward pressure, twist and rotate the biopsy punch back and forth until it pops through to the fat.
5. Cut the base of the specimen with a scissors. Care should be taken not to crush the tissue with forceps.
6. Place the specimen in formalin fixative for routine histopathologic examination.
7. Specimens for culture should be placed on a sterile gauze soaked with nonbacteriostatic saline in a sterile container.
8. Close the defect by placing a simple interrupted suture (using 4/0 prolene or nylon).
9. Apply antibiotic ointment and adhesive bandage (Band-Aid).
10. Remove sutures in 7–10 days.

Box 6-5 Biopsy technique for direct immunofluorescence

1. Biopsy the freshest, most recent lesion.
2. Perilesional (normal) skin is most desirable. Never biopsy the base of an ulcer or the center of a blister.
3. If the epidermis and dermis become detached during the procedure, submit both in separately labeled containers.
4. Place specimens in transport medium (Michel's transport medium or Zeus's fixative). Never place the specimen in formalin.
5. If transport medium is not available, cover the biopsy with saline-soaked gauze and transport it immediately to immunofluorescence laboratory for processing.

antibodies directed against basement membrane components may also be used.[34]

As with specimens obtained for electron microscopy, clinically normal skin is sampled and subjected to rotary traction. The specimen should be placed in an immunofluorescence transfer medium (Michel's, Zeus's) and forwarded to a reference laboratory experienced in antigenic mapping. Immunofluorescence antigenic mapping may offer several advantages over electron microscopy for the diagnosis of EB. The transport medium used for immunofluorescence is inexpensive and readily available, and specimens can be evaluated several weeks after biopsy if necessary. Immunofluorescence antigenic mapping can be completed rapidly, within 2 hours of receipt of a given specimen, unlike EM examination, which can take up to several weeks to complete.[32]

Immunohistochemistry/Cell Typing

In general, immunohistochemical procedures require fresh tissue, as formalin fixation and subsequent tissue processing may damage antigens localized to the cell membrane.[35] However, there are several antibodies that can be used on formalin-fixed, paraffin-embedded tissue.[36] The use of monoclonal and polyclonal antibodies can be helpful to determine the origin of a cell, especially if the cell appears anaplastic. However, false-negative staining can occur as a result of outdated or poorly diluted antibody preparations.[37] Furthermore, a cell may be so highly anaplastic that it loses the antigenic marker and does not stain positively. There is currently no antibody that uniformly distinguishes benign from malignant cells.

SURGICAL/PROCEDURAL ISSUES IN NEONATES

EMLA

EMLA cream is an eutectic mixture of local anesthetics (2.5% lidocaine and 2.5% prilocaine) in an oil-in-water emulsion that induces topical anesthesia of intact skin. Its use in infants is well established and generally safe if caution is exercised. EMLA is very useful for reducing the pain of local anesthetic infiltration, lumbar puncture, subcutaneous drug reservoir punctures, intravenous catheter placement, venepuncture, and as anesthesia for superficial dermatologic procedures.[38,39] It induces anesthesia at a maximum depth of 5 mm, making its use alone inadequate for excisional surgery or punch biopsy. The degree, depth, and onset of anesthesia are related to the duration of application. Mucous membranes, genital skin, and inflamed skin absorb the product more rapidly, allowing for shorter application times (5–40 minutes) in these anatomic areas. EMLA should be used cautiously in infants less than 3 months of age because of the risk of associated methemoglobinemia. The development of methemoglobinemia from prilocaine is caused by two of its metabolites, 4-hydroxy-2-methylaniline and 2-methylanaline (o-toluidine), which lead to oxidation of hemoglobin. Young infants are more susceptible to drug-induced methemoglobinemia because they have lower levels of reduced nicotinamide adenine dinucleotide (NADH)-methemoglobin reductase, catalase, and glutathione peroxidase; higher levels of hemoglobin F, which is more susceptible to oxidation; and because the dose of lidocaine and prilocaine is usually greater per kilogram of body weight.[41-44] Patients with hemoglobinopathies or glucose-6-

phosphate dehydrogenase (G6PD) deficiency may also be at greater risk.[45] Clinical cyanosis becomes apparent with a methemoglobin level at about 15%.[46] A few small studies of EMLA use in preterm infants and those less than 3 months of age have failed to detect methemoglobinemia in the absence of the concomitant medication use, but caution is warranted.[47] Short application times, and limited quantities of EMLA (<2 g) are recommended in young infants to reduce the risk of methemoglobinemia (Table 6-3). Medications that induce a methemoglobin stress and might increase the risk of EMLA-associated methemoglobinemia include sulfonamides, acetaminophen, benzocaine, dapsone, phenobarbital, antimalarials, and phenytoin.[48,49] Use of EMLA in infants less than 3 months is therefore not advised in the presence of the above medications.

The use of EMLA is generally well tolerated and safe. Local side effects from EMLA use include transient blanching, erythema, eye irritation, edema, and dermatitis. Allergic contact dermatitis has been reported, with prilocaine as the implicated allergen in most studies.[50,51] A petechial or purpuric eruption has been observed after EMLA use in neonates, children, and adults[52,53] (Fig. 6-5). The eruption does not seem to be related to either dose or duration of application. It appears during or immediately after EMLA application as early as 30 minutes after application. The purpura resolves spontaneously over days. Purpura may be more common in premature infants,

TABLE 6-3 Parameters for the safe use of EMLA in children*

Body weight requirements	Maximum total dose of EMLA (g)	Maximum application area (cm²)
<5 kg	1	10
5–10 kg	2	20

*These guidelines are applicable to infants with intact, nondiseased skin.

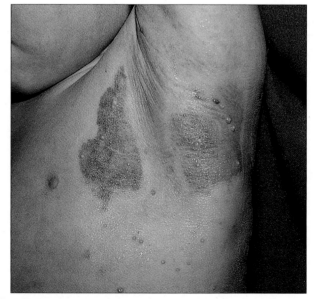

FIG. 6-5 Petechial eruption after application of EMLA cream.

especially those younger than 32 weeks' gestational age, and in patients with atopic dermatitis.[53] Patch testing to EMLA cream, prilocaine, lidocaine, emollient base, and Tegaderm plaster was negative in all patients tested in one study.[54] A direct toxic effect to capillary endothelium has been postulated. Rechallenge with EMLA after this reaction has been negative. Nevertheless, EMLA should be used cautiously, if at all, in infants with a history of this reaction.

To be effective, the use of an occlusive dressing for at least 1–2 hours is necessary to allow the lidocaine/prilocaine mixture to absorb into the skin, with the exception of genital and mucosal sites. Applications with nonairtight adhesive bandages (Band-Aids), gauze wraps, or other nonocclusive dressings will result in suboptimal anesthesia.

Newer lidocaine containing topical anesthetics including 4% liposomal lidocaine are commercially available. This product is free of prilocaine and therefore eliminates the risk of anesthetic-induced associated methemoglobinemia. As with all topical anesthetics in infants, short application times and limited quantities are recommended to avoid lidocaine toxicity. Further studies are warranted to evaluate this potentially useful topical anesthetic, especially in neonates, owing to the proposed diminished risk of methemoglobinemia.

Lidocaine Toxicity

The two most widely used local anesthetics are lidocaine and bupivacaine (Marcaine/Sensorcaine). For most skin surgery, the recommended anesthetic is 1% lidocaine with epinephrine (adrenaline). Advantages of this drug combination include a negligible incidence of allergy, virtually instantaneous onset of anesthesia, and minimal bleeding caused by the epinephrine. The most common commercial preparation contains 1% lidocaine (10 mg/mL) and 1 : 100 000 epinephrine. Toxicity from lidocaine is extremely rare if dosed appropriately. Maximum recommended doses are listed in Table 6-4.

Although data on lidocaine pharmacokinetics in neonates are limited, it appears that the elimination half-life of lidocaine is prolonged compared to that in adults.[55,56] The volume of distribution of lidocaine in neonates is at least twofold higher than in adults, partially because of lidocaine's diminished binding to plasma proteins.[55,56] In neonates, only 20% of lidocaine is protein bound, compared to 60–70% protein binding in adults.[57,58] This increased bioavailability may make neonates more susceptible to lidocaine toxicity than older patients at a given serum concentration.[59]

In general, lidocaine has a low incidence of systemic toxicity. Toxic reactions can occur, however, and can range from cardiovascular or central nervous system reactions to death. Central nervous system toxicity may begin with agitation and progress to convulsions, unconsciousness, and respiratory depression. Early detection of lidocaine toxicity in infants can be difficult because of problems detecting early signs, such as lightheadedness, dizziness, and confusion. The safe use of viscous lidocaine in neonates has been questioned because of reports of seizures following its use.[60,61] Furthermore, a recent report of recurrent seizures in a neonate after intravenous lidocaine administration at a standard dose suggests that lidocaine may have greater toxicity in neonates and infants with a developing central nervous system.[59] Additional pharmacokinetic studies are indicated to better define appropriate lidocaine dosing in this population.

Preoperative Care and Complications

Postoperative wound care in the neonate is usually straightforward and uncomplicated, but requires adequate parental instruction. It is best to teach wound care to the patient's family after the surgical procedure, as beforehand they are usually preoccupied and anxious, and unable to pay attention to information. Written and verbal instructions for postoperative wound care should be provided. If daily cleansing of the wound is recommended, the family should be encouraged to look at the wound before the dressing is applied, so that they are prepared for its postoperative appearance.

There is great variability in recommendations for wound care in dermatology.[62–64] The need for daily cleansing of a sterilely induced sutured wound is debatable.[65] Although laboratory studies have suggested that hydrogen peroxide is toxic to epithelial cells,[66] it is unclear whether this has any clinical relevance, as most wounds cleansed with this agent heal without difficulty. Despite its global acceptance and use as a wound cleanser, hydrogen peroxide is a poor antiseptic.[67] Its benefits are probably a consequence of the debridement induced by its effervescence rather than its antimicrobial properties.[67] Therefore, the use of hydrogen peroxide for wound cleansing is best reserved for those wounds that are crusted and in need of gentle debridement.

The goal of wound management is to minimize bacterial colonization while providing a moist environment.[68] For most surgical wounds in pediatric patients a nonsensitizing topical antibiotic, such as bacitracin or polymyxin B and bacitracin, covered by a nonadherent dressing will suffice. Because of the risk of allergic contact dermatitis, topical antibiotics without neomycin are generally recommended. Enhanced wound healing with topical antibiotics is probably a result of the moist environment provided and not a result of their antimicrobial activity. Wounds treated with petrolatum alone re-epithelialize faster than untreated wounds.[69,70]

The use of topical silver sulfadiazine (Silvadene) in neonates is probably best avoided because of reports of transient leukopenia following application.[71] Because neonatal skin, especially that of young premature infants, is more fragile than that of older children or adults, adhesive dressings should be used as sparingly as possible.

OTHER DIAGNOSTIC TESTS

Nikolsky's Sign

Nikolsky first defined this clinical sign in 1927, in a description of a patient with pemphigus foliaceus.[72] It has since become a clinical tool for evaluating blistering diseases. Gentle

TABLE 6-4 Maximum doses of 1% lidocaine with and without epinephrine		
Type of lidocaine	Maximum dose	Maximum dose for 5 kg infant
1% Lidocaine without epinephrine	4.5 mg/kg	2.3 mL
1% Lidocaine with epinephrine	7 mg/kg	3.5 mL

lateral pressure is applied to the normal skin surface, or adjacent to a bulla, vesicle, or erosion, either with the thumb or with an object such as a pencil eraser. Separation of the epidermis from the dermis with this lateral pressure is considered a positive Nikolsky's sign, indicating altered structural integrity of the skin, either at the dermoepidermal junction or within the epidermis. A similar lack of skin attachment can be demonstrated by applying vertical pressure with the thumb on the top of an intact bulla or vesicle, causing extension of the bulla into apparently normal skin.

Although Nikolsky's sign was classically applied to pemphigus, it occurs in several diseases, including toxic epidermal necrolysis, bullous erythema multiforme, staphylococcal scalded skin syndrome,[73] bullous impetigo, and EB. Some authors have suggested that several of the disorders characterized by a positive Nikolsky's sign can be further distinguished by examining the skin at the base of the bulla.[74] If this is dry, referred to as a dry Nikolsky's sign, this implies a subcorneal blistering process such as pemphigus foliaceus or staphylococcal scalded skin. If the base of the bulla is moist, glistening, and exudative, referred to as a wet Nikolsky's sign, the level of split of the skin is deeper in an intraepidermal or subepidermal location, such as toxic epidermal necrolysis, bullous erythema multiforme, or pemphigus vulgaris. The exception to this rule is bullous impetigo, where the subcorneal split is very wet because of the presence of severe inflammation.

Darier's Sign

Gentle stroking of skin lesions in mastocytosis or urticaria pigmentosa produces edema, erythema, induration, and sometimes vesiculation of the skin surface, called a Darier's sign. Changes in the skin reflect mast cell degranulation from rubbing and the effect of potent mediators released from these cells on the blood vessels in the surrounding skin. Caution should be taken to rub gently in the case of a suspected solitary mastocytoma because blistering is not uncommon following manipulation. A history of a positive Darier's sign can often be obtained from the parents, helping to confirm the diagnosis.

Insect bites and papular urticaria can also produce a positive Darier's sign as a result of release of histamine into the skin. Recent reports have described a positive Darier's sign in non-Hodgkin's lymphoma,[75] leukemia cutis,[76] and cutaneous T-cell lymphoma.[77]

A pseudo-Darier's sign can be observed in patients with cutaneous smooth muscle hamartomas.[78–80] Smooth muscle hamartomas comprise a collection of arrector pili muscles. Rubbing of the surface of these lesions produces piloerection and temporary induration that can appear similar to a Darier's sign. This feature can be very useful in distinguishing smooth muscle hamartomas from congenital nevi because both are pigmented congenital lesions with hypertrichosis.

Darkfield Examination

Darkfield examination is an infrequently performed examination used to detect *Treponema pallidum*, the pathologic organism in syphilis. The spirochete is most likely to be detected in nasal discharge or scrapings from moist mucocutaneous lesions, but specimens from the mouth should be avoided because of the presence of normal oral spirochetes, which can be mistaken for *T. pallidum*. With a special condenser (dark-field) and a funnel stage for the lens, any microscope can be converted to a darkfield microscope. This technique uses an oblique beam of light, which refracts off small particles undetectable with conventional optics. Considerable experience is needed to master this technique. The key to successful diagnosis with a darkfield examination is in the collection of the specimen. The procedure is described in Box 6-6.[81]

Wood's Light Examination

A Wood's lamp is helpful in the clinical evaluation of cutaneous pigmentary disease, selected cutaneous infections, and porphyria. Long-wave ultraviolet radiation, or black light, is emitted from a high-pressure mercury lamp fitted with a filter made of nickel oxide and silica. The resulting light is emitted with wavelengths ranging from 320 to 400 nm. Melanin is absorbed at these wavelengths, so that minor losses of melanin in skin are accentuated. Hypopigmentation appears somewhat paler than surrounding normal skin, and, depending on baseline normal pigmentation, depigmentation is starkly contrasted with surrounding skin.[82]

Early subclinical hypopigmented macules of tuberous sclerosis and streaky hypopigmentation seen in hypomelanosis of Ito,[83] for example, are often detected with the Wood's lamp, making this an essential tool in the evaluation of infants with possible tuberous sclerosis and pigmentary disease. Use of the lamp is often extended to examination of the parents of infants with possible incontinentia pigmenti or tuberous sclerosis.

Wood's lamp examination can also be extended to nonpigmentary cutaneous pathology. For example, various dermatologic conditions have characteristic fluorescent patterns, including yellow-green fluorescence of hair in selected dermatophyte infections (e.g. *Microsporum canis*), yellow-green fluorescence of skin in *Pseudomonas* infection, and pinkish-red fluorescence of urine in porphyria.

Specific Genetic and Metabolic Testing
Polymerase Chain Reaction
The polymerase chain reaction (PCR) is one of the most significant breakthroughs for medical diagnosis of the 20th century.[84,85] First described in 1985,[86] PCR is an efficient, economic, and sensitive method used to detect even minute amounts of DNA. Specific DNA sequences are amplified using repetitive automated cycling.[87] At the end of one cycle, the quantity of DNA present is doubled. Expansion of a particular genetic sequence is therefore exponential ($2n$, with n representing the number of cycles). Twenty cycles of PCR results in a theoretic yield of approximately 1 million copies of the original DNA sequence. This allows detection of a specific

---

Box 6-6 Technique for darkfield examination

1. While wearing gloves, clean the surface of the lesion with dry gauze.
2. Touch a cover slip to serous fluid expressed from a lesion.
3. Drop the cover slip on a drop of saline on a glass slide.
4. Examine immediately (if possible at the bedside); do not let the specimen dry out.
5. Spirochetes, if present, will be seen as undulating and rotating corkscrew-shaped organisms.

DNA sequence, even if present in minute amounts, in any specimen.[88]

Detection of foreign DNA is important in the diagnosis of infectious diseases. Practical dermatologic applications include the identification of infectious agents, which is especially helpful in neonates for whom serologic methods may be unreliable, viral cultures unproductive, and results delayed.[89–92]

PCR is also useful to detect genetic mutations for diagnosis of genetic diseases, and for oncology. The technique has been used to detect chromosomal translocations in leukemias and lymphomas in children.[93] PCR is 100 000 times more sensitive than cytogenetic studies and 10 000 times more sensitive than flow cytometry or Southern blotting techniques in detecting chromosomal translocations.[94]

PCR is proving to be of immense value in the prenatal diagnosis of a number of genetic disorders, including dermatologic diseases. Any genetic diseases in which the defective gene is known can potentially be diagnosed using PCR technology. PCR can be used to analyze minute amounts of fetal genetic material. Because the genes for many inherited skin conditions have been or are in the process of being identified, the future applications of PCR are many. PCR has also been performed on single cells removed at the blastomere stage, allowing identification of defective genes in in-vitro fertilization programs[95] (see later section on Prenatal Diagnosis).

The remarkable sensitivity of PCR makes testing under the most stringent of laboratory conditions essential. Contaminations of minute amounts of extraneous DNA can be disastrous and lead to potentially erroneous results. Appropriate positive and negative controls are essential. False-negative results can also occur. Rarely, DNA sequences may be lost because the material sought may be denatured by the use of inappropriate tissue fixatives.[96]

A major advantage of PCR is that it can be performed on minimal amounts of tissue. Both the quantity of the sample and the transport medium requirements for PCR are liberal.[97] For the identification of herpes simplex virus DNA, for example, the amount of tissue used for a Tzanck smear is sufficient. Viral culture medium is effective for transport and is often readily available at the bedside.[97] Fresh, fresh-frozen, formalin-fixed, and even paraffin-embedded specimens are acceptable for PCR testing.[98]

Fluorescence in situ Hybridization

Fluorescence in situ hybridization (FISH) represents a unique technology in which molecular biologic and histochemical techniques are used to evaluate gene expression in tissue sections and cytologic preparations. With FISH, specific regions of the genome can be detected by applying complementary labeled nucleic acid probes.[99] After denaturation of the DNA, the probes can hybridize to target sequences on chromosomes and form a new DNA duplex. The hybridized probes are identified using fluorescence microscopy. With this technique, also referred to as interphase cytogenetics, karyotype changes can be detected at the single cell level. This allows for examination of chromosomal aberrations among morphologically or immunologically deficient cell populations present within a tumor sample, for example.

FISH methods have unlimited applications for clinical medicine and diagnostic pathology. For example, DNA probes can be used to identify foreign genes, including bacteria, viruses, and fungi. Detection of infectious agents with FISH techniques has been reported for human immunodeficiency virus (HIV),

cytomegalovirus, herpes simplex virus, hepatitis B virus, and Epstein–Barr virus, among others.

PRENATAL DIAGNOSIS

Knowledge of specific gene defects for many genodermatoses has led to the development of DNA-based prenatal diagnosis, which has largely superseded older techniques such as fetoscopy and fetal skin biopsy. For example, PCR-based prenatal diagnosis of dystrophic and junctional EB has been performed through analysis of type VII collagen and laminin-5 genes of dystrophic and junctional EB, respectively,[100,101] and of keratin 10 for epidermolytic hyperkeratosis[102] and others. DNA may be derived through chorionic villus sampling (CVS) at 10–15 weeks' gestation, or by amniocentesis at 12–15 weeks' gestation in families at risk for recurrence of EB. Periumbilical vein blood samples during the early weeks of pregnancy may provide an even earlier source of fetal DNA without any increased risk to the fetus.[103] In most cases, fetal cells are also cultured, and the test can be confirmed approximately 2 weeks later from the cultured cells. Thus DNA-based prenatal diagnosis offers an early, expedient, and accurate method of prenatal testing for genodermatoses with known underlying disorders. It must be emphasized, however, that use of molecular techniques for prenatal diagnosis requires that the molecular defect is known. Although prenatal cytogenetic diagnosis based on amniocytes or chorionic villus cells is accurate, the procedure carries a risk of miscarriage. Because of this, CVS- or amniocentesis-based prenatal testing should be reserved for women at high risk for chromosomal abnormalities.

Preimplantation genetic diagnosis (PGD) is an alternative to conventional approaches to prenatal diagnosis. With this technique, the genetic abnormality in question is diagnosed before implantation of the fetus, allowing for selection of non-affected, normal fetuses. DNA analysis and in vitro fertilization are utilized to select for a normal genotype before implantation. At the 6–10 cell stage one cell is removed for DNA extraction and PCR amplification. Removal of one or two cells at this stage does not affect viability or the rate of development of the embryo(s). After analysis, only the embryos with normal DNA are implanted, theoretically ensuring that the implanted fetus will be normal. This technique has been used in families at risk for cystic fibrosis[104] and EB.

The field of prenatal diagnosis is developing at an astounding pace. New molecular, enzymatic, and ultrastructural markers will be available in the future, which will aid in the accuracy and utility of in-utero or preimplantation diagnosis. Readers are referred to their local genetic centers for information regarding prenatal diagnosis of specific genetic diseases. The internet is a valuable resource for current information on specific dermatologic conditions and their prenatal diagnosis. The Online Mendelian Inheritance in Man website, http://www.ncbi.nlm.nih.gov/Omim, is a database of human genes and genetic disorders. It contains textual information, pictures, and valuable reference information, as well as extensive links to the National Center for Biotechnical Information's Entrez database of MEDLINE articles and genetic sequencing information. For more clinically based genetic information, http://www.geneclinics.org may be helpful. Genedx is an invaluable resource for the diagnosis of rare genetic disorders of the skin. The reader is referred to www.genedx.com for mutation testing in rare disorders for the purpose of diagnosis, carrier detection and prenatal testing.

REFERENCES

1. Martin AG, Kobayashi GS. Superficial fungal infections: Dermatophytosis, tinea nigra, piedra. In: Fitzpatrick TB, Eisen AZ, Wolff K, et al. Dermatology in general medicine, 4th edn. New York: McGraw-Hill, 1993; 2337–2359.
2. Truhan AP, Hebert AA, Esterly NB. The double-edge knife. Arch Dermatol 1985; 121: 970.
3. Crissey JT. Common dermatophyte infections. A simple diagnostic test and current management. Postgrad Med 1998; 103: 191–2, 197–200, 205.
4. Friedlander SF, Pickering B, Cunningham BB, et al. Use of the cotton swab method in diagnosing tinea capitis. Pediatrics 1999; 104: 276–279.
5. Machler BC, Kirsner RS, Elgart GW. Routine histologic examination for the diagnosis of onychomycosis: an evaluation of sensitivity and specificity. Cutis 1998; 61: 217–219.
6. Bourgeois SD, Bourgeois MH. Use of the rapid streptococcus test in extracellular sites. Am Fam Phys 1996; 54: 1634–1636.
7. Tzanck A. Le cyto-diagnostic immédiat en dermatologie. Ann Dermatol Venereol 1947; 7: 68–70.
8. Buslau M, Biermann H, Shah PM. Gram-positive septic-toxic shock with bullae. Intraepidermal splitting as an indication of toxin effect. Hautarzt 1996; 47: 783–789.
9. Skeete MV. Evaluation of the usefulness of immunofluorescence on Tzanck smears in pemphigus as an aid to diagnosis. Clin Exp Dermatol 1977; 2: 57–63.
10. Colon-Fontanez F, Eichenfield LE, Krous HF, Friedlander SF. Congenital Langerhans' cell histiocytosis: The utility of the Tzanck test as a diagnostic screening tool. Arch Dermatol 1998; 134: 1039–1040.
11. Solomon AR, Rasmussen JE, Varani J, et al. The tzanck smear in the diagnosis of cutaneous herpes simplex. JAMA 1984; 251: 633–635.
12. Zirn JR, Tompkins SD, Huie C, Shea CR. Rapid detection and distinction of cutaneous herpesvirus infections by direct immunofluorescence. J Am Acad Dermatol 1995; 33: 724–728.
13. Bryson YJ, Conant MA, Solomon AR, et al. Questions and answers. J Am Acad Dermatol 1988; 18: 222–223.
14. Solomon AR. New diagnostic tests for herpes simplex and varicella zoster infections. J Am Acad Dermatol 1988; 18: 218–221.
15. Erlich KS. Laboratory diagnosis of herpesvirus infections. Clin Lab Med 1987; 7: 759–776.
16. Detlefs RL, Frieden IJ, Berger TG, Weston D. Eosinophil fluorescence: a cause of false positive slide tests for herpes simplex virus. Pediatr Dermatol 1987; 4: 129–133.
17. Lo JY, Lim WW, Tam BK, Lai MY. Vancomycin and amikacin in cell cultures for virus isolation. Pathology 1996; 28: 366–369.
18. Crumpacker CS, Gulick RM. Herpes simplex. In: Fitzpatrick TB, Eisen AZ, Wolff K, et al. eds. Dermatology in general medicine, 4th edn. New York: McGraw-Hill, 1993; 2414–2450.
19. Chen CL, Chow KC, Wong CK, et al. A study on Epstein–Barr virus in erythema multiforme. Arch Dermatol Res 1998; 290: 446–449.
20. Chang YT, Liu HN, Chen CL, et al. Detection of EBV and HTL V-1 in T cell lymphoma of skin in Taiwan. Am J Dermatopathol 1998; 20: 250–254.
21. Drago F, Ranieri E, Malaguti F, et al. Human herpesvirus 7 in patients with PR. Electron microscopy investigations and PCR in mononuclear cells, plasma and skin. Dermatology 1997; 195: 374–378.
22. Hidalgo F, Melon S, de Ona M, et al. Diagnosis of herpetic keratoconjunctivitis by nested polymerase chain reaction in human tear film. Euro J Clin Microbiol Infect Dis 1998; 17: 120–123.
23. Tremblay C, Coutlee F, Weiss J, et al. Evaluation of a non-isotopic polymerase chain reaction assay for detection in clinical specimens of herpes simplex virus type 2 DNA. Canadian Women's HIV Study Group. Clin Diagn Virol 1997; 8: 53–62.
24. Tanphaichitr A, Brodell RT. How to spot scabies in infants. Postgrad Med 1999; 105: 191–192.
25. Elenitsas R, Jaworsky C, Murphy GF. Diagnostic methodology: Immunofluorescence. In: Murphy GF, ed. Dermatopathology a practical guide to common disorders. Philadelphia: WB Saunders, 1995; 29–45.
26. Rogers M. Hair shaft abnormalities: Part II. Australas J Dermatol 1996; 37: 1–11.
27. Netherton EW. A unique case of trichorrhexis nodosa 'bamboo hairs' Arch Dermatol 1958; 78; 483.
28. Wilkinson RD, Curtis GH, Hawk WA. Netherton's disease. Trichorrhexis invaginata (bamboo hair), congenital ichthyosiform erythroderma and the atopic diathesis: A histopathologic study. Arch Dermatol 1964; 89: 106.
29. De Berker DA, Paige DG, Harper J, Dawber RPR. Golf tee hairs: A new sign in Netherton's syndrome. Br J Dermatol 1992; 127: 30.
30. Hurwitz S. Hair disorders. In: Schachner LA, Hansen RC, eds. Pediatric dermatology, 2nd edn. New York: Churchill Livingstone, 1995; 583–614.
31. Mancini AJ, Chan LS, Paller AS. Partial albinism with immunodeficiency: Griselli syndrome: Report of a case and review of the literature. J Am Acad Dermatol 1998; 38: 295–300.
32. Fine JD. Laboratory tests for epidermolysis bullosa. Dermatol Clin 1994; 12: 123–132.
33. Nisengard RJ, Blazczyk M, Chorzelski T, et al. Immunofluorescence of biopsy specimens: Comparison of methods of transportation. Arch Dermatol 1978; 114; 1329–1332.
34. Fine JD, Gay S. LDA-1 monoclonal antibody: An excellent reagent for immunofluorescence mapping studies in patients with epidermolysis bullosa. Arch Dermatol 1986; 122: 48–51.
35. Kurban RS, Mihm MC. Dermatopathology: Cutaneous reaction patterns and the use of specialized laboratory techniques. In: Moshella SL, Hurley HJ, eds. Dermatology, 3rd edn. Philadelphia: WB Saunders, 1992; 125–148.
36. Hood AF, Kwan TH, Mihm MC, Horn TD. Primer of dermatopathology. Boston: Little Brown, 1993; 40–43.
37. Lever WF, Schaumburg-Lever, eds. Histopathology of the skin, 7th edn. Laboratory Methods. Philadelphia: JB Lippincott, 44–54.
38. Gajraj NM, Pennant JH, Watcha MF. Eutectic mixture of local anesthetics (EMLA). Anesth Analg 1994; 78: 574–583.
39. Halperin DL, Koren G, Attias D, et al. Topical skin anesthesia for venous subcutaneous drug reservoir and lumbar punctures in children. Pediatrics 1989; 84: 281–284.
40. Chang PC, Goresky GV, O'Connor G, et al. A multicentre randomized study of single-unit dose package of EMLA patch vs. EMLA 5% cream for venepuncture in children. Can J Anesth 1994; 41: 59–63.
41. Reynolds F. Adverse effects of local anesthetics. Br J Anaesth 1987; 59: 78–95.
42. Jakobson B, Nilsson A. Methaemoglobinemia associated with prilocaine–lidocaine cream and trimethoprim–sulphamethoxazole. A case report. Acta Anaesthesiol Scand 1985; 453–455.
43. Kumar AR, Dunn N, Naqvi M. Methemoglobinemia associated with a prilocaine–lidocaine cream. Clin Pediatr 1997; 36: 239–240.
44. Frayling IM, Addison GM, Chattergee K, Meakin G. Methemoglobinaemia in children treated with prilocaine–lignocaine cream. Br Med J 1990; 301: 153–154.
45. Olson ML, McEvoy GK. Methemoglobinemia induced by local anesthetics. Am J Hosp Pract 1981; 38: 89–93.
46. Hall AH, Kulig KW, Rumack BH. Drug and chemical induced methemoglobinemia: clinical features and management. Med Toxicol 1986; 1: 253–260.
47. Archarya AB, Bustani PC, Phillips JD, et al. Randomised controlled trial of

eutectic mixture of local anaesthetics cream for venepuncture in healthy preterm infants. Arch Dis Child Fetal Neonatol 1998; 78: F138–F142.

48. EMLA: Prescribing information. Astra Pharmaceutical Products, Inc. 1998 Westborough, MA 01581.

49. Nilsson A, Engberg, Henneberg S, et al. Inverse relationship between age-dependent erythrocyte activity of methaemoglobin ductase and prilocaine-induced methaemoglobinemia during infancy. Br J Anaesth 1990; 64: 72–76.

50. Van Den Hove J, Decroix J, Tennstedt D, Lachapelle JM. Allergic contact dermatitis from prilocaine, one of the local anaesthetics in EMLA cream. Contact Dermatitis 1994; 30: 239.

51. le Coz CJ, Cribier BJ, Heid E. Patch testing in suspected allergic contact dermatitis due to EMLA cream in haemodialyzed patients. Contact Dermatitis 1996; 35: 316–317.

52. deWaard-van der Spek FB, van den Berg GM, Oranje AP. EMLA cream an improved local anesthetic: review of current literature. Pediatr Dermatol 1992; 9: 126–131.

53. Juhlin L, Rollman O. Vascular effects of a local anesthetic mixture in atopic dermatitis. Acta Dermatol Venereol 1984; 64: 439–440.

54. de Waard-van der Spek FB, Oranje AP. Purpura caused by EMLA is of toxic origin. Contact Dermatitis 1997; 36: 11–13.

55. Mofenson HC, Caraccio TR, Miller H, Greensher J. Lidocaine toxicity from topical mucosal application: with a review of the clinical pharmacology of lidocaine. Clin Pediatr 1983; 22: 190–192.

56. Milhaly GW, Moore CR, Thomas J, et al. The pharmacokinetics and metabolism of the anilide local anesthetics in neonates. Eur J Clin Pharmacol 1978; 13: 143–152.

57. Morselli PL. Clinical pharmocokinetics in neonates. Clin Pharmacokinet 1976; 1: 81–98.

58. Boyes RN, Scott DB, Jebson PJ, et al. Pharmacokinetics of lidocaine in man. Clin Pharmacol Ther 1971; 12; 105–116.

59. Resar LM, Helfaer MA. Recurrent seizures in a neonate after lidocaine administration. J Perinatol 1998; 18: 193–195.

60. Rothstein P, Dornbusch J, Shaywitz BA. Prolonged seizures associated with the use of viscous lidocaine. J Pediatr 1982; 101: 461–163.

61. Wehner D, Hamilton GC. Seizures following topical application of local anesthetics to burns patients. Ann Emerg Med 1984; 13: 456–458.

62. Marshall DA, Mertz PM, Eaglstein WH. Occlusive dressings: Does dressing type influence the growth of common bacterial pathogens? Arch Surg 1990; 125: 1136–1139.

63. Telfer N, Moy R. Wound care after office procedures. J Dermatol Surg Oncol 1993; 19: 722–731.

64. Noe, JM, Keller M. Can stitches get wet? Plast Reconstruct Surg 1988; 81: 82–84.

65. Lineaweaver W, Howard R, Soucy D, et al. Topical antimicrobial toxicity. Arch Surg 1985; 120: 267–270.

66. Niedner R, Schopf E. Inhibition of wound healing by antiseptics. Br J Dermatol 1986; 115; 41–44.

67. Cunningham BB, Bernstein L, Woodley DT. Wound dressings. In: Roenigk HH, Roenigk RK, eds. Dermatologic surgery principles and practice, 2nd edn. New York: Marcel Dekker, 1996; 131–148.

68. Zitelli J. Wound healing by first and second intention. In: Roenigk HH, Roenigk RK, eds. Dermatologic surgery principles and practice, 2nd edn. New York: Marcel Dekker, 1996; 101–130.

69. Eaglstein W, Mertz P. Inert vehicles do affect wound healing. J Invest Dermatol 1980; 74: 90–91.

70. McGrath MH. How topical dressings salvage questionable flaps: Experimental study. Plast Reconstruct Surg 1981; 67; 653.

71. Viala J, Simon L, Le Pommelet C, et al. Agranulocytosis after application of silver sulfadiazine in a 2-month old infant. Arch Pediatr 1997; 4; 1103–1106.

72. Doubleday CW. Who is Nikolsky and what does his sign mean? [letter]. J Am Acad Dermatol 1987; 16: 1054–1055.

73. Moss C, Gupta E. The Nikolsky sign in staphylococcal scalded skin syndrome. Arch Dis Child 1998; 79: 290.

74. Salopek TG. Nikolsky's sign: is it 'dry' or is it 'wet'? Br J Dermatol 1997; 136: 762–767.

75. Lewis FM, Colver GB, Slater DN. Darier's sign associated with non-Hodgkin's lymphoma. Br J Dermatol 1994; 130: 126–127.

76. Yen A, Sanchez R, Oblender M et al. Leukemia cutis: Darier's sign in a neonate with acute lymphoblastic leukemia. J Am Acad Dermatol 1996; 34: 375–378.

77. Ollivaud L, Cosnes A, Wechsler J, et al. Darier's sign in cutaneous large T-cell lymphoma. J Am Acad Dermatol 1996; 34: 506–507.

78. Zvulunov A, Rotem A, Merlob P, et al. Congenital smooth muscle hamartoma. Prevalence and clinical findings in 15 patients. Am J Dis Child 1990; 144: 782–784.

79. Johnson MD, Jacobs AH. Congenital smooth muscle hamartoma. A report of six cases and a review of the literature. [Review] Arch Dermatol 1989; 125: 820–822.

80. Berberian BJ, Burnett JW. Congenital smooth muscle hamartoma: a case report. Br J Dermatol 1986; 115: 711–714.

81. Felman YM, Nikitas, JA. Syphilis serology today. Arch Dermatol 1980; 116; 84–89.

82. Gilchrest BA, Fitzpatrick TB, Anderson RR, et al. Localization of melanin pigment on the skin with a Wood's lamp. Br J Dermatol 1977; 96: 245.

83. Pini G, Faulkner LB. Cerebellar involvement in hypomelanosis of Ito. Neuropediatrics 1995; 26: 208–10.

84. Bluestone M. Where is Roche taking PCR? Bio/Technology 1991; 9: 1028–1030.

85. Lo A C, Feldman SR. Polymerase chain reaction: Basic concepts and clinical applications in dermatology. J Am Acad Dermatol 1994; 30: 250–260.

86. Saiki RK, Scharf S, Faloona F, et al. Enzymatic amplification of beta-globin genomic sequences and restriction site analysis for diagnosis of sickle-cell anemia. Science 1985; 230: 1350–1354.

87. Mullis KB, Faloona FA. Specific synthesis of DNA in vitro via a polymerase-catalyzed chain reaction. Meth Enzymol 1987; 155; 335–350.

88. Eisenstein BI. The polymerase chain reaction: a new method of using molecular genetics for medical diagnosis. N Engl J Med 1990: 322: 178–183.

89. Ou CY, Kwok S, Mitchell SW, et al. DNA amplification for direct detection of HIV-1 in DNA of peripheral blood mononuclear cells. Science 1988; 239: 295–297.

90. Rogers MF, Ou CY, Rayfield M, et al. Use of the polymerase chain reaction for the early detection of the proviral sequences of human immunodeficiency virus in infants born to seropositive mothers. New York City collaborative study of maternal HIV transmission and Montefiore Medical Center HIV Perinatal Transmission Study Group. N Engl J Med 1989; 320: 1649–1654.

91. Shoji H, Koga M, Kusuhara, T, et al. Differentiation of herpes simplex virus 1 and 2 in cerebrospinal fluid of patients with HSV encephalitis and meningitis by stringent hybridization of PCR-amplified DNAs. J Neurol 1994; 241: 526–530.

92. Schlesinger Y, Tebas P, Gaudreault-Keener M, et al. Herpes simplex virus type 2 meningitis in the absence of genital lesions: Improved recognition with use of the polymerase chain reaction. Clin Infect Dis 1995; 20: 842–848.

93. Kawasaki ES, Clark SS, Coyne MY, et al. Diagnosis of chronic myeloid and acute lymphocytic leukemias by detection of leukemia-specific mRNA sequences amplified in vitro. Proc Natl Acad Sci 1988; 85: 5698–5702.

94. Wright PA, Wynford-Thomas D. The polymerase chain reaction: Miracle or mirage? A critical review of its uses and limitations in diagnosis and research. J Pathol 1990; 162: 99–117.

95. McGrath JA, Handyside AH. Preimplantation genetic diagnosis of

severe inherited skin diseases Exp Dermatol 1998; 7: 65–72.

96. Goltz RW. Polymerase chain reaction in dermatology. West J Med 1994; 160: 362.

97. Nahass GT, Goldstein BA, Zhu WY, et al. Comparison of Tzanck smear, viral culture, and DNA diagnostic methods in detection of herpes simplex and varicella-zoster infection. JAMA 1992; 268: 2541–2544.

98. Greer CE, Peterson SL, Kiviat NB, et al. PCR amplification from paraffin-embedded tissues. Effects of fixative and fixation time. Am J Clin Pathol 1991; 95: 117–124.

99. Werner M, Wilkens L, Aubele M, et al. Interphase cytogenetics in pathology: principles, methods, and applications of fluorescence in situ hybidization (FISH). Histochem Cell Biol 1997 108: 381–390.

100. Christiano AM, LaForgia S, Paller AS, et al. Prenatal diagnosis for recessive dystrophic epidermolysis bullosa in 10 families by mutation and haplotype analysis in the type VII collagen gene (coc 7A1). Mol Med 1996; 2: 59–76.

101. Christiano AM, Pulkkinen L, McGrath JA, et al. Mutation based prenatal diagnosis of Herlitz junctional epidermolysis bullosa. Prenatal Diagn 1997; 17: 343–354.

102. Rothnagel JA, Longley MA, Holder RA, et al. Prenatal diagnosis of epidermolytic hyperkeratosis by direct gene sequencing. J Invest Dermatol 1994; 102: 13–16.

103. Bianchi DW. Prenatal diagnosis by analysis fetal cells in maternal blood. J Pediatr 1995; 127: 847–856.

104. Handyside AH, Lesko JG, Tarin JJ, et al. Birth of a normal girl after in vitro fertilization and preimplantation diagnostic testing for cystic fibrosis. N Engl J Med 1992; 327: 905–909.

7

Transient Benign Cutaneous Lesions in the Newborn

Anne W. Lucky

Transient benign cutaneous lesions in the newborn are important to recognize. Not only can parents be reassured, but unnecessary and erroneous evaluation and treatment of presumed serious diseases can be prevented. This chapter discusses the most common transient benign conditions seen in neonates. Table 7-1 summarizes eight studies of the incidences of transient benign cutaneous lesions.[1-8] In some instances, racial and ethnic background may determine significant differences in the incidence of a disorder. Several excellent reviews of these conditions are also available.[9-16]

PAPULES AND PUSTULES

Milia

Milia are common papules that occur primarily on the face and scalp (Fig. 7-1). Clinically, they are tiny (up to 2 mm), white, smooth-surfaced papules, which are usually discrete, but their numbers may vary from a few to several dozen. They may be present at birth or appear later in infancy. Although they usually occur on the face, they may be found anywhere. Milia are tiny inclusion cysts within the epidermis that contain concentric layers of trapped keratinized stratum corneum. Primary milia are associated with pilosebaceous units arising from the infundibula of vellus hairs. Secondary milia usually appear after trauma and originate from a variety of epithelial structures, such as hair follicles, sweat ducts, sebaceous ducts, or epidermis.[17] Neonatal milia are presumably primary. The diagnosis is a clinical one. If confirmation is needed, a small incision with the tip of a #11 blade can release the contents, which appear either as a smooth, white ball or keratinous debris.

The most important differential diagnosis of milia is from sebaceous hyperplasia (see the following discussion), which also presents with small white papules. However, sebaceous hyperplasia tends to be clustered around the nose and a bit more yellow, and occurs in large plaques. Milia may be associated with certain syndromes, including junctional and dystrophic epidermolysis bullosa, where lesions appear in sites of healing erosions, and in orofacial–digital syndrome type I, which features congenital mouth malformations, distinct facial features, and brachydactyly.[18] In these cases milia are numerous and persistent.

Milia usually resolve spontaneously over several months without treatment. If persistent, lesions can be incised and

expressed, but this is rarely necessary. Why they occur with increased frequency in the newborn period is unknown.

Oral Mucosal Cysts of the Newborn (Palatal Cysts or Epstein's Pearls, and Alveolar Cysts or Bohn's Nodules)

Epstein's pearls and Bohn's nodules are actually both similar to milia, being microkeratocysts[19,20,21] located in the mouth. They are 1–2 mm, smooth, yellow to gray-white papules found singly or in clusters, most commonly on the median palatal raphe (68–81%). They also occur on the alveolar ridges (22%), more on the maxillary than the mandibular ridge, but rarely on both. They occur in 64–89% of normal neonates and are more common in Caucasian infants. A recent study from Taiwan of 420 neonates up to 3 days old examined by one dentist revealed a 94% incidence of oral cysts.[22]

When on the palate they have been called Epstein's pearls, and when on the alveolar ridges, Bohn's nodules. Although Bohn and others had presumed that these were mucous gland cysts, more recent studies have shown them to be keratin cysts derived from the dental lamina. Both of these epidermal cysts occur in keratinized mucous membranes and form in embryonic lines of fusion. Epstein's pearls originate from epithelial remnants after fusion of palatal shelves. In a recent study of 1021 Swedish neonates,[21] most of the palatal cysts had discharged spontaneously and resolved by age 5 months. Interestingly, 17 children developed new palatal cysts postnatally. However, most of the alveolar cysts regressed. A study of 60 premature compared to 60 term infants showed a lower prevalence in the prematures (9% vs 30%).[23] The diagnosis is clinical. Other congenital papules in the mouth include gingival (alveolar) cysts of the newborn, dental lamina cysts, congenital epulis (granular cell tumor), lymphangiomas, mucoceles, and ranulas[19] (see also Chapter 27.)

Perineal Median Raphe Cysts and Foreskin Cysts

Other common locations for epidermal inclusion cysts are in the foreskin and along the ventral surface of the penis and scrotum[24] (see Fig. 9.8) These lesions tend to be larger than the milia that appear on the head and neck, and may represent a developmental abnormality of fusion with entrapment of epidermal or urethral cells. Histologically, they usually have a

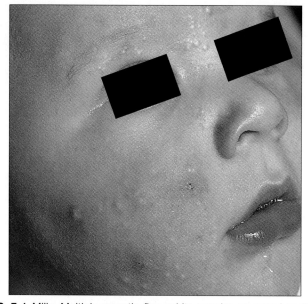

FIG. 7-1 Milia. Multiple smooth, firm, white papules are noted on the bridge of the nose; an acneiform eruption on the cheek is also evident in this young infant.

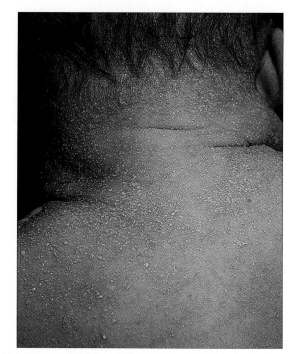

FIG. 7-2 Tiny superficial vesicles seen on the back and neck of this newborn are characteristic of miliaria crystallina.

TABLE 7-1 Incidence of common transient benign lesions in the neonate[1-8]	
Epstein's pearls	56–89%
Sebaceous hyperplasia	32–48%
Erythema toxicum	21–41%
Miliaria crystallina	3–15%
Mongolian spot	
African-American	64–96%
Asian	84–86%
Latino	46–65%
Caucasian	3–13%
Salmon patch	
African-American	59%
Asian	22%
Latino	68%
Caucasian	70%

stratified squamous epithelial lining, but may have pseudostratified columnar epithelium or ciliated or mucus-secreting cells as well, depending on from which part of the urethra they are derived. They often will enlarge throughout infancy and/or seem to appear after the newborn period, often in young men.[25] Some may be pigmented due to the presence of melanocytes and melanophages in the cyst lining.[26] They are benign and asymptomatic, although they may require surgical removal because of their large size or if they become infected.

Miliaria

Miliaria is a general term for describing obstructions of the eccrine duct.[27] Miliaria occurs in infants in warm climates, or those who are being kept warm or are febrile. It is thus more common in nonair-conditioned nurseries and in hot rather than in temperate climates.[4,6] The clinical manifestations of miliaria vary, depending on the level of the obstruction.

In the immediate newborn period the most common form of miliaria is the most superficial, miliaria crystallina (sudamina). In miliaria crystallina, ductal obstruction is subcorneal or intracorneal. Obstruction at this level leads to very superficial trapping of sweat under the stratum corneum, producing typical small, crystal-clear vesicles that resemble water droplets on the skin (Fig. 7-2). These vesicles are extremely fragile and may be wiped away on cleansing of the skin. Miliaria crystallina usually appears in the first few days of life, but there are reports of congenital lesions.[28-31] Occasionally there will be many neutrophils within the lesions, giving them a more pustular than vesicular appearance. The causes of ductal blockage or leakage are not known. Some authors, however, favor the hypothesis that the ductal occlusion is caused by extracellular polysaccharide substance (EPS) from *Staphylococcus epidermidis*.[32] Miliaria crystallina is precipitated by environmental overheating or fever, with consequent superficial retention of sweat in the obstructed ducts and surrounding epidermis. The diagnosis is clinical, although a smear of the clear fluid contents of the vesicles shows an absence of cellular material or, at most, a few neutrophils. Reducing the ambient temperature or treating the fever will prevent and/or treat miliaria. Miliaria crystallina is benign, but could be mistaken for more serious vesicular or pustular disorders such as herpes simplex.

Miliaria rubra is also common in overheated or febrile infants. Other terms for this disorder include 'heat rash' and 'prickly heat.' Miliaria rubra presents as erythematous, 1–3 mm papules or papulopustules on the head, neck, face, scalp, and trunk (Fig. 7-3). It can occur anywhere, but has a predilection for the forehead, upper trunk, and flexural or covered surfaces. The lesions are not follicular. When there is inflammation with multiple neutrophils in the lesions, as may be

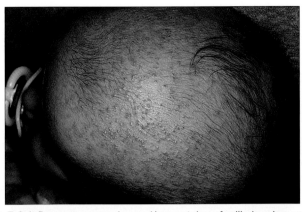

FIG. 7-3 Inflammatory papules and/or pustules of miliaria rubra are nonfollicular in distribution and are seen here on the scalp of an overheated newborn infant.

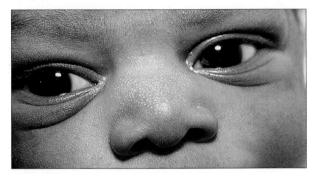

FIG. 7-4 Sebaceous hyperplasia is typically located on and surrounding the nose, with sheets of tiny white-yellow follicular papules without inflammation.

found under occlusion beneath monitor leads or bandages, miliaria rubra may look pustular and mimic worrisome conditions such as neonatal infections. Some authors subclassify this pustular form as miliaria pustulosa. Histologically, there is dermal inflammation around occluded eccrine ducts. The sweat duct obstruction is lower than in miliaria crystallina, but still intraepidermal. The diagnosis is made clinically, but if there is any doubt a biopsy will confirm eccrine duct occlusion. The erythematous papules of miliaria rubra may mimic a variety of neonatal conditions, such as neonatal acne, as well as candidal, staphylococcal, or herpes simplex infections. Correcting the overheating is usually sufficient to manage miliaria.

Miliaria profunda, the third and deepest level of sweat duct obstruction, has occlusion at or below the dermoepidermal junction. It is rare in the newborn period. In older children and adults, this deep obstruction causes white papules representing dermal edema and can actually prevent adequate sweating, leading to hyperthermia.

Sebaceous Hyperplasia

Sebaceous hyperplasia is most prominent on the face, especially around the nose and upper lip, where the density of sebaceous glands is highest. Sebaceous hyperplasia appears as follicular, regularly spaced, smooth white-yellow papules grouped into plaques (Fig. 7-4). There is no surrounding erythema. Hormonal (androgen) stimulation in utero, which comes from either the mother or the infant, causes hypertro-

phy of sebaceous glands. Premature infants are less affected, but sebaceous hyperplasia occurs in nearly half of term newborns.[6,7] Sebaceous hyperplasia gradually involutes in the first few weeks of life. The papules differ from milia, which are epidermal inclusion cysts, and are usually discrete, solitary, and whiter in color.

Erythema Toxicum Neonatorum (Toxic Erythema of the Newborn, 'Flea Bite' Dermatitis)

Erythema toxicum is unquestionably the best-known benign eruption in the newborn period, occurring in approximately half of term newborns.[29,32,33] Estimates of the incidence in large series range from 21% to 41%, but frequencies as high as 72% have been reported.[33] The discrepancies in estimates of incidence may be due to the length of time these infants were observed. The presence of erythema toxicum has been well correlated with birthweight and gestational age.[34] Other apparently associated environmental factors include first pregnancy, summer or autumn season, milk powder feedings, vaginal delivery, and duration of labor.[35] It is virtually never seen in premature infants or those weighing less than 2500 g. There is no sexual or racial predilection.[36] Congenital lesions can occur,[37-39] but the majority of cases have their onset between 24 and 48 hours of life. Lesions wax and wane, usually lasting a week or less, but cases lasting beyond 7 days have been reported. Occasionally very atypical presentations are seen (i.e. onset as late as 10 days of age) and pustules contain predominantly neutrophils,[36,40] but such cases require careful evaluation and skin biopsy to exclude other causes.

The classic eruption consists of barely elevated yellowish papules or pustules measuring 1–3 mm in diameter, with a surrounding irregular macular flare or wheal of erythema measuring 1–3 cm. The irregular shape of the flare has been likened to that of a flea bite (Fig. 7-5A). Although the characteristic lesions of erythema toxicum are usually discrete and scattered (Fig. 7-5B), extensive cases with either clusters of pustules, confluent papules, or pustules with surrounding erythema forming huge erythematous plaques can occur and be more difficult to diagnose (Fig. 7-5C). Lesions may appear first on the face and spread to the trunk and extremities, but may appear anywhere on the body except on the palms and soles.

Histologically, the lesions are eosinophilic pustules and characteristically intrafollicular, occurring subcorneally above the entry of the sebaceous duct.[41] This follicular location explains the absence of lesions on the palms and soles. Peripheral eosinophilia has also been associated in a minority (about 15%) of cases. The etiology of erythema toxicum is unknown: a graft-versus-host reaction against maternal lymphocytes has been postulated as a possible mechanism,[42] but there are no data to substantiate this claim. Another theory proposes an immune response to microbial colonization through the hair follicles as early as 1 day of age.[43] Immunohistochemical analysis of lesions from 1-day-old infants supports the accumulation and activation of immune cells in erythema toxicum lesions.[44]

The diagnosis of erythema toxicum can usually be made by clinical appearance alone, but simple scraping of the pustule, smearing the contents onto a glass slide, and staining with Wright or Giemsa stain will reveal sheets of eosinophils with a few scattered neutrophils. Skin biopsy is rarely needed.

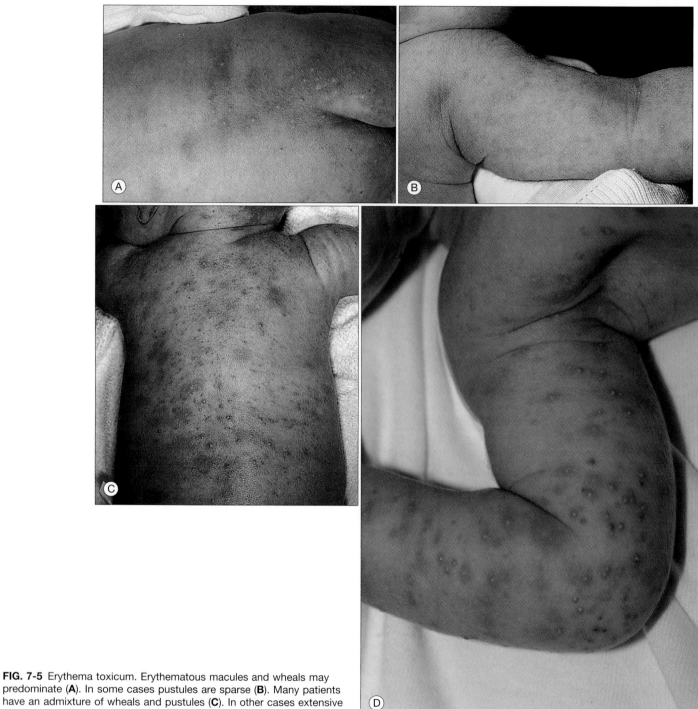

FIG. 7-5 Erythema toxicum. Erythematous macules and wheals may predominate (**A**). In some cases pustules are sparse (**B**). Many patients have an admixture of wheals and pustules (**C**). In other cases extensive pustules predominate (**D**).

The differential diagnosis of erythema toxicum includes other pustular disorders of the newborn: infantile acropustulosis has a more acral rather than truncal distribution; herpes simplex has a more vesicular character, with subsequent crusting; staphylococcal impetigo has more well-developed pustules; congenital candidiasis has a positive KOH and can be more scaly. Transient neonatal pustular melanosis (TNPM) (see the following discussion) has primarily neutrophils in the infiltrate and is present at birth, and the pustules quickly disappear, leaving pigmented macules, but erythema toxicum and TNPM may appear together in some infants. Miliaria rubra can also present with erythematous papulopustules, but these favor the head and neck and are smaller lesions without the erythematous flare. No therapy is needed for erythema toxicum except for parental reassurance.

Transient Neonatal Pustular Melanosis

This disorder was first described in 1976,[45] although it had undoubtedly occurred before that time. In fact, an abstract in 1961[46] is likely to be the first description of TNPM, which was then called 'lentigines neonatorum.' It occurs primarily in full-term African descent infants in both sexes. In the 1976 report, 4.4% of African-American and 0.6% of Caucasian infants were affected.[45] Lesions were always present at birth.

TNPM has three phases and hence three types of lesion. First, very superficial vesicopustules, ranging in size from 2 mm to as large as 10 mm, may be present in utero and are virtually always evident at birth (Fig. 7-6A). Because they are intracorneal and subcorneal, and thus very fragile, the pustules may be easily wiped away during the initial cleaning of the infant to remove vernix caseosa, so that the pustular phase may not be evident (Fig. 7-6B). The second phase is represented by a fine collarette of scale around the resolving pustule (Fig. 7-6C). The third phase consists of hyperpigmented brown macules at the site of previous pustulation (Fig. 7-6D). Although these macules have been called 'lentigines' (because of their resemblance to lentils), they are not true lentigines but appear to represent transient postinflammatory hyperpigmentation. They may last for up to several months before they fade. Some infants are born with these macules, the pustular phase having presumably occurred in utero. The most common location for TNPM has been under the chin, on the forehead,

at the nape, and on the lower back and shins, although the face, trunk, palms, and soles are also affected.

The etiology of TNPM is unknown. However, some authors[47,48] have postulated that TNPM is a precocious form of erythema toxicum neonatorum, with clinical and histologic overlap. They have proposed the term sterile transient neonatal pustulosis to describe this overlap entity. It is more likely, however, that these two conditions, which are both common, may coexist. In most infants there is little confusion based either on clinical appearance or time of onset.

Smears of the contents of the pustules stained with Giemsa or Wright stain show predominantly neutrophils, although a few eosinophils have also been reported. A biopsy is rarely needed for diagnosis. Histologically, these lesions consist of subcorneal pustules filled with neutrophils, fibrin, and rare eosinophils.[47] The differential diagnosis of TNPM includes the following:

- Erythema toxicum neonatorum, which appears a few days after birth and is inflammatory, and whose vesicles contain primarily eosinophils
- Staphylococcal impetigo, which shows Gram-positive cocci on smear and positive cultures

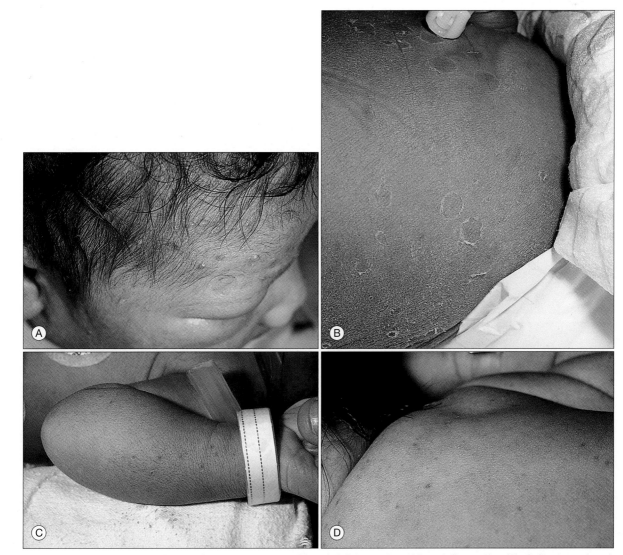

FIG. 7-6 Transient neonatal pustular melanosis first appears as small, superficial pustules without inflammation (**A**). Collarettes of scale, typical of the second stage, are occasionally seen at birth without evident pustules (**B**), or may develop after pustules have ruptured (**C**). The final stage is that of small hyperpigmented macules resembling lentils, which gradually fade over weeks to months (**D**).

- Neonatal candidiasis, which reveals pseudohyphae and spores on KOH examination
- Miliaria crystallina or rubra, which would not leave post-inflammatory hyperpigmentation
- Acropustulosis of infancy, which usually appears later and predominates on the hands and feet.

Although the pustules of TNPM resolve rapidly, the pigmented macules may take weeks to months to fade away. No treatment is needed except parental reassurance.

Neonatal and Infantile Acne

Neonatal and infantile acne are distinct entities distinguishable by time of onset and clinical features. Neonatal acne may occur at birth and usually appears within the first 2–3 weeks of life. This disorder is currently under close scrutiny as to its existence and/or etiology: is it acne or another pustular disorder of infancy? The term "neonatal cephalic pustulosis" has been proposed to replace the term neonatal acne. Classically, neonatal acne has been described as inflammatory, erythematous papules and pustules, located primarily on the cheeks, but scattered over the face and often extending onto the scalp[49–52] (Fig. 7-7). Comedonal lesions are absent. There has been a recent hypothesis that these erythematous papulopustules seen in the first month of life may be an inflammatory reaction to *Pityrosporum* (*Malassezia*) species, both *M. furfur* and *M. sympodialis*.[53–57] In addition, clinical differentiation between neonatal acne and miliaria rubra may be impossible. Biopsies would aid in diagnosis, but they are not justified as both conditions are benign and transient.

A later form of acne has been termed infantile acne.[49–51] This may be due to a persistence of neonatal acne or a later onset of true acne at 2–3 months of age. Infantile acne shows typical acneiform lesions, including open and closed comedones, as well as papules, pustules, and occasionally nodules (Fig. 7-8). It is found primarily on the face.

Infantile acne has been considered to be an androgen-driven condition with hyperplasia of sebaceous activity.[58] It may rarely be a sign of underlying androgen excess, such as in congenital adrenal hyperplasia, steroid-producing gonadal or adrenal tumor, or true precocious puberty. There is usually spontaneous resolution in the first 6–12 months of life. This would correlate well with what is known about neonatal androgens. The fetal adrenal gland is really an enlarged zona reticularis, which is the androgen-producing zone of the adrenal, producing pubertal levels of dehydroepiandrosterone (DHEA) and its sulfate (DHEAS), which wane over the first 6

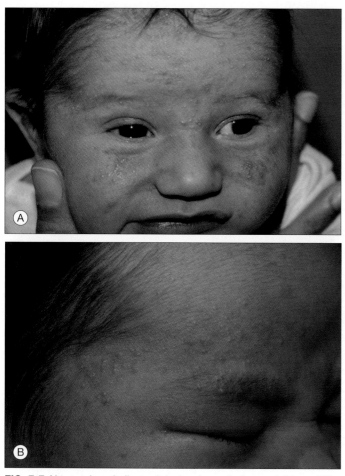

FIG. 7-7 Neonatal cephalic pustulosis, also called neonatal 'acne' (**A, B**), is usually found on the cheeks and scalp in the first 2–4 weeks of life; small red papules and pustules without comedones are evident.

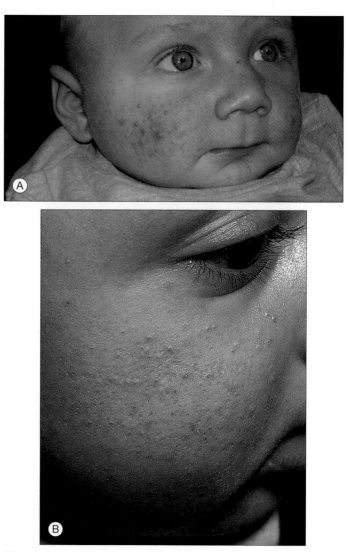

FIG. 7-8 True infantile acne (**A, B**). This is a form of acne vulgaris with the features of adolescent acne, including open and closed comedones and inflammatory papules.

months of life in both male and female infants. In the male, testicular testosterone is also elevated for the first 6–12 months of life, perhaps explaining the observation that males are more affected with infantile acne than are females.

Whereas neonatal acne resolves spontaneously without treatment, infantile acne may be more persistent and even cause scarring, and can benefit from treatment. Small inflammatory papules and pustules respond to topical benzoyl peroxide or erythromycin. Topical tretinoin in low concentrations (0.01% gel or 0.025% cream) can be used for open and closed comedones. Erythromycin is the only appropriate systemic antibiotic for larger papules or pustules that may scar. Tetracyclines are contraindicated because they cause permanent tooth staining. In rare cases of severe, scarring nodular infantile acne, systemic isotretinoin has been used safely and effectively.[59–64]

SUCKING BLISTERS, EROSIONS, PADS, AND CALLUSES

Sucking blisters, erosions, and calluses on the hands and forearms are present at birth and can be solitary or bilateral.[65] Although the primary lesion from sucking is usually a tense, fluid-filled blister on normal-appearing skin (Fig. 7-9), when the blister has ruptured an erosion may result, or if the sucking has been less vigorous and more chronic, the lesion may become a callus. These lesions appear to result from repetitive vigorous sucking in utero at one particular spot. Often when the neonate is presented after birth with the affected extremity, he/she will immediately demonstrate sucking behavior on that area. Sucking blisters on the extremities may be mistaken for other serious disorders such as herpes simplex, but their solitary, asymmetric nature and characteristic location should help to establish the correct diagnosis.

In infants who are vigorous suckers postnatally, sucking pads or calluses can also occur on the lips (see Fig. 27-9). These occur postnatally and should be differentiated from the lesions on the extremities. Sucking calluses appear on the mucosa caudal to the closure line of infants' lips and are hyperkeratotic pads which eventually desquamate over 3–6 months.[66] Histologically, there is epithelial hyperplasia and intracellular edema secondary to friction. No therapy is required.

UMBILICAL GRANULOMA, PATENT URACHUS AND OMPHALOMESENTERIC DUCT REMNANT (UMBILICAL POLYP)

In some neonates, granulation tissue develops at the umbilical stump after the cord dries up and falls off, usually 6–8 days after birth. In most infants the raw surface of the umbilicus heals within 12–15 days.[67,68] Umbilical granulomata are grayish-pink papules on the umbilical stump. They are extremely friable and bleed easily to touch. They have a 'velvety' feel to the surface.

The etiology of umbilical granulomas is failure of the surface of the proximal portion of the cord to heal and subsequent proliferation of endothelial cells without atypia.[69] The term granuloma is misleading, because these lesions are composed of proliferating endothelial cells, like pyogenic granulomas, and are not true granulomas.

The diagnosis is clinical (Fig. 7-10). However, it is important to distinguish umbilical granulomas from other embryonic remnants. The normal umbilical cord consists of two umbilical arteries, one umbilical vein, a rudimentary allantois attached to the bladder (urachus), and a remnant of the vitelline (omphalomesenteric duct) attached to the ileum.[67] The proximal end of the vitelline duct creates Meckel's diverticulum. A patent urachus will intermittently discharge urine. A persistent vitelline duct will have a malodorous discharge. An umbilical polyp is a distal remnant of the vitelline duct that creates an erythematous papule similar in appearance to an umbilical granuloma, but the surface is sticky because of mucus secreted from the intestinal mucosa (see Figs 9-28 and 9-29).[70] These developmental lesions all require surgical therapy. When talc-containing powders are used on the umbilical stump, talc granulomas can also form and look identical to umbilical granulomas.

The traditional treatment of umbilical granulomas is topical application of silver nitrate. Care must be taken to very lightly touch only the granulomas; otherwise burns may occur on the surrounding normal skin.[71] If lesions fail to respond to one or two treatments, then serious consideration should be given to alternative diagnoses. Most umbilical granulomas are seen and treated by pediatricians and rarely come to the attention of the dermatologist.

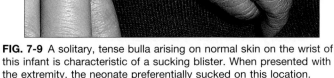

FIG. 7-9 A solitary, tense bulla arising on normal skin on the wrist of this infant is characteristic of a sucking blister. When presented with the extremity, the neonate preferentially sucked on this location.

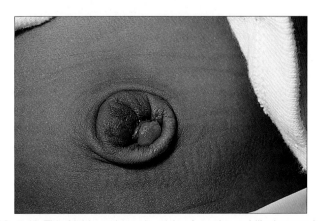

FIG. 7-10 This friable, red papule arising from the umbilical stump is a typical umbilical granuloma.

COLOR CHANGES IN THE NEWBORN

Pigmentary Abnormalities Resulting from Abnormalities of Melanin Dermal Melanosis (Mongolian Spots)

Mongolian spots are collections of melanocytes located in the dermis. They are macules or patches that may be solitary and measure a few millimeters, or multiple and several centimeters in size. They are a distinctive slate blue, gray, or black (Fig. 7-11) and are most commonly located over the buttocks and sacrum, but often occur elsewhere.[2,72] Over the buttocks, Mongolian spots are seen in up to 96% of African-American, 86% of Asian, and 13% of Caucasian neonates (Box 7-1). In

---

Box 7-1 Color changes in the neonate

Pigmentary
1. Melanin
   a. Dermal melanosis (Mongolian spots)
   b. Hyperpigmentation
   c. Hypopigmentation
2. Nonmelanin
   a. Bilirubin
   b. Meconium
   c. Vernix

Vascular
1. Vasomotor instability
   a. Cutis marmorata
   b. Acrocyanosis
   c. Harlequin color change
2. Rubor
3. Twin transfusion
4. Transient capillary vascular malformations

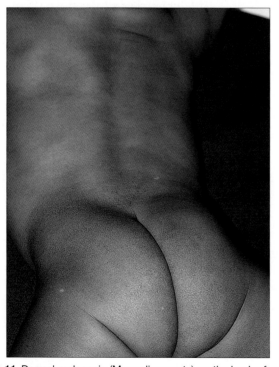

FIG. 7-11 Dermal melanosis (Mongolian spots) on the back of an African-American infant, which will most likely fade over several years.

this location they usually resolve over several years. Similarly appearing dermal melanosis in other locations such as the arms and shoulders (nevus of Ito) or around the cheek and eye, including the sclera (nevus of Ota), may not resolve at all. The blue color of dermal melanosis is a result of the Tyndall effect, in which red wavelengths of light are absorbed and blue wavelengths are reflected back from the brown melanin pigment located deep in the dermis. The pathogenesis is postulated to be a defect in migration of pigmented neural crest cells, which usually reside at the dermoepidermal junction. Histologically, spindle-shaped melanocytes are dispersed within dermal collagen. No treatment is recommended for dermal melanosis. Extensive Mongolian spots have been described in infants with GM1 gangliosidosis (see Chapter 22).

The pigmentation of nevus of Ota has been successfully treated with the Q-switched ruby laser.[73] A small risk of melanoma exists for a nevus of Ota. It is most important to distinguish dermal melanosis from bruising, which would undergo a sequential color change from blue-black to green to yellow, so that there is no confusion about possible child abuse.

Epidermal Hyperpigmentation

In more darkly pigmented neonates, transient, nearly black hyperpigmentation can be observed in the genital areas on the labia and scrotum (Fig. 7-12A, B), in a linear fashion on the lower abdomen (linea nigra), around the areolae, in the axillae, on the pinnae, and at the base of the fingernails (Fig. 7-12C).[13] This is believed to be due to stimulation by melanocyte-stimulating hormone (MSH) in utero, but the mechanism is unclear.

Other nonhormonal patterns of brown hyperpigmentation have also been reported. Horizontal bands of hyperpigmentation corresponding to creases in the abdomen (Fig. 7-13A)[74] or on the back seem to reflect flexion in utero. They are transient and are thought to be a result of mechanical trauma from hyperkeratosis within the folds. Transient reticulated or linear pigmentation on the back and knees has also been reported (Fig. 7-13B),[75] presumably as a result of posttraumatic hyperpigmentation in utero.

The most important differential diagnosis of the neonate with hormonally induced hyperpigmentation is congenital adrenal hyperplasia (CAH). In this life-threatening condition there is massive stimulation by adrenocorticotropic hormone (ACTH) resulting from an enzyme block in the synthesis of cortisol. The hyperpigmentation is believed to be due to cross-reactivity of ACTH with MSH receptors. Children with CAH also have ambiguous genitalia and will die if not promptly diagnosed and treated with replacement cortisol.

Hypopigmentation

African-American and Asian infants often have much lighter overall pigmentation in the newborn period, which gradually darkens over the first year of life. Generalized hypopigmentation is also seen in genetic conditions such as phenylketonuria (PKU), Menkes' syndrome, Chediak–Higashi syndrome, and albinism (see Chapter 21).

Pigmentary Changes not Caused by Melanin

Physiologic jaundice results from transient elevation of serum bilirubin, resulting in a generalized yellow discoloration of the

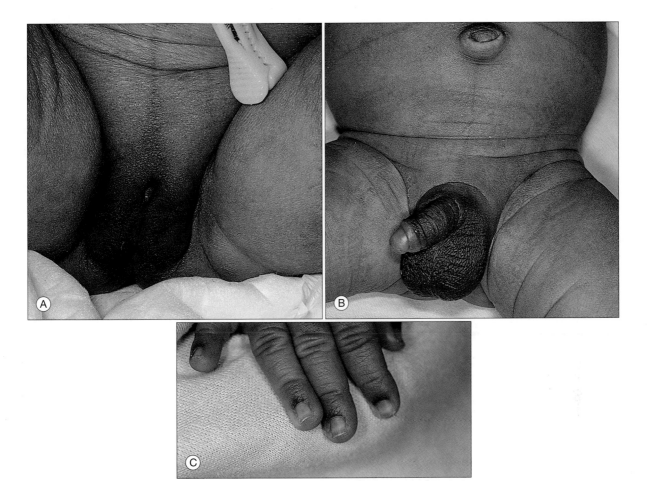

FIG. 7-12 Intense hyperpigmentation. In neonates with dark skin, transient accentuation of nearly black pigmentation can be seen in several locations on the vulva (**A**), scrotum (**B**), lower abdomen (linea nigra) (**A**, **B**), and base of the fingernails (**C**).

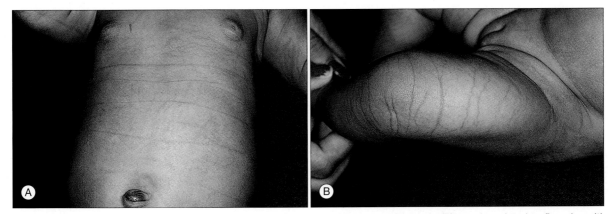

FIG. 7-13 Horizontal linear hyperpigmentation in the creases on the abdomen (**A**) or over the knees (**B**) may be related to flexed positions and hyperkeratosis in utero.

skin in the first few days of life (Fig. 7-14). With jaundice, in contrast to carotenemia, which may occur later in infancy at age 1–2 years, there is yellow discoloration of the sclerae as well as the skin. Physiologic jaundice fades after the bilirubin returns to normal.

Meconium staining often will darken the vernix caseosa but can also leave patchy, yellow-brown pigmentation, especially on desquamating epidermis.

Color Changes Resulting from Vascular Abnormalities
Cutaneous Vasomotor Instability
The ability of neonates to adjust to extrauterine surroundings is at first immature, and they can exhibit distinct cutaneous blood flow abnormalities. When neonates are cold, their constricted capillaries and venules may produce a reticulated, mottled, blanchable, violaceous pattern termed cutis marmo-

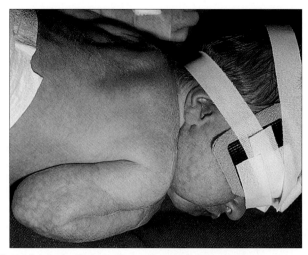

FIG. 7-14 Infant with jaundice undergoing phototherapy.

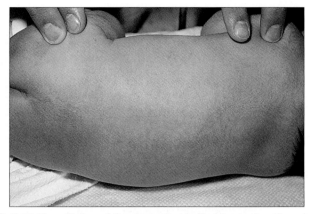

FIG. 7-17 Vasodilation of the dependent half of the body with a sharp midline cutoff is typical of a harlequin color change.

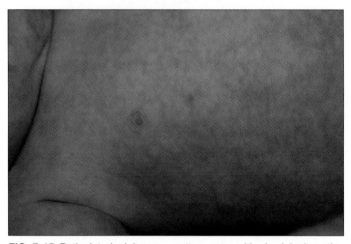

FIG. 7-15 Reticulated, violaceous pattern seen with physiologic cutis marmorata. A small accessory nipple, a common anomaly, is noted.

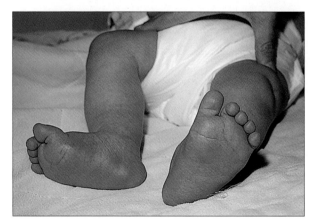

FIG. 7-16 Acrocyanosis. Purplish discoloration of the feet on exposure to cold.

rata (Fig. 7-15). Exposure to cold temperatures may also induce more vasoconstriction in acral than central areas of the body, resulting in deep violaceous to blue coloration of the hands, feet and lips, termed acrocyanosis (Fig. 7-16). Both of these conditions occur more often in premature infants.

These transient conditions rapidly improve upon rewarming of the infant, and the tendency to occur diminishes with age. Cutis marmorata should not be confused with cutis marmorata telangiectatica congenita, a vascular malformation that persists for several years and occurs in large, well-defined patches.

The so-called 'harlequin' color change is a rare physiologic phenomenon whereby the amount of blood flow differs markedly on the right and left sides of the body, with a sharp cutoff at the midline.[76] This is most often seen when a child is lying on one side, the dependent side exhibiting vasodilation and being strikingly redder than the upper half of the body (Fig. 7-17). The face and genitalia may be spared. Episodes last from seconds to minutes and are rapidly reversible with a change in position or increased activity. It is more common in premature infants, but can affect up to 10% of full-term babies. Its onset is at 2–5 days of age, and the phenomenon lasts up to 3 weeks. There is no pathologic significance.

Rubor Resulting from Excessive Hemoglobin

Because newborns have high levels of hemoglobin in the first weeks of life there is generalized rubor, which fades as the hemoglobin physiologically drops to normal levels. Twin transfusion may occur in twins as a result of shunting of blood from one to the other, resulting in a major color difference at birth, reflecting a marked discrepancy in hemoglobin levels between the two infants.

Capillary Ectasias (Nevus Simplex, Salmon Patch)

Erythematous macules and patches occurring over the occiput, eyelids, glabella, and, to a lesser extent, the nose and upper lip are minor vascular malformations consisting of ectatic capillaries in the upper dermis with normal overlying skin (Fig. 7-18). They occur in 70% of white, 59% of African-American, 68% of Latino, and 22% of Asian newborns,[3] and have been given the common designations 'angel's kisses' (eyelids) or 'stork bites' (nape) (see Table 7-1). Most resolve over several months to years, but 25–50% of nuchal lesions and a much smaller percentage of the glabellar lesions may persist into adult life. The primary differential diagnosis of these benign transient lesions is port-wine stains, which are usually more lateral in location, do not resolve, and often continue to darken and thicken with age. These stains, particularly the glabellar ones, are often inherited as an autosomal dominant trait.

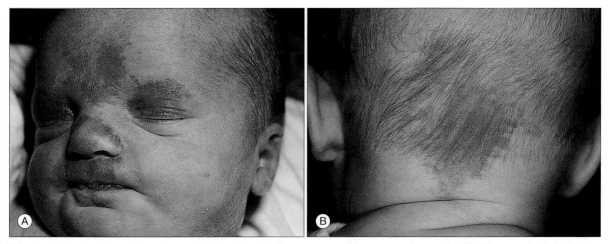

FIG. 7-18 Salmon patch. An infant with salmon patch on the glabella, nevus, eyelids, nose and upper lip (**A**). The nape is the most common location for a salmon patch (**B**).

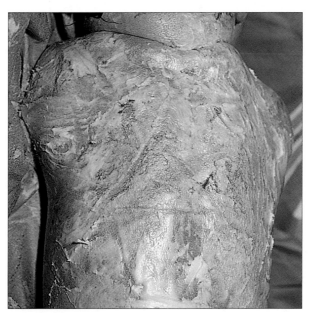

FIG. 7-19 The vernix caseosa is a white to grey, cheesy, greasy layer of sebum, keratin, and hair which has protected the fetus in utero.

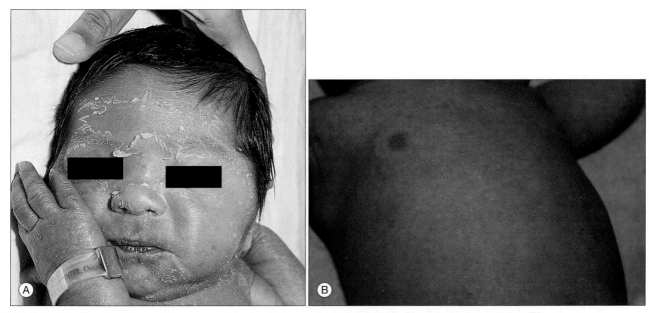

FIG. 7-20 Extensive desquamation can be a normal finding in the postmature infant (**A**). Physiologic dequamation (**B**).

VERNIX CASEOSA

Vernix caseosa is notable on the surface of the skin at birth as a chalky-white mixture of shed epithelial cells, sebum, and sometimes hair (Fig. 7-19). The vernix presumably serves as a lubricant to protect the infant skin from amniotic fluid. It enhances skin hydration and provides a natural barrier.[77] Recent studies support its role in natural defense from microbes because it contains antimicrobial peptides and lipids.[78,79] It becomes thicker with advancing gestational age, although postmature infants usually have no vernix.[12] In infants who have prepartum passage of meconium the vernix may be stained yellow-brown, and this can be a clue to fetal distress.

DESQUAMATION

Most full-term infants will have fine desquamation of the skin at 24–48 hours of age. Premature infants do not show desquamation until 2–3 weeks of life. The postmature infant, however, is often born with cracking and peeling of the skin that is much greater in intensity than in full-term or premature infants (Fig. 7-20). The differential diagnosis of physiologic desquamation includes various forms of ichthyosis, as well as hypohidrotic ectodermal dysplasia. These are discussed in detail in Chapters 18 and 26.

REFERENCES

1. Jacobs AH, Walton RG. The incidence of birthmarks in the neonate. Pediatrics 1976; 58: 218–222.
2. Cordova A. The Mongolian spot: A study of ethnic differences and a literature review. Clin Pediatr Phil 1981; 20: 714–719.
3. Alper JC, Holmes LB. The incidence and significance of birthmarks in a cohort of 4641 newborns. Pediatr Dermatol 1983; 1: 58–68.
4. Hidano A, Purwoko R, Jitsukawa K. Statistical survey of skin changes in Japanese neonates. Pediatr Dermatol 1986; 3: 140–144.
5. Osburn K, Schosser RH, Everett MA. Congenital pigmented and vascular lesions in newborn infants. J Am Acad Dermatol 1987; 16: 788–792.
6. Nanda A, Kaur S, Bhakoo ON, Dhall K. Survey of cutaneous lesions in Indian newborns. Pediatr Dermatol 1989; 6: 39–42.
7. Rivers JK, Frederiksen PC, Dibdin C. A prevalence survey of dermatoses in the Australian neonate. J Am Acad Dermatol 1990; 23: 77–81.
8. Tsai FJ, Tsai CH. Birthmarks and congenital skin lesions in Chinese newborns. J Formos Med Assoc 1993; 92: 838–841.
9. Hodgman JE, Freedman RI, Levine NE. Neonatal dermatology. Pediatr Clin North Am 1971; 18: 713–756.
10. Solomon LM, Esterly NB. Transient cutaneous lesions. In: Neonatal dermatology. Philadelphia: WB Saunders, 1973; 43–48.
11. Schachner L, Press S. New clinical, diagnostic and therapeutic aspects of vesiculo bullous disorders in infancy and childhood. Pediatr Ann 1982; 11: 213–224.
12. Wagner AM, Hansen RC. Neonatal skin and skin disorders. In: Schachner LA, Hansen RC, eds. Pediatric dermatology, 2nd edn. New York: Churchill Livingstone, 1995; 263–283.
13. Rudolph AJ. Dermatology and perinatal infection. In: Atlas of the newborn. Hamilton, Ontario: BC Decker, 1997.
14. Treadwell PA. Dermatoses in newborns. Am Fam Phys 1997; 56: 443–450.

15. Van Praag MG, Van Rooij RG, Folkers E, et al. Diagnosis and treatment of pustular disorders in the neonate. Pediatr Dermatol 1997; 14: 131–143.
16. Wagner A. Distinguishing vesicular and pustular disorders in the neonate. Curr Opin Pediatr 1997; 9: 396–405.
17. Lever WF, Schaumberg-Lever G. Histology of the skin. Philadelphia: JB Lippincott, 1990; 536.
18. Larralde de Luna M, Raspa ML, Ibargoyen J. Oral-facial-digital type 1 syndrome of Papillon-Leage and Psaume. Pediatr Dermatol 1992; 9: 52–56.
19. Eisen D, Lynch DP. Developmental disorders. In: The mouth: Diagnosis and treatment. St Louis: Mosby, 1998: pp 37–57.
20. Jorgenson RJ, Shapiro SD, Salinas CF, Levin LS. Intraoral findings and anomalies in neonates. Pediatrics 1982; 69: 577–582
21. Flinck A, Paludan A, Matsson L, et al. Oral findings in a group of newborn Swedish children. Int J Paediatr Dentis 1994; 4: 67–73.
22. Liu MH, Huang. Oral abnormalities in Taiwanese newborns. J Dent Child 2004; 71: 118–120.
23. Donley CL, Nelson LP. Comparison of palatal and alveolar cysts of the newborn in premature and full term infants. Pediatr Dent 2000; 22: 321–324.
24. LeVasseur JG, Perry VE. Perineal median raphe cyst. Pediatr Dermatol 1997; 5: 391–392.
25. Nagor E, Sanchez-Motilla WH, Febrer JM, et al. Median raphe cysts of the penis: a report of five cases. Pediatr Dermatol 1998; 15: 191–193.
26. Urahashi J, Hara H, Yamaguchi ZI, Morishima T. Pigmented median raphe cysts of the penis. Acta Dermatol Venereol 2000; 80: 297–298.
27. Feng E, Janniger C. Miliaria. Cutis 1995; 55: 213–216.
28. Straka BF, Cooper PH, Greer KE. Congenital miliaria crystallina. Cutis 1991; 47: 103–106.
29. Arpey CJ, Nagashima-Whalen LS, Chren MM, et al. Congenital miliaria crystallina: Case report and literature review. Pediatr Dermatol 1992; 9: 283–287.

30. Haas, N, Henz, BM, Weigel, H, Congenital miliaria crystallina. J Am Acad Dermatol 2002; 47: S270–S272.
31. Gan VN, Hoang MP. Generalized vesicular eruption in a newborn. Pediatr Dermatol 2004; 21: 171–173.
32. Mowad CM, McGinley KJ, Foglia A, et al. The role of extracellular polysaccharide substance produced by *Staphylococcus epidermidis* in miliaria. J Am Acad Dermatol 1995; 33: 729–733.
33. Harris JR, Schick B. Erythema neonatorum. Am J Dis Child 1956; 92: 27–33.
34. Carr JA, Hodgman JE, Freedman RI, et al. Relationship between toxic erythema and infant maturity. Am J Dis Child 1966; 112: 129–134.
35. Liu C, Feng J, Qu R, et al. Epidemiologic study of the predisposing factors in erythema toxicum neonatorum.
36. Chang MW, Jiang SB, Orlow SJ. Atypical erythema toxicum neonatorum of delayed onset in a term infant. Pediatr Dermatol 1999; 16: 137–141.
37. Levy HL, Cothran F. Erythema toxicum neonatorum present at birth. Am J Dis Child 1962; 103: 125–127.
38. Marino LJ. Toxic erythema present at birth. Arch Dermatol 1965; 92: 402–403.
39. Maffei FA, Michaels MG. An unusual presentation of erythema toxicum: scrotal pustules present at birth. Arch Pediatr Adolesc Med 1996; 150: 649–650.
40. Berg FJ, Solomon LM. Erythema neonatorum toxicum. Arch Dis Child 1987; 62: 327–328.
41. Luders D. Histologic observations in erythema toxicum neonatorum. Pediatrics 1960; 26: 219–224.
42. Bassukus ID. Is erythema toxicum neonatorum a mild self-limited acute cutaneous graft-versus-host-reaction from maternal-to-fetal lymphocyte transfer? Med Hypotheses 1992; 38: 334–338.
43. Marchini G, Nelson A, Edner J, et al. Erythema toxicum neonatorum is an innate immune response to commensal microbes penetrated into the skin of the newborn infant.

44. Marchini G, Ulfgrcn AK, Lore K, et al. Erythema toxicum neonatorum: an immunohistochemical analysis. Pediatr Dermatol 2001; 18: 177–187.

45. Ramamurthy RS, Reveri M, Esterly NB, et al. Transient neonatal pustular melanosis. J Pediatr 1976; 88: 831–835.

46. Perrin E, Sutherland J, Baltazar S. Inquiry onto the nature of lentigines neonatorum: Demonstration of a statistical relationship with squamous metaplasia of the amnion. Am J Dis Child 1961; 102: 648–649.

47. Barr RJ, Globerman LM, Werber FA. Transient neonatal pustular melanosis. Int J Dermatol 1979; 18: 636–638.

48. Ferrandiz C, Coroleu W, Ribera M, et al. Sterile transient neonatal pustulosis is a precocious form of erythema toxicum neonatorum. Dermatology 1992; 185: 18–22.

49. Jansen T, Burgdorf WHC, Plewig G. Pathogenesis and treatment of acne in childhood. Pediatr Dermatol 1997; 14: 17–21.

50. Lucky AW. A review of infantile and pediatric acne. Dermatology 1998; 196: 95–97.

51. Lucky AW. Acne therapy in infancy and childhood. Dermatol Ther 1998; 6: 74–81.

52. Cunliffe WJ, Baron SE, Coulson IH. A clinical and therapeutic study of 29 patients with infantile acne. Br J Dermatol 2001; 145: 463–466.

53. Rapelanoro R, Mortureux P, Couprie B, et al. Neonatal *Malassezia furfur* pustulosis. Arch Dermatol 1996; 132: 190–193.

54. Bordazzi F. Transient cephalic neonatal pustulosis. Arch Dermatol 1997; 133: 528–529.

55. Niamba P, Weill FX, Sarlangue J, et al. Is common neonatal cephalic pustulosis (neonatal acne) triggered by *Malassezia sympodialis*? Arch Dermatol 1998; 134: 995.

56. Bernier V, Weill FX, Hirigoyen V, et al. Skin colonization by *Malassezia* species in neonates. Arch Dermatol 2002; 138: 215–218.

57. Bergman, JN, Eichenfield, LF, Neonatal acne and cephalic pustulosis: is *Malassezia* the whole story? Arch Dermatol 2002; 138: 255–256.

58. MacFarlane JT, Davies D. Infantile acne associated with transient increases in plasma concentrations of luteinising hormone, follicle-stimulating hormone and testosterone. Br Med J 1981; 282: 1275–1276.

59. Burket JM, Storrs FJ. Nodulocystic infantile acne occurring in a kindred of steatocystoma. Arch Dermatol 1987; 123: 432–433.

60. Arbegast KD, Braddock SW, Lamberty LF, et al. Treatment of infantile cystic acne with oral isotretinoin: a case report. Pediatr Dermatol 1991; 2: 166–168.

61. Horne HL, Carmichael AJ. Juvenile nodulocystic acne responding to systemic isotretinoin [letter]. Br J Dermatol 1997; 136: 796–797.

62. Mengesha YM, Hansen R. Toddler-age nodulocystic acne. J Pediatr 1999; 134: 644–648.

63. Barnes CJ, Eichenfield LF, Lee J, Cunningham BB. A practical approach for the use of oral isotretinoin for infantile acne. Pediatr Dermatol 2005; 22: 166–169.

64. Torrelo A, Pastor MA, Zambrano A. Severe acne infantum successfully treated with isotretinoin. Pediatr Dermatol 2005; 22: 357–359.

65. Murphy WF, Langly AN. Common bullous lesions – presumably self-inflicted – occurring in utero in the newborn infant. Pediatrics 1963; 32: 1099–1100.

66. Heyl T, Raubenheimer EJ. Sucking pads (sucking calluses) of the lips in neonates: A manifestation of transient leukoedema. Pediatr Dermatol 1987; 4: 123–128.

67. McCallum DI, Hall GFM. Umbilical granuloma with particular reference to talc granuloma. Br J Dermatol 1970; 83: 151–156.

68. Andreassi L. Diseases of the umbilicus. In: Ruiz-Maldonado R, Parish LC, Beane JM, eds. Textbook of pediatric dermatology. Philadelphia: Grune & Stratton, 1989; 820–822.

69. Johnson BL, Honig PG, Jaworsky C. Pediatric dermatopathology. Boston: Butterworth –Heinemann, 1994; 16–17.

70. Pomeranz, A, Anomalies, abnormalities and care of the umbilicus. Pediatr Clin North Am 2004; 819–827.

71. Daniels J, Craig F, Wajed R, Meates M. Umbilical granulomas: a randomized controlled trial. Arch Dis Child Fetal Neonatal Ed 2003; 88: F255–258.

72. Levine N. Pigmentary abnormalities. In: Schachner LA, Hansen RC, eds. Pediatric dermatology, 2nd edn. New York: Churchill Livingstone, 1995; 546–547.

73. Geronemus RG. Q-switched ruby laser therapy of nevus of Ota. Arch Dermatol 1992; 128: 1618.

74. Gibbs RC. Unusual striped hyperpigmentation of the torso. Arch Dermatol 1967; 95: 385–386.

75. Halper S, Rubenstein D, Prose N, Levy ML. Pigmentary lines of the newborn. J Am Acad Dermatol 1993; 28: 893–894.

76. Selimoglu MA, Dilmen U, Karakelleoglu C, et al. Harlequin color change. Arch Pedatr Adolesc Med 149: 1171–1172, 1995.

77. Visscher MO, Narendran V, Pickens WL, et al. Vernix caseosa in neonatal adaptation. J Perinatol 2005; 25: 440–446.

78. Akinbi HT, Narendran V, Pass AK, et al. Host defense proteins in vernix caseosa and amniotic fluid. Am J Obstet Gynecol 2004; 191: 2090–2096.

79. Bergsson TM, Kai-Larsen G, Lengqvist J, et al. Vernix caseosa as a multi-component defence system based on polypeptides, lipids and their interactions. Cell Mol Life Sci 2005; 62: 2390–2399.

8

Iatrogenic and Traumatic Injuries

Sheila S. Galbraith, Nancy B. Esterly

A variety of untoward events may befall the developing infant while in utero or postpartum. Some of these perinatal problems are inherent in the birth process. Others are related to technologic advances that have become standard obstetric and nursery practice. Although these diagnostic and therapeutic procedures have reduced morbidity and mortality, some also pose a significant risk for iatrogenic complications.

PUNCTURE WOUNDS

Amniocentesis Scars

Amniocentesis is currently the most widely used technique for the antenatal diagnosis of genetic disorders. Although routinely a second-trimester procedure, it may also be performed in the third trimester for management of isoimmunization or evaluation of fetal maturity, or late in the first trimester for fetal karyotyping and DNA analysis.[1] The risk of damage to the fetus is quite low, particularly in the middle trimester; nevertheless, needle puncture of the skin and sometimes of the underlying structures is a possible complication. Estimates of the incidence of cutaneous scarring ranged as high as 9% in the 1970s;[2,3] however, with increased experience and the advent of real-time ultrasonography, this figure has dropped to less than 1%.[4] Despite the benignity of the procedure, the incidence of fetal injury rises dramatically with an increasing number of needle passages at amniocentesis.

Amniocentesis scars are depressed, dimple-like lesions that usually measure 1–5 mm in diameter, although scars as large as 12 mm in diameter and 8 mm in depth have been documented[5] (Fig. 8-1). They may be solitary or multiple, and are often inconspicuous. Shallow linear lesions have also been described.[3,4,6] Although sometimes present at birth, they are often not noticed until the infant is several weeks to months old.[2,5] The most frequent sites of injury are the extremities, followed by the head, neck, and chest.[6] Usually the scars are innocuous; however, the possibility of penetration of the underlying tissues must always be considered. Complications include damage to peripheral nerves, blindness secondary to ocular penetration, ileocutaneous and arteriovenous fistulization, gangrene of the arm, and exsanguination of the fetus.[5,6] Midtrimester amniocentesis has the lowest risk of puncture because the fetus occupies only about 50% of the amniotic cavity; in both the first and third trimesters there is less room to maneuver, and sudden movements of the fetus may make injury unavoidable.

Amniocentesis scars must be differentiated from congenital sinus tracts, aplasia cutis, focal dermal dysplasia, amniotic band syndrome, accessory nipples, and dimples associated with congenital rubella, diastematomyelia, Bloom syndrome, and cerebrohepatorenal syndrome.

Chorionic Villus Sampling

Chorionic villus sampling (CVS), which can be performed early in the first trimester, is the preferred procedure for patients at risk for certain single gene disorders. The technique yields mitotically active cells suitable for rapid DNA analysis and permits detection of placental mosaicism. Of concern, however, are reports of increased risk of limb and jaw malformations, particularly in fetuses undergoing CVS at less than 9 weeks of age.[1,7] An analysis of 138 996 outcomes in a multicenter study disputes this notion[8] but is not universally accepted,[9,10] and thus the issue remains a controversial area still under study. A distinctive defect of absent distal third fingers with tapering of other digits was more recently reported to be associated with exposure to CVS in a review by Golden et al.[11]

An increased incidence of hemangiomas has been noted in infants born following chorionic villus sampling compared to those undergoing amniocentesis. In a questionnaire survey by Burton et al.[12] a threefold increase in hemangiomas occurred in the total CVS group; however, affected infants were largely confined to the subset who had CVS by the transcervical route, as opposed to the transabdominal approach. One-third of the infants with hemangiomas had multiple lesions, and all but one were cutaneous in location. Other studies have found no increased risk of hemangiomas associated with CVS, and this association is now considered controversial.[13,14] Only one vas-

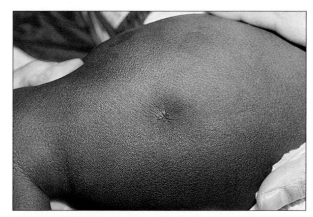

FIG. 8-1 Deep dimple and scar on the buttock of an infant whose mother had an amniocentesis.

cular malformation, a port wine stain, was reported in the CVS group. No correlation was observed between the incidence of these neoplasms and gestational age at sampling, sample size, or number of sampling attempts. Whether or not the development of hemangiomas is related to CVS limb disruption defects is currently unknown.

Fetal Monitoring

Intrauterine electronic monitoring of the fetal heart rate via a spiral electrode attached to the presenting part has become standard obstetric practice. Complications are infrequent and consist mainly of minor lacerations, ulcerations, scalp abscesses, and herpetic infections.[15,16] Herpetic infections are extremely rare; however, incidence figures for scalp abscesses in monitored infants due to other agents range from 0.1% to 5.4%,[17–21] with most in the 0.3–0.5% range.

Scalp abscesses are localized collections of suppurative material that present as erythematous, indurated masses with or without fluctuance in the area of electrode application. Usually solitary, they vary in size from 1 to several centimeters. Onset can be as early as the first day or as late as the third week, but they are most frequently noted on the third or fourth day of life. Enlarged posterior cervical lymph nodes often accompany the abscess. Usually the inflammation remains confined to the skin, but osteomyelitis of the underlying bone[17,18,22] and sepsis[22] have been documented in a few infants.

Contributing factors in some series (but not others) appear to be high-risk pregnancy (prematurity), prolonged rupture of the membranes, and long duration of fetal heart rate monitoring. The presence of amnionitis[15,19,21,23] does not seem to be correlated. Although an infectious cause has been disputed, because cultures obtained from some infants have been sterile, data from large series do not support the concept of a noninfectious etiology. Okada et al.[19] reported on 42 infants with scalp abscess, 100% of whom had positive cultures: 85% were polymicrobial, 58% grew both aerobes and anaerobes, 33% grew aerobes only, and 9% grew anaerobes only. The predominant aerobic organisms were *Staphylococcus epidermidis* and *Streptococcus* groups A and B; the predominant anaerobes were *Streptococcus* and *Peptococcus*. A confirmatory study by Brook et al.[24] demonstrated similar findings in 23 infants.

It is critical to distinguish infants with intrapartum inoculation of herpes simplex virus (HSV) from neonates with a bacterial scalp abscess. Although HSV infection as a complication of scalp monitoring is distinctly uncommon, the outcome can be devastating, with permanent neurologic damage[25] or death from systemic disease.[26] Both type 1[26] and type 2 infections[16] have been documented; unfortunately, this complication may occur with asymptomatic shedding of the virus and in the absence of a history of overt clinical disease.

Scalp abscesses usually heal uneventfully but may leave minor degrees of scarring, hypopigmentation, and alopecia, causing confusion with aplasia cutis, nevus sebaceus, or focal dermal hypoplasia in later years.

Fetal Blood Gas Sampling

Scalp puncture for fetal blood gas sampling, a procedure performed more infrequently than electrode monitoring, usually causes larger lacerations in the scalp than the do electrodes, but does not seem to be associated with abscess formation.[23]

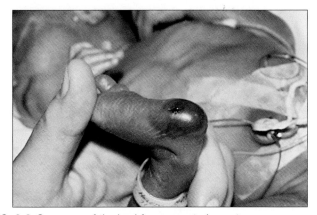

FIG. 8-2 Gangrene of the heel from repeated punctures.

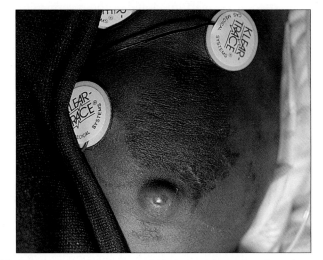

FIG. 8-3 Area of anetoderma noted at several months of age in an infant born prematurely.

Needle Marks and Scars

Needle marks consisting of hypopigmented pinhead-size lesions, when presenting in large numbers, may impart a speckled appearance to the skin.[27] These marks are due to venepuncture, arterial punctures, and catheter insertion, and are most commonly seen on the hands, wrists, feet, ankles, arms, and legs. Fox and Rutter[28] reported an improvement in the appearance of needle marks by 9 years of age in their cohort of 90 patients. Heel pricks from blood sampling may cause dimpling or, rarely, calcified nodules (see the following discussion), hypertrophic scars, or even gangrene (Fig. 8-2).

Anetoderma of Prematurity

This recently described entity consists of atrophic patches of skin that result from thinning of the dermis. Prerequisites appear to be extreme prematurity (24–29 weeks) and a lengthy stay in the neonatal intensive care unit,[29] although one report suggests that low birthweight may be a more important factor than young gestational age.[30] The lesions are absent at birth and lack an identifiable antecedent inflammatory phase, developing de novo between 6 weeks and 10 months of age. The patches are confined to the anterior trunk and proximal limbs, are oval or circular, appear depressed, and measure a few millimeters to several centimeters in diameter (Fig. 8-3). Often

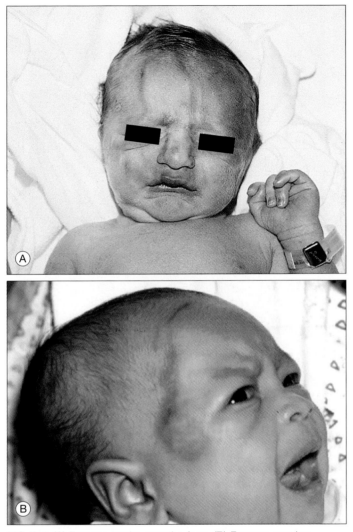

FIG. 8-4 (A) Forceps marks over the face. (B) Forceps causing subcutaneous fat necrosis, an unusual association.

they develop at sites of application of adhesives and placement of monitoring devices. Histopathologic examination of a skin biopsy specimen demonstrates a reduction or absence of dermal elastic tissue.[29]

The cause is unknown. It has been postulated that the decrease in elastic tissue might be attributable to a subclinical inflammatory reaction or, alternatively, to a transient metabolic derangement in the skin. Presumably the atrophic patches persist indefinitely, but as yet there are no long-term observational studies. A report of congenital anetoderma in premature twins may represent the same entity.[31]

PERINATAL SOFT TISSUE INJURY

Injury to the soft tissues may occur in the setting of a prolonged labor because of cephalopelvic disproportion, or in the case of a forceps delivery. Erythema, abrasions, and forceps marks are most common over the face, but rarely cause significant injury and usually resolve spontaneously (Fig. 8-4A, B).

Petechiae on the head, neck, and upper body are likely to be caused by pressure differences that occur during passage of

the chest through the birth canal. It is important to exclude the possibility of an underlying infection or hematologic disorder with appropriate laboratory studies. Petechiae caused by trauma are innocuous and usually fade within 2–3 days.

Ecchymoses may be extensive following a traumatic or breech delivery. Large areas of bruising may result in hyperbilirubinemia, requiring phototherapy. Ecchymoses resolve gradually, but may take up to several days to disappear completely.

CAPUT SUCCEDANEUM

Diffuse edematous swelling of the scalp, when it is the presenting part, is known as caput succedaneum. Extravasation of blood or serum above the periosteum occurs as a result of venous congestion caused by pressure of the uterus, cervix, and the vaginal wall on the infant's head during a prolonged or difficult labor and delivery. Because the accumulation of fluid is external to the periosteum, it crosses the midline and is not limited by the suture lines. If labor is prolonged, petechiae, purpura, and ecchymoses, as well as molding of the head and overriding sutures, may be prominent features. Unlike cephalhematoma, with which a caput is occasionally confused, the skin findings resolve within a few days. The molding may take a few weeks to disappear. Treatment is not indicated except in the rare instance when severe hemorrhage requires blood transfusions.

HALO SCALP RING

Alopecia in an annular configuration, presumably the consequence of localized injury during the birth process, has been referred to as halo scalp ring.[32] The hair loss is manifest at birth or shortly thereafter as a band of alopecia ranging in width from 1 to 4 cm, usually located over the vertex (Fig. 8-5A). There is an associated caput succedaneum and in some instances frank tissue necrosis (Fig. 8-5B). If the injury is mild, the alopecia is usually temporary;[32,33] however, scarring alopecia may result if the injury is severe (Fig. 8-5C).[34,35] The defect can be corrected by plastic surgery, with excellent cosmetic results.

ALOPECIA FROM ISCHEMIA

Scarring alopecia of the occipital scalp has been documented as a consequence of ischemia and compromised oxygenation, or as a complication of extracorporeal membrane oxygenation (ECMO) therapy in neonates.[36] During a 6-month period, five infants in a neonatal intensive care unit were observed to develop erythema and edema that progressed to crusted ulcerations (Fig. 8-6A) and resulted in a patch of scarring alopecia (Fig. 8-6B). The ulcers were believed to be the result of prolonged pressure in a setting of hypoperfusion, acidosis, and hypoxemia. The institution of a protocol requiring frequent repositioning of the head and use of a temperature-stable gel pad as preventive measures eliminated this problem.

CEPHALHEMATOMA

Cephalhematoma is caused by rupture of the diploic veins of the skull during a prolonged or difficult labor or delivery. The result of subperiosteal hemorrhage, it differs clinically from caput succedaneum in that it is almost always unilateral. The

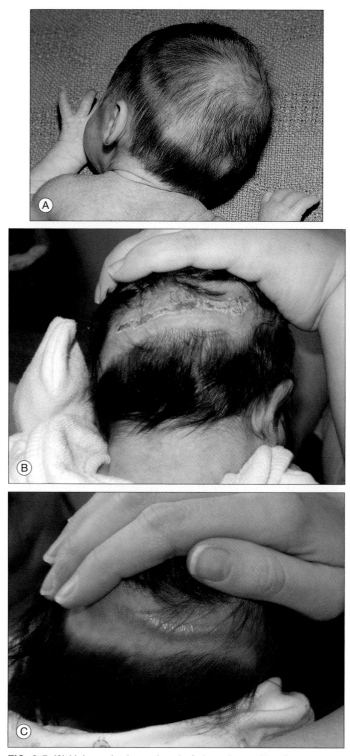

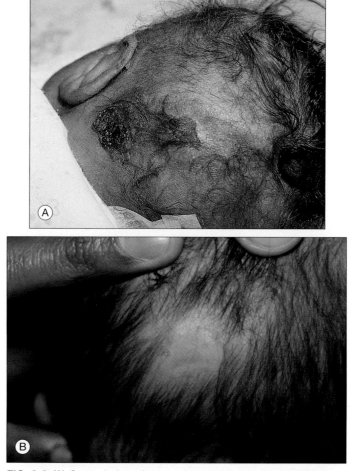

FIG. 8-6 (A) Crusted ulcerations on the posterior scalp associated with ECMO therapy. (B) Scarring alopecia 6 months after cardiac surgery with prolonged anesthesia.

FIG. 8-5 (A) Halo scalp ring: a band of alopecia resulting from localized injury during the birth process. (Courtesy of John Hall, MD.) (B) Halo scalp ring with tissue necrosis 1 week after birth. (C) Halo scalp ring healed with scarring alopecia.

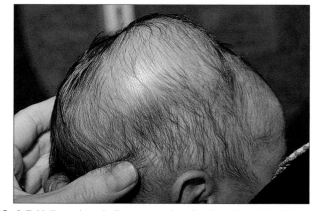

FIG. 8-7 Unilateral cephalhematoma localized to the parietal bone.

hematoma is localized most often to the area over the parietal bone, and the mass is confined by the periosteum, which adheres to the margin of the bone (Fig. 8-7). Cephalhematoma less frequently involves the occipital bones, and only rarely the frontal bones. If both parietal bones are involved, the hematomas are sharply delimited and separated by a midline depres-

sion corresponding to the intervening suture. The overlying scalp is not discolored.

Cephalhematomas are seen more commonly in vacuum-assisted vaginal deliveries than in forceps or spontaneous births.[37,38] The swelling may not become apparent until several hours to days after birth. As the hematoma ages it develops a calcified rim and is gradually completely overlaid with bone. Estimates of underlying skull fractures have ranged from 5.4%

to 25%.[39,40] Differential diagnosis includes caput succedaneum and cranial meningocele.[41] Meningoceles can be differentiated by the presence of pulsations, increased pressure when crying, and the presence of a bony defect on X-rays. Infection of the mass and severe hemorrhage resulting in anemia and hyperbilirubinemia are rare complications for which antibiotics, blood transfusions, and phototherapy may be required.[42] Treatment is unnecessary for uncomplicated lesions. Most cephalhematomas are resorbed during the first few weeks of life and are of no consequence.[37] Occasionally they calcify and persist for months to years.

UNTOWARD EFFECTS OF VACUUM EXTRACTION[43]

The formation of some type of hematoma is a common occurrence with the use of a vacuum extractor, although with the introduction of softer silicone cups the risk has been reduced. A 'chignon,' or artificial caput succedaneum, is created by adherence of the cup to the scalp and is most obvious immediately following removal of the cup. However, the swelling usually disperses relatively rapidly after birth. If a chignon is formed in the presence of a natural caput, the scalp may have a boggy sensation suggesting subgaleal hemorrhage, a potentially lethal event.[44]

Cephalhematomas (Fig. 8-7), a ring of suction blisters, lacerations, and abrasions may also result from the use of the vacuum extractor.[45] The latter are usually the result of prolonged traction and sudden detachment of the cup. Subcutaneous emphysema of the scalp has been attributed to vacuum extraction in an infant with a coexistent scalp electrode wound.[46]

LACERATIONS

Scalpel lacerations to the infant during cesarean section represent a potential form of injury. Smith et al.[47] found an incidence of fetal injury of 1.9% in a series of 896 cesarean deliveries. Lacerations were much more common in those deliveries where the indication was nonvertex presentation (breech or transverse lie). In these infants the injuries were almost always located on the lower portion of the body, whereas infants in a vertex presentation usually sustained their lacerations on the head. Failure to recognize the injury in the delivery room was a common occurrence.

BURNS

Chemical burns from concentrated disinfectants or other solvents have been reported following their use in the neonatal intensive care nursery (see Chapter 5). Isopropyl alcohol has caused second- and third-degree burns when substituted for electrode paste beneath electrocardiograph (ECG) leads[48] or used as a preparation for the umbilical area.[49] Alcohol-based skin cleansers, including chlorhexidine gluconate, have also been reported to cause extensive burns in neonates.[50,51] Small premature infants are particularly predisposed to skin damage because of an immature epidermal barrier, and their vulnerability may be accentuated by hypoxia and hypothermia. Burns are evident as intense erythema associated with blister formation and sloughing of the damaged skin (Fig. 8-8). Tissue damage can be prevented if the skin is dried immediately and protected from prolonged contact with these substances.

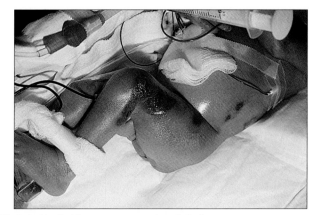

FIG. 8-8 Alcohol burn on a premature infant.

Scald injury and contact burns must be considered in the differential diagnosis of bullous lesions of unknown etiology. Inadvertent immersion injury was described in one such instance where the temperature of the hospital water supply was raised for purposes of infection control.[52] Contact with a disposable warmer causing cicatricial alopecia and a cranial defect requiring bone grafts was reported in another neonate.[53] Reports of deep burn injuries with relatively low-temperature (42°C) warming bottles have also been reported in the neonatal period.[54,55]

ULCERATIONS

Pressure ulcers occur in hospitalized or critically ill patients who have reduced mobility or sensation. Neonates, for the most part, are dependent on their caregivers for mobility. Premature infants often require prolonged hospitalization and are therefore at risk for developing pressure ulcers. Pressure ulcers in children are poorly documented, however. In a recent multicenter survey the prevalence of pressure ulcers in pediatric inpatients was found to be 4%, with infants under 3 months old comprising 26% of reported pressure ulcers and 45% of other types of skin breakdown.[56] Thirty-one per cent of these infants had pressure ulcers on their head, which was thought to be related to the large body surface area of the head in infants.[56]

UMBILICAL ARTERY CATHETERIZATION

Catheterization of the umbilical arteries has become standard practice in the neonatal intensive care unit for monitoring intravascular pressures, chemistries, pH, and blood gases, and for administering fluids and medications to critically ill neonates. However, this procedure is fraught with risk of serious complications, even in experienced hands. Thrombosis is the most frequent problem, as documented by aortography.[57] Other potential complications include vasospasm, blanching of the limbs, embolism, perforation of the vessels, vascular damage from hypertonic solutions, hemorrhage, infections, and ischemic and chemical necrosis of the abdominal viscera.[58,59] These untoward events are usually caused by incorrect placement of the catheter, or to unduly rapid infusion of hazardous drugs or hypertonic solutions, rather than vessel injury.[60]

Vasospasm may occur during placement of the catheter in the umbilical artery. It is manifest by temporary blanching or

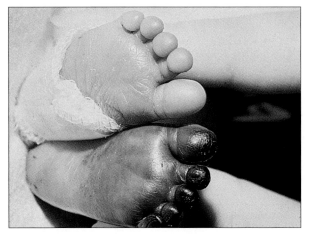

FIG. 8-9 Gangrene of the foot secondary to umbilical artery catheterization and thrombosis.

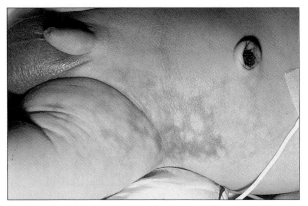

FIG. 8-10 Early skin changes of reticulated erythema resulting from attempted umbilical artery catheterization.

cyanosis of the leg and foot. Prompt removal of the catheter is indicated, and if this procedure is followed sequelae are unlikely.

Thromboses and multiple small emboli can cause infarcts of the toes. Depending on the location of the thrombus, unilateral or bilateral gangrene of the feet, lower extremities, or buttocks can occur (Fig. 8-9).[59,61,62] Gangrene of the distal upper extremity with loss of fingers has also been documented secondary to similar events following percutaneous radial artery catheterization.[63] Early skin changes include erythema, transient blanching, vesicles, and bulla formation (Fig. 8-10). These lesions may abate or may progress to extensive skin and subcutaneous tissue necrosis, demarcation, and gangrene.[62]

PERINATAL GANGRENE OF THE BUTTOCK

This alarming and fortunately rare occurrence is usually attributed to iatrogenic causes[64] but has also been documented as an apparently spontaneous event.[65,66] The onset is heralded by the sudden appearance of an erythematous patch involving the buttock, perineum, and genitalia. Within hours the involved area rapidly becomes edematous and then rock hard and cold to the touch, with well-defined black borders. Bullae may form on the surface. Generally the lower limbs are spared and remain warm and normal in color, with palpable femoral pulses. Over the subsequent several days the necrotic tissue

demarcates and sloughs, leaving a deep ulcer that heals by secondary intention with scarring.

The diagnosis is made on the basis of the abrupt onset and clinical findings. The differential diagnosis is mainly that of an infectious process, but cultures are invariably negative, as are biochemical and hematologic laboratory studies. Chemical or thermal injury must also be considered.

The presumed cause is an occlusive vascular event involving the internal iliac artery. This artery, which feeds into the umbilical artery, splits into two terminal branches, the inferior gluteal and the internal pudendal arteries; these two vessels supply the buttock, perineum, vulva, and scrotum. Vasospasm followed by thrombus formation resulting from a variety of pathogenetic factors, such as injury to the umbilical cord or obstruction by a misdirected umbilical catheter, is thought to account for this condition. Despite the extent of the gangrenous process, the lesions generally heal without complications and the sphincters remain intact.[64,65]

COMPLICATIONS OF PHOTOTHERAPY

Visible light phototherapy has become standard therapy in the newborn nursery for infants with significant indirect hyperbilirubinemia. Visible light energy isomerizes unconjugated bilirubin to more polar forms, which are excreted into the bile and ultimately into the stool within minutes of exposure. Bilirubin absorbs light maximally in the blue portion of the spectrum (420–500 nm). Daylight fluorescent bulbs have an emission spectrum from 320 to 700 nm, which includes small amounts of ultraviolet A (UVA), as well as the therapeutic blue wavelengths. High-energy blue lamps emit light in a narrower range and exclude light in the ultraviolet spectrum; however, they are used less frequently because the hue produced by them makes it difficult to assess skin color in jaundiced infants, and also may cause nausea and dizziness in nursery personnel.

Because phototherapy is not standardized, response and outcome may vary from one setting to another. Daylight, cool white, and special blue fluorescent lights can be used separately or in combination, or tungsten–halogen lamps may be used. Likewise, the energy output, or irradiance, of the phototherapy unit may vary depending on the positioning of the lamps and the amount of skin surface area exposed to the light. Therapy may be intermittent or continuous, and most recently, fiberoptic phototherapy has been introduced using a halogen light source transmitted to a blanket that is wrapped around the infant. Adverse effects of phototherapy are few, but include erythematous, purpuric, and vesicular transient eruptions (see Chapters 5 and 19), bronze baby syndrome, and rarely, ultraviolet light burns.

Ultraviolet Light Burns

Burns have been reported in only a few instances and have been a result of misadventure causing prolonged exposure to inadequately shielded phototherapy lights. Siegfried et al.[67] reported two premature infants who developed generalized erythema, one with blistering, on exposure to fluorescent daylight bulbs. The burns were from the UVA wavelengths and were sustained because of inadvertent failure to place Plexiglas covers over the banks of bulbs.[67] The erythema was most intense in areas of the body closest to the light source and spared the shielded areas. The authors point out that it is important to recognize that infants cared for in beds other than Plexiglas isolettes are not protected from UVA transmission unless these shields are in place. They also caution that plastic wrap and plastic shell vapor barriers do not protect against this type of injury.

Phototherapy-Induced Drug Eruptions

Apart from burns, erythematous and vesiculobullous eruptions may be associated with phototherapy under other circumstances. Drug-induced phototoxicity eruptions have been documented in neonates receiving certain therapeutic agents (e.g. furosemide or fluorescein dye for a radiologic procedure) or exposed to methylene blue dye prenatally.[68–70] These eruptions have occurred in infants given a photosensitizing drug and exposed to light of the appropriate wavelength to cause photoactivation of the chemical compound. As with true burns, these bullae develop only on light-exposed skin. Discontinuation of therapy usually results in an uneventful recovery.

Transient Porphyrinemia and Phototherapy Eruptions

Transient porphyrinemia in combination with phototherapy has also been documented as a cause of blisters and erosions,[71] as well as erythematous and purpuric lesions[72,73] in several neonates with hemolytic disease (Fig. 8-11). The eruptions in all cases were confined to exposed areas, sparing the sites protected from the lights (e.g. skin under leads, dressings, and temperature probes). Onset was between 1 and 4 days after initiation of phototherapy, although one infant had a more delayed response.[71] Reactions ranged from violaceous discoloration resembling sunburn[72] to frank purpura.[73] One infant had blisters with erosions and skin fragility instead.[71]

Skin biopsy specimens from the purpuric lesions showed only extravasation of erythrocytes[73] without epidermal changes, thus distinguishing the eruption from a burn. In the infant who blistered, the cleavage plane occurred at the level of the lamina lucida (subepidermal), and there was an associated minimal dermal infiltrate.[71]

The porphyrin levels in affected infants differed somewhat in that one infant had elevated free erythrocyte protoporphyrin and zinc protoporphyrin levels,[72] whereas the others had mainly increased amounts of both coproporphyrin and protoporphyrin in their plasma.[71,73] Although the cause of the elevated porphyrin levels in these infants was not clear, it was postulated that multiple factors, including cholestasis, altered hepatic function, concomitant administration of photosensitizing drugs and transfused blood products, and renal failure, might be responsible. In addition, a prolonged course of phototherapy at a relatively high level of irradiance was thought to be a contributing factor in one instance.[71]

Differential diagnosis includes infections, epidermolysis bullosa, neonatal lupus erythematosus, metabolic photosensitivity eruptions, true porphyria, and drug eruptions. Both the cutaneous eruption and the transient porphyrinemia clear spontaneously within a few weeks, and there are no significant sequelae.

Bronze Baby Syndrome

In this rare complication of phototherapy the infant's skin, serum, and urine become a gray-brown color after several hours under the phototherapy lamps (Fig. 8-12). All of the infants who have developed this disorder have had prior evidence of hepatic dysfunction, marked by conjugated hyperbilirubinemia and retention of bile acids.[74–76] The serum acquires a dark brown color and shows a nonspecific absorbance from 380 to 520 nm on spectroanalysis.[76] The peculiar color has been attributed to the formation of a photo-oxidation product of bilirubin or to copper-bound porphyrins, which yield brown photoproducts in the presence of bilirubin.[77,78] It has also been suggested that biliverdin pigments may contribute to the bronzing effect.[79] The odd hue is easily distinguished from that of cyanosis or typical neonatal jaundice. The discoloration fades over time after phototherapy is discontinued, and there are no significant sequelae.

CALCINOSIS CUTIS

Calcification of the skin occurs as a consequence of deposition of hydroxyapatite crystals and amorphous calcium phosphate in the soft tissues. Based on the pathophysiologic mechanisms, calcinosis cutis is usually classified as idiopathic (normal tissue and a normal calcium/phosphorus ratio); dystrophic (damaged tissue and a normal calcium/phosphorus ratio); or metastatic (normal tissue and an abnormal calcium/

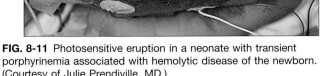

FIG. 8-11 Photosensitive eruption in a neonate with transient porphyrinemia associated with hemolytic disease of the newborn. (Courtesy of Julie Prendiville, MD.)

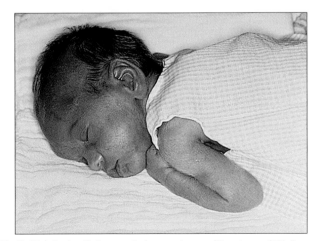

FIG. 8-12 Infant with bronze baby syndrome. (Courtesy of Walter Burgdorf, MD.)

phosphorus ratio). Iatrogenic calcinosis cutis in neonates is usually of the dystrophic type and is most often the result of an intravenous infusion of calcium gluconate or calcium chloride for treatment of neonatal hypocalcemia.[80–82] It may also occur following the application of electrode paste containing calcium chloride for electroencephalography, electromyography, or brainstem auditory evoked potentials, particularly if applied to abraded skin[83] and in association with subcutaneous fat necrosis.

Calcinosis Cutis from Infusion of Calcium Salts

Visible evidence of soft tissue calcification develops on average 13 days after infusion of the calcium solution, with a range of 2 hours to 24 days (Fig. 8-13). There may be marked swelling with an intense inflammatory response, even in the absence of extravasation of fluid, and occasionally there is soft tissue necrosis. The calcification takes the form of papules, nodules, an annular plaque, or a large subcutaneous plaque, or may have a linear configuration conforming to the vein in which the solution is administered. The lesions are firm, erythematous, and brown, yellow, or white; when extravasation has occurred they may be tender, warm, and fluctuant, resembling an abscess.[80]

Radiographic changes can be detected as early as 4–5 days following the infusion.[81,84] Three patterns have been described: (1) a calcified mass localized to or near the site of injection; (2) more diffuse calcification along fascial planes; and (3) a pattern of vascular or perivascular calcification.[81,85,86] Skin biopsy specimens contain calcium deposits in the dermal papillae, as well as amorphous masses of calcium intermingled with degenerated collagen and a lymphohistiocytic infiltrate in the deeper dermis. Stains for calcium (e.g. von Kossa) demonstrate focal calcium deposits in the walls of the vessels, both arteries and veins.

Several factors are believed to contribute to this reaction, which peaks at about 2 weeks. In some instances, tissue damage results from leakage of infusate from the vein at the puncture site or the development of frank phlebitis, particularly if the infusion is given over a prolonged period. However,

calcinosis cutis may occur even in the absence of obvious extravasation of fluid.[82] Precipitation of calcium salts is also facilitated by an alkaline pH that results from tissue damage, or when bicarbonate or certain drugs (e.g. amphotericin, prednisolone sodium phosphate) are infused through the same intravenous line.

The diagnosis of calcinosis cutis can be made clinically based on the distinctive appearance of the skin lesions and confirmed by skin biopsy and/or radiographs. Differential diagnosis includes cellulitis, osteomyelitis, periostitis, hematoma, abscess, and subcutaneous fat necrosis.[84]

Treatment is generally symptomatic, and spontaneous resolution occurs over several months by transepidermal elimination of the calcified material. An animal study has suggested that intralesional injection of triamcinolone may be effective in reducing inflammation and facilitating the resorption of calcium.[87]

Calcinosis Cutis associated with Subcutaneous Fat Necrosis

Subcutaneous fat necrosis may develop in infants who experience perinatal iatrogenic problems such as obstetric trauma, asphyxia, or hypothermia (see also Chapter 24). Hypercalcemia occasionally complicates the course in these infants.[88] Rarely, there is accompanying soft tissue calcification identifiable by biopsy or radiography.[89–93] The presence of soft tissue calcification does not seem to portend a more ominous prognosis and eventually resolves.

Calcified Nodules of the Heels

These lesions have been seen in association with heel prick marks, principally in infants of low birthweight and young gestational age who as neonates received numerous heel sticks in the nursery.[27,94] Rho et al.,[95] however, reported a calcified heel nodule after a single heel stick. Onset is usually between 4 and 12 months after birth and is marked by the appearance of multiple tiny white or yellow specks within depressed areas on the heels (Fig. 8-14). The papulonodules enlarge and become elevated and firm, but are neither inflamed

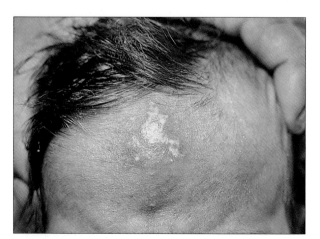

FIG. 8-13 Calcified plaque on the forehead secondary to extravasation of calcium gluconate.

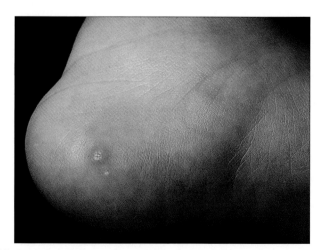

FIG. 8-14 Calcified papules nodules on the heel secondary to heel sticks.

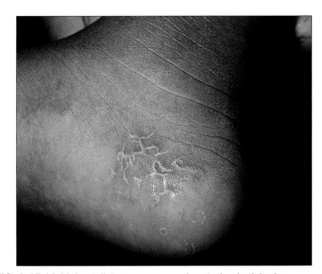

FIG. 8-15 Multiple stellate scars secondary to heel sticks in a premature infant.

nor symptomatic. The accumulated calcified material is eventually extruded spontaneously through the epidermis, or can be manually expressed. There is no associated underlying biochemical abnormality, and metabolic studies are not indicated. Linear or stellate scarring without calcification may also be seen secondary to heel sticks in neonates (Fig. 8-15).

On histologic examination the nodules consist of a cystic-like space with irregular calcification around the margins, but no epithelial lining. The calcification is surrounded by fibrous connective tissue and a patchy mononuclear infiltrate. The pathogenesis is poorly understood, although undoubtedly trauma plays a role. Differential diagnosis includes subepidermal calcified nodule (of Winer). The process is self-limiting and does not require intervention.

EXTRAVASATION INJURIES

Extravasation of intravenous fluids into subcutaneous tissue can lead to tissue necrosis and scar formation, particularly in premature infants who have fragile skin and minimal subcutaneous tissue. Wilkins and Emmerson[96] recently reported the prevalence of extravasation injuries in neonatal intensive care units in the United Kingdom to be 38 per 1000 babies, with 70% of injuries occurring in infants 26 weeks' gestation or less. The majority of extravasation injuries occur with peripheral catheters, and the extent of damage is dependent on the volume and physicochemical characteristics of the infiltrated solution.[97] Clinically, extravasation injuries are characterized by pain and swelling near the intravenous site, which may progress to blanching, signs of impaired profusion, blistering, discoloration, ulceration, and eschar formation. Calcinosis cutis can develop after infiltration of calcium solutions, as discussed in the previous section. Scar formation is related to the degree of tissue damage and can result in cosmetically or functionally disfiguring lesions, although the scars do tend to improve with age.[28] There is no consensus on treatment for extravasation injuries in neonates. Elevation, warm or cold compresses, multiple puncture technique, saline flushing or liposuction, and hyaluronidase have been reported to be helpful, although further studies are needed in neonates.[97] Wound care with hydrocolloid or hydrogel dressings may promote healing and help to avoid significant scar formation.

COMPLICATIONS OF BLOOD GAS AND SKIN TEMPERATURE MONITORING

The use of noninvasive techniques for skin surface monitoring of blood gases and temperature has become routine practice in the newborn intensive care nursery.[98] Transcutaneous measurements of oxygen and carbon dioxide tension and pulse oximetry for assessment of arterial saturation levels provide accurate, reproducible information facilitating clinical management of premature and sick infants. Infant skin temperature probes are also used to monitor infants in radiant warmers. Although these techniques are widely used, they do pose some risk of damage to the infant's skin at sites of contact with the sensors and electrodes.

Pulse Oximetry

Pulse oximetry relies on the spectrophotometric analysis of light to measure the oxygen saturation of hemoglobin. The technique employs a sensor that wraps around a hand, foot, or finger, or an ear probe that clips to the antihelix. It requires no calibration and no skin heating and provides almost continuous measurement of oxygen saturation. Tight application of a probe may cause a first-degree thermal burn, skin erosion, hyperpigmentation, blister, or pressure necrosis.[99] Second- and third-degree burns have also been observed, particularly in instances where sensors and oximeters from different companies were paired and found to be incompatible.[100,101] Because pulse oximetry does not require tight contact with the skin, this complication is avoidable by frequent inspection of the probe site.[99]

Transcutaneous Oxygen Monitoring

Although also considered a noninvasive procedure, transcutaneous oxygen monitoring poses a greater risk for local skin damage because the electrode must be heated to 42–45°C to promote adequate blood flow.[27,98,102–104] The heated electrode produces local hyperthermia and vasodilation, arterializing the vascular bed at the electrode site. As one might expect, thermal injury is a frequent problem and is directly related to the temperature of the sensor, the sensitivity of the infant's skin, and the duration of placement of the monitoring device at a single skin site. Indeed, it is usual with this device to induce a first-degree burn, although the erythema is likely to fade by 12 hours (Fig. 8-16). Second- and third-degree burns have also been documented.[98]

In a study by Boyle and Oh[102] all infants monitored with these sensors developed blanchable erythema, the equivalent of a first-degree burn. A smaller number of infants, more often those born prematurely, sustained a more severe thermal reaction evidenced by nonblanchable erythema, which lasted from 60 hours to 6 days.[102] These reactions were interpreted as mild second-degree burns. Vesicles have been noted when the electrode is applied for extended periods.

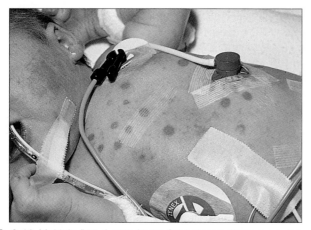

FIG. 8-16 Multiple first-degree burns from transcutaneous oxygen monitoring device.

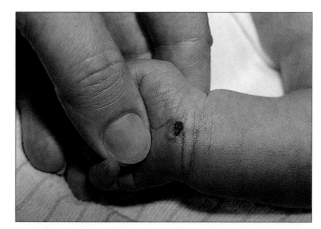

FIG. 8-18 Thermal burns from a transillumination unit causing blisters in a neonate. (Courtesy of Sheila Fallon-Friedlander, MD.)

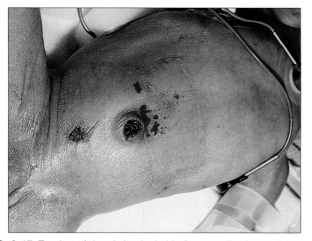

FIG. 8-17 Erosion of the abdominal skin from application and removal of adhesives.

Transillumination Blisters

Thermal burns may occur as a complication of the use of transillumination devices for the detection of hydrocephalus, subdural effusions, cystic hygroma, and pneumomediastinum, or for localization of arteries and veins for blood sampling. Typical lesions are small (<5 mm), round, discrete blisters with a necrotic base that develop at sites of transillumination (Fig. 8-18).[105] It is thought that specific wavelengths of the high-intensity fiberoptic light are converted to heat energy in the skin, causing thermal damage. Infrared and ultraviolet filters within the light source, usually a quartz halogen lamp, eliminate wavelengths of less than 570 nm, reducing the risk of thermal injury. A defect in the transilluminator unit, missing filters,[106] or failure of the filter to function properly have accounted for the occurrence of these blisters in neonates.

Infant Skin Temperature Probes

Infant skin temperature probes are used to monitor infant temperatures in radiant warmers. A heat-reflective adhesive patch is used to attach the probe to a soft area on the infant, such as the abdomen. Although relatively safe, there have been several reports of blister formation related to improper use of skin temperature probes.[107]

MEATAL ULCERATION FOLLOWING CIRCUMCISION

Thermal damage caused by the electrode can be compounded by yet another type of injury due to application and removal of the adhesive ring that secures the sensor in place. Stripping of the stratum corneum occurs with removal of the sensor, which is placed in a new site every 4 hours (Fig. 8-17). This epidermal damage is particularly perilous in premature infants under 30 weeks of age because it compromises an already fragile and incompetent barrier, putting the infant at increased risk for fluid and electrolyte imbalance and loss of temperature control. Furthermore, if a large surface area is denuded, these infants may be more vulnerable to infectious organisms and chemicals placed on the skin.[98,103] The use of a copolymer acrylic dressing (OpSite) has been shown to protect the skin from adhesive trauma and does not interfere with transcutaneous oxygen measurements.[103]

A rare complication described in two infants is the development of circular hyperpigmented macules at monitoring sites, which over several months became crateriform and remained as permanent marks. Biopsy of one affected infant revealed focal dermal cicatricial fibrosis.[104] Interestingly, the craters did not develop until several months of age, a course reminiscent of that of anetoderma of prematurity.

Mackenzie[108] has proposed that meatal ulceration is a frequently unrecognized consequence of neonatal circumcision. He has suggested that removal of the prepuce subjects the epithelium of the glans penis to undue irritation from the diaper, which may result in erosions followed by healing with stenosis. Because the erosions do not necessarily occur in the immediate postoperative period, the cause-and-effect relationship is not appreciated. Other rare complications include direct injury to the glans and urethra, bleeding, and infection.

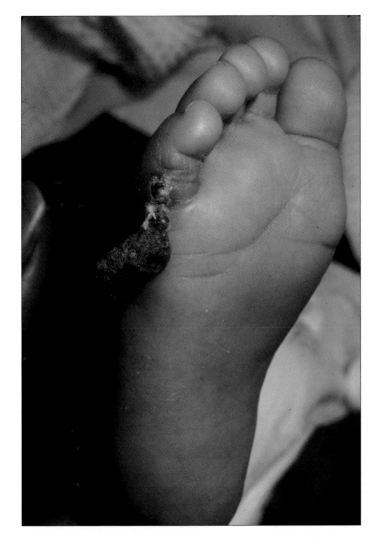

FIG. 8-19 Necrosis of a supernumerary digit after suture ligation.

CUTANEOUS NECROSIS FOLLOWING SUTURE LIGATION OF SUPERNUMERARY DIGITS AND ACCESSORY TRAGI

Supernumerary digits and accessory tragi (which may erroneously be referred to as 'tags') are sometimes removed with suture ligation rather than surgical excision. This method, by it nature, constricts the blood flow to the skin and leads to skin necrosis. If the appendage is not tiny, the amount of necrosis can be considerable (Fig. 8-19) and can even serve as a potential nidus for infection. Accessory tragi have associated cartilage and for this reason are not well suited to this technique.[109] Supernumerary digits treated in this manner may result in traumatic neuroma and chronic pain.[110]

REFERENCES

1. Jauniaux E, Rodeck C. Use, risks and complications of amniocentesis and chorionic villous sampling for prenatal diagnosis in early pregnancy. Early Pregnancy Biol Med 1995; 1: 245–252.
2. Karp LE, Hayden PW. Fetal puncture during midtrimester amniocentesis. Obstet Gynecol 1977; 49: 115–117.
3. Epley SL, Hanson JW, Cruikshank DP. Fetal injury with mid-trimester diagnostic amniocentesis. Obstet Gynecol 1979; 53: 77–80.
4. Cambiaghi S, Restano L, Cavalli R, et al. Skin dimpling as a consequence of amniocentesis. J Am Acad Dermatol 1998; 39: 888–890.
5. Bruce S, Duffy JO, Wolf JE, Jr. Skin dimpling associated with mid-trimester amniocentesis. Pediatr Dermatol 1984; 2: 140–142.
6. Raimer SS, Raimer BG. Needle puncture scars from midtrimester amniocentesis. Arch Dermatol 1984; 120: 1360–1362.
7. Stoler JM, McGuirk CK, Lieberman E, et al. Malformations reported in chorionic villus sampling exposed children: A review and analytic synthesis of the literature. Genet Med 1999; 1: 315–322.
8. Froster UG. Limb defects and chorionic villus sampling: results from an international registry, 1992–94. Lancet 1996; 347: 489–1494.
9. Firth H, Boyd PA, Chamberlain P, et al. Limb defects and chorionic villus sampling. Lancet 1996; 347: 1406.
10. Mastroiacovo P, Botto LD. Limb defects and chorionic villus sampling. Lancet 1996; 347: 1407–1408.
11. Golden CM, Ryan LM, Homes LB. Chorionic villus sampling: a distinctive teratogenic effect on fingers? Birth Defects Res A Clin Mol Teratol 2003; 67: 557–562.
12. Burton BK, Schulz CJ, Angle B, et al. An increased incidence of haemangiomas in infants born following chorionic villus sampling

(CVS). Prenat Diagn 1995; 15: 209–214.

13. Schaap AH, van der Pol HG, Boer K, et al. Long-term follow-up of infants after transcervical chorionic villus sampling and after amniocentesis to compare congenital abnormalities and health status. Prenat Diagn 2002; 22: 598–604.

14. Alfirevic Z. Early amniocentesis versus transabdominal chorion villus sampling for prenatal diagnosis. Cochrane Database of Systemic Reviews 4, 2005.

15. Ashkenazi S, Metzker A, Merlob P, et al. Scalp changes after fetal monitoring. Arch Dis Child 1985; 60: 267–269.

16. Amann ST, Fagnant RJ, Chartrand SA, et al. Herpes simplex infection associated with short-term use of a fetal scalp electrode. J Reprod Med 1992; 37: 372–374.

17. Feder HM Jr, MacLean WC Jr, Moxon R. Scalp abscess secondary to fetal scalp electrode. J Pediatr 1976; 89: 808–809.

18. Plavidal FJ, Werch A. Fetal scalp abscess secondary to intrauterine monitoring. Am J Obstet Gynecol 1976; 125: 65–70.

19. Okada DM, Chow AW, Bruce VT. Neonatal scalp abscess and fetal monitoring: Factors associated with infection. Am J Obstet Gynecol 1977; 129: 185–189.

20. Wagener MM, Rycheck RR, Yee RB, et al. Septic dermatitis of the neonatal scalp and maternal endomyometritis with intrapartum internal fetal monitoring. Pediatrics 1984; 74: 81–85.

21. Winkel CA, Snyder DL, Schlaerth JB. Scalp abscess: A complication of the spiral fetal electrode. Am J Obstet Gynecol 1976; 126: 720–722.

22. Overturf GD, Balfour G. Osteomyelitis and sepsis: Severe complications of fetal monitoring. Pediatrics 1975; 55: 244–247.

23. Cordero L, Anderson CW, Zuspan FP. Scalp abscess: A benign and infrequent complication of fetal monitoring. Am J Obstet Gynecol 1983; 146: 126–130.

24. Brook I, Frazier EH. Microbiology of scalp abscess in newborns. Pediatr Infect Dis J 1992; 11: 766–768.

25. Katz M, Greco A, Antony L, et al. Neonatal herpesvirus sepsis following internal monitoring. Int J Gynecol Obstet 1980; 17: 631–633.

26. Goldkrand JW. Intrapartum inoculationof herpes simplex virus by fetal scalp electrode. Obstet Gynecol 1982; 59: 263–265.

27. Cartlidge PHT, Fox PE, Rutter N. The scars of newborn intensive care. Early Hum Dev 1990; 21: 1–10.

28. Fox PE, Rutter N. The childhood scars of newborn intensive care. Early Hum Dev 1998; 51: 171–177.

29. Prizant TL, Lucky AW, Frieden IJ, et al. Spontaneous atrophic patches in extremely premature infants. Arch Dermatol 1996; 132: 671–674.

30. Todd DJ. Anetoderma of prematurity. Arch Dermatol 1997; 133: 789.

31. Zeyllman GL, Levy ML. Congenital anetoderma in twins. J Am Acad Dermatol 1997; 36: 483–485.

32. Neal PR, Merk PF, Norins AL. Halo scalp ring: A form of localized scalp injury associated with caput succedaneum. Pediatr Dermatol 1984; 2: 52–54.

33. Tanzi EL, Hornung RL, Silverberg NB. Halo scalp ring: a case series and review of the literature. Arch Pediatr Adolesc Med 2002; 156: 188–190.

34. Beutner KR. Halo ring scarring alopecia. Pediatr Dermatol 1985; 3: 83.

35. Prendiville JS, Esterly NB. Halo scalp ring: A cause of scarring alopecia. Arch Dermatol 1987; 123: 992–993.

36. Gershan LA, Esterly NB. Scarring alopecia in neonates as a consequence of hypoxemia–hypoperfusion. Arch Dis Child 1993; 68: 591–593.

37. Bofill JA, Rust OA, Davidas M. et al. Neonatal cephalohematoma from vacuum extraction. J Reprod Med 1997; 42: 565–569.

38. Johnson JH, Figueroa R, Garry D, et al. Immediate maternal and neonatal effects of forceps and vacuum-assisted deliveries. Obstet Gynecol 2004; 103: 513–518.

39. Kendall N, Woolshin H. Cephalhematoma associated with fracture of the skull. J Pediatr 1952; 41: 125–127.

40. Zelson C, Lee SJ, Pearl M. The incidence of skull fractures underlying cephalhematomas in newborn infants. J Pediatr 1974; 85: 371–373.

41. Winter TC, Mack LA, Cyr DR. Prenatal sonographic diagnosis of scalp edema/cephalhematoma mimicking an encephalocele. Am J Roentgenol 1993; 161: 1247–1248.

42. Tan KL, Lim GC. Phototherapy for neonatal jaundice in infants with cephalhematomas. Clin Pediatr 1995; 34: 7–11.

43. Vacca A. Birth by vacuum extraction: Neonatal outcome. J Paediatr Child Health 1996; 32: 204–206.

44. Benaron DA. Subgaleal hematoma causing hypovolemic shock during delivery after failed vacuum extraction: A case report. J Perinatol 1993; 13: 228–231.

45. Metzker A, Brenner S, Merlob P. Iatrogenic cutaneous injuries in the neonate. Arch Dermatol 1999; 135: 697–703.

46. Birenbaum E, Robinson G, Mashiach S, et al. Skull subcutaneous emphysema – a rare complication of vacuum extraction and scalp electrode. Eur J Obstet Gynecol Reprod Biol 1986; 22: 257–260.

47. Smith JF, Hernandez C, Wax JR. Fetal laceration injury at cesarean delivery. Obstet Gynecol 1997; 90: 344–346.

48. Schick JB, Milstein JM. Burn hazard of isopropyl alcohol in the neonate. Pediatrics 1981; 68: 587–588.

49. Weintraub Z, Iancu TC. Isopropyl alcohol burns. Pediatrics 1982; 69: 506.

50. Watkins AM, Keogh EJ. Alcohol burns in the neonate. J Paediatr Child Health 1992; 28: 306–308.

51. Reynolds PR, Banerjee S. Meek JH. Alcohol burns in extremely low birthweight infants: still occurring. Arch Dis Child Fetal Neonatal Ed 2005; 90: F10.

52. Mirowski GW, Frieden IJ, Miller C. Iatrogenic scald burn: a consequence of institutional infection control measures. Pediatrics 1996; 98: 963–965.

53. Matsumura H, Shigehara K, Ueno T, et al. Cranial defect and decrease in cerebral blood flow resulting from deep contact burn of the scalp in the neonatal period. Burns 1996; 22: 560–565.

54. Mohrenschlager M, Weigl LB, Haug S, et al. Iatrogenic burns by warming bottles in the neonatal period. J Burn Care Rehab 2003; 24: 52–55.

55. Rimdeika R, Bagdonas R. Major full thickness skin burn injuries in premature neonate twins. Burns 2005; 31: 76–84.

56. McLane KM, Bookout K, McCord S, et al. The 2003 national pediatric pressure ulcer and skin breakdown prevalence survey: a multisite study. J Wound Ostomy Continence Nurs 2004; 31: 168–178.

57. Neal WA, Reynolds JW, Jarvis CW, et al. Umbilical artery catheterization: Demonstration of arterial thrombosis by aortography. Pediatrics 1972; 50: 6–13.

58. Kitterman JA, Phibbs RH, Tooley WH. Catheterization of umbilical vessels in newborn infants. Pediatr Clin North Am 1970; 17: 895–912.

59. Cutler VE, Stretcher GS. Cutaneous complications of central umbilical artery catheterization. Arch Dermatol 1977; 113: 61–63.

60. Marsh JL, King W, Barrett C, et al. Serious complications after umbilical artery catheterization for neonatal monitoring. Arch Surg 1975; 110: 1203–1208.

61. deSanctis N, Cardillo G, Rega AN. Gluteoperineal gangrene and sciatic nerve palsy after umbilical vessel injection. Clin Orthop Rel Res 1995; 316: 180–184.

62. Letts M, Blastorah B, Al-Azzam S. Neonatal gangrene of the extremities. J Pediatr Orthop 1997; 17: 397–401.

63. Cartwright GW, Schreiner RL. Major complication secondary to percutaneous radial artery catherization in the neonate. Pediatrics 1980; 65: 139–141.

64. Rudolph N, Wang HH, Dragutsky D. Gangrene of the buttock: A complication of umbilical artery

catheterization. Pediatrics 1974; 53: 106–109.

65. Serrano G, Aliaga A, Febrer I, et al. Perinatal gangrene of the buttock: A spontaneous condition. Arch Dermatol 1985; 121: 23–24.

66. Bonifazi E, Meneghini C. Perinatal gangrene of the buttock: An iatrogenic or spontaneous condition? J Am Acad Dermatol 1980; 3: 596–598.

67. Siegfried EC, Stone MS, Madison KC. Ultraviolet light burn: a cutaneous complication of visible light phototherapy of neonatal jaundice. Pediatr Dermatol 1992; 9: 278–282.

68. Kearns GL, Williams BJ, Timmons OT. Fluorescein phototoxicity in a premature infant. J Pediatr 1985; 107: 796–798.

69. Burry JN, Lawrence JR. Phototoxic blisters from high furosimide dosage. Br J Dermatol 1976; 94: 495–499.

70. Porat R, Gilbert S, Magilner D. Methylene blue-induced photosensitivity: an unrecognized complication. Pediatrics 1996; 97: 717–721.

71. Mallon E, Wojnarowska F, Hope P, et al. Neonatal bullous eruption as a result of transient porphyrinemia in a premature infant with hemolytic disease of the newborn. J Am Acad Dermatol 1995; 33: 333–336.

72. Crawford RI, Lawlor ER, Wadsworth LD, et al. Transient erythroporphyria of infancy. J Am Acad Dermatol 1996; 35: 833–834.

73. Paller AS, Eramo LR, Farrell EE, et al. Purpuric phototherapy-induced eruption in transfused neonates: Relation to transient porphyrinemia. Pediatrics 1997; 100: 360–364.

74. Tan KL, Jacob E. The bronze baby syndrome. Acta Pediatr Scand 1982; 71: 409–414.

75. Rubaltelli FF, Jori G, Reddi E. Bronze baby syndrome: A new porphyrin-related disorder. Pediatr Res 1983; 17: 327–330.

76. Ashley JR, Littler CM, Burgdorf WC, et al. Bronze baby syndrome. J Am Acad Dermatol 1985; 12: 325–328.

77. Onishi S, Itoh S, Isobe K, et al. Mechanism of development of bronze baby syndrome in neonates treated with phototherapy. Pediatrics 1982; 69: 273–276.

78. Jori G, Reddi E, Rubaltelli FF. Bronze baby syndrome: An animal model. Pediatr Res 1990; 27: 22–25.

79. Purcell SM, Wians FH Jr, Ackerman NB Jr, et al. Hyperbiliverdinemia in the bronze baby syndrome. J Am Acad Dermatol 1987; 16: 172–177.

80. Ramamurthy RS, Harris V, Pildes RS. Subcutaneous calcium deposition in the neonate associated with intravenous administration of calcium gluconate. Pediatrics 1975; 55: 802–806.

81. Sahn EE, Smith DJ. Annular dystrophic calcinosis cutis in an infant. J Am Acad Dermatol 1992; 26: 1015–1017.

82. Weiss Y, Ackerman,C, Shmilovitz A. Localized necrosis of scalp in neonates due to calcium gluconate infusions: A cautionary note. Pediatrics 1975; 56: 1084–1086.

83. Puig L, Rocamora V, Romani J, et al. Calcinosis cutis following calcium chloride electrode paste application for auditory-brainstem evoked potentials recording. Pediatr Dermatol 1998; 15: 27–30.

84. Berger PE, Heidelberger KP, Poznanski AK. Extravasation of calcium gluconate as a cause of soft tissue calcification in infancy. Am J Roentgenol 1974; 121: 109–116.

85. Lee FA, Gwinn JL. Roentgen patterns of extravasation of calcium gluconate in the tissues of the neonate. J Pediatr 1975; 86: 598–601.

86. Hironaga M, Fujigaki T, Tanaka S. Calcinosis cutis in a neonate following extravasation of calcium gluconate. J Am Acad Dermatol 1982; 6: 392–395.

87. Ahn SK, Kim KT, Lee SH, et al. The efficacy of treatment with triamcinolone acetonide in calcinosis cutis following extravasation of calcium gluconate: a preliminary study. Pediatr Dermatol 1997; 14: 103–109.

88. Hicks MJ, Levy ML, Alexander J, et al. Subcutaneous fat necrosis of the newborn and hypercalcemia: Case report and review of the literature. Pediatr Dermatol 1993; 10: 271–276.

89. Norwood-Galloway A, Lebwohl M, Phelps RG, et al. Subcutaneous fat necrosis of the newborn with hypercalcemia. J Am Acad Dermatol 1987; 16: 435–439.

90. Sharlin DN, Koblenzer P. Necrosis of subcutaneous fat with hypercalcemia, a puzzling and multifaceted disease. Clin Pediatr 1970; 9: 290–294.

91. Thomsen RJ. Subcutaneous fat necrosis of the newborn and idiopathic hypercalcemia. Arch Dermatol 1980; 116: 1155–1158.

92. Duhn R, Schoen EJ, Siu M. Subcutaneous fat necrosis with extensive calcification after hypothermia in two newborn infants. Pediatrics 1968; 41: 661–664.

93. Gu LL, Daneman A, Binet A, et al. Nephrocalcinosis and nephrolithiasis due to subcutaneous fat necrosis with hypercalcemia in two full-term asphyxiated neonates: sonographic findings. Pediatr Radiol 1995; 25: 142–144.

94. Sell EJ, Hansen RC, Struck-Pierce S. Calcified nodules on the heel: A complication of neonatal intensive care. J Pediatr 1980; 96: 473–475.

95. Rho NK, Youn SJ, Park HS, et al. Calcified nodules on the heel of a child following a single heel stick in the neonatal period. Clin Exp Dermatol 2003; 28: 502–503.

96. Wilkins CE, Emmerson AJB. Extravasation injuries on regional neonatal units. Arch Dis Child Fetal Neonatal Ed 2004; 89: F274–F275.

97. Ramasethu, J. Prevention and management of extravasation injuries in neonates. NeoReviews 2004; 5: e491–e497.

98. Peabody JL, Emery JR. Noninvasive monitoring of blood gases in the newborn. Clin Perinatol 1985; 12: 147–160.

99. Miyasaka K, Ohata J. Burn, erosion, and 'sun'tan with the use of pulse oximetry in infants. Anesthesiol 1987; 67: 1008–1009.

100. Sobel DB. Burning of a neonate due to a pulse oximeter: arterial saturation monitoring. Pediatrics 1992; 89: 154–155.

101. Murphy KG, Secunda JA, Rockoff MA. Severe burns from a pulse oximeter. Anesthesiology 1990; 73: 350–352.

102. Boyle RJ, Oh W. Erythema following transcutaneous PO_2 monitoring. Pediatrics 1980; 65: 333–334.

103. Evans NJ, Rutter N. Reduction of skin damage from transcutaneous oxygen electrodes using a spray on dressing. Arch Dis Child 1986; 61: 881–884.

104. Golden SM. Skin craters – a complication of transcutaneous oxygen monitoring. Pediatrics 1981; 67: 514–516.

105. Sajben SF, Gibbs NF, Fallon-Friedlander S. Transillumination blisters in a neonate. J Am Acad Dermatol 1999; 41: 264–265.

106. Keroack MA, Kotilainen HR, Griffin BE. A cluster of atypical skin lesions in well-baby nurseries and a neonatal intensive care unit. J Perinatol 1996; 16: 370–373.

107. Woo EK. Infant skin temperature probes. Nursing 1998; 28: 31.

108. Mackenzie AR. Meatal ulceration following neonatal circumcision. Obstet Gynecol 1966; 28: 221–223.

109. Frieden IJ, Chang MW, Lee I. Suture ligation of supernumerary digits and 'tags': an outmoded practice? Arch Pediatr Adolesc Med 1995; 149: 1284.

110. Leber GE, Gosain AK. Surgical excision of pedunculated supernumerary digits prevents traumatic amputation neuromas. Pediatr Dermatol 2003; 20: 108–112.

9

Developmental Abnormalities

Liborka Kos, Beth Ann Drolet

Developmental abnormalities of the skin are a diverse group of anomalies that represent errors in morphogenesis. By definition they are present at birth, and most are diagnosed in infancy. They vary in severity from the inconsequential to the serious, and in some instances represent a marker for significant extracutaneous problems.

SUPERNUMERARY MAMMARY TISSUE

Accessory mammary tissue (supernumerary nipples, accessory nipple, polythelia, polymastia) may consist of true glandular tissue (accessory breasts), areola, nipples, or a combination thereof. It is often bilateral and found along the course of the embryologic breast lines, which run from the axilla to the inner thigh. Accessory nipples are the most common variant and occur in as many as 2% of females, manifesting clinically as a soft, brown, pedunculated papule (Fig. 9-1). In the newborn the lesions are often very subtle, appearing as a light brown or pearly 1–3 mm macule. Familial occurrence has been reported.

Extracutaneous Findings
It has been suggested that renal and urogenital malformations occur with increased frequency in infants with polythelia. However, the results of published studies are conflicting: incidence figures range from zero to approximately 10%.[1–6] Ultrasound has been employed to evaluate these infants, and as this procedure is noninvasive it should be considered in infants with worrisome clinical findings or if there is concern regarding an occult developmental defect.

Diagnosis
The diagnosis is usually made clinically but can be confirmed by histologic demonstration of mammary tissue. An accessory nipple will show epidermal thickening, pilosebaceous structures, and smooth muscle, with or without true mammary glands.[7] The differential diagnosis includes melanocytic nevus, neurofibroma, verruca, or skin tag.

Treatment
Complete surgical excision is usually recommended if there is glandular tissue because enlargement at puberty may cause pain and embarrassment. Small accessory nipples need not be excised. Breast carcinoma has also been reported in ectopic mammary tissue.[8]

PREAURICULAR PITS AND SINUSES

The auricle is formed by fusion of six tubercles derived from the first and second branchial arches. Incomplete fusion may lead to entrapment of epithelium, forming cysts that communicate to the surface through sinuses.[9] If the cyst and sinus are obliterated, a pit is left behind. Preauricular pits are common and may be inherited in an autosomal dominant fashion. They manifest as small depressions at the anterior margin of the ascending limb of the helix (Fig. 9-2).

Preauricular cysts manifest as tender swellings in the preauricular region; occasionally they are bilateral. If there is a sinus tract, fluid or pus may drain from a small opening just anterior to the ascending portion of the helix (Fig. 9-3). Most patients with preauricular cysts will have a history of recurrent infections.

Extracutaneous Findings
The purported association of preauricular pits, accessory tragi, and sinuses with renal abnormalities is controversial.[10] The most recent recommendations reserve renal ultrasound screening for patients with additional dysmorphic features, a family history of deafness, auricular and/or renal malformations, or a maternal history of gestational diabetes.[11] Patients with preauricular pits or tags may have a higher incidence of hearing

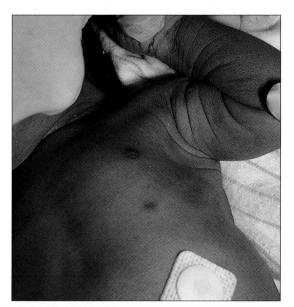

FIG. 9-1 Accessory nipple.

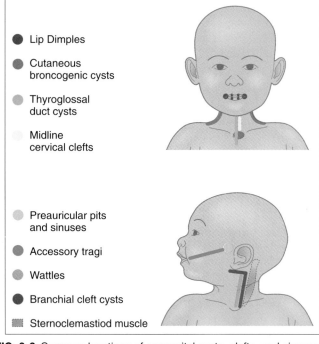

- ● Lip Dimples
- ● Cutaneous broncogenic cysts
- ○ Thyroglossal duct cysts
- ○ Midline cervical clefts
- ○ Preauricular pits and sinuses
- ○ Accessory tragi
- ○ Wattles
- ● Branchial cleft cysts
- ▧ Sternoclemastiod muscle

FIG. 9-2 Common locations of congenital cysts, clefts, and sinuses.

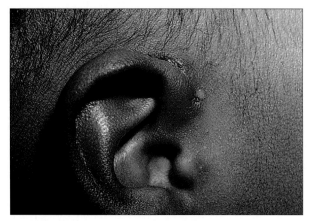

FIG. 9-3 Preauricular sinus with superinfection.

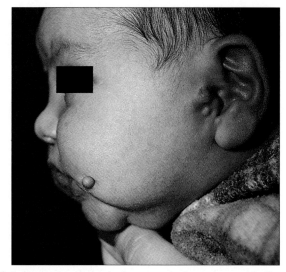

FIG. 9-4 Accessory tragus in the preauricular region and in the much less common region of the lateral commissure of the mouth.

Box 9-1 Genetic disorders associated with preauricular anomalies

Preauricular pits/sinuses
Branchio-otorenal syndrome
Goldenhar syndrome
Cat eye syndrome

Accessory tragi
Goldenhar syndrome
Treacher–Collins syndrome
Townes–Brock syndrome
VACTERL
Wolf–Hirschhorn syndrome (4p deletion syndrome)
Delleman syndrome

---

impairment, although studies are conflicting. Most studies do suggest screening for hearing deficits if the universal newborn hearing screen is not routinely performed.[12]

Diagnosis and Treatment

The diagnosis is usually apparent clinically. The sinuses and cysts are lined by stratified squamous epithelium. Surgical excision of preauricular cysts and sinuses is indicated to prevent secondary infection. An experienced surgeon should perform the excision because the procedure may be complicated by multiple cysts along a tract that ends at the periosteum of the auditory canal.

ACCESSORY TRAGI

The tragus is derived from the dorsal portion of the first branchial arch. Accessory tragi (erroneously referred to as preauricular 'tags') are pedunculated, flesh-colored, soft, round papules usually arising on or near the tragus. They may occur anywhere from the preauricular region to the corner of the mouth, following the line of fusion of the mandibular and maxillary branches of the first branchial arch (Fig. 9-4). They may be bilateral or multiple. The same hearing and renal screening recommendations discussed above regarding preauricular pits should be followed. Accessory tragi are usually isolated defects, but may be associated with other developmental abnormalities of the first branchial arch.[13] Goldenhar syndrome (oculoauriculovertebral syndrome) manifests as epibulbar dermoids, vertebral anomalies, and accessory tragi (Box 9-1).[14]

Diagnosis and Treatment

The diagnosis is usually clinically apparent. Histologically, there are numerous tiny hair follicles with prominent connective tissue. A central core of cartilage is usually present.[15] Accessory tragi should be removed by careful surgical dissection because most contain cartilage that may extend deeply, contiguous with the external ear canal. They are *not* skin tags and should not be tied off with suture material.[16]

CERVICAL TABS/WATTLES/CONGENITAL CARTILAGINOUS RESTS OF THE NECK

Cervical tabs are soft, pedunculated, irregular nodules occurring on the neck along the anterior border of the sternocleidomastoid muscle. They are thought to be remnants of branchial arches and tend to occur along branchial arch fusion lines (Fig. 9-5). Histologically they show lobules of mature cartilage embedded in collagen. The lesions do not extend deeply, but complete surgical excision is the treatment of choice because ligation may result in complications.[17,18]

SUPERNUMERARY DIGITS (RUDIMENTARY POLYDACTYLY)

Supernumerary digits arise from the lateral surface of a normal digit. They are most common on the ulnar surface of the fifth digit, but may occur on any finger. They may be bilateral or multiple. Some are small pedunculated papules, whereas others are normal-sized digits containing both cartilage and nail (Fig. 9-6). These lesions should be surgically excised and the associated nerve dissected if present. Ligating the supernumerary digit with suture material without completely removing the nerve may result in skin necrosis, infection, and painful neuromas in adult life.[16]

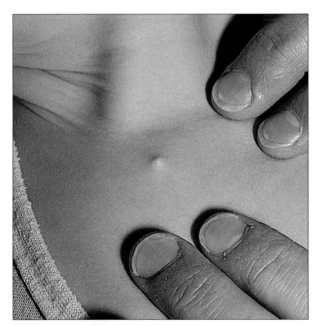

FIG. 9-5 Cartilaginous rest of the neck.

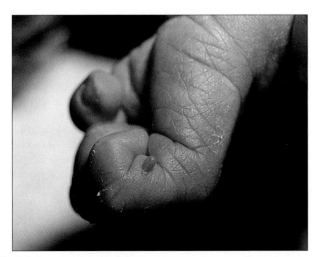

FIG. 9-6 Supernumerary digit.

BRANCHIAL CYSTS, BRANCHIAL CLEFTS, AND BRANCHIAL SINUSES

Branchial cysts are congenital malformations; however, they are not often apparent clinically until the first or second decade of life. They are painless, mobile, cystic swellings in the neck. Most measure 1–2 cm, although they may be as large as 10 cm. They may enlarge during respiratory tract infections. Branchial cysts derived from the second branchial arch are the most common and are found on the lateral aspect of the upper neck, along the sternocleidomastoid muscle (Fig. 9-7). Branchial cleft cysts derived from the first branchial arch are very rare and are located in the periauricular area or on the upper neck anterior to the sternocleidomastoid muscle. Definitive diagnosis is made by histologic examination of the lesions. Branchial cysts are lined by stratified squamous epithelium, or rarely by ciliated columnar epithelium. There is often abundant lymphoid tissue. Squamous cell carcinomas arising in these cystic lesions have been described in adults.[19]

Branchial sinuses and branchial clefts are thought to be remnants of the branchial cleft depressions. They are usually present at birth or noted during the first few years of life. The most common location is along the lateral lower third of the neck. Often a skin tag with a small amount of cartilage is associated with the pit. Branchial cleft anomalies should be surgically excised to prevent infection, with careful attention to the possibility of a true fistula connecting to the tonsillar oropharynx. Preoperative imaging may be necessary to exclude the possibility of true fistulae.

THRYOGLOSSAL DUCT CYSTS

Thryoglossal duct cysts are the most common etiology of a congenital neck mass. They result from the persistence of a tract formed during the migration of the rudimentary thyroid gland from the base of the tongue to the anterior cervical regions. The most common location is on or just off of the midline neck in the area of the hyoid bone, but they can be found anywhere from the posterior tongue to the suprasternal

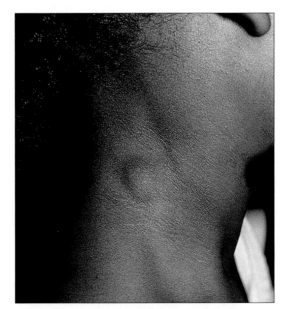

FIG. 9-7 Branchial cyst on the lateral region of the neck.

notch. Most thyroglossal duct cysts present in childhood as an asymptomatic mass that moves upward with tongue protrusion or swallowing. Occasionally, ectopic thyroid tissue can be found in these cysts, and an association with thyroid cancer has been reported. The treatment is complete surgical excision to prevent growth and infection. Preoperative imaging with high-resolution ultrasound is important to confirm the diagnosis and identify the presence of a normal thyroid gland.[20]

CUTANEOUS BRONCHOGENIC CYSTS AND SINUSES

Bronchogenic cysts are usually found within the chest or mediastinum but may also occasionally be found in the skin. The most common cutaneous location is in the subcutaneous tissue at the suprasternal notch, but other locations include the lateral neck, scapula, and presternal area. Thus, these cysts should be included in the differential of both lateral and midline neck masses. The cysts are congenital and usually apparent at birth. They are asymptomatic, small cystic swellings that will gradually enlarge over time and may discharge a mucoid material. These lesions are not usually associated with other malformations and do not connect to underlying structures.[21,22] The diagnosis is made by histologic examination of the nodule or sinus. Bronchogenic cysts are lined by lamina propria and a pseudostratified columnar ciliated epithelium with goblet cells.[23] The cyst wall may contain smooth muscle, mucus glands, and cartilage. Lymphatic tissue may or may not be present.

The differential diagnosis includes branchial arch cysts, thyroglossal duct cysts, teratomas, and heterotopic salivary gland tissue. The treatment is complete surgical excision to prevent infection.

MEDIAN RAPHE CYSTS

Median raphe cysts (congenital sinus and cysts of the genitoperineal raphe, mucous cysts of the penile skin, parameatal cysts) are the consequence of incomplete fusion of the ventral aspect of the urethral or genital folds. In most cases they remain asymptomatic unless superinfection occurs. They are small, soft, flesh-colored papules along the ventral aspect of the penis in the line of the median raphe (Fig. 9-8). The cysts are lined with pseudostratified columnar epithelium, except at the distal penis, where they have stratified epithelium.[24]

VENTRAL MIDLINE CLEFTS/DEFECTS

Supraumbilical Cleft

Disruption of abdominal wall fusion causes midline defects of variable degree, often involving the heart and sternum, as well as the abdominal wall. Supraumbilical raphes are linear, midline clefts that occur anterior to the umbilicus. A well-described association of supraumbilical raphe and/or sternal clefting has been described in association with hemangiomas and PHACE(S) (see Chapter 20).[25–27]

Midline Cervical Clefts

This rare abnormality of the midline ventral neck presents as a small skin tag superiorly with a linear, vertically oriented atrophic patch. At the inferior aspect of the patch there is often

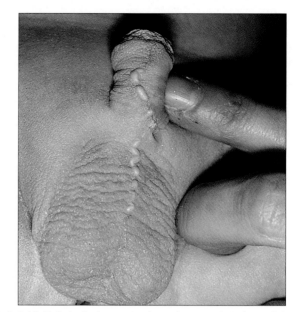

FIG. 9-8 Multiple inclusion cysts along the ventral surface of the penis.

a small sinus containing ectopic salivary tissue.[28] Midline cervical clefts can be associated with cleft lip, palate, mandible, chin, tongue or midline neck hypoplasia.[29] Excision with serial Z-plasties is the treatment of choice.

CUTANEOUS SIGNS OF NEURAL TUBE DYSRAPHISM

The skin and the nervous system share a common ectodermal origin. Separation of the neural and cutaneous ectoderm occurs early in gestational life at about the same time as the neural tube is fusing. This embryologic association may explain simultaneous malformations of the skin and nervous system. The neural tube is no longer believed to fuse in a zipper-like fashion, but rather in a segmental, noncontiguous pattern.[30] This theory is supported by the clinical observation of cutaneous 'hotspots' for dysraphic conditions. Each hotspot corresponds to a fusion point of the various segments of the neural tube (Fig. 9-9). This discussion will be limited to cutaneous markers of occult neural tube dysraphic conditions in the cranial region (calvarial defects) and those along the spinal axis.

Cranial Dysraphism

Cephaloceles/Cutaneous Neural Heterotopias

The term cutaneous neural heterotopia was introduced to describe leptomeningeal or glial tissue which is found in the subcutaneous tissue or dermis of the skin. These malformations are the result of incomplete or faulty closure of the neural tube and are not a malignancy. Cephalocele is the general term for congenital herniation of intracranial structures through a scalp defect. Encephalocele is herniation of both glial and meningeal tissue. Meningoceles are congenital cephaloceles in which only the meninges and cerebrospinal fluid herniate through a calvarial defect. Large encephaloceles and meningoceles pose no diagnostic problem and are usually easily diagnosed prenatally or at birth. Smaller or atretic encephaloceles

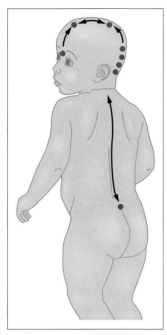

FIG. 9-9 Cutaneous 'hotspots' for neural tube dysraphism are depicted by the circles. The arrows represent the direction of fusion of each neural tube segment.

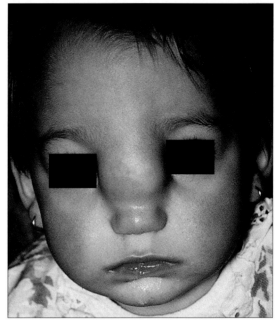

FIG. 9-10 Frontal encephalocele. (Courtesy of Dr Odile Enjolras.)

Box 9-2 Terms used to describe cutaneous neural heterotopias

Heterotopic meningeal nodules

Ectopic brain tissue

Heterotopic brain tissue/nodules

Meningioma

Rudimentary encephalocele/meningocele

Atretic encephalocele/meningocele

Vestigial encephalocele/meningocele

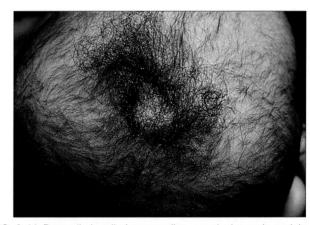

FIG. 9-11 Dense 'hair collar' surrounding a vesicular scalp nodule found to be a meningocele.

and meningoceles may be mistaken for cutaneous lesions such as hematomas, hemangiomas, aplasia cutis, dermoid cysts, or inclusion cysts. Several terms have been used to describe these smaller lesions (Box 9-2). These labels were derived from the amount and type of neural tissue present, as well as the degree of connection to the CNS. Unfortunately, it is not possible to predict the degree of CNS connection on clinical grounds alone. Therefore, all congenital exophytic scalp nodules should be evaluated thoroughly, as 20–37% of congenital, nontraumatic scalp nodules connect to the underlying central nervous system.[31,32]

Cutaneous Findings

Cephaloceles occur in the frontal, parietal, and occipital regions. They are usually midline, although they may also be found 1–3 cm lateral to the midline. Small cephaloceles are clinically heterogeneous, their appearance dictated by the type and amount of cutaneous ectoderm overlying the lesion. They may be covered with normal skin (Fig. 9-10), or have a blue, translucent, or glistening surface. There is usually a disruption of the surrounding and overlying normal hair pattern. They are soft, compressible, round, or pedunculated nodules that

increase in size when the baby cries or with a Valsalva maneuver.

The association of a cephalocele with certain other cutaneous abnormalities makes the diagnosis of cranial dysraphism highly suspicious. Stigmata include hypertrichosis, or the 'hair-collar sign,' capillary malformations, hemangiomas, and cutaneous dimples and sinuses.[33,34] The hypertrichosis may overlie the nodule, surround a small sinus, or encircle the nodule (hair collar). A hair collar is defined as a congenital ring of hair that is usually denser, darker, and coarser than the normal scalp hair. When found encircling an exophytic scalp nodule, it is highly suggestive of cranial dysraphism (Figs 9-11 and 9-12).[33,34] The hair-collar sign may be found in association with encephaloceles, meningoceles, atretic encephaloceles, atretic meningoceles, and heterotopic brain tissue. A hair collar may also be seen with some lesions of aplasia cutis; thus this sign is not entirely specific.[35] Cranial neural tube defects may also be associated with overlying red, blanchable patches that represent capillary malformations. The combination of a

117

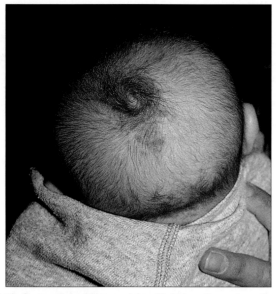

FIG. 9-12 Congenital midline nodule with hair collar and capillary malformation. MRI confirmed an atretic encephalocele.

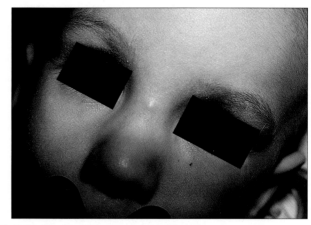

FIG. 9-13 Small midline nasal dermoid cyst.

hair collar sign and capillary malformation surrounding a congenital scalp lesion is almost always indicative of a dysraphic condition (Fig. 9-11).[34]

Extracutaneous Findings and Diagnosis

From a clinical standpoint, encephaloceles, meningoceles, atretic cephaloceles, and heterotopic brain tissue are virtually impossible to differentiate. All congenital midline scalp nodules carry a significant risk of intracranial connection and should have radiologic imaging studies performed before surgical removal to prevent complications such as meningitis. Membranous aplasia cutis congenita (ACC) has many overlapping clinical features (including the hair-collar sign); in addition, the loose fibroconnective tissue seen histologically is very similar to the changes observed surrounding encephaloceles.[33] The presence of a palpable nodule within a lesion of ACC, however, is uncommon and should always prompt further evaluation. Magnetic resonance imaging (MRI) is the most sensitive modality for detecting small cephalocoeles with intracranial connections.

Differential Diagnosis and Management

Included in the differential diagnosis of congenital scalp nodules are pilomatrixoma, epidermoid cyst, lipoma, osteoma, eosinophilic granuloma, hemangioma, sinus pericranii, dermoid cyst, leptomeningeal cyst, and cephalohematoma.[36] Surgical correction is indicated for all cephaloceles.

Nasal Gliomas

Gliomas are rests of ectopic neural tissue and differ from frontal encephaloceles in that they do not have a patent intracranial communication. The lesions may be external, intranasal, or combined. Clinically they are firm, noncompressible, nontender, skin-colored to red-purple nodules at the root of the nose. They do not transilluminate. Gliomas may be covered with nasal mucosa or normal skin; they are often associated with telangiectasia and misdiagnosed as a hemangioma. They may widen the nasal bone, giving the appearance

of hypertelorism. They are congenital and do not proliferate, which helps to differentiate them from hemangiomas. Immediate neurosurgical referral is required for surgical removal and reconstruction.

Cranial Dermoid Cysts and Sinuses

Dermoid cysts are congenital subcutaneous lesions that are distributed along embryonic fusion lines. The cysts may occur within the fusion lines of the facial processes or along the neural axis. They represent faulty development and may include both epidermal and dermal elements.

Cutaneous Findings

Although dermoid cysts are always congenital, they may not be noted until early childhood, when they begin to enlarge. They can occur anywhere on the face, scalp, or spinal axis but are most frequently seen overlying the anterior fontanelle, at the junction of the sagittal and coronal sutures on the scalp, on the upper lateral region of the forehead within or near the eyebrow, and in the submental region.[37–41] They are nontender, noncompressible, nonpulsatile, firm blue or skin-colored nodules measuring 1–4 cm (Figs 9-13, 9-14). They do not transilluminate or enlarge with a Valsalva maneuver. The overlying skin is normal, unless there is an external connection in the form of a pit or a sinus. Dermoid cysts may adhere to the underlying periosteum.

Dermal sinuses are 1–5 mm tracts that typically connect a dermoid cyst to the skin surface. They are usually midline and are found on the nose, occipital scalp, and anywhere along the spinal axis. They may become clinically apparent when they become infected and drain purulent material. A small tuft of hair is often found protruding from the orifice. If the sinus and/or cyst communicates directly with the central nervous system, the patient is at risk for meningitis. The sinus serves as an occult portal of entry for bacteria, often causing a recurrent meningitis that is culture positive for skin flora. *Staphylococcus aureus* meningitis should be considered secondary to a dermal sinus until proved otherwise, and a thorough search for a cutaneous fistula should be carried out, which may necessitate shaving the scalp hair.[42] All midline dermal sinuses should have radiologic imaging prior to surgical excision. Probing these lesions is contraindicated, given the potential risk of meningitis.

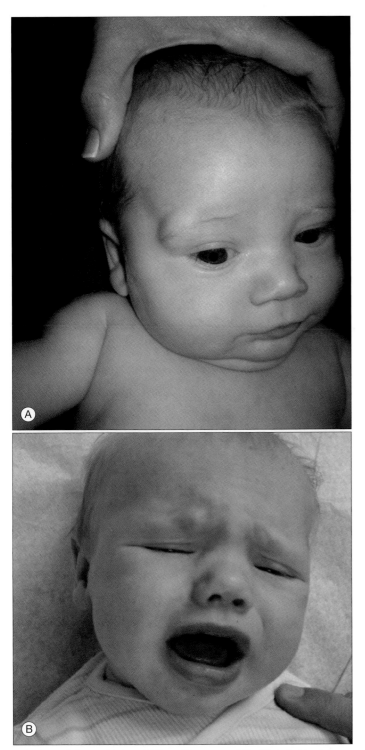

FIG. 9-14 A Lateral Dermoid Cyst (Courtesy of Dr. Victoria Barrio). **B** Medial eyebrow dermoid cyst.

gliomas, the patient may have the appearance of hypertelorism if the cyst has widened the nasal bones. Nasal dermoids should always be excised, because over time they enlarge and damage the nasal bones. Dermoid cysts that are not midline should also be excised because they have the potential for infection. Dermoids of the lateral eyebrow area do not have central nervous system connections and may be surgically excised, either directly or using an endoscopic approach via a scalp incision to avoid facial scarring (Fig. 9-14). Lateral brow dermoids appear deceptively superficial, but most are actually located beneath muscle, so that either removal must be via an endoscopic approach or the surgeon must be prepared to dissect through the muscle to remove the cyst.

Diagnosis

Definitive diagnosis is made by histologic examination of the lesions. Dermoids cysts are usually found in the subcutaneous tissue and are lined by stratified squamous epithelium that often contains hair follicles, sebaceous glands, and sweat glands. The lumen may contain keratin, lipid, and hair. Radiologic imaging is a very sensitive screening method and should be undertaken prior to surgical intervention. Currently the most sensitive study is MRI. Computed tomography (CT) may better delineate bony defects and may also be necessary for surgical planning, especially in the nasal region. Plain radiographs were used extensively in the past but are not sensitive and should not be used for screening.

SPINAL DYSRAPHISM

Spinal dysraphism, or incomplete closure of the spinal axis, encompasses many congenital anomalies of the spine. Larger defects, such as meningomyeloceles, are usually obvious at birth and fall within the purview of the neurosurgeon. However, small or occult malformations causing tethering of the spinal cord may have subtle signs and be asymptomatic. Early diagnosis is imperative, as it may prevent irreversible neurologic damage in these patients. A diagnosis of occult spinal dysraphism is often suspected solely on the basis of overlying cutaneous findings, particularly in the newborn. Cutaneous markers are found in 50–90% of these patients.[43–52]

Cutaneous Findings

The cutaneous lesions that should alert the physician to an underlying occult spinal dysraphism are listed in Box 9-3. Most are found on or near the midline in the lumbosacral region; however, similar markers in the cervical or thoracic regions may also be indicative of an underlying malformation. The literature suggests that certain skin lesions are more indicative than others of underlying malformation.[43–54] Tavafoghi[52] reviewed 200 cases of spinal dysraphism and found that 102 had cutaneous signs. Other studies have documented an even higher incidence of cutaneous malformations (71–100%). Unfortunately, no prospective studies have been carried out to determine what percentage of children with cutaneous anomalies overlying the spinal axis have occult dysraphism.

These cutaneous markers should also be evaluated in the context of a full history and physical examination, particularly in the older child. The history should include questions about additional congenital malformations, family history of neural tube defects, weakness or pain in the lower extremities, abnormal gait, scoliosis, difficulties with toilet training or incontinence, recurrent urinary tract infections, and recurrent

Extracutaneous Findings

Midline or nasal dermoid cysts are of the greatest concern because 25% have an intracranial connection.[38] Nasal dermoid cysts may occur anywhere from the glabella to the tip of the nose; a nasal pit or sinus is present in about half the cases.[37] The pit often leads caudally to a dermal sinus and eventuates in a cyst that may be either external or within the nasal bones. If the dermoid cyst connects to the central nervous system, cerebrospinal fluid may drain from the sinus. As with nasal

> **Box 9-3 Cutaneous lesions associated with spinal dysraphism**
>
> **High index of suspicion**
> Hypertrichosis
>
> Dimples (large, >2.5 cm from the anal verge, atypical)
>
> Acrochordons/pseudotails/true tails
>
> Lipomas
>
> Hemangiomas
>
> Aplasia cutis or scar
>
> Dermoid cyst or sinus
>
> **Low index of suspicion**
> Telangiectasia
>
> Capillary malformation (port-wine stain)
>
> Hyperpigmentation
>
> Melanocytic nevi
>
> Small sacral dimples 2.5 cm from anal verge
>
> Teratomas

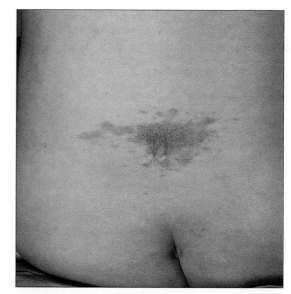

FIG. 9-15 Subtle patch of hypertrichosis with an overlying capillary malformation in a patient with a dermal sinus.

meningitis. The vertebrae should be palpated for any defects or abnormalities. Examination of the rectum and genitalia is also indicated, as there are often associated congenital abnormalities of the urogenital system.[55–57] The gluteal cleft should be examined carefully for small acrochordons or sinuses; it should be straight and the buttocks symmetric. If the gluteal cleft deviates, it is suggestive of an underlying mass such as a lipoma or meningocele. Examination of the lower extremities is important in older children because they may have trophic changes secondary to nerve damage.

Hypertrichosis

Localized lumbosacral hypertrichosis, or 'hairy patch,' is usually present at birth. The hair may be dark or light. The texture of the hair can vary but is frequently described as silky (faun tail nevus). The hypertrichosis is often V-shaped and poorly circumscribed (Fig. 9-15). Prominent hypertrichosis is commonly associated with other cutaneous stigmata of spinal dysraphism and is highly indicative of a spinal defect. Hypertrichosis in the lumbosacral region can be a normal finding, however, especially in certain ethnic or racial groups, and it may be difficult to decide whether or not further evaluation is indicated. Referral to a neurologist or neurosurgeon for a more complete neurologic examination may be a prudent measure in these cases.

Lipomas

Lipomas associated with spinal dysraphism are thought to be congenital and are also highly indicative of an underlying defect. Unlike acquired lipomas, they may be poorly circumscribed and feel more like an area of increased subcutaneous fat than a discrete lesion. The lipoma may lie in the dermis or the spinal canal, and often penetrates from the dermis through a vertebral defect into the intraspinal space (lipomyelomeningocele). Intraspinal lipomas are a common cause of tethered cord. Appropriate radiologic investigation of lumbosacral lipomas must be performed before surgical excision, and a neurosurgeon should be involved because small intraspinal

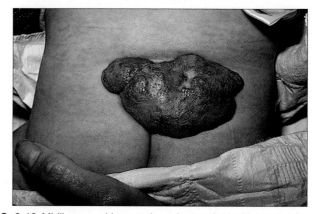

FIG. 9-16 Midline sacral hemangioma in a patient with an occult lipomyelomeningocele.

connections may be missed, even with the most sensitive radiologic imaging.

Hemangiomas, Telangiecstasias, and Capillary Malformations

Hemangiomas are proliferative vascular tumors that may be present at birth or develop in the first months of life. In 1986 Goldberg et al. described five children with large sacral hemangiomas and several other associated abnormalities.[56] Three of the five had lipomyelomeningoceles. In 1989 Albright et al.[43] reported seven infants with lumbar hemangiomas and a tethered spinal cord. Several subsequent reports have supported this association. Hemangiomas associated with spinal dysraphism are usually large (>4 cm) and overlie the midline (Figs 9-16, 9-17). There is often a skin defect or ulceration within the hemangioma. The hemangiomas may be associated with other cutaneous stigmata, such as lipoma, acrochordon, or dermal sinus. These patients are difficult to manage because the hemangiomas can ulcerate, and surgical repair of the tethered cord often may have to be delayed until the hemangioma partially regresses.

Reports of telangiectatic patches are probably describing nascent or partially regressed hemangiomas. Enjolras et al.[58]

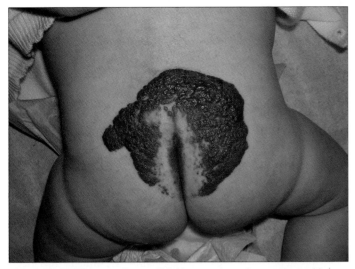

FIG. 9-17 Midline sacral superficial hemangioma in a patient with an underlying lipoma and tethered spinal cord.

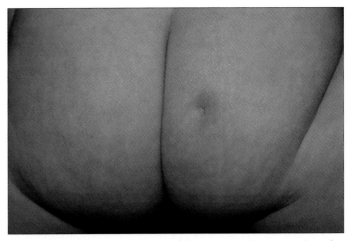

FIG. 9-19 Dimple on buttock with bluish discoloration suggestive of a lateral congenital spinal dermal sinus.

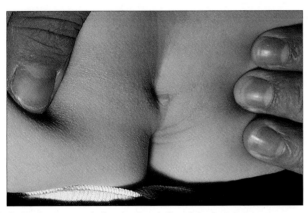

FIG. 9-18 Deep sacral dimple above the gluteal crease.

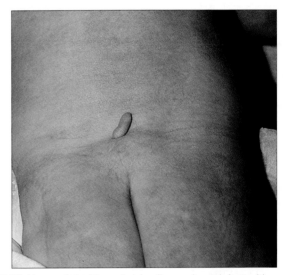

FIG. 9-20 Human tail with underlying lipoma in an infant with lipomyelomeningocele.

reported two patients with cervical spinal dysraphism with an overlying capillary malformation (port-wine stain), but spinal dysraphism associated with a midline, lumbosacral capillary malformation without additional clinical findings is probably uncommon. Two small studies have shown a low but real incidence of spinal dysraphism associated with a solitary capillary malformation of the lumbosacral region.[59,60] Further investigation is needed to completely clarify the need for imaging in these infants. A neurologic consultation may be warranted.

Dimples, Sinuses, Aplasia Cutis, and Congenital Scars

Lumbosacral dimples are common, but can occasionally be a sign of spinal dysraphism.[61,62] Most infants with sacral dimples that fall within the gluteal crease are normal.[63] Dimples that are deep, large (≥0.5 cm), located in the superior portion or above the gluteal crease (>2.5 cm from the anal verge), or associated with other cutaneous markers should be radiologically imaged (Fig. 9-18).[60] Deep dimples may actually be dermal sinuses, communicating directly with the spinal canal. They may also be located off of the midline, on the buttock (Fig. 9-19).[64] These lesions should not be probed, but instead should prompt MR imaging studies and neurosurgical consultation.

Aplasia cutis has rarely been reported in the lumbosacral region and in that site may be associated with underlying spinal dysraphism.[44] Scar-like defects have also been described in patients with spinal dysraphism, and may in fact be a variant of aplasia cutis.[56] The scar-like regions found in lumbosacral hemangiomas may represent a similar phenomenon.

Acrochordons, Tails, and Pseudotails

Acrochordons are small skin-covered sessile or pedunculated papules or nodules (Fig. 9-20). Histologically they are composed of epidermis and a dermal stalk. A true human tail (persistent vestigial tail) is rare and is differentiated from a pseudotail and an acrochordon by the presence of a central core of mature fatty tissue, small blood vessels, bundles of muscle fibers, and nerve fibers. A pseudotail is a stump-like structure considered to be a hamartoma composed of fatty tissue and often cartilage. Clinically these lesions are difficult to distinguish, and all have been associated with spinal dysraphism.[46,48,52,56,65] Preoperative radiologic investigation is indicated in all cases.

Diagnosis

A definitive diagnosis of spinal dysraphism is made only at surgery. Radiologic imaging provides a sensitive screening method. Three radiologic modalities are currently used for the preoperative diagnosis of spinal dysraphism. MRI remains the gold standard, but high-resolution ultrasound is an excellent noninvasive alternative in an infant less than 6 months of age.[66-71] An infant's vertebrae are not yet completely ossified, and ultrasound serves as a relatively inexpensive screening tool. If abnormalities are found, MRI is required preoperatively.[71] Also used in the past, myelograms have been replaced by MRI. It is often useful to speak to the radiologist before ordering the examination because the technology is changing rapidly and will vary by institution. Urodynamic studies are increasingly being used as another modality for assessing spinal cord function in settings where radiologic findings are equivocal.[72]

APLASIA CUTIS

Aplasia cutis is a general term that is used to describe focal, congenital defects of the skin. The condition is rare and its true incidence is unknown. Several theories have been proposed as to its pathogenesis, but most authors believe that aplasia cutis has no single underlying cause but is rather a clinical finding that results from a variety of events that occur in utero. Several classifications of aplasia cutis have been proposed (Table 9-1).[73]

When evaluating a newborn with aplasia cutis, particular attention should be given to the morphology and the distribution of the defects because this may be helpful in determining the etiology, possible associated malformations, and prognosis (Table 9-2). For example, infants with large defects of aplasia cutis on the bilateral extremities have generalized increased skin fragility, the result of a genetic deficiency, and almost all have been classified as having epidermolysis bullosa. This is a lifelong affliction and will have immediate implications for the care of the infant. Large defects may be seen with trisomy 13 (Fig. 9-21). Table 9-3 correlates the clinical findings with the proposed etiology and associations.

Cutaneous Findings

Membranous aplasia cutis is the most common form. It occurs primarily on the scalp, but may also be seen on the lateral aspects of the face (focal facial dermal hypoplasia). The lesions are usually small, oval, or round and measure 2–5 cm. They are well circumscribed, with a 'punched-out' appearance (Fig. 9-22). At birth, the surface is atrophic, often thin, glistening, and membrane-like. Scar-like lesions in the same configuration are more common in older children. Rarely the lesions may be bullous at birth, containing a thick, clear fluid (Fig. 9-23). The bullous lesions may drain spontaneously and reform, eventually flattening to the more typical appearance. Defects of membranous aplasia cutis are often multiple, occurring in a linear configuration. The most common location is at the vertex of the scalp, but they may also be found anterior to the vertex, 1–2 cm off the midline on the parietal scalp, or even extending down onto the forehead along a line from the lateral forehead to the lateral edge of the eyebrows. Rarely, lesions of membranous aplasia cutis occur on the face in a line extending from the preauricular region to the angles of the mouth.[74] The term focal facial dermal hypoplasia has been used to describe these lesions (Fig. 9-24). Lesions of temporal aplasia cutis may be associated with Setleis syndrome and found with additional facial anomalies. Most reports of membranous aplasia cutis are sporadic; however, there are well-documented patients with autosomal dominant and autosomal

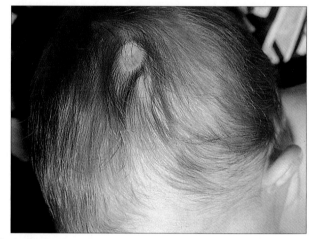

FIG. 9-22 Membranous aplasia cutis with a subtle hair-collar sign.

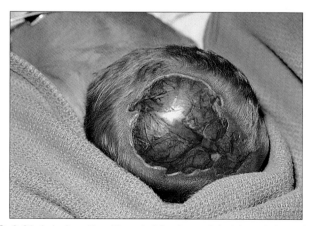

FIG. 9-21 Aplasia cutis with underlying bone defect in an infant with trisomy 13.

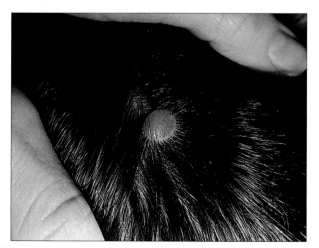

FIG. 9-23 Bullous aplasia cutis in a newborn.

TABLE 9-1 A classification of aplasia cutis congenita

Category	Body area affected	Associated abnormalities	Inheritance
Group 1: scalp ACC without multiple anomalies	Scalp, usually vertex	Cleft lip and palate; tracheoesophageal fistula; double cervix and uterus; patent ductus arteriosus; omphalocele; polycystic kidney; mental retardation; cutis marmorata telangiectatica congenita	Autosomal dominant or sporadic
Group 2: scalp ACC with associated limb abnormalities (most cases are Adams-Oliver syndrome)	Midline scalp	Limb reduction abnormalities; 2–3 syndactyly; clubfoot; nail absence or dystrophy; skin tags on toes; persistent cutis marmorata; encephalocele; woolly hair; hemangioma; heart disease; cryptorchidism; postaxial polydactyly (1 family)	Autosomal dominant
Group 3: Scalp ACC with associated epidermal and organoid nevi	Membranous scalp lesions, may be asymmetric, solitary or multiple	Cephaloceles; corneal opacities; scleral dermoids; eyelid colobomas; psychomotor retardation; seizures	Sporadic
Group 4: ACC overlying embryologic malformations	Abdomen, lumbar skin, scalp; any site	Meningomyeloceles; spinal dysraphia; cranial stenosis; congenital midline porencephaly; leptomeningeal angiomatosis; ectopia of ear; omphalocele; gastroschisis	Depends on underlying condition
Group 5: ACC with associated fetus papyraceus or placental infarcts	Multiple, symmetric areas, often stellate or linear, on scalp, chest, flanks, axillae, and extremities	Single umbilical artery; developmental delay; spastic paralysis; nail dystrophy; clubbed hands and feet; amniotic bands; gastrointestinal atresia	Sporadic
Group 6: ACC associated with EB: Blistering, usually localized, without multiple congenital anomalies	Extremities	Blistering of skin and/or mucous membranes; absent or deformed nails; metatarsus varus; congenital absence of kidney (seen in cases of recessive, dystrophic EB; dominant, dystrophic EB; and EB simplex)	Depends on EB type: may be autosomal dominant or recessive
Junctional EB with pyloric atresia	Large areas on extremities and torso	Pyloric or duodenal atresia; abnormal ears and nose; ureteral stenosis; renal abnormalities; arthrogryposis	Autosomal recessive
Group 7: ACC localized to extremities without blistering	Pretibial areas; dorsal aspects of hands and feet; extensor areas of wrists	None	Autosomal dominant or recessive
Group 8: ACC caused by specific teratogens	Scalp (with methimazole); any area (with varicella and herpes simplex infections)	Imperforate anus (methimazole); signs of intrauterine infection with varicella and herpes simplex infections	Not inherited
Group 9: ACC associated with malformation syndromes (see also Table 9-2)	Scalp; any location	Trisomy 13; 4p – syndrome; many ectodermal dysplasias; Johanson-Blizzard syndrome; focal dermal hypoplasia; amniotic band disruption complex; XY gonadal dysgenesis	Varies, depending on specific syndrome

ACC, *Aplasia cutis congenita*; EB, *epidermolysis bullosa*.
Modified from Frieden IJ. *J AM Acad Dermatol* 1986;14:646–660.

recessive patterns of inheritance.[75,76] Although the exact etiology of these lesions is unknown, the configuration, distribution, and clinical appearance would suggest incomplete closure of embryonic fusion lines, rather than vascular interruption or trauma to the skin.[74] A case of membranous aplasia cutis was detected by prenatal ultrasound at 27 weeks' gestation. A protruding, round, cystic lesion was noted at the vertex of the scalp. The lesion resolved spontaneously at 37 weeks' gesta-tion, and a small oval lesion of membranous aplasia cutis was found in the identical location at birth.[77]

Irregular, large, or stellate scalp defects of aplasia cutis are much less common but may occur along the midline of the scalp (Fig. 9-25). These defects are more commonly familial and often associated with large underlying bony defects.[78] They have a risk of infection and sagittal sinus thrombosis or hemorrhage Abnormalities of the underlying venous system

TABLE 9-2 Associated malformations and chromosomal defects reported with aplasia cutis

Syndrome	Clinical phenotype	Associated features	Inheritance
Opitz syndrome	Membranous aplasia cutis	Hypertelorism, cleft lip/palate, hypospadias, cryptorchidism	–
Adams-Oliver syndrome	Large, ill-defined, irregular scalp defects	Distal limb reduction abnormalities	Autosomal dominant
Oculocerebrocutaneous syndrome	Membranous aplasia cutis	Orbital cysts, cerebral malformations, facial skin tags, seizures, developmental delay	–
Trisomy D(13–15)	Membranous aplasia cutis	Holoprosencephaly, seizures, ocular abnormalities, deafness, neural tube defects	–
4p(–) syndrome	Not specified	Mental retardation, deafness, seizures, ocular abnormalities	–
Johanson-Blizzard syndrome	Small stellate defects of frontal scalp and membranous aplasia cutis	Dwarfism, mental retardation, deafness, hypothyroidism, pancreatic insufficiency	–
X-p22 microdeletion syndrome	Bilateral linear reticulated defects of the malar region of the face	Microphthalmia, sclerocornea	–
Chromosome 16–18 defect	Large scalp defects	Scalp arteriovenous malformation with underlying bony defect	–

TABLE 9-3 Correlation of clinical findings with proposed etiology and associations in aplasia cutis

Clinical phenotype	Proposed etiology	Associations
Cranial and facial membranous aplasia cutis	Developmental	Organoid nevi
Truncal, stellate aplasia cutis	Vascular disruption	Fetus papyraceus, placental insufficiency, gastrointestinal atresia
Extremity, angulated defects	Increased skin fragility	Epidermolysis bullosa
Small scar like defects	Maternal infections	Varicella, herpes simplex virus infections
Cranial large, midline irregular defects	Developmental, genetic	Bone defects, hydrocephalus, arteriovenous fistula, sinus thrombosis
Reticulated facial lesions	Chromosomal abnormality	X-p22 deletion syndrome

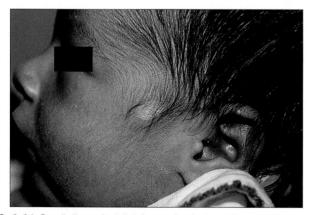

FIG. 9-24 Small, linear facial defects of aplasia cutis.

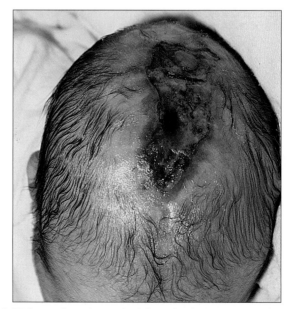

FIG. 9-25 Large, irregular scalp defect of aplasia cutis.

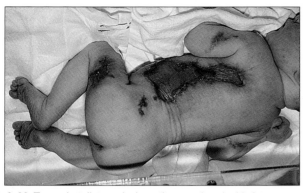

FIG. 9-26 Truncal stellate aplasia cutis associated with fetus papyraceus.

and arteriovenous malformations may be associated with these types of defect. Radiologic imaging with particular attention to the vasculature is recommended before surgical intervention, as hemorrhagic complications and death have been reported.[79]

Aplasia Cutis of the Trunk

When the term aplasia cutis is used in the most literal sense, this condition is found overlying abdominal malformations such as gastroschisis and omphalocele. Extensive truncal and limb defects have been associated with fetus papyraceus.[80,81] These defects differ clinically from membranous aplasia cutis. They are large, linear, or stellate erosions involving the lateral aspects of the trunk and extensor surfaces of the extremities (Fig. 9-26). Frequently they are bilateral and symmetric. It is theorized that these defects are the result of placental infarction after the death of a twin fetus, which would explain their symmetric distribution. These types of cutaneous lesion may also be associated with gastrointestinal malformations, particularly bowel atresia, which is also thought to be a consequence of early ischemia.[82] Additional extracutaneous findings include neurodevelopmental delay, intracranial hemorrhage, cardiac and arterial anomalies, renal cortical necrosis, and neonatal Volkmann ischemic contracture.[83,84] Similar truncal defects have been seen in patients with pale or small placentas, and several have also been reported without mention of the placenta.[83] Irregular defects of the extremities and trunk have been reported with blistering of the skin (Bart's syndrome); however, these are now considered to be a form of epidermolysis bullosa.[73,85]

Reticulated linear skin defects of the malar region of the face have been reported as part of the X-p22 microdeletion syndrome (see Chapter 26). All reported cases have been female, suggesting that the deletion may be lethal in males. Severity varies in females from relatively mild facial scarring to major organ malformations. It is associated with microphthalmia and sclerocornea.[86–88]

Pathogenesis

Several theories have been proposed as to the etiology of aplasia cutis. Incomplete closure of the neural tube may explain midline lesions, and incomplete closure of embryonic fusion lines may explain the lateral membranous aplasia cutis lesions.[74] Vascular insufficiency to the skin may result from placental insufficiency or thromboplastic material from a fetus papyraceus. Amniotic membrane adhesions, teratogenic agents, and intrauterine infections have also been implicated.

The heterogeneity of the associated findings makes a unifying theory unlikely.

Extracutaneous Findings

The lesions of membranous aplasia cutis most commonly occur as an isolated defect and usually require no further investigation. Even small underlying bony defects usually heal spontaneously. However, there are exceptions. Any lesion of aplasia cutis with a palpable lump within it should prompt further evaluation (see discussion of dermoids above). Midline lesions occurring at sites between the vertex and occiput are less common, and may have a greater risk of underlying defects and/or connections. Larger lesions of aplasia cutis with large underlying bony defects need prompt imaging studies to assess for underlying CNS defects or connections, as well as evidence of close proximity to the sagittal sinus, as life-threatening hemorrhage has been reported in this setting and prompt surgical intervention may be required. Interpreting reports of associated abnormalities is difficult because most authors do not specify the morphology of the lesion. Tables 9-2 and 9-3 list some of the associated malformations and chromosomal defects reported with aplasia cutis.[89]

Diagnosis

The diagnosis is usually based on clinical data; however, histologic examination of the defects may help to confirm the diagnosis. Membranous aplasia cutis has the most characteristic histologic findings: the epidermis is atrophic and flattened, and the normal superficial dermis is replaced by loose connective tissue.[74] The normal adnexal structures are small or completely absent.[90] If a hair collar is present, then the edge of the specimen will have clustered, hypertrophic hair follicles. Other subtypes of aplasia cutis show superficial scarring with loss of normal adnexal structures. Increased levels of acetylcholinesterase and α-fetoprotein have been reported in the amniotic fluid of mothers with children with aplasia cutis.[91,92]

Differential Diagnosis

Postnatal trauma from forceps or monitoring devices, Goltz syndrome, epidermolysis bullosa, and incontinentia pigmenti can be confused with aplasia cutis.

Prognosis and Management

If the lesion is ulcerated at birth, the area should be cleansed daily and a topical antibiotic ointment applied until complete healing has occurred. Secondary infection is uncommon except in cases of extensive scalp aplasia cutis. Small superficial skin ulcers usually heal in the first months of life. Likewise, small defects of the underlying bone usually ossify completely without treatment.[93] Most small defects will become inconspicuous as the child's scalp grows, but larger lesions may cause significant visible deformity, and almost all will result in localized alopecia. Surgical excision may be considered later in life. Very large stellate scalp defects do not heal completely and will require early surgical intervention. Large, irregular stellate defects often have underlying cranial defects and abnormalities of the intracranial vascular system. Radiologic investigation is required before surgical correction is undertaken because severe hemorrhage and even death has been reported after repair of large defects.[94,95] The defects associated with fetus papyraceus heal remarkably well, leaving hypopigmented scars, and do not usually require surgical correction.

CUTANEOUS DIMPLES

Cutaneous dimples are small depressions or pits in the skin that measure 1–4 mm. Dimples may occur at any location, but are more common over bony prominences such as the elbow, knee, acromion, and sacral region.[96] Cutaneous dimples may be normal, particularly in some locations such as the face. Symmetric shoulder dimples over the acromion or supraspinous fossae may be familial and inherited in an autosomal dominant pattern.[96–99] Cutaneous dimples have been associated with a wide variety of genetic disorders (Box 9-4).[100–103] Dimples may be the result of aberrant fetal positioning in early gestation in patients with congenital skeletal dysplasia.[103] Lip dimples or lip pits may be an isolated defect or associated with Van der Woude syndrome, where they are bilateral, on the lower lip, and associated with cleft lip or palate. Usually dimples do not require treatment as they are small and not cosmetically disfiguring. Surgical excision may be indicated for lip dimples, as they can communicate with underlying minor salivary glands and have recurrent inflammation. Deep dimples in certain locations such as overlying the spine or on the buttock may actually represent superficial manifestations of an underlying sinus tract, requiring evaluations as discussed above.

ADNEXAL POLYP

Adnexal polyp is a small, congenital papule found on the chest, usually on or just medial to the areola of the nipple. The lesions are small (1–2 mm), flesh-colored, firm, pedunculated papules with a smooth surface (Fig. 9-27). Older lesions may have a superficial crust. Histologically the lesions are composed of adnexal structures. Hair follicles, vestigial sebaceous glands, and eccrine glands are present in the center of the lesion.[102] The lesions appear to fall off spontaneously soon after birth.

DEVELOPMENTAL ANOMALIES OF THE UMBILICUS

The umbilicus is a scar that represents the site of attachment of the umbilical cord in the fetus. After birth it has no function but contains embryonic remnants, the urachus, the omphalomesenteric duct, and the round ligament of the liver, all of which may give rise to medical complications.

Anomalies of the Urachus

The urachus is the remnant of the regressed allantois that runs from the apex of the bladder to the umbilicus. If this structure fails to regress, leaving complete patency, a fistula forms between the bladder and the umbilicus. This is manifest by urine draining from the umbilicus. Partial patency of the urachus will result in a cystic dilation in which both ends are obliterated, forming a urachal cyst. Urachal cysts may occur at any point along the course of the urachus but do not communicate with the umbilicus or bladder. They present as tender, midline swellings between the umbilicus and the symphysis pubis. If the urachus is only patent at the umbilicus a urachal sinus forms, which is usually associated with a proximal urachal cyst presenting as a cystic swelling at the umbilicus (Fig. 9-28).

Box 9-4 Genetic disorders associated with cutaneous dimples

Dimples associated with aberrant positioning during fetal life
Arthrogryposis
Metaphyseal chondrodysplasia
Camptomelic dysplasia
Khyphomelic dysplasia
Mesomelic dysplasia
Hypophosphatasia

Facial dimples
Cheeks
Chin
'Whistling face' syndrome
Simosa craniofacial syndrome
Weaver syndrome

Lip dimples
Van der Woude syndrome
Kabuki make-up syndrome
Oral–facial–digital syndrome type 1
Popliteal pterygium syndrome
Branchio-oto-renal syndrome

Shoulder dimples
Autosomal dominant dimples
18q deletion syndrome
Trisomy 9p
Russell–Silver syndrome
Popliteal pterygium syndrome

Pretibial dimples
Oral–facial–digital syndrome
Osteoglophonic syndrome
Kyphomelic dysplasia

Sacral dimples
Spina bifida
Bloom syndrome
Carpenter syndrome
FG syndrome
Robinow syndrome
Smith–Lemli–Opitz syndrome
Dubowitz syndrome
Zellweger syndrome
Wolf–Hirschhorn syndrome (4p deletion syndrome)
X-linked dysmorphic syndrome with mental retardation

Other
Maternal rubella syndrome
Amniocentesis
Joubert syndrome
Caudal dysplasia sequence

Anomalies of the Omphalomesenteric Duct

The omphalomesenteric duct connects the ileum to the umbilicus. This duct usually regresses during the 5th to 9th weeks of gestation, leaving a fibrous cord. Failure of normal obliteration will result in a range of congenital anomalies, depending

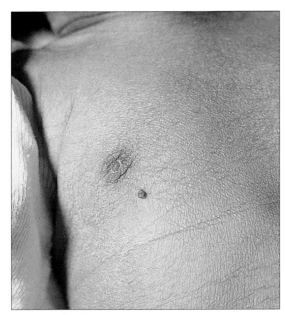

FIG. 9-27 Adnexal polyp.

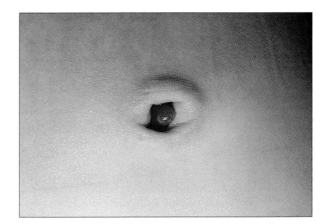

FIG. 9-29 Umbilical polyp (omphalomesenteric duct cyst).

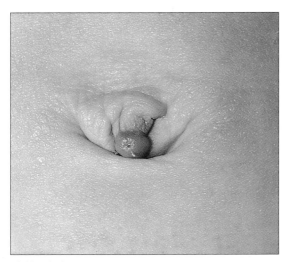

FIG. 9-28 Urachal cyst.

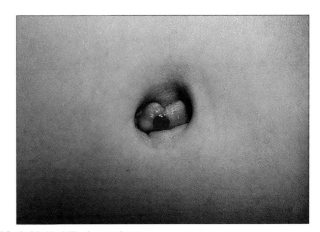

FIG. 9-30 Umbilical granuloma.

not usually present at birth. They can be distinguished from umbilical polyps by the lack of serous, mucoid, or bloody discharge (Fig. 9-30), and their response to treatment with topical silver nitrate.

AMNION RUPTURE MALFORMATION SEQUENCE/AMNIOTIC BANDS

A variety of disorders results from premature rupture of the amniotic sac. The clinical features will vary depending on the stage of development of the fetus at the time of rupture.[105] The defects are thought to result from early rupture of the amniotic membrane, which subsequently results in failure of growth of the amniotic sac and the formation of fibrous strands from the outer surface of the amnion and the chorion. The fetus may become entangled in these strands if it passes through the defect. There may also be compression of the fetus secondary to oligohydramnios. Maternal trauma, dietary deficiencies, and teratogens have all been associated with amniotic rupture sequence.

Cutaneous Findings

The most classic cutaneous finding is that of a constriction band of the distal extremity (Fig. 9-31). The band is usually circumferential and may be deep enough to cause lymphedema, compression of nerves, or even ischemia with resultant

on the extent and the site of persistent patency. The entire duct may be patent, forming a fistula between the ileum and the umbilicus; this presents during infancy with a red nodule at the umbilicus with a surrounding fistula. Fecal material may discharge from the fistula, often resulting in irritation of the surrounding skin. If intermediate portions of the duct remain patent, an omphalomesenteric cyst forms. If the cyst is located toward the periphery of the duct (i.e. near the umbilicus), it will give rise to a bright red, glistening polypoid nodule usually referred to as an umbilical polyp (Fig. 9-29). Meckel's diverticulum, the most common anomaly of the omphalomesenteric duct, results from incomplete regression of the most proximal (enteric) portion.

Umbilical Granuloma

These are small, bright red papules that develop if the umbilicus does not re-epithelialize completely; therefore they are

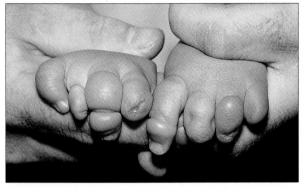

FIG. 9-31 Multiple anomalies of the feet secondary to the amniotic band sequence.

amputation.[106] Aplasia cutis, irregular patches of alopecia, abnormal palmar creases, and alteration in dermatoglyphic pattern are also cutaneous features of the amnion rupture malformation syndrome.

Extracutaneous Findings

Rupture early in gestation, during organogenesis, will lead to the most severe deformities. Severe craniofacial abnormalities, such as neural tube defects, and facial, chest, and abdominal wall clefts, have all been reported.

Treatment

Surgical correction is the only treatment option for these deformities and is often very challenging.[104]

REFERENCES

1. Armoni M, Filk D, Schlesinger M, et al. Accessory nipples: any relationship to urinary tract malformation? Pediatr Dermatol 1992; 9: 239–240.
2. Mimouni F, Merlob P, Reisner SH. Occurrence of supernumerary nipples in newborns. Am J Dis Child 1983; 137: 952–953.
3. Cohen PR. The significance of polythelia. J Am Acad Dermatol 1995; 32: 688.
4. Meggyessy V, Mehes K. Association of supernumerary nipples and renal anomalies. J Pediatr 1987; 111: 412–413.
5. Urbani CE, Betti R. Accessory mammary tissue associated with congenital and hereditary nephrourinary malformations. Int J Dermatol 1996; 35: 349–352.
6. Grotto I, Browner-Elhanan K, Mimouni D, et al. Occurrence of supernumerary nipples in children with kidney and urinary tract malformations. Pediatr Dermatol 2001; 18: 291–294.
7. Hrabovszky T, Schneider I, Zombai E. Axillare akzessorische brustdruson Hautarzt 1995; 46: 576–578.
8. Kao GF, Graham JH, Helwig EB. Paget's disease of the ectopic breast with an underlying intraductal carcinoma: A report of a case. J Cutan Pathol 1986; 13: 59–66.
9. Jacobs PH, Shafer JC, Higdon RS. Congenital branchigenous anomalies. J Am Med Assoc 1959; 169: 442–446.
10. Leung AK, Robson WL. Association of preauricular sinuses and renal anomalies. Urology 1992; 40: 259–261.
11. Wang RY, Earl DL, Ruder RO, et al. Syndromic ear anomalies and renal ultrasounds. Pediatrics 2001; 108: 32–39.
12. Kugelman A, Hadad B, Ben-David J, et al. Preauricular tags and pits in newborn: The role of hearing tests. Acta Pediatr 1997; 86: 170–172.
13. Resnick KI, Soltani K, Berstein JE, et al. Accessory tragi and associated syndromes involving the first branchial arch. J Dermatol Surg Oncol 1981; 7: 39–41.
14. Zelante L, Gasparini P, Scanderbeg AC, et al. Goldenhar complex: A further case with uncommon associated anomalies. Am J Med Genet 1997; 69: 418–421.
15. Satoh T, Tokura Y, Katsumata T, et al. Histologic diagnostic criteria for accessory tragi. J Cutan Pathol 1990; 17: 206–210.
16. Frieden IJ, Chang MW, Lee I. Suture ligation of supernumerary digits and 'tags': An outmoded practice? Arch Pediatr Adolesc Med. 1995; 149: 1284.
17. Sperling LC. Congenital cartilaginous rests of the neck. Int J Dermatol 1986; 3: 186–187.
18. Hogan D, Wilkinson RD, Williams. Congenital anomalies of the head and neck. Int J Dermatol 1980; 19: 479–486.
19. Maran AGD, Buchanan DR. Branchial cysts, sinuses and fistulae. Clin Otolaryngol 1978; 3: 77–92.
20. Ahuja AT, Wong KT, King AD, et al. Imaging for thyroglossal duct cysts: the bare essentials. Clin Radiol 2005; 60: 141–148.
21. Muramatsu T, Shirai T, Sakamoto K. Cutaneous bronchogenic cyst. Int J Dermatol 1990; 29: 143–144.
22. Jona JZ, Extramediastinal bronchogenic cysts in children. Pediatr Dermatol 1995; 12: 304–306.
23. Patterson JW, Pittman DL, Rich JD. Presternal ciliated cyst. Arch Dermatol 1984; 120: 240–242.
24. Asarch RG, Golitz LE, Sausker WF, et al. Median raphe cysts of the penis. Cutis 1981; 27: 170–172.
25. Carmi R, Boughman JA. Pentalogy of Cantrell and associated midline anomalies: A possible ventral midline developmental field. Am J Med Genet 1992; 42: 90–95.
26. Hersh JH, Waterfill D, Rutledge J, et al. Sternal malformation/vascular dysplasia association. Am J Med Genet 1985; 21: 117–186.
27. Kaplan LC, Kurnit DM, Welch KJ, Anterior midline defects: Association with ectopic cordis or vascular dysplasia, defines two distinct entities. Am J Med Genet 1985; 21: 203.
28. Gargon R, McKinnon M, Mulliken J. Midline cervical cleft. Plast Reconstruct Surg 1985; 76: 226–229.
29. Eastlack JP, Howard RM, Frieden IJ. Congenital midline cervical cleft: case report and review of the English language literature. Pediatr Dermatol 2000; 17: 118–122.
30. Golden JA, Chernoff GF. Multiple sites of anterior neural tube closure in humans: evidence from anterior neural tube defects (anencephaly). Pediatrics 1995; 95: 506–510.
31. Peter J, Sinclair-Smith C, deVilliers J. Midline dermal sinuses and cysts and their relationship to the central nervous system. Eur J Pediatr Surg 1991; 1: 73–79.
32. Powell K, Cherry J, Hougen T, et al. A prospective search for congenital dermal abnormalities of the craniospinal axis. J Pediatr 1975; 87: 744–750.
33. Commens C, Rogers M, Kan A. Heterotopic brain tissue presenting as bald cysts with a collar of hypertrophic hair; the hair collar sign. Arch Dermatol 189; 125: 1253–1256.
34. Drolet B, Clowry Jr L, McTigue K, et al. The hair collar sign: A cutaneous marker for neural tube dysraphism. Pediatrics 1995; 96: 309–313.
35. Drolet B, Prendiville J, Golden J, et al. Membranous aplasia cutis with hair collars: Congenital absence of the skin or neuroectodermal defect? Arch Dermatol 1995; 131: 1427–1429.
36. Howard R. Congenital midline lesions: Pits and protuberances. Pediatr Ann 1998; 27: 150–160.
37. Nocini P, Barbaglio A, Dolci M, et al. Dermoid cyst of the nose: A case report and review of the literature. J Oral Maxillofac Surg 1996; 54: 357–362.
38. Peter J, Sinclair-Smith C, deVillies J. Midline dermal sinuses and cysts and their relationship to the central

nervous system. Eur J Pediatr Surg 1991; 1: 73–79.

39. Paller AS, Pensler J, Tomita T. Nasal midline masses in infants and children. Dermoids, encephaloceles, and nasal gliomas. Arch Dermatol 1991; 127: 362–366.

40. Martinez-Lage JF, Capel A, Costa TR, et al. The child with a mass on its head: Diagnostic and surgical strategies. Childs Nerv Syst 1992; 8: 247–252.

41. Hattori H, Higuchi Y, Tashiro Y. Dorsal dermal sinus and dermoid cysts in occult spinal dysraphism. J Pediatr 1999; 134: 793.

42. Kriss T, Kriss V, Warf B. Recurrent meningitis: The search for the dermoid or epidermoid tumor. Pediatr Infect Dis J 1995; 14: 697–700.

43. Albright A, Gartner J, Weiner E. Lumbar cutaneous hemangiomas as indicators of tethered spinal cords. Pediatrics 1989; 83: 977–980.

44. Higginbottom M, Jones K, James H, et al. Aplasia cutis congenita: A cutaneous marker of occult spinal dysraphism. J Pediatr 1980; 96: 687–689.

45. Anderson F. Occult spinal dysraphism: A series of 73 cases. Pediatrics 1975; 55: 826–835.

46. Assaad A, Mansy A, Kotb M, et al. Spinal dysraphism: Experience with 250 cases operated upon. Child's Nerv Syst 1989; 5: 324–329.

47. Burrows F. Some aspects of occult spinal dysraphism: A study of 90 cases. Br J Radiol 1968; 41: 487–491.

48. Hall D, Udvarhelyi G, Altman J. Lumbosacral skin lesions as markers of occult spinal dysraphism. JAMA 1981; 246: 2606–2608.

49. Lemire R, Graham C, Beckwith J. Skin-covered sacrococcygeal masses in infants and children. J Pediatr 1971; 79: 948–954.

50. Sattar M, Bannister C, Turnbull I. Occult spinal dysraphism – the common combination of lesions and the clinical manifestations in 50 patients. Eur J Pediatr Surg 1997; 6: 10–14.

51. Scatliff J, Kendall B, Kingsley D, et al. Closed spinal dysraphism: Analysis of clinical, radiological and surgical findings in 104 consecutive patients. Am J Roentgenol 1989; 10: 269–277.

52. Tavafoghi V, Ghandchi A, Hambrick G, et al. Cutaneous signs of spinal dysraphism: report of a patient with a tail-like lipoma and review of 200 cases in the literature. Arch Dermatol 1978; 114: 573–577.53.

53. Keim HA, Greene AF. Diastematomyelia and scoliosis. J Bone Joint Surg [Am] 1973; 55: 1425–1434.

54. Guggisberg D, Hadj-Rabia S, Viney C, et al. Skin markers of occult spinal dysraphism in children: a review of 54 cases. Arch Dermatol 2004; 140: 1109–1115.

55. Karrer F, Flannery A, Nelson, M, et al. Anorectal malformations. Evaluation of associated spinal dysraphic syndromes. J Pediatr Surg 1988; 23: 45–48.

56. Goldberg N, Hebert A, Esterly N. Sacral hemangiomas and multiple congenital abnormalities. Arch Dermatol 1986; 122: 684–687.

57. Rivosecchi M, Luchetti M, Zaccara A, et al. Spinal dysraphism detected by MRI in patients with anorectal abnormalities: Incidence and clinical significance. J Pediatr Surg 1995; 30: 383–388.

58. Enjolras O, Boukobza M, Jdid R. Cervical occult spinal dysraphism: MRI findings and the value of a vascular birth mark. Pediatr Dermatol 1995; 12: 256–259.

59. Ben-Amitai D, Davidson S, Schwartz M, et al. P16 The role of imaging in the evaluation of sacral nevus flammeus simplex: A prospective neonatal study. Eur J Pediatr Dermatol Int Congress Dermatol 1998; 8: 40.

60. Kriss VM, Desal NS. Occult spinal dysraphism in neonates: Assessment of high-risk cutaneous stigmata on sonography. Am J Roentgenol 1998; 171: 1687–1692.

61. McAtee-Smith J, Hebert A, Rapini R, et al. Skin lesions of the spinal axis and spinal dysraphism. Arch Pediatr Adolesc Med 1994; 148: 740–748.

62. Harrist T, Gang D, Kleinman G, et al. Unusual sacrococcygeal embryologic malformations with cutaneous manifestations. Arch Dermatol 1982; 118: 643–648.

63. Weprin BE, Oakes WJ. Coccygeal pits. Pediatrics 2000; 105: 69–73.

64. Carrillo R, Carreira LM, Prada JJ, Rosas C. Lateral congenital spinal dermal sinus. A new clinical entity. Childs Nerv Syst 1985; 1: 238–240.

65. Dao A, Netsky M. Human tails and pseudotails. Hum Pathol 1984; 15: 449–453.

66. Barnes P, Lester P, Yamanashi W, et al. Magnetic resonance imaging in infants and children with spinal dysraphism. Am J Neuroradiol 1986; 7: 465–472.

67. Byrd S, Darling C, Melone D, et al. MR imaging of the pediatric spine. Magn Reson Imag Clin North Am 1996; 4: 797–833.

68. Rindahl M, Colletti P, Zee C, et al. Magnetic resonance imaging of pediatric spinal dysraphism. Magn Reson Imag 1989; 7: 217–224.

69. Tracy P, Hanigan W. Spinal dysraphism: Use of magnetic resonance imaging in evaluation. Clin Pediatr 1990; 29: 228–233.

70. Raghavendra B, Epstein F, Pinto R, et al. The tethered spinal cord: Diagnosis by high-resolution real time ultrasound. Radiology 1983; 149: 123–128.

71. Rohrschneider U, Forsting M, Darge K, et al. Diagnostic value of spinal ultrasound: Comparative study with MR imaging in pediatric patients. Radiology 1996; 200: 383–388.

72. Myerat BJ, Tercier S, Lutz N, et al. Introduction of a urodynamic score to detect pre- and postoperative neurological deficits in children with a primary tethered cord. Childs Nerv Syst 2003; 19: 716–721.

73. Frieden IJ. Aplasia cutis congenita: A clinical review and proposal for classification. J Am Acad Dermatol 1986; 14: 646–660.

74. Drolet BA, Baselga E, Gosain AK, et al. Preauricular skin defects: A consequence of a persistent ectodermal groove. Arch Dermatol 1997; 133: 1551–1554.

75. Pap GS. Congenital defect of the scalp and scull in three generations of one family. Plast Reconstruct Surg 1970; 46: 194–196.

76. Sybert V. Aplasia cutis congenita. A report of 12 new families and review of the literature. Pediatr Dermatol 1985; 3: 1–14.

77. Cambiaghi S, Gelmetti C, Nicolini U. Prenatal findings in membranous aplasia cutis. J Am Acad Dermatol 1998; 39: 638–640.

78. Baselga E, Torrelo A, Drolet BA. Familial nonmembranous aplasia cutis of the scalp. Pediatr Dermatol 2005; 22: 213–217.

79. Singman R, Asaikan S, Hotson G, et al. Aplasia cutis congenita and arteriovenous fistula. Arch Neurol 1990; 47: 1255–1258.

80. Saier F, Burden L, Cavanagh D. Fetus papyraceus: An unusual case with congenital anomaly of the surviving fetus. Obstet Gynecol 1975; 45: 217–220.

81. Mannino F, Jones K, Benirschke K. Congenital skin defects and fetus papyraceus. J Pediatr 1977; 91: 559–564.

82. Branspiegel N. Aplasia cutis congenita and intestinal lymphangiectasia: an unusual association. Am J Dis Child 1985; 139: 509–513.

83. Dowler VB. Congenital defect of the skin in a newborn infant. Am J Dis Child 1932; 44: 1279–1284.

84. Leaute-Lebreze C, Depaire-Duclos F, Sarlangue J, et al. Congenital cutaneous defects as complications of surviving co-twins; aplasia cutis congenita and neonatal Volkmann ischemic contracture of the forearm. Arch Dermatol 1998; 134: 1121–1124.

85. Bart B, Garlin R, Anderson V, et al. Congenital absence of the skin and associated abnormalities resembling epidermolysis bullosa. Arch Dermatol 1966; 93: 296–304.

86. Al-Gazali Li, Mueller RF, Caine A, et al. Two 46, xxt(X:Y) females with linear skin defects and congenital microphthalmia: a new syndrome at Xp2.3. J Med Genet 1990; 27: 59–63.

87. Temple K, Hurst JA, Hings S, et al. De novo deletion of Xp22.2pter in a female with linear skin lesions on the face and neck, microphthalmia, and

anterior chamber eye anomalies. J Med Genet 1990; 27: 56–58.

88. Allanson J, Richter S. Microphthalmia: A new syndrome at Xp22.2. J Med Genet 1991; 28: 143–144.

89. Evers MJ, Steijlen PM, Hamel BJ. Aplasia cutis congenita and associated disorders: An update. Clin Genet 1995; 47: 295–301.

90. Lever WF. Aplasia cutis. In: Lever WF, Schaumburg-Lever G. eds. Histopathology of the skin, 7th edn. Philadelphia: JB Lippincott, 1990; 65–66.

91. Farine D, Maidman J, Rubin S, et al. Elevated alpha-fetoprotein in pregnancy complicated by aplasia cutis after exposure to methimazole. Obstet Gynecol 1988; 71: 996–997.

92. Bick DP, Balkite MS, Baumgarten JC, et al. The association of congenital skin disorders with acetylcholinesterase in amniotic fluid. Prenat Diagn 1987; 7: 543–549.

93. Wexler A, Harris M, Lesavoy M. Conservative treatment of cutis aplasia. Plast Reconstruct Surg 1990; 86: 1066–1071.

94. Glasson DW, Duncan GM. Aplasia cutis congenita: Delayed closure complicated by massive hemorrhage. Plast Reconstruct Surg 1985; 75: 423–425.

95. Schneider BM, Berg RA, Kaplan AM. Aplasia cutis complicated by sagittal sinus thrombosis. Pediatrics 1980; 66: 948–950.

96. Samlaska CP. Congenital supraspinous fossae. J Am Acad Dermatol 1991; 25: 1078–1079.

97. Weidemann Hr. Cheek dimples. Am J Med Genet 1990; 36: 376.

98. Biachine JW. Acromial dimples: A benign familial trait. Am J Hum Genet 26: 412–413.

99. Wood VE. Congenital skin fossae about the shoulder. Plast Reconstruct Surg 1990; 85: 798–800.

100. DiRocco, M. On Saraiva and Baraister and Joubert syndrome: A review. Am J Med Genet 1993; 46: 732–733.

101. Jones KL. Smith's recognizable patterns of human malformations, 4th edn. Philadelphia: WB Saunders, 1988; 42–44, 94–95,112–113,104–15,178–179,182–183,240–241, 370–371, 575–576.

102. Squires LA, Raymond G, Neumeyer AM, et al. Dysmorphic features of Joubert syndrome. Dysmorph Clin Genet 1991; 5: 72.

103. Kozlowski K, Baca L, Brachimi L, et al. Mesomelic dysplasia of the upper extremities associated with other abnormalities: A new syndrome? Pediatr Radiol 1993; 23: 108–110.

104. Higginbottom MC, Jones KL, Hall BD, et al. The amniotic band disruption complex: Timing of amniotic rupture and variable spectra of consequence of defects. J Pediatr 1979; 95: 544–549.

105. Rossillon D, Rombouts JJ, Verellen-Dumoulin C, et al. Congenital ring-constriction syndrome of the limbs; a report of 19 cases. Br J Plast Surg 1988; 41: 270–277.

106. Hidano A, Kobayashi T. Adnexal polyp of neonatal skin. Br J Dermatol 1975; 92: 659.

10

Vesicles, Pustules, Bullae, Erosions, and Ulcerations

Renee Howard, Ilona J. Frieden

Vesiculopustular and bullous disorders are common in the neonatal period. Accurate and prompt diagnosis is essential because several of the conditions presenting with these skin findings are truly life-threatening. In contrast, many conditions causing blisters and pustules are innocuous and self-limited, and inaccurate diagnosis of a more serious condition can lead to iatrogenic complications, expense, and parental anguish. A prospective study in India evaluated 100 neonates to determine the causes of pustular eruptions. They found that 58% had infectious causes, predominantly impetigo, infectious intertrigo, scabies, and viral diseases. The most common non-infectious causes of pustules were miliaria and erythema toxicum neonatorum. Though no comparable study has been performed in a developed country, it is likely that the results would be quite different, with infectious causes comprising a distinct minority.[1]

Several articles have reviewed an approach to infants with these cutaneous findings.[2–4] There is also considerable overlap with the subject matter in several other chapters of this book, most notably Chapter 7 (Transient Cutaneous Lesions) and Chapters 12 through 14 (Bacterial, Viral, and Fungal Infections), and the main discussion of the specific disorders discussed are in those chapters. Chapter 11 is devoted to a discussion of the diagnosis and management of epidermolysis bullosa, an important group of diseases presenting with bullae and erosions in the neonatal period. This chapter discusses not only pustules, vesicles, and bullae (Boxes 10-1, 10-2), but also erosions and ulcerations (Box 10-3). Although vesicles, pustules, and bullae are *primary* skin lesions, they can result in *secondary* skin lesions (erosions and/or ulcerations) as their sequelae. In certain conditions primary lesions evolve very rapidly or occur in utero, such that secondary skin changes may be the predominant morphology at the time of presentation. Examples include staphylococcal scalded skin syndrome, where erythema and skin erosions predominate over blisters, and *Pseudomonas* skin infection, where pustules rapidly evolve into necrotic ulcers.

Because of the wide array of conditions in the differential diagnosis, newborns and young infants with vesicles, pustules, bullae, ulcers, or erosions should always be evaluated with a thorough history and physical examination (Box 10-4). Laboratory evaluation(s) must be tailored to the specific clinical setting. Table 10-1 summarizes the differential diagnoses of vesiculopustular diseases, and Table 10-2 the differential diagnoses of conditions where bullae, erosions, and ulcerations

predominate. The decision to list infectious diseases first in each category is a deliberate one. When examining newborns it is always important to ask whether the skin eruption could be due to an infection, as certain infections in the newborn period can lead to severe morbidity and even death. Conversely, the large number of entities discussed in this chapter emphasizes that whereas infections should be considered, they should not preclude consideration of other diagnoses or investigations.

Box 10-1 Conditions where pustules and/or vesicles predominate

Common causes
Superficial staphylococcal infection
Erythema toxicum neonatorum
Neonatal pustular melanosis
Miliaria crystallina and rubra
Neonatal 'acne' (benign cephalic pustulosis)
Neonatal candidiasis

Uncommon causes
Congenital candidiasis
Herpes simplex infection
Scabies
Acropustulosis of infancy
Incontinentia pigmenti

Rare causes
Listeria monocytogenes infection
H. influenzae infection
Group A streptococcal infection
Pseudomonas infection
Neonatal varicella
Cytomegalovirus infection
Aspergillus infection
Eosinophilic pustular folliculitis
Erosive pustular dermatosis of the scalp
Langerhans' cell histiocytosis
Hyperimmunoglobulin E syndrome
Pustular eruption in Down syndrome
Pustular psoriasis
Neonatal Behçets' disease

Box 10-2 Conditions where bullae may predominate

Common causes
Bullous impetigo
Sucking blisters

Uncommon causes
Staphylococcal scalded skin syndrome
Epidermolysis bullosa

Rare causes
Group B streptococcal infection
Pseudomonas infection
Congenital syphilis infection
Neonatal varicella infection
Bullous mastocytosis
Maternal bullous disease
   Pemphigus vulgaris
   Herpes gestationis
   Pemphigus foliaceus
Chronic bullous dermatosis of childhood (linear IgA disease)
Bullous pemphigoid
Toxic epidermal necrolysis
Epidermolytic hyperkeratosis
Acrodermatitis enteropathica
Membranous aplasia cutis congenita
Absent dermal ridge patterns, milia, and blisters of fingertips and soles

Box 10-3 Conditions where erosions or ulcerations may predominate

Common causes
Sucking blisters
Skin changes due to perinatal/neonatal trauma
   Diaper erosions
   Scalp electrode injury
   Skin trauma due to adhesives, etc.

Uncommon causes
Staphylococcal scalded skin syndrome
Herpes simplex, especially congenital
Epidermolysis bullosa
Aplasia cutis congenita

Rare causes
Group B streptococcus infection
Pseudomonas (ecthyma gangrenosum)
Intrauterine varicella infection
Congenital syphilis
Aspergillus infection
Zygomyocosis/trichosporosis
Neonatal lupus erythematosus
Toxic epidermal necrolysis
Intrauterine epidermal necrosis
Congenital erosive and vesicular dermatosis
Erosive pustular dermatosis of the scalp
Pyoderma gangrenosum
Noma neonatorum
Acrodermatitis enteropathica
Methylmalonic acidemia and other metabolic disorders
Bullous congenital ichthyosiform erythroderma
Restrictive dermopathy
Hemangiomas and vascular malformations
Aplasia cutis congenita
Linear porokeratosis
Giant congenital melanocytic nevi
Focal dermal hypoplasia
Porphyrias
   Transient porphyrinemia
   Erythropoietic porphyria
Perinatal gangrene of the buttock
Congenital deficiency of protein C, S, or fibrinogen

BACTERIAL INFECTIONS (See also Chapter 12)

Staphylococcus Aureus Infections

Skin infections caused by *S. aureus* are relatively common in newborns, and epidemic outbreaks are occasionally seen in newborn nurseries. In recent years, methicillin-resistant *S. aureus* infections have been increasingly reported in hospital nursery and maternity units, paralleling a trend toward such infections in other settings. Interestingly, most have had the molecular fingerprint of community-acquired, rather than nosocomial MRSA.[5] Two forms of *S. aureus* infection involving the skin can occur: direct skin infection and staphylococcal scalded skin syndrome, produced by staphylococcal toxins.

Staphylococcus Aureus Pyoderma

Superficial skin infections with *S. aureus* (staphylococcal pyoderma) can result in crusted impetigo, bullous impetigo, and pustular folliculitis. Deeper skin infections can result in furunculosis, cellulitis, and abscesses. Infection is virtually never present at birth, but often develops in the first days to weeks of life. It usually presents with vesicles, pustules, or, in the case of toxin-producing *S. aureus*, with tense, fragile bullae. Fluid inside the vesicles and bullae may be clear or yellow, but often becomes turbid or purulent with time. As vesicles and bullae rupture, they leave moist superficial erosions or thinly crusted areas with a collarette of scale. Superficial staphylococcal infection can also present with crusted impetigo without clinically obvious vesicles, pustules, or bullae.[6]

Common sites of involvement include the neck folds, diaper area, and axillae.[7] More extensive cases of generalized bullous impetigo are occasionally seen.[8] Infants are usually otherwise well, without signs of more generalized infection. Diagnosis and management are discussed in Chapter 12.

Staphylococcal Scalded Skin Syndrome

Staphylococcal scalded skin syndrome (SSSS) is an acute, potentially life-threatening disease caused by exotoxin-producing *S. aureus*, usually phage types 1, 2, or 3. Although epidemics as well as sporadic outbreaks of SSSS have been reported,[9] it is still a relatively uncommon to rare condition. A recent population-based study in Germany found an incidence of approximately 0.1 cases per million inhabitants per year (including all ages) with a bimodal distribution of ages from young children to adults.[10] Only one case of congenital SSSS has been reported; the vast majority present between 3

Box 10-4 Key points of obstetrical and neonatal history and examination

Maternal, family, and obstetric history
Maternal history of skin or mucous membrane diseases

Family history of birthmarks, blistering, skin fragility, or ectodermal defect

History of previous pregnancies/miscarriages

Prenatal care

Results of maternal serologies (including syphilis, rubella, and HIV)

History of maternal illnesses, surgery, fever, rash, or medications during pregnancy

History of maternal fever during delivery

Length of ruptured amniotic membranes

Method of delivery

History of intrauterine monitoring

Presence of meconium in the amniotic fluid

Placental abnormalities

Neonatal history
Apgar scores

Gestational age at birth

Birthweight relative to gestational age (i.e. small, average, or large)

Illnesses during the newborn period

Past history of surgery, sepsis, anatomic/structural abnormalities

Recent history of lethargy, irritability, temperature instability, and/or poor feeding

Medications: past or present

Neonatal examination
Weight, length, head circumference

Complete examination of the skin, mucous membranes, hair and nails

Accurate definition of the morphology and distribution of skin lesion(s)

Head circumference (percentile for age)

Ophthamologic abnormalities

Adenopathy

Liver or spleen enlargement

Skeletal abnormalities

Neurologic abnormalities

and 7 days of age or older, with an abrupt onset of cutaneous erythema, tenderness, and widespread areas of skin fragility, superficial blistering, and/or erosions.[11] The erythema often begins on the face, especially around the mouth, and spreads rapidly. Flaccid blisters usually appear within 24–48 hours and quickly erode, producing areas of superficially denuded skin. These erosions are particularly prominent in areas of mechanical stress, such as the shoulders, buttocks, body folds, feet, and hands. When firmly rubbed, the skin is easily separated from the underlying epidermis (Nikolsky's sign). A milder form of SSSS, characterized by a scarlatiniform rash with periorificial scaling, is often seen in older infants and children.

Temperature instability, irritability, and/or lethargy are common. Perioral or periocular edema and mucopurulent con-junctivitis are sometimes present. Although the primary site of *S. aureus* infection is usually not the skin, occasionally a primary skin infection, such as an abscess, purulent umbilicus, or localized area of impetigo, may be the source of disease.[6,9,12,13]

Diagnosis is made by skin biopsy, which demonstrates a cleavage plane in the upper epidermis with acantholytic cells and minimal dermal inflammation. To speed diagnosis, a snip biopsy of exfoliating portions of the skin can be sent for frozen section. The differential diagnosis includes toxic epidermal necrolysis, epidermolysis bullosa, boric acid poisoning, and certain metabolic disorders such as methylmalonic academia.[14,15] The management of SSSS is discussed in Chapter 12.

Streptococcal Infection

Several epidemics of group A streptococcus (GAS) have been reported in the newborn period. Although most infants present with omphalitis or a moist umbilical cord stump, in rare cases isolated pustules may be the presenting sign of GAS infection. GAS can also cause a form of intertrigo in infancy.[16] Generalized sepsis, cellulitis, meningitis, or pneumonia are occasionally seen.[17–19] Because neonatal group A streptococcal infection can result in an invasive infection, parenteral antibiotics should be considered, and infants should be observed closely for signs of systemic illness. Although bacterial cultures are the 'gold standard' for diagnosis, rapid antigen testing for GAS has been shown to have a high level of sensitivity and specificity and can be used while awaiting culture.[20] Two other presentations of GAS infection, not typically in newborns but in somewhat older infants, are streptococcal intertrigo and atopic dermatitis with secondary streptococcal infection. In streptococcal intertrigo, moist eroded areas may be present in the folds of the neck, axilla, groin, or perianal area.[16]

In atopic dermatitis, crusting and/or pustules due to *S. aureus* infection can occur even in very young infants. In cases where secondary infection is due to GAS, however, pustules are often more deep-seated.[21]

Infection with group B β-hemolytic streptococci (GBS) is one of the most common causes of neonatal sepsis, but skin lesions resulting from GBS infection are very rare. In a few cases vesicles, bullae, erosions, and honey-crusted lesions resembling GAS impetigo have been described,[6,22,23] either at the time of birth or later in the neonatal period.[23,24] Many areas of the body, including the scalp, face, torso, and extremities, can be affected, with lesion size varying from a few millimeters to several centimeters. Other manifestations of group B streptococcal disease (including bacteremia, pneumonia, and meningitis) should be sought.

Listeria Infection

Listeria monocytogenes is an uncommon cause of a rare form of sepsis in the newborn period, typically acquired via vertical transmission from an affected mother. Epidemics and sporadic cases due to inadequately pasteurized dairy products have been reported.[25,26] Skin disease, when it occurs, is associated with an early-onset form of infection which is present at birth or develops in the first few days of life (so-called granulomatosis infantiseptica). The rash, which is usually present at birth, consists of discrete but widespread pustules and petechiae over the trunk and extremities. In less severely affected infants,

Table 10-1 Differential diagnosis of vesiculopustular diseases

Disease	Usual age of onset	Skin: morphology	Skin: usual distribution	Clinical: other	Diagnosis/findings
Infectious causes					
Staphylococcal pyoderma	Few days to weeks	Pustules, bullae, occasional vesicles	Mainly diaper area, periumbilical	Boys more than girls; may be in epidemic setting	Gram stain: PMNs Gram-positive cocci in clusters. Bacterial culture
Group A streptococcal disease	Few days to weeks	Isolated pustules, honey-crusted areas	No specific site predisposed	Moist umbilical stump; occasional cellulitis, meningitis, pneumonia	Gram stain: Gram-positive cocci in chains; bacterial culture
Group B streptococcal infection	At birth or first few days	Vesicles bullae, erosions, honey-crusted lesions	Any area	Pneumonia, bacteremia, meningitis	Gram stain: Gram-positive cocci in chains; bacterial culture
Listeriosis	Birth, first few hours	Hemorrhagic pustules and petechiae	Generalized, especially trunk and extremities	Sepsis; respiratory distress; Maternal fever and premature labor	Gram-positive rods; bacterial culture skin and other sites
Haemophilus influenzae infection	Birth or first few days	Vesicles, crusted areas	No specific site predisposed	Bacteremia, meningitis may be present	Gram-negative bacilli; bacterial culture
Pseudomonas infection	Days to weeks	Erythema, pustules, hemorrhagic bullae, necrotic ulcerations	Any area, but especially diaper, periorificial	History of illness in neonatal period	Skin or tissue Gram stain: Gram-negative rods; cultures skin, blood
Congenital candidiasis	Birth or first few days	Erythema, small papules and pustules	Any part of body; palms, soles often involved	Prematurity; Foreign body in cervix/uterus are risk factors	KOH: hyphae, budding yeast; Placental lesions
Neonatal candidiasis	Days or older	Scaly red patches with satellite pustules and papules	Diaper or other intertriginous area	Usually otherwise healthy	KOH: hyphae, budding yeast if pustules are present
Aspergillus infection	Few days to weeks	Pustules often clustered rapidly evolve to ulcers	Any area	Extreme prematurity usually present	Skin biopsy: septate hyphae; tissue fungal culture
Neonatal herpes simplex	Usually 5–14 days	Vesicles, pustules, crusts, erosions	Any site; especially scalp, torso; may involve mucosa	Signs of sepsis; irritability, lethargy	Tzanck; FA or immunoperoxidase slide test, PCR, viral culture
Intrauterine herpes simplex	Birth	Vesicles, pustules, widespread erosions, scars, areas of missing skin	Any site	Low birthweight; microcephaly, chorioretinitis	Tzanck; FA or immunoperoxidase slide test, PCR, viral culture
Neonatal varicella	0–14 days	Vesicles on erythematous base	Generalized distribution	Maternal primary varicella infection 7 days before to 2 days after delivery	Tzanck, FA, viral culture
Herpes zoster	Usually 2 weeks or older	Vesicles on erythematous base	Dermatomal pattern	Maternal primary varicella infection during pregnancy or few days after delivery	Tzanck; FA, viral culture
Scabies	Usually 3–4 weeks or older	Papules, nodules, wheals, crusted areas, vesicles, burrows	Accentuated axillae, feet, wrists, may occur anywhere	Usually family members with itching, rash	Scabies prep demonstrating mites, eggs, or feces; clinical
Transient skin lesions					
Erythema toxicum neonatorum	Usually 24–28 hours, but can be birth to 2 weeks	Erythematous macules, papules, pustules, wheals	Anywhere except palms, soles	Term infants >2500 g	Clinical; Wright's stain: eosinophils
Neonatal pustular melanosis	Birth	Pustules without erythema; collarettes of scale; hyperpigmented macules	Anywhere; most often forehead, ears, back, fingers, toes	Term infants; more common in black infants	Clinical; Wright's stain: PMNs, occasional eosinophil, cellular debris
Miliaria crystallina	Birth or early infancy	Fragile vesicles without erythema	Forehead, upper trunk, arms most common	May be a history of overwarming or fever	Clinical; Wright, Gram and Tzanck preparations negative

Table 10-1 Differential diagnosis of vesiculopustular diseases—cont'd					
Disease	Usual age	Skin: morphology	Skin: usual distribution	Clinical: other	Diagnosis/findings
Miliaria rubra	Days to weeks	Erythematous papules with superimposed pustules	Forehead, upper trunk, arms most common	Sometimes history of overwarming, fever	Clinical; Wright, Gram and Tzanck preps negative
Neonatal 'acne': Benign cephalic pustulosis	Days to weeks	Papules and pustules on erythematous base	Cheeks, forehead, eyelids, neck, upper chest, scalp	Otherwise well	Usually clinical; Giemsa: negative or fungal spores, neutrophils
Uncommon and rare causes					
Acropustulosis of infancy	Birth or days to weeks	Vesicles and pustules	Hands and feet, occasional lesion elsewhere	Severe pruritus; lesions come in crops	Clinical; skin biopsy: intraepidermal vesicle/pustule
Eosinophilic pustular folliculitis	Birth or days to weeks	Pustules	Mainly scalp and face; occasionally trunk, extremities	Pruritus; waxing and waning course with recurrent crops	Skin biopsy: dense perifollicular mixed infiltrate with eosinophils
Erosive pustular dermatosis of the scalp	Weeks to months	Crusting, pustules, scaly erythema	Scalp, in association with areas of persistent alopecia	Severe scalp edema or necrosis of delivery	Clinical setting
Incontinentia pigmenti	Birth to days	Vesicles, hyperkeratosis in linear array	Most common trunk, scalp, extremities	Extracutaneous involvement common but often not evident at birth. Family history sometimes positive	Skin biopsy: eosinophilic spongiosis with dyskeratosis
Hyperimmuno-globulin E syndrome	Days to months	Single or grouped pustules, vesicles, or crusting	Face, scalp, upper torso	Blood eosinophilia; Note: IgE levels often become elevated *after* neonatal period.	Skin biopsy: intraepidermal vesicle with eosinophils or eosinophilic folliculitis
Neonatal Behçet's disease	First week of life	Oral and genital ulcerations and vesicles, necrotic skin lesions on	Mucosal lesions; Skin lesions mainly on hands and feet	Maternal history of Behçet's disease; diarrhea, vasculitis in 1 case	Clinical and maternal history
Pustular psoriasis	First weeks or months of life	Pustules generalized, but especially palms, soles; may have underlying erythroderma	Generalized	Irritability, occasionally fever	Skin biopsy: epidermal microabcesses & acanthosis, parakeratosis, dilated capillaries

erythematous macules may progress to pustules with an erythematous halo. Salmon-colored papules concentrated on the trunk have also been described.[25,26] Typically, maternal fever, fetal tachycardia, and meconium staining of amniotic fluid are present before delivery, and premature delivery is common.[26] Affected infants are usually gravely ill, with respiratory distress, meningitis, and other signs of sepsis.

The differential diagnosis includes several other infections, including congenital candidiasis, intrauterine herpes infection, and *Haemophilus influenzae* infection. Further details of diagnosis and management are discussed in Chapter 12.

Haemophilus Influenzae Infection

Haemophilus influenzae is a very rare cause of neonatal skin disease. Findings have included vesicles, pustules, crusted areas, and abscesses.[27,28] Halal et al. provided the best descriptions of skin lesions in an infant with discrete vesicles on an erythematous base, as well as several 2–3 mm crusted areas, present at birth. Gram stains and culture from skin lesions

confirmed the presence of *H. influenzae* type B, but cultures from sites other than the ear canal were negative.[28] Onset of symptoms is at birth or in the first few days of life.

If *H. influenzae* is suspected, diagnostic evaluation should include Gram stain and culture of skin lesions, and cultures of the infant's blood, urine, cerebrospinal fluid (CSF), and nasopharynx. Cultures of the placenta (if available) and of the maternal cervix and lochia should also be performed. The differential diagnosis includes other infections. A Gram stain demonstrating pleomorphic Gram-negative bacilli is strong evidence for *H. influenzae* infection. Treatment is discussed in Chapter 12.

Pseudomonas Infection

Pseudomonas aeruginosa in newborns is nearly always occurs after 5 days of age, most commonly in infants weighing <1500 g at birth. Risk factors include feeding intolerance, parenteral nutrition, prolonged intravenous antibiotics, and necrotizing enterocolitis.[29] Skin lesions are usually a result of

TABLE 10-2 Differential diagnosis of bullae, erosions, and ulcerations

Disease	Usual age	Skin: morphology	Skin: usual distribution	Clinical: other	Diagnosis/findings
Infectious causes					
Staphylococcal scalded skin syndrome	Few days to weeks; one congenital case	Widespread erythema, fragile bullae, erosions	Generalized with periorificial accentuation	Irritability; temperature instability	Biopsy: epidermal separation at granular cell layer Cultures of blood, urine or other sites demonstrates *S. aureus*
Group B streptococcal infection	At birth or first few days	Vesicles bullae, erosions, honey-crusted lesions	Any area	Pneumonia, bacteremia, meningitis	Gram stain: Gram-positive cocci in chains; bacterial culture
Pseudomonas infection	Days to weeks	Erythema, pustules, hemorrhagic bullae, necrotic ulcerations	Any area, but especially diaper, periorificial	History illness in neonatal period	Skin or tissue Gram stain: Gram-negative rods; cultures skin, blood
Congenital syphilis	Birth or first few days	Bullae or erosions	Especially hands, feet, and periorificial	Lack of prenatal care, organomegaly; bony lesions on X-ray, etc.	Darkfield exam of skin; FA; syphilis serologies, skin biopsy.
Aspergillus infection	Few days to weeks	Pustules often clustered rapidly evolve to ulcers	Any area	Extreme prematurity usually present	Skin biopsy: septate hyphae; Tissue fungal culture
Zygomyocosis/ trichosporosis	Days to weeks	Generalized peeling and skin breakdown or cellulitis evolving into necrotic ulcer	Any area	Extreme prematurity	Skin biopsy and tissue fungal culture
Intrauterine herpes simplex infection	Birth	Vesicles, pustules, widespread erosions, scars, areas of missing skin	Any site	Low birthweight; microcephaly, chorioretinitis; history of maternal fever, discordance of HSV infection mother and father	Tzanck; FA or immunoperoxidase slide test, PCR, viral culture
Fetal varicella infection	At birth	Scarring, limb hypoplasia, erosions	Any site but often extremity	Maternal chickenpox first trimester	Tzanck, FA, viral culture
Transient skin lesions					
Sucking blisters	At birth	Flaccid bulla or linear erosion – occasionally 2 symmetric lesions	Fingers, wrists, occasionally foot	Sucks on affected areas	Clinical
Perinatal trauma/ Iatrogenic injury	At birth or neonatal period	Erosions, ulcerations	Depends on cause of trauma	Perinatal history of monitoring, prolonged labor and /or vacuum or forceps delivery; other monitoring; more common in premature infants	History and clinical findings
Uncommon and rare causes					
Epidermolysis bullosa	At birth or first few days	Bullae and skin fragility; depending on type: mucosal erosions, aplasia cutis of anterior leg, milia, nail dystrophy, etc.	May be widespread or limited depending on type: most often extremities, especially hands, feet	Pain, irritability and difficulty feeding Occasionally corneal, respiratory tract, or gastrointestinal (pyloric atresia); anemia	Skin biopsy of blister <24 hours or induced with friction; Specific type diagnosed with electron microscopy or immunofluorescent mapping
Mastocytosis	Birth or weeks to months	Localized form: infiltrated nodular area with intermittent superimposed wheal or bullae; Generalized form: blistering usually superimposed on infiltrated skin	Any site: often on torso	Variably present: hives, flushing, irritability, sudden pallor, diarrhea	Biopsy demonstrating increased Mast cells in dermis

TABLE 10-2 Differential diagnosis of bullae, erosions, and ulcerations—cont'd

Disease	Usual age	Skin: morphology	Skin: usual distribution	Clinical: other	Diagnosis/findings
Maternal bullous disease	Birth	Depends on type of maternal disease: tense or flaccid bullae or erosions	Usually generalized	Maternal history of blistering disease but occasionally inactive at time of pregnancy	Maternal history; Skin biopsy and direct immunofluorescence with results depending on maternal type
Chronic bullous dermatosis of childhood	1 case at birth; Most in later infancy, childhood	Tense blisters often form rosette or sausage shapes	Generalized but often concentrated growing, buttocks, thighs; Usually spares mucosa	Usually absent	Skin biopsy: Subepidermal bullae; Direct immunofluorescence: Linear pattern IgA DEJ
Bullous pemphigoid	2 months of age or older	Tense blisters	Often accentuated on hands and feet but may be generalized	Usually absent	Skin biopsy: Subepidermal bullae; Direct immunofluorescence: Linear pattern IgG DEJ
Toxic epidermal necrolysis	Usually 6 weeks of age or older except for cases due to intrauterine graft vs host disease	Erythema, erosions, bullae and cutaneous tenderness usually with mucosal involvement	Generalized, evolving rapidly over hours to days	Usually associated with gram negative sepsis or due to Intrauterine graft vs host disease in infant with congenital immunodeficiency	Superpidermal blister with widespread epidermal necrosis (usually full-thickness)
Intrauterine epidermal necrosis	Birth	Widespread erosions and ulceration without vesicles or pustules	Generalized, spares mucous membranes	Prematurity and rapid mortality	Skin biopsy: epidermal necrosis and calcification pilosebaceous follicles
Congenital erosive and vesicular dermatosis	Birth	Erosions, vesicles, crusts, erythematous areas	Generalized, usually sparing face, palms, soles	Prematurity, Variably: collodion membrane, transparent skin, reticulated vascular pattern	Clinical diagnosis, often retrospective. Skin biopsy: neutrophilic infiltrate; exclusion of other etiologies of erosions, vesicles
Pyoderma gangrenosum	1 case report neonate at 2 days of age	Sharply demarcated ulcerations with undermined borders	Any site, but usually groin, buttock in infancy	Many associations, mainly inflammatory bowel disease	Clinical, exclusion of other etiologies; skin biopsy with neutrophilic infiltration without vasculitis, infection, etc.
Noma neonatorum	Days to weeks	Deep ulcerations, with bone loss, mutilation in some cases	Nose, lips, intraoral, anus, genitalia	Some cases due to *Pseudomonas*; Others due to malnutrition, immunodeficiency	Clinical; Exclusion of other etiologies especially infection
Acrodermatitis enteropathica	Weeks to months	Sharply demarcated crusted plaques; occasionally vesicles, bullae, erosions	Periorificial, i.e. mouth, nose, eyes, genitalia as well as neck folds, hands, and feet	Premature, breast-fed infants with low maternal milk zinc; prolonged parenteral hyperalimentation	Low serum zinc levels (less than 50 µg/dL)
Methylmalonic acidemia	Days to weeks	Erosive erythema	Periorificial accentuation	Lethargy, hypotonia, neutropenia, low platelets	Characteristic abnormalities plasma amino acids
Restrictive dermopathy	Birth	Rigid tense skin with erosions, linear ulcerations	Generalized skin abnormalities	Joint contractures, micrognathia, natal teeth	Clinical; distinguish from Neu–Laxova syndrome
Infantile hemangiomas and other vascular birthmarks	Birth or first few days to weeks	Ulceration without initial vesicle or bullae	Any site, but often lip or perineum	Underlying vascular anomaly – may not always be initially evident in evolving hemangiomas	Clinical
Aplasia cutis congenita	Birth	'Bullous' form: sharply demarcated with overlying membrane; other types with raw, full-thickness defect skin	Scalp or face most common; other sites depending on etiology	Depends on etiology: CNS defects, trisomy 13, limb-reduction abnormalities	Usually clinical; imaging studies to evaluate underlying bone, CNS

TABLE 10-2 Differential diagnosis of bullae, erosions, and ulcerations—cont'd

Disease	Usual age	Skin: morphology	Skin: usual distribution	Clinical: other	Diagnosis/findings
Linear porokeratosis and Porokeratotic eccrine and ostial dermal duct nevus	Birth	Linear erosions	Leg, face, but any site possible	Eventual risk squamous CA skin	Skin biopsy: coronoid lamella – may not be evident in newborn period
Erosions overlying giant nevi	Birth, first few days	Erosions, ulcerations	Superimposed on giant nevi	In some cases neurocutaneous melanosis	Clinical and biopsy to exclude melanoma if persistence or other unusual features present
Focal dermal hypoplasia	Birth	Occasional blisters, but more often hypolasia, aplasia of skin	Linear and whorled pattern, often arms, legs, scalp	Skeletal, eye, and CNS abnormalities to varying degree	Clinical; family history; skin biopsy
Absent dermal ridges and congenital milia syndrome	Birth	Multiple bullae	Fingers, soles of feet	Absent dermal ridge patterns, multiple milia	Clinical; family history (autosomal dominant)
Porphyrias	Days to weeks	Photosensitive blistering	May be in sun-exposed areas or more generalized if exposed to phototherapy for hyperbilirubinemia	Transient form usually due to hemolytic disease; Rarer: erythropoietic porphyria (EP)	Transient: elevated plasma porphyrins. EP: pink urine; elevated urine, fecal and plasma porphyrins
Perinatal gangrene of the buttock	Days	Sudden onset erythema, cyanosis, and gangrenous ulcerations	Buttocks	Umbilical artery catheterization in some cases	Clinical
Neonatal purpura fulminans	Days	Initially purpura or cellulitis-like areas evolving to necrotic bullae or ulcers	Buttocks, extremities, trunk and scalp most common sites	Other sites of DIC	Prolonged PT, PTT, low fibrinogen, elevated FDPs, Low protein C or S levels

septicemia and hematogenous spread of infection to the skin. However, in older infants, ulcerative skin lesions of *Pseudomonas* have been reported in the diaper area and in young infants in the absence of documented bloodborne infection.[30] The skin lesions of *Pseudomonas* infection are known as 'ecthyma gangrenosum,' but in the newborn period they have sometimes been referred to as 'noma neonatorum'.[31] They typically evolve from areas of erythema to hemorrhagic bullae or pustules. The pus may be green, caused by a dye produced by the bacteria. Lesions rapidly erode, becoming punched-out necrotic ulcerations with an indurated base (so-called ecthyma gangrenosum).[32] A single case report of fatal ecthyma gangrenosum has been reported in an infant with harlequin ichthyosis.

In septicemic forms the affected neonates are usually gravely ill, and prompt diagnosis and rapid institution of treatments are necessary to prevent death from overwhelming sepsis.[32] Gram staining of fluid from a pustule or bulla will reveal Gram-negative rods. If lesions are eroded, biopsy and tissue Gram staining should be performed to expedite diagnosis. Cultures of both the skin and blood will confirm the diagnosis. Treatment of suspected infection must take into account the local patterns of antibiotic resistance and is discussed in Chapter 12.

Congenital Syphilis

Congenital syphilis is a very rare neonatal infection in the United States and most often occurs in the setting of inadequate prenatal care.[33] Rarer still is presentation with blistering or ulcerations. These findings occur almost exclusively in early-onset disease and are present in approximately 3% of cases, usually at the time of birth.[34] Bullae are most often located on the palms, soles, knees, or abdomen, superimposed on dusky, hemorrhagic, or erythematous skin.[35] Moist areas of eroded skin may also occur around the mouth, nose, and anogenital area.

Because syphilis affects many organ systems, a variety of other clinical features may be present, as discussed in Chapter 12. The diagnosis can be confirmed by examining bullous or erosive skin lesions via a darkfield examination or direct fluorescent antigen (FA) for treponemal antigen, because such skin lesions are usually teeming with spirochetes. If FA or darkfield examination is negative and the skin lesions are very suggestive, a skin biopsy can be performed to demonstrate a dense inflammatory infiltrate of plasma cells. Spirochetes may be visible with a silver or Warthin–Starry stain.

Blistering congenital syphilis must be differentiated from other disorders causing blistering on the palms and soles, including congenital candidiasis, acropustulosis of infancy, scabies, and epidermolysis bullosa. The clinical findings, as well as serologies, potassium hydroxide (KOH) preparation, and skin biopsy when necessary, help in this differentiation. The details of the evaluation and therapy of congenital syphilis are discussed in Chapter 12.

INFECTIOUS CAUSES – FUNGAL
(See also Chapter 14)

Nosocomially acquired fungemia has increasingly been recognized as a cause of morbidity and mortality in neonates, particularly very low-birthweight infants. Most cases are due to *Candida* spp., but infections from *Aspergillus, Trichosporon,* and other fungi have been reported.[36]

Congenital and Neonatal Candidiasis

Several candidal species can cause infections in neonates. Depending on the case series, *C. albicans, C. parapsilosis,* and to a lesser degree *C. tropicalis* are the most frequent isolates.[37] The cutaneous signs associated with candidal infections have been most clearly described for infection due to *Candida albicans*. Congenital candidiasis, an uncommon condition, is due to exposure to *C. albicans,* in utero or during delivery, resulting in a generalized skin eruption. The condition is usually present at birth but may have its onset at any time in the first week of life. Risk factors include a foreign body in the uterus or cervix (such as a retained intrauterine device or cervical suture), premature delivery, and a maternal history of vaginal candidiasis.[38–40] Several types of skin lesions may be present, including erythematous papules, diffuse erythema, vesicopustules, and fine scaling. Typically, a fine erythematous papular eruption is first noted, which over time evolves into a more pustular and scaly eruption. In milder cases, sparse papules and incipient pustules are scattered over the upper chest, back, and extremities. Virtually any part of the skin may be involved, and unlike many pustular eruptions (such as erythema toxicum and miliaria), the palms and soles are often involved.[41] Nail dystrophy and oral thrush are occasionally present.

Invasive fungal dermatitis is a term used to describe a generalized eruption very similar, if not identical, to congenital candidiasis. It usually develops in the first 2 weeks of life but onset may be somewhat later, predominantly in very low-birthweight infants. Diffuse erythema and scaling with superficial erosions resembling a first-degree burn have been reported and may evolve into full-thickness skin infection and necrosis. These skin lesions are associated with high rates of positive blood cultures, as well as pulmonary and other sites of infection.[42–44] Skin abscesses have been reported as an early finding of systemic candidosis.[45]

Diagnosis can often be confirmed with potassium hydroxide (KOH) preparation and/or culture from involved skin, demonstrating budding yeast and pseudohyphae. Organisms are often present in large numbers even in cases where pustules are relatively sparse, but if necessary, skin biopsy can also help confirm the diagnosis. Candida may also be present in the gastric aspirate. If the placenta is examined, characteristic yellow-white papules may be found on the umbilical cord, with evidence of infection also found at the periphery of the cord in Wharton's jelly.[6,46]

Differential diagnosis includes *Listeria* and intrauterine herpes simplex infections, erythema toxicum neonatorum, pustular miliaria rubra, and neonatal pustular melanosis. KOH preparation or tissue stains for fungi will help differentiate congenital candidiasis from these conditions.

Treatment of congenital candidiasis and invasive fungal dermatitis depends on the gestational age and weight of the infant. Premature infants weighing <1500 g have a much greater risk of disseminated candidiasis and need further investigations, such as blood, spinal fluid, and urine cultures, and immediate institution of systemic therapy as discussed in Chapter 14.

Infants with a higher birthweight and gestational age without evidence of disseminated disease must be observed closely because on rare occasions systemic infection, with respiratory distress or other organ involvement, may develop;[47] however, they are usually cured with topical therapy such as an imidazole cream.

Postnatally acquired *mucocutaneous candidiasis* is common after 1 week of age in both term and preterm infants. Colonization occurs in approximately one-quarter of infants <1500 g birthweight, and nearly one-third of those colonized develop mucocutaneous disease.[48] The most common sites of involvement are the diaper area and the oral mucous membranes, but other intertriginous areas may be affected (including the face), particularly if the infant has been intubated.[6] Typically, beefy red scaly patches with satellite papules at the periphery are the presenting findings. Pustules at the periphery of lesions can be seen, but are less frequent findings. Topical therapy with an imidazole cream or nystatin ointment is usually sufficient because dissemination does not develop in immunocompetent infants. Very low-birthweight infants with evidence of postnatally acquired candidiasis should be observed closely, and blood, urine, and CSF cultures should be obtained if signs of systemic infection are present.[44]

Aspergillus Infection

Primary cutaneous aspergillosis has been reported in more than a dozen neonates, most of whom were very premature. *Aspergillus fumigatus, A. niger,* and *A. flavus* can all cause skin disease. The age at diagnosis typically ranges from 1 week to 1 month.[49] Predisposing factors in addition to prematurity include prior treatment with systemic antibiotics or, less commonly, use of systemic corticosteroids. Skin lesions are usually the result of primary cutaneous disease, where the skin is the initial or only site of infection. This form is often preceded by skin maceration or injury and/or abrasions from adhesive tape. Hospital renovations or construction are a risk factor in some cases. Secondary cutaneous disease, where another organ, most commonly the lungs, is the primary site of infection, can also occur. In this case skin lesions are via hematogenous spread. In both primary and secondary skin disease a variety of skin lesions have been reported, including pustules and ulcerations, often superimposed on indurated plaques. In some cases the most prominent clinical feature is a necrotic eschar. In secondary disease lesions may be more extensive. Common sites of skin infection include the perineum and buttock, but any skin site can be affected.[49–51] A third form of aspergillosis reported in immunocompromised individuals is infection of a cavity such as a sinus with contiguous mucocutaneous spread, similar to that seen in other fungal infections such as mucormycosis.

Skin biopsies, which demonstrate dermal inflammation and broad anastomosing septate hyphae on special stains, are usually necessary for diagnosis, with culture for confirmation. Management is discussed in Chapter 14. The prognosis is guarded, both because of possible systemic aspergillosis and because of other diseases associated with prematurity.[50,51]

Trichosporosis and Zygomycosis (See Chapter 14)

More than a dozen cases of *Trichosporon* infection have been reported in neonates, most of whom were very low birthweight due to prematurity. Infection can be associated with generalized skin breakdown, peeling, and oozing without vesicles or pustules as well as necrotic eschar formation.[52,53] More than a dozen cases of mucormycosis have been reported, again nearly all in very low-birthweight infants. The age at diagnosis varied from 4 to 33 days. Damage to the skin from adhesive tape and/or invasive catheters is felt to be an important risk factor. This, combined with prematurity, broad-spectrum antibiotics, and in some the systemic use of corticosteroids, is a factor conducive to these opportunistic pathogens. Mucormycosis in this setting typically presents as either a cellulitis or an area of skin discoloration, which evolves into a black necrotic ulcer with surrounding erythema. Skin biopsy is usually needed for diagnosis.[54,55] Both types of infection have a poor prognosis, but treatment with amphotericin B (with or without surgical debridement) has been successful in some cases.

Malassezia Infections (See Neonatal Acne)

INFECTIOUS CAUSES – VIRAL

Herpes Simplex Infection (See Chapter 13)

Herpes simplex (HSV) infection is one of the most feared causes of blisters and pustules in the newborn. Subtle or inconspicuous skin lesions may herald the onset of infection, and the failure to promptly recognize and treat neonatal HSV infection can worsen the prognosis of this potentially devastating disease. Skin lesions are present in both intrauterine and neonatal herpes simplex infection, and although there is considerable overlap, the time of onset and many of the clinical features of the skin disease differ.

In intrauterine HSV infection skin lesions are usually present at the time of birth, or develop within 24–48 hours in 90% of affected infants. In addition to the characteristic vesicular eruption, widespread bullae and erosions resembling epidermolysis bullosa,[56,57] absence of skin on the scalp (resembling aplasia cutis congenita), and scars on the scalp, face, trunk, or extremities have been reported.[58] Affected infants are often premature, weighing less than 2500 g, and most have microcephaly, chorioretinitis, and abnormalities in the brain detected with imaging studies.

In contrast, neonatal HSV infection has three characteristic patterns of neonatal infection: mucocutaneous disease (limited to the skin, eyes, or mouth); disseminated disease (with evidence of visceral organ involvement, including liver, lungs, or disseminated intravascular coagulation); and central nervous system disease (where CSF or brain abnormalities are present in the absence of other visceral disease). Skin lesions may occur in all three types.[59]

Skin disease is the most characteristic finding in neonatal HSV infection, but it often lags behind other symptoms in onset and is noted in less than half of infants with disseminated and CNS disease at presentation. Feeding problems and lethargy are the most common presenting complaints.[60,61] The average age at onset of symptoms is 6–8 days, but the average age at diagnosis is 11–13 days, owing at least in part to the lack of specific symptoms or characteristic skin lesions early in the disease course.

Most infants will have vesicular skin lesions at some point in the course of disease. The most characteristic skin lesions are vesicles, which evolve over time into pustules, crusts, or erosions. Another important form of presentation is a poorly healing fetal scalp monitor site. Although grouped vesicles on an erythematous base are a hallmark of herpetic infection, lesions in neonatal herpes frequently lack such grouping, and in some cases a widespread vesicular exanthem or zoster-like blistering localized to one or two dermatomes may occur. Oral ulcerations are present in nearly one-third of cases.[62]

A maternal history of primary herpes simplex infection (or new-onset genital ulcerations, even if not specifically diagnosed) is an important clue to infection, but the majority of cases occur in women who are either asymptomatic or whose symptoms go unrecognized.[63] Other signs and symptoms of infection in neonates include lethargy, temperature instability, jaundice, coagulopathy, hepatitis, and neurologic deterioration.[60]

If skin lesions suggest herpes infection, prompt diagnosis and institution of treatment is imperative. Skin scrapings for Tzanck preparation are helpful in experienced hands, but direct immunofluorescent stains are increasingly being used for rapid detection; polymerase chain reaction (PCR) is used as a rapid way to obtain preliminary confirmation of HSV infection.[64] False positive immunofluorescent studies have occasionally been reported.[65] Viral cultures remain the gold standard of diagnosis, and cultures of the skin, conjunctiva, throat, cerebrospinal fluid, and urine should be obtained.[62]

The differential diagnosis of herpetic skin lesions depends on the specific clinical presentation (see Boxes 10-1 and 10-2, Tables 10-1 and 10-2). Vesicular lesions may resemble incontinentia pigmenti, congenital varicella, and acropustulosis of infancy. Dermatomal lesions may mimic herpes zoster. Pustular lesions may resemble congenital candidiasis, erythema toxicum neonatorum, congenital self-healing histiocytosis, listeriosis, and so on. Widespread blistering or erosions may mimic epidermolysis bullosa, although some vesicles or pustules are usually present in HSV infection.

There are some clinical presentations that are unlikely to represent herpes simplex infection. In particular, a vigorous term infant with a widespread pustular eruption presenting at birth is unlikely to have herpes simplex infection because its presence at birth implies intrauterine infection, which is typically associated with low birthweight or other findings. A premature infant with a widespread vesiculopustular eruption involving the palms and soles could have herpes infection, but is more likely to have congenital candidiasis. Although a high index of suspicion for herpes infection is appropriate, fear of this disease should not preclude a rational and systematic approach to differential diagnosis. The management of the infant presumed to have herpes simplex infection includes strict isolation and prompt institution of intravenous antiviral therapy[62] while awaiting cultures, and is discussed in more detail in Chapter 13.

Fetal and Neonatal Varicella

Cutaneous stigmata of varicella infection may occur in the newborn period as a result of early intrauterine infection, also referred to as the 'fetal varicella syndrome,' 'congenital varicella,' and 'varicella embryopathy.' Varicella can also occur as a result of intrauterine exposure just prior to delivery. This condition, which should more properly called 'neonatal varicella,' is often referred to in the literature as 'congenital varicella.'

The fetal varicella syndrome may occur as a result of primary varicella infection in the mother, almost always during the first trimester of pregnancy.[66] Cutaneous features include dermatomal scarring and occasional skin ulcerations, but blisters and pustules are not usually present in the neonatal period.[66–68] Herpes zoster in the newborn period can also result from exposure to varicella in utero, including infection later in pregnancy.[69–71]

Primary varicella in the neonatal period occurs in one-quarter of infants exposed to maternal varicella during the last 3 weeks of pregnancy, and can be especially severe if exposure occurs between 7 days before and 2 days after delivery.[72,73] Onset is usually at 5–10 days of age. When maternal infection occurs between 1 and 3 weeks before delivery, partial transplacental immunity results in earlier onset of infection and milder disease.

The skin lesions in neonatal varicella begin as vesicles superimposed on an erythematous base, gradually becoming cloudy and then crusted. The clinical pattern often resembles that seen in immunocompromised hosts. Lesions may be extremely numerous, widespread, and monomorphic, with all lesions occurring at the same stage of development instead of varying. They may also be hemorrhagic and enlarge into bullae.

The most life-threatening complication of neonatal varicella is pneumonia. The diagnosis is usually obvious because of the maternal history. A positive Tzanck preparation and viral cultures are confirmatory. Management is discussed in Chapter 13.

Other Viruses

Cytomegalovirus (CMV) is a relatively common cause of intrauterine and perinatal infection, but presentations with vesicles or ulcerations are quite rare.[74,75] In one case report, a premature and growth-retarded infant with hepatitis had two vesicles on the forehead, and blister fluid, as well as saliva and urine, produced a cytopathic effect characteristic of CMV in cell culture.[74] In another infant, perineal ulcers developed at 1 month of age and were biopsied after lack of response to numerous topical therapies. This biopsy demonstrated intranuclear inclusions and positive immunoperoxide staining for CMV.[75] Enteroviruses are well-recognized causes of vesicular eruptions in infants and children. Enterovirus infections may occur congenitally or during neonatal life, particularly in the summer months.[76] Reports of such infections describe maculopapular rashes, but vesicular eruptions have not been mentioned. One infant with fatal neonatal echovirus 19 infection developed a hemorrhagic bulla associated with gangrene and necrosis of a portion of her hand and fingers.[77]

Cutaneous Infestations: Scabies

Scabies (see also Chapter 14) is a cutaneous infestation caused by the mite Sarcoptes scabiei. Clinically recognizable infection in infants less than 3–4 weeks old is rare, but becomes relatively common thereafter.[78–80] Vesicles and pustules are a more common presentation in infants than in older children or adults, and are often concentrated on the medial feet, wrists, palms, and soles. These areas may also demonstrate erythematous papules, nodules, and burrows. The eruption may also be concentrated in the axillae, periumbilical area, and groin. Secondary bacterial infection can occur and should be suspected if bullae or significant honey-crusted areas are present. Young infants often lack significant pruritus.

The diagnosis can be suspected on clinical morphology. In most cases, a history of itching or rash in other family members can be elicited. Whenever possible, the diagnosis should be confirmed with skin scrapings, which demonstrate a mite, eggs, or feces. The best lesions for scraping are burrows, intact vesicles, and pustules, but in young infants mites are also found in crusted areas.[81] The diagnosis and management are discussed in Chapter 14.

TRANSIENT SKIN LESIONS (See also Chapter 7)

Erythema Toxicum Neonatorum

Erythema toxicum neonatorum (toxic erythema of the newborn; see Chapter 7) is a common condition of term infants, but is rare in premature infants and those weighing less than 2500 g.[82,83] Most cases occur between 24 and 48 hours of age, with 11% occurring before 24 hours and 25% with onset after 48 hours of life. Cases of presentation at birth[83–85] or onset as late as 10–14 days of life have been reported, but are unusual and should prompt consideration of alternative diagnoses.[83,86]

Four distinct skin lesions occur in varying combinations: erythematous macules, wheals, papules, and pustules (Fig. 10-1). Occasionally, lesions appear as small vesicles before becoming pustular. The face, buttocks, torso, and proximal extremities are common sites of involvement. The palms and soles are virtually never affected. Erythematous macules and wheals may vary in size from a few millimeters to several centimeters, with papules and pustules 1–2 mm in size superimposed on erythematous macules or wheals. The rash waxes and wanes, with previously involved skin returning to normal in a few hours to 1–2 days, with new lesions continuing to develop for several days.[87] Mechanical irritation of the skin can precipitate the onset of new lesions.

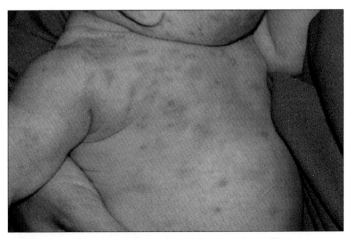

FIG. 10.1 Pustules in an infant with erythema toxicum. Note numerous papules and pustules scattered over the torso, arms, and face.

The diagnosis of erythema toxicum is usually based on the clinical appearance of the rash in an otherwise healthy term infant. The diagnosis can be confirmed with Wright's stain of a pustule, which demonstrates numerous eosinophils. Peripheral eosinophilia is present in a small percentage of cases.[4] Skin biopsy, usually unnecessary, demonstrates eosinophilic infiltration of the outer root sheath of the hair follicle epithelium. In pustular lesions, eosinophils coalesce into an intraepidermal or subcorneal pustule, adjacent to a hair follicle. An upper dermal and perivascular eosinophilic infiltrate is also present.[88]

The differential diagnosis of erythema toxicum includes neonatal pustular melanosis, congenital candidiasis, miliaria rubra, incontinentia pigmenti, and eosinophilic pustular folliculitis. The latter two conditions have eosinophilic inflammation, but can be differentiated by their distribution, their more chronic course, and with histopathology. The associated erythema and typical postnatal onset may help to distinguish erythema toxicum from pustular melanosis, but overlapping features and simultaneously occurrence have been reported.[89] Once the diagnosis has been established, no specific treatment is necessary. Parents can be reassured about the benign and noninfectious nature of the condition.

Transient Neonatal Pustular Melanosis (See also Chapter 7)

Transient neonatal pustular melanosis (TNPM) is a relatively common condition of unknown etiology. Like erythema toxicum, it is more common in term infants and is unassociated with other abnormalities.[90] Unlike erythema toxicum, lesions are virtually always present at birth.

Three types of lesions occur in TNPM: pustules with little or no underlying erythema; ruptured pustules manifesting as slightly hyperpigmented macules with a surrounding collarette of scale; and hyperpigmented macules without scale. Lesions vary in size from 1 to 10 mm, but are typically 2–3 mm. They may be solitary or grouped. Small satellite pustules may be present at the periphery of larger pustules (Fig. 10-2). More than one type of lesion may be present at the same time. The eruption may occur on virtually any part of the skin, but is most common on the forehead, behind the ears, under the

chin, on the neck and back, and on the hands and feet. The palms and soles may be affected.

The diagnosis of pustular melanosis is usually based on lesional morphology, time of onset, and the absence of other findings. Clues to clinical diagnosis are the extremely superficial nature of the pustules and the absence of underlying erythema.

Wright's stain often demonstrates polymorphonuclear neutrophils (PMN), with an occasional eosinophil, but in rare cases eosinophils may predominate.[91] Gram staining demonstrates PMNs but no bacteria. Skin biopsy, rarely necessary for diagnosis, demonstrates hyperkeratosis, acanthosis, and an intracorneal or subepidermal pustule filled with PMNs, occasional eosinophils, and variable amounts of keratinous debris, serous fluid, and fragmented hair shafts.[90]

The differential diagnosis of TNPM includes erythema toxicum, staphylococcal impetigo and other bacterial infections, congenital candidiasis, acropustulosis of infancy, and miliaria. These conditions can nearly always be differentiated by time of onset, lesional morphology, demonstration of PMNs on Wright's stain, and the absence of organisms on Gram stain and KOH preparations.

Once the diagnosis of TPNM has been established, no treatment is necessary. Pustules usually resolve over a few days, but hyperpigmented macules may last for several weeks to months before resolving.

Sterile Transient Neonatal Pustulosis

The term sterile transient neonatal pustulosis was introduced by Ferrandiz et al.[89] to describe infants with clinical and histologic features of both erythema toxicum neonatorum and TNPM. They proposed that a clear-cut differentiation between these two conditions is not always possible. Although there may be overlap in some cases, most authors continue to use the diagnostic categories of erythema toxicum neonatorum and TNPM rather than lump the two together.

Miliaria

Miliaria (prickly heat; see Chapter 7) is a relatively common finding in newborns. In warm climates without air-conditioned nurseries, miliaria may be present in up to 15% of newborns,[92,93] but it is less common in temperate climates.[94] Two types of miliaria occur in the newborn period. Miliaria crystallina is due to blockage of the sweat duct at the level of the stratum corneum. Sweat accumulates beneath the stratum corneum, causing tiny flaccid vesicles that resemble dewdrops. Miliaria rubra is also due to blockage of the sweat duct in the stratum corneum, but the obstruction leads to focal leakage of sweat into the dermis, resulting in an inflammatory response, evident in the erythematous papules and pustules that are present clinically (Fig. 10-3).[95] Both may follow excessive warming in an incubator, fever, occlusive dressings, or inappropriately warm clothing. Miliaria crystallina is occasionally present at the time of birth, whereas miliaria rubra is more common after the first week of life.[96]

The most common locations are the forehead and upper trunk. Lesions often become confluent and this, combined with location, time of onset, and a history of excessive warming, may help distinguish miliaria from other vesicular and pustular eruptions. Miliaria crystallina is also easily recognized because the dewdrop-like vesicles rupture easily with only slight pressure.

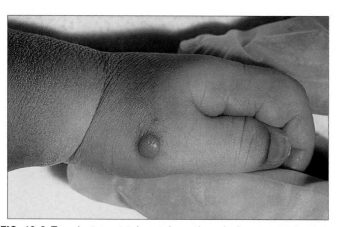

FIG. 10-2 Transient neonatal pustular melanosis. Large pustule on the hand with tiny 'satellite' pustules may mimic infection. (From Frieden IJ. Blisters and pustules in the newborn. Curr Probl Pediatr 1989; 19: 587.)

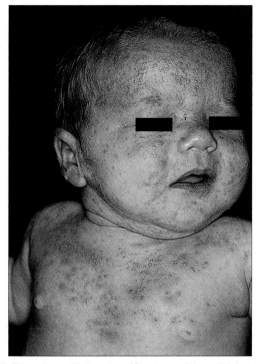

FIG. 10-3 Extensive miliaria rubra. (Courtesy of Anne W. Lucky.)

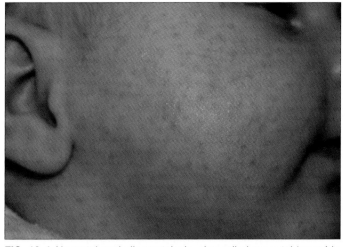

FIG. 10-4 Neonatal cephalic pustulosis, also called neonatal 'acne,' is characterized by papules and small, superficial pustules.

Although the precise cause of miliaria is not known, recent evidence supports the concept that an extracellular polysaccharide substance produced by some strains of *Staphylococcus epidermidis* may obstruct sweat delivery.[97]

In cases where the diagnosis is uncertain, a skin biopsy can be performed. In miliaria crystallina, subcorneal vesicles are contiguous with underlying sweat ducts. In miliaria rubra, intraepidermal vesicles are due to epidermal edema. These vesicles, which are also in contiguity with a sweat duct, have an intravesicular and dermal chronic inflammatory infiltrate.[95] No specific treatment is necessary for miliaria; the condition will disappear spontaneously if overheating is avoided.

Sucking Blisters

Sucking blisters result from vigorous sucking by the infant during fetal life. The lesions are always present at birth; they occur in approximately 1 in every 250 live births, and are not associated with other abnormalities.[98,99] These bullae are usually flaccid, vary in size from 5 to 15 mm, and may evolve rapidly to become superficial linear or round erosions. Characteristic locations include the radial forearm, wrist, and hand, including the dorsal thumb and index fingers. The lesions may be unilateral or bilateral and symmetric.

The diagnosis can be suspected if typical skin changes are present at characteristic sites, without evidence of vesicles or bullae on other areas of the body. The infant usually confirms the diagnosis by demonstrating 'an insatiable appetite for the skin of their own forearms, wrists, and fingers.'[98] The lesions resolve without specific treatment within days to weeks.

Neonatal Cephalic Pustulosis (Neonatal 'Acne')

Although neonatal 'acne' has been considered common, the term 'neonatal cephalic pustulosis' has been proposed for this condition. This is at least in part to distinguish it from the infantile form of acne vulgaris, which usually presents after a month of age, with comedones and its associated inflammatory lesions[100] (see also Chapter 7).

The condition is characterized by a papulopustular facial eruption usually concentrated on the cheeks, but the forehead, chin, eyelids, neck, upper chest, and scalp may also be affected (Fig. 10-4). The mean age of onset is 2–3 weeks, with some cases beginning as early as 1 week of life. It is usually asymptomatic and generally unassociated with other medical conditions, although prolonged true acne and seborrheic dermatitis have been described.[101] Several authors have proposed *Malassezia furfur* and *M. sympodialis* as causes of this condition.[101,102] Cultures of pustules have demonstrated both *M. furfur* and *M. sympodialis*, especially in severe cases. Because these organisms are found on the skin under normal conditions, their role in causing this disease is still somewhat controversial.

The diagnosis is usually made clinically, but Giemsa-stained smears can demonstrate fungal spores, as well as neutrophils and occasionally other inflammatory cells.[101] Special growth media are necessary to culture *Malassezia* species. Treatment with topical imidazole creams such as ketoconazole can result in resolution of the eruption, but the condition also frequently improves with low-potency topical corticosteroids such as hydrocortisone and also remits spontaneously after several weeks.

Diaper Erosions

Rapidly healing superficial erosions have been noted in the diaper area between 1 and 14 days of life in several otherwise healthy infants who were being studied prospectively as part of a study of diaper dermatitis. The erosions were attributed to either perinatal trauma or the minor trauma of normal diaper care. The findings suggest that term infants may have increased skin fragility compared to older infants, where such erosions are not typically seen.[103] This and other causes of skin disease that occur specifically in the diaper area are discussed in Chapter 16.

Iatrogenic Causes of Erosions and Ulcerations
(See also Chapter 8)

Many iatrogenic interventions can cause cutaneous erosions or, less commonly, ulcerations.[104] Scalp erosions can be due to intrauterine placement of fetal scalp electrodes for monitoring purposes. One prospective study of 535 monitored newborns found that 21% had very minor superficial lacerations that healed before discharge, and 18.7% had superficial lacerations still present at discharge. A rarer finding, scalp ulcerations, was present in 1.3% of cases.[105] These lesions are usually only a few millimeters in diameter, but occasionally measure up to 1–1.5 cm. They are sometimes confused with the lesions of aplasia cutis congenita. Persistent scalp erosions, ulcerations, or crusting should always lead to consideration of possible neonatal herpes infection.[62]

Transcutaneous pulse oximetry may rarely lead to blistering or erosions, particularly if a defective device results in overheating of the skin leading to a thermal burn, or from sustained pressure from a probe left in one location for over 24 hours.[106] Erosions or crusted areas may also occur on the heel, following multiple heel punctures to draw blood.

Scald burns represent a relatively common form of childhood injury. They can also occur in neonates or young infants as a result of child abuse or misinformed parenting. Scald burns with blistering were reported in a 1-day-old infant bathed in inappropriately hot water. The water temperature had recently been raised by the hospital because of a nosocomial outbreak of *Legionella*.[107]

UNCOMMON AND RARE CAUSES OF VESICLES AND PUSTULES

Infantile Acropustulosis

Infantile acropustulosis is a condition of unknown etiology characterized by the development of extremely pruritic vesicles and pustules concentrated on the hands and feet. Lesions may be present at birth, but more often develop in the first weeks or months of life.[108,109] The condition is more common in black people, but occurs in all races.[110] An association with atopy has been reported in some patients and families.[111] Lesions occur in crops every 2–4 weeks, and individual lesions usually last for 5–10 days. Boys are more commonly affected. Intensely pruritic vesicles and pustules are located on the palms and soles, dorsal hands and feet, as well as the sides of the fingers and toes (Fig. 10-5). Scattered lesions may also be located on the ankles and wrists. Occasionally papules occur at more distant sites, such as the chest, back, and abdomen. Lesions are initially tense, then flatten, developing scale and postinflammatory hyperpigmentation. Infants who are too young to scratch may instead seem irritable and rub their feet vigorously against the bedding.

A second, more common form of infantile acropustulosis has also been described, occurring after scabies infestation. This condition, called postscabetic acropustulosis, is also concentrated on the insteps and hands, but lesions on the torso can also be present. Postscabetic acropustulosis usually follows scabies infestation that has been either severe in degree or present for a prolonged period.

The diagnosis can be clinical, but also may be confirmed with either direct smears from vesicles and/or pustules or skin biopsy. Scrapings of lesions show numerous PMNs and occa-

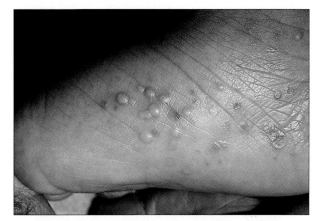

FIG. 10-5 Acropustulosis of infancy. (From Frieden IJ. Blisters and pustules in the newborn. Curr Probl Pediatr 1989; 19: 591.)

sional eosinophils.[112] Skin biopsy demonstrates an intraepidermal or subcorneal pustule filled with neutrophils, eosinophils, or both. The earliest histopathologic changes are focal vesiculation and degeneration of keratinocytes with cell necrosis.[113] Peripheral eosinophilia is occasionally present.[114]

The major differential diagnosis of infantile acropustulosis is actual scabies infestation. Careful physical examination, family history, and multiple skin scrapings may be necessary to differentiate the two. As mentioned, the condition may actually be preceded by an episode of scabies, even after adequate antiscabetic treatment.[115] Other conditions in the differential diagnosis include dyshidrotic eczema and pustulosis palmaris et plantaris, which are rare in infancy; congenital candidiasis, which is usually more widespread; and neonatal pustular melanosis, which is not pruritic and does not occur beyond the immediate newborn period. An association with eosinophilic pustular folliculitis has also been reported.[116]

Acropustulosis of infancy spontaneously remits within 1–2 years; postscabetic cases resolve more quickly. Very potent topical corticosteroids (class I or II) are fairly effective in halting early lesions and/or controlling symptoms, but should be used cautiously to avoid localized atrophy or systemic absorption.[115] If symptoms are severe, oral antihistamines at maximum doses can be used to control pruritus. Dapsone 1–2 mg/k/day has been used for severe cases, but should be used with caution because of the risk of methemoglobinemia and other adverse effects.[108]

Eosinophilic Pustular Folliculitis

Eosinophilic pustular folliculitis (EPF) is a rare disorder. Several cases have been reported in young infants, including a few cases with onset at birth or in the first few days of life.[117–120] In the neonatal cases, the children were born with or developed pustules primarily on the scalp and face but also intermittently on the trunk or extremities (Fig. 10-6). The pustules are usually very itchy; they may evolve with crusting and heal with scarring. Recurrent crops of lesions appear, leading to a waxing and waning course that lasts from a few months up to 5 years.[120] Peripheral eosinophilia is present in some patients. The pattern of recurrences, extreme pruritus, involvement of the extremities, and similar histology has led the authors in at least one report to speculate that infantile acropustulosis

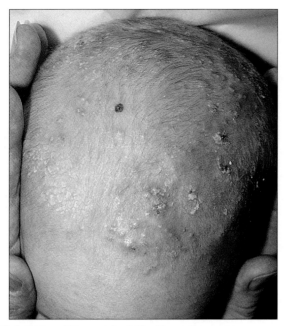

FIG. 10-6 Eosinophilic pustular folliculitis on the scalp.

and EPF may be part of the same clinical spectrum,[116] but in neither case is the etiology known.

Histopathology demonstrates a dense diffuse periadnexal and perifollicular eosinophilic dermal infiltrate. Some authors argue that this nonspecific histopathologic reaction pattern should not be attributed to one distinctive clinical entity.[121] However, when one considers the biopsy findings with the clinical context, a specific diagnosis can usually be made and parents reassured about the benign nature of the process. The differential diagnosis in neonates includes hyperimmunoglobulin E syndrome, transient neonatal pustular melanosis, erythema toxicum neonatorum, Langerhans' cell histiocytosis, and acropustulosis of infancy. There is no specific treatment for the condition, but oral antihistamines and potent topical corticosteroids may help control the symptoms temporarily.

Erosive Pustular Dermatosis of the Scalp

Erosive pustular dermatosis of the scalp is rare in neonates. Siegel et al.[122] reported a series of neonates who developed necrotic caput succedaneum or so-called halo-scalp ring injury from damage to the scalp and hair follicles during a difficult delivery (see also Chapter 8). Infants typically have had scalp edema or frank scalp necrosis at the time of birth. Over the next several days to weeks the inflammation continues, with pustules, scaling, and crusting developing in scarred areas of the scalp. The clinical features of erosive pustular dermatosis of the scalp have also been described in adults with either severe scalp injuries or severe chronic sun damage. Infants with this condition improve with application of potent topical steroids. Complications include bacterial superinfection. Scarring alopecia is present in all of the affected infants.[122]

Langerhans' Cell Histiocytosis

Langerhans' cell histiocytosis (LCH) can be present in the newborn period, either as a generalized eruption or as a solitary nodule (see also Chapter 25). The most dramatic form has been called variously 'congenital self-healing reticulohistiocytosis' or Hashimoto–Pritzker disease. Although some reports initially described it as a distinct histiocytic disorder, further evaluations, including immunohistochemical stains, have confirmed its place as part of the disease spectrum of LCH, with few exceptions.[123–126] In congenital LCH skin lesions are virtually always present at birth, and new lesions may continue to erupt over the first several weeks. The eruption may be present on any area of the body, including the palms and soles. Numerous morphologic characteristics have been reported, including erythematous papules, hemangioma-like papules, nodules, pustules, vesicles, bullae, necrotic and hemorrhagic bullae, discrete erosions, widespread eroded patches, and ulcerations.[127–131] Lesions vary in size from a few millimeters to several centimeters, but in most cases with vesicles or pustules small lesions predominate. Petechiae, atrophy, and milia may occasionally be present, and anetoderma-like scarring has been reported.[132]

If suspected, a preliminary diagnosis can be obtained via Tzanck preparation, which demonstrates histiocytes with reniform nuclei and abundant cytoplasm,[133] and can then be confirmed with skin biopsy. An infiltrate of histiocytes, with large cells and irregularly shaped vesicular nuclei and eosinophilic cytoplasm, is present in the upper dermis. The histiocytes may also invade the epidermis focally. Occasional lymphocytes and eosinophils may be present. The diagnosis should be further confirmed with an S-100 stain, immunohistochemical markers, and/or electron microscopy to evaluate for the presence of Langerhans' cells.[134] The differential diagnosis of congenital self-healing histiocytosis includes intrauterine herpes simplex infection, congenital candidiasis, neonatal varicella, and intrauterine graft-versus-host disease.

Most cases remain confined to the skin and resolve without treatment, but eye and lung involvement in the neonatal period has been reported. In both cases extracutaneous disease remitted spontaneously.[135,136] Because cutaneous or even systemic relapse may occur months to years later, long-term follow-up and monitoring is required.[137,138] In addition, infants with acute disseminated LCH (formerly called Letterer–Siwe disease) can present with similar skin changes in the first few weeks to months of life, further emphasizing the need for ongoing clinical surveillance in newborns and young infants with LCH.

Incontinentia Pigmenti

Incontinentia pigmenti (IP) (see Chapter 26) is a multisystem disease, inherited as an X-linked dominant condition that is usually lethal in males. Located at Xq28, the mutation responsible for IP in most cases involves the NFκB essential modulator (NEMO) gene.[139,140] Skin lesions are present at birth in 50% of cases and occur within 2 weeks in 90%, usually beginning a vesicular eruption that evolves into linear streaks of clear or yellow confluent vesicles, following the lines of Blaschko[141] (Fig. 10-7). These lines, presumably derived from embryonal migration patterns, are not dermatomal, but instead form linear patterns on the extremities and curvilinear, whorled patterns on the torso. The eruption is most common on the trunk, extremities, and scalp, often sparing the face. The vesicular phase may wax and wane for up to a year and occasionally recur, but individual lesions usually resolve within 1–2 weeks. As the initial vesicular phase subsides, a verrucous stage consisting of hyperkeratotic streaks usually occurs, followed by a

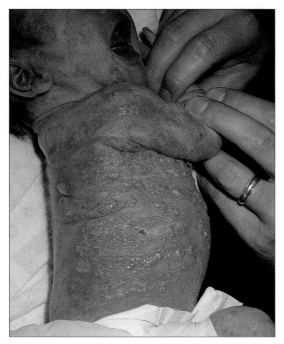

FIG. 10-7 Incontinentia pigmenti. The extensive linear blistering in this case – more pronounced than is usually seen – can resemble other causes of neonatal vesicles and bullae.

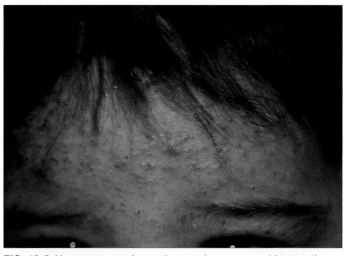

FIG. 10-8 Numerous papules and crusted areas are evident on the forehead of this young infant with hyper-IgE syndrome. (Courtesy of Dr Sarah Chamlin.)

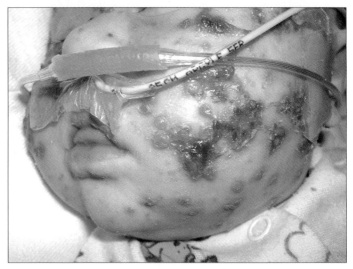

FIG. 10-9 Extensive vesiculopustular eruption in the setting of leukemoid reaction associated with Down Syndrome. (Courtesy of Drs Alanna Bree and Elaine Siegfried.)

pigmented stage with streaky, reticulated pigment forming a 'marble-cake pattern' that fades over many years. The final stage is that of hypopigmented, atrophic patches, usually on the extremities, which may be subtle and unappreciated. Because these stages may overlap in time, as well as occurring in utero, vesicular lesions may be seen in conjunction with verrucous or hyperpigmented lesions. Additional cutaneous changes include patchy, scarring alopecia, woolly hair nevus, nail dystrophy and abnormalities in sweating.[139,142]

Diagnosis is made by skin biopsy, which demonstrates an edematous (spongiotic) epidermis with eosinophilic infiltration, dyskeratosis, and eosinophilic microabscesses.[95] Herpes simplex infection is often confused with the vesicular phase of IP,[143] but coexistent neonatal HSV infection and IP have been reported.[144,145] One should carefully examine the entire skin surface for grouped vesicles and perform direct immunofluorescence and viral cultures on any suspicious areas. Other entities in the differential diagnosis of vesicular IP include erythema toxicum neonatorum, bullous impetigo, and diffuse cutaneous mastocytosis. IP is also discussed in Chapter 26.

Hyperimmunoglobulin E Syndrome

Hyperimmunoglobulin E syndrome (HIES) is a primary immunodeficiency that can present in the newborn period with skin findings but is typically diagnosed later in infancy. In one retrospective study, the average age of rash onset was 7 days. The eruption begins as pink papules that evolve over days into pustules, primarily located on the face and scalp (Fig. 10-8).[146,147] The rash during the newborn period is nonspecific, and differential diagnosis at this age includes several other conditions, including neonatal cephalic pustulosis, erythema toxicum neonatorum, and eosinophilic pustular folliculitis. Clues to diagnosis include the persistent – albeit fluctuating – nature of the rash, the propensity for recurrent *Staphylococcus aureus* infection, pruritus, and spread to other body sites. Over time the eruption may evolve into a chronic atopic dermatitis-

like condition.[147] Two additional clues to diagnosis are peripheral eosinophilia and skin biopsy demonstrating an eosinophilic folliculitis. Other features of HIES, seen in older children and adults, include chronic folliculitis, abscesses, recurrent pneumonia and pneumatocele formation, osteomyelitis, osteopenia, retention of deciduous teeth, and mucocutaneous candidiasis. Although the disease has been named and defined by high IgE levels, levels during the newborn period, although higher than in normal age-matched controls, are often less than 2000 IU/mL and may not rise until after 1 year of age.[147,148] In addition, infants with severe atopic dermatitis without HIES may actually have higher levels of IgE.

Pustular Eruption in Association with Leukemoid Reaction in Down Syndrome

Several infants with trisomy 21 and transient myeloproliferative disorders have been reported with widespread vesiculopustular eruptions. The pustules begin on the face in the first few days of life, spread to the upper body, and resolve spontaneously. They may show pathergy, the tendency to aggregate at areas of skin injury (Fig. 10-9).[149,150] In some cases, Wright's stain showed immature myelocytes and promyelocytes; cultures were sterile.[150] In another case, skin biopsy revealed an intraepidermal spongiotic vesicopustule and a perivascular infiltrate of immature myeloid cells, reminiscent of leukemia cutis. This infant was subsequently diagnosed with myelodysplasia and developed acute myelogenous leukemia at 2 years of age.[151] This condition can even occur in infants without obvious Down syndrome. In one case report, a phenotypically normal neonate who had transient myeloproliferative disorder and vesiculopustular eruptions was later found to have trisomy 21 in the leukemic cells and disomy 21 in buccal cells.[152]

Pustular Psoriasis

At least one case of pustular psoriasis has been described in a 20-day-old infant presenting with an exfoliative dermatitis with onset in the first few days of life. Pustules were present on the palms and soles. Skin biopsies helped confirm the diagnosis.[153] Pustular psoriasis with onset in infancy and early childhood has also been reported (Fig. 10-10). In many cases it presents as an annular pustular eruption mimicking tinea corporis, which can develop into more generalized pustular psoriasis.[154]

Neonatal Behçet's Disease

Behçet's disease rarely presents in the neonatal period: in one French study, four out of 55 pediatric cases had onset of symptoms before age 1 year.[155] A few cases of neonatal Behçet's disease acquired transplacentally from affected mothers have been described. Skin manifestations develop within 1 week of life and generally resolve by 2–3 months of age. These infants present with oral and/or genital ulcerations, and may develop pustular or necrotic skin lesions, primarily on the hands and feet and at sites of trauma.[156] Although most infants have no systemic symptoms, two cases with severe systemic manifestations have been described.[157,158] One child of a mother with known Behçet's disease died of neurological complications at 9 days of age. Another infant had bloody diarrhea and vasculitis, which responded to systemic corticosteroids. Of note, the mother of this infant had not been diagnosed with Behçet's disease prior to her delivery. She had developed oral and genital

ulcerations during pregnancy that resolved and then recurred when the infant was 24 days old.[157] With this exception, infants with neonatal-onset Behçet's disease were diagnosed because of a known diagnosis in the mother. The primary consideration in the differential diagnosis of neonatal Behçet's disease is HSV infection; viral cultures and maternal history of the disease can help distinguish these entities.

DISORDERS PRESENTING PRIMARILY WITH BULLAE, EROSIONS, OR ULCERATIONS

Although there is some overlap between those conditions that present with vesicles and pustules, several disorders feature mainly bullae, erosions, and/or ulcerations. One of the most common causes of widespread bullae in the newborn period, epidermolysis bullosa, is discussed in Chapter 11. It should always be considered as a possible diagnosis when bullae or large erosions or ulcers occur in the neonatal period.

Mastocytosis (See Chapter 25)

Mast cell disease causing blisters of the skin in infants occurs in three forms: (1) discrete nodules, or mastocytomas (2) multiple papules and plaques (so-called urticaria pigmentosa) and (3) widespread infiltration of the skin (so-called diffuse cutaneous mastocytosis), which is quite rare. In all three types blisters can develop superimposed on lesional skin. In diffuse cutaneous mastocytosis, blisters also may develop on apparently uninvolved skin.

Mastocytomas may be solitary or multiple. When a child has multiple lesions, the condition is sometimes referred to as urticaria pigmentosa. Mastocytomas may be present at birth or develop in early infancy. Typically, lesions have an orange-red or brown color and may have a *peau d'orange* surface texture. They vary in size from 1 to 5 cm. With friction, vasoactive substances including histamine are released, leading to erythema, wheal formation (so-called Darier sign), and occasionally blisters or erosions on the surface of the lesion[159,160] (Fig. 10-11A, B). The lesions of urticaria pigmentosa typically present mainly as pigmented spots with subtle elevation. Blistering is relatively uncommon in this form of mast cell disease. Diffuse cutaneous mastocytosis is a rare condition, characterized by large collections of mast cells that infiltrate the skin over large areas. Lesions may be present at birth[161] but usually develop in the first few weeks to months of life [162–164]. Initially, blisters can develop on normal-appearing skin, making the clinical diagnosis difficult until thickened, leathery skin develops (Fig. 10-12). Conversely, the skin can be so thickened that so-called pachydermia with extensive skin folding has been reported.[165] Blisters may occur anywhere on the body, including the scalp. Acute episodes of sudden, massive blistering may lead to erosions and desquamation.[146,166] Dermographism is usually prominent. Wheezing, urticaria, diarrhea, and hypotension may also occur. Other complications include coagulation abnormalities, myeloproliferative disorder, syncope, hypotension, and shock.[166] Familial cases with apparent autosomal dominant inheritance have been reported.[167] The differential diagnosis of bullous mastocytosis includes staphylococcal scalded skin syndrome, toxic epidermal necrolysis, and erythema multiforme. Management depends on the degree of systemic symptoms and is discussed in Chapter 25. Systemic corticosteroids can control blistering and can be used in severe cases.[166,168]

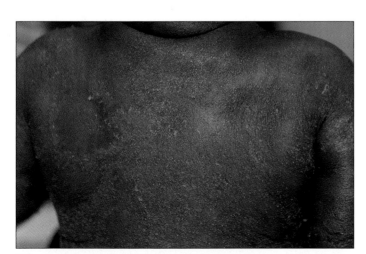

FIG. 10-10 Generalized pustules and desquamation in an infant with pustular psoriasis. (Courtesy of Dr Brandon Newell.)

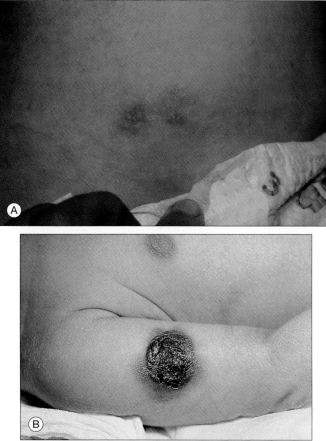

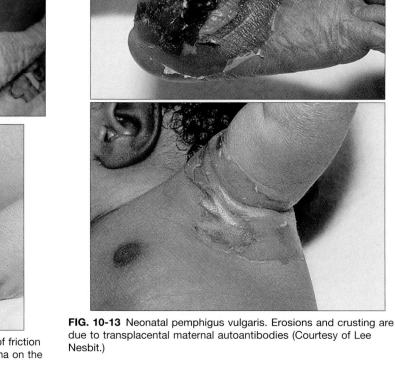

FIG. 10-13 Neonatal pemphigus vulgaris. Erosions and crusting are due to transplacental maternal autoantibodies (Courtesy of Lee Nesbit.)

FIG. 10-11 Small blisters evident in a mastocytoma in area of friction from a diaper (**A**) and blistering and crusting in a mastocytoma on the arm (**B**). (Courtesy of Neil Prose.)

Blistering Caused by Maternal Bullous Disease

Blistering may occur in the newborn whose mother has an autoimmune blistering disease mediated by IgG. IgG crosses the placenta and causes a similar disease in the fetus. This finding has been reported in three IgG-mediated diseases: pemphigoid gestationis (formerly called herpes gestationis), pemphigus vulgaris, and very rarely in pemphigus foliaceus.[169–177]

Blistering is virtually always present at birth. Lesional morphology depends on which autoimmune disease affects the mother, and ranges from tense or flaccid bullae to widespread areas of erosion (Fig. 10-13). There may be a few lesions or many. Infants may be born prematurely; before the advent of corticosteroids there was an increased incidence of stillbirths in pemphigoid gestationis.

The diagnosis is usually obvious because of a maternal history of an autoimmune blistering disease. Most mothers have active disease during their pregnancy, but there have been rare reported of affected infants born to women with inactive disease.[178,179]

The diagnosis can be confirmed with skin biopsy and direct immunofluorescence on the infant's skin. In pemphigoid gestationis, a subepidermal bulla with eosinophils in the bulla fluid and dermis is usually present, and direct immunofluorescence demonstrates a linear pattern of complement (C3) at the dermoepidermal junction. Lesions in pemphigus vulgaris demonstrate an intraepidermal blister, acantholysis of keratinocytes, and a mild inflammatory infiltrate of eosinophils and occasional plasma cells;[95] immunofluorescence shows IgG and

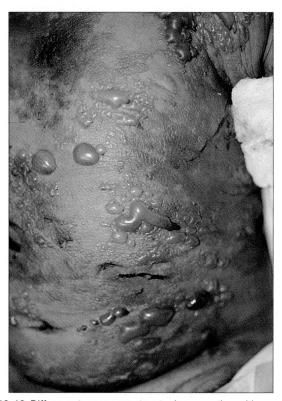

FIG. 10-12 Diffuse cutaneous mastocytosis presenting with widespread blistering (Courtesy of Dr Sarah Chamlin.)

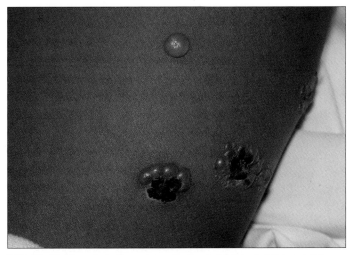

FIG. 10-14 Chronic bullous dermatosis of childhood: blisters with rosettes or sausage-like shapes are often seen. (Courtesy of Albert Yan.)

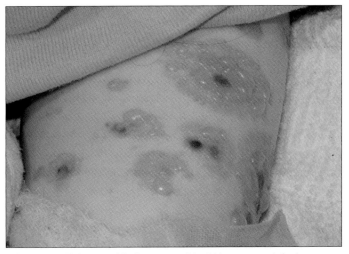

FIG. 10-15 Widespread bullous pemphigoid in a young infant.

C3 staining of the intraepidermal cement substance. In pemphigus foliaceus, intraepithelial vesicles are evident, and immunofluorescence demonstrates intercellular IgG and C3 in the superficial epidermis.

A major differential diagnosis is epidermolysis bullosa, but a maternal history of an immunobullous skin helps in diagnosis. Once the diagnosis is made no specific therapy is needed, but topical petrolatum and/or antibiotics may help avoid secondary infection.[169] New blisters do not usually occur after the newborn period. If blistering is extensive, the infant should be watched closely for signs of cutaneous or systemic infection. Systemic corticosteroids should be considered only in extremely severe cases.

Chronic Bullous Dermatosis of Childhood (Linear IgA Disease)

The most common autoimmune blistering disease in children, chronic bullous dermatosis of childhood (CBDC), is not usually seen in the newborn period,[180] but at least one severe case has been reported in a neonate. This child had two blisters at birth and was diagnosed with CBDC at 2 weeks of age. His course was complicated by multiple infections. Other atypical features of this case included permanent ocular scarring, swallowing difficulties, and recurrent asthma.[181]

Typically, the disease is characterized by onset between 1 and 6 years of age, with widespread, tense blisters having the greatest concentration on the groin, buttocks, and thighs. Blisters often form rosettes or sausage-like shapes (Fig. 10-14). A subepidermal bulla and linear deposition of IgA at the dermoepidermal junction are the key diagnostic findings. Treatment options include prednisone 1–2 mg/kg/ day, dapsone 1–2 mg/kg/day, and sulfapyridine 65 mg/kg/day.[182]

Bullous Pemphigoid

Bullous pemphigoid does not usually occur during the neonatal period, but cases with onset as young as 2 months of age have been reported.[183,184] Tense, generalized blisters characterize the disease (Fig. 10-15). Involvement of the hands and feet appears to be more common in infancy.[185] The diagnosis is suspected if skin biopsy demonstrates a subepidermal bulla with eosinophils; it is confirmed by demonstration of linear staining of IgG and C3 along the basement membrane zone.[185] Treatment regimens vary: in some cases potent topical corticosteroids can control disease, whereas in others systemic corticosteroids are necessary.

Neonatal Lupus Erythematosus

Neonatal lupus erythematosus (NLE) (see also Chapter 19) is an uncommon disorder caused by the fetal and neonatal effects of transplacental maternal autoantibodies, particularly SS-A (Ro), but also SS-B (La) and RNP. Blistering is virtually never seen with NLE, but the disease can present with widespread erosions or crusting.[186–188] These erosions may have resulted from the shearing of atrophic epidermis from the underlying dermis during the birth process.

The diagnosis can be suspected because, in addition to erosions, areas of atrophic or discoid skin lesions are also present. Skin biopsy shows epidermal atrophy and a vacuolar interface dermatitis, which may have associated increased dermal mucin. The mothers of affected infants are usually asymptomatic. Serology tests of both mother and infant should be obtained, looking specifically for anti-SS-A, -SS-B, and -RNP antibodies. If NLE is suspected, infants should be carefully examined and an ECG, CBC, platelet count, and liver function tests should be obtained.

Toxic Epidermal Necrolysis and Bullous Erythema Multiforme

Toxic epidermal necrolysis (TEN) and erythema multiforme (EM) are extremely rare in the newborn period. Scattered cases of EM have been described, but most have no associated blistering. A 25-day-old neonate was reported with biopsy-proven erythema multiforme preceded by upper respiratory infection. Clinical features included bullae on the face and erosions on the palate, but without a generalized, confluent eruption.[189]

The few cases of TEN reported in early infancy have been in premature infants and caused by Gram-negative infections.[190] Graft-versus-host disease can also cause TEN and may occur at birth because of intrauterine passage of maternal cells to an immunodeficient fetus.[191,192] Infants with TEN may present with irritability, temperature instability, and diffuse cutaneous erythema, followed by flaccid blisters and erosions (Fig. 10-16). The diagnosis can be confirmed by skin biopsy, which demonstrates extensive, full-thickness epidermal necrosis and minimal to absent dermal inflammation. The epidermal cleavage is located at the dermoepidermal junction or in the mid to lower epidermis. A frozen section can be performed for rapid diagnosis.[193] TEN is a potentially life-threatening condition at any age, because the skin necrosis causes the functional equivalent of severe first- and second-degree burns. The situation is even worse in the newborn period because of decreased immune defenses and a more tenuous balance of fluids and electrolytes. The prognosis is poor in the neonatal period: most affected neonates have died either from TEN or other causes.

The differential diagnosis includes staphylococcal scalded skin syndrome and intrauterine epidermal necrosis.[194] Management of TEN at any age is difficult, and the mortality is high, especially in young infants. The cause of the eruption should be identified and, in the case of graft-versus-host disease or sepsis, treated appropriately. Treatment of the skin parallels that of patients with widespread epidermolysis bullosa (see Chapter 11). The prognosis is extremely grave.[190]

Intrauterine Epidermal Necrosis

This rare condition is characterized by widespread epidermal necrosis. It has been described in a few premature infants. Skin changes were present at the time of delivery, and all affected infants have died shortly after birth.[194] Widespread areas of erosion and ulceration were noted, without vesicles or pustules, and mucous membranes were spared. Histopathology of the skin demonstrated extensive epidermal necrosis and pilosebaceous follicular calcification. Autopsy study demonstrated brain infarcts and leukomalacia, as well as cardiomegaly and renal tubular necrosis. The etiology of this condition in these cases is unknown. A fourth case with similar clinical and histopathologic findings was associated with congenital herpes

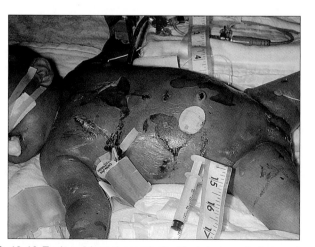

FIG. 10-16 Toxic epidermal necrolysis. Most documented cases in very young infants are due to Gram-negative infections, but this case was as a result of intrauterine graft-versus-host disease. (Courtesy of Mary L. Williams.)

simplex infection.[195] The differential diagnosis includes intrauterine infection, epidermolysis bullosa, acute graft-versus-host disease with TEN, and congenital erosive and vesicular dermatosis.

Congenital Erosive and Vesicular Dermatosis

More than a dozen cases of this condition have been reported.[196–199] Nearly all of the infants were premature. Reports from the neonatal period describe erosions and vesicles at birth, as well as crusting, 'scalded skin-like,' and erythematous areas which eventually healed with reticulate and supple scarring. Additional variably reported features include collodion membrane, transparent areas of skin, and a reticulated vascular pattern with subsequent ulcerations. In some cases the face, palms, and soles are spared. Erosions and ulcerations heal with scarring, usually by 1–2 months of age. The resulting scarring is reticulated and often covers the majority of the skin surface. Ongoing but milder, nonscarring blistering can continue for years.[198,200] Other more variable mucocutaneous findings include scarring alopecia of the scalp and eyelashes, scarring of the tongue, absent or hypoplastic nails, and heat intolerance. Mental retardation, cerebral atrophy, hemiparesis, and retinal scars have also been described.

The cause of the condition is unknown, although some have speculated that an intrauterine infection, as yet unidentified, might result in these findings. The diagnosis has usually been made in retrospect, with biopsy specimens demonstrating scar formation and loss of eccrine structures. There are few cases with histology during the neonatal period. Those reports have demonstrated an eroded epidermis with a dense neutrophilic infiltrate[201] or discrete vesicles in the superficial papillary dermis with mildly increased dermal collagen.[198] The differential diagnosis includes the erosive form of neonatal lupus, acute intrauterine graft-versus-host disease, bullous ichthyosis, intrauterine epidermal necrosis, and a variety of intrauterine infections, especially HSV and varicella. All neonates with the clinical findings of vesicles and atrophy in the newborn period should have thorough investigations, including cultures, biopsies, and serologic evaluations for infection, and should be followed closely, especially for neurologic deficits. There is no specific treatment.

Pyoderma Gangrenosum

Pyoderma gangrenosum (PG), a disorder characterized by the spontaneous onset of skin ulcerations, has rarely been reported in children less than 1 year of age. To date only one case with neonatal onset has been reported. In this infant the ulcers began to develop at 2 days of age. Lesions were most prominent in the groin and buttocks, as has been the case in most other infants[202] (Fig. 10-17). The lesions are sharply demarcated ulcerations, which usually arise without prior vesiculation or pustules, and have characteristically undermined borders. PG has been associated with inflammatory bowel disease, leukemia, arthritis, and less commonly immunodeficiency. The diagnosis, which is one of exclusion, is made by correlating typical clinical features with histopathology demonstrating a neutrophilic infiltrate without evidence of infection, vasculitis, or other causes of ulceration. The differential diagnosis includes noma neonatorum, HSV infection, and ulcerations arising in hemangioma precursors.

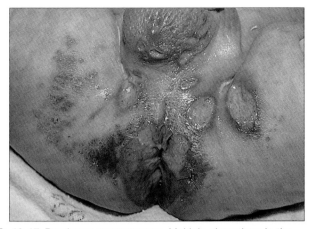

FIG. 10-17 Pyoderma gangrenosum. Multiple ulcerations in the perineum are evident.

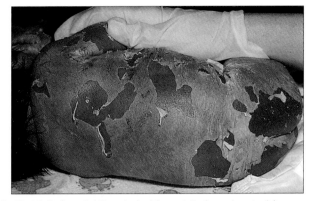

FIG. 10-18 Bullous ichthyosis (epidermolytic hyperkeratosis) presenting with widespread blistering.

The initial treatment of choice is intralesional or systemic corticosteroids, but cytotoxic agents and sulfones are sometimes needed to control disease.

Noma Neonatorum

Noma neonatorum is a gangrenous disease that has been described mainly in developing countries, with *Pseudomonas aeruginosa* septicemia implicated as a causative agent in the majority of cases.[203] The clinical features in these cases include the abrupt onset of gangrenous, ulcerative skin lesions affecting the nose, lips, mouth, anus, scrotum, and eyelids. In severe cases the ulcerations can be mutilating, resulting in bone loss and extensive deformity. Predisposing factors include prematurity, low birthweight, malnutrition, and previous illness. There is some controversy about whether this is an entity distinct from neonatal ecthyma gangrenosum.[31] Although many neonatal cases undoubtedly represent primary *Pseudomonas* infection of the skin, other etiologies may be responsible in some cases. Similar ulcerations have been described in several Native American children with severe combined immunodeficiency.[204] The presence of oral and perineal ulcerations in newborns and young infants should prompt a thorough search for infectious and immunologic causes as possible etiologies.

Acrodermatitis Enteropathica

Acrodermatitis enteropathica (AE) (see Chapter 17) is caused by zinc deficiency and can present in the first few weeks to months of life, but usually not before 4 weeks of age. It can result either from inadequate zinc intake or as an autosomal recessively inherited defect in the transport and absorption of zinc. The most common form in young infants is the nongenetic form, most commonly seen in breastfed premature infants. Zinc stores are lower in preterm infants. Their rapid postnatal growth is occurring at a time when maternal breast milk zinc levels are declining, and this can result in an imbalance between the supply and demand for zinc.[205] Rash, and diarrhea are the most characteristic findings in this form of AE, but alopecia is rarely present early in the course.[206] The rash is usually periorificial and acrally located, although the neck folds and inguinal creases maybe involved. Typically, sharply demarcated, scaly, crusted plaques are located around the eyes, nose, mouth, anus, and genitalia, and these may be erosive in some cases. Acral lesions are often bullous or vesicular. Occasional cutaneous findings include paronychia, nail dystrophy, and edema.[206,207] Irritability and diarrhea are almost always present. The diagnosis is confirmed by low serum zinc levels, although occasional false-positive and -negative results have been reported.[208] The gene for the genetic form of AE, *SLC39A4*, has been localized to 8q and is thought to affect a transmembrane protein involved in zinc transport, hZIP4.[209,210]

Methylmalonic Acidemia and other Metabolic Disorders

The term methylmalonic acidemia (MMA; see Chapter 17) refers to a group of defects in the metabolism of isoleucine and valine. Skin rashes can result from the metabolic perturbations or the dietary restrictions used to manage these inherited disorders of amino acid metabolism. An erosive erythema with periorificial accentuation resembling staphylococcal scalded skin syndrome and a periorificial rash resembling acrodermatitis enteropathica have both been described in MMA.[14,211] Other symptoms in early-onset disease include lethargy, hypotonia, neutropenia, and thrombocytopenia. The diagnosis is made by documenting characteristic abnormal levels of plasma amino acids. Treatment with dietary restrictions may be helpful in some cases, and intramuscular hydroxocobalamin is also helpful in some cases.[14]

Disorders of Cornification: Epidermolytic Hyperkeratosis and Ichthyosis Bullosa of Siemens)

Bullous ichthyosis (epidermolytic hyperkeratosis, EHK; see Chapter 18) is an uncommon form of ichthyosis which is inherited as an autosomal dominant trait. At birth the epidermis is thickened, macerated, and erythematous, and bullae or raw denuded areas are present (Fig. 10-18). In some cases bullae are the prominent or exclusive morphology at birth, leading to diagnostic confusion with epidermolysis bullosa.[212] Spontaneous or mechanically induced bullae continue to form throughout infancy and early childhood, especially on the hands and feet, but generalized blistering usually resolves. Individuals with the condition are otherwise healthy.[213,214]

Ichthyosis bullosa of Siemens can also present in the first months of life and resemble EHK, although blistering is milder and more localized, with sparing of palms and soles.[215]

Restrictive Dermopathy

Restrictive dermopathy (see Chapter 18) is a rare autosomal recessive disease characterized by rigid, tense skin with erosions and ulcerations that may be linear. Infants born with this condition are often premature, have multiple joint contractures, a fixed facial expression, micrognathia, microstomia, and more variably blepharophimosis, absent eyelashes, natal teeth, and cardiac defects. The etiology of the condition is unknown. Most infants die in the newborn period.[216–218]

Vascular tumors and Malformations
(See Chapter 20)

In rare cases, ulcerations develop in infantile hemangiomas just before or at the onset of their rapid proliferative phase. Precursor lesions with macular erythema or a blanched, bruised-like area are usually present as a clue to diagnosis. Such early ulcerations are most common on the pinna, the lip, and in the perineal area, but can occur at other sites (Fig. 10-19).[219] The presence of an ulceration either superimposed on or in direct contiguity with a vascular lesion is a key clue to the diagnosis.[220] Ulcerations are also occasionally present in fully formed congenital hemangiomas, or so-called rapidly involuting congenital hemangiomas (RICH).[221] Ulcerated hemangiomas are treated with wound care, topical antibiotics, topical and intralesional steroids. In severe cases becaplarmin gel or pulsed dye laser have been used effectively.[219,222,223]

Similarly, ulcerations may develop in the vascular malformations of cutis marmorata telangiectatica congenita (CMTC) without preceding blistering or other inciting event. The diagnosis can be suspected if ulcerations occur over patches of mottled and reticulated vascularity. Localized areas of cutaneous atrophy may also be present.[224] One case of life-threatening ulceration in an infant CMTC was reported that presented with bleeding leading to hypovolemic shock at 1 day of age, and later gangrene.[225]

Aplasia Cutis Congenita

Aplasia cutis congenita (ACC; see Chapter 9) is a heterogeneous group of disorders characterized by absent areas of skin at birth. The many causes include an autosomal dominant genetically inherited trait; intrauterine herpes simplex or varicella infection; placental infarctions; absence of skin overlying structural malformations; chromosomal abnormalities; epidermolysis bullosa; and several other genetic conditions. In most cases it is easy to distinguish ACC from blistering conditions causing erosions at birth, because the absence of skin in ACC is usually full-thickness, involving both epidermis and dermis, whereas in most blistering disorders it is less deep.[226,227]

The scalp is the most common location of ACC. Lesions usually present as raw, ulcerated stellate patches, but some have a membranous covering, are fluid-filled, and thus appear blister-like (Fig. 10-20). This latter type, known as membranous ACC, is often associated with an increase in hair at the periphery, the so-called hair collar sign. The location on the scalp, the membranous covering, and the usual concave nature of the underlying defect help distinguish this condition from other forms of blistering. The membranous form of ACC is often a sign of an atretic cephalocele and occasionally has deeper intracranial connections and/or bony defects.[228] Associated vascular stains may be present.[229,230]

Linear Porokeratosis

At least two forms of porokeratosis can present with erosions and/or ulcerations in the newborn period: linear porokeratosis and porokeratotic eccrine ostial and dermal duct nevus (PEODDN). Linear porokeratosis can rarely present with extensive linear erosions at the time of delivery.[231] Establishing the diagnosis in the newborn period may be difficult, as initial biopsies can be nondiagnostic, but after the lesions heal more the diagnosis may become more obvious, both clinically and histologically. Infants with linear porokeratosis have a risk of eventually developing squamous cell carcinoma in affected skin, but this does not usually happen during childhood.[231] Cases of PEODDN with similar findings have also been described (unpublished observations) (Fig. 10-21). The differential diagnosis includes Goltz syndrome and intrauterine varicella infection.

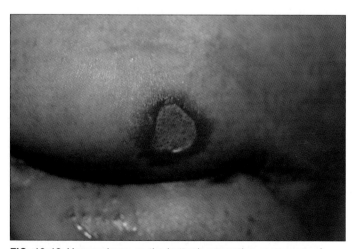

FIG. 10-19 Hemangioma on the buttock presenting as an area of skin ulceration. Note the rim of bright erythema which suggests an evolving hemangioma.

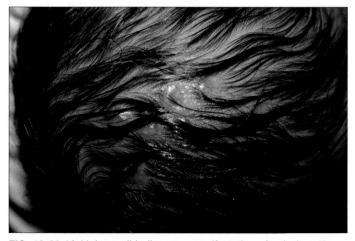

FIG. 10-20 Multiple small bullae as a manifestation of aplasia cutis congenita.

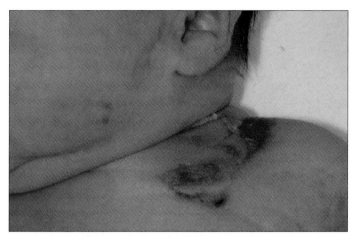

FIG. 10-21 Porokeratotic eccrine and ostial dermal duct nevus presenting with erosions on the neck in a newborn.

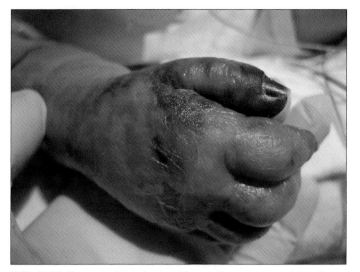

FIG. 10-22 Erosions, blistering, and impending cutaneous infarction as a result of disseminated intravascular coagulation due to congenital hypercoagulability (Courtesy of Sarah Arron.)

Erosions and Ulcerations Overlying Giant Melanocytic Nevi

Several cases of erosions or ulcerations overlying giant melanocytic nevi have been reported.[232–234] The mechanism of these ulcerations is uncertain, but is possibly due to weakening of the dermoepidermal junction as a result of the large number of melanocytes present.[232] Although ulceration overlying nevi can herald malignant melanoma, the finding does not appear to be as ominous in the neonatal period. Such infants should be followed closely, but no cases of malignant melanoma have been diagnosed in these ulcerated areas.[232–234]

Ectodermal Dysplasia Syndromes (See also Chapter 26)

Blistering in the newborn period or early infancy has been reported in several forms of ectodermal dysplasia. In focal dermal hypoplasia (Goltz syndrome) blistering is an occasional feature, but the more striking cutaneous features are widespread hypoplasia and aplasia of the skin in linear and whorled patterns following Blaschko's lines. Hair and nail dystrophy is common, as are skeletal and ophthalmologic abnormalities.[235] The condition is inherited as an X-linked dominant condition and is usually lethal in males.[236]

Basan syndrome (OMIM 129200) is characterized by absent dermal ridge patterns, congenital milia, and blisters of the fingertips and soles. Blistering is present at birth and was said to resemble multiple sucking blisters. Other features of the condition include decreased sweating on the hands and feet, increased heat tolerance, and painful fissures on the fingertips in affected adults.[237]

Ankyloblepharon–ectodermal dysplasia–cleft palate (AEC, Hay Wells syndrome) presents in the newborn period with congenital erythroderma and linear erosions of the skin resembling a collodion membrane.[238] Extensive scalp erosions are reported in 70% of patients and are often present at birth.[239] Over the first months of life a severe erosive dermatitis of the scalp and body develops, associated with bacterial and fungal infections and resulting in scarring alopecia.[238,240] Cribriform atrophy of the scrotum has also been described.[241] In two cases presenting in the newborn period with extensive scalp erosions, two novel mutations were found in the *TP63* gene.[242] Both AEC and ectrodactyly–ectodermal dysplasia–clefting syn-

drome (EEC) have now been linked to mutations in the *P63* gene.[239]

Porphyrias

Photosensitive blistering can occur the newborn period in several porphyrin disorders (see Chapters 8 and 19), including transient porphyrinemia, resulting from hemolytic disease in the newborn period,[243] and erythropoietic porphyria (Gunther's disease), an extremely rare and severe form of porphyria caused by an inborn deficiency of the enzyme uroporphyrinogen cosynthetase. In two cases diagnosed prenatally, blistering developed at 10 and 15 days of age, respectively.[244] In both cases hemolytic anemia leads to hyperbilirubinemia, and the use of phototherapy to control hyperbilirubinemia can result in generalized blistering.

Perinatal Gangrene of the Buttock

Perinatal gangrene of the buttock (see Chapter 8) is a rare condition characterized by the sudden onset of erythema and cyanosis of the buttocks, followed by the progressive development of gangrene and ulcerations. Some cases have been attributed to therapeutic injections via an umbilical artery catheter, but other cases are apparently spontaneous.[245,246] The distribution of the cutaneous infarction suggests occlusion or spasm of the internal iliac artery.[245] The differential diagnosis includes congenital protein C deficiency, and clotting disorders or forms of disseminated intravascular coagulation.

Neonatal Purpura Fulminans

Neonatal purpura fulminans is a rare condition in which severe purpura fulminans occurs within the first days of life. It can present in infants with congenital deficiency of protein S and protein C, or other hypercoagulable states. Bullae, when present, are typically hemorrhagic. They are the result of disseminated intravascular coagulation (DIC leading to edema and bullae due to ischemia and impending skin infarction (Fig. 10-22). Evaluation and management are discussed in Chapter 19.

REFERENCES

1. Nanda S, Reddy BS, Ramji S, Pandhi D. Analytical study of pustular eruptions in neonates. Pediatr Dermatol 2002; 19: 210–215.
2. Frieden IJ. The dermatologist in the newborn nursery: approach to the neonate with blisters, pustules, erosions, and ulcerations. Curr Probl Dermatol 1992: 123–168.
3. Wagner A. Distinguishing vesicular and pustular disorders in the neonate. Curr Opin Pediatr 1997; 9: 396–405.
4. Van Praag MC, Van Rooij RW, Folkers E, et al. Diagnosis and treatment of pustular disorders in the neonate. Pediatr Dermatol 1997; 14: 131–143.
5. Regev-Yochay G, Rubinstein E, Barzilai A, et al. Methicillin-resistant Staphylococcus aureus in neonatal intensive care unit. Emerg Infect Dis 2005; 11: 453–456.
6. Hebert AA, Esterly NB. Bacterial and candidal cutaneous infections in the neonate. Dermatol Clin 1986; 4: 3–21.
7. Speck WT, Driscoll JM, Polin RA, et al. Staphylococcal and streptococcal colonization of the newborn infant: effect of antiseptic cord care. Am J Dis Child 1977; 131: 1005–1008.
8. Sandhu K, Kanwar AJ. Generalized bullous impetigo in a neonate. Pediatr Dermatol 2004; 21: 667–669.
9. Faden H. Neonatal staphylococcal skin infections. Pediatr Infect Dis J 2003; 22: 389.
10. Mockenhaupt M, Idzko M, Grosber M, et al. Epidemiology of staphylococcal scalded skin syndrome in Germany. J Invest Dermatol 2005; 124: 700–703.
11. Loughead JL. Congenital staphylococcal scaled skin syndrome: report of a case. Pediatr Infect Dis J 1992; 11: 413–414.
12. Curran JP, Al-Salihi FL. Neonatal staphylococcal scalded skin syndrome: massive outbreak due to an unusual phage type. Pediatrics 1980; 66: 285–290.
13. Shinefield H. Staphococcal infections. In: Remington JS, Klein JO, eds. Infectious diseases of the fetus and newborn infant. Philadelphia: WB Saunders, 1995; 1105–1141.
14. Howard R, Frieden IJ, Crawford D, et al. Methylmalonic acidemia, cobalamin C type, presenting with cutaneous manifestations. Arch Dermatol 1997; 133: 1563–1566.
15. Rubenstein AD, Musher DM. Epidemic boric acid poisoning simulating staphylococcal toxic epidermal necrolysis of the newborn infant: Ritter's disease. J Pediatr 1970; 77: 884–887.
16. Honig PJ, Frieden IJ, Kim HJ, Yan AC. Streptococcal intertrigo: an underrecognized condition in children. Pediatrics 2003; 112: 1427–1429.
17. Isenberg HD, Tucci V, Lipsitz P, RR FA. Clinical laboratory and epidemiological investigations of a Streptococcus pyogenes cluster epidemic in a newborn nursery. J Clin Microbiol 1984; 19: 366–370.
18. Lehtonen OP, Kero P, Ruuskanen O, et al. A nursery outbreak of group A streptococcal infection. J Infect 1987; 14: 263–270.
19. Nelson J, Dillon HJ, Howard J. A prolonged nursery epidemic associated with a newly recognized type of group A streptococcus. J Pediatr 1976: 792–796.
20. Clegg HW, Dallas SD, Roddey OF, et al. Extrapharyngeal group A Streptococcus infection: diagnostic accuracy and utility of rapid antigen testing. Pediatr Infect Dis J 2003; 22: 726–731.
21. Akiyama H, Yamasaki O, Kanzaki H, et al. Streptococci isolated from various skin lesions: the interaction with Staphylococcus aureus strains. J Dermatol Sci 1999; 19: 17–22.
22. Lopez JB, Gross P, Boggs TR. Skin lesions in association with beta-hemolytic Streptococcus group B. Pediatrics 1976; 58: 859–861.
23. Guha A, Eisenhut M, Shears P, Dalzell M. Impetigo neonatorum associated with late onset group B streptococcal meningitis. J Infect 2003; 47: 185–7.
24. Franciosi RA, Knostman JD, Zimmerman RA. Group B streptococcal neonatal and infant infections. J Pediatr 1973; 82: 707–718.
25. Evans JR, Allen AC, Stinson DA, et al. Perinatal listeriosis: report of an outbreak. Pediatr Infect Dis 1985; 4: 237–241.
26. Bortolussi R, Hawkins A, Evans J, Albretton W. Listeriosis. In: Feign RD, Cherry JD, eds. Textbook of pediatric infectious diseases. Vol. 1. Philadelphia: WB Saunders, 1999; 1330–1336.
27. Khuri-Bulos N, McIntosh K. Neonatal Haemophilus influenzae infection. Report of eight cases and review of the literature. Am J Dis Child 1975; 129: 57–62.
28. Halal F, Delorme L, Brazeau M, Ahronheim G. Congenital vesicular eruption caused by Haemophilus influenzae type b. Pediatrics 1978; 62: 494–496.
29. Foca MD. Pseudomonas aeruginosa infections in the neonatal intensive care unit. Semin Perinatol 2002; 26: 332–339.
30. Boisseau AM, Sarlangue J, Perel Y, et al. Perineal ecthyma gangrenosum in infancy and early childhood: septicemic and nonsepticemic forms. J Am Acad Dermatol 1992; 27: 415–418.
31. Freeman AF, Mancini AJ, Yogev R. Is noma neonatorum a presentation of ecthyma gangrenosum in the newborn? Pediatr Infect Dis J 2002; 21: 83–85.
32. Hughes JR, Newbould M, du Vivier AW, Greenough A. Fatal Pseudomonas septicemia and vasculitis in a premature infant. Pediatr Dermatol 1998; 15: 122–124.
33. Edozien A, Heffelfinger J, Weinstock H, et al. Congenital syphilis – United States, 2002. MMWR Weekly 2004; 53: 716–719.
34. Wilfert C, Gutman L. Syphilis. In: Feign RD, Cherry JD, eds. Textbook of pediatric infectious disease. Vol. 2. Philadelphia: WB Saunders, 1987; 1724–1743.
35. Mallory SB, Krafchik BR. Syphilis. Pediatr Dermatol 1989; 6: 51–52.
36. Kaufman D. Fungal infection in the very low birthweight infant. Curr Opin Infect Dis 2004; 17: 253–259.
37. Roilides E, Farmaki E, Evdoridou J, et al. Neonatal candidiasis: analysis of epidemiology, drug susceptibility, and molecular typing of causative isolates. Eur J Clin Microbiol Infect Dis 2004; 23: 745–750.
38. Kam LA, Giacoia GP. Congenital cutaneous candidiasis. Am J Dis Child 1975; 129: 1215–1218.
39. Darmstadt GL, Dinulos JG, Miller Z. Congenital cutaneous candidiasis: clinical presentation, pathogenesis, and management guidelines. Pediatrics 2000; 105: 438–444.
40. Rudolph N, Tariq AA, Reale MR, et al. Congenital cutaneous candidiasis. Arch Dermatol 1977; 113: 1101–1103.
41. Resnick SD, Greenberg RA. Autoinoculated palmar pustules in neonatal candidiasis. Pediatr Dermatol 1989; 6: 206–209.
42. Brian Smith P, Steinbach WJ, Benjamin DK, Jr. Invasive Candida infections in the neonate. Drug Resist Update 2005; 8: 147–162.
43. Chapman RL. Candida infections in the neonate. Curr Opin Pediatr 2003; 15: 97–102.
44. Baley JE. Neonatal candidiasis: the current challenge. Clin Perinatol 1991; 18: 263–280.
45. Leibovitz E. Neonatal candidosis: clinical picture, management controversies and consensus, and new therapeutic options. J Antimicrob Chemother 2002; 49: 69–73.
46. Dvorak A, Gavaller B. Congenital systemic candidiasis. Report of a case. N Engl J Med 1966: 540–543.
47. Cosgrove BF, Reeves K, Mullins D, et al. Congenital cutaneous candidiasis associated with respiratory distress and elevation of liver function tests: a case report and review of the literature. J Am Acad Dermatol 1997; 37: 817–823.
48. Baley JE, Kliegman RM, Boxerbaum B, Fanaroff AA. Fungal colonization in the very low birth weight infant. Pediatrics 1986; 78: 225–232.
49. Woodruff CA, Hebert AA. Neonatal primary cutaneous aspergillosis: case report and review of the literature. Pediatr Dermatol 2002; 19: 439–444.
50. Groll AH, Jaeger G, Allendorf A, et al. Invasive pulmonary aspergillosis in a

critically ill neonate: case report and review of invasive aspergillosis during the first 3 months of life. Clin Infect Dis 1998; 27: 437–452.

51. Roth JG, Troy JL, Esterly NB. Multiple cutaneous ulcers in a premature neonate. Pediatr Dermatol 1991; 8: 253–255.

52. Salazar GE, Campbell JR. Trichosporonosis, an unusual fungal infection in neonates. Pediatr Infect Dis J 2002; 21: 161–165.

53. Maheshwari A, Stromquist CI, Pereda L, Emmanuel PJ. Mixed infection with unusual fungi and staphylococcal species in two extremely premature neonates. J Perinatol 2004; 24: 324–326.

54. Linder N, Keller N, Huri C, et al. Primary cutaneous mucormycosis in a premature infant: case report and review of the literature. Am J Perinatol 1998; 15: 35–38.

55. Oh D, Notrica D. Primary cutaneous mucormycosis in infants and neonates: case report and review of the literature. J Pediatr Surg 2002; 37: 1607–1611.

56. Harris HH, Foucar E, Andersen RD, Ray TL. Intrauterine herpes simplex infection resembling mechanobullous disease in a newborn infant. J Am Acad Dermatol 1986; 15: 1148–1155.

57. Honig PJ, Brown D. Congenital herpes simplex virus infection initially resembling epidermolysis bullosa. J Pediatr 1982; 101: 958–960.

58. Hutto C, Arvin A, Jacobs R, et al. Intrauterine herpes simplex virus infections. J Pediatr 1987; 110: 97–101.

59. Whitley R, Arvin A, Prober C, et al. Predictors of morbidity and mortality in neonates with herpes simplex virus infections. The National Institute of Allergy and Infectious Diseases Collaborative Antiviral Study Group. N Engl J Med 1991; 324: 450–454.

60. Jacobs RF. Neonatal herpes simplex virus infections. Semin Perinatol 1998; 22: 64–71.

61. Elder DE, Minutillo C, Pemberton PJ. Neonatal herpes simplex infection: keys to early diagnosis. J Paediatr Child Health 1995; 31: 307–311.

62. Kohl S. Neonatal herpes simplex virus infection. Clin Perinatol 1997; 24: 129–150.

63. Riley LE. Herpes simplex virus. Semin Perinatol 1998; 22: 284–292.

64. Cohen PR. Tests for detecting herpes simplex virus and varicella-zoster virus infections. Dermatol Clin 1994; 12: 51–68.

65. Detlefs RL, Frieden IJ, Berger TG, Westrom D. Eosinophil fluorescence: a cause of false positive slide tests for herpes simplex virus. Pediatr Dermatol 1987; 4: 129–133.

66. Paryani SG, Arvin AM. Intrauterine infection with varicella-zoster virus after maternal varicella. N Engl J Med 1986; 314: 1542–1546.

67. Alkalay AL, Pomerance JJ, Rimoin DL. Fetal varicella syndrome. J Pediatr 1987; 111: 320–323.

68. Bai PV, John TJ. Congenital skin ulcers following varicella in late pregnancy. J Pediatr 1979; 94: 65–67.

69. Brunell PA, Kotchmar GS, Jr. Zoster in infancy: failure to maintain virus latency following intrauterine infection. J Pediatr 1981; 98: 71–73.

70. Querol I, Bueno M, Cebrian A, Gonzalez-Echeverria FJ. Congenital herpes zoster. Cutis 1996; 58: 231–234.

71. Mogami S, Muto M, Mogami K, Asagami C. Congenitally acquired herpes zoster infection in a newborn. Dermatology 1997; 194: 276–277.

72. Nathwani D, Maclean A, Conway S, Carrington D. Varicella infections in pregnancy and the newborn. A review prepared for the UK Advisory Group on Chickenpox on behalf of the British Society for the Study of Infection. J Infect 1998; 36: 59–71.

73. Miller E, Cradock-Watson JE, Ridehalgh MK. Outcome in newborn babies given anti-varicella-zoster immunoglobulin after perinatal maternal infection with varicella-zoster virus. Lancet 1989; 2: 371–373.

74. Blatt J, Kastner O, Hodes DS. Cutaneous vesicles in congenital cytomegalovirus infection. J Pediatr 1978; 92: 509.

75. Hancox JG, Shetty AK, Sangueza OP, Yosipovitch G. Perineal ulcers in an infant: an unusual presentation of postnatal cytomegalovirus infection. J Am Acad Dermatol 2006; 54: 536–539.

76. Cherry J. Enteroviruses. In: Remington JS, Klein JO, eds. Infectious diseases of the fetus and newborn infant. Philadelphia: WB Saunders, 1995; 404–446.

77. Arnon R, Naor N, Davidson S, et al. Fatal outcome of neonatal echovirus 19 infection. Pediatr Infect Dis J 1991; 10: 788–789.

78. Burns B, Lampe R, Hansen G. Neonatal scabies. Am J Dis Child 1979: 1031–1034.

79. Hurwitz S. Scabies in babies. Am J Dis Child 1973; 126: 226–228.

80. Sterling GB, Janniger CK, Kihiczak G, et al. Scabies. Am Fam Phys 1992; 46: 1237–1241.

81. Madsen A. Mite burrows in crusts from young infants. Acta Dermatol Venereol 1970; 50: 391–392.

82. Berg FJ, Solomon LM. Erythema neonatorum toxicum. Arch Dis Child 1987; 62: 327–328.

83. Carr JA, Hodgman JE, Freedman RI, Levan NE. Relationship between toxic erythema and infant maturity. Am J Dis Child 1966; 112: 129–134.

84. Marino LJ. Toxic erythema present at birth. Arch Dermatol 1965; 92: 402–403.

85. Levy HL, Cothran F. Erythema toxicum neonatorum present at birth. Am J Dis Child 1962; 103: 617–619.

86. Chang MW, Jiang SB, Orlow SJ. Atypical erythema toxicum neonatorum of delayed onset in a term infant. Pediatr Dermatol 1999; 16: 137–141.

87. Harris JR, Schick B. Erythema neonatorum. AMA J Dis Child 1956; 92: 27–33.

88. Luders D. Histologic observations in erythema toxicum neonatorum. Pediatrics 1960; 26: 219–224.

89. Ferrandiz C, Coroleu W, Ribera M, et al. Sterile transient neonatal pustulosis is a precocious form of erythema toxicum neonatorum. Dermatology 1992; 185: 18–22.

90. Ramamurthy RS, Reveri M, Esterly NB, et al. Transient neonatal pustular melanosis. J Pediatr 1976; 88: 831–835.

91. Coroleu Lletget W, Natal Pujol A, Ferrandiz Foraster C, Prats Vinas J. [Transient neonatal pustular melanosis]. An Esp Pediatr 1990; 33: 117–119.

92. Hidano A, Purwoko R, Jitsukawa K. Statistical survey of skin changes in Japanese neonates. Pediatr Dermatol 1986; 3: 140–144.

93. Nanda A, Kaur S, Bhakoo ON, Dhall K. Survey of cutaneous lesions in Indian newborns. Pediatr Dermatol 1989; 6: 39–42.

94. Esterly NB. Vesicopustular eruptions in the neonate. Australas J Dermatol 1991; 32: 1–12.

95. Cohen L, Skopicki B, Harrist T, et al. Noninfectious vesiculobullous and vesiculopustular diseases. In: Elder D, Elenitsas R, Jaworsky C, Johnson B, eds. Lever's histopathology of the skin. Philadelphia: Lippincott Raven, 1997; 209–252.

96. Straka BF, Cooper PH, Greer KE. Congenital miliaria crystallina. Cutis 1991; 47: 103–106.

97. Mowad CM, McGinley KJ, Foglia A, Leyden JJ. The role of extracellular polysaccharide substance produced by Staphylococcus epidermidis in miliaria. J Am Acad Dermatol 1995; 33: 729–733.

98. Murphy WF, Langley AL. Common bullous lesions – presumably self-inflicted – occurring in utero in the newborn infant. Pediatrics 1963; 32: 1099–1101.

99. Libow LF, Reinmann JG. Symmetrical erosions in a neonate: a case of neonatal sucking blisters. Cutis 1998; 62: 16–17.

100. Mengesha YM, Hansen RC. Toddler-age nodulocystic acne. J Pediatr 1999; 134: 644–648.

101. Rapelanoro R, Mortureux P, Couprie B, et al. Neonatal Malassezia furfur pustulosis. Arch Dermatol 1996; 132: 190–193.

102. Niamba P, Weill FX, Sarlangue J, et al. Is common neonatal cephalic pustulosis (neonatal acne) triggered by Malassezia sympodialis? Arch Dermatol 1998; 134: 995–998.

103. Lane AT, Rehder PA, Helm K. Evaluations of diapers containing absorbent gelling material with conventional disposable diapers in newborn infants. Am J Dis Child 1990; 144: 315–318.

104. Metzker A, Brenner S, Merlob P. Iatrogenic cutaneous injuries in the neonate. Arch Dermatol 1999; 135: 697–703.

105. Ashkenazi S, Metzker A, Merlob P, et al. Scalp changes after fetal monitoring. Arch Dis Child 1985; 60: 267–269.

106. Cartlidge PH, Fox PE, Rutter N. The scars of newborn intensive care. Early Hum Dev 1990; 21: 1–10.

107. Mirowski GW, Frieden IJ, Miller C. Iatrogenic scald burn: a consequence of institutional infection control measures. Pediatrics 1996; 98: 963–965.

108. Kahn G, Rywlin AM. Acropustulosis of infancy. Arch Dermatol 1979; 115: 831–833.

109. Jarratt M, Ramsdell W. Infantile acropustulosis. Arch Dermatol 1979; 115: 834–836.

110. Jennings JL, Burrows WM. Infantile acropustulosis. J Am Acad Dermatol 1983; 9: 733–738.

111. Lowy G, Serapiao CJ, Oliveira MM. [Childhood acropustulosis. A study of 10 cases]. Med Cutan Ibero Lat Am 1986; 14: 171–176.

112. Lucky AW, McGuire JS. Infantile acropustulosis with eosinophilic pustules. J Pediatr 1982; 100: 428–429.

113. Vignon-Pennamen MD, Wallach D. Infantile acropustulosis. A clinicopathologic study of six cases. Arch Dermatol 1986; 122: 1155–1160.

114. Falanga V. Infantile acropustulosis with eosinophilia. J Am Acad Dermatol 1985; 13: 826–828.

115. Mancini AJ, Frieden IJ, Paller AS. Infantile acropustulosis revisited: history of scabies and response to topical corticosteroids. Pediatr Dermatol 1998; 15: 337–341.

116. Vicente J, Espana A, Idoate M, et al. Are eosinophilic pustular folliculitis of infancy and infantile acropustulosis the same entity? Br J Dermatol 1996; 135: 807–809.

117. Lucky AW, Esterly NB, Heskel N, et al. Eosinophilic pustular folliculitis in infancy. Pediatr Dermatol 1984; 1: 202–206.

118. Giard F, Marcoux D, McCuaig C, et al. Eosinophilic pustular folliculitis (Ofuji disease) in childhood: a review of four cases. Pediatr Dermatol 1991; 8: 189–193.

119. Larralde M, Morales S, Santos Munoz A, et al. Eosinophilic pustular folliculitis in infancy: report of two new cases. Pediatr Dermatol 1999; 16: 118–120.

120. Buckley DA, Munn SE, Higgins EM. Neonatal eosinophilic pustular folliculitis. Clin Exp Dermatol 2001; 26: 251–255.

121. Ziemer M, Boer A. Eosinophilic pustular folliculitis in infancy: not a distinctive inflammatory disease of the skin. Am J Dermatopathol 2005; 27: 443–455.

122. Siegel D, Holland K, Phillips R, et al. Erosive pustular dermatosis of the scalp after perinatal scalp injury. Pediatr Dermatol (in press).

123. Hertz CG, Hambrick GW, Jr. Congenital Letterer–Siwe disease. A case treated with vincristine and corticosteroids. Am J Dis Child 1968; 116: 553–556.

124. Valderrama E, Kahn LB, Festa R, Lanzkowsky P. Benign isolated histiocytosis mimicking chicken pox in a neonate: report of two cases with ultrastructural study. Pediatr Pathol 1985; 3: 103–113.

125. Herman LE, Rothman KF, Harawi S, Gonzalez-Serva A. Congenital self-healing reticulohistiocytosis. A new entity in the differential diagnosis of neonatal papulovesicular eruptions. Arch Dermatol 1990; 126: 210–212.

126. Oranje AP, Vuzevski VD, de Groot R, Prins ME. Congenital self-healing non-Langerhans' cell histiocytosis. Eur J Pediatr 1988; 148: 29–31.

127. Morgan KW, Callen JP. Self-healing congenital Langerhans' cell histiocytosis presenting as neonatal papulovesicular eruption. J Cutan Med Surg 2001; 5: 486–489.

128. Huang CY, Chao SC, Ho SF, Lee JY. Congenital self-healing reticulohistiocytosis mimicking diffuse neonatal hemangiomatosis. Dermatology 2004; 208: 138–141.

129. Kim KJ, Jee MS, Choi JH, et al. Congenital self-healing reticulohistiocytosis presenting as vesicular eruption. J Dermatol 2002; 29: 48–49.

130. Inuzuka M, Tomita K, Tokura Y, Takigawa M. Congenital self-healing reticulohistiocytosis presenting with hemorrhagic bullae. J Am Acad Dermatol 2003; 48: S75–77.

131. Thong HY, Dai YS, Chiu HC. An unusual presentation of congenital self-healing reticulohistiocytosis. Br J Dermatol 2003; 149: 191–192.

132. Brazzola P, Schiller P, Kuhne T. Congenital self-healing Langerhans' cell histiocytosis with atrophic recovery of the skin: clinical correlation of an immunologic phenomenon. J Pediatr Hematol Oncol 2003; 25: 270–273.

133. Colon-Fontanez F, Eichenfield LE, Krous HF, Friedlander SF. Congenital Langerhans' cell histiocytosis: the utility of the Tzanck test as a diagnostic screening tool. Arch Dermatol 1998; 134: 1039–1040.

134. Rowden G, Connelly EM, Winkelmann RK. Cutaneous histiocytosis X. The presence of S-100 protein and its use in diagnosis. Arch Dermatol 1983; 119: 553–559.

135. Zaenglein AL, Steele MA, Kamino H, Chang MW. Congenital self-healing reticulohistiocytosis with eye involvement. Pediatr Dermatol 2001; 18: 135–137.

136. Chunharas A, Pabunruang W, Hongeng S. Congenital self-healing Langerhans' cell histiocytosis with pulmonary involvement: spontaneous regression. J Med Assoc Thai 2002; 85 Suppl 4: S1309–1313.

137. Longaker MA, Frieden IJ, LeBoit PE, Sherertz EF. Congenital 'self-healing' Langerhans' cell histiocytosis: the need for long-term follow-up. J Am Acad Dermatol 1994; 31: 910–916.

138. Larralde M, Rositto A, Giardelli M, et al. Congenital self-healing Langerhans' cell histiocytosis: the need for a long term follow up. Int J Dermatol 2003; 42: 245–246.

139. Bruckner AL. Incontinentia pigmenti: a window to the role of NF-kappaB function. Semin Cutan Med Surg 2004; 23: 116–124.

140. Berlin AL, Paller AS, Chan LS. Incontinentia pigmenti: a review and update on the molecular basis of pathophysiology. J Am Acad Dermatol 2002; 47: 169–187; quiz 188–190.

141. Cohen BA. Incontinentia pigmenti. Neurol Clin 1987; 5: 361–377.

142. Francis JS, Sybert VP. Incontinentia pigmenti. Semin Cutan Med Surg 1997; 16: 54–60.

143. Faloyin M, Levitt J, Bercowitz E, et al. All that is vesicular is not herpes: incontinentia pigmenti masquerading as herpes simplex virus in a newborn. Pediatrics 2004; 114: e270–272.

144. Fromer ES, Lynch PJ. Neonatal herpes simplex and incontinentia pigmenti. Pediatr Dermatol 2001; 18: 86–87.

145. Stitt WZ, Scott GA, Caserta M, Goldsmith LA. Coexistence of incontinentia pigmenti and neonatal herpes simplex virus infection. Pediatr Dermatol 1998; 15: 112–115.

146. Chamlin SL, Cowper SE, Longley BJ, Williams ML. Generalized bullae in an infant. Arch Dermatol 2002; 138: 831–836.

147. Eberting CL, Davis J, Puck JM, et al. Dermatitis and the newborn rash of hyper-IgE syndrome. Arch Dermatol 2004; 140: 1119–1125.

148. Kamei R, Honig PJ. Neonatal Job's syndrome featuring a vesicular eruption. Pediatr Dermatol 1988; 5: 75–82.

149. Burch JM, Weston WL, Rogers M, Morelli JG. Cutaneous pustular leukemoid reactions in trisomy 21. Pediatr Dermatol 2003; 20: 232–237.

150. Nijhawan A, Baselga E, Gonzalez-Ensenat MA, et al. Vesiculopustular eruptions in Down syndrome neonates with myeloproliferative disorders. Arch Dermatol 2001; 137: 760–763.

151. Lerner LH, Wiss K, Gellis S, Barnhill R. An unusual pustular eruption in an infant with Down syndrome and a congenital leukemoid reaction. J Am Acad Dermatol 1996; 35: 330–333.

152. Solky BA, Yang FC, Xu X, Levins P. Transient myeloproliferative disorder

causing a vesiculopustular eruption in a phenotypically normal neonate. Pediatr Dermatol 2004; 21: 551–554.

153. Chang SE, Choi JH, Koh JK. Congenital erythrodermic psoriasis. Br J Dermatol 1999; 140: 538–539.

154. Liao PB, Rubinson R, Howard R, et al. Annular pustular psoriasis – most common form of pustular psoriasis in children: report of three cases and review of the literature. Pediatr Dermatol 2002; 19: 19–25.

155. Kone-Paut I, Gorchakoff-Molinas A, Weschler B, Touitou I. Paediatric Behçet's disease in France. Ann Rheum Dis 2002; 61: 655–656.

156. Lewis MA, Priestley BL. Transient neonatal Behçet's disease. Arch Dis Child 1986; 61: 805–806.

157. Stark AC, Bhakta B, Chamberlain MA, Dear P, Taylor PV. Life-threatening transient neonatal Behçet's disease. Br J Rheumatol 1997; 36: 700–702.

158. Jog S, Patole S, Koh G, Whitehall J. Unusual presentation of neonatal Behçets disease. Am J Perinatol 2001; 18: 287–292.

159. Golkar L, Bernhard JD. Mastocytosis. Lancet 1997; 349: 1379–1385.

160. Heide R, Tank B, Oranje AP. Mastocytosis in childhood. Pediatr Dermatol 2002; 19: 375–381.

161. Harrison PV, Cook LJ, Lake HJ, Shuster S. Diffuse cutaneous mastocytosis: a report of neonatal onset. Acta Dermatol Venereol 1979; 59: 541–543.

162. Golitz LE, Weston WL, Lane AT. Bullous mastocytosis: diffuse cutaneous mastocytosis with extensive blisters mimicking scalded skin syndrome or erythema multiforme. Pediatr Dermatol 1984; 1: 288–294.

163. Shah PY, Sharma V, Worobec AS, et al. Congenital bullous mastocytosis with myeloproliferative disorder and c-kit mutation. J Am Acad Dermatol 1998; 39: 119–121.

164. Oranje AP, Soekanto W, Sukardi A, et al. Diffuse cutaneous mastocytosis mimicking staphylococcal scalded-skin syndrome: report of three cases. Pediatr Dermatol 1991; 8: 147–151.

165. Walker T, von Komorowski G, Scheurlen W, et al. Neonatal mastocytosis with pachydermic bullous skin without c-Kit 816 mutation. Dermatology 2006; 212: 70–72.

166. Has C, Misery L, David L, Cambazard F. Recurring staphylococcal scalded skin syndrome-like bullous mastocytosis: the utility of cytodiagnosis and the rapid regression with steroids. Pediatr Dermatol 2002; 19: 220–223.

167. Oku T, Hashizume H, Yokote R, et al. The familial occurrence of bullous mastocytosis (diffuse cutaneous mastocytosis). Arch Dermatol 1990; 126: 1478–1484.

168. Verma KK, Bhat R, Singh MK. Bullous mastocytosis treated with oral betamethasone therapy. Indian J Pediatr 2004; 71: 261–263.

169. Walker DC, Kolar KA, Hebert AA, Jordon RE. Neonatal pemphigus foliaceus. Arch Dermatol 1995; 131: 1308–1311.

170. Bonifazi E, Meneghini CL. Herpes gestationis with transient bullous lesions in the newborn. Pediatr Dermatol 1984; 1: 215–218.

171. Storer JS, Galen WK, Nesbitt LT Jr, DeLeo VA. Neonatal pemphigus vulgaris. J Am Acad Dermatol 1982; 6: 929–932.

172. Merlob P, Metzker A, Hazaz B, et al. Neonatal pemphigus vulgaris. Pediatrics 1986; 78: 1102–1105.

173. Krusinski PA, Saurat JH. Transplacentally transferred dermatoses. Pediatr Dermatol 1989; 6: 166–177.

174. Chen SH, Chopra K, Evans TY, et al. Herpes gestationis in a mother and child. J Am Acad Dermatol 1999; 40: 847–849.

175. Campo-Voegeli A, Muniz F, Mascaro JM, et al. Neonatal pemphigus vulgaris with extensive mucocutaneous lesions from a mother with oral pemphigus vulgaris. Br J Dermatol 2002; 147: 801–805.

176. Avalos-Diaz E, Olague-Marchan M, Lopez-Swiderski A, et al. Transplacental passage of maternal pemphigus foliaceus autoantibodies induces neonatal pemphigus. J Am Acad Dermatol 2000; 43: 1130–1134.

177. Hirsch R, Anderson J, Weinberg JM, et al. Neonatal pemphigus foliaceus. J Am Acad Dermatol 2003; 49: S187–189.

178. Tope WD, Kamino H, Briggaman RA, et al. Neonatal pemphigus vulgaris in a child born to a woman in remission. J Am Acad Dermatol 1993; 29: 480–485.

179. Chowdhury MM, Natarajan S. Neonatal pemphigus vulgaris associated with mild oral pemphigus vulgaris in the mother during pregnancy. Br J Dermatol 1998; 139: 500–503.

180. Esterly NB, Furey NL, Kirschner BS, et al. Chronic bullous dermatosis of childhood. Arch Dermatol 1977; 113: 42–46.

181. Hruza LL, Mallory SB, Fitzgibbons J, Mallory GB, Jr. Linear IgA bullous dermatosis in a neonate. Pediatr Dermatol 1993; 10: 171–176.

182. Chorzelski TP, Jablonska S. IgA linear dermatosis of childhood (chronic bullous disease of childhood). Br J Dermatol 1979; 101: 535–542.

183. Amos B, Deng JS, Flynn K, Suarez S. Bullous pemphigoid in infancy: case report and literature review. Pediatr Dermatol 1998; 15: 108–111.

184. Voltan E, Maeda JY, Muniz Silva MA, et al. Childhood bullous pemphigoid: report of three cases. J Dermatol 2005; 32: 387–392.

185. Fisler RE, Saeb M, Liang MG, et al. Childhood bullous pemphigoid: a clinicopathologic study and review of the literature. Am J Dermatopathol 2003; 25: 183–189.

186. Scheker LE, Kasteler JS, Callen JP. Neonatal lupus erythematosus mimicking Langerhans' cell histiocytosis. Pediatr Dermatol 2003; 20: 164–166.

187. Crowley E, Frieden IJ. Neonatal lupus erythematosus: an unusual congenital presentation with cutaneous atrophy, erosions, alopecia, and pancytopenia. Pediatr Dermatol 1998; 15: 38–42.

188. Kaneko F, Tanji O, Hasegawa T, et al. Neonatal lupus erythematosus in Japan. J Am Acad Dermatol 1992; 26: 397–403.

189. Johnston GA, Ghura HS, Carter E, Graham-Brown RA. Neonatal erythema multiforme major. Clin Exp Dermatol 2002; 27: 661–664.

190. Scully MC, Frieden IJ. Toxic epidermal necrolysis in early infancy. J Am Acad Dermatol 1992; 27: 340–344.

191. Oranje AP, de Groot R. Letter to the Editor. Pediatr Dermatol 1985: 83.

192. Alain G, Carrier C, Beaumier L, et al. In utero acute graft-versus-host disease in a neonate with severe combined immunodeficiency. J Am Acad Dermatol 1993; 29: 862–865.

193. Honig PJ, Gaisin A, Buck BE. Frozen section differentiation of drug-induced and staphylococcal-induced toxic epidermal necrolysis. J Pediatr 1978; 92: 504–505.

194. Ruiz-Maldonado R, Duran-McKinster C, Carrasco-Daza D, et al. Intrauterine epidermal necrosis: report of three cases. J Am Acad Dermatol 1998; 38: 712–715.

195. Allee JE, Saria EA, Rosenblum D, et al. Intrauterine epidermal necrosis. J Cutan Pathol 2001; 28: 383–386.

196. Cohen BA, Esterly NB, Nelson PF. Congenital erosive and vesicular dermatosis healing with reticulated supple scarring. Arch Dermatol 1985; 121: 361–367.

197. Sidhu-Malik NK, Resnick SD, Wilson BB. Congenital erosive and vesicular dermatosis healing with reticulated supple scarring: report of three new cases and review of the literature. Pediatr Dermatol 1998; 15: 214–218.

198. Metz BJ, Hicks J, Levy M. Congenital erosive and vesicular dermatosis healing with reticulated supple scarring. Pediatr Dermatol 2005; 22: 55–59.

199. Vun YY, Malik MM, Murphy GM, O'Donnell B. Congenital erosive and vesicular dermatosis. Clin Exp Dermatol 2005; 30: 146–148.

200. Stein S, Stone S, Paller AS. Ongoing blistering in a boy with congenital erosive and vesicular dermatosis healing with reticulated supple scarring. J Am Acad Dermatol 2001; 45: 946–948.

201. Sadick NS, Shea CR, Schlessel JS. Congenital erosive and vesicular dermatosis with reticulated, supple scarring: a neutrophilic dermatosis.

J Am Acad Dermatol 1995; 32: 873–877.

202. Graham JA, Hansen KK, Rabinowitz LG, Esterly NB. Pyoderma gangrenosum in infants and children. Pediatr Dermatol 1994; 11: 10–17.

203. Ghosal SP, Sen Gupta PC, Mukherjee AK, et al. Noma neonatorum: Its aetiopathogenesis. Lancet 1978; 2: 289–291.

204. Rotbart HA, Levin MJ, Jones JF, et al. Noma in children with severe combined immunodeficiency. J Pediatr 1986; 109: 596–600.

205. Chew AL, Chan I, McGrath JA, Atherton DJ. Infantile acquired zinc deficiency resembling acrodermatitis enteropathica. Clin Exp Dermatol 2005; 30: 594–595.

206. Perafan-Riveros C, Franca LF, Alves AC, Sanches JA, Jr. Acrodermatitis enteropathica: case report and review of the literature. Pediatr Dermatol 2002; 19: 426–431.

207. Kumar SP, Anday EK. Edema, hypoproteinemia, and zinc deficiency in low-birth-weight infants. Pediatrics 1984; 73: 327–329.

208. Van Wouwe JP. Clinical and laboratory diagnosis of acrodermatitis enteropathica. Eur J Pediatr 1989; 149: 2–8.

209. Wang F, Kim BE, Dufner-Beattie J, et al. Acrodermatitis enteropathica mutations affect transport activity, localization and zinc-responsive trafficking of the mouse ZIP4 zinc transporter. Hum Mol Genet 2004; 13: 563–571.

210. Nakano A, Nakano H, Nomura K, et al. Novel SLC39A4 mutations in acrodermatitis enteropathica. J Invest Dermatol 2003; 120: 963–966.

211. Bodemer C, De Prost Y, Bachollet B, et al. Cutaneous manifestations of methylmalonic and propionic acidaemia: a description based on 38 cases. Br J Dermatol 1994; 131: 93–98.

212. Klein I, Bergman R, Indelman M, Sprecher E. A newborn presenting with congenital blistering. Int J Dermatol 2004; 43: 295–297.

213. Ammirati CT, Mallory SB. The major inherited disorders of cornification. New advances in pathogenesis. Dermatol Clin 1998; 16: 497–508.

214. Traupe H, Kolde G, Hamm H, Happle R. Ichthyosis bullosa of Siemens: a unique type of epidermolytic hyperkeratosis. J Am Acad Dermatol 1986; 14: 1000–1005.

215. Akiyama M, Tsuji-Abe Y, Yanagihara M, et al. Ichthyosis bullosa of Siemens: its correct diagnosis facilitated by molecular genetic testing. Br J Dermatol 2005; 152: 1353–1356.

216. Nijsten TE, De Moor A, Colpaert CG, et al. Restrictive dermopathy: a case report and a critical review of all hypotheses of its origin. Pediatr Dermatol 2002; 19: 67–72.

217. Smitt JH, van Asperen CJ, Niessen CM, et al. Restrictive dermopathy. Report of 12 cases. Dutch Task Force on Genodermatology. Arch Dermatol 1998; 134: 577–579.

218. Wesche WA, Cutlan RT, Khare V, et al. Restrictive dermopathy: report of a case and review of the literature. J Cutan Pathol 2001; 28: 211–218.

219. Kim HJ, Colombo M, Frieden IJ. Ulcerated hemangiomas: clinical characteristics and response to therapy. J Am Acad Dermatol 2001; 44: 962–972.

220. Liang MG, Frieden IJ. Perineal and lip ulcerations as the presenting manifestation of hemangioma of infancy. Pediatrics 1997; 99: 256–259.

221. Boon LM, Enjolras O, Mulliken JB. Congenital hemangioma: evidence of accelerated involution. J Pediatr 1996; 128: 329–335.

222. Metz BJ, Rubenstein MC, Levy ML, Metry DW. Response of ulcerated perineal hemangiomas of infancy to becaplermin gel, a recombinant human platelet-derived growth factor. Arch Dermatol 2004; 140: 867–870.

223. Sugarman JL, Mauro TM, Frieden IJ. Treatment of an ulcerated hemangioma with recombinant platelet-derived growth factor. Arch Dermatol 2002; 138: 314–316.

224. Mulliken J. Capillary (port-wine) and other telangiectatic stains. In: Mulliken JB, Young AE, eds. Vascular birthmarks. Philadelphia: WB Saunders, 1988; 170–195.

225. Hu IJ, Chen MT, Tai HC, et al. Cutis marmorata telangiectatica congenita with gangrenous ulceration and hypovolaemic shock. Eur J Pediatr 2005; 164: 411–413.

226. Frieden IJ. Aplasia cutis congenita: a clinical review and proposal for classification. J Am Acad Dermatol 1986; 14: 646–660.

227. Baselga E, Torrelo A, Drolet BA, et al. Familial nonmembranous aplasia cutis of the scalp. Pediatr Dermatol 2005; 22: 213–217.

228. Drolet B, Prendiville J, Golden J, et al. 'Membranous aplasia cutis' with hair collars. Congenital absence of skin or neuroectodermal defect? Arch Dermatol 1995; 131: 1427–1431.

229. Fujita Y, Yokota K, Akiyama M, et al. Two cases of atypical membranous aplasia cutis with hair collar sign: one with dermal melanocytosis, and the other with naevus flammeus. Clin Exp Dermatol 2005; 30: 497–499.

230. Herron MD, Coffin CM, Vanderhooft SL. Vascular stains and hair collar sign associated with congenital anomalies of the scalp. Pediatr Dermatol 2005; 22: 200–205.

231. Fisher CA, LeBoit PE, Frieden IJ. Linear porokeratosis presenting as erosions in the newborn period. Pediatr Dermatol 1995; 12: 318–322.

232. Giam YC, Williams ML, Leboit PE, et al. Neonatal erosions and ulcerations

in giant congenital melanocytic nevi. Pediatr Dermatol 1999; 16: 354–358.

233. Borbujo J, Jara M, Cortes L, Sanchez de Leon L. A newborn with nodular ulcerated lesion on a giant congenital nevus. Pediatr Dermatol 2000; 17: 299–301.

234. Gonzalez J, Palangio M, Fialkoff CN, et al. Giant congenital melanocytic nevus with a large ulceration at birth: a 5-year follow-up. J Am Acad Dermatol 2003; 49: 752–754.

235. Goltz RW, Henderson RR, Hitch JM, Ott JE. Focal dermal hypoplasia syndrome. A review of the literature and report of two cases. Arch Dermatol 1970; 101: 1–11.

236. Mianda SB, Delmaestro D, Bertoli R, et al. Focal dermal hypoplasia with exuberant fat herniations and skeletal deformities. Pediatr Dermatol 2005; 22: 420–423.

237. Reed T, Schreiner RL. Absence of dermal ridge patterns: genetic heterogeneity. Am J Med Genet 1983; 16: 81–88.

238. Vanderhooft SL, Stephan MJ, Sybert VP. Severe skin erosions and scalp infections in AEC syndrome. Pediatr Dermatol 1993; 10: 334–340.

239. Siegfried E, Bree A, Fete M, Sybert VP. Skin erosions and wound healing in ankyloblepharon–ectodermal defect–cleft lip and/or palate. Arch Dermatol 2005; 141: 1591–1594.

240. Steele JA, Hansen H, Arn P, Kwong PC. Spectrum of phenotypic manifestations from a single point mutation of the p63 gene, including new cutaneous and immunologic findings. Pediatr Dermatol 2005; 22: 415–419.

241. Hill VA, Nischal KK, Collin JR, Harper JI. An unusual ectodermal dysplasia with unique eye defects. Br J Dermatol 2005; 152: 365–367.

242. Payne AS, Yan AC, Ilyas E, et al. Two novel TP63 mutations associated with the ankyloblepharon, ectodermal defects, and cleft lip and palate syndrome: a skin fragility phenotype. Arch Dermatol 2005; 141: 1567–1573.

243. Mallon E, Wojnarowska F, Hope P, Elder G. Neonatal bullous eruption as a result of transient porphyrinemia in a premature infant with hemolytic disease of the newborn. J Am Acad Dermatol 1995; 33: 333–336.

244. Lazebnik N, Lazebnik RS. The prenatal presentation of congenital erythropoietic porphyria: report of two siblings with elevated maternal serum alpha-fetoprotein. Prenat Diagn 2004; 24: 282–286.

245. Bonifazi E, Meneghini C. Perinatal gangrene of the buttock: an iatrogenic or spontaneous condition? J Am Acad Dermatol 1980; 3: 596–598.

246. Serrano G, Aliaga A, Febrer I, et al. Perinatal gangrene of the buttock: a spontaneous condition. Arch Dermatol 1985; 121: 23–24.

Epidermolysis Bullosa

Anna L. Bruckner

Epidermolysis bullosa (EB) is a family of rare, inherited disorders characterized by fragility of the skin and sometimes the mucosa in response to minor mechanical trauma. Frictional forces on epithelia lead to blisters and erosions, and so EB is often referred to as a mechanobullous disease. EB is caused by mutations in various genes that encode proteins that form the basement membrane zone (BMZ) of the skin (Fig. 11-1). BMZ proteins are structural molecules that function to allow adhesion of the epidermis and dermis. When one of these proteins is absent or abnormal, adhesion strength is diminished and blistering occurs as a response to frictional stress. Data from the recent National Epidermolysis Bullosa Registry (NEBR) estimates the incidence of all forms of EB in the United States as 20 cases per million live births.[1]

EB is classified into three major types based on the ultrastructural level of blistering: in EB simplex (EBS) cleavage occurs in the basal epidermal cells above the BMZ; in junctional EB (JEB) it occurs through the BMZ; and in dystrophic EB (DEB) cleavage arises in the superficial dermis.[2] Each type is further divided into subtypes based on inheritance pattern, clinical findings, and the implicated molecular and genetic defects.[3] The current classification of EB types, subtypes, and their molecular defects is listed in Table 11-1. Some experts advocate a fourth type, hemidesmosomal EB, referring to those forms of EBS and JEB that are caused by defects in the molecular components of the hemidesmosome.[4,5] Although this makes sense from a molecular perspective, the three-type classification system is conceptually elegant and widely accepted and will be used in this chapter.

The prospect of evaluating and caring for a newborn with presumed EB often induces anxiety in both parents and care providers. Diagnosing the type and subtype of EB in the neonatal period on clinical findings alone is often impossible, leaving parents and care providers with uncertainty regarding the infant's prognosis. In addition, many activities integral to the newborn period, such as diapering, feeding, or simply picking up the infant, can induce more blisters, thereby compounding anxieties. Thus, the approach to the diagnosis and management of a newborn with suspected EB differs slightly from that of an older infant or child with a known diagnosis of EB. Within the neonatal period, there are three imperative goals: the prompt institution of nontraumatic handling of the baby to minimize further skin trauma; the initiation of non-adherent bandaging of the skin to promote healing, prevent infection, and keep the baby comfortable; and rapid and accurate diagnosis of the EB type and subtype in order to better counsel and educate parents on the baby's prognosis and guide future therapy.

CLINICAL FEATURES OF EB

Friction-induced blisters and erosions are the cardinal cutaneous features of EB. The distribution and extent of blistering varies depending on the disease subtype. Some forms of EB, such as EBS and dominant DEB (DDEB), are stereotyped as mild and often localized forms, whereas blistering in recessive DEB (RDEB) and JEB is often severe and generalized. It is important to remember that these generalizations best apply to older infants and children in whom a 'mature' EB phenotype has developed. In contrast, neonates with any type of EB may present with marked blistering and erosions. Mucosal erosions and absent or dystrophic nails can also be seen in neonates with all forms of EB. Thus, diagnosing the specific type and subtype based on clinical findings alone can be difficult, if not impossible, in the first weeks of life. Likewise, certain EB subtypes are associated with extracutaneous manifestations and complications, but these most often become significant after the neonatal period. This section will first discuss the common clinical features seen in neonates with EB, and the following sections will review EB subtypes and their specific characteristics.

Neonatal Features

Neonates with EB may present at birth with large ulcers, usually on the lower extremities, called congenital localized absence of skin (CLAS) (Fig. 11-2). The edges of such ulcers are well demarcated and the base is red and shiny. Bart and

TABLE 11-1 The classification of EB		
EB type (abbreviation)	Major subtypes (abbreviation)	Molecular defect
Simplex (EBS)	Weber–Cockayne (EBS-WC)	Keratin 5 and 14
	Koebner (EBS-K)	Keratin 5 and 14
	Dowling–Meara (EBS-DM)	Keratin 5 and 14
	Mottled pigmentation (EBS-MP)	Keratin 5
	Muscular dystrophy (EBS-MD)	Plectin
Junctional (JEB)	Herlitz (JEB-H)	Laminin-5
	Non-Herlitz (JEB-nH)	Laminin-5; collagen XVII
	Pyloric atresia (JEB-PA)	α6β4 integrin
Dystrophic	Dominant (DDEB)	Collagen VII
	Recessive (RDEB)	Collagen VII

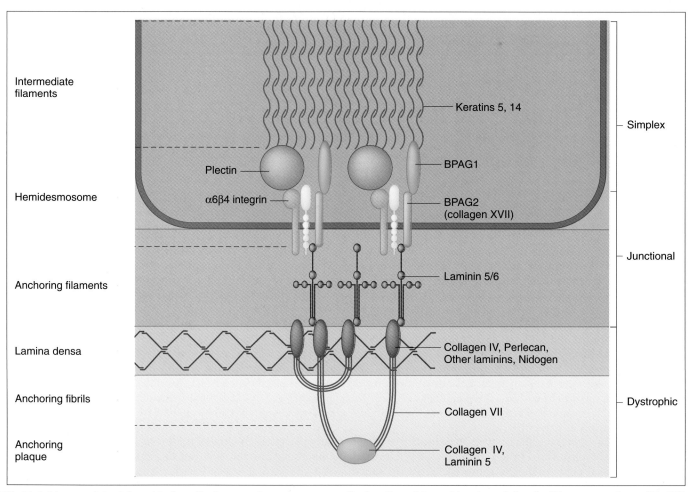

FIG. 11-1 Many proteins interact to form the basement membrane zone, the junction of the epidermis and dermis. (Diagram courtesy of Dr MP Marinkovich.)

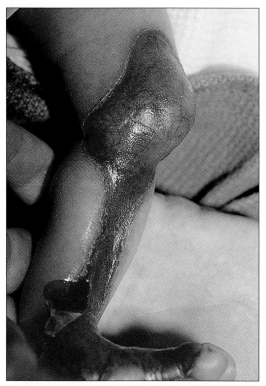

FIG. 11-2 Congenital localized absence of skin can be seen in all types of EB.

colleagues[6] originally described the association of CLAS, mucosal blistering, and nail dystrophy and proposed that this triad represented a distinct syndrome, later termed Bart's syndrome. Since that description, however, CLAS has been reported as a presenting sign in all EB types.[7-14] In addition, Bart's original kindred was examined with current molecular and genetic diagnostic techniques and found to have DDEB.[15,16] CLAS probably results from intrauterine friction, such as the leg rubbing against the uterine wall, and is not specific for any one type of EB.[7] In fact, the use of the term Bart's syndrome is now discouraged.[3]

With or without CLAS, neonates with EB develop friction-induced blistering and erosions after birth. Skin changes may initially correlate with areas traumatized during the birth process, such as the scalp and face in cases of vaginal birth. In many instances, blistering may be generalized. After birth, areas that are most subject to friction, such as the hands, diaper area, extensor extremities, and back, are most likely to blister (Fig. 11-3). Intact blisters are filled with serous or hemorrhagic fluid. In JEB and RDEB the bullae can be quite large, and the pressure of fluid within the blister cavity can cause the lesion to extend (Fig. 11-4). More superficial blisters may rupture easily, leaving open erosions.

The blisters in EBS and JEB often heal without scarring, but macular hypo- or hyperpigmentation may be a transient change after blisters heal. DEB blisters heal with scarring that is often atrophic. Healing with milia (Fig. 11-5) suggests DEB, but

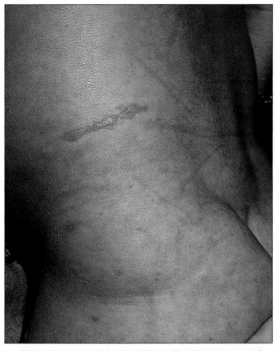

FIG. 11-3 Blistering caused by the edge of a diaper in an infant with a milder form of EB.

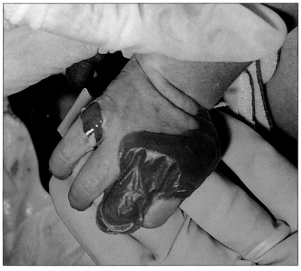

FIG. 11-4 Tense, fluid-filled blisters rapidly enlarge in patients with severe EB phenotypes.

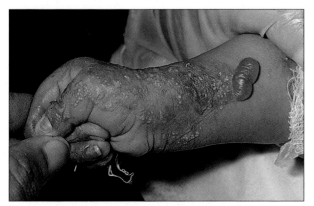

FIG. 11-5 Healing with milia most often occurs in DEB.

milia can be seen in all forms of EB.[17] Recurrent blistering on the scalp can produce scarring alopecia. Blisters and erosions are at risk of becoming infected. Signs of infection include the formation of crusts and foul-smelling or purulent drainage. Granulation tissue, which is often described as 'exuberant' in JEB, can be seen in any EB erosion that has been slow to heal but is not often seen in the neonatal period.

Oral involvement is most often seen in neonates with JEB or DEB but can be seen in EBS as well. Open erosions or intact vesicles can occur on the lips, gums, and palate. These probably result from the trauma of sucking and may result in pain with feeding. In any form of EB, trauma to the periungual skin can result in nails that are absent, dystrophic, or may be shed.

Neonates with EB and extensive erosions are at risk for developing fluid and electrolyte abnormalities as well as sepsis. Although uncommon, neonates with EB, particularly EB associated with pyloric atresia, may present with gastrointestinal obstruction at birth.[9,18] In these cases, polyhydramnios and gastric distension may have been noted on prenatal ultrasound.[18–20] Genitourinary strictures and obstruction are often present as well.[9,18] Airway involvement is uncommon in neonates with EB, but can occur. Although it is most often associated with JEB, laryngeal involvement has been described in infants with certain forms of EBS.[21] An early sign of blisters and erosions of the larynx is hoarseness, which can progress to stridor as airway obstruction worsens.[22–24]

SPECIFIC EB SUBTYPES

Epidermolysis Bullosa Simplex

EBS is the most common and often the mildest form of EB. Most forms are transmitted in an autosomal dominant manner. Individuals with localized forms of EBS may not present for medical evaluation, thus precise estimates of the true prevalence of EBS are lacking. For example, using data from 1990 the NEBR calculated the prevalence of EBS to be 4.60 cases per million, but also acknowledged that the registry probably captured only 10% of all individuals affected with EBS.[1] Population-based data from Scotland show a prevalence of 28.6 cases per million in 1992.[25]

EBS Weber–Cockayne (EBS-WC) is the most common form of EB and is characterized as the mildest. The estimated prevalence in the United States may be as high as 26 cases per million.[1] Blisters are usually localized to the hands and feet. Extracutaneous involvement does not occur. Patients may first develop blisters at any age, including birth, but it is common for the first signs to present in the toddler years, or sometimes as late as adolescence, after a period of marked frictional stress.

EBS Koebner (EBS-K) is also a common and relatively mild form of EB. It presents at birth and is characterized by intraepidermal blistering in a generalized distribution that is most pronounced on the extremities. Oral involvement can be seen in infancy but improves with age. Atrophic scarring and nail dystrophy may be seen. Extracutaneous involvement in this type of EB is extremely uncommon. For both EBS-WC and EBS-K, life expectancy is normal and the overall prognosis is good. Affected adults report that acral blistering can be painful and limits daily activities such as walking, thereby affecting quality of life.[26,27]

In contrast, another form of generalized EBS, EBS Dowling–Meara (EBS-DM), is more severe and can even be fatal in the newborn period.[8,27–29] Blistering presents at birth or within the first days of life. In severe cases the skin involvement is generalized, whereas in milder cases blisters and erosions are localized to areas of friction, such as the acral extremities and periungual areas. EBS-DM is often called EB herpetiformis because blisters characteristically occur in a grouped or annular configuration (Fig. 11-6). This feature, however, is not always reliable and may not be present until after 1 year of age. Milia and atrophic scarring may occur, and nail dystrophy is fairly common in this form of EBS. Nails may be thickened, ridged, or shed. In childhood, a confluent palmoplantar keratoderma develops and becomes more prominent with age, persisting into adulthood. This hyperkeratosis can interfere with ambulation, and joint contractures may be a subsequent complication.[27,29] Oral blistering is often present and varies in severity. Laryngeal involvement, presenting as hoarseness, has been reported, but unlike in JEB does not signal a poor prognosis.[21] Extracutaneous involvement does not occur otherwise. The severity of EBS-DM generally decreases over time, with less blistering in adolescence, and rare blistering in adulthood in many cases. Patients may also report reduced blistering during febrile illnesses.

EBS with mottled pigmentation (EBS-MP) is a rare subtype of autosomal dominant EBS. It is characterized by acral, non-scarring blistering that presents in infancy. In addition, 2–5 mm hypo- and hyperpigmented macules occur in a reticulate pattern around the neck, axillary, and groin areas.[30] The mottled pigmentation may be congenital or can develop later in infancy.[30,31]

Unlike other forms of EBS, EBS with muscular dystrophy (EBS-MD) is inherited recessively. This rare disease begins at or shortly after birth with generalized blistering and mucous membrane involvement. Other cutaneous findings include milia, atrophic scarring, and nail dystrophy.[32] Respiratory involvement in infancy has also been described.[24,33] In addition, dental enamel hypoplasia with caries is seen after infancy. In most cases, progressive muscle weakness begins in adolescence or adulthood, although onset in infancy has been reported.[32,34]

Genetics and Pathogenesis

The Weber–Cockayne, Koebner, and Dowling–Meara forms of EBS are almost always dominantly inherited and are caused

by mutations in the genes that encode keratins 5 and 14.[35–38] Rare cases of autosomal recessive inheritance are reported.[39–41] Keratins 5 and 14 are complementary intermediate filaments expressed in basal keratinocytes. They are crucial components of the cytoskeleton involved in maintaining structural integrity. In addition, they function in the adhesion of these cells to the BMZ by attaching to the hemidesmosome via plectin (see Fig. 11-1).[42] Mutations in these keratin genes lead to abnormal keratin intermediate filaments with reduced ability to withstand frictional stress, resulting histologically in basal cell cytolysis and in blistering clinically. Recent studies have better defined genotype–phenotype correlations for specific mutations in K5 and 14, but this correlation is not always straightforward.[5,42,43] Generally speaking, mutations in the highly conserved boundary domains of the α-helical rod domain lead to the Dowling–Meara phenotype, whereas mutations in the less conserved regions produce the Koebner phenotype, and the Weber–Cockayne phenotype is caused by mutations in the nonhelical linker region of the gene.[43,44]

A point mutation in the nonhelical amino-terminal head domain of K5 produces EBS-MP.[31,45,46] Exactly how this mutation leads to disruption of keratin intermediate filaments or pigmentation is currently unclear.

EBS-MD is caused by homozygous mutations in plectin.[34,47,48] As mentioned above, plectin anchors basal keratins to the hemidesmosome and is also expressed in the sarcolemma of muscle. Thus, one mutation leads to both the skin and the muscular findings in this disease. Studies of genotype–phenotype correlations suggest that mutations producing premature termination codons, resulting in loss of functional plectin, are associated with disabling muscular dystrophy and other extracutaneous manifestations, whereas less common, minor mutations (such as in-frame deletions) lead to milder phenotypes.[33,34]

Junctional Epidermolysis Bullosa

JEB is the least common type of EB. Data from the NEBR suggests an incidence of two cases per million live births.[1] Inheritance of all forms of JEB is autosomal recessive. As with other forms, a spectrum of clinical phenotypes ranging from mild and localized to generalized and severe can be seen. However, JEB is the one type that is most likely to be associated with a poor outcome in infancy, as two subtypes, JEB–Herlitz and JEB with pyloric atresia, are often not compatible with long term survival.

JEB–Herlitz (JEB-H) is characterized by generalized skin and mucosal erosions with a propensity for the skin to form exuberant granulation tissue. Other associated findings include nail dystrophy, dental enamel hypoplasia, and involvement of the respiratory epithelium (Fig. 11-7). Blistering and erosions are seen at or shortly after birth and can be large and extensive (Fig. 11-8). The amount of blistering is not predictive of outcome, as infants with little skin involvement can do poorly. Although not pathognomonic, severe involvement of the back and buttocks is common (Fig. 11-9). Neonates who survive into infancy often develop exuberant granulation tissue within their ulcers, a finding with high specificity for JEB-H.[49] The central face, especially the periorificial areas (Fig. 11-10), periungual skin (paronychial inflammation), and nape of the neck are most commonly affected. Absent nails, dystrophic nails, or nail shedding are often present. Ocular erosions can occur as well.[50,51] Oral blistering and erosions are often present in

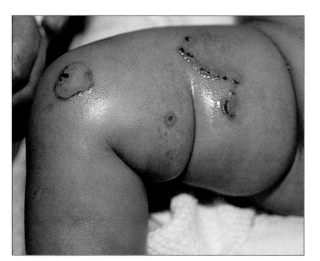

FIG. 11-6 Annular blistering is characteristic of EBS-DM.

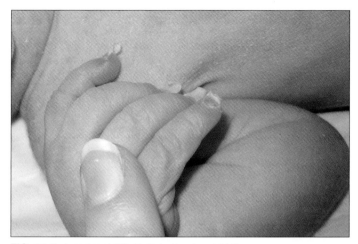

FIG. 11-7 Junctional EB. Nail dystrophy at birth.

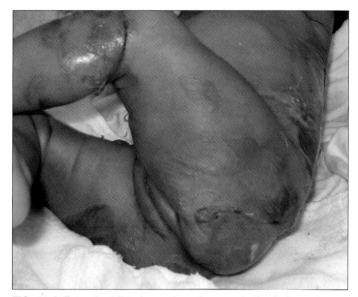

FIG. 11-9 Extensive blistering and erosions on the back, buttocks, and legs of an infant with JEB-H.

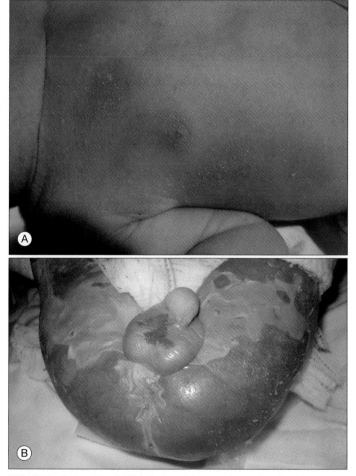

FIG. 11-8 A Junctional EB infant at 2 hours of age; localized erythema and erosions. B Same infant 1 week later with diffuse erosions.

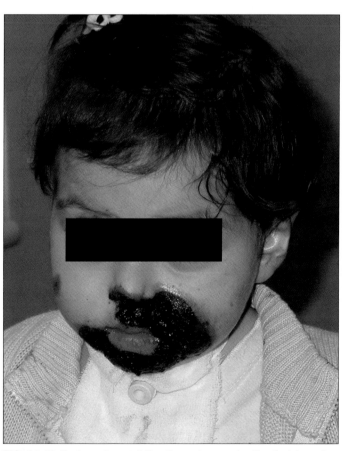

FIG. 11-10 Exuberant granulation tissue in a nonhealing facial erosion in a toddler with JEB-H. A tracheostomy tube is also in place.

the neonatal period and can make feeding difficult. The laryngeal and respiratory epithelia may also be affected, often presenting as a hoarse cry. Stridor suggests worsening airway obstruction, which can be fatal.[22,23] Involvement of the gastrointestinal and urinary epithelia also occurs.[52,53]

Extensive erosions are a risk for sepsis, which is a common cause of death in infants with JEB; pneumonia and other causes of respiratory failure may be fatal as well.[54] Although the true likelihood of death in JEB-H patients is difficult to assess, the prognosis for any affected neonate is guarded at best. The NEBR reported that, as of 1 December 1995, nine of 22 (40.9%) enrolled JEB-H patients had died, and nearly 90% of those deaths occurred before 1 year of age.[54] These figures may underreport actual mortality, as infants with rapid demise may not have been referred to the registry. Neonates with JEB-H who survive into infancy develop failure to thrive that is often refractory to treatment. Anemia, probably due to a combination of iron deficiency and chronic inflammation, also occurs.

The term JEB-non-Herlitz (JEB-nH) now includes those disorders formerly referred to as JEB-mitis and generalized atrophic benign epidermolysis bullosa (GABEB), a reflection of the clinical heterogeneity within this subtype.[55-57] JEB-nH is a generalized form of JEB with similar features to JEB-H, although it is generally less severe and its prognosis tends to be better. In the neonatal period, clinical signs and pathologic analysis may not fully distinguish between JEB-H and JEB-nH, and a final diagnosis is often based on the long-term outcome of the patient. Generalized blistering and oral involvement are seen in the neonatal period, and both improve as the child ages. Healing with granulation tissue is less common and less pronounced than in JEB-H, but can occur. Erosions may heal with atrophy and pigmentary alterations. In hair-bearing areas, alopecia may result. Nail dystrophy is prominent. Laryngeal involvement may occur, sometimes resulting in respiratory failure. The overall prognosis for JEB-nH is generally better than for JEB-H; nevertheless, some affected infants fare poorly.

Infants with JEB with pyloric atresia (JEB-PA) present at birth with upper gastrointestinal obstruction, most often affecting the pylorus. The degree of skin involvement is variable and ranges from extensive CLAS to normal skin, with the onset of blistering at several months of age.[58] Prenatal signs of an affected fetus include polyhydramnios and abdominal masses appreciated on ultrasound.[18-20] The ocular, respiratory, and urogenital epithelia are often affected. The prognosis for neonates with JEB-PA is generally poor, but nonlethal cases are reported in the literature.[58] Infants with extensive erosions often die rapidly because of fluid and electrolyte imbalances as well as sepsis. If surgical correction of the pyloric atresia is successful, infants may still succumb to sepsis, feeding intolerance and failure to thrive, and respiratory or renal disease before 1 year of age.[59]

Genetics and Pathogenesis

JEB-H and a subset of JEB-nH are caused by mutations in three genes, *LAMA3*, *LAMB3*, and *LAMC2*, which encode the constitutive subunits of the basement membrane protein laminin-5.[60,61] As a component of the basal lamina, laminin-5 plays a critical role in the adhesion of keratin intermediate filaments to the basement membrane. Absent or abnormal laminin-5 leads to structural instability, manifesting as blistering through the lamina lucida.[62] In the majority of JEB-H cases studied, mutations that result in premature termination codons have been found.[60,61] These mutations lead to an absence of laminin-5 in skin and other epithelia, a condition incompatible with long-term survival. In the case of JEB-nH, less deleterious mutations result in an abnormal laminin-5 protein that retains some degree of function.[60,61] The remaining cases of JEB-nH are caused by mutations in the gene encoding type XVII collagen/bullous pemphigoid antigen 2, a component of the hemidesmosome.[60] Mutations resulting in premature termination codons and less deleterious mutations seem to produce the same phenotype.

JEB-PA most often results from mutations in the genes encoding the hemidesmosomal proteins α6β4 integrin.[58,60] Most mutations have been found in the β4 integrin gene. A limited study of genotype–phenotype correlations suggests that patients with lethal disease have homozygous mutations producing premature termination codons, whereas those rarer cases with milder phenotypes result from a combination of missense mutations.[58] Mutations in the plectin gene have been reported recently in a minority of patients with EB and pyloric atresia.[63,64]

Dystrophic Epidermolysis Bullosa

In DEB, blistering occurs in the superficial dermis, below the lamina densa of the BMZ. DEB may be inherited in an autosomal dominant or recessive fashion. In both forms there is a range of phenotypes. DDEB is often characterized as mild, and both localized and generalized variants exist. Milder forms of RDEB resemble DDEB, but in general, RDEB is severe, generalized, and associated with significant complications.

Like the milder forms of EBS, DDEB may be more common than reported, as individuals with mild phenotypes may not seek medical attention. The NEBR estimated the prevalence of DDEB to be approximately 1 per million,[1] and Scottish data suggests a prevalence of 14.6 per million.[25] Infants with DDEB may present with CLAS or, more commonly, with blistering in the newborn period. Affected areas heal well, and as the child grows older the tendency for blistering decreases. Blistering most commonly affects those areas predisposed to trauma, such as the hands, feet, elbows, and knees, and heals with atrophy and milia. Oral erosions occur but are often mild. Nail dystrophy is common and may be the only clinical sign of disease.[65] Extracutaneous complications such as esophageal strictures are uncommon. Transient bullous dermolysis of the newborn is a distinctive variant of DDEB that is benign and self-limited. Blistering begins at birth or in the newborn period and dramatically improves or even remits completely, usually within the first year of life.[66,67] Most reported cases are sporadic, but familial cases also occur.[68]

RDEB occurs in approximately one to two individuals per million.[1,25] It is divided into two subtypes but is best thought of as a spectrum of disease severity. The term RDEB-Hallopeau–Siemens (RDEB-HS) is given to those most severely affected, whereas those with milder phenotypes are classified as RDEB-non-Hallopeau–Siemens (RDEB-nHS). In RDEB blistering begins at birth and may be quite extensive. Affected areas heal with marked scarring that can lead to the development of joint contractures over time (Fig. 11-11). Recurrent scarring of the hands and feet leads to the loss of the interdigital spaces and eventual contracture of the digits, called pseudosyndactyly or 'mitten' deformities.[69] Pseudosyndactyly is pathognomonic of RDEB. Joint contractures and pseudosyndactyly may begin in the first year of life.[69] As with other forms of EB nail involvement is also common, and many affected individuals will have loss of the nails over time.

Extracutaneous involvement is the rule in RDEB. Mucosal involvement includes the gastrointestinal tract, ocular mucosa, and genitourinary system. Oral ulcers are painful and make eating difficult, limiting the ability of the patient to take in adequate calories. Oral scarring leads to microstomia, ankyloglossia, and loss of the vestibules.[70] Esophageal involvement is extremely common and does not necessarily correlate with the extent of skin disease.[71,72] Erosions and strictures produce dysphagia and also limit adequate caloric intake. Furthermore, intestinal erosions may lead to poor absorption of nutrients. Anal erosions make defecation painful, exacerbating constipa-

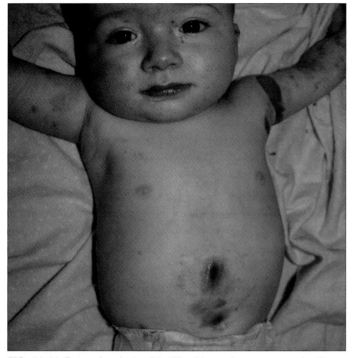

FIG. 11-11 Recessive dystrophic EB with erosions, scars and milia

tion.[71,72] The cornea and conjunctiva are frequent sites of ocular injury. Recurrent abrasions and ulcers lead to scarring that can affect visual acuity.[50,51] Urinary tract involvement may present with dysuria, hematuria, meatal stenosis, or even sepsis. Ureterovesical obstruction and hydronephrosis can occur.[52,53]

Failure to thrive is another common complication of RDEB and results from unmet nutritional needs. Chronic wound healing, blood and protein losses from erosions, and infection increase the body's need for calories. At the same time, oral and esophageal involvement hinders adequate intake. In addition to causing growth failure, chronic malnutrition contributes to poor wound healing, the development of anemia, deficiencies of essential minerals and trace elements, and increased susceptibility to infection.[73–75] Anemia is another chronic complication of RDEB and probably results from both iron deficiency and poor iron utilization due to chronic inflammation.[76]

During the neonatal period sepsis is the most worrisome complication and can lead to death. However, infants with RDEB generally do fairly well, especially compared to infants with JEB. RDEB patients need lifelong monitoring as complications from their disease are common and expected. Aggressive squamous cell carcinomas may develop in adulthood and are the leading cause of death in RDEB patients.[54]

Genetics and Pathogenesis

All forms of DEB are caused by mutations in the gene *COL7A1*, which encodes type VII collagen, the major component of anchoring fibrils.[77] Each collagen VII molecule is made of three polypeptide chains that associate and assemble into a triple helix. Two collagen VII molecules align in an antiparallel fashion, and groups of these dimers form the anchoring fibrils that connect the lamina densa to anchoring plaques in the dermis. As with other forms of EB, genotype–phenotype correlations have begun to emerge. In the case of RDEB-HS,

homozygous mutations resulting in premature termination codons and lack of collagen VII are most commonly found.[77] This correlates with an absence of anchoring fibrils in the skin. Less deleterious homozygous mutations, such as missense mutations or the combination of a missense mutation and a premature termination codon, are found in RDEB-nHS.[77] An abnormal collagen VII product is made, but its function is significantly decreased. Finally, DDEB is caused by heterozygous mutations resulting in glycine substitutions.[77] In this case, a full-length protein is formed, but the substitution leads to conformational instability of the triple helix. Thus, the DDEB phenotype results from a dominant negative mutation.

Although only limited studies are available, three different mutations in the *COL7A1* gene have been identified in patients with transient bullous dermolysis of the newborn.[68,78,79] In addition, a *COL7A1* mutation that results in a glycine substitution has been identified in patients with EBS superficialis (EBSS).[80] EBSS was described by Fine and colleagues[81] in two families with erosions and crusts that healed with milia and atrophic scarring; nail dystrophy and oral erosions were also seen. Ultrastructural studies showed cleavage arising in the superficial epidermis below the stratum corneum, leading to its classification as a variant of EBS. However, based on genetic analysis of one kindred, EBSS is actually DDEB.[80]

Laboratory Evaluation

Because an accurate diagnosis of the type and subtype of EB based on clinical findings alone is often impossible in the neonatal period, laboratory evaluation is crucial. The diagnosis is best made by skin biopsy analyzed by a combination of transmission electron microscopy (TEM) and immunofluorescence (IF) studies. Routine light microscopy yields nonspecific results, but is helpful in differentiating EB from other diagnoses that must be considered.

In order for an accurate diagnosis to be made, it is imperative that a freshly induced blister is biopsied. Existing blisters, even if intact, may show signs of re-epithelialization that interfere with proper interpretation. The steps involved in inducing a blister are outlined in Box 11-1. The decision of whether to use a punch or shave technique for biopsy depends on the pathologist's preference, but at least two biopsies (one for TEM and one for IF studies) should be taken. Each should include a portion of the induced blister and a portion of normal skin. Specimens sent for TEM should be stored in glutaraldehyde, whereas IF specimens are placed in IF media such as Zeus or Michel's fixative.

IF testing is advantageous because of its rapid turnaround time. IF immunomapping, a fairly common procedure, uses a limited panel of antibodies to basement membrane proteins to map the level of the blister, rapidly diagnosing the EB type.[82] More specific results are obtained by using antibodies directed at the specific molecules involved in EB, effectively diagnosing the subtype. Absent or attenuated staining for a particular antigen is diagnostic for that EB subtype (Table 11-2).[3,83,84] As an example, if initial testing suggests a diagnosis of JEB, subsequent testing with antibodies against plectin, α6β4 integrin, collagen XVII, and laminin-5 can be performed. Absent staining for laminin-5 correlates with a diagnosis of JEB-H, whereas absent staining for plectin is diagnostic for EBS-MD, and so forth. Unfortunately, many dermatopathology services may not have the antibodies needed for EB-specific IF studies. In such cases, referral to a laboratory experienced in diagnosing EB, such as the Stanford Dermatopathology Service (dermatopathology.stanford.edu, 650-723-6736) or Beutner Laboratories (www.beutnerlabs.com, 1-800-288-0549) is recommended.

TEM has been considered the gold standard for diagnosing EB as it clearly elucidates the ultrastructural level of the blister, thereby categorizing the EB type.[2] In some cases, morphologic changes on TEM are diagnostic for certain EB subtypes (see Table 11-2).[3] TEM is often available at academic institutions, but it is time- and labor-intensive, making it less effective than IF when a rapid diagnosis is needed.

DNA mutation analysis can be used to confirm the clinical and pathologic diagnosis. It is most accurate when testing can be directed toward a particular gene, therefore it is recommended that the EB subtype be diagnosed by IF analysis before genetic testing is ordered. Genetic testing may be helpful in cases where the clinical and pathologic findings are indistinguishable, such as distinguishing mild RDEB from DDEB. Knowing a child's mutation also helps guide genetic counseling and facilitates prenatal diagnosis in future pregnancies. Gene testing is time-consuming, however, and results will probably not be available until several weeks after the test is ordered. Thus, it is not reasonable at this time to rely on genetic testing for diagnostic or prognostic counseling in the neonatal period. DNA analysis for EB is available through the commercial company GeneDx (www.genedx.com, 301-519-2100).

Prenatal diagnosis of EB was formerly available only by fetal skin biopsy, but is now more commonly performed using DNA mutation analysis.[85] In these cases, knowing the DNA mutations in previously affected siblings and the parents guides testing and decision-making regarding the fetus. Fetal tissue is acquired by chorionic villus sampling or amniocentesis. The DNA in these tissues is then screened for the suspected mutation. Preimplantation genetic diagnosis for potentially lethal EB phenotypes is also possible.[84]

Differential Diagnosis

The differential diagnosis of blisters and erosions in the newborn is discussed in detail in Chapter 10. The most critical immediate task is to exclude infection, especially intrauterine herpes simplex infection. Other potential infectious etiologies include neonatal varicella and bacterial infections. Noninfec-

TABLE 11-2 Laboratory evaluation for EB: Characteristic immunofluorescence and transmission electron microscopy findings

EB subtype	Immunofluorescence	Electron microscopy
EBS-WC	Normal	Basal cytolysis
EBS-K	Normal	Basal cytolysis
EBS-DM	Normal	Basal cytolysis, clumped KF
EBS-MD	Absent to reduced plectin	Basal cytolysis, KF not attached to HD
JEB-H	Absent laminin-5	Cleavage in lamina lucida, reduced to absent HD
JEB-nH	Reduced laminin-5; absent to reduced collagen XVII	Cleavage in lamina lucida, rudimentary HD
JEB-PA	Absent α6β4 integrin	Cleavage in stratum basale or lamina lucida, small HD, reduced attachment of KF to HD
DDEB	Normal	Sub-lamina densa cleavage, normal to decreased AF
DDEB-TBDN	Intraepidermal, granular collagen VII	Sub-lamina densa cleavage, stellate bodies in basal keratinocytes, reduced AF
RDEB-HS	Absent collagen VII	Sub-lamina densa cleavage, absent AF
RDEB-nHS	Normal to reduced collagen VII	Sub-lamina densa cleavage, reduced or rudimentary AF

AF, anchoring fibril; HD, hemidesmosome; KF, keratin filament; TBDN, transient bullous dermolysis of the newborn.

tious causes must also be considered. Infants with disorders of cornification, particularly epidermolytic hyperkeratosis, can present neonatally with widespread erosions. Other genetic causes of blistering or erosions in neonates include incontinentia pigmenti and Kindler syndrome (KS). KS is a rare, autosomal recessive disorder in which trauma-induced blistering begins at birth or early in infancy. Based on clinical and laboratory features, it is often diagnosed as a form of EB in the neonate. However, patients with KS also have photosensitivity and later develop poikiloderma and cutaneous atrophy that persist into adulthood.[86] KS is caused by defects in the actin–extracellular matrix linker protein kindlin-1.[87,88] Immune-mediated blistering disorders, such as bullous pemphigoid and linear IgA disease, must also be considered. Infants born to mothers with immune-mediated blistering disorders may also manifest transient blisters and erosions as neonates. Diffuse cutaneous mastocytosis may also produce extensive blistering and erosion in newborns.

Management of EB in Infancy

No specific therapy is yet available for EB. Treatment therefore consists of supportive measures aimed at maintaining the physical health of the infant and the psychosocial well-being of the family.

EB can be a great management challenge in the neonatal period, especially when the infant has widespread blistering or significant extracutaneous complications. Newborns with presumed EB are best cared for in a nursery or neonatal intensive care unit with experience in treating EB. A neonatologist or pediatrician may oversee the care, with the dermatologist providing guidance on the diagnostic work-up, wound care, and other disease-specific aspects of treatment. Other specialists may also be needed, depending on the baby's particular complications. A skilled nurse, particularly one with experience in wound care, is another critical component of the EB care team.

The goals of EB management in the newborn period are outlined in Table 11-3. In addition, attention should be paid to basic needs such as fluid and electrolyte balance and temperature control. Skin erosions may result in increased fluid loss and electrolyte alterations, such as hypernatremia. Intravenous fluids are often needed in the first few days, and electrolytes should be checked regularly until stable. Temperature control can be aided initially by the use of a radiant warmer or isolette. However, the environment should not be too warm, as this may promote blistering.[89,90] Temperature probes or other monitoring devices should not be taped to the skin.

Given the nature of EB, it is impossible to completely prevent new blisters from forming, but by minimizing trauma to the skin and mucosa it is possible to limit their frequency and severity. As even minimal trauma can produce blisters, careful handling of the baby is paramount.[89,90] Tape or adhesives should not be used on EB skin as their removal produces blistering. If medical devices need to be secured, they may be fastened to dressings or a self-adhesive compression wrap (e.g. Coban, 3M) can be used. Mepitac (Mölnlycke Health Care), a silicone 'tape' that does not contain adhesives, can be used on fragile skin, but should be used with care in those EB subtypes with excessive skin fragility. Friction often occurs where clothes or diapers rub the skin. Cloth diapers may be less traumatic around the waistband and thigh areas. Alternatively, the elastic cuffs can be cut out of disposable diapers, minimizing blistering on the thighs. Seams from clothing may also

TABLE 11-3 Goals of EB management in the neonatal period

Goal	How achieved
Minimize new blisters and erosions	Gentle handling, reduce friction No tape or adhesives on skin
Promote wound healing	Wound care Thoroughly wash hands or use alcohol-based hand sanitizers before and after patient care Daily bathing and wound care Vigilant inspection of wounds
Prevent infection	Topical or systemic antibiotics if needed
Promote comfort	Wound care Use nonadherent dressings Oral sucrose with dressing changes
Reduce procedural pain	Acetaminophen or opiate agonist for extreme discomfort
Optimize caloric intake	Fortify breast milk or formula Use soft nipples or cleft lip and palate feeder Sucralfate for oral ulcers to reduce pain Treat gastroesophageal reflux

TABLE 11-4 An example of the items needed for daily dressing changes

Item	Purpose
Warm water and mild cleanser	To clean the skin
Sterile needles and sterile gauze	To lance and drain intact blisters
Sterile sharp scissors	To trim excess or hanging skin
Preservative-free, petrolatum-based ointment	Emolliates the skin, provides moisture to wounds, prevents bandages from adhering to wounds
Petrolatum-impregnated gauze (or Mepitel)	Contact layer, applied over wounds
Rolled cotton dressing	Absorbent layer, soaks up exudate and protects non-injured skin
Elastic tubular dressing	Holds dressings in place

produce blistering. Clothing should be soft and loose fitting, and if covered seams are not available the clothing should be turned inside out. The baby should not be lifted under the arms; instead, the head and buttocks should be supported at all times. To minimize blistering on the back, soft padding such as a sheepskin should be used to line the bed (which should remain flat), and a disposable underpad covered with a thin layer of petroleum jelly or a similar ointment will help minimize friction.

For existing blisters and erosions, good wound care is essential to promoting healing and preventing infection. Bandaging also provides protection to the skin and helps limit future blistering.[91,92] Wound care should be performed daily. The complete task of bathing and redressing the baby can take up to 2 hours to complete and needs two people working together to run smoothly. Having all the necessary materials prepared ahead of time (Table 11-4) greatly speeds the task.

To minimize trauma to exposed skin, it is best to clean and bandage the baby one part at a time. For instance, wound care can be performed on each extremity, followed by the torso and then the face and scalp. Bandages should be removed gently. If they are adherent to the wound, they should be soaked off with water or dabbed with a petrolatum-based ointment until soft. Bandages should never be forcibly removed: this is both painful and disrupts the healing process.[91] The skin should then be cleaned with a mild soap or cleanser and water, and gently patted dry with a soft towel. The skin should not be rubbed. Existing erosions should be assessed for signs of infection and for evidence of healing. Intact blisters should be slit open on their dependent side using a sterile needle, to prevent extension of the lesion (Fig. 11-12).[89–91] Gentle pressure is then applied to the blister while sterile gauze wicks away blister fluid. The blister roof should be left in place unless it hangs freely. Redundant skin or crust can be gently trimmed away with clean, sharp scissors.

The skin should then be covered with dressings. Ideal dressings for EB patients should be nonadherent and promote a moist, healthy wound bed.[91,92] Many products fulfill these criteria, and the ultimate decision as to which are used depends on their availability, cost, and physician (and later parent) preference. The first bandage to cover the wound, the contact layer, should be a nonstick dressing over which other dressings may be applied. Examples of common contact layers include petrolatum-impregnated gauze and Telfa clear (Kendall). If these products are used, wounds should be liberally covered with an emollient such as petroleum jelly or Aquaphor ointment (Biersdorf) first. This prevents the wound from drying out and reduces the likelihood of the bandage sticking to the wound. Mepitel (Mölnlycke Health Care) is another excellent choice for a contact layer. This is a fenestrated silicone product that clings gently to noninjured skin. As it is hydrophobic, it is easily removed by moistening it with water. Mepitel should be applied over the ulcer first, and ointments are used on top of it. If wounds have no signs of infection, the use of topical antibiotics is not recommended.[93] If topical antibiotics are used to control bacterial load they should be discontinued when the wound appears clean, or rotated every 1–3 months to prevent resistance.[91,94] Bathing with dilute bleach may also be useful to reduce the bacterial load on the skin and may help minimize reliance on topical antibiotics. Two teaspoons of undiluted bleach per gallon of water is one recommended concentration.

Absorptive dressings are then applied over the contact layer. These soak up exudate and provide padding and protection for the child. Rolled gauze, with additional gauze pads as needed, is frequently used. Wound care products that are both non-adherent and absorptive may be helpful for highly exudative wounds.[91] One such product is EXU-DRY (Smith & Nephew), which combines a nonadherent contact layer and absorbent padding. Foam dressings such as Mepilex (Mölnlycke Health Care) and Allevyn (Smith & Nephew) are less bulky and can be applied directly to the wound. Dressings should then be secured with a thin layer of conformable rolled gauze or stretchable burn netting. In the case of infants with RDEB and digital erosions, separating the digits with strips of petrolatum-impregnated gauze and wrapping the fingers individually may help delay the onset of webbing and pseudosyndactyly (Fig. 11-13). With good wound care, even extensive erosions will show excellent healing within 1–2 weeks (Fig. 11-14).

Signs of wound infection include increased erythema, drainage, odor, crusting, or tenderness. Drainage may be yellow or green. If infection is suspected, a wound culture should be obtained and the results used to guide therapy. Minor wound infections often improve with the use of topical antibiotics and dressings that help to wick away excess exudate. Common topical antibiotics include bacitracin, mupirocin, and gentamicin ointments. As mentioned previously, it is best to limit the

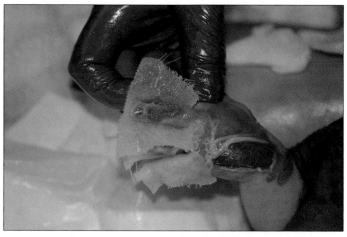

FIG. 11-13 Infant with recessive dystrophic epidermolysis bullosa having digits wrapped with petrolatum-impregnated gauze.

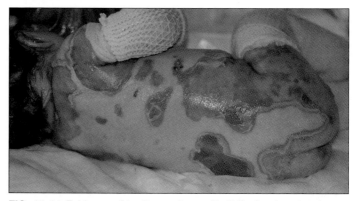

FIG. 11-14 Evidence of healing and re-epithelialization in extensive ulcers after 2 weeks of wound care.

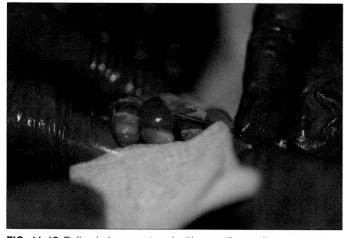

FIG. 11-12 Bullae being punctured with a sterile needle to prevent lesion extension.

duration of use of topical antibiotics to periods of suspected infection. If redness extends beyond the wound, cellulitis must be suspected. Open erosions act as portals of entry for bacteria, and sepsis is a complication of EB in the neonatal period. Neonates with presumed cellulitis or sepsis should be treated with broad-spectrum systemic antibiotics, which should be subsequently narrowed based on wound and blood culture results.

In addition to the calories needed for normal growth, infants with extensive erosions have added metabolic demands due to wound healing. Failing to account for this contributes to failure to thrive in children with JEB and RDEB. However, obtaining adequate nutrition in the newborn period can be a management challenge, especially when oral erosions and ulcers make feeding painful and laborious. Mothers who choose to breast-feed should apply ointment to their nipples beforehand. However, in those infants at high risk for failure to thrive it may be preferable to express and then fortify the breast milk. Likewise, high-calorie formulas should be used for infants with JEB and RDEB that are formula fed.[95] Nipples should be soft and preferably high flow, so that the infant does not need to suck vigorously. A cleft lip and palate nurser, such as the Haberman feeder (Medela) may also be helpful. The input of the gastroenterology and nutrition team can be very helpful. An occupational therapist may also be helpful in cases where oral feeding is difficult.

The blisters and erosions of EB, both on the skin and internally, are painful, and most patients report living with chronic pain.[96] In addition, pain is often exacerbated by procedures such as dressing changes. Pain management in EB is a challenge, owing to the chronic nature of the disease. Proper wound care is the mainstay of pain control.[91–93] In infants with extensive erosions systemic pain medications may be needed initially, especially with dressing changes. Medications should be given 20–30 minutes before beginning bandaging. Acetaminophen may be tried first, and if this is not sufficient an opiate agonist can be added.[93] However, the long-term use of narcotics is not recommended because of their adverse effects and risk of dependency.[92] Oral sucrose is effective to control procedural pain in neonates and may also be used,[97] although it has not been specifically evaluated for EB. Oral discomfort may be controlled with topical analgesics before feeding. The use of sucralfate to coat ulcers is also effective.[98] The use of eye ointments to prevent and treat corneal erosions reduces eye pain. Gastroesophageal reflux may also be painful, especially if the baby has esophageal erosions. The use of an H_2 blocker or proton-pump inhibitor in these cases reduces pain.

In those cases where neonates present with extracutaneous manifestations requiring surgical intervention, such as pyloric stenosis or respiratory distress in the case of suspected JEB-H, the risks and benefits of surgical intervention must be weighed against the child's overall prognosis. With careful attention, patients with EB can tolerate intubation (either nasopharyngeal or endotracheal) and anesthesia for procedures.[93] Repair of pyloric atresia[59] and early placement of tracheostomy tubes[23] have been performed successfully in EB patients, but these infants often succumb to other complications of their disease. Thus, palliative care alone is a valid treatment option for infants with EB subtypes that carry a poor prognosis, such as JEB-PA and JEB-H.[99]

Having a newborn with EB is a life-altering experience, and the medical team must be able to provide psychosocial support for the family. This is important both during the uncertain period before the diagnosis is known and afterwards when discussions about prognosis and future expectations are critical. An excellent resource for families affected by EB is the Dystrophic Epidermolysis Bullosa Research Association of America (DEBRA, www.debra.org). In addition to providing excellent information geared toward a lay audience, DEBRA offers consultation with an EB nurse specialist.

In order to be discharged home, infants with EB need to be medically stable. From a dermatologic standpoint, a reasonable goal is no more than 10% skin involvement, minimal development of new blisters, and evidence of adequate feeding and weight gain. In addition, parents or care providers should demonstrate comfort with and competence at changing the baby's dressings, and support services such as a home health nurse and sufficient medical supplies need to be in place. Infants should follow up with care providers who are experienced in managing EB. A multidisciplinary approach is needed to monitor for and treat the many complications that may develop as the child ages.

Finally, families should be encouraged to maintain hope that disease-specific treatments for EB may one day be available. Much has been learned about EB in recent years, and scientists continue to add to that knowledge. There has been initial success in correcting the cutaneous manifestations of JEB-H and RDEB via gene or protein transfer in mouse models.[100–102] Additionally, in a recent landmark study keratinocyte stem cells from an adult patient with JEB-nH were genetically corrected and successfully transplanted back to affected areas of the legs, resulting in normal, robust skin during the 1-year follow-up period.[103] Although it is difficult to predict when this technology will be widely available for all EB subtypes, the future remains promising.

ACKNOWLEDGMENTS

The author would like to thank Drs Renee Howard and Ilona J. Frieden for their contributions from the previous edition, and Drs Phuong Khuu and Alfred Lane for their thoughtful review and comments.

REFERENCES

1. Fine J-D, Johnson LB, Suchindran C, et al. The epidemiology of epidermolysis bullosa. In: Fine J-D, Bauer EA, McGuire J, et al., eds. Epidermolysis bullosa: clinical, epidemiologic, and laboratory advances and the findings of the National Epidermolysis Bullosa Registry. Baltimore: Johns Hopkins University Press, 1999; 101–113.
2. Pearson RW. Clinicopathologic types of epidermolysis bullosa and their nondermatological complications. Arch Dermatol 1988; 124: 718–725.
3. Fine J-D, Eady RA, Bauer EA, et al. Revised classification system for inherited epidermolysis bullosa: report of the Second International Consensus Meeting on diagnosis and classification of epidermolysis bullosa. J Am Acad Dermatol 2000; 42: 1051–1066.
4. Pai S, Marinkovich MP. Epidermolysis bullosa: new and emerging trends. Am J Clin Dermatol 2002; 3: 371–380.
5. Uitto J, Richard G. Progress in epidermolysis bullosa: from eponyms

to molecular genetic classification. Clin Dermatol 2005; 23: 33–40.

6. Bart BJ, Gorlin RJ, Anderson VE, et al. Congenital localized absence of skin and associated abnormalities resembling epidermolysis bullosa: a new syndrome. Arch Dermatol 1966; 93: 296–304.

7. Kanzler MH, Smoller B, Woodley DT. Congenital localized absence of the skin as a manifestation of epidermolysis bullosa. Arch Dermatol 1992; 128: 1087–1090.

8. Furumura M, Imayama S, Hori Y. Three neonatal cases of epidermolysis bullosa herpetiformis (Dowling–Meara type) with severe erosive skin lesions. J Am Acad Dermatol 1993; 28: 859–861.

9. Puvabanditsin S, Garrow E, Kim DU, et al. Junctional epidermolysis bullosa associated with congenital localized absence of skin, and pyloric atresia in two newborn siblings. J Am Acad Dermatol 2001; 44: 330–335.

10. Maman E, Maor E, Kachko L, et al. Epidermolysis bullosa, pyloric atresia, aplasia cutis congenita: histopathological delineation of an autosomal recessive disease. Am J Med Genet 1998; 78: 127–133.

11. Skovan I, Drzewiecki KT. Congenital localized skin defect and epidermolysis bullosa hereditaria letalis. Acta Dermatol Venereol 1979; 59: 533–537.

12. Wakasugi S, Mizutari K, Ono T. Clinical phenotype of Bart's syndrome seen in a family with dominant dystrophic epidermolysis bullosa. J Dermatol 1998; 25: 517–522.

13. Butler DF, Berger TG, James WD, et al. Bart's syndrome: microscopic, ultrastructural, and immunofluorescent mapping features. Pediatr Dermatol 1986; 3: 113–14.

14. Wojnarowska FT, Eady RA, Wells RS. Dystrophic epidermolysis bullosa presenting with congenital localized absence of skin: report of four cases. J Dermatol 1983; 108: 477–483.

15. Zelickson B, Matsumura K, Kist D, et al. Bart's syndrome: ultrastructure and genetic linkage. Arch Dermatol 1995; 131: 663–668.

16. Christiano AM, Bart BJ, Epstein EH, et al. Genetic basis of Bart's syndrome: a glycine substitution mutation in the type VII collagen gene. J Invest Dermatol 1996; 106: 1340–1342.

17. Devries DT, Johnson LB, Weiner M, et al. Relative extent of skin involvement in inherited epidermolysis bullosa (EB): composite regional anatomic diagrams based on the findings of the National EB Registry, 1986 to 2002. J Am Acad Dermatol 2004; 50: 572–581.

18. Puvabanditsin S, Garrow E, Samransamraujkit R, et al. Epidermolysis bullosa associated with congenital localized absence of skin, fetal abdominal mass, and pyloric atresia. Pediatr Dermatol 1997; 14: 359–362.

19. Azarian M, Dreux S, Vuillard E, et al. Prenatal diagnosis of inherited epidermolysis bullosa in a patient with no family history: a case report and literature review. Prenat Diagn 2006; 26: 57–59.

20. De Jenlis Sicot B, Deruelle P, Kacet N, et al. Prenatal findings in epidermolysis bullosa with pyloric atresia in a family not known to be at risk. Ultrasound Obstet Gynecol 2005; 25: 607–609.

21. Shemanko CS, Horn HM, Keohane SG, et al. Laryngeal involvement in the Dowling–Meara variant of epidermolysis bullosa simplex with keratin mutations of severely disruptive potential. Br J Dermatol 2000; 142: 315–320.

22. Gonzalez C, Roth R. Laryngotracheal involvement in epidermolysis bullosa. Int J Pediatr Otorhinolaryngol 1989; 17: 305–311.

23. Lyos AT, Levy ML, Malpica A, et al. Laryngeal involvement in epidermolysis bullosa. Ann Otol Rhinol Laryngol 1994; 103: 542–546.

24. Mellerio JE, Smith FJ, McMillan JR, et al. Recessive epidermolysis bullosa simplex associated with plectin mutations: infantile respiratory complications in two unrelated cases. Br J Dermatol 1997; 137: 898–906.

25. Horn HM, Priestley GC, Eady RA, et al. The prevalence of epidermolysis bullosa in Scotland. Br J Dermatol 1997; 136: 560–564.

26. Horn HM, Tidman MJ. Quality of life in epidermolysis bullosa. Clin Exp Dermatol 2002; 27: 707–710.

27. Horn HM, Tidman MJ. The clinical spectrum of epidermolysis bullosa simplex. Br J Dermatol 2000; 142: 468–472.

28. Buchbinder LH, Lucky AW, Ballard E, et al. Severe infantile epidermolysis bullosa simplex. Dowling–Meara type. Arch Dermatol 1986; 122: 190–198.

29. McGrath JA, Ishida-Yamamoto A, Tidman MJ, et al. Epidermolysis bullosa simplex (Dowling–Meara). A clinicopathological review. Br J Dermatol 1992; 126: 421–430.

30. Fisher T, Gedde-Dahl T Jr. Epidermolysis bullosa simplex and mottled pigmentation: a new dominant syndrome. I. Clinical and histological features. Clin Genet 1979; 15: 228–238.

31. Moog U, de Die-Smulders CEM, Scheffer H, et al. Epidermolysis bullosa simplex with mottled pigmentation: clinical aspects and confirmation of the P24L mutation in the KRT5 gene in further patients. Am J Med Genet 1999; 86: 376–379.

32. Fine JD, Stenn J, Johnson L, et al. Autosomal recessive epidermolysis bullosa simplex. Generalized phenotypic features suggestive of junctional or dystrophic epidermolysis bullosa, and association with neuromuscular diseases. Arch Dermatol 1989; 125: 931–938.

33. Schara U, Tucke J, Mortier W, et al. Severe mucous membrane involvement in epidermolysis bullosa simplex with muscular dystrophy due to a novel plectin gene mutation. Eur J Pediatr 2004; 163: 218–222.

34. Shimizu H, Takizawa Y, Pulkkinen L, et al. Epidermolysis bullosa simplex associated with muscular dystrophy: phenotype–genotype correlations and review of the literature. J Am Acad Dermatol 1999; 41: 950–956.

35. Bonifas JM, Rothman AL, Epstein EH, Jr. Epidermolysis bullosa simplex: evidence in two families for keratin gene abnormalities. Science 1991; 254: 1202–1205.

36. Coulombe PA, Hutton ME, Letai A, et al. Point mutations in human keratin 14 genes of epidermolysis bullosa simplex patients: genetic and functional analyses. Cell 1991; 66: 1301–1311.

37. Lane EB, Rugg EL, Navsaria H, et al. A mutation in the conserved helix termination peptide of keratin 5 in hereditary skin blistering. Nature 1992; 356: 244–246.

38. Chan Y-M, Yu Q-C, Fine J-D, et al. The genetic basis of Weber–Cockayne epidermolysis bullosa simplex. Proc Natl Acad Sci USA 1993; 90: 7414–7418.

39. Fine JD, Johnson L, Wright T, et al. Epidermolysis bullosa simplex: identification of a kindred with autosomal recessive transmission of the Weber–Cockayne variety. Pediatr Dermatol 1989; 6: 1–5.

40. Chan Y, Anton-Lamprecht I, Yu QC, et al. A human keratin 14 'knockout': the absence of K14 leads to severe epidermolysis bullosa simplex and a function for an intermediate filament protein. Genes Dev 1994; 8: 2574–2587.

41. Batta K, Rugg EL, Wilson NJ, et al. A keratin 14 'knockout' mutation in recessive epidermolysis bullosa simplex resulting in less severe disease. Br J Dermatol 2000; 143: 621–627.

42. Irvine AD. Inherited defects in keratins. Clin Dermatol 2005; 23: 6–14.

43. Fuchs EV. The molecular biology of epidermolysis bullosa simplex. In: Fine J-D, Bauer EA, McGuire J, et al., eds. Epidermolysis bullosa: clinical, epidemiologic, and laboratory advances and the findings of the National Epidermolysis Bullosa Registry. Baltimore: Johns Hopkins University Press, 1999; 280–299.

44. Irvine AD, McLean WHI. Human keratin diseases: the increasing spectrum of disease and subtlety of the phenotype–genotype correlation. Br J Dermatol 1999; 140: 815–828.

45. Uttam J, Hutton E, Coulombe PA, et al. The genetic basis of epidermolysis bullosa simplex with mottled pigmentation. Proc Natl Acad Sci USA 1996; 93: 9079–9084.

46. Irvine AD, Rugg EL, Lane EB, et al. Molecular confirmation of the unique phenotype of epidermolysis bullosa simplex with mottled pigmentation. Br J Dermatol 2001; 144: 40–45.

47. Pulkkinen L, Smith FJD, Shimizu H, et al. Homozygous deletion mutations in the plectin gene (PLEC1) in patients with epidermolysis bullosa simplex associated with late-onset muscular dystrophy. Hum Mol Genet 1996; 5: 1539–1546.

48. Smith FJ, Eady RA, Leigh IM, et al. Plectin deficiency results in muscular dystrophy with epidermolysis bullosa. Nature Genet 1996; 13: 450–457.

49. Fine J-D, Johnson LB, Suchindran C, et al. Cutaneous and skin-associated musculoskeletal manifestations of inherited epidermolysis bullosa. In: Fine J-D, Bauer EA, McGuire J, et al., eds. Epidermolysis bullosa: clinical, epidemiologic, and laboratory advances and the findings of the National Epidermolysis Bullosa Registry. Baltimore: Johns Hopkins University Press, 1999; 114–146.

50. Tong L, Hodgkins PR, Denyer J, et al. The eye in epidermolysis bullosa. Br J Ophthalmol 1999; 83: 323–326.

51. Fine JD, Johnson LB, Weiner M, et al. Eye involvement in inherited epidermolysis bullosa: experience of the National Epidermolysis Bullosa Registry. Am J Ophthalmol 2004; 138: 254–262.

52. Glazier DB, Zaontz MR. Epidermolysis bullosa: a review of the associated urological complications. J Urol 1998; 159: 2122–2125.

53. Fine J-D, Johnson LB, Weiner M, et al. Genitourinary complications of inherited epidermolysis bullosa: experience of the National Epidermolysis Bullosa Registry and review of the literature. J Urol 2004; 172: 2040–2044.

54. Fine J-D, Johnson LB, Suchindran C, et al. Premature death and inherited epidermolysis bullosa. In: Fine J-D, Bauer EA, McGuire J, et al., eds. Epidermolysis bullosa: clinical, epidemiologic, and laboratory advances and the findings of the National Epidermolysis Bullosa Registry. Baltimore: Johns Hopkins University Press, 1999; 206–224.

55. Hintner H, Wolff K. Generalized atrophic benign epidermolysis bullosa. Arch Dermatol 1982; 118: 375–384.

56. Paller AS, Fine J, Kaplan S, et al. The generalized atrophic benign form of junctional epidermolysis bullosa. Arch Dermatol 1986; 122: 704–710.

57. Darling TN, Bauer JW, Hintner H, et al. Generalized atrophic benign epidermolysis bullosa. Adv Dermatol 1997; 13: 87–119.

58. Nakano A, Pulkkinen L, Murrell D, et al. Epidermolysis bullosa with congenital pyloric atresia: novel mutations in the β4 integrin gene (ITGB4) and genotype/phenotype correlations. Pediatr Res 2001; 49: 618–626.

59. Dank JP, Kim S, Parisi MA, et al. Outcome after surgical repair of junctional epidermolysis bullosa–pyloric atresia syndrome. Arch Dermatol 1999; 135: 1243–1247.

60. Pulkkinen L, Uitto J, Christiano AM. The molecular basis of the junctional forms of epidermolysis bullosa. In: Fine J-D, Bauer EA, McGuire J, et al., eds. Epidermolysis bullosa: clinical, epidemiologic, and laboratory advances and the findings of the National Epidermolysis Bullosa Registry. Baltimore: Johns Hopkins University Press, 1999; 300–325.

61. Nakano A, Chao S-C, Pulkkinen L, et al. Laminin 5 mutations in junctional epidermolysis bullosa: molecular basis of Herlitz vs non-Herlitz phenotypes. Hum Genet 2002; 110: 41–51.

62. McGowan KA, Marinkovich MP. Laminins and human disease. Microsc Res Tech 2000; 51: 262–279.

63. Pfender E, Uitto J. Plectin gene mutations can cause epidermolysis bullosa with pyloric atresia. J Invest Dermatol 2005; 124: 111–115.

64. Nakamura H, Sawamura D, Goto M, et al. Epidermolysis bullosa simplex associated with pyloric atresia is a novel clinical subtype caused by mutations in the plectin gene (PLEC1). J Mol Diagn 2005; 7: 28–35.

65. Dharma B, Moss C, McGrath JA, et al. Dominant dystrophic epidermolysis bullosa presenting as familial nail dystrophy. Clin Exp Dermatol 2001; 26: 93–96.

66. Hashimoto K, Matsumoto M, Iacobelli D. Transient bullous dermolysis of the newborn. Arch Dermatol 1985; 121: 1429–1438.

67. Hashimoto K, Burk JD, Bale GF, et al. Transient bullous dermolysis of the newborn: Two additional cases. J Am Acad Dermatol 1989; 21: 708–713.

68. Fassihi H, Diba VC, Wessagowit V, et al. Transient bullous dermolysis of the newborn in three generations. Br J Dermatol 2005; 153: 1058–1063.

69. Fine JD, Johnson LB, Weiner M, et al. Pseudosyndactyly and musculoskeletal contractures in inherited epidermolysis bullosa: experience of the National Epidermolysis Bullosa Registry, 1986–2002. J Hand Surg 2005; 30: 14–22.

70. Wright JT. Oral manifestations of epidermolysis bullosa. In: Fine J-D, Bauer EA, McGuire J, et al., eds. Epidermolysis bullosa: clinical, epidemiologic, and laboratory advances and the findings of the National Epidermolysis Bullosa Registry. Baltimore: Johns Hopkins University Press, 1999; 236–256.

71. Ergun GA, Lin AN, Dannenberg AJ, et al. Gastrointestinal manifestations of epidermolysis bullosa. A study of 101 patients. Medicine 1992; 71: 121–127.

72. Fine J-D, Johnson LB, Suchindran C, et al. Extracutaneous manifestations of inherited epidermolysis bullosa. The National Epidermolysis Bullosa Registry experience. In: Fine J-D, Bauer EA, McGuire J, et al., eds. Epidermolysis bullosa: clinical, epidemiologic, and laboratory advances and the findings of the National Epidermolysis Bullosa Registry. Baltimore: Johns Hopkins University Press, 1999; 147–174.

73. Fine JD, Tamura T, Johnson L. Blood and trace metal levels in epidermolysis bullosa. Arch Dermatol 1989; 125: 374–379.

74. Allman S, Haynes L, MacKinnon P, et al. Nutrition in dystrophic epidermolysis bullosa. Pediatr Dermatol 1992; 9: 231–238.

75. Ingen-Housz-Oro S, Blanchet-Bardon C, Vrillat M, et al. Vitamin and trace metal levels in recessive dystrophic epidermolysis bullosa. J Eur Acad Dermatol Venereol 2004; 18: 649–653.

76. Fridge JL, Vichinsky EP. Correction of the anemia of epidermolysis bullosa with intravenous iron and erythropoietin. J Pediatr 1998; 132: 871–873.

77. Uitto J, Pulkkinen L, Christiano AM. The molecular basis of the dystrophic forms of epidermolysis bullosa. In: Fine J-D, Bauer EA, McGuire J, et al., eds. Epidermolysis bullosa: clinical, epidemiologic, and laboratory advances and the findings of the National Epidermolysis Bullosa Registry. Baltimore: Johns Hopkins University Press, 1999; 326–350.

78. Christiano AM, Fine JD, Uitto J. Genetic basis of dominantly inherited transient bullous dermolysis of the newborn: a splice site mutation in the type VII collagen gene. J Invest Dermatol 1997; 109: 811–814.

79. Hammami-Hauasli N, Raghunath M, Kuster W, et al. Transient bullous dermolysis of the newborn associated with compound heterozygosity for recessive and dominant COL7A1 mutations. J Invest Dermatol 1998; 111: 1214–1219.

80. Martinez-Mir A, Liu J, Gordon D, et al. EB simplex superficialis resulting from a mutation in the type VII collagen gene. J Invest Dermatol 2002; 118: 547–549.

81. Fine JD, Johnson L, Wright T. Epidermolysis bullosa simplex superficialis. A new variant of epidermolysis bullosa characterized by subcorneal skin cleavage mimicking peeling skin syndrome. Arch Dermatol 1989; 125: 633–638.

82. Fine J-D, Smith LT. Nonmolecular diagnostic testing of inherited epidermolysis bullosa: current techniques, major findings, and relative sensitivity and specificity. In: Fine J-D, Bauer EA, McGuire J, et al., eds. Epidermolysis bullosa: clinical, epidemiologic, and laboratory advances and the findings of the National Epidermolysis Bullosa Registry.

Baltimore: Johns Hopkins University Press, 1999; 48–78.

83. Bergman R. Immunohistopathologic diagnosis of epidermolysis bullosa. Am J Dermatopathol 1999; 21: 185–192.

84. Hanson SG, Fine J-D, Levy ML. Three new cases of transient bullous dermolysis of the newborn. J Am Acad Dermatol 1999; 40: 471–476.

85. Fassihi H, Eady RAJ, Mellerio JE, et al. Prenatal diagnosis for severe inherited skin disorders: 25 years' experience. Br J Dermatol 2006; 154: 106–113.

86. Ashton GHS. Kindler syndrome. Clin Exp Dermatol 2004; 29: 116–121.

87. Siegel DH, Ashton GH, Penagos HG, et al. Loss of kindling-1, a human homolog of the *Caenorhabditis elegans* actin-extracellular-matrix linker protein UNC-112, causes Kindler syndrome. Am J Hum Genet 2003; 73: 174–187.

88. Jobard F, Bouadjar B, Caux F, et al. Identification of mutations in a new gene encoding a FERM family protein with a pleckstrin homology domain in Kindler syndrome. Hum Mol Genet 2003; 12: 925–935.

89. Bello YM, Falabella AF, Schachner LA. Management of epidermolysis bullosa in infants and children. Clin Dermatol 2003; 21: 278–282.

90. Schachner L, Feiner A, Samisulli S. Epidermolysis bullosa: management principles for the neonate, infant, and young child. Dermatol Nurs 2005; 17: 56–59.

91. Schober-Flores C. Epidermolysis bullosa: the challenges of wound care. Dermatol Nurs 2003; 15: 135–138, 141–144.

92. Weiner MS. Pain management in epidermolysis bullosa: an intractable problem. Ostomy Wound Manage 2004; 50: 13–14.

93. Herod J, Denyer J, Goldman A, et al. Epidermolysis bullosa in children: pathophysiology, anaesthesia and pain management. Paediatr Anaesth 2002; 12: 388–397.

94. Lin AN. Management of patients with epidermolysis bullosa. Dermatol Clin 1996; 14: 381–387.

95. Birge K. Nutrition management of patients with epidermolysis bullosa. J Am Diet Assoc 1995; 95: 575–579.

96. Fine JD, Johnson LB, Weiner M, et al. Assessment of mobility, activities and pain in different subtypes of epidermolysis bullosa. Clin Exp Dermatol 2004; 29: 122–127.

97. Stevens B, Yamada J. Ohlsson A. Sucrose for analgesia in newborn infants undergoing painful procedures.

Cochrane Database Syst Rev 2004; 3: CD001069.

98. Marini I, Vecchiet F. Sucralfate: a help during oral management in patients with epidermolysis bullosa. J Periodontol 2001; 72: 691–695.

99. Yan EG, Paris JJ, Ahluwalia J, et al. Treatment decision-making for patients with the Herlitz subtype of junctional epidermolysis bullosa. J Perinatol 2007; 27: 307–311.

100. Sawamura D, McMillan JR, Akiyama M, et al. Epidermolysis bullosa: directions for future research and new challenges for treatment. Arch Dermatol Res 2003; 295: S34–S42.

101. Ferrari S, Pellegrini G, Mavilio F, et al. Gene therapy approaches for epidermolysis bullosa. Clin Dermatol 2005; 23: 43–436.

102. Hengge UR. Progress and prospects of skin gene therapy: a ten year history. Clin Dermatol 2005; 23: 107–114.

103. Mavilio F, Pellegrini G, Ferrari S, et al. Correction of junctional epidermolysis bullosa by bransplantion of genetically modified epidermal stem cells. Nat Med 2006; 12: 1397–1402.

12

Bacterial Infections

James G. H. Dinulos, Nicole C. Pace

Bacterial skin infections vary in both their clinical presentation and their propensity for the development of systemic sequelae in the neonate as a result of several factors: (1) the nature of the pathogen; (2) the developmental stage of the infant when infection is acquired, that is, early (first or second trimester) or late (third trimester) in gestation, early (first few days) or late (2–8 weeks) postnatal life; and (3) the manner in which inoculation occurs (i.e. congenitally, at the time of birth via an infected mother, or postnatally). Disease present at birth that results from hematogenous penetration of the placental barrier, for example, is often devastating, involving multiple organ systems in addition to the skin, because of the vulnerable state of the developing neonate. Even postnatally acquired infections are potentially more serious than in older children because of the immature immune defenses of the neonate.

The development of skin infection involves a complex interaction between environmental and local ecologic factors, such as:

- Alterations in the normal bacterial flora
- Predisposing tissue factors, such as local trauma with breach of the epidermal barrier
- Competence of systemic and local tissue defenses of the host
- Expression of bacterial virulence factors and synergism.

Organisms that normally colonize the skin are the major agents of sepsis in very low-birthweight infants, suggesting that sepsis may be a consequence of bacterial penetration at sites of skin injury or through their immature epidermal barrier. Susceptibility to systemic complications of skin infection, resulting from the immaturity of immune defenses, is especially problematic in the premature infant.[1] Consequently, neonatal cutaneous infections mandate a prompt and thorough evaluation and aggressive treatment. Furthermore, these infections sometimes signify the presence of congenital immunodeficiency.

SUPERFICIAL INFECTIONS

Impetigo

Impetigo is the single most common primary skin infection in children,[2] and impetiginous infection of atopic dermatitis is the most important secondary skin infection.[3] Nonbullous impetigo is a superficial infection localized to the subcorneal portion of the epidermis. Bullous impetigo occurs when an infant is infected with coagulase-positive *Staphylococcus aureus*, most commonly phage group 2 (types 71 and 55) which elaborates toxins.[4] These toxins cause epidermolysis and subsequent blister formation. Bullous impetigo is thought to be a localized form of staphylococcal scalded skin syndrome (SSSS).[5]

Cutaneous Findings

Nonbullous impetigo is characterized by erythematous, honey-colored crusted plaques. Lesions tend to be localized in primary impetigo, but may become more widespread when superimposed secondarily on diseased skin. Moist intertriginous and periumbilical areas are commonly involved in both nonbullous and bullous impetigo. Bullous impetigo often presents during the first 2 weeks of life with flaccid, transparent, subcorneal bullae, which may be single or clustered, and often lack underlying cutaneous erythema. The bullae may contain pus that layers out in the dependent portion. The lesions rupture easily, leaving a shallow erosion surrounded by a narrow rim of scale that heals without scarring (Fig. 12-1). However, postinflammatory pigmentary changes may persist for weeks to months. Multiple small pustules on the abdomen and diaper area are characteristic of staphylococcal pustulosis (Fig. 12-2).[6]

Extracutaneous Findings

Most cases of impetigo, including neonatal bullous impetigo, are unaccompanied by constitutional signs of illness. Occasionally, hematogenous spread may result in osteomyelitis, septic arthritis, pneumonia, or septicemia, particularly in neonates with bullous impetigo.[2,7]

Etiology/Pathogenesis

S. aureus is isolated from approximately 85% of impetigo lesions and in 50–60% of cases is the sole pathogen. *Streptococcus pyogenes* causes the remainder of cases. Bullous impetigo is always caused by coagulase-positive *S. aureus*; 80% are from phage group 2.[7] The staphylococcal organisms that cause nonbullous impetigo are variable, but are generally not from phage group 2. Locally produced exfoliative or epidermolytic toxins (ETA and ETB) induce bulla formation by cleaving desmoglein I within desmosomes, via serine proteases.[8] Epidermolytic toxin A is more commonly associated with bullous impetigo than is epidermolytic toxin B. High titers of neutralizing antibodies against ETA and/or the inability of ETA to penetrate through the epidermis may explain why ETA does not commonly cause SSSS.[9]

Diagnosis

Gram staining showing Gram-positive cocci in clusters, and culture of fluid from a vesicle or pustule or from beneath the

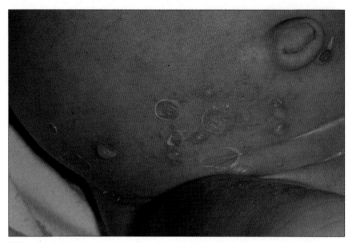

FIG. 12-1 Flaccid bullae seen in bullous impetigo that easily rupture, leaving a fine collarette of scale.

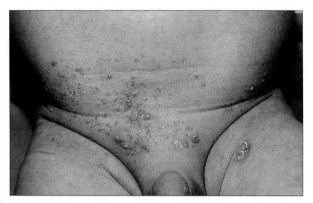

FIG. 12-2 Multiple vesicles and bullae of staphylococcal pustulosis.

lifted edges of a crusted plaque of impetigo, are usually sufficient to establish a diagnosis. When the diagnosis is in question, and Gram stain and culture are negative, a skin biopsy can be useful, although this is seldom necessary. Histologically, early lesions of impetigo show a vesicle or pustule in the subcorneal or granular region of the epidermis with marked dermal inflammation; the cavity is larger in the bullous form.

Differential Diagnosis
Staphylococcal impetigo is clinically indistinguishable from streptococcal impetigo.[2] Bullous impetigo may be confused with several other infectious vesiculobullous or pustular disorders, such as herpes simplex virus (HSV), varicella, enterovirus, congenital cutaneous candidiasis, listeriosis, and scabies, as well as noninfectious disorders such as erythema toxicum neonatorum, transient neonatal pustular melanosis, eosinophilic pustulosis, chronic bullous disease of childhood, incontinentia pigmenti, epidermolysis bullosa, pemphigus, and pemphigoid.

Course/Management/Treatment/Prognosis
The most common complication is cellulitis, which has been reported in up to 10% of cases, although this is probably an overestimate. In the absence of fever or local soft-tissue involvement such as lymphadenitis or cellulitis, localized nonbullous impetigo in neonates may be managed with oral β-

lactamase-resistant antibiotics, such as cephalexin, cloxacillin, or dicloxacillin.[10] Second-line oral agents that may be considered for the treatment of uncomplicated impetigo include erythromycin, cefadroxil, cefprozil, loracarbef, clarithromycin, azithromycin, and amoxicillin/clavulanate. Recently, there has been a trend towards using topical mupirocin and fusidic acid for localized forms of impetigo and reserving oral antibiotics for those patients with more diffuse involvement or resistant organisms.[11]

Bullous impetigo may advance rapidly if not treated. Consequently, most experts recommend that therapy be initiated parenterally in neonates, usually with nafcillin, oxacillin, or methicillin. Clindamycin, a protein synthesis inhibitor, may be advantageous for decreasing epidermolytic toxin production, and a first-generation cephalosporin such as cefazolin is also suitable. Once signs of infection have begun to subside, and if constitutional signs are absent, therapy may be completed orally. In older infants, oral therapy similar to that used for nonbullous impetigo may be adequate. Topical antibiotics (e.g. mupirocin) are not appropriate for the treatment of bullous impetigo. A 7-day course of therapy may be sufficient, but because a 10-day course of treatment has been studied, it is the usual recommended duration.

The antibiotic susceptibility profile must be considered when treating methicillin-resistant strains of *S. aureus* (MSRA). Vancomycin remains a reliable agent for treatment of MRSA, although other agents to which the organism is susceptible in vitro may be effective (see Methicillin-resistant *Staphylococcus aureus*).

Folliculitis
Bacterial folliculitis is a superficial infection of the hair follicle ostium.

Cutaneous Findings
Folliculitis presents as discrete, dome-shaped pustules with an erythematous base located at the ostia of the pilosebaceous canals. The lesions are usually asymptomatic, but may be pruritic or painful. Occasionally, a lesion may extend to involve deeper tissues and form an abscess (e.g. furuncle, carbuncle).

Extracutaneous Findings
Extracutaneous findings are not typically present.

Etiology/Pathogenesis
Folliculitis is caused predominantly by *S. aureus*, although coagulase-negative staphylococci are occasionally involved. A moist environment, maceration, poor hygiene, application of an occlusive emollient, and drainage from adjacent wounds and abscesses can be provoking factors.

Diagnosis
The causative organism of folliculitis can be identified by Gram stain and culture of purulent material from the follicular orifice.

Differential Diagnosis
Candida albicans, Pityrosporum ovale, and *Malassezia furfur* can cause follicular papules and/or pustules. Diagnosis may be made by potassium hydroxide examination of lesion scrapings or by skin biopsy. Several other conditions may mimic folliculitis, including miliaria, eosinophilic pustular folliculitis, acne

neonatorum, tinea corporis, congenital cutaneous candidiasis, scabies, and erythema toxicum neonatorum.

Course/Management/Treatment/Prognosis
An attempt should be made to identify and eliminate predisposing factors. Localized uncomplicated folliculitis may be managed by removing causative factors, antiseptic cleansing (e.g. chlorhexidine), and topical antibiotics. Severe or refractory folliculitis should be managed with oral therapy: cephalexin, dicloxacillin, or cloxacillin for 2 weeks is usually curative. Recurrent episodes should warrant investigation into asymptomatic nasal carriage of *S. aureus* by the patient and immediate caregivers.[12]

Paronychia

Paronychia is a localized inflammation of the nail fold, which can be classified as congenital or acquired (acute or chronic).[13]

Cutaneous Findings
Paronychia presents with the lateral nail fold becoming warm, erythematous, edematous, and painful (Fig. 12-3). A purulent exudate may develop. Dermatitis often occurs around the affected area and may contribute to initiation and/or perpetuation of the problem.

Extracutaneous Findings
Extracutaneous findings generally are absent.

Etiology/Pathogenesis
Although the primary disorder is separation of the eponychium from the nail plate, secondary infection is common. *S. aureus* and *S. pyogenes* are the most common aerobic organisms. Occasionally, Gram-negative organisms such as *Pseudomonas* spp., *Proteus* spp., and *Escherichia coli* are involved.[14]

Diagnosis
The diagnosis is made clinically; in acute cases both aerobic and anaerobic cultures of purulent material are recommended.

Differential Diagnosis
The differential diagnosis includes *Candida albicans*, a frequent cause of acute and chronic paronychia in neonates, and

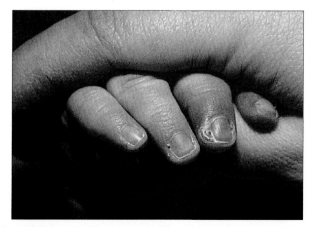

FIG. 12-3 Paronychia, presenting with erythema and edema of the lateral nail fold, was due to *Staphylococcus aureus* in this case.

HSV infection. Zidovidine-induced neutropenia has been reported to be associated with severe paronychia in a neonate.[15]

Course/Management/Treatment/Prognosis
Attention must be directed toward eliminating or reducing predisposing factors of nail-fold maceration and trauma. Warm compresses generally are curative for superficial lesions. Drainage of the abscess may be facilitated by gently pushing the nail fold away from the nail plate. In addition to incision and drainage, antibiotics are needed for treatment of deeper lesions. Dicloxacillin, cloxacillin, or cephalexin are the antibiotics of choice for treatment of infections caused by *S. aureus*, whereas amoxicillin plus clavulanic acid is preferred for empiric treatment as a result of the emergence of β-lactamase-producing anaerobes.

Funisitis/Omphalitis

Funisitis is inflammation of the umbilical cord or stump characterized by increased secretions and a foul odor. Funisitis may accompany chorioamnionitis. Omphalitis is infection of the umbilical stump. Low-birthweight infants and those with complicated deliveries are at increased risk for omphalitis.[16]

Cutaneous Findings
Excessive exudate from the umbilical stump, as seen in funisitis, may be a harbinger of subsequent infection. The exudate may be accompanied by bleeding from the umbilical vessels caused by a delay in closure. Omphalitis shows periumbilical erythema, edema, and tenderness, with or without discharge. On average, signs of infection occur on the third day of life. The infection may extend subcutaneously to cause cellulitis, or along abdominal wall fascial planes to cause necrotizing fasciitis. Black discoloration or crepitus of the periumbilical tissues suggests a mixed infection and more advanced disease.

Extracutaneous Findings
The umbilical cord of the newborn infant is a particularly common portal of entry for invasive bacterial pathogens. Invasion may occur directly into the peritoneal cavity, with resultant peritonitis. Ascending infection along the umbilical vein is a particularly serious complication. Septic umbilical arteritis or suppurative thrombophlebitis of umbilical or portal veins, portal vein thrombosis, and liver abscesses may occur. Septic embolization from infected umbilical vessels (arteries or the vein) is uncommon, but may seed various organs, including the lungs, pancreas, kidneys, heart (i.e. endocarditis) or skin.

Etiology/Pathogenesis
Omphalitis is caused by a variety of organisms, but *S. aureus*, *S. pyogenes* and Gram-negative organisms are most common.[17] The umbilical cord stump may become highly colonized with pathogenic bacteria shortly after birth, including vaginal flora and bacteria from carer givers' hands. Candidal funisitis has been reported.

Diagnosis
Gram stain and culture of moist umbilical stump material may show organisms and be helpful in the early diagnosis of omphalitis, although correlation with clinical signs is neces-

sary to determine true infection. Culture results are helpful for guiding antimicrobial therapy.

Differential Diagnosis

The serous secretions of funisitis/omphalitis must be distinguished from those of a vitelline duct remnant, umbilical papilloma, or urachal remnant.

Course/Management/Treatment/Prognosis

Most cases are responsive to broad-spectrum antimicrobial coverage against Gram-positive and Gram-negative organisms. Ampicillin and gentamicin administered together are an effective therapy for initial coverage. With either suspicion for or microbiologic evidence of anaerobic infection, the addition of metronidazole or substitution with clindamycin for ampicillin is usually effective. Intravenous antibiotics should be continued until the erythema and drainage subside. Complications include evisceration, umbilical hernia, necrotizing fasciitis, cellulitis, peritonitis, superficial abscess, liver abscess and peritoneal adhesions.[18] Predictors of poor outcome include early onset of the infection, unplanned home delivery, and temperature instability. Patients should be monitored closely for signs of necrotizing fasciitis, which has a high mortality rate.

Cellulitis

Cellulitis is characterized by infection and inflammation of loose connective tissue, with limited involvement of the dermis and relative sparing of the epidermis. A break in the skin resulting from trauma, surgery, or an underlying skin lesion predisposes to cellulitis. Cellulitis may be seen with vascular malformations such as Klippel–Trénaunay syndrome and lymphatic malformations, and in immunodeficiency disorders, but it also occurs in healthy infants.

Cutaneous Findings

Cellulitis presents as an area of edema, warmth, erythema, and tenderness. The lateral margins tend to be indistinct because the process is deep in the skin. Application of pressure may produce pitting. Cellulitis caused by *S. aureus* tends to be more localized and may be suppurative, whereas infections caused by *S. pyogenes* tend to spread more rapidly and may be associated with lymphangitis, but this distinction is not generally clear-cut.

Extracutaneous Findings

Regional adenopathy and constitutional signs and symptoms of fever, chills, and malaise are common. Complications of cellulitis include osteomyelitis, septic arthritis, thrombophlebitis, and bacteremia. Glomerulonephritis also can follow infection with *S. pyogenes*.

Etiology/Pathogenesis

Besides *S. aureus* and *S. pyogenes*, causal organisms can include group G or C streptococci, *Streptococcus pneumoniae*, and group B streptococci or *E. coli*. In premature newborns or newborns with immunologic defects a number of other bacterial or fungal agents may be involved. *Pasteurella multocida* is implicated in cellulitis that follows dog or cat bites, whereas human bites may become infected with *Eikenella corrodens*. Immunization against *Haemophilus influenzae* type B has significantly reduced the incidence of cellulitis due to this organism.[19]

Diagnosis

Aspirates from the leading edge of inflammation, skin biopsy, and blood cultures collectively allow for identification of the causal organism in approximately 25% of cellulitis cases. An aspirate taken from the point of maximum inflammation yields the causal organism more often than does a leading-edge aspirate.[20] Lack of success in isolating an organism stems primarily from the low number of organisms present within the lesion.

Differential Diagnosis

Congenital Wells syndrome, insect bites, drug reactions, contact dermatitis, and cold panniculitis may resemble cellulitis.

Course/Management/Treatment/Prognosis

Empiric therapy for cellulitis should be directed by the history of the illness, the location and character of the cellulitis, and the age and immune status of the patient. Cellulitis in the neonate should prompt a sepsis workup, followed by initiation of empiric therapy intravenously with a β-lactamase-stable antistaphylococcal antibiotic such as methicillin, oxacillin, or nafcillin, and an aminoglycoside such as gentamicin or a cephalosporin such as cefotaxime. Once the regional erythema, warmth, edema, and fever have decreased significantly, a 10-day course of treatment may be completed on an outpatient basis provided that other sites of infection (e.g. the CSF) have been excluded.

Periorbital/Orbital Cellulitis

Infection of the soft tissues surrounding the eye is classified as periorbital (preseptal) cellulitis or orbital (postseptal) cellulitis.

Cutaneous Findings

The orbital septum connects the orbital periosteum to the upper and lower eyelid structures. This tough fibrous band acts to prevent harmless superficial infections from extending into the orbit and threatening vision. Periorbital cellulitis is a superficial infection that presents with redness, swelling, and tenderness of soft tissues anterior to the orbital septum. Orbital cellulitis involves deeper structures behind the orbital septum. Orbital cellulitis can be associated with sinusitis or direct penetrating trauma to the orbital septum. Orbital cellulitis presents with eyelid erythema, edema, and conjunctival hyperemia, and is distinguished clinically from periorbital cellulitis by ocular involvement.

Extracutaneous Findings

Periorbital cellulitis can be associated with bacteremia, particularly when *Streptococcus pneumoniae* is involved. Orbital cellulitis is associated with proptosis, limited painful eye movement, decreased vision, and loss of corneal sensation. Constitutional signs such as fever can be seen with both periorbital and orbital cellulitis.

Etiology/Pathogenesis

Orbital cellulitis is most commonly caused by an extension of ethmoiditis into the surrounding soft tissue. *Streptococcus* and *Staphylococcus* spp. are the most common pathogens among newborns.[21] Methicillin-resistant *S. aureus* and anaerobes less commonly cause orbital cellulitis in newborns.[22,23]

Diagnosis

Tissue cultures are useful to detect causal organisms. Blood cultures are positive in up to 33% of children. Ultrasound does not reliably detect deep soft tissue infection. Computed tomography (CT) is the most appropriate imaging study to define the extent of infection. Prompt imaging should be undertaken in any infant with proptosis and limited eye movement, as a delay in diagnosing orbital cellulitis can threaten vision and result in death.[23]

Differential Diagnosis

Adenoviral conjunctivitis may mimic preseptal and septal cellulitis. Orbital pseudotumor, rhabdomyosarcoma, and *Aspergillus* fungal sinusitis must be excluded in the patient with periorbital swelling.

Course/Management/Treatment/Prognosis

Deep soft tissue infection in the orbital region is a medical emergency. Initial therapy should include intravenous cefuroxime and metronidazole. Most pain can be managed adequately with decongestants and analgesics. Prompt consultation with ophthalmologists and otolaryngologists should be obtained. Signs of optic nerve compression, such as decreased visual acuity, require urgent surgical decompression of the orbital space and infected sinuses.[23] Intravenous antibiotic therapy should be continued for at least 5 days following abscess drainage, and either oral or IV antibiotic should be continued for at least 14–21 days.

SUBCUTANEOUS/SYSTEMIC INFECTIONS

Abscesses

An abscess is a localized collection of pus in a cavity formed by the disintegration or necrosis of tissue, resulting in a firm, tender, erythematous nodule that becomes fluctuant (Fig. 12-4). In the neonatal period an abscess is a potentially serious infection because of the higher risk for bacterial dissemination. Overall, *S. aureus* is the single most common pathogen causing abscesses. Abscesses can be seen in normal newborns, but multiple abscesses are characteristic of immunodeficiency syndromes such as hyper-IgE syndrome and leukocyte adhesion deficiency. Identification of organisms not typically associated with abscess formation, especially organisms of low virulence, should raise concerns about underlying immunodeficiency. The principal organisms causing abscesses vary with the location of the lesion on the body.

Breast Abscess

Breast abscesses develop in full-term neonates during the first 1–6 weeks of life, most commonly during the 4th and 5th weeks.[24] The incidence is approximately equal in males and females during the first 2 weeks of life, but thereafter the incidence in girls is nearly twice that in boys.

Cutaneous Findings

Breast abscesses present initially with breast enlargement, accompanied by varying degrees of erythema, induration, and tenderness. Fluctuance may or may not occur, depending in part on how early antibiotic therapy is initiated. Bilateral infection occurs in less than 5% of cases. Breast abscess caused by *S. aureus* is accompanied by cutaneous pustules or bullae on

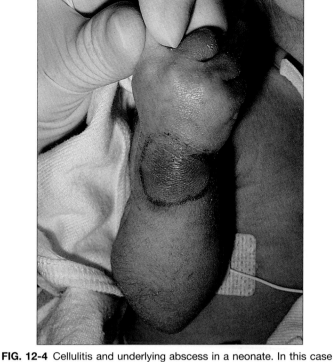

FIG. 12-4 Cellulitis and underlying abscess in a neonate. In this case the abscess was due to an intravenous line. 'Inking' the margin, as was done in this case, is one way to determine response to treatment.

the trunk, particularly in the perineal region, in 25–50% of patients. The symptoms, age at presentation, and clinical findings of infants with breast abscess caused by Gram-negative bacilli, or those that harbor anaerobes, are similar to those of infants infected with *S. aureus*, except that infants infected with *Salmonella* sp. generally also have gastrointestinal illness.

Extracutaneous Findings

Affected infants usually lack fever (present in approximately one-third) or constitutional symptoms such as irritability or toxicity. Leukocytosis (>15 000/mm³) is found in approximately half to two-thirds of patients. Bacteremia, pneumonia, osteomyelitis, or sepsis are unusual.

Etiology/Pathogenesis

Breast abscess is usually due to *S. aureus*, but occasionally is caused by group B streptococcus, *E. coli*, *Salmonella* sp., *Proteus mirabilis*, *Pseudomonas aeruginosa*, or *Ureaplasma urelyticum*.[25] Although anaerobic organisms can be isolated from up to 40% of infections, their pathogenic role in neonates is questionable, and therapy directed specifically against them is generally unnecessary. The increased incidence in girls after 2 weeks of age (when breast gland development is more pronounced in girls than boys) and the lack of the disorder in the underdeveloped breast of premature infants suggest that increased ductal tissue may be a factor in pathogenesis. Breast manipulation has also been suggested as a predisposing factor. Infants with *S. aureus* breast abscesses are typically colonized with the same organism in the nose or pharynx. It seems likely that *S. aureus* spreads from the nasopharynx to colonize the skin of the nipple, moving up the ducts of the physiologically enlarged, predisposed breast, perhaps facilitated by breast manipulation, to infect deeper tissues.

Diagnosis

Gram stain of material expressed from the nipple or obtained by needle aspiration or incision and drainage can help to guide initial antibiotic therapy. The presence of cutaneous vesicles or bullae may help in identifying *S. aureus* as the causal agent. Blood cultures should be obtained, but unless the infant is febrile or appears ill, cultures of urine and cerebrospinal fluid (CSF) are unnecessary.

Course/Management/Treatment/Prognosis

Typically, breast abscesses remain localized and resolve with appropriate therapy. If fluctuance is absent, systemic anti-staphylococcal antibiotic therapy may be curative and prevent abscess development. If fluctuance is present, the abscess must be drained by needle aspiration, by gently expressing pus from the nipple, or surgically, and Gram stain and culture obtained. Antibiotic therapy with a β-lactamase-resistant anti-staphylococcal antibiotic should be given systemically. If Gram-negative bacilli are seen, or the infant has constitutional symptoms or appears ill, initial therapy should be administered parenterally. An aminoglycoside or cefotaxime should be given while awaiting culture results. Once infection has begun to subside, oral therapy may be considered. In most instances, a total of 5–7 days of therapy is sufficient, although many experts continue treatment for 10–14 days. The most common complication of breast abscess is cellulitis, which develops in approximately 5–10% of affected infants. The cellulitis is generally localized, but can extend rapidly to involve the shoulder and/or abdomen. Scar formation leading to decreased breast size following puberty can occur as a late complication.

Scalp Abscess

Scalp abscess develops in neonates at the insertion site of a fetal scalp monitoring electrode. The reported incidence of scalp abscess is between 0.1% and 5.2%.[26]

Cutaneous Findings

Presentation occurs most commonly on the third or fourth days of life, but may be as early as the first day and as late as 3 weeks. The lesion initially appears as a localized, erythematous area of induration 0.5–2 cm in diameter. The site may become fluctuant or pustular.

Extracutaneous Findings

Regional lymphadenopathy may be present, but other more serious complications, such as cranial osteomyelitis, subgaleal abscess, necrotizing fasciitis of the scalp, bacteremia, sepsis, and death, are rare.

Etiology/Pathogenesis

Scalp abscess is typically a polymicrobial infection and includes both aerobes and anaerobes. The anaerobic flora present reflects that found in the normal cervix during labor. The most common organisms are *Streptococcus* sp., *Staphylococcus epidermidis*, and *E. coli*.[27] The most plausible hypothesis for the pathogenesis of scalp abscess is that the infection occurs via the ascent of normal cervical flora into the uterus following rupture of membranes, aided by procedures that access the uterine cavity. Placement of the electrode breaks the skin

barrier, providing a foreign-body nidus for infection in the subcutaneous tissue. Risk factors include longer duration of ruptured membranes, longer duration of monitoring, monitoring for high-risk indications, amnionitis, and endometritis. In general, it appears that procedures that serve to provide increased access of vaginal flora to the infant or more trauma to the scalp may increase the risk of abscess development.

Diagnosis

Infants who are subjected to scalp electrode monitoring in utero should be followed closely during the first weeks of life for evidence of infection. Parents should be instructed in surveillance, and if an abscess is noted it is advisable to remove the hair directly around the lesion to allow for closer observation. Culture for both aerobic and anaerobic organisms can be obtained by swabbing the exudate from the puncture site or by needle aspiration.

Differential Diagnosis

Differential diagnosis includes cephalohematoma and HSV infection. A cephalhematoma is typically seen at birth and does not demonstrate erythema, warmth, or tenderness. It resolves spontaneously over 3 weeks and generally requires no treatment. Cutaneous HSV infection can mimic scalp abscess and occurs with a peak onset between 4 and 10 days of life. Prompt diagnosis and treatment of HSV is essential to prevent systemic dissemination. Aplasia cutis congenita can have clear drainage and resemble a scalp abscess.

Course/Management/Treatment/Prognosis

Most scalp abscesses resolve spontaneously, but if fluctuance develops without spontaneous suppuration, incision and drainage are appropriate. In infants with signs of infection, culture and sensitivities should be obtained and the appropriate antibiotic instituted.

Necrotizing Fasciitis

Necrotizing fasciitis is a rare, rapidly progressive, and potentially life threatening infection of the superficial fascia and subcutaneous tissue.[28]

Cutaneous Findings

Local swelling, erythema, tenderness, and heat are typical and develop most commonly in the abdominal wall or back (Fig. 12-5). Skin changes may progress over 24–48 hours as nutrient vessels are thrombosed and cutaneous ischemia develops. Because the infection advances along the superficial fascial plane, there may be few initial cutaneous signs to herald the serious nature and extent of the subcutaneous tissue necrosis that is occurring. Late cutaneous signs include the formation of bullae, initially filled with straw-colored and later bluish to hemorrhagic fluid. There is also darkening of affected tissues from red to purple to blue. Skin anesthesia, followed by frank tissue gangrene, develops as a result of the ischemia and necrosis. Infections resulting from one organism or a combination of organisms cannot be distinguished clinically, although the development of crepitus signals the presence of *Clostridium* sp. or Gram-negative bacilli such as *E. coli*, *Klebsiella*, *Proteus*, and *Aeromonas*.

Extracutaneous Findings

In necrotizing fasciitis, fever, tachycardia and leukocytosis are usually present.[29] Bacteremia and thrombocytopenia are

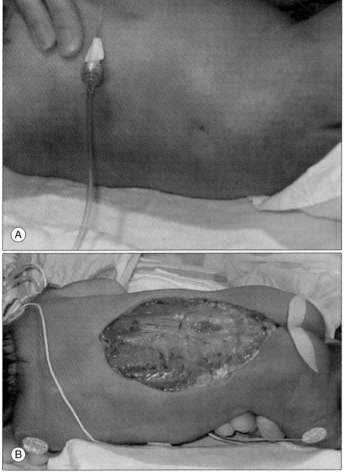

FIG. 12-5 A: Erythema and firm skin of early necrotizing fasciitis **B:** Necrotizing fascitis: Perioperative image of extent of debridement (Courtesy of Angela Medina)

present in approximately half of patients. Significant systemic toxicity may develop, including shock and multiorgan failure. The advance of infection in this setting can be rapid, progressing to death within hours.

Etiology/Pathogenesis

Common predisposing factors in neonates include omphalitis,[17,18] circumcision,[30] balanitis,[30] breast and scalp abscesses,[31] necrotizing enterocolitis (NEC),[32] Hirschsprung enterocolitis,[33] staphylococcal folliculitis, bullous impetigo,[34] fetal monitoring,[35] and surgery.[36] Most cases in newborns are polymicrobial, involving a mixture of anaerobic bacteria and aerobic and/or facultative bacteria that act together to cause tissue necrosis. The predominant aerobic bacteria include *S. aureus* and *S. pyogenes*. Fungi of the order Mucorales, particularly *Rhizopus* sp., *Mucor* sp., and *Absidia* sp., rarely can cause necrotizing fasciitis.[37]

Diagnosis

Fever, tachycardia, and leukocytosis may be the first signs of an evolving necrotizing fasciitis. A definitive diagnosis is made by surgical exploration, which must be undertaken as soon as the diagnosis is suspected. Although magnetic resonance imaging (MRI), CT scanning or ultrasound may aid in delineating the extent and tissue planes of involvement, these imaging studies should not delay surgical intervention. Frozen

section incisional biopsy taken early in the course of the infection can aid management by decreasing the time to diagnosis and helping to establish margins of involvement.[38] Histopathologically, necrotizing fasciitis shows necrosis and suppuration of the superficial fascia, edema, and an acute inflammatory infiltrate in the deep dermis, subcutaneous fat, and fascia. Microorganisms within destroyed tissue and thrombosis of arteries and veins are seen at all levels.

Differential Diagnosis

Distinguishing between nonnecrotizing (e.g. cellulitis) and necrotizing infection is the most important management decision, because necrotizing soft tissue infection will not respond to antibiotics alone and requires prompt surgical removal of all devitalized tissue. Pain out of proportion to the cutaneous findings, rapidly progressive tissue necrosis, and systemic toxicity distinguish necrotizing fasciitis from cellulitis, which does not destroy subcutaneous tissue.

Course/Management/Treatment/Prognosis

Prompt supportive care, surgical debridement, and parenteral antibiotic administration are mandatory.[37] All devitalized tissue must be removed to freely bleeding edges, and repeat exploration is generally indicated within 24–36 hours to confirm that no necrotic tissue remains. Surgery may need to be repeated on several occasions until devitalized tissue has ceased to form. Daily meticulous wound care also is paramount. Broad-spectrum, parenteral antibiotic therapy must be initiated as soon as possible. Most experts recommend initial empiric therapy with a combination of a broad-spectrum antistaphylococcal penicillin, an aminoglycoside such as gentamicin, and metronidazole.[32] The reported mortality rate is close to 50%.[28]

Ecthyma Gangrenosum

Ecthyma gangrenosum refers to necrotic skin lesions caused by *Pseudomonas* infection.[39]

Cutaneous Findings

The lesion begins as a painful red or purpuric macule, which develops a pustular or vesicular center with a surrounding rim of pink or violaceous skin that rapidly ulcerates (Fig. 12-6A). The infection also may present with bullae. The ulcer develops raised edges with a necrotic, dense, black, depressed, and crusted center. Erythema multiforme-like lesions also have been described at onset. Lesions may be single or multiple, and sometimes cluster around areas of moisture such as the mouth or perineum (Fig. 12-6B).

Extracutaneous Findings

Most infants with ecthyma gangrenosum are septic, and skin lesions result from bacteremic spread of infection; however, only 1.3–13% of patients with sepsis with *Ps. aeruginosa* develop cutaneous lesions.[40] There have been nonsepticemic variants described in newborns.

Etiology/Pathogenesis

Ecthyma gangrenosum is due to *Ps. aeruginosa*, a Gram negative bacillus. During septicemia, the organism tends to multiply in the walls of small blood vessels, which results in arterial and venous thrombosis, and ultimately dermal necrosis.[40] Risk factors in neonates and young infants include prematurity,

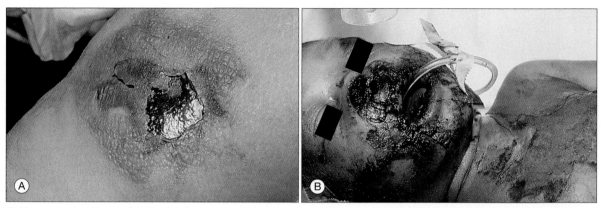

FIG. 12-6 (A) Hemorrhagic, ulcerated bulla of ecthyma gangrenosum due to *Pseudomonas aeruginosa*. **(B)** *Pseudomonas* septicemia with periorificial accentuation of ecthyma gangrenosum.

prolonged illness, necrotizing enterocolitis, previous bowel surgery, and an immunocompromised state, especially neutropenia. Ecthyma grangrenosum arises from direct inoculation of organisms.

Diagnosis/Differential Diagnosis

Lesions of ecthyma gangrenosum mandate a full sepsis work-up, tissue examination for Gram stain and culture, and histopathology. Gram stain is best performed on scrapings from the base of the ulceration. Histopathologic examination allows distinction of this entity from streptococcal ecthyma. A pauci-inflammatory vasculitis, particularly of the veins, with surrounding edema, hemorrhage, and necrosis, is seen. Bacteria may be seen in the perivascular tissue and occasionally in the vessel walls, particularly the adventitia and media of dermal veins, but not the arteries; the intima and lumina generally are spared. Similar lesions rarely can develop as a result of infection with other agents, such as *Aeromonas hydrophila*, *Enterobacter* spp., *E. coli*, *Proteus* spp., *Pseudomonas cepacia*, *S. marcescens*, *Xanthomonas maltophilia*, *Aspergillus* spp., Mucorales, and *C. albicans*.

Course/Management/Treatment/Prognosis

Ecthyma gangrenosum in association with bacteremia is a grave sign. Aggressive empiric therapy should be initiated with an extended-spectrum penicillin (e.g. ticarcillin or piperacillin) or ceftazidime in combination with an aminoglycoside. Once the culture and susceptibility results are available, therapy may be narrowed. If the infection proves to be caused by *Pseudomonas*, combination therapy (i.e. ticarcillin, piperacillin, or ceftazidime plus an aminoglycoside) should be continued for the duration of treatment.

Purpura Fulminans

Purpura fulminans (PF) is a potentially disabling and life-threatening disorder characterized by an acute onset of progressive cutaneous hemorrhage and necrosis caused by dermal vascular thrombosis, and disseminated intravascular necrosis (DIC).[41] Purpura fulminans usually arises in previously healthy neonates who become systemically ill, especially from meningococcal sepsis, varicella, pneumococcal sepsis, and meningitis.[42]

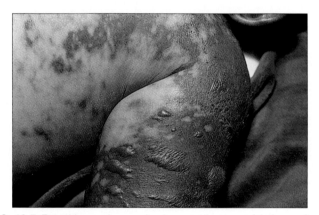

FIG. 12-7 Petechiae and purpuric plaques of purpura fulminans due to *N. meningitidis*.

Cutaneous Findings

Cutaneous erythema with or without edema and petechiae develops first. Sites of involvement appear transiently to resemble ecchymoses, and up to this point the pathologic process in the skin is reversible without progression to necrosis. Lesions evolve rapidly into painful, indurated, well-demarcated, irregularly bordered purpuric papules and plaques surrounded by a thin, advancing erythematous border. Late findings in necrotic areas are the formation of vesicles and bullae, which mark the development of hemorrhagic necrosis (Fig. 12-7), and finally firm eschar, which ultimately sloughs. The distal extremities are often the most severely involved, usually in a symmetric manner. This is probably a result of fewer collateral channels for tissue perfusion, and the relatively greater impact of circulatory collapse on perfusion of distal vascular beds. Acute infectious PF tends to progress proximally to form purpuric plaques of various sizes and shapes in a patchy distribution.

Extracutaneous Findings

Shock is characteristic of acute infectious PF, and the development of systemic consumptive coagulopathy (i.e. DIC) is a defining feature. Thrombohemorrhagic manifestations may be found in multiple vascular beds and organ systems, and multiple organ dysfunction syndromes are common. Massive non-traumatic subdural hematoma can occur in extremely premature infants. Fibrinogen, coagulation factors (e.g. factors V and VIII), and platelets are consumed in ongoing thrombosis and fibrinolysis. Prothrombin time (PT) and partial thromboplastin time (PTT) are prolonged; fibrin degradation products (e.g. D-dimers) are elevated; and protein C, protein S, and antithrombin III levels are reduced.

Etiology/Pathogenesis
Purpura fulminans develops in 15–25% of individuals with meningococcemia.[43] In the neonate, acute infectious PF may be caused by early- or late-onset group B streptococcus (GBS) disease, or occasionally a number of other Gram-positive and Gram-negative pathogens. PF results from an imbalance between anticoagulant and procoagulant activities of endothelial cells, shifting to a state of increased coagulation. This shift to a procoagulant state is triggered by endotoxin, producing an increase in interleukin (IL)-2, interferon-γ, tumor necrosis factor (TNF)-β, and IL-1, and leading to consumption of proteins C and S and antithrombin III.[41]

Diagnosis
Neisseria meningitidis can sometimes be identified as the cause of PF initially by finding the Gram-negative diplococci on Gram stain of material obtained by needle aspiration of a petechial skin lesion,[44] or by scraping the lesion with a needle and making a smear of blood.[45] The histopathologic hallmarks of PF are dermal vascular thrombosis and secondary hemorrhagic necrosis.[46] Vasculitis, including a perivascular neutrophilic infiltrate, is a characteristic feature.

Differential Diagnosis
Purpura fulminans in the neonatal period may be a manifestation of inherited, homozygous protein C, or rarely, protein S deficiency.[47] Congenitally acquired infection with rubella, toxoplasmosis, and cytomegalovirus, and postnatally acquired infection with herpes simplex virus, viral hepatitis, Coxsackie-A virus, enterovirus, and respiratory syncytial virus, can produce PF. Purpura fulminans can develop from birth trauma, blood group incompatibility, neonatal isoimmune thrombocytopenia, maternal idiopathic thrombocytopenia purpura, maternal lupus erythematosus, drugs administered to the mother, Kasabach–Merritt syndrome, thrombocytopenia absent radius (TAR) syndrome, congenital Letterer–Siwe disease, disseminated intravascular coagulation (DIC), congenital leukemia, and child abuse.[48]

Course/Management/Treatment/Prognosis
The size of the skin hemorrhage increases with disease severity, and the presence of purpura, particularly when generalized, is associated with high morbidity and mortality.[49] Many who survive PF have cutaneous and/or skeletal deformities resulting from gangrene. Initial management of the patient with acute infectious PF must be focused on preserving life through respiratory and hemodynamic support and prompt broad-spectrum intravenous antibiotic coverage. Antibiotic therapy can be adjusted after the organism has been recovered and its susceptibility profile determined. Third-generation cephalosporins are the drugs of choice for susceptible isolates of N. meningitidis.[50] Surgical consultation should be sought early in the course to monitor compartment pressures and intervene in compartment syndrome. Nutritional support is also important and should be continued during the rehabilitative phase.

Therapeutic interventions that should be initiated for all patients with PF and DIC include vitamin K and fresh frozen plasma (FFP, 8–12 mg/kg every 12 hours) to correct possible deficiencies of vitamin K-dependent coagulation factors, antithrombin III, protein C, and protein S. A number of other newer, nonconventional treatment modalities are available in some centers, including concentrates of protein C or antithrombin III, recombinant tissue-type plasminogen activator, prostacyclin, plasmapheresis, hyperbaric oxygen, and a host of targeted immunotherapies (e.g. IL-1 receptor antagonist, monoclonal antibody to TNF-β, anti-endotoxin antibodies, platelet-activating factor receptor antagonist, and pentoxifylline).[41]

Close contacts of patients with invasive meningococcal disease should receive prophylaxis with rifampin (or possibly ciprofloxacin for those aged 18 or over) as soon as possible. Patients with complement or properdin deficiency should be vaccinated with tetravalent meningococcal vaccine (A/C/Y/W135) after the age of 2 years.

OTHER INFECTIOUS AGENTS

Group B Streptococcus

Group B streptococcus or Streptococcus agalactiae, a Gram-positive coccus, is one of the most common causes of neonatal septicemia in developed countries. As with listeriosis, there are early and late forms of GBS disease. Early-onset disease presents within the first 6 days of life, although signs of infection are typically present at birth or within hours of delivery; preterm infants are particularly susceptible. Late-onset disease occurs from 7 days to 3 months of life, with a median age at onset of 27 days.

Cutaneous Findings
Cutaneous manifestations of GBS infection are rare.[51] Skin lesions, however, may be an early sign of bacteremia or, alternatively, may provide a focus of infection from which bacteremia may occur. Cellulitis is the most common cutaneous manifestation of GBS infection and characteristically develops in late-onset disease. GBS cellulitis has a predilection for the face, submental, and submandibular regions in infants less than 12 weeks of age. A rapidly progressive facial cellulitis with ipsilateral submandibular adenitis and pulmonary consolidation,[52] and inguinal, scrotal, prepatellar, or retropharyngeal cellulitis may also occur. This organism can cause vesicles, bullae, and erosions that resemble impetigo. The lesions may be present at birth and appear anywhere on the body. Additional cutaneous manifestations of GBS infection include abscesses of the scalp, breast, submandibular gland, and subcutaneous tissue; erythema nodosum-like lesions; conjunctivitis; necrotizing fasciitis; acute necrotizing cellulitis of the scrotum; and purpura fulminans.

Extracutaneous Findings
Early-onset disease is characterized by septicemia, respiratory distress, apnea, shock, pneumonia, and less commonly meningitis (5–15%). Bacteremia without a focus of infection (40–50%) is the most common presentation of late-onset disease, although other foci such as osteomyelitis, septic arthritis, and cellulitis/adenitis may be found. Cellulitis usually is associated with bacteremia (90%).

Etiology/Pathogenesis

Cutaneous manifestations of GBS infection may be due to primary infection of the skin, often in association with surgery (e.g. circumcision) or cutaneous trauma (e.g. fetal scalp monitoring), or as a result of tertiary infection of the skin during bacteremia. Colonization of the neonate as a prelude to infection is thought to occur either in utero via the ascent of organisms, or during delivery. Approximately 30% of women are carriers of GBS, yet only 1–2% of their infants develop early-onset disease, indicating that neonatal infection reflects a complex interaction between host defenses and bacterial virulence factors. In general, the likelihood of neonatal infection increases with greater bacterial inoculum, duration of exposure, and immaturity of the host. A viral infection commonly precedes the development of late-onset disease, suggesting that alteration of epithelial surfaces may promote transepithelial entry of GBS into the bloodstream. Infants who develop either early- or late-onset disease have low levels of antibody to type III polysaccharide, one of the organism's major virulence factors.[53]

Diagnosis

The organisms may be visualized on Gram stain and recovered in cultures from skin lesions. Because skin findings may be an early indicator of occult bacteremia, evaluation should include blood and CSF cultures and a chest radiograph.

Differential Diagnosis

Other bacterial organisms producing nonnecrotizing (e.g. impetigo, cellulitis, abscesses), necrotizing (e.g. necrotizing fasciitis) soft tissue infections or purpura fulminans in the neonate can mimic GBS infection.

Course/Management/Treatment/Prognosis

Parenteral penicillin remains the drug of choice, but initial therapy for suspected GBS infection should consist of ampicillin and an aminoglycoside such as gentamicin, because this regimen provides broad coverage for the important pathogens in neonatal septicemia as well as synergic action against GBS. Once GBS has been identified as the pathogen and the bloodstream and CSF have been shown to be sterile for 24–48 hours, penicillin G alone can be given.[54] The duration of therapy required for treatment of GBS skin infections depends on the nature and severity of the infection and the involvement of other sites (e.g. bloodstream, meninges), but typically will be at least 10 days. Interestingly, many infants who present with facial cellulitis have been treated previously with systemic antibiotics, suggesting there may be sanctuary sites that harbor organisms.[55] When there is GBS-induced meningitis, 30–50% of the neonates will have permanent neurologic defects.[56] Overall mortality has improved greatly, from 50% in the 1970s to 5–6% in recent years.[57] Vaccination against GBS is potentially the most effective method of prevention, but is currently not universally available.[58]

Coagulase-Negative Staphylococcus

The normal human flora includes 13 species of coagulase-negative staphylococci (CONS). These colonize the skin of most neonates within 2–4 days of birth,[59] are of relatively low virulence, and typically do not cause infection. However, they are an important cause of sepsis in preterm infants and may cause cutaneous infection. *Staphylococcus epidermidis* is the most prevalent member of this group, making up 60–90% of the CONS on the skin. The most virulent and most important causes of clinical disease are *S. epidermidis* and *Staphylococcus haemolyticus*.

Cutaneous Findings

S. epidermidis is the most important cause of indwelling catheter-related infections. Infection can occur at the catheter exit site, along the tunnel, or at its site of insertion into the vessel. Occurrence at the latter two sites can lead to bacteremia. Signs of catheter-related cutaneous infection include erythema, tenderness, and the presence of exudate at the exit site. The most common cutaneous infections in neonates resulting from CONS are omphalitis and abscesses, particularly of the breast and scalp (see earlier sections). Skin abscesses have been reported in a significant proportion (e.g. 40% in one series) of low-birthweight infants with septicemia due to CONS.[60] Postoperative wound infections and purulent exudative conjunctivitis also may occur.

Extracutaneous Findings

These organisms typically cause indolent disease, although they are capable of producing fulminant infections. In developed countries the CONS are the principal agents of sepsis in premature neonates.[60,61] They also are an important cause of septicemia in neonates in many developing countries. Additional extracutaneous infections caused by CONS include infective endocarditis, CSF shunt infections, necrotizing enterocolitis, pneumonia, urinary tract infection, and osteomyelitis.

Etiology/Pathogenesis

Infection occurs in those with disruption of host defense mechanisms resulting from surgery, placement of an indwelling medical device, or immunosuppression. Overall, CONS infections are most important in preterm neonates, particularly those with an indwelling medical device, and in febrile immunocompromised oncology patients. Colonization of the skin is a prerequisite for infection, and development of disease generally requires compromise of the epidermal barrier. Heavy skin colonization is a risk factor for the development of catheter-related infection. The increased incidence of infection in preterm infants is probably due to the defective neutrophil oxidative burst compared to term infants.[62]

Diagnosis

Gram stain and cultures of skin and blood are required. Because this organism colonizes the skin, clinical correlation is necessary to determine whether it is the cause of the clinical disease.

Differential Diagnosis

Skin infections resulting from CONS must be differentiated from infections caused by other bacterial pathogens.

Course/Management/Treatment/Prognosis

Strict handwashing is essential to limit the spread of CONS within the neonatal nursery. Vancomycin is generally begun empirically when infection is suspected or demonstrated, because resistance to penicillin, methicillin (approximately 60%), and gentamicin is common among hospital-acquired isolates. All severe infections should be treated with vancomycin. The treatment regimen can be modified appropriately once antibiotic susceptibility results are available. Infections resulting from penicillin-susceptible, β-lactamase-negative organisms can be treated with penicillin. Nafcillin is effective for treatment of penicillin-resistant strains that are susceptible to penicillinase- resistant penicillins. Penicillinase-resistant isolates should also be considered cross-resistant to cephalosporins.

Methicillin-Resistant *Staphylococcus Aureus*

In 1961, the first strains of *Staphylococcus aureus* resistant to methicillin (MRSA) were identified in hospitalized patients. Since that time, there has been a steady increase in such strains in the USA. During the late 1990s, MRSA emerged in the community setting in individuals with no known nosocomial risk factors. Over the last several years, community-acquired MRSA has significantly increased in prevalence and has become a major public health concern. Because of antibiotic resistance patterns, virulence factors, and clinical patterns of disease, community-acquired MRSA is thought to have evolved from methicillin-sensitive strains of *S. aureus*. These strains have recently surfaced in neonatal intensive care units.[63,64] This 'reverse penetration' of community-acquired strains into the hospital setting is being seen with increased frequency, leading some authors to suggest that it is more important to consider an organism's virulence factors, rather than where an infection was acquired (i.e. community versus hospital).[65] Patients should classified as having community-onset MRSA without healthcare-associated risk factors, community-onset MRSA with healthcare-associated risk factors, or hospital-acquired MRSA infection.[65]

Cutaneous Findings

MRSA causes superficial and deep infections and toxin-mediated disease similar to methicillin-sensitive strains. MRSA causes impetigo (Fig. 12-8), bullous impetigo, orbital cellulitis,[22] abscesses, scalded skin syndrome, necrotizing fasciitis and toxic shock syndrome. Furunculosis with deep abscess formation is characteristic for community-acquired MRSA.

Extracutaneous Findings

In the neonatal period, bacteremia without cutaneous signs is the most frequently encountered disorder. Necrotizing pneu-

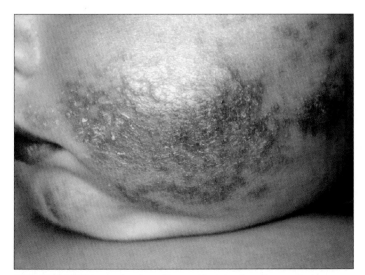

FIG. 12-8 MRSA causing impetigo on the cheeks of a newborn.

monia and osteomyelitis are two more common extracutaneous findings.

Etiology/Pathogenesis

Strains of MRSA have been grouped primarily by the type of resistance genes that they carry in a genetic element referred to as the cassette chromosome element called SCCMEC (SCCmec). Nosocomial MRSA contains types 1, 2, and 3 SCCmec, conferring multidrug resistance to non-β-lactam antibiotics. Community-acquired MRSA contains type 4 or 5 SCCmec, making this strain more susceptible to antimicrobial agents.[63,65] MRSA carries many virulence factors that are essential in determining the type and extent of disease. Panton–Valentine leukocidin (PVL) is a common virulence factor associated with community-acquired MRSA. Patients infected with MRSA strains carrying the PVL virulence factor are susceptible to tissue necrosis, resulting in epidemic furunculosis, deep abscesses, and necrotizing pneumonia. Other virulence factors are described in the sections covering SSSS and TSS.

Diagnosis

A neonate with suspected MRSA infection should have appropriate cultures taken from the blood, skin, and soft tissues.

Differential Diagnosis

Late-onset MRSA bacteremia must be differentiated from late-onset GBS infection.

Course/Management/Treatment/Prognosis

Outbreaks in neonatal nurseries and intensive care units (NICU) are difficult to contain, leading to a high likelihood of cross-contamination within the nursery. For superficial skin infections such as impetigo the course is self-limited, often resolving with topical antibiotic therapy such as mupirocin. Infants should be followed closely for deeper infections such as furuncles, abscesses, cellulitis, osteomyelitis, endocarditis, and pneumonia. Infants with deeper cutaneous infections require parenteral therapy with vancomycin for at least 10 days after documentation of a negative blood culture. Linezolid also shows excellent activity against MRSA. The mortality rate in NICUs due to MRSA infection has been as high as 38% in some cohorts. Mortality rates are highest in infants developing bacteremia and septic shock.[63–65] Late-onset neonatal sepsis, occurring 2–3 weeks after birth, has been seen with nosocomial MRSA infections. Thus, patients should be followed closely, even if they appear healthy.

Listeria Monocytogenes

Listeria monocytogenes is an uncommon cause of infection in newborn infants, with an incidence of 5.2 cases per 100 000 live births. Worldwide, however, it is one of the three major causes of neonatal meningitis.[66] Similar to infection with group B streptococcus, affected infants present with disease shortly after birth, or with a late-onset form that generally develops between 2 and 5 weeks of life. Skin lesions, however, have only been described in early-onset disease.

Cutaneous Findings

Lesions usually are evident at birth. Generalized petechiae and erythematous macules progress to erythematous pustules.[67] Purulent conjunctivitis may also occur. Focal infection may occur from direct skin inoculation. Granulomatosis infantisepticum are widely disseminated granulomas that are characteristic of severe Listerial disease.[66] These lesions are not only on the skin but can be seen in the liver, placenta, brain, spleen, kidneys, lungs, and GI tract.

Extracutaneous Findings
Neonates with early-onset disease generally are delivered prematurely to mothers with a febrile illness and are septicemic (80%). Other symptoms include acute respiratory distress, pneumonia, meningitis, and myocarditis. Late-onset disease is usually seen days to weeks after an uncomplicated full-term delivery, with signs of sepsis or meningitis, including irritability, fever, lethargy, and diarrhea.

Etiology/Pathogenesis
L. monocytogenes is a Gram-positive, motile coccobacillus that may resemble diphtheroids, cocci, or diplococci. The organism is usually transmitted via the consumption or aspiration of contaminated meat, dairy products, or raw vegetables.[66] Affected pregnant women develop an influenza-like illness that may include vertical transmission to the fetus via hematogenous spread to the placenta, from an ascending vaginal infection, or during passage through the birth canal.[68] Rarely, infection may result from cross-contamination in the delivery suite or nursery. The highest concentrations of organisms are found in the lungs and gut of the neonate, suggesting that infection may be acquired in utero via infected amniotic fluid. The organism has a predilection for the placenta and, once invasive disease has occurred, the central nervous system.

Diagnosis
A full sepsis evaluation should be performed in infants with suspected listeriosis, including bacterial cultures of the blood, urine, and CSF. The diagnosis may be aided by obtaining Gram stains and cultures from the mother's vagina, the amniotic fluid, and the infant's meconium, gastric washings, skin, posterior pharynx, and conjunctivae. Gram staining of meconium may be particularly revealing in granulomatosis infantisepticum. Cutaneous pustules show Gram-positive rods, but the organism may appear as cocci in pairs and simulate pneumococcus. L. monocytogenes also can produce white plaques on the surface of the cord. Serologic tests are not useful because of lack of sensitivity.

Differential Diagnosis
Other pathogens that can cause a generalized vesiculopustular eruption must be excluded (see Chapter 10). The other pathogen that characteristically shows involvement of the umbilical cord is Candida sp.

Course/Management/Treatment/Prognosis
Infection acquired in utero may result in death of the fetus or congenital listeriosis. Early-onset Listeria infection in the first 2 days of life carries a 30% mortality rate, although mortality rates up to 38–60% have been reported.[68,69] L. monocytogenes is sensitive to many antibiotics, including penicillin, ampicillin, erythromycin, sulfamethoxazole, trimethoprim, chloramphenicol, rifampim, tetracyclines and aminoglycosides, but it is always resistant to cephalosporins.[70] Initial therapy is parenteral ampicillin and an aminoglycoside, such as gentamicin, which provides synergy against L. monocytogenes. After an

adequate clinical response has been achieved, a course of therapy (10–14 days for invasive disease without meningitis, 2–3 weeks if meningitis is present) can be completed with ampicillin or penicillin alone.[66]

Treponema Pallidum
Congenital syphilis (CS) occurs in infants born to mothers infected with the spirochete T. pallidum. In the 1980s and 1990s, the number of reported cases of CS and maternal syphilis in the United States increased, but since 1991 they have declined every year. Between 28% and 35% of neonates with CS had mothers who did not receive prenatal care.[71] The lack of historical and laboratory data to make a diagnosis of CS in these cases emphasizes the importance of recognizing the dermatologic features of the disease.

Congenital syphilis is divided into early and late disease. Early disease usually presents before 3 months of age, although signs can appear anytime in the first 2 years of life. Late disease appears after age 2 years.

Cutaneous Findings
Overall, approximately half of newborns with CS are asymptomatic at birth. Cutaneous findings, although highly variable, are present in only 38% of those affected.[72] The palmar/plantar, perioral, and anogenital regions are classically involved. Mucous membrane involvement may present as snuffles (syphilitic rhinitis), which is often the first sign of CS. Syphilitic rhinitis begins as clear nasal discharge that may be mistaken clinically for a viral upper respiratory infection and may become profuse, chronic, and/or bloody. Associated inflammation and ulceration of the nasal mucosa can result in perforation of the nasal septum, with subsequent alteration of the nasal cartilage (saddle nose deformity). Condyloma lata refers to the highly infectious flat-topped papules and plaques that occur at the mucocutaneous junctions of the nares, angles of the mouth, and in the anogenital region; chronic induration in these areas leads to rhagades, or linear scars, which fan out from the corners of the mouth and the affected orifices. Mucous patches may also occur on the lips, tongue, and palate. Other early findings include petechiae (usually from thrombocytopenia), hemorrhagic vesicles and bullae (pemphigus syphiliticus), and erythematous macular, papulosquamous, annular, or polymorphous eruptions (Fig. 12-9). The papulosquamous eruption is most common on the posterior aspects, particularly the buttocks, back, and thighs, in addition to the soles. Although the papulosquamous rash resembles the coppery-red eruption of acquired secondary syphilis, pemphigus syphiliticus is unique to the newborn. Bullae form on an indurated, red base and rupture easily, leaving a macerated area that may form crusts. Changes on the palms and soles include erythema with a polished appearance; superficial peeling; indurated fissures; and oval ham-colored macules and papules that acquire a coppery-brown color as they age. Nail deformities, paronychia, and alopecia may occur. Untreated skin lesions resolve in 1–3 months with postinflammatory hyperpigmentation and/or hypopigmentation, but dyspigmentation is infrequent in the newborn period.

Extracutaneous Findings
CS commonly presents with extracutaneous findings that include low birthweight, hepatomegaly with elevation of serum alkaline phosphatase, splenomegaly, anemia, thrombocytope-

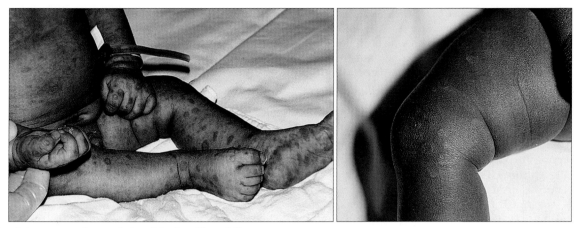

FIG. 12-9 Papulosquamous plaques in two infants with syphilis.

nia, jaundice, osteochondritis, generalized lymphadenopathy, respiratory distress, hydrops fetalis, meningitis, meningoencephalitis, nephrotic syndrome, chorioretinitis, and pseudoparalysis.[72] Late manifestations (i.e. appearing after 2 years of age) involve the central nervous system (neurosyphilis, which may be asymptomatic), bones (frontal bossing, saddle nose, concave central face, saber shins, Clutton's joints), teeth (Hutchinson peg-shaped notched central incisors, mulberry multicuspid first molars), skin (rhagades, nodular syphilides, gummata), eyes (interstitial keratitis, optic atrophy), and ears (eighth-nerve deafness). Hutchinson's triad of defects includes interstitial keratitis, defects of the incisors, and sensorineural hearing loss.

Etiology/Pathogenesis

Infection occurs via invasion of the placenta by the spirochete *T. pallidum*. The organism enters the bloodstream directly and invades the liver, with subsequent invasion of other organs, principally the skin, mucous membranes, bones, and central nervous system. Infection can occur at any time during pregnancy or at birth. Spirochetes preferentially adhere to endothelial cells and induce vasculitis. Nearly all neonates born to mothers with primary or secondary syphilis have congenital infection, but only about 50% are clinically symptomatic at birth.[73] A high percentage will be preterm and at high risk for neurologic complications. As many as 25–40% of infected fetuses die in utero.[74] Neonates infected during the third trimester typically are normal at birth, may become ill during the first weeks of life, but most commonly show signs at 2–6 weeks of age.

Diagnosis

The laboratory diagnosis of CS may be difficult because false-positive and -negative serologies confound interpretation and because *T. pallidum* cannot be cultured on artificial media.[75] Maternal nontreponemal and treponemal IgG antibodies are present in the fetus as a result of transplacental transfer even if the mother was adequately treated during pregnancy. Serum should be taken from the infant, rather than from cord blood, to increase the accuracy of serologic test results.[76] The diagnosis can be made by demonstration of spirochetes within a clinical specimen, obtained by scraping the base of a mucocutaneous lesion, using darkfield microscopy or direct fluorescent antibody testing. Specimens from mouth lesions require direct fluorescent antibody techniques to distinguish *T. pallidum* from commensal oral spirochetes. Histopathologic exam-

ination of the placenta and umbilical cord using specific fluorescent antitreponemal antibody staining also is recommended. If a serum nontreponemal titer (VDRL, RPR) in the infant is four times the mother's level, then the diagnosis of congenital syphilis is made; a titer less than four times that of the mother, however, does not exclude CS. Nontreponemal tests in both an infected mother and her congenitally infected infant may be falsely negative if the mother acquired the disease late in pregnancy, or in the case of a prozone phenomenon. False-positive reactivity of nontreponemal tests can be caused by certain infectious diseases (e.g. hepatitis, varicella, measles, infectious mononucleosis, tuberculosis, malaria, endocarditis), malignancies (e.g. lymphoma), and connective tissue disease (e.g. systemic lupus erythematosus). The nontreponemal tests are useful for screening, and, if reactive, should always be confirmed using a treponemal test. Treponemal tests (FTA-ABS, MHA-TP) also are not 100% specific for syphilis because reactivity may occur in patients with other spirochetal diseases, such as yaws, pinta, bejel, leptospirosis, rat-bite fever, and Lyme disease. The most helpful specific serologic test is serum IgM against *T. pallidum* (IgM FTA-ABS). A CSF VDRL test should be performed on all neonates evaluated for CS, remembering that a negative result does not exclude neurosyphilis. A false-positive result, however, may occur in an uninfected newborn with a transplacentally acquired high serum VDRL titer. Newer techniques may improve our diagnostic capabilities, including immunoblotting to detect IgM against a 47 kDa membrane protein and PCR amplification of the genomic region encoding this same membrane protein.[77] A skin biopsy is helpful in the evaluation of CS and shows swelling and proliferation of endothelial cells, and a predominantly perivascular infiltrate composed of lymphoid cells and plasma cells. Radiographic abnormalities are particularly important, as they are present in up to 95% of symptomatic and 20% of asymptomatic neonates with CS.[78] Several long bones tend to be affected symmetrically, particularly the lower extremities. The metaphyseal lesions of osteochondritis vary from radio-opaque bands to punctate lucencies to mottled regions. Diaphyseal lesions appear as periosteal new bone formation.

Differential Diagnosis

As a result of the variable morphology of the lesions and the broad differential diagnosis it engenders, syphilis has been called 'the great imitator.' Blistering in CS must be differentiated from that in other vesiculobullous conditions that involve the palms and soles, including but not limited to congenital candidiasis, acropustulosis of infancy, scabies, and epidermolysis bullosa (see Chapter 10). Congenital Lyme borreliosis has been described.[79] Nontreponemal tests can be used to differentiate Lyme disease from syphilis because in the former the VDRL test is nonreactive.

Course/Management/Treatment/Prognosis

If an infant cannot be fully evaluated, or if adequate follow-up is uncertain, then empiric treatment is recommended.[76] For infants with proven or probable CS (see Centers for Disease Control and Prevention (CDC) guidelines),[76] a 10-day course of parenteral aqueous crystalline penicillin G is the treatment of choice. A sustained fourfold decrease in titer of the nontreponemal test is indicative of successful treatment; the nontreponemal test usually becomes nonreactive within 2 years of successful treatment in CS. It is recommended that infants treated for CS have follow-up examinations at 1, 2, 4, 6, and 12 months of age, including nontreponemal tests at 3, 6, and 12 months after treatment, or until they become nonreactive. If the infant was not infected and nontreponemal tests were initially positive as a result of transplacentally acquired maternal antibody, then the antibody titer should decline by 3 months of age and be nonreactive at age 6 months. A fourfold increase in titer following treatment suggests reinfection or relapse; patients with persistent, stable low titers also should be considered for retreatment. Treated infants should be followed with a CSF examination at 6-month intervals until the examination becomes nonreactive. A reactive CSF VDRL at 6 months, or cell counts that are abnormal or not steadily decreasing, are indications for retreatment.[76] Positive MHA-TP and FTA-ABS treponemal tests usually remain reactive for life, despite successful treatment. The prognosis in promptly treated early congenital syphilis is excellent.

Mycobacterium Tuberculosis

The risk of congenital tuberculosis (CT) has increased in the 1990s because of an increase in the number of tuberculosis cases in women of childbearing age. This reflects an increase in the incidence of tuberculosis overall, due in part to the human immunodeficiency virus (HIV) epidemic, as well as increased international adoption and lack of nonemergency medical care to illegal immigrants. An infant is considered to have CT if proven tuberculous lesions and one of the following criteria are present: tuberculous lesions in the first week of life; a primary hepatic complex or hepatic granulomas; tuberculous infection of the maternal genital tract or placenta; or exclusion of postnatal transmission of tuberculosis by a thorough investigation of contacts.[80] Distinguishing neonatal tuberculosis from congenital tuberculosis is not always possible. Even though the distinction is not important for treatment, identification of the person infecting the infant postnatally is important to halt the spread of infection in the community.

Cutaneous Findings

Cutaneous findings in CT are unusual and include scaly, erythematous, umbilicated papules and subcutaneous nodules.[81] Infants with postnatal genital tuberculosis following circumcision may present with firm, nontender, enlarged, inguinal lymph nodes that progress to ulcerated, suppurative, bilateral, inguinal lymphadenopathy with sinus tract formation. Exten-

sive ulceration of the penis and scrotum and varicella-like cutaneous lesions also have been described.[82]

Extracutaneous Findings

Newborns with CT are frequently premature and have low birthweight. They may be symptomatic at birth, but illness more commonly presents during the 2nd to 4th weeks of life with poor feeding, listlessness, respiratory distress, fever, hepatosplenomegaly, abdominal distension, ear discharge, and lymphadenopathy.[80] Most infected infants have abnormal chest radiographs (e.g. hilar lymphadenopathy, parenchymal infiltrates), and approximately 50% have a miliary pattern. Meningitis is present in about 20% of cases. Infants with postnatally acquired tuberculosis may present with fever, lethargy, respiratory distress, cough, vomiting, weight loss, lymphadenopathy, anemia, and hepatosplenomegaly at 4 weeks to several months after birth.[82]

Etiology/Pathogenesis

Although acid-fast bacilli can be identified in the placenta of 50% of women with tuberculosis,[80] congenital infection is quite rare. Infected mothers with miliary tuberculosis are most apt to transmit the disease. The mother of an affected infant also may have tuberculous pleural effusion, meningitis, or endometritis. Women with only pulmonary tuberculosis are unlikely to infect the infant until after birth. CT is thought to be acquired primarily via transplacental spread of *M. tuberculosis* through the umbilical vein. Transplacental spread may produce a primary focus of infection in the liver, with involvement of the periportal lymph nodes and secondary hematogenous spread to the lungs, spleen, other viscera, and the central nervous system.[80] In the neonate, tuberculosis can be acquired after birth by inhalation or ingestion of infected droplets, ingestion of infected milk, or contamination of traumatized skin or mucous membranes. Inhalation is the most common route of postnatal infection, but may be impossible to distinguish from infection acquired in utero. Infection of the skin of the head and neck or the oral mucous membranes, associated with regional lymphadenopathy, may occur by kissing. In the past, tuberculosis of the skin and mucous membranes of the male genitalia was reported 1–4 weeks after ritual circumcision by an infected operator.

Diagnosis

CT should be suspected in any infant who presents with a sepsis-like syndrome, negative bacterial cultures, and lack of response to antibiotic therapy. Diagnosis is confirmed by identification of *M. tuberculosis* in tissue (e.g. liver, lymph node, bone marrow, skin) or fluid from the stomach, trachea, urinary tract, bone marrow, middle ear, or pleural spaces. False-positive smears from gastric aspirates in a newborn are rare. The CSF frequently is negative. Acid-fast stains are helpful if they are positive. Because *M. tuberculosis* is slow growing, it may take up to 10 weeks to detect the organism on solid media; use of a DNA probe may allow earlier detection. The Mantoux skin test, performed with 5 TU PPD (tuberculin purified protein derivative) is usually negative and may take 3 weeks to 3 months to become positive. The placenta should be examined and cultured, and the mother evaluated for the presence of tuberculosis, including uterine infection.

Course/Management/Treatment/Prognosis

The course of CT may vary from acute and fulminant to subacute and insidious. The overall mortality is 38% without

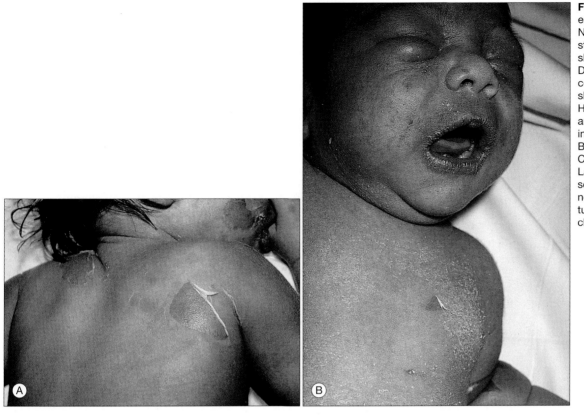

FIG. 12-10 (A) Diffuse erythroderma and Nikolsky's sign in staphylococcal scalded skin syndrome. (From Darmstadt GL. Staphylococcal and streptococcal skin infections. In: Harahap M, ed. Diagnosis and treatment of skin infections. Oxford: Blackwell Science, 1997; Courtesy of Alfred T. Lane.) (B) Staphylococcal scalded skin syndrome: note the perioral accentuation which is characteristic.

treatment and 22% with treatment.[80] Treatment for CT and postnatally acquired disease is the same and should be initiated promptly, regardless of skin test results, with isoniazid, rifampin, pyrazinamide, and streptomycin or kanamycin. Information on the drug susceptibility of the isolate from the infant and/or mother will help direct therapy. Identification of the source for infection of the neonate is important to prevent infection of others.

TOXIN-MEDIATED DISEASE

Exotoxin-mediated diseases are caused by the effects of extracellular toxins produced at a focus of infection or colonization. The site of bacterial replication is typically inconspicuous in relation to the clinical effects of the toxins. Toxins can act locally, as in bullous impetigo, or can cause widespread clinical signs resulting from hematogenous spread, as seen in scalded skin syndrome.

Staphylococcal Scalded Skin Syndrome

Staphylococcal scalded skin syndrome (SSSS) is a staphylococcal epidermolytic toxin-mediated disease characterized by cutaneous tenderness and superficial, widespread blistering and/or desquamation.[83] In the neonatal period, it can result in nursery outbreaks.[84]

Cutaneous Findings

Exquisite tenderness of the skin may herald the onset of SSSS. Generalized macular erythema evolves rapidly into a scarlatiniform eruption that is accentuated in flexural and periorificial areas (Fig. 12-10). The brightly erythematous skin acquires a

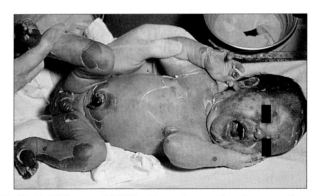

FIG. 12-11 Widespread SSSS with erosions and scaly areas of desquamation.

wrinkled appearance, leading to thick flaky desquamation, particularly in the flexures, over approximately 2–5 days. In severe cases, the erythrodermic phase is followed by the development of diffuse, sterile, flaccid blisters and erosions, and diffuse, bullous desquamation of large sheets of skin (Fig. 12-11; see also Fig. 16-12). At this stage, areas of epidermis may separate in response to a gentle shear force (Nikolsky's sign). As large sheets of epidermis peel away, moist, glistening, denuded areas become apparent, initially in the flexures and subsequently over much of the body surface. As the exposed denuded skin dries, it develops a crusted, flaky appearance. Distinctive radial crusting and fissuring around the eyes, mouth, and nose develop approximately 2–5 days after the onset of erythroderma. Secondary cutaneous infection, cellulitis, omphalitis, and severe surgical wound infections may occur.

Extracutaneous Findings

Complications may include excessive fluid loss, electrolyte imbalance, faulty temperature regulation, pneumonia, endocarditis, and septicemia. Mortality, due predominantly to sepsis, is unusual, but is highest in the severe generalized form of the disease.

Etiology/Pathogenesis

SSSS is caused predominantly by phage group II staphylococci, particularly strains 71 and 55; occasionally, a group I or III isolate is involved.[85] Foci of infection include the nasopharynx, or less commonly the umbilicus, urinary tract, a cutaneous wound, conjunctivae, blood, and rarely through breastfeeding.[86] These bacteria produce epidermolytic (i.e. exfoliative or exfoliating) toxins A, B, and/or D.[87,88] ETB is more frequently associated with generalized SSSS than ETA. A reduced concentration of antibodies directed against ETB and an increased ability to penetrate into the bloodstream may explain why ETB is associated more frequently with SSSS.[9] These epidermolytic toxins induce bulla formation by cleaving desmoglein I within desmosomes, via serine proteases. The severity of the disease is related to the toxin load, rather than the nature of the focal infection, and this load may be particularly high in neonates owing to reduced renal clearance.[85]

Diagnosis

Recovery of a toxin-producing strain of *S. aureus* in an infant with widespread blistering establishes the diagnosis of SSSS.[83] Although intact bullae on the skin are sterile, cultures should be obtained from multiple sites, including the blood, cerebrospinal fluid, nasopharynx, urine, umbilicus, and any suspected sites of localized infection, in an attempt to identify the source of the epidermolytic toxins. Histopathologically, subcorneal bulla formation through the granular layer without an inflammatory infiltrate is characteristic (Fig. 12-12). In cases that demand a rapid diagnosis, the exfoliated corneal layer can be seen on a frozen biopsy specimen of the desquamating epidermis. Scattered acantholytic cells that are evident histopathologically in the cleft-like bullae can also be seen in a Tzanck preparation.

Differential Diagnosis

SSSS may be mistaken for a number of other blistering and exfoliating disorders, including scarlet fever, bullous impetigo, Kawasaki disease, epidermolysis bullosa, diffuse cutaneous mastocytosis, familial peeling skin syndrome with eosino-philia, epidermolytic hyperkeratosis, viral exanthema, drug eruption, erythema multiforme, and drug-induced toxic epidermal necrolysis (TEN; Lyell's disease). TEN often can be distinguished by a history of drug ingestion, the presence of Nikolsky's sign only at sites of erythema, and absence of perioral crusting. The differentiation of TEN from SSSS may occasionally require a skin biopsy. TEN results in full-thickness epidermal necrosis, with a blister cleavage plane in the lowermost epidermis. Distinguishing between these conditions is particularly important because mortality rates as high as 30% have been reported with TEN, and avoidance of the offending drug is crucial to prevent recurrence.

Course/Management/Treatment/Prognosis

Recovery usually is rapid once appropriate antibiotic therapy is begun. Parenteral nafcillin or methicillin should be given promptly. Strict isolation is imperative to avoid the spread of infection. See Chapters 10 and 11 for skin care recommendations in blistering diseases. General principles include minimizing the handling of the infant, and the use of emollients (e.g. petrolatum and petroleum jelly gauze) and semiocclusive dressings to provide lubrication and minimize pain. Corticosteroids are detrimental and should be avoided. Healing occurs without scarring in 10–14 days.

Toxic Shock Syndrome

Streptococcal toxic shock syndrome (STSS) is characterized by acute onset of shock and multisystem organ failure, caused by *Streptococcus pyogenes* infection at a normally sterile site.[89] It is very rare in newborns.

Etiology/Pathogenesis

STSS is associated with an invasive infection. Most patients are bacteremic and/or have focal tissue infection at the time of presentation. Streptococcal toxic shock syndrome develops most often in the setting of a minor, focal skin and/or soft tissue infection, which presumably provides a portal of entry.[90] There is production of an exotoxin, which acts as a superantigen that can activate the immune system by bypassing the usual antigen-mediated immune response system.[91] Lack of antibody against exotoxin appears to be a risk factor for severe, invasive disease and STSS.[91] Most isolates of *S. pyogenes* that cause STSS are M protein types 1, 3, 12, and 28 that produce streptococcal pyrogenic exotoxins A and/or B.[90,92,93]

Cutaneous Findings

Most patients have localized swelling and erythema at a site of exquisite pain. The development of vesicles and bullae (5%) is a late, ominous sign of tissue devitalization.[94,95] Patients without soft tissue infection have a variety of focal infections, including endophthalmitis, osteomyelitis, myositis, pneumonia, perihepatitis, peritonitis, myocarditis, and sepsis.[95] Other cutaneous signs in a minority of patients include a petechial, maculopapular, or diffuse scarlatiniform eruption.

Extracutaneous Findings

Streptococcal TSS is characterized by acute onset and early, frequently fulminant progression to shock and multiorgan compromise or failure. The most common presenting sign is fever, generally accompanied by tachycardia and hypotension. Patients rapidly develop hypotensive shock, often accompanied by early renal impairment and onset of respiratory dis-

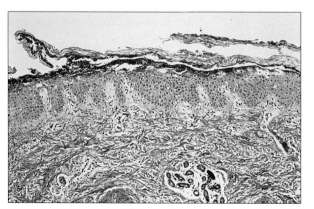

FIG. 12-12 Skin biopsy of SSSS reveals a subcorneal split at the level of the stratum granulosum.

tress syndrome. Renal impairment tends to progress for the first few days regardless of therapy, often necessitating dialysis, but function generally is regained. Toxic cardiomyopathy is a life-threatening complication that is characterized by decreased contractility and cardiac output and refractory shock. Laboratory abnormalities, including hemoglobinuria, elevation of serum creatinine, and leukocytosis with a marked left shift develop early and reflect the multiorgan system dysfunction. As the disease progresses, most patients display hypoalbuminemia, hypocalcemia, anemia, and thrombocytopenia. Soft tissue infection, particularly the development of necrotizing fasciitis and myositis, is reflected in an elevation of creatine phosphokinase.[90,95]

Diagnosis

A definitive diagnosis of STSS requires isolation of *S. pyogenes* from a normally sterile site in a patient with hypotension and multiorgan failure.

Course/Management/Treatment/Prognosis

Patients suspected of having STSS should be managed in an intensive care setting because of the rapidly progressive, fulminant nature of the syndrome. Management consists of aggressive intravenous fluid resuscitation, culture of potential sites of infection, early surgical exploration of suspected deep-seated infections with debridement of devitalized tissue, and prompt administration of antibiotics. Inotropic agents may be necessary to manage shock due to toxic cardiomyopathy. The use of epinephrine (adrenaline) in patients with intractable hypotension may be complicated by gangrene of digits. The use of intravenous immunoglobulins is still controversial. While ruling out septic shock from Gram-negative bacilli or polymicrobial necrotizing fasciitis, broad-spectrum antimicrobial therapy should be initiated, as discussed for necrotizing fasciitis. Once a diagnosis of STSS is made, therapy can be tailored. Clindamycin has advantages over penicillin, although many experts recommend the concurrent use of both agents.[96]

REFERENCES

1. Larson AA, Dinulos JG. Cutaneous bacterial infections in the newborn. Curr Opin Pediatr 2005; 17: 481–485.
2. Darmstadt GL, Lane AT. Impetigo: an overview. Pediatr Dermatol 1994; 11: 293–303.
3. Leyden JJ, Marples RR, Kligman AM. *Staphylococcus aureus* in the lesions of atopic dermatitis. Br J Dermatol 1974; 90: 525–530.
4. Florman AL, Holzman RS. Nosocomial scalded skin syndrome. Ritter's disease caused by phage group 3 *Staphylococcus aureus*. Am J Dis Child 1980; 134: 1043–1045.
5. Sandhu K, Kanwar AJ. Generalized bullous impetigo in a neonate. Pediatr Dermatol 2004; 21: 667–669.
6. Hebert AA, Esterly NB. Bacterial and candidal cutaneous infections in the neonate. Dermatol Clin 1986; 4: 3–21.
7. Watkins P. Impetigo: aetiology, complications and treatment options. Nurs Stand 2005; 19: 50–54.
8. Hanakawa Y, Schechter NM, Lin C, et al. Molecular mechanisms of blister formation in bullous impetigo and staphylococcal scalded skin syndrome. J Clin Invest 2002; 110: 53–60.
9. Yamasaki O, Yamaguchi T, Sugai M, et al. Clinical manifestations of staphylococcal scalded-skin syndrome depend on serotypes of exfoliative toxins. J Clin Microbiol 2005; 43: 1890–1893.
10. Darmstadt GL. Antibiotics in the management of pediatric skin disease. Dermatol Clin 1998; 16: 509–525.
11. Koning S, van der Wouden JC. Treatment for impetigo. Br Med J 2004; 329: 695–696.
12. Sladden MJ, Johnston GA. More common skin infections in children. Bmj 2005; 330: 1194–1198.
13. Wollina U. Acute paronychia: comparative treatment with topical antibiotic alone or in combination with corticosteroid. J Eur Acad Dermatol Venereol 2001; 15: 82–84.
14. Brook I. Aerobic and anaerobic microbiology of paronychia. Ann Emerg Med 1990; 19: 994–996.
15. Russo F, Collantes C, Guerrero J. Severe paronychia due to zidovudine-induced neutropenia in a neonate. J Am Acad Dermatol 1999; 40: 322–324.
16. Guvenc H, Aygun AD, Yasar F, et al. Omphalitis in term and preterm appropriate for gestational age and small for gestational age infants. J Trop Pediatr 1997; 43: 368–372.
17. Manzar S, Nair AK, Pai MG, Al-Khusaiby SM. Omphalitis and necrotizing fasciitis in neonates. Saudi Med J 2004; 25: 2044–2045.
18. Ameh EA, Nmadu PT. Major complications of omphalitis in neonates and infants. Pediatr Surg Int 2002; 18: 413–416.
19. Sadow KB, Chamberlain JM. Blood cultures in the evaluation of children with cellulitis. Pediatrics 1998; 101: E4.
20. Howe PM, Eduardo Fajardo J, Orcutt MA. Etiologic diagnosis of cellulitis: comparison of aspirates obtained from the leading edge and the point of maximal inflammation. Pediatr Infect Dis J 1987; 6: 685–686.
21. Molarte AB, Isenberg SJ. Periorbital cellulitis in infancy. J Ophthalm Nurs Techn 1990; 9: 106–109.
22. Anari S, Karagama YG, Fulton B, Wilson JA. Neonatal disseminated methicillin-resistant *Staphylococcus aureus* presenting as orbital cellulitis. J Laryngol Otol 2005; 119: 64–67.
23. Howe L, Jones NS. Guidelines for the management of periorbital cellulitis/abscess. Clin Otolaryngol Allied Sci 2004; 29: 725–728.
24. Stricker T, Navratil F, Sennhauser FH. Mastitis in early infancy. Acta Paediatr 2005; 94: 166–169.
25. Brook I. The aerobic and anaerobic microbiology of neonatal breast abscess. Pediatr Infect Dis J 1991; 10: 785–786.
26. Cordero L, Anderson CW, Zuspan FP. Scalp abscess: a benign and infrequent complication of fetal monitoring. Am J Obstet Gynecol 1983; 146: 126–130.
27. Brook I, Frazier EH. Microbiology of scalp abscess in newborns. Pediatr Infect Dis J 1992; 11: 766–768.
28. Nazir Z. Necrotizing fasciitis in neonates. Pediatr Surg Int 2005; 21: 641–644.
29. Krebs VL, Koga KM, Diniz EM, et al. Necrotizing fasciitis in a newborn infant: a case report. Rev Hosp Clin Fac Med Sao Paulo 2001; 56: 59–62.
30. Bliss DP, Jr, Healey PJ, Waldhausen JH. Necrotizing fasciitis after Plastibell circumcision. J Pediatr 1997; 131: 459–462.
31. Bodemer C, Panhans A, Chretien-Marquet B, et al. Staphylococcal necrotizing fasciitis in the mammary region in childhood: a report of five cases. J Pediatr 1997; 131: 466–469.
32. Ignacio RC, Falcone RA, Jr, Warner BW. Necrotizing fasciitis: a rare complication of neonatal necrotizing enterocolitis. J Pediatr Surg 2005; 40: 1805–1807.
33. Epps C, Brown M. Necrotizing fasciitis: a case study. Neonatal Netw 1997; 16: 19–25.
34. Weinberger M, Haynes RE, Morse TS. Necrotizing fasciitis in a neonate. Am J Dis Child 1972; 123: 591–594.
35. Siddiqi SF, Taylor PM. Necrotizing fasciitis of the scalp. A complication of fetal monitoring. Am J Dis Child 1982; 136: 226–228.
36. Farrell LD, Karl SR, Davis PK, et al. Postoperative necrotizing fasciitis in children. Pediatrics 1988; 82: 874–879.
37. Sawin RS, Schaller RT, Tapper D, et al. Early recognition of neonatal abdominal wall necrotizing fasciitis. Am J Surg 1994; 167: 481–484.
38. Stamenkovic I, Lew PD. Early recognition of potentially fatal necrotizing fasciitis. The use of frozen-section biopsy. N Engl J Med 1984; 310: 1689–1693.

39. Hughes JR, Newbould M, du Vivier AW, Greenough A. Fatal *Pseudomonas* septicemia and vasculitis in a premature infant. Pediatr Dermatol 1998; 15: 122–124.

40. Gunes T, Akcakus M, Kurtoglu S, et al. Harlequin baby with ecthyma gangrenosum. Pediatr Dermatol 2003; 20: 529–530.

41. Darmstadt GL. Acute infectious purpura fulminans: pathogenesis and medical management. Pediatr Dermatol 1998; 15: 169–183.

42. Gurgey A, Aytac S, Kanra G, et al. Outcome in children with purpura fulminans: report on 16 patients. Am J Hematol 2005; 80: 20–25.

43. Wong VK, Hitchcock W, Mason WH. Meningococcal infections in children: a review of 100 cases. Pediatr Infect Dis J 1989; 8: 224–227.

44. van Deuren M, van Dijke BJ, Koopman RJ, et al. Rapid diagnosis of acute meningococcal infections by needle aspiration or biopsy of skin lesions. Br Med J 1993; 306: 1229–1232.

45. Periappuram M, Taylor MR, Keane CT. Rapid detection of meningococci from petechiae in acute meningococcal infection. J Infect 1995; 31: 201–203.

46. Adcock DM, Hicks MJ. Dermatopathology of skin necrosis associated with purpura fulminans. Semin Thromb Hemost 1990; 16: 283–292.

47. Ezer U, Misirlioglu ED, Colba V, et al. Neonatal purpura fulminans due to homozygous protein C deficiency. Pediatr Hematol Oncol 2001; 18: 453–458.

48. Katier N, Traen M, De Dooy J, Geyskens L, Mahieu L. Neonatal purpura due to *Neisseria meningitidis* serogroup C infection. Eur J Pediatr 2003; 162: 283–284.

49. Brandtzaeg P, van Deuren M. Meningococcal infections at the start of the 21st century. Adv Pediatr 2005; 52: 129–162.

50. Leclerc F, Noizet O, Dorkenoo A, et al. [Treatment of meningococcal purpura fulminans]. Arch Pediatr 2001; 8: 677s–688s.

51. Lopez JB, Gross P, Boggs TR. Skin lesions in association with beta-hemolytic *Streptococcus* group B. Pediatrics 1976; 58: 859–861.

52. Baker CJ. Group B streptococcal cellulitis–adenitis in infants. Am J Dis Child 1982; 136: 631–633.

53. Shet A, Ferrieri P. Neonatal and maternal group B streptococcal infections: a comprehensive review. Indian J Med Res 2004; 120: 141–150.

54. Gibbs RS, Schrag S, Schuchat A. Perinatal infections due to group B streptococci. Obstet Gynecol 2004; 104: 1062–1076.

55. Rand TH. Group B streptococcal cellulitis in infants: a disease modified by prior antibiotic therapy or hospitalization? Pediatrics 1988; 81: 63–65.

56. El Beitune P, Duarte G, Maffei CM. Colonization by *Streptococcus agalactiae* during pregnancy: maternal and perinatal prognosis. Brazil J Infect Dis 2005; 9: 276–282.

57. Puopolo KM, Madoff LC, Eichenwald EC. Early-onset group B streptococcal disease in the era of maternal screening. Obstet Gynecol Surv 2005; 60: 637–639.

58. Law MR, Palomaki G, Alfirevic Z, et al. The prevention of neonatal group B streptococcal disease: a report by a working group of the Medical Screening Society. J Med Screen 2005; 12: 60–68.

59. D'Angio CT, McGowan KL, Baumgart S, et al. Surface colonization with coagulase-negative staphylococci in premature neonates. J Pediatr 1989; 114: 1029–1034.

60. Patrick CC. Coagulase-negative staphylococci: pathogens with increasing clinical significance. J Pediatr 1990; 116: 497–507.

61. Hall RT, Hall SL, Barnes WG, et al. Characteristics of coagulase-negative staphylococci from infants with bacteremia. Pediatr Infect Dis J 1987; 6: 377–383.

62. Bjorkqvist M, Jurstrand M, Bodin L, et al. Defective neutrophil oxidative burst in preterm newborns on exposure to coagulase-negative staphylococci. Pediatr Res 2004; 55: 966–971.

63. Regev-Yochay G, Rubinstein E, Barzilai A, et al. Methicillin-resistant *Staphylococcus aureus* in neonatal intensive care unit. Emerg Infect Dis 2005; 11: 453–456.

64. Healy CM, Hulten KG, Palazzi DL, et al. Emergence of new strains of methicillin-resistant *Staphylococcus aureus* in a neonatal intensive care unit. Clin Infect Dis 2004; 39: 1460–1466.

65. Zetola N, Francis JS, Nuermberger EL, Bishai WR. Community-acquired methicillin-resistant *Staphylococcus aureus*: an emerging threat. Lancet Infect Dis 2005; 5: 275–286.

66. Posfay-Barbe KM, Wald ER. Listeriosis. Pediatr Rev 2004; 25: 151–159.

67. Smith KJ, Yeager J, Skelton HG, 3rd, Angritt P. Diffuse petechial pustular lesions in a newborn. Disseminated *Listeria monocytogenes*. Arch Dermatol 1994; 130: 245, 248.

68. Evans JR, Allen AC, Stinson DA, et al. Perinatal listeriosis: report of an outbreak. Pediatr Infect Dis 1985; 4: 237–241.

69. McLauchlin J. Human listeriosis in Britain, 1967–85, a summary of 722 cases. 1. Listeriosis during pregnancy and in the newborn. Epidemiol Infect 1990; 104: 181–189.

70. Espaze EP, Reynaud AE. Antibiotic susceptibilities of *Listeria*: in vitro studies. Infection 1988; 16: S160–164.

71. Congenital syphilis – United States, 2002. MMWR Morb Mortal Wkly Rep 2004; 53: 716–719.

72. Chawla V, Pandit PB, Nkrumah FK. Congenital syphilis in the newborn. Arch Dis Child 1988; 63: 1393–1394.

73. Wendel GD. Gestational and congenital syphilis. Clin Perinatol 1988; 15: 287–303.

74. Evans HE, Frenkel LD. Congenital syphilis. Clin Perinatol 1994; 21: 149–162.

75. Woods CR. Syphilis in children: congenital and acquired. Semin Pediatr Infect Dis 2005; 16: 245–257.

76. Sexually transmitted diseases treatment guidelines 2002. Centers for Disease Control and Prevention. MMWR Recomm Rep 2002; 51(RR-6): 1–78.

77. Sanchez PJ. Laboratory tests for congenital syphilis. Pediatr Infect Dis J 1998; 17: 70–71.

78. Brion LP, Manuli M, Rai B, et al. Long-bone radiographic abnormalities as a sign of active congenital syphilis in asymptomatic newborns. Pediatrics 1991; 88: 1037–1040.

79. Trevisan G, Stinco G, Cinco M. Neonatal skin lesions due to a spirochetal infection: a case of congenital Lyme borreliosis? Int J Dermatol 1997; 36: 677–680.

80. Cantwell MF, Shehab ZM, Costello AM, et al. Brief report: congenital tuberculosis. N Engl J Med 1994; 330: 1051–1054.

81. McCray MK, Esterly NB. Cutaneous eruptions in congenital tuberculosis. Arch Dermatol 1981; 117: 460–464.

82. Kendig EL, Jr. Tuberculosis in the very young; report of three cases in infants less than one month of age. Am Rev Tuberc 1954; 70: 161–165.

83. Shwayder T, Akland T. Neonatal skin barrier: structure, function, and disorders. Dermatol Ther 2005; 18: 87–103.

84. Saiman L, Jakob K, Holmes KW, et al. Molecular epidemiology of staphylococcal scalded skin syndrome in premature infants. Pediatr Infect Dis J 1998; 17: 329–334.

85. Melish ME, Glasgow LA. Staphylococcal scalded skin syndrome: the expanded clinical syndrome. J Pediatr 1971; 78: 958–967.

86. Raymond J, Bingen E, Brahimi N, et al. Staphylococcal scalded skin syndrome in a neonate. Eur J Clin Microbiol Infect Dis 1997; 16: 453–454.

87. Amagai M, Matsuyoshi N, Wang ZH, et al. Toxin in bullous impetigo and staphylococcal scalded-skin syndrome targets desmoglein 1. Nature Med 2000; 6: 1275–1277.

88. Amagai M, Yamaguchi T, Hanakawa Y, et al. Staphylococcal exfoliative toxin B specifically cleaves desmoglein 1. J Invest Dermatol 2002; 118: 845–850.

89. Working Group on Severe Streptococcal Infections. Defining the group A streptococcal toxic shock syndrome. Rationale and consensus definition. JAMA 1993; 269: 390–391.

90. Stevens DL. Invasive group A streptococcal disease. Infect Agents Dis 1996; 5: 157–166.

91. Chuang YY, Huang YC, Lin TY. Toxic shock syndrome in children:

epidemiology, pathogenesis, and management. Paediatr Drugs 2005; 7: 11–25.

92. Belani K, Schlievert PM, Kaplan EL, Ferrieri P. Association of exotoxin-producing group A streptococci and severe disease in children. Pediatr Infect Dis J 1991; 10: 351–354.

93. Stevens DL. Streptococcal toxic-shock syndrome: spectrum of disease, pathogenesis, and new concepts in treatment. Emerg Infect Dis 1995; 1: 69–78.

94. Wolf JE, Rabinowitz LG. Streptococcal toxic shock-like syndrome. Arch Dermatol 1995; 131: 73–77.

95. Stevens DL, Tanner MH, Winship J, et al. Severe group A streptococcal infections associated with a toxic shock-like syndrome and scarlet fever toxin A. N Engl J Med 1989; 321: 1–7.

96. Bisno AL, Stevens DL. Streptococcal infections of skin and soft tissues. N Engl J Med 1996; 334: 240–245.

13

Viral Infections

Sheila Fallon Friedlander, John S. Bradley

Viral infections can induce a remarkable variety of cutaneous manifestations in the neonate. The form of response that occurs from any infection depends on the virulence of the pathogen, the tissue tropism of the virus, and the time of gestation at which the infection is acquired. Infections may occur in utero, perinatally (acquired between the onset of labor and the delivery), or postnatally. Skin pathology may be a direct consequence of skin infection or an indirect effect resulting from viral infection of other tissues. Diagnosis of infection is based on morphology and the distribution of the skin lesions in the context of the overall clinical presentation of the infant, supported by specific laboratory studies. Rapid diagnosis and appropriate antiviral therapy maximize the possibility of a positive outcome for the infant.

HERPES SIMPLEX VIRUS

Herpes simplex virus (HSV) types 1 and 2 are pathogens for the fetus and newborn infant, leading to a spectrum of clinical disease in which manifestations depend on the time of exposure, the route of exposure, and the presence or absence of maternal immunity (primary versus recurrent maternal infection). Herpes simplex virus is a large, double-stranded DNA virus that can produce an acute primary infection in the susceptible host. In addition, HSV-1 and -2, like other herpes viruses, have the ability to integrate into host DNA and establish latency. Poorly understood host and environmental factors can cause reactivation of virus within latently infected sensory ganglia, leading to a recurrent, active infection. Neonatal infection occurs most often as a direct result of active maternal infection, usually from primary infection acquired during pregnancy. The rate of neonatal disease has been shown to parallel the rate of genital herpes in a community.[1]

Epidemiology

Neonatal infection is estimated to occur at a rate of 0.2–0.5 per 1000 live births. Infection of the fetus or newborn may occur during gestation (in utero), at the time of labor and delivery (perinatally), or following the delivery (postnatally). Although the majority of neonatal infections (80–90%) are considered to be acquired perinatally, both in utero infections (4%) and postnatal infections (10%) have been well documented.[2]

The majority of neonates acquire infection from exposure to infectious genital secretions or lesions present at the time of vaginal delivery. Although primary infection in the pregnant woman usually leads to symptomatic illness, a significant proportion of women with primary infection do not have rec-ognizable systemic or local disease.[3] Primary maternal infection is usually associated with prolonged shedding (2–3 weeks) of high titers of virus from lesions while the maternal immune response develops, in contrast to the more limited viral shedding and much shorter duration of lesions (2–5 days) that accompanies recurrent disease in women with specific humoral and cellular immunity. Neonatal infection occurs in up to 50% of infants born to mothers during primary infection, compared to 5% or less of infants born to mothers during recurrent infection. Active maternal infection at the time of delivery, based on viral culture, is thought to occur in approximately 1–7 per 1000 births.[4] However, data based on polymerase chain reaction (PCR) techniques from genital specimens at delivery suggest that active maternal infection may occur up to eight times more frequently than previously appreciated.[5] Prospective studies have documented that the majority of women with active infection at the time of delivery are asymptomatic, suggesting that improved rapid laboratory diagnosis and careful examination will be necessary to identify the at-risk mother and infant. The optimal strategy for preventing neonatal HSV infection is controversial. Discordant HSV status of sexual partners is a risk factor if the female is susceptible, and queries regarding partner status are appropriate, as is advice regarding abstinence near term for susceptible women with infected partners. There is no consensus regarding the use of weekly cultures near term in high-risk women. Although caesarian section delivery is used by some experts for women with active disease near term, universal recommendations are not available. Maternal antiviral therapy is employed by some when the mother has active disease, but the risk–benefit ratio of treatment must be weighed in each case.[6] Postnatal infections may be transmitted from both maternal, nongenital sites (including transmission from breast lesions) and nonmaternal sources. These include other family members and nosocomial transmission from healthcare workers.

Intrauterine Infection

Congenital (intrauterine) infection was described in 1966 by Sieber et al.[7] in an infant with culture-positive lesions, seizures, and evidence of immunity at the time of a normal delivery in which the amniotic membranes were ruptured at birth. In 1969 South[8] described an infant with microcephaly, microphthalmia, seizures, and vesicular lesions on the fingers and toes following a maternal primary HSV-2 genital infection during the first month of pregnancy. Subsequent studies of congenital infection have documented the presence of specific cell-mediated immunity to HSV in the newborn at birth, whereas infants infected during labor and delivery do not usually develop cellular immunity until the second week of the infection.[9]

Infection in utero may occur either as a result of ascending infection through apparently intact membranes, or potentially as a result of viremia occurring with a primary maternal infection. Fetal infection often leads to fetal death; however, if the fetus survives, delivery may occur at term with late sequelae in both skin and central nervous system (CNS).

Cutaneous Findings

Skin manifestations at delivery are the result of residua from primary fetal infection in addition to latent virus reactivation at previous cutaneous sites of fetal infection. Skin lesions are common in the neonatal period (Fig. 13-1). In one study, 70% of infected infants had vesicular lesions, and 30% also had evidence of scar formation on the face, trunk, or extremities.[10] Lesions characteristic of epidermolysis bullosa have also been described, as well as aplasia cutis congenita-like lesions.[11] Atrophic limbs, previously reported with congenital varicella virus infection, have also been documented with congenital HSV infection.[12]

Extracutaneous Findings

Infections acquired in utero in which the infant completes a normal gestation are almost invariably associated with CNS damage, which is easily detected by computed tomography (CT). Changes in the CNS indicate longstanding destruction of neuronal tissue without acute inflammation. Microcephaly is present in over 50%, and chorioretinitis is present in 60% of infants with congenital infection. Although skin and CNS abnormalities are present at birth, infected infants often do not show the signs of systemic toxicity and overwhelming sepsis that may occur with primary perinatal or postnatal infection.

Diagnosis

The diagnosis of a herpes virus infection can be made in several ways (Table 13-1). Histologic staining of epithelial cells obtained by scraping the base of a vesicle or mucosal ulceration (Tzanck preparation) will demonstrate multinucleate giant epithelial cells containing intranuclear viral inclusions (see Chapter 6). A biopsy is usually not required to arrive at a diagnosis, but will show the characteristic intraepidermal vesicle with ballooning degeneration of epithelial cells, resulting in acantholysis. Eosinophilic inclusion bodies may be seen in the degenerating epithelial cells. In the adjacent dermis, an inflammatory cell infiltrate of variable severity reflects the nature of the infant's response to the viral infection (primary versus recurrent).

A specific diagnosis of herpes simplex virus can be obtained rapidly by antibody-specific stains (such as direct fluorescent antibody for HSV-1 or HSV-2). Viral culture can be performed on skin or mucous membrane lesions. Cultures generally take from 2 to 7 days to develop cytopathic effects. The PCR technique for diagnosis of HSV takes several hours and is currently not well standardized for biologic samples other than cerebrospinal fluid. Attempting to identify the type of herpes simplex virus responsible for the infection is important because the epidemiology of acquisition of virus and the course of the infection differ between HSV-1 and HSV-2.

The serologic status of an infant should be obtained to assess pre-existing and ongoing antibody response. In perinatal infection, anti-HSV antibody present at birth is maternal in origin, with transplacental antibody decreasing as the infant's humoral immunity to HSV increases, a response pattern that is distinct from early congenital infection, in which antibody present at birth is derived from both fetal and maternal production.

Differential Diagnosis

Other congenital infections associated with skin lesions and CNS injury should be investigated, such as congenital varicella syndrome and syphilis. Noninfectious entities such as incontinentia pigmenti and other disorders producing vesicular lesions (Chapters 10 and 24) should also be considered.

Management/Prognosis

Infants are treated with intravenous acyclovir at 60 mg/kg/day divided every 8 hours, based on current protocols for infants with perinatal CNS infection.[13] No prospective data exist on the required treatment course for congenitally infected infants, although pre-existing immunity should allow for a shorter course of therapy than in infants with primary infection. The neurologic prognosis for infants with congenital infection is poor, with virtually all demonstrating significant developmental delay.

Neonatal (Perinatal) Herpes Simplex Infection

Neonatal disease occurs in three clinically recognized syndromes, all acquired in the perinatal period: disseminated infection; infection localized to the skin, eyes, or mouth; and CNS infection. Exposure to maternal primary infection at the time of delivery may lead to overwhelming infection in the neonate, with a high mortality rate, or a more slowly progressive, insidious disease in which the infant has only mucocutaneous manifestations or develops slowly progressive neurologic symptoms. The incubation period varies substantially, from clinical symptoms at delivery due to presumed ascending infection, through nonintact membranes, to infection presenting as late as 3 weeks of age. The variability of the incubation period is dependent on the integrity of the amniotic membranes, the inoculum of virus, the tissue site inoculated (e.g. skin, mucous membrane), and the presence or absence of transplacental specific antibody.

Cutaneous Manifestations

The infection may manifest clinically with cutaneous or mucosal lesions (mouth, nose, eye), with or without signs of

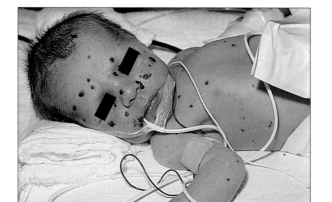

FIG. 13-1 Congenital herpes simplex. Generalized necrotic crusted papules.

TABLE 13-1 Diagnosis of infection

Virus	Culture	Histology of skin lesion	PCR	Serology
HSV	Widely available; reliable; culture skin lesions; eyes, mouth, CSF, rectum, urine or blood	Tzanck stain of epithelial cells from the bottom of a vesicle: specific for herpesviruses HSV and VZV; direct fluorescent antibody stains for HSV 1 or 2 are specific; DFA stains are specific and sensitive	Highly sensitive; best studied on CSF (sensitivity of skin lesions not well studied)	Rising antibody titer to HSV IgG is a sensitive and specific test; HSV IgM is not a sensitive test in the newborn
VZV	Available in many reference laboratories; culture skin lesions	Tzanck stain (see above): specific stains available for VZV	Highly sensitive, but not well studied on skin lesions; not widely available	Rising antibody titer to VSV IgG is a sensitive and specific test; VZV IgM is not a sensitive test in the newborn
CMV	Widely available; reliable; culture urine, saliva; shell vial technique yields results in 48–72 hours	Skin lesions are due to extramedullary hematopoiesis, not due to viral replication in skin	Highly sensitive; well studied in plasma as a marker of disseminated CMV infection in immune compromised hosts	Rising antibody titer to CMV IgG is a sensitive and specific test; CMV IgM is not a sensitive test in the newborn
Rubella	Not usually available; culture pharynx; respiratory secretions, CSF, tissue	Skin lesions are due to extramedullary hematopoiesis, not due to viral replication in skin	Not well studied	Rising antibody titer to rubella IgG is a sensitive and specific test; rubella IgM is not a sensitive test in the newborn. Compare mother's prenatal serology test results with those at the time of birth
Enterovirus	Available in reference laboratories; culture vesicular lesions, pharynx (during the acute phase of illness), and stool (up to 6 weeks following the illness)	Nonspecific	Highly sensitive; widely available	Not usually helpful, as no class-specific antibody response can be measured and type-specific serologies are not widely available
Parvovirus B19	Not available in standard cell culture	Placental and fetal tissues—intranuclear inclusions in nucleated erythroid cells EM and immunohistochemistry may be helpful	Highly sensitive; can be used on amniotic fluid, fetal blood, and tissues	IgM or IgG seroconversion helpful in pregnant female Fetal IgM specific but not sensitive
HIV	Available; not highly sensitive in newborn not recommended	Nonspecific	Sensitive means of diagnosis, can be repeated at 1–2 months and 4–6 months of age prn	Nonspecific passive maternal antibody present at birth persists, 18 month evaluation preferred with PCR

sepsis or encephalitis. Infants with skin, eye, or mouth disease account for 40% of all neonatal cases of HSV infection. The skin lesions appear as small, 2–4 mm vesicles, with surrounding erythema, often in herpetiform (zosteriform) clusters (Fig. 13-2). They usually occur on the part of the body in prolonged contact with the cervix. Often, lesions will occur at sites where the skin integrity has been breached. One of the most common sites of cutaneous infection is on the scalp vertex at the site of placement of fetal scalp monitor electrodes (Fig. 13-3). Vesicular lesions usually develop within the first 1–2 weeks of life following inoculation at this site. They may progress locally, or disseminate (Fig. 13-4). In areas of mucosal involvement, a shallow ulceration with moderate inflammation is most often seen. The ulceration may be focal, with the lesion size closely resembling that of a cutaneous vesicle, or ulcerations may spread irregularly, coalescing over a much larger area. Lesions tend to follow the clinical stages of vesicle resolution seen in the older child, with pustulation 24–72 hours after the appearance of the vesicle, followed by eschar formation. Skin lesions are present in most neonates with disseminated disease (77%), and in 60% of infants who present with CNS disease. In any newborn with skin or mucosal lesions of HSV, even without a history of symptomatic illness, an investigation

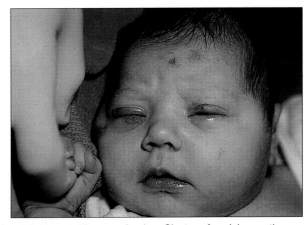

FIG. 13-2 Neonatal herpes simplex. Cluster of vesicles on the forehead and periocular area.

must be undertaken to rule out disseminated or CNS disease.

Extracutaneous Manifestations

Dissemination is the most devastating manifestation, presenting in the more premature infant (average gestational age at

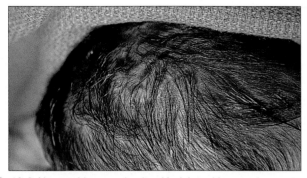

FIG. 13-3 Neonatal herpes simplex. Vesicles with central necrotic plaque at site of fetal monitor electrode placement.

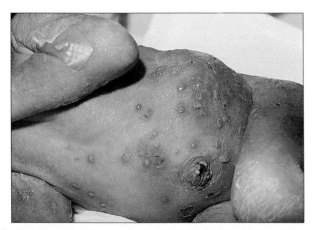

FIG. 13-4 Neonatal herpes simplex virus. Multiple vesicles and crusted papules on an erythematous base in the periumbilical area and left flank.

birth of 36.5 weeks) at an average chronologic age of 11 days. Multisystem involvement is analogous to overwhelming bacterial sepsis. Shock, disseminated intravascular coagulation, and multiple organ system failure are characteristic. Involvement of the lung, liver, and brain is common. The mortality is high. Without antiviral therapy approximately 75% of infants will die, and even with specific antiviral therapy mortality is 50%. Neurologic sequelae in survivors are also common, occurring in approximately 40%. Statistically, these infants have the lowest average circulating concentration of antibody to HSV.

In as many as 40% of infants ultimately diagnosed with disseminated or CNS infection, clinical disease begins with skin lesions only. Clinical and laboratory evidence of dissemination or CNS involvement not obvious at the time of presentation may develop during the first days of treatment, despite antiviral therapy.

Infants with encephalitis present at a slightly older age (mean 17 days) and tend to be full term, in contrast with newborns with other clinical presentations. Antibody titers are higher in this group, leading to speculation that antibody may modify the progression of disease, with virus inoculated at delivery producing a clinically undetectable initial infection with spread from mucosal sites to the CNS. Subtle neurologic symptoms are often present for days before the parent recognizes that the infant requires medical attention. As the child becomes more irritable and seizures become more pronounced, infants are hospitalized and evaluated. Skin lesions are only present in 60% of infants with HSV encephalitis, making the diagnosis difficult in many.

Diagnosis

Rapid diagnosis of herpes virus infection can be made on the basis of a Tzanck-stained smear, but for infants without skin or mucous membrane lesions, the diagnosis is more difficult. Laboratory and radiographic evidence of multisystem involvement is supportive, but not diagnostic. Viral cultures of cutaneous lesions, nasopharynx, conjunctiva, urine, plasma, and CSF can provide a specific diagnosis but take several days for results. Direct fluorescent antibody testing can provide a more rapid analysis but is not 100% sensitive or specific. Cerebrospinal fluid examination is important because pleocytosis, elevated protein, and a high CSF red blood cell count can suggest necrotizing encephalitis. Culture of CSF is positive for HSV in up to 20% of infants with encephalitis. Rapid diagnosis of encephalitis by HSV PCR may be attempted, but the sensitivity of this assay is only about 70% in the newborn.[14]

CT of the brain may be helpful in the diagnosis of encephalitis but is not considered sensitive until after 5 days of CNS symptoms. Magnetic resonance imaging (MRI) is more sensitive for CNS inflammation of the temporal lobes, the preferred sites of viral replication, and may be diagnostic within 3 days of onset of symptoms. EEG can also be helpful in CNS infections localized to the temporal lobe and may be positive earlier than any imaging study.

Differential Diagnosis

Disseminated infection with HSV produces a clinical picture similar to that of early-onset neonatal sepsis caused by group B streptococcus, enteric Gram-negative bacilli, and *Listeria*. Empiric therapy with antibiotics (standard management for the hospitalized ill neonate) will have no effect on the progression of HSV disease. For infants with progressive clinical symptoms of sepsis and sterile bacterial cultures of blood, urine, and CSF, HSV should be considered as a potential pathogen.

Other viral infections in the newborn period may also be confused with HSV. Enteroviral infection can cause a wide spectrum of clinical signs in the neonate, from fever and irritability to overwhelming sepsis with multiple organ system failure, to aseptic meningoencephalitis with minimal symptoms of systemic toxicity. Enteroviral infections may be associated with cutaneous vesiculopustular lesions. Neonatal seizures caused by enteroviral infections are the result of diffuse CNS irritation, in contrast to the focal temporal lesions of early HSV disease. Destructive changes of HSV that are appreciated on serial imaging studies of the CNS (by either CT or MRI) are not generally seen with enteroviral disease.

Perinatal varicella may produce overwhelming sepsis in the newborn. The density of cutaneous lesions in neonatal varicella usually far exceeds that seen with HSV infections, which characteristically produce a focal cluster of lesions at the site of inoculation with minimal cutaneous dissemination. However, both demonstrate the identical findings of multinucleate giant cells on Tzanck preparations. Only virus-specific staining techniques, PCR, or culture will be able to differentiate between these viruses.

Other viral pathogens occasionally cause severe acute disease in the newborn, including influenza A and B, parainfluenza 1, 2, and 3, and adenovirus. In general, the seasonal context of the infection, exposure history, and a predominance of respiratory tract symptoms help differentiate these infections. Viral cultures of the respiratory tract will assist in the identification of these pathogens.

Incontinentia pigmenti may present with localized vesicles, which may be mistaken for herpes simplex infections. These infants often have peripheral eosinophilia. Biopsy will reveal increased numbers of eosinophils, and cultures will be negative for HSV. Vesicular lesions that appear herpetic can occur in Langerhans' cell histiocytosis. Tzanck preparation will reveal histiocytes, and biopsy will show large numbers of histiocytes and an absence of multinucleate giant cells.

Management and Prognosis

The treatment of choice in neonatal herpes infections is acyclovir administered intravenously, regardless of the clinical presentation.[15] Although the dose originally studied for skin or mucosal surface infection was 15 mg/kg/day divided into 8-hourly doses, data collected in infants treated at 30 mg/kg/day for disseminated infection and encephalitis suggest that this dose may safely be used in mild to moderate neonatal herpes simplex infections.[16] Clinical trials of 60 mg/kg/day for dissemination and encephalitis suggest a small incremental improvement in efficacy, with safety that is equivalent to the 30 mg/kg/day dose.[13] In infants with renal failure, the doses should be reduced accordingly.

Varicella

Varicella (chicken pox) is usually a benign, self-limited disease when it occurs in immunocompetent individuals during childhood. Unfortunately, the developing fetus and neonate are at higher risk for an adverse outcome following infection. Approximately 95% of women acquire the varicella infection before the childbearing years and are immune, thereby conferring immunity to the fetus. This percentage will hopefully approach even closer to 100% in the near future as a result of the widespread vaccination of young children with the Merck OKA varicella vaccine introduced in 1995. A booster dose of vaccine at 4–6 years of age with catch-up vaccination of all at-risk children before age 13, as well as efforts to vaccinate all women prior to pregnancy, should lead to a lower incidence of disease in the general population as well as in neonates. However, the vaccine is not 100% effective, and healthcare practitioners must be aware of the possible manifestations of varicella infection in neonates, as well as appropriate therapy.

The exact incidence of varicella during pregnancy is unknown, but three to 10 cases per 10 000 pregnancies have been documented.[17–25] Fetal or early neonatal exposure may result in a variety of manifestations, ranging from minimal cutaneous lesions to significant morbidity and death. Three distinct disorders may occur following intrauterine or neonatal exposure to VZV: fetal varicella syndrome, neonatal varicella, and infantile herpes zoster.

Fetal Varicella Syndrome

Congenital defects predominantly involving the skin, nervous system, and musculoskeletal system can occur following fetal exposure to varicella virus. Other terms for the fetal varicella syndrome include varicella embryopathy and congenital varicella syndrome.

Cutaneous Findings

Specific anomalies include cicatricial skin lesions that correspond to a dermatomal distribution, often with hypoplasia of underlying tissues. These lesions may initially appear as

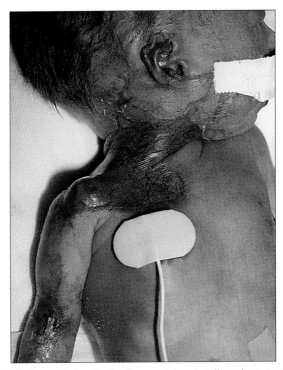

FIG. 13-5 Congenital varicella. Segmental and stellate deep scars on the right ear, head, shoulder, and arm, which appear to follow a dermatome.

denuded areas and subsequently develop stellate or angular scars (Fig. 13-5).

Extracutaneous Findings

Low birth-weight is a common finding in affected infants. The varied extracutaneous manifestations of this syndrome can be grouped as neurologic, musculoskeletal, ophthalmologic, gastrointestinal, and genitourinary. Limb paresis and hypoplasia of the extremities are common findings, as is chorioretinitis. Less common findings include microphthalmia, cataracts, nystagmus, hydrocephalus, and mental retardation (Table 13-2).[20]

Etiology and Pathogenesis

Varicella zoster (VZV) is a herpes virus consisting of double-stranded DNA. The incubation period is usually 14 days, but extends from 10 to 21 days after exposure. Most fetuses exposed to VZV during gestation will have no discernible sequelae. The greatest risk for fetal varicella syndrome occurs in the first 20 weeks of gestation, with the highest risk (2%) between 13 and 20 weeks.[25] A lower rate before 13 weeks (0.4%) may reflect underreporting or a higher rate of spontaneous abortion. Rare cases in the second half of pregnancy have been reported.[24,26] A prospective study carried out in Germany and the United Kingdom between 1980 and 1993 identified 1373 women who had varicella and 366 who had zoster during the first 36 weeks of gestation. Nine cases of congenital varicella syndrome occurred overall, and all occurred after maternal varicella infection in the first 20 weeks of pregnancy. The highest risk occurred between 13 and 20 weeks of gestation, with seven cases noted in this subset. No cases of congenital varicella were noted following maternal herpes zoster during pregnancy. Herpes zoster in infancy was identified in 10 children whose mothers had varicella during pregnancy. Although 97 women who received varicella zoster immunoglobulin

TABLE 13-2 Features of varicella syndrome

Characteristic organ system	Common (>50%)	Uncommon (<50%, >10%)	Rare (<10%)
Skin	Cicatricial lesions	Hydrocephalus and cortical atrophy vesicles	Cerebellar hypoplasia
Neurologic	Limb paresis	Seizures Horner syndrome Bulbar dysphagia Mental retardation Optic nerve atrophy Anal sphincter malfunction Microcephaly Phrenic nerve palsy Developmental delay and encephalomyelitis	Auditory nerve palsy Facial nerve palsy
Eye	Chorioretinitis	Anisocoria Nystagmus Microphthalmia Cataract	Corneal opacity Heterochromia
Skeletal	Hypoplasia of upper or lower extremities	Hypoplasia of fingers or toes Equinovarus or calcaneovalgus Hypoplasia of scapulae or clavicles Hypoplasia of ribs	Hypoplasia of mandible Scoliosis Lacunar skull
Gastrointestinal	Low birth weight		Gastroesophageal reflux Duodenal stenosis Dilated jejunum Small left colon Sigmoid atresia
Genitourinary			Absence of kidney Hydronephrosis Hydroureter Undescended testes Bladder abnormalities

(VZIG) developed varicella, no cases of congenital varicella occurred in this group.[25] Some believe that the failure to identify congenital varicella in late pregnancy reflects the limited statistical power of epidemiologic efforts, but nonetheless late pregnancy is clearly a time of lower risk for the development of the classic stigmata of congenital disease.[27]

It has been postulated that the severe segmental anomalies that can be seen in fetal varicella syndrome are the result of reactivation of primary varicella in the developing fetus at a time when the immune system is not sufficiently developed to modify the severity of infection. Maternal herpes zoster does not appear to pose a significant risk to the fetus. No cases of congenital varicella occurred in a prospective study of 366 women who had zoster during pregnancy, and no serological evidence of transplacental transmission was noted.[25]

Approximately 18 cases of congenital anomalies occurring in association with maternal herpes zoster infection have been reported; however, it is not clear that these anomalies were a result of maternal zoster infection.[28] A case of cutaneous lesions and limb hypoplasia in a fetus whose mother developed disseminated herpes zoster at 12 weeks' gestation did appear consistent with fetal varicella syndrome, but localized maternal zoster has not been clearly implicated as a cause of fetal disease.[29]

Diagnosis

The denuded or scarred areas seen with fetal varicella syndrome may be mistaken for aplasia cutis congenita or Bart syndrome. Other congenital viral infections should be considered in any infant presenting with microcephaly, ophthalmologic, or neurologic abnormalities.

Prenatal diagnosis of fetal varicella syndrome using viral or immunologic methods is unreliable.[30] IgM may be undetectable, even in infants with classic clinical findings. Infection before 18 weeks' gestation may lead to a suboptimal or altered immune response resulting from immaturity of the fetal immune system. Prenatal diagnosis of intrauterine exposure to varicella may be accomplished by means of cordocentesis, amniocentesis, and chorionic villus sampling.[30] IgM may be detected in cord blood as early as 19–22 weeks' gestation. Virus can be grown from amniotic fluid and fetal blood samples, and DNA probes can be utilized to evaluate placental tissue.[31,32] However, transplacental transfer of virus can occur without any significant sequelae to the fetus, and the degree of fetal involvement cannot be determined by immunologic or viral evaluation. Thus, although the above-mentioned evaluations may be useful in diagnosing fetal varicella syndrome, they are neither sensitive nor specific enough to accurately determine which fetuses will suffer untoward effects.

High-quality ultrasound at 20–22 weeks' gestation has been used as a means of surveying at-risk fetuses. Sonographic abnormalities include fetal hydrops, polyhydramnios, abnormal foci within the liver, microcephaly, and limb hypoplasia.[33] Unfortunately, some findings may not be apparent until later in pregnancy. A recent report of a fatal case of varicella embryopathy that used ultrasonography and MRI at 26 and 32 weeks of gestation found a high correlation between fetal imaging and subsequent pathologic findings, including limb involvement and even dermatologic features; however, MRI scanning was required to identify CNS abnormalities. The authors recommend combining prenatal ultrasonography with MRI in any woman noted to have varicella seroconversion during pregnancy.[34] Varicella virus is not usually isolated from live-borne infants with congenital infection, and other findings must be used to confirm the diagnosis.

Criteria useful in confirming the diagnosis include clinical, virologic, or serologic evidence of maternal varicella infection during pregnancy; skin lesions in a dermatomal distribution; and immunologic evidence of varicella infection in the infant, including IgM antibody or persistence of IgG antibody beyond 1 year of life in the absence of clinical varicella infection.[30] The development of herpes zoster in the first year of life without a prior history of varicella infection is also good evidence that the infant was exposed to varicella zoster during gestation. In rare instances, herpes virus particles have been detected by means of electron microscopy in skin samples obtained at or near birth.[31]

Treatment

Prevention by eliminating natural infection during pregnancy is the best approach to this disease, and should be facilitated by the increasing use of the varicella vaccine in childhood. Ideally, preconception evaluation should identify at-risk women, who should then receive the varicella vaccine before conceiving. No fetal anomalies have been reported in infants born to pregnant women who have received the vaccine inadvertently. Nonetheless, the vaccine, which is a live attenuated virus, is contraindicated in pregnancy.

Therapeutic abortion is not automatically recommended to at-risk mothers as the risk of a fetal anomaly following exposure is so small.[35] At-risk mothers known to have recent exposure to varicella during the first 20 weeks of pregnancy should have varicella serologic evaluation. Complement fixation tests are insensitive; however, latex agglutination (LA), immunofluorescent (IFA), fluorescent antibody-to-membrane antigen assays (FAMA), and enzyme-linked immunoabsorbent assays (ELISA) are sensitive and specific.[30] The LA test is also rapid and simple, making it quite useful in evaluating at-risk pregnant women.[30]

Varicella zoster immunoglobulin postexposure prophylaxis may be offered to varicella-susceptible pregnant women. It may be administered within 96 hours of exposure, but is most efficacious within the first 48 hours. It does not reliably prevent maternal illness, but does modify the severity of infection. It is unclear whether VZIG prevents fetal varicella syndrome or neonatal infection, but there were no cases of fetal infection in 97 pregnancies complicated by maternal exposure and treated with postexposure VZIG prophylaxis.[25,36] Because fetal varicella syndrome is so rare, larger studies would be required to confirm protection. Exposed pregnant women who are seropositive for VZV do not require VZIG.

Treatment with acyclovir should be considered in any pregnant women with varicella, particularly those in the third trimester, because of the risk of severe maternal disease, and to minimize the risk of neonatal disease in case delivery occurs during or soon after acute infection. The drug is usually well tolerated with little toxicity to the mother, but the risks and benefits to the mother and fetus have not yet been clearly delineated.[37] The International Registry of Acyclovir Use During Pregnancy has followed at least 1,246 fetal exposures to the drug thus far, and no increased incidence of fetal abnormalities in exposed infants has been noted.[38] It has not been determined whether such treatment will eliminate the risk of varicella embryopathy or infantile zoster in exposed fetuses. Ophthalmologic and neurologic evaluation of the infant born

to a mother with varicella during pregnancy is indicated, as is careful examination of the musculoskeletal, genitourinary, and gastrointestinal systems for underlying anomalies.

Neonatal Varicella

Neonatal varicella may result if a mother develops chicken pox before or immediately after delivery. If maternal varicella occurs from 5 days before to 2 days after delivery, the in utero-inoculated fetus is at high risk for severe disseminated disease.

Cutaneous Findings

The clinical course of neonatal varicella can be quite variable. Those who are more likely to develop severe illness generally develop skin lesions within 5–10 days after delivery. Some children will develop a few cutaneous lesions, but otherwise remain well. Lesions often appear initially as small pink to red macules that relatively rapidly become papular and subsequently develop a teardrop-shaped vesicle. Other patients initially develop crops of cutaneous lesions that may evolve into hemorrhagic and/or necrotic vesicles (Fig. 13-6).

Extracutaneous Findings

Disseminated infection with widespread cutaneous and visceral involvement may develop and lead to severe morbidity. The mortality rate for neonatal varicella before the use of acyclovir has been estimated at 10–30%.[35,36] Death from severe pneumonitis and respiratory distress often occurs 4–6 days after onset of lesions. Hepatitis and encephalitis may also develop. A study from Thailand in 1999, evaluating 26 children with neonatal varicella, reported no mortality. Twelve of the 26 children received intravenous acyclovir.[40]

Etiology/Pathogenesis

Infants may develop lesions from 1 to 16 days after birth if the mother experiences active disease near the time of birth (Fig. 13-7). Administration of VZIG may prolong the incubation period to 28 days.[38] The usual onset of rash is 9–15 days after onset of maternal rash. Infection later in gestation is more likely to lead to zoster in infancy or neonatal chicken pox. In aggregate data from two studies, 23–62% of infants whose mothers developed varicella in the last 3 weeks of pregnancy developed neonatal varicella.[25] The risk of severe neonatal varicella is related to the time maternal infection occurs, presumably because of a critical period when transmission of

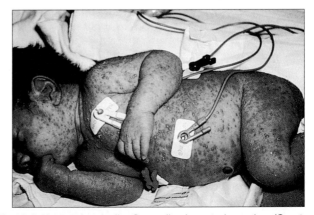

FIG. 13-6 Neonatal varicella. Generalized crusted papules. (Courtesy of Dr Gerald Goldberg.)

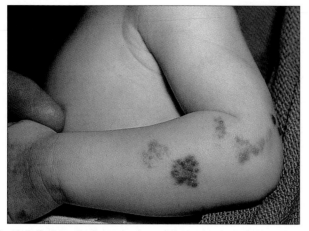

FIG. 13-7 Early varicella zoster in an infant whose mother contracted varicella during pregnancy.

virus to the infant occurs prior to the development and transplacental transfer of maternal antibodies, which modify expression of the infection in the neonate.

Diagnosis

Smears of vesicles using a Tzanck preparation will demonstrate multinucleate giant cells and margination of the nucleoplasm. Direct fluorescent antibody testing and VZV PCR evaluation are also helpful and are more specific for VZV. Fluorescent antibody tests are occasionally false positive in disorders such as incontinentia pigmenti and Langerhans' cell histiocytosis; therefore positive viral culture remains the best, most reliable means of diagnosis.[41] A history of maternal varicella infection during pregnancy is also helpful but not necessary to confirm the diagnosis because infants may also contract the disease from siblings, carers, and other close contacts.

The differential diagnosis of vesiculopustular lesions is discussed in Chapter 10.

Treatment

Prevention is the best intervention. Delaying delivery until sufficient time has elapsed for transplacental transfer of maternal antibody is one approach; this generally occurs 5–7 days after the onset of maternal illness. Neonates born to mothers who have developed varicella from 5 days before to 2 days after delivery should receive VZIG intramuscularly as soon as possible after delivery.[38] Direct contact between the infant and maternal skin lesions should be avoided, but breastfeeding is not prohibited if such contact can be avoided. Neonates who develop lesions or signs of infection should be treated with intravenous acyclovir, 20 mg/kg every 8 hours for a minimum of 10 days. More prolonged therapy of 14–21 days may be necessary for disseminated or CNS infection.[39] Aggressive supportive therapy is sometimes also required. The use of prophylactic acyclovir in high-risk infants has also been suggested by some authors.[38]

It should be borne in mind that any infant born to a woman who has had varicella within 3 weeks of delivery may be infectious at birth or shortly thereafter. If onset of maternal infection is within 1–2 weeks of delivery, many experts recommend that the child be isolated (from at-risk hospital personnel and other babies) from birth. If onset of disease occurs in the mother within 1 week of delivery, or following the birth of the infant, the infant should be isolated 7 days after the onset of maternal disease.[38]

If a mother develops a varicella rash 3 or more days after delivery, the infant may well contract varicella but this will more likely be via the respiratory route, which theoretically leads to a smaller systemic inoculum and less severe disease. However, serious illness has been reported in the first 4 weeks of life when infants contract disease from their mother or siblings during this period. Severe infantile disease may occasionally occur even in infants born to immune mothers.[42] If the mother is seronegative and the infant is exposed to an infectious sibling, many experts would recommend VZIG postexposure prophylaxis for the infant. Postexposure prophylaxis with acyclovir may be effective in older infants, but no data exist for its efficacy or safety in neonates.[38] Although the mortality rate following noncongenital infantile varicella (0.008%) is higher than that in older children, it is still lower than the rate in immunocompromised individuals (7%) or following intrauterine exposure (10–30%).[33]

Infantile Herpes Zoster

Following primary infection, the varicella zoster virus persists in the sensory dorsal root ganglia and is kept in check by cell-mediated host immune mechanisms. Reactivation of the virus can occur and generally leads to localized involvement of skin and nerves in a dermatomal pattern corresponding to the ganglion in which reactivation took place. This disease, termed herpes zoster, has been recognized since antiquity. The term zoster ('girdle' in Greek) refers to the tendency of the lesions to involve the trunk in a 'girdle-like' pattern. Infants may develop classic herpes zoster without prior evidence of primary varicella if exposed to varicella virus in utero. Pediatric herpes zoster is more common in immunocompromised children, and in immunocompetent children within the first year of life who have been exposed to varicella in utero.[24] Neonatal herpes zoster has only rarely been reported. It is generally a benign disease without significant morbidity or sequelae for the infant unless the infant is immunocompromised.

Cutaneous Findings

Affected infants usually have discrete papular lesions that involve predominantly the thoracic dermatomes. The lesions initially appear as a group of small pink to erythematous papules that subsequently vesiculate and crust (Fig. 13-7). Occasionally lesions become hemorrhagic and develop necrotic eschars. Scarring may occur in the involved area. Although the disease may disseminate, immunocompetent children usually have a benign course and an excellent outcome.

Diagnosis

The diagnosis is usually straightforward when the lesions assume a dermatomal distribution. A Tzanck preparation is the most rapid means to evaluate suspicious vesicular lesions. Zoster lesions may be initially mistaken for arthropod bites or impetigo. Herpes simplex infections may mimic herpes zoster but are usually more localized, with the potential to recur. Direct fluorescent antibody testing and PCR evaluation are also relatively rapid diagnostic techniques (see discussion in Infantile Varicella). Varicella virus can be isolated from vesicular lesions of herpes zoster.

Etiology/Pathogenesis

Pediatric herpes zoster is more common in immunocompromised children, and in immunocompetent children within the first year of life who have been exposed to varicella in utero.[24] Neonatal herpes zoster has only rarely been reported. The risk of infantile herpes zoster increases if exposure to varicella zoster virus occurs in the second half of pregnancy.[25] Approximately 2% of fetuses exposed to VZV during the second half of pregnancy will develop herpes zoster during infancy.[25]

Treatment

Many infectious disease experts treat zoster in neonates with systemic aciclovir. Immunocompetent infants with zoster generally do well and do not require antiviral therapy. Patients who develop severe hemorrhagic disease, as well as those with disseminated lesions, are likely to benefit from systemic therapy. Supportive therapy in all cases should include good hygiene at the blister sites, compresses as needed, and treatment for secondary bacterial infection if indicated.

Special Concerns for the Neonatal Nursery and Intensive Care Unit

Varicella Exposure in the Neonatal Intensive Care Unit

Recommendations regarding prophylaxis vary. The UK Advisory Group on Chickenpox recommends routine administration of VZIG to all neonates following exposure.[26] If sensitive and rapid testing is available, exposed infants may be tested and the use of VZIG avoided for those with passive antibody to VZV. Others recommend concentrating prophylactic measures on those infants less than 30 weeks old and weighing less than 1 kg. The Red Book Report of the Committee on Infectious Diseases of the AAP recommends VZIG for all exposed, hospitalized premature infants who were less than 28 weeks' gestation, or who weighed 1 kg or less at birth. In addition, those exposed, hospitalized premature infants of 28 weeks or more gestation, born to mothers who are seronegative or lack a history of varicella infection, should also be given VZIG.[39]

CYTOMEGALOVIRUS

Cytomegalovirus (CMV), one of the most common viral infections of the newborn, is acquired congenitally, perinatally, or postnatally. CMV is a double-stranded DNA virus, a member of the herpes virus family. It represents the most frequently recognized cause of congenital infection, occurring in 1–2% of all births.[43]

Cutaneous Findings

The principal cutaneous manifestations of CMV infection are similar to those of congenital rubella syndrome and consist of skin lesions of extramedullary hematopoiesis ('blueberry muffin' spots) and petechiae secondary to thrombocytopenia, which resolves during the first weeks of life.

Extracutaneous Findings

Other manifestations of congenital CMV infection syndrome include intrauterine growth retardation, microcephaly with chorioretinitis, hepatosplenomegaly, and pneumonitis.

Etiology/Pathogenesis

Congenital infection occurs most often following reactivation of a latent maternal infection during pregnancy, resulting in viremia and/or transplacental transmission of lymphocyte-associated virus to the fetus. The vast majority of infected infants born to immune mothers with reactivation of CMV are normal and have no stigmata of congenital infection. However, seronegative mothers may acquire a primary CMV infection during pregnancy, leading to a far greater incidence of symptomatic disease in the neonate.[44] The severity of infection depends on the trimester in which fetal infection has occurred, with infections early in gestation leading to more pronounced clinical findings and a poorer prognosis than those sustained during the third trimester. Infection may also occur at the time of delivery following exposure to infectious secretions during the process of vaginal birth. The infection is acquired perinatally in 40% of infants born to culture-positive mothers. Postnatal transmission has also been well documented in breastfed infants following the ingestion of culture-positive breast milk.

Diagnosis

Viral culture of urine or saliva is the easiest, most widely available method of diagnosis. Infants with congenital infection are, by definition, culture positive at the time of birth. For a diagnosis of congenital infection, cultures should be obtained within the first 2 weeks of life. If cultures are positive in the infant beyond 1–2 weeks of age, it is not possible to differentiate between congenital and perinatal CMV infection. This distinction is often critical, however, as the prognosis for perinatal CMV is uniformly good, whereas that of congenital CMV is not. Skin biopsies do not usually reveal evidence of active CMV infection, although specimens from liver, lung, or kidney will show clear evidence of CMV inclusions in infected parenchymal tissues. A spun sample of urine may demonstrate viral inclusions in tubular epithelial cells in up to 50% of culture-positive samples, and may demonstrate CMV by electron microscopy in up to 93% of culture-positive urine samples.[45] Serologic studies can also be used to make a diagnosis of congenital/perinatal CMV infection, either by demonstrating specific CMV-IgM antibody produced by the neonate or by documenting a persistent, increasing titer of IgG antibody during the first 4–6 months of life. Although the presence of specific CMV-IgM in cord blood will verify congenital infection, the sensitivity of this test as currently performed in reference laboratories may be less than 50%. PCR testing for CMV-DNA is accepted as a very sensitive diagnostic technique for plasma and certain tissue fluids in immunocompromised hosts, and is a highly sensitive test in the newborn.[43]

Treatment

Vaccines have been in development for several years but have not demonstrated sufficiently adequate protection from CMV infection to justify their extensive use.[46] Currently, treatment of CMV infections is primarily accomplished with ganciclovir, a nucleoside analog with potent activity against most strains of CMV.[47] The antiviral is available in both intravenous and oral formulations, but is associated with significant bone marrow toxicity. Clinical trials of intravenous ganciclovir for congenital CMV demonstrated a significant reduction in hearing loss at 6 months in infants with CNS (central nervous system) manifestations of congenital infection.[48] Unfortunately, congenital CMV infections cannot be cured but only suppressed during the period of antiviral administration. Limited data exist on the use of oral ganciclovir and valganciclovir in the neonate.[49]

RUBELLA

The association of maternal rubella infection with congenital disease of the newborn was first recognized in 1941. Extensive investigations have resulted in delineation of the congenital rubella infection syndrome, typified by a small-for-gestational age infant with microcephaly, deafness, cataracts, heart defects, chorioretinitis, hepatosplenomegaly, and a papular rash on the face, trunk, and extremities.

Cutaneous Findings

The rash can be mild or extensive, and is a manifestation of intradermal sites of extramedullary hematopoiesis (EMH). It often becomes hemorrhagic secondary to thrombocytopenia present at birth in these infants. The initial 'cranberry muffin' character of these 2–20 mm raised, erythematous, soft, spongy lesions changes to the more characteristic appearance of 'blueberry muffin' spots following intralesional hemorrhage. Petechiae may also be present in addition to the lesions of EMH. The lesions of EMH are not specific for rubella infection, and may also occur with congenital cytomegalovirus and toxoplasma infections. Petechial and purpuric lesions are evident in up to 60% of infants with congenital rubella.

Extracutaneous Findings

Associated clinical findings, beyond those listed previously, include congenital heart disease (patent ductus arteriosus, pulmonic stenosis, aortic stenosis), cataracts, and pneumonia, which may actually develop and progress after birth. Psychomotor retardation and deafness occur in up to 50% of infants with documented congenital rubella syndrome.[50]

Etiology/Pathogenesis

Maternal infection gives rise to viremia, which is transmitted to the fetus, affecting rapidly dividing fetal tissues most prominently during the first 12 weeks of gestation. This single-stranded RNA virus usually causes a noncytolytic infection of cells, leading to cell dysfunction and defects in organogenesis. Although fetal infection may occur at any time during gestation, visible consequences of infection are most common following first-trimester infection, rare with a second-trimester infection, and virtually nonexistent following infection late in pregnancy.[51]

Diagnosis

Viral culture of the pharynx is the definitive method of confirming the diagnosis of rubella infection (see Table 13-1), as virus shedding continues for several weeks to months after birth. Assessing the maternal serologic status can be helpful, but many 'prenatal' serologies are actually performed at the end of the first trimester and therefore do not truly represent the mother's immune status before pregnancy and cannot rule out infection at week 12 of gestation. If the infant is believed to have been infected, acute (cord blood) and convalescent (obtained at 4–6 months of age) blood samples should be obtained to determine antibody titers for rubella. These titers are diagnostic, as virtually all maternal transplacental antibody will have disappeared from the infant by 6 months of age. Evaluation of the cutaneous lesions will lead only to the non-specific diagnosis of EMH.

Prevention and Treatment

No specific antiviral therapy exists for rubella virus. In the United States universal immunization of children is specifically designed to prevent congenital rubella infection. Prenatal screening of women during early pregnancy should detect susceptible individuals, and immunization immediately following the pregnancy is indicated.

ACQUIRED IMMUNODEFICIENCY SYNDROME

Acquired immunodeficiency syndrome (AIDS) is a multisystem disorder characterized by T-lymphocyte depletion and recurrent opportunistic infections. It results from infection with the human immunodeficiency virus (HIV), an RNA retrovirus that infects CD4 T lymphocytes as well as other immune cells. Transmission can occur in utero, perinatally, or via breast milk. Characteristics of the infection include a variable latency period and an extremely high mortality rate. Perinatal transmission from infected mothers is the most common cause of childhood infection.[52] The number of pediatric cases decreased by 90% in 2002 compared to 1992, mainly because of a decrease in perinatal transmission due to screening for HIV during pregnancy, with antiretroviral treatment of the mother at the end of pregnancy and treatment of the newborn for the first 6 weeks of life.[52,53] Most infected infants are asymptomatic in the first few months, but severe disease can occur within this timeframe. Cutaneous abnormalities are among the earliest findings, and may be infectious, inflammatory, or neoplastic in nature. Failure to thrive, recurrent infections, and pulmonary disease (relating to Pneumocystis jiroveci or lymphoid interstitial pneumonia) are common findings in infants. These children are also at risk for gastrointestinal disorders, including malabsorption, hepatosplenomegaly, and CMV-mediated organ involvement such as hepatitis and marrow failure.

Cutaneous Findings

Cutaneous and mucous membrane disease is very common in infants with symptomatic HIV infection. Frequently the first indication that an infant is infected is the development of a severe or recurrent bacterial or fungal infection. In other instances, widespread and protracted seborrheic dermatitis may be the first clue to the patient's underlying immunodeficiency. Cutaneous infections that are extensive, progressive, or difficult to treat should raise suspicion for HIV infection. The type of cutaneous involvement that occurs with disease is generally related to the degree of immunosuppression.

Infectious Disorders

Mucocutaneous candidiasis is the most common dermatologic manifestation of pediatric HIV infection and occurs in the overwhelming majority of symptomatic children.[54] The disease is more severe and chronic than in the immunocompetent host and frequently persists beyond the first 6 months of life. White, cheesy patches or plaques overlying an erythematous base are found on the buccal mucosa, tongue, and palate. The lesions are friable and in severe cases may extend to involve the esophagus. The diaper area is commonly involved, with a beefy-red erythema involving the convex surfaces and creases, along with satellite papules or pustules. There may be angular cheilitis and extensive, generalized cutaneous involvement. Severe dermatophyte infections of the nails, hair, and skin may develop, and other unusual fungi such as cryptococcus and Aspergillus may cause systemic, as well as cutaneous disease.[55]

Bacterial infections of the skin may take the form of severe and recurrent staphylococcal impetigo, folliculitis, cellulitis, or abscesses. Other more unusual pathogens may be noted, particularly when the patient is severely immunosuppressed. Although polymorphonuclear (PMN) function against bacteria is not altered, T/B-cell cooperation leading to opsonizing antibacterial function may be severely affected.

Viral infections are also atypical in course and lesion morphology. The lesions of varicella zoster infection may become chronic, hemorrhagic, ulcerating, and/or hyperkeratotic.[56] Herpes zoster occurs earlier and more frequently in HIV-infected children. Herpes simplex infections may also be severe, prolonged, and/or recurrent. Molluscum contagiosum and papilloma virus infections are more frequent and may be relatively refractory to therapy.

Scabies can occur in early infancy and may present in a severe crusted form, often referred to as Norwegian scabies. Such cases are highly infectious because the affected infant usually possesses numerous generalized crusted papules that harbor large numbers of organisms.

Neoplastic Disease

Cancer is the presenting sign for AIDS in only 2% of children, compared to 15% of adults.[57] Kaposi's sarcoma (KS) is significantly less common in childhood than in adult AIDS. However, a report from Zambia noted a significant increase in the incidence of pediatric KS since 1987.[58]

Kaposi's sarcoma has been described in a 6-day-old infant, but is rare in the neonatal period.[59] Non-Hodgkin's lymphomas, which are sometimes limited to the CNS, occur with increased frequency in children with AIDS, as do leiomyomas and leiomyosarcomas.[60]

Inflammatory Disease

Confluent beefy erythema with superimposed greasy thin scale first noted on the scalp and face is characteristic of seborrheic dermatitis in children with AIDS. It spreads to involve the axillae and diaper area, and occasionally may progress to a severe generalized erythroderma. Atopic dermatitis and psoriasis can also occur in HIV-infected patients, but are not commonly diagnosed in the neonatal period. Drug eruptions, particularly from trimethoprim-sulfamethoxazole, are more frequent in children with AIDS.[61] The rash usually develops within 7–10 days after the start of therapy and is a pink, papular or morbilliform eruption. Evolution to TEN (toxic epidermal necrolysis) may occur, but most eruptions resolve following discontinuation of the offending agent.

Extracutaneous Manifestations

An HIV-related embryopathy described in 1986, and characterized by microcephaly and dysmorphic facial features, has not been substantiated. The papular exanthem/enanthem that develops shortly after HIV infection in adults has not been noted in perinatally acquired disease.[62]

Clinical conditions that should raise suspicion for HIV infection include failure to thrive, recurrent severe bacterial or opportunistic infections, hepatitis, lymphoid interstitial pneumonia, parotitis, lymphadenopathy, and hepatosplenomegaly. *Pneumocystis jiroveci* pneumonia is the most common serious opportunistic infection in HIV-infected children and usually develops between 3 and 6 months of age; however infection can occur in infants as young as 4–6 weeks. Patients may also develop severe wasting, encephalopathy, developmental delay, nephropathy, cardiomyopathy, and diarrhea.

Etiology/Pathogenesis

HIV is a human retrovirus containing RNA. Two forms exist: HIV-1, most prevalent in the United States, and HIV-2, a related virus more commonly seen in West Africa. The virus has a predilection for CD4 lymphocytes, glial cells, macrophages and monocytes, and infection generally leads to significant impairment in cell-mediated immunity.

HIV is transmitted by contaminated blood, semen, human milk, and cervical secretions. The virus has also been isolated from saliva, tears, urine, cerebrospinal fluid, and pleural fluid, but these have not been shown to routinely transmit infection.

Many sources have documented that perinatal transmission of HIV accounts for the overwhelming majority of pediatric cases in the United States.[52,63] Infection may be transmitted to the infant in utero, at the time of delivery, or through breastfeeding. The risk of infection for an infant whose mother did not receive interventions to prevent transmission is approximately 13–39%.[53] The risk of intrapartum transmission is higher than for intrauterine spread. In areas with high rates of breastfeeding one-third to half of maternal transmissions occur through breastfeeding. It is thought that the majority of infections are transmitted close to or at the time of delivery. Routine prenatal screening for HIV infection and treatment of infected women and their infants with antiviral agents such as zidovudine, and other retrovirds, are recommended. If an infected mother is compliant with antiretroviral medications and her viral load is <1.00 copies/mL, her risk of vertical HIV transmission decreases to 1%. Cesarean section delivery decreases the risk of HIV transmission to the fetus by approximately 50%, presumably because the infant has a reduced exposure to maternal blood and cervical secretions.[64] The combined use of maternal antiviral therapy and caesarian section delivery can theoretically reduce the risk of transmission to approximately 0.5%.

The incubation period for HIV infection is quite variable. Infants are generally asymptomatic during the first few months of life. The median age of onset for perinatally acquired untreated disease is 12–18 months. Conversely, severe illness can develop in the first few months of life. Approximately 10–15% of children will die before 4 years of age.[65]

Diagnosis

Diagnosis during infancy requires the detection of virus or viral nucleic acid, as almost all infants born to HIV-seropositive mothers will have transplacentally acquired antibodies, which may persist for up to 18 months. It is therefore necessary to document infection using other methods in the newborn and young infant. A positive viral culture is diagnostic; however, only 25–50% of infected children will be identified at birth by means of culture. In addition, viral culture is expensive, not widely available, and requires up to a month for results. PCR evaluation is a very sensitive and widely available method for the detection of HIV infection in the neonatal period, and is currently recommended.

Approximately 30% of HIV-infected infants will have positive PCR studies within the first 48 hours of life, and 93% will be positive by 2 weeks of age.[66] If initial evaluation within the first 48 hours is negative, repeat tests should be performed at 1–3 months, and then again at 4–6 months if necessary.[66]

Laboratory findings suspicious for HIV infection include a decreased ratio of helper to suppressor T cells, and hypergammaglobulinemia. One study suggested that elevated IgG levels and oral candidiasis in children less than 15 months of age had a high (98%) specificity for the diagnosis, but low sensitivity (37%).[66] Lymphopenia is not usually seen in infants and children. Microcytic, hypochromic anemia is common, and thrombocytopenia may also be present. Because cutaneous disease in HIV-infected patients often presents in an atypical fashion, culture and biopsy of any suspicious lesion should be obtained if the diagnosis is in doubt.

Treatment

Treatment with zidovudine of the HIV-infected pregnant woman and the newborn infant can significantly decrease perinatal transmission, as can caesarian section delivery (see above). Oral administration of zidovudine to the infant for 6 weeks significantly reduces the risk of perinatal transmission. CDC guidelines are continuously updated, are available on the CDC website, and represent the most current consensus on treatment. (See *www.aidsinfo.nih.gov* for updates regarding interventions). Most infected pregnant women are on combination antiretroviral therapy. Short-term adverse effects of the drug include anemia, neutropenia, and hepatitis. No long-term adverse side effects have been noted.[67] Infected infants should be referred to an HIV specialist as recommendations for therapy are developing. Breastfeeding by HIV-infected women is not recommended in areas where safe alternative options are available.

Chemoprophylaxis with TMP/SMX (trimethoprim-solfamethoxazole) reduces the risk of infection with *Pneumocystis jiroveci* and may reduce the incidence of cutaneous bacterial infections. Cutaneous infections with fungi, bacteria, and viruses should be treated as appropriate for each disease. Candidiasis usually requires systemic therapy, and fluconazole has proved particularly useful for this purpose. Acyclovir therapy is appropriate for the treatment of herpes simplex and zoster infections, but chronic use may lead to acyclovir resistance, which is more common in the AIDS population. Foscarnet and ganciclovir have both proved to be efficacious antiviral agents in immunocompromised patients.

HUMAN PARVOVIRUS B19 INFECTIONS

Parvovirus B19 infection is classically associated with a benign viral exanthem of childhood (erythema infectiosum) consisting of a distinctive 'slapped cheek' appearance, followed by a reticulate, lacy truncal eruption. The virus can also less commonly manifest other findings in children and adults (see Table 13-3), as well in the developing fetus and infant.[68] The entire range of clinical manifestations caused by parvovirus B19 continues to expand, and the list of associated findings is remarkable for its diversity. This virus has a particular propensity for red blood progenitor cells, but can also affect skin, liver, and myocardial cells.[67] Although the majority of healthy individuals who are infected have few or no symptoms, the fetus is at particular risk for significant morbidity. Infection during pregnancy has been associated with an increased risk of miscarriage, fetal hydrops, intrauterine growth retardation, and isolated pleural and pericardial effusions.[69] The risk of fetal death is approximately 1–9%, with the greatest risk occurring

TABLE 13-3 Manifestations of human Parvovirus B19 infection

Host	Findings
Immunocompetent children	Erythema infectiosum, papular purpuric gloves and socks syndrome
Immmunocompetent adults	Transient arthritis
Individuals with increased hemolysis, e.g. sickle cell disease	Transient aplastic crisis
Immunodeficient patients	Chronic anemia
Fetus (first 20 weeks' gestation)	Hydrops fetalis, pleural, pericardial, peritoneal effusion, anemia
Infant	Persistent anemia, red cell aplasia; blueberry muffin lesions (rare)

TABLE 13-4 Recommendations for pregnant women exposed to parvovirus B19*

Obtain titers; if IgG positive, check for IgM; if IgM negative, patient is immune with no risk
If titers are negative, recheck in 2 mos; if IgM then positive offer serial ultrasound follow-up

Highest risk present in first 20 weeks of pregnancy.

during the first half of pregnancy (Table 13-4). Recommendations for management of exposed pregnant women are summarized in Table 13-4. Symptomatic neonatal disease is rare and usually consists of persistent anemia following congenital infection.[70]

Fetal/Congenital and Neonatal Disease

Cutaneous Findings

The most common findings in affected abortuses are pallor, maceration, and subcutaneous edema, all consistent with the diagnosis of hydrops. Blueberry muffin lesions showing extramedullary hematopoiesis have also been reported.

Extracutaneous Findings

Increased fluid may develop in the pericardial, peritoneal and pleural cavities. The exact risk of congenital anomalies following B19 infection is controversial, but is thought to be extremely low. Significant ocular abnormalities involving the globe, retina, and cornea have been reported in one case.[71] Bilateral cleft lip and palate, micrognathia, subcutaneous hemorrhage, and congestion of internal organs have been found in fetuses in association with characteristic nuclear inclusions within erythroid precursor cells, endothelial, and smooth muscle cells.[72] Three live-born infants with severe neurologic defects whose mothers had serologically documented parvovirus infection during pregnancy have also been described.[73] Large prospective studies have failed to note any significant risk of congenital abnormalities following maternal parvovirus infection.[74] Current consensus is that the risk of congenital infection from parvovirus is less than 1% and is not yet clearly determined.[75]

Most cases of documented neonatal infection consist of persistent anemia following congenital infection.[65] Isolated congenital red cell aplasia, which may mimic Diamond–Blackfan anemia, may be caused by parvovirus B19 infection.[75] Relapsing erythroid hypoplasia in a 2-month-old infant has also been attributed to parvoviral infection. Multisystem disease in an infant who presented at birth with petechiae and thrombocytopenia and developed edema, cardiomegaly, bradycardia, and hypotension on day 2 has also been reported.[76] True neonatal disease is thought to be rare, but it is possible that it may be unrecognized and underreported. Unfortunately, technical problems in identifying neonatal infection make it difficult to ascertain the true incidence (see the following discussion).

Etiology/Pathogenesis

Parvovirus is one of the smallest known DNA viruses to infect humans. It is a global pathogen with increased prevalence in the late winter and early spring in temperate climates. Periodic epidemics occur.[77] The most common mode of transmission is person-to-person contact via respiratory secretions. The incubation period is 4–14 days, but can be as long as 21 days.[74] B19 can also be transmitted vertically from mother to fetus, and during transfusion with contaminated blood products.[78] Since 2002, quantitative DNA measurement has been used to screen plasma products and thus reduce the risk of transmission through blood products.

Infection is rare in the first year of life, and the highest rate of infection occurs among children of school age. The prevalence of IgG antibodies in pregnant women is approximately 65%.[68] Secondary attack rates are highest with household contact. Pregnant women with a child aged 5–7 years in the household appear to have a higher risk of becoming infected than do those with children under 2 years of age. Of particular concern is the risk to seronegative women in day-care and school settings, because infection in the first 20 weeks of gestation can lead to increased fetal wastage and fetal hydrops. The greatest risk occurs during epidemics, and nursery school teachers appear to have a threefold increased risk of acute infection compared to other pregnant women.[68] Nonetheless, routine exclusion of pregnant women from the workplace is not recommended, as risk of infection from other contacts is also likely during epidemics.

Parvovirus B19 propagates in human erythroid cells. In normal hosts, the cytotoxic effect of the virus leads to cessation of red blood cell production for approximately 4–8 days, creating a significant stress in patients with a rapidly expanding red cell mass (e.g. second-trimester fetus), or decreased red cell survival (e.g. underlying hemolytic anemia). The cellular receptor for parvovirus B19 (globoside or blood group P antigen) is located predominantly on the surface of erythroid precursor cells, thus explaining the virus's affinity for this cell line. It is also present on myocardial cells, megakaryocytes, and endothelial cells, which may explain the thrombocytopenia, vasculitis, and myocarditis that are occasionally noted in affected fetuses and individuals.[67] Immunocompromised hosts, presumably including fetuses, may have persistent viral infection and resultant chronic anemia.

The pathogenesis of hydrops secondary to parvovirus may be multifactorial. Severe anemia is almost always present and may lead to hypoxic injury and high output cardiac failure. Ascites, effusions, and skin edema may result. Myocarditis and diminished fetal cardiac output have also been noted in some cases, and may contribute to hydrops.

The exact risk to any pregnant woman (and her fetus) following exposure is not precisely known, although there appears to be a risk only if infection develops within the first 20 weeks of gestation. Various studies have estimated the risk of adverse fetal outcome following maternal infection to be from 1% to 9%.[68] Prospective studies have shown an excess rate of fetal loss of 9%, confined to exposure during the first 20 weeks of gestation, and an incidence of fetal hydrops of 2.9% with maternal infection between 11 and 18 weeks' gestation.[74,79] No significant risk for congenital anomalies has been noted. Spontaneous resolution of hydrops has been documented and complicates the issue of when and if intrauterine transfusion should be carried out (see Treatment, below).

Diagnosis

The diagnosis of acute parvovirus infection in pregnant women using IgM antibodies or IgG seroconversion is straightforward. Using radioimmunoassay or ELISA, over 90% of cases can be documented at the time of rash.[78] The presence of IgM indicates that infection probably occurred within the previous 2–4 months. IgG levels are helpful to determine past exposure, and hence immunity, but are not helpful in detecting acute infection, as more than 50% of adults are seropositive. Fetuses, neonates, and immunocompromised patients may not mount an appropriate immune response following infection, and other methods may be required to document infection in these patients.

Virus may be identified using DNA hybridization techniques and PCR assays for B19.[72] Routine histopathologic evaluation may reveal the presence of characteristic intranuclear inclusions in nucleated erythroid cells in placental or fetal tissue. Immunohistochemistry may detect viral antigen by staining techniques. Electron microscopy has been used to detect virus particles in serum, and prenatally in amniotic fluid, fetal blood, and ascitic fluid, as well as in postmortem tissue.[69]

Serologic evidence of infection in infants may be reevaluated at 1 year of age, at which time maternal antibody should have disappeared and immunoglobulin detection will indicate true fetal or neonatal infection. Viral studies may fail to reveal acute infection if carried out subsequent to resolution of the infection. Viremia persists only 2–4 days in the immunocompetent host, and is generally absent by the time the classic rash develops.

Differential Diagnosis

Nonimmune fetal hydrops can result from a number of diverse etiologies. It has been associated with many cardiac, infectious, hematologic, and genetic abnormalities, including anemias of diverse origins, CMV, toxoplasmosis, and syphilis.

Treatment

Management of the Exposed Pregnant Woman

Serologic evaluation should be offered; if the woman has high IgG titers to parvovirus B19 and lacks IgM, she is immune and not at risk. If she is seronegative, titers should be rechecked in 2 weeks for the presence of specific IgM. If evidence of acute infection exists, serial ultrasonographic evaluation is suggested.[80,81] α-Fetoprotein levels have also been used as a screening tool.[80,81] The risk of adverse outcome is minimal if infection occurs after 20 weeks' gestation, and low even if the mother becomes infected in the first two trimesters.

Management of Fetal Hydrops

Fetal intrauterine digitalization and transfusion may be useful if significant fetal hydrops is observed.[81] Although studies have shown reduced mortality with transfusion, its use is controversial because cases with spontaneous resolution of intrauterine hydrops can occur, and the procedure poses some risk to the fetus.

Congenital and Neonatal Infection

Neonates with congenital infection attributed to parvovirus may respond to intravenous immunoglobulin therapy. Supportive care, including transfusion, may be required.

Prophylaxis

A candidate recombinant vaccine composed of capsid proteins has been evaluated in phase I trials and appears both immunogenic and safe.[82]

ENTEROVIRUS

The enteroviruses are a group of common, single-stranded RNA viruses that include the polioviruses, Coxsackie viruses A and B, and echoviruses. Enteroviral infection in the neonate occurs most frequently during summer and early fall.

Cutaneous Findings

Perinatal disease occurs within the first few weeks of life and results in the nonspecific clinical symptoms of sepsis (fever, irritability, poor feeding), accompanied by skin findings in approximately one-third to two-thirds of infants.[83,85] The rash is most often maculopapular (morbilliform), macular, or petechial (Fig. 13-8). The vesicopustular lesions that occur on intact skin (lesions analogous to those seen in hand, foot, and mouth disease) develop secondary to viremia, not from local inoculation as is seen in HSV infections. The pharynx is often erythematous, but usually without lesions. However, ulcers consistent with herpangina may appear on the soft palate. These early lesions may be indistinguishable from those of HSV infection. With progression of the infection, oral lesions remain circular (2–4 mm in diameter), confined to the soft palate, and exhibit a 'punched-out' appearance surrounded by a rim of erythema. Unlike those of HSV, they do not continue to enlarge or involve the hard palate, buccal mucosa, or gingival sulci.

Extracutaneous Findings

Systemic manifestations of infection may be mild or severe. Disseminated infection involving the lungs, liver, and CNS (in addition to the upper respiratory tract and skin) occurs more often in the premature than in the full-term infant. The degree of transplacental antibody present is likely to affect the severity of the infection; therefore the most overwhelming infections occur in premature infants who lack significant amounts of specific maternal antibody for the infecting type of enterovirus.

In utero disease may occur rarely, with insufficient numbers of cases reported to consider a 'congenital infection syndrome.' Findings in the neonate appear to result from residual damage to the heart, gastrointestinal tract, urogenital tract, muscle, or cutaneous tissue, rather than ongoing infection or latent infection with reactivation of virus, with an apparent high intrauterine mortality rate.[86]

Etiology/Pathogenesis

Estimated rates of neonatal infection are between 2 and 38 cases per 1000 births.[83,87] Modes of transmission to the infant

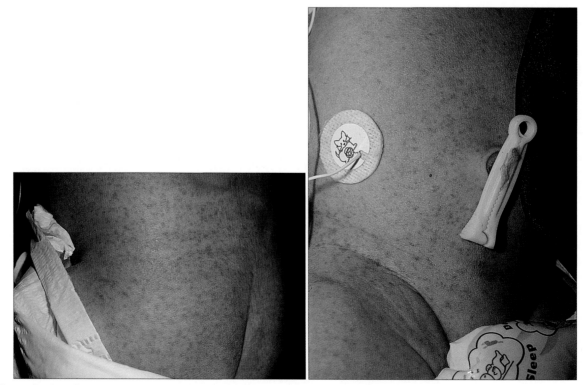

FIG. 13-8 Generalized erythematous papular eruption associated with enterovirus infection.

are similar to those for HSV. Acquisition from maternal sources at the time of delivery occurs in the majority of neonatal infections, with congenital infection being reported only rarely.[88] Postnatal infection from sources other than the mother is also very common, leading to illness and frequent hospitalization of symptomatic infants during the first few months of life.

Diagnosis

Definitive diagnosis of enteroviral infection is most often achieved PCR or by viral culture of the pharynx or stool (see Table 13-1). During acute infection, cultures of the pharynx are the most likely to yield the pathogen, whereas intestinal excretion of virus from gut-associated lymphoid tissue increases following clinical recovery. Fecal shedding of virus may continue for up to 6 weeks after acute infection, despite the presence of neutralizing antibody in serum. The PCR technique has been exceptionally useful in the diagnosis of enteroviral meningitis, and may be performed on the CSF of an infant whose rash is suspected to be enteroviral in origin.[83,89] PCR of material from the pharynx, stool, or lesions has not been systematically evaluated. Histologic examination of the morbilliform skin eruptions does not yield specific cytologic information on the viral etiology of the rash. Serologies are not usually helpful, as no class-specific antibody response occurs with enteroviral infections, and at least 72 serotypes of enterovirus have been identified to date.

Treatment

Traditionally, only supportive care has been given; however, some experts recommend the administration of intravenous immunoglobulin to infants with overwhelming systemic infection.[90] Specific antiviral therapy with a novel antipicorna agent, pleconaril, is currently in clinical trials in newborn infants with disseminated infection and has the potential to offer effective therapy for serious enteroviral infections.[83]

HUMAN PAPILLOMA VIRUS INFECTIONS

Infection with the human papilloma virus (HPV) can lead to cutaneous infections that commonly manifest as warts on the skin or mucous membranes. Lesions may be spread by direct sexual or nonsexual contact. Mother to infant transmission can be transplacental or via exposure to cervical or genital lesions. Autoinoculation or transmission via sexual abuse can also occur. There is some evidence that fomite spread is possible through the use of bidets, shared towels and undergarments.[91] The incubation period for HPV has been estimated at 1–20 months, but latency periods may be in excess of 2 years.[92] Although the vast majority of HPV disease results in transient lesions with a benign course, infection with certain subtypes of HPV (16, 18, 31, 33) can eventually lead to malignant metaplasia of the infected tissue.

Clinical lesions associated with HPV infections are only rarely present at birth or during the early neonatal period. Such lesions include anogenital warts (condyloma acuminata) and laryngeal papillomatosis. These lesions are more likely to become evident from 6 months to 2 years of age, and are believed to result from perinatal infection with a long latency period preceding clinical expression. A recent epidemiologic study of anogenital and laryngeal lesions in children under 13 years of age noted that the mean age of children with HPV was 4.5 years.[94] Given that the majority of cases of anogenital

HPV occur beyond 2 years of age, and that only a minority of these are sexually transmitted, it appears that many anogenital and laryngeal HPV infections in children are the result of horizontal transmission that is nonsexual. In general, in preadolescents the older the child, the higher the risk of sexual abuse. Nonetheless, it is still generally recommended that every case of anogenital warts be evaluated to ascertain the likelihood of sexual abuse, with appropriate follow-up investigations as deemed necessary.

Cutaneous Findings

Condyloma acuminata favor the mucocutaneous junctions and are soft, papillomatous pink to flesh-colored lesions that may be discrete or confluent, pedunculated or flat-topped (Fig. 13-9). Areas most frequently affected in infants include the perianal skin, glans penis, vulva, and vaginal introitus (Fig. 13-10). The usual interval between exposure and the development of lesions appears to be 1–8 months, with an average of 3 months; however it is believed that much longer latency periods, perhaps up to 2 years, can occur.[95,96] Lesions presenting in the neonatal period may represent in utero or perinatal exposure. Laryngeal papillomas may affect the larynx, and less commonly the trachea, bronchial, and pulmonary epithelia. They are thought to be acquired by aspiration of infectious

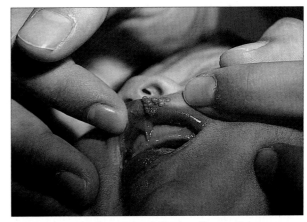

FIG. 13-9 Human papilloma virus infection. Congenital verrucous, filiform papules of the upper lip.

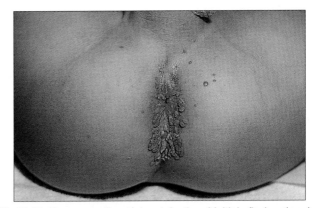

FIG. 13-10 Human papilloma virus infection. Multiple flesh-colored, discrete, and coalescent verrucous papules in the perianal region. Several smaller, ovoid flat lesions can be seen peripheral to the perianal site.

maternal vaginal and cervical secretions during labor. Such lesions usually present in infancy with hoarseness and respiratory distress.

Etiology/Pathogenesis

HPV is a small (55 nm), nonenveloped, circular, double-stranded DNA virus. It is expressed exclusively in fully differentiated keratinocytes and cannot be perpetuated in tissue culture. Over 130 different subtypes possessing varied oncogenic potential and tissue tropism have been identified.[97] Although the papilloma viruses are categorized as to mucosal or cutaneous tropism, this classification is not strict, as genital types may be found on the skin, and cutaneous subtypes have been identified in anogenital lesions, particularly in children.[97] The viruses have also been classified as to their malignant potential. HPV 6 and 11 are considered low-risk subtypes, whereas HPV 16, 18, 31, and 33 have been associated with anogenital cancer. HPV 30 has been associated with oral and laryngeal carcinoma, as well as anogenital carcinoma.[97]

HPV is currently one of the most common sexually transmitted diseases, and the increasing incidence in infants and children that has been noted by clinicians probably reflects the increasing prevalence in the adult population.[98] Most anogenital warts are subclinical and asymptomatic. The prevalence of genital lesions (condyloma) in the adult population is 0.6–13%, but molecular diagnostic studies show evidence of HPV infection in 11–80% of asymptomatic, sexually active young women.[99,100] Polymerase chain reaction studies have found a prevalence of genital HPV infection to be up to 80% among young women who are sexually active.[101] Anogenital and laryngeal involvement in children has risen in parallel with the increasing rate among adults. Transmission of infection may occur through vertical, innocent, and sexual contact. Subclinical infection of the cervix or vagina of a pregnant woman may lead to infection in her infant.[102] The virus can be transmitted from mother to fetus before or during birth, and the rate of perinatal transmission from genital HPV-positive mothers to the pharyngeal mucosa of their infants is approximately 30–50%.[103,104] However, studies of mother–neonate pairs have demonstrated that even when there is transmission of virus, it is most often only transiently positive and clinical disease is unlikely to occur.[103–105]

Neonates appear to be at higher risk for exposure to HPV during vaginal delivery than during cesarean section.[104] However, infants born by cesarean section have been found to be HPV DNA positive for the same type as their mothers.[106] Rare cases of anogenital warts present at birth following cesarean section delivery would support the possibility of ascending infection.[103] Transplacental exposure would explain such findings, as would small amniotic tears or leaks. The risk of a child contracting laryngeal papillomatosis is quite small.

HPV DNA has been identified in hepatic tissue from four infants with extrahepatic biliary duct atresia and three with neonatal giant cell hepatitis. Concordant HPV types were found in the infants' mothers, supporting vertical transmission of the virus and its role in the pathologies noted in these infants.[107]

Diagnosis

The clinical appearance of anogenital warts is usually diagnostic. A careful maternal history, including prior genital lesions and abnormal PAP smears, should be obtained. However, a negative history and normal maternal examination do not rule out the possibility of HPV disease. A spontaneous remission rate as high as 67% has been reported for HPV infections,[98] and subclinical infection of the cervix or vagina may be present.

Histopathologic examination of anogenital HPV lesions demonstrates a slightly thickened stratum corneum, papillomatosis, and acanthosis of the epithelium, and thickening and elongation of the rete ridges. The presence of large vacuolated cells (koilocytes) in the epithelium is a characteristic sign, but is absent in approximately 50% of biopsies. HPV typing using probes against the most commonly encountered types (6, 11, 16, 18, and 33) may be useful. Such typing can now be performed using paraffin sections from routinely fixed tissue samples. PCR evaluation of suspicious areas has also been performed using specimens obtained by swabbing the site with a simple cotton swab.[108]

Differential Diagnosis

Sexual abuse must be considered in childhood HPV disease but is much less likely in the small infant. Condyloma lata should always be considered in the differential diagnosis.

Syphilitic lesions are usually moister, wider based, and frequently larger than anogenital HPV lesions. Infantile pyramidal protrusion consists of a soft tissue swelling covered by smooth erythematous skin on the perineal median raphe. These may be congenital, tend to be larger than anogenital HPV lesions, and possess a smoother surface and a broad base. Molluscum contagiosum lesions are generally smoother, with a dome-shaped configuration, and central umbilication. Pseudoverrucous papules and nodules occur following a chronic irritant diaper dermatitis and can be mistaken for condylomata. Skin tags may resemble condyloma acuminata, but are uncommon in the neonatal period, are flesh-colored, discrete, and do not spread.

Treatment

Prevention is the optimal approach, and the development of at least two human papilloma virus vaccines has increased the likelihood of success of this goal. One of these vaccines is effective against HPV types 6, 11, 16, and 18, and has shown excellent safety and efficacy in a number of phase II and III randomized, double-blinded placebo-controlled trials.[109] The Merck vaccine is FDA approved, and vaccination of all females from 9-25 has been recommended. This vaccine is effective only if given prior to exposure to the particular HPV subtypes represented, and therefore vaccination prior to full sexual intercourse is recommended.

Many experts believe that treatment of these viral lesions may not always be necessary because warts are relatively asymptomatic, the spontaneous remission rate is quite high, and the cure rate with therapy low.[110] However, it must be kept in mind that oncogenic forms (HPV 16, 18, 31, 33) can lead to genital and clinical causes later in life. Fortunately, these sub-types are not usually found in childhood lesions. No easy, universally effective treatment exists. A number of therapeutic modalities have been used in adults and older children. These include liquid nitrogen, podophyllin resin, trichloroacetic acid, cantharidin, podofilox, imiquimod 5% cream, and interferon. Physical destruction, including electrodesiccation, laser therapy, and simple excision, is an alternative therapy. The failure rate for treatment of HPV infections has been estimated at 25–50%, regardless of the method used.[110] Vaccination to prevent acquisition of these strains with reoplastic potential would be the optimal approach.

Most experts opt for simple, less painful means of treatment in infants and young children. Topical agents frequently used include podophyllin resin, trichloroacetic acid and imiquimod cream. The family must be aware that frequent treatments are often required and that subclinical lesions in surrounding skin may become evident over time, despite the eradication of currently existing lesions.

MOLLUSCUM CONTAGIOSUM

Molluscum contagiosum is a viral infection of the skin that most commonly affects young children, but can occur at any age. This disease is only rarely noted in the neonatal period, but lesions have been documented within the first week of life.[111] A recent retrospective chart review of 302 patients found that less than 1% of affected patients were under 1 year; 28% of all affected patients were less than 36 months of age. The majority of patients who contracted the disease had less than 15 lesions, and children with atopic dermatitis were at higher risk for an increased number of lesions.[112]

Cutaneous Findings
Molluscum lesions initially appear as small pink or flesh-colored pinpoint papules, which gradually enlarge and assume a pearly or white dome-shaped appearance. The papules are usually 1–5 mm in size, but giant lesions in excess of 1 cm can occur. The lesions tend to cluster, and more commonly appear on the trunk and in intertriginous areas such as the antecubital and popliteal fossae and axillae. Rarely lesions may develop on the palms, soles, or mucous membranes. An eczematoid, red, scaling patch may surround the papules and is termed molluscum dermatitis. Autoinoculation from scratching or shaving may occur.[111]

There are rare reports of neonatal disease in the literature. Mandel and Lewis[111] reported an infant who developed two thigh papules at 1 week of life, and another author documented multiple scalp lesions in a 6-week-old.[113] Wilkin[114] described five women who had genital lesions at the time of delivery; none of their infants developed molluscum.

Etiology/Pathogenesis
Molluscum contagiosum is caused by a large, approximately 300 nm, brick-shaped poxvirus which contains double-stranded DNA. At least 43 different DNA subtypes have been identified. The entire genetic sequence of MCV type 1 has been determined, and there appears to be considerable protein homology with the smallpox virus.[115] The virus does not grow in tissue culture, and an animal model does not exist.

Molluscum has a worldwide distribution, but is most common in tropical countries. Spread is through direct (including sexual) contact with infected persons, contaminated items, or by means of autoinoculation. The incubation period is estimated at 2 weeks to 6 months. The duration of disease is quite variable and may last just a few weeks or more than a year.[116] Two peaks in incidence occur, one in early childhood and the other in young adults as a result of sexual transmission. An increased incidence has been noted in wrestlers and swimmers, and outbreaks have occurred in pools and water parks.[117] The disease has only rarely been noted in neonates, and it has been hypothesized that transplacental maternally derived antibody may be protective. The immunocompromised, especially those with HIV infection, are subject to particularly extensive and prolonged infections that commonly involve the face. Patients with atopic dermatitis also appear to have more prolonged infections.

Diagnosis
The diagnosis is easily established when classic dome-shaped opalescent lesions with central umbilication are present. A curd-like material can be expressed from the central core and examined for the presence of molluscum bodies. These appear as monomorphous ovoid granular structures, and are best visualized with Wright's or Giemsa stains, (KOH) potassium hydroxide staining is also an option. Histopathologic evaluation of a lesion will reveal large intracytoplasmic inclusion bodies within suprabasilar epithelial cells and lobular proliferation of the epidermis.

Differential Diagnosis
Cutaneous cryptococcal lesions are occasionally mistaken for molluscum contagiosum in immunocompromised patients. Small lesions may be mistaken for common or flat warts. Giant molluscum lesions can resemble juvenile xanthogranuloma or Langerhans' cell histiocytosis. Large inflamed lesions may resemble furuncles. The differential diagnosis for atypical giant lesions includes a number of neoplastic disorders, and biopsy is indicated in such cases.

Treatment
Molluscum is generally self-limited and frequently does not require therapy.[118] Instances where intervention may be necessary include conjunctival lesions, which may damage the cornea, irritated, bleeding, or rapidly spreading lesions, and cosmetically disfiguring lesions, particularly in the immunosuppressed patient. Genital lesions are usually treated to prevent spread. A number of therapeutic modalities are used, including physical agents such as cryotherapy and curettage. Topical chemical treatments include cantharidin 0.7% in collodion, imiquimod 5%, podophyllin, salicylic acid, tretinoin, and silver nitrate. Cantharidin is commonly used, and is applied with a wooden applicator to each site, taking care to avoid mucosal, intertriginous, and facial areas. The site is not occluded, and the family is instructed to wash the area in 2–6 hours, depending on previous sensitivity to the agent. Repeat treatments are sometimes required. Adhesive tape occlusion and systemic cimetidine therapy have been utilized, all with variable results. A local anesthetic consisting of topical lidocaine (LMX-4) may be applied prior to curettage. Families should be advised that multiple visits and treatments may be required and that spread of infection may occur through shared baths, towels, and swimming pools. Genital lesions are not uncommon in young children and are thought to be the result of autoinoculation. The issue of sexual abuse may be raised in older children, but supporting evidence should be documented prior to referral, as nonsexually transmitted genital involvement is often seen in childhood infections.[118]

REFERENCES

1. Sullivan-Bolyai J, Hull HF, Wilson C, et al. Neonatal herpes simplex virus infection in King County, Washington. JAMA 1983; 250: 3059–3062.
2. Overall JC. Herpes simplex virus infection of the fetus and newborn. Pediatr Ann 1994; 23: 131–136.
3. Brown ZA, Benedetti J, Ashley R, et al. Neonatal herpes simplex virus infection in relation to asymptomatic maternal infection at the time of labor. N Engl J Med 1991; 324: 1247–1252.
4. Brown ZA, Wald A, Ahsley R, et al. Effect of serologic status and cesarean delivery on transmission rates of herpes simplex virus from mother to infant. JAMA 2003; 289; 203–209.
5. Cone RW, Hobson AC, Brown Z, et al. Frequent detection of genital herpes simplex virus DNA by polymerase chain reaction among pregnant women. JAMA 1994; 272: 792–796.
6. Brown Z. Preventing herpes simplex virus transmission to the neonate. Herpes 2004; 11: 175A–186A.
7. Sieber OF, Fulginiti VA, Brazie J, et al. In utero infection of the fetus by herpes simplex virus. J Pediatr 1966; 69: 30–34.
8. South MA, Tompkins WAF, Morris CP, et al. Congenital malformation of the central nervous system associated with genital (type 2) herpes virus. J Pediatr 1969; 75: 13–18.
9. Sullender WM, Miller JL, Yasukawa LL, et al. Humoral and cell-mediated immunity in neonates with herpes simplex virus infection. J Infect Dis 1987; 155: 28–37.
10. Hutto C, Arvin A, Jacobs R, et al. Intrauterine herpes simplex virus infections. J Pediatr 1987; 110: 97–101.
11. Honig PJ, Brown D. Congenital herpes simplex infection initially resembling epidermolysis bullosa. J Pediatr 1982; 101: 958–960.
12. Johansson A, Rassart A, Blum D, et al. Lower-limb hypoplasia due to intrauterine infection with herpes simplex virus type-2: possible confusion with intrauterine varicella-zoster syndrome. Clin Infect Dis 2004; 38: e57–62.
13. Kimberlin DW, Jacobs RF, Powell DA, et al. The safety and efficacy of high-dose (HD) intravenous aciclovir (ACV) in the management of neonatal herpes simplex virus (HSV) infections. Pediatr 2001; 108; 230–238.
14. Kimberlin DW. Diagnosis of herpes simplex virus infections of the CNS. Expert Rev Mol Diagn 2005; 5: 537–547.
15. Kimberlin, DW. Herpes simplex virus infections in neonates and early childhood. Semin Pediatr Infect Dis 2005; 16: 271–281.
16. Whitley R, Arvin A, Prober C, et al. A controlled trial comparing vidarabine with acyclovir in neonatal herpes simplex virus infection. N Engl J Med 1991; 324: 444.
17. Sever J, White LR. Intrauterine viral infections. Annu Rev Med 1968; 19: 471–486.
18. Dufour P, de Bievre P, Vinatier D, et al. Varicella and pregnancy. Eur J Obstet Gynecol Reprod Biol 1996; 66: 119–123.
19. McIntosh D, Isaacs D. Varicella-zoster virus infection in pregnancy. Arch Dis Child 1993; 68: 1–2.
20. Kellner B, Kitai I, Krafchik B. What syndrome is this? Congenital varicella syndrome. Pediatr Dermatol 1996; 13: 341–344.
21. Paryani SG, Arvin AM. Intrauterine infection with varicella-zoster virus after maternal varicella. N Engl J Med 1986; 314: 1542–1546.
22. Enders G. Varicella-zoster virus infection in pregnancy. Prog Med Virol 1984; 29: 166–196.
23. Pastuszak AL, Levy M, Schick B, et al. Outcome after maternal varicella infection in the first 20 weeks of pregnancy. N Engl J Med 1994; 330: 901–905.
24. Kadourouo T, Theodoridou M, Mostrou G, et al. Herpes zoster in children. J Am Acad Dermatol 1998; 39: 207–210.
25. Enders G, Miller E, Craddock-Watson J, et al. Consequences of varicella and herpes zoster in pregnancy: Prospective study of 1739 cases. Lancet 1994; 343: 1548–1551.
26. Salzman MB, Sood SK. Congenital anomalies resulting from maternal varicella at 25½ weeks of gestation. Pediatr Infect Dis J 1992; 11: 504–505.
27. Koren G Congenital varicella syndrome in the third trimester. Lancet 2005; 366: 1591–1592.
28. Birthistle K, Carrington D. Fetal varicella syndrome – a reappraisal of the literature. A review prepared for the UK Advisory Group on Chickenpox on behalf of the British Society for the Study of Infection. J Infect 1998; 36: 25–29.
29. Harris RE, Rhoades ER. Varicella pneumonia complicating pregnancy: Report of a case and review of literature. Obstet Gynecol 1965; 25: 734–740.
30. Chapman SJ. Varicella in pregnancy. Semin Perinatol 1998; 22: 339–346.
31. Hartung J, Enders G, Chaoui R, et al. Prenatal diagnosis of congenital varicella syndrome and detection of varicella-zoster virus in the fetus: A case report. Prenat Diagn 1999; 19: 163–166.
32. Mouly F, Mirlesse V, Meritet JF, et al. Prenatal diagnosis of fetal varicella-zoster virus infection with polymerase chain reaction of amniotic fluid in 107 cases. Am J Obstet Gynecol 1997; 177: 894–898.
33. Pretorius DH, Hayward I, Jones KL, et al. Sonographic evaluation of pregnancies with maternal varicella infection. J Ultrasound Med 1992; 11: 459–463.
34. Berstraelen H, Banzieleghem B Defoort P et al. Prenatal ultrasound and magnetic resonance imaging in fetal varicella syndrome: correlation with pathology findings. Prenat Diagn 2003; 23: 705–709.
35. Gershon AA. Chicken Pox, measles, and mumps. Infect Dis Fetus Newborn 1995; 4: 578–583.
36. Miller E, Cradock-Watson JE, Ridehalgh MK. Outcome in newborn babies given anti-varicella zoster immunoglobin after perinatal maternal infection with varicella zoster virus. Lancet 1989; 2: 371–373.
37. Eldridge R, Tillson HH. Pregnancy outcome following systemic prenatal acyclovir exposure. Arch Dermatol 1994; 130: 153–154.
38. Stone KM, Reiff-Eldridge R, White AD, et al. Pregnancy Outcomes following Systemic Prenatal Acyclovir Exposure. Conclusions from the International Prenatal Acyclovir Exposure Registry 1984–89. Birth Defects Research Part A Clinical & Molecular Teratology 2004; 70: 201–207.
39. American Academy of Pediatrics. Varicella zoster infections. In: Pickering LK, ed. Red Book: Report of the Committee on Infectious Diseases, 27th edn. Elk Grove Village, IL: 2006; 711–725.
40. Singalavanija S, Limpongsanurak W, Horpoapan S, et al. Neonatal varicella: a report of 26 cases. J Med Assoc Thai 1999; 82: 957–962.
41. Frieden IJ, Berger TG, Westrom D. Eosinophil fluorescence: A cause of false positive slide tests for herpes simplex virus. Pediatr Dermatol 1987; 4: 129–133.
42. Bendig JA, Meurisse EV, Anderson F, et al. Neonatal varicella despite maternal immunity. Lancet 1998; 352: 1985–1986.
43. Ross SA, Boppana SB. Congenital cytomegalovirus infection: outcome and diagnosis. Semin Pediatr Infect Dis 2005; 16: 44–49.
44. Stagno S, Pass RF, Dworsky ME, et al. Congenital cytomegalovirus infection: the relative importance of primary and recurrent maternal infection. N Engl J Med 1982; 306: 945–949.
45. Demmler GJ. Summary of a workshop on surveillance for congenital cytomegalovirus disease. Rev Infect Dis 1991; 13: 315–329.
46. Arvin AM, Fast P, Myers M, et al. Vaccine development to prevent cytomegalovirus disease: report from the national vaccine advisory committee. Clin Infect Dis 2004; 39: 233–239.

47. Schleiss MR. Antiviral therapy of congenital cytomegalovirus infection. Semin Pediatr Infect Dis 2005; 16: 50–59.

48. Kimberlin DW, Lin CY, Sanchez PJ, et al. Effect of ganciclovir therapy on hearing in symptomatic congenital cytomegalovirus disease involving the central nervous system. J Pediatrics 2003 July; 143(1): 16–25.

49. Acosta EP, Brundage RC, King JR, et al. Ganciclovir population pharmacokinetics in neonates following intravenous administration. Clin Pharm Therapy 2007 Jun; 81: 867–872.

50. Cooper LZ, Preblud SR, Alford CA, et al. Rubella. In: Remington JS, Kln JO, Baber C, Wilson C, eds. Infectious diseases of the fetus and newborn infant, 6th edn. Philadelphia: WB Saunders, 2006.

51. Sanchez P. Viral infections of the fetus and neonate. In: Feigin RD, Cherry JD, Demmler GJ, Kaplan SL, eds. Textbook of pediatric infectious diseases, 6th edn. Philadelphia: WB Saunders, 2004; 881–885.

52. Burchett SK, Pizzo PA. HIV infection in infants, children and adolescents. Pediatr Rev 2003; 24: 186–194

53. American Academy of Pediatrics. Human Immunodeficiency Virus Infection Committee on Infectious Diseases. Red Book 2003; 360–382.

54. Pahwa S, Kaplan M, Fikrig S, et al. Spectrum of human T-cell lymphotropic virus type III infection in children. Recognition of symptomatic, asymptomatic, and seronegative patients. JAMA 1986; 255: 2299–2305.

55. Shetty D, Giri N, Gonzalez CE, et al. Invasive aspergillosis in human immunodeficiency virus-infected children. Pediatr Infect Dis J 1997; 16: 216–221.

56. Prose NS. Cutaneous manifestations of HIV infection in children. Dermatol Clin 1991; 9: 543–550.

57. Centers for Disease Control. HIV/AIDS surveillance report. Cancer as AIDS-defining illness. 1993; 1–18.

58. Athale UH, Patil PS, Chintu C, et al. Influence of HIV epidemic on the incidence of Kaposi's sarcoma in Zambian children. J AIDS Hum Retrovirol 1995; 8: 96–100.

59. Gutierrez-Ortega P, Hierro-Orozco S, Sanchez-Cisneros R, et al. Kaposi's sarcoma in a 6-day-old infant with human immunodeficiency virus. Arch Dermatol 1989; 125: 432–433.

60. Mueller BU, Butler KM, Higham MC, et al. Smooth muscle tumors in children with human immunodeficiency virus infection. Pediatrics 1992; 90: 460–463.

61. Straka BF, Whitaker DL, Morrison SH, et al. Cutaneous manifestations of the acquired immunodeficiency syndrome in children. J Am Acad Dermatol 1988; 18: 1089–1102.

62. Marion RW, Wiznia AA, Hutcheon RG, et al. Fetal AIDS syndrome score. Correlation between severity of dysmorphism and age at diagnosis of immunodeficiency. Am J Dis Child 1987; 141: 429–431.

63. Luzuriaga K, Sullivan JL. Pediatric HIV-1 infections advances and challenges. AIDS Rev 2002; 4: 21–26.

64. Gelber RD, Shapiro DE. Mode of delivery and the risk of vertical transmission of HIV-1. N Engl J Med 1999; 15: 341: 206–207.

65. American Academy of Pediatrics. Human Immunodeficiency Virus In: Pickering L, ed. 2003 Red Book: Report of the Committee on Infectious Diseases, 26th edn. Elk Grove Village, IL: American Academy of Pediatrics, 2003; 367.

66. Meyer MP, Latief Z, Haworth C, et al. Symptomatic HIV infection in infancy – clinical and laboratory markers of infection. S Africa Med J 1997; 87: 158–162.

67. Culnane M, Fowler M, Lee SS, et al. Lack of long-term effects of in utero exposure to zidovudine among uninfected children born to HIV-infected women. Pediatric AIDS Clinical Trials Group Protocol 219/076 Teams. JAMA 1999; 13: 281: 151–157.

68. Vogel H, Kornman M, Ledet SC, et al. Congenital parvovirus infection. Pediatr Pathol Lab Med 1997; 17: 903–912.

69. Valeur-Jensen AK, Pedersen CB, Westergaard T, et al. Risk factors for parvovirus B19 infection in pregnancy. JAMA 1999; 281: 1099–1105.

70. Brown KE, Green SW, Antunez de Mayolo J, et al. Congenital anaemia after transplacental B19 parvovirus infection. Lancet 1994; 343: 895–896.

71. Van Elsacker-Niele AM, Salimans MM, Weiland HT, et al. Fetal pathology in human parvovirus B19 infection. Br J Obstet Gynaecol 1989; 96: 768–775.

72. Tiessen RG, van Elsacker-Niele AM, Vermeij-Keers C, et al. A fetus with a parvovirus B19 infection and congenital anomalies. Prenat Diagn 1994; 14: 173–176.

73. Conroy JA, Torok T, Andrews PI. Perinatal encephalopathy secondary to inutero human parvo B19 infection [abstract 7365]. Neurology 1993; 43: A346.

74. Miller E, Fairley CK, Cohen BJ, et al. Immediate and long-term outcome of human parvovirus B19 infection in pregnancy. Br J Obstet Gynaecol 1998; 105: 174–178.

75. Auerbach AD, Verlander PC, Brown KE, et al. New molecular diagnostic tests for two congenital forms of anemia. J Clin Lab Anal 1997; 11: 17–22.

76. Minowa H, Nishikubo T, Uchida Y, et al. Neonatal erythema infectiosum. Acta Paediatr Jpn 1998; 40: 88–90.

77. Brown KE, Young NS. Parvovirus B19 in human disease. Annu Rev Med 1997; 48: 59–67.

78. American Academy of Pediatrics. Paruovirus B19 In: Pickering L, ed. Red Book: Report of the Committee on Infectious Diseases, 26th edn. Elk Grove Village, IL: American Academy of Pediatrics, 2003; 459–461.

79. Public Health Laboratory Service Working Party on Fifth Disease. Prospective study of human parvovirus (B19) infection in pregnancy. Br Med J 1990; 300: 1166–1170.

80. Levy R, Weissman A, Blomberg G, et al. Infection by parvovirus B 19 during pregnancy: A review. Obstet Gynecol Surv 1997; 52: 254–259.

81. Fairley CK, Smoleniec JS, Caul OE, et al. Observational study of effect of intrauterine transfusions on outcome of fetal hydrops after parvovirus B19 infection. Lancet 1995; 346: 1335–1337.

82. Ballou WR, Reed JL, Noble W et al. Safety and immunogenicity of a recombinant parvovirus B19 vaccine formulated with MF59C.1. J Infect Dis 2003; 187: 675–678.

83. Abzug MJ. Presentation, diagnosis, and management of enterovirus infections in neonates. Pediatr Drugs 2004; 6: 1–10.

84. Lake AM, Lauer BA, Clark JC, et al. Enterovirus infections in neonates. J Pediatr 1976; 89: 787–791.

85. Abzug MJ, Levin MJ, Rotbart HA. Profile of enterovirus disease in the first two weeks of life. Pediatr Infect Dis J 1993; 12: 820–824.

86. Nuovo GJ, Cooper LD, Bartholomew D. Histologic, infectious, and molecular correlates of idiopathic spontaneous abortion and perinatal mortality. Diagn Mol Pathol 2005; 14: 152–158.

87. Sanchez P. Viral infections of the fetus and neonate. In: Feigin RD, Cherry JD, Demmler GJ, Kaplan SL, eds. Textbook of pediatric infectious diseases, 5th edn. Philadelphia: WB Saunders, 2004; 895–897.

88. Modlin JF. Update on enterovirus infections in infants and children. Adv Pediatr Infect Dis 1997; 12: 155–180.

89. Sawyer MH. Enterovirus infections: Diagnosis and treatment. Pediatr Infect Dis J 1999; 18: 1033–1040.

90. Abzug MJ, Keyserling HL, Lee ML, et al. Neonatal enterovirus infection: Virology, serology, and effects of intravenous immune globulin. Clin Infect Dis 1995; 20: 1201–1206.

91. Pacheco B, DiPaola G, Ribs J et al. Vulvar infections caused by human papilloma virus in children and adolescents without sexual contact. Adolesc Pediatr Gynecol 1991; 4: 136–142.

92. Siegfried EC. Warts on children: An approach to therapy. Pediatr Ann 1996; 25: 79–90.

93. Frasier LD. Human papillomavirus infections in children. Pediatr Ann 1994; 23: 354–360.
94. Sinclair KA, Woods CR, Kirse DJ, Sinal SH. Anogenital and respiratory tract human papillomavirus infections among children: Age, gender, and potential transmission through sexual abuse. Pediatrics 2005; 116: 815–825.
95. Barrett TJ. Genital warts: A venereal disease. J Am Acad Dermatol 1954: 333–334.
96. Oriel JD. Natural history of genital warts. Br J Venereal Dis 1971; 47: 1–13.
97. Majewski S, Jablonska S. Human papillomavirus-associated tumors of the skin and mucosa. J Am Acad Dermatol 1997; 36: 659–685; quiz 686–688.
98. Allen AL, Siegfried EC. The natural history of condyloma in children. J Am Acad Dermatol 1998; 39: 951–955.
99. Schneider A, Koutsky LA. Natural history and epidemiological features of genital HPV infection. IARC Sci Publ 1992; 265: 472–477.
100. Moscicki AB. Human papillomavirus infections. Adv Pediatr 1992; 39: 257–281.
101. Brown DR, Shew ML, Qadadri B et al. A longitudinal study of genital human papillomavirus infection in a cohort of closely followed adolescent women. J Infect Dis 2005; 191: 182–192.
102. Mazzatenta C, Fimiani M, Rubegni P, et al. Vertical transmission of human papillomavirus in cytologically normal women. Genitourinary Med 1996; 72: 445–446.
103. Tseng CJ, Liang CC, Soong YK, et al. Perinatal transmission of human papillomavirus in infants: Relationship between infection rate and mode of delivery. Obstet Gynecol 1998; 91: 92–96.
104. Sedlacek TV, Lindheim S, Eder C, et al. Mechanism for human papillomavirus transmission at birth. Am J Obstet Gynecol 1989; 161: 55–59.
105. Tenti P, Zappatore R, Migliora P, et al. Perinatal transmission of human papillomavirus from gravidas with latent infections. Obstet Gynecol 1999; 93: 475–479.
106. Puranen MH, Yliskoski MH, Saarikoski SV, et al. Exposure of an infant to cervical human papillomavirus infection of the mother is common. Am J Obstet Gynecol 1997; 176: 1039–1045.
107. Drut R, Gomez MA, Drut RM, et al. Acta Gastroenterol Latinoam 1998; 28: 27–31 [Spanish].
108. Siegfried EC, Frasier LD. Anogenital warts in children. Adv Dermatol 1997; 12: 141–166; discussion 167.
109. Villa LL, Costa RL, Andrade RP et al. Prophylactic quadrivalent human papillomavirus L1 virus-like particle vaccine in young women: a randomized double-blind placebo-controlled multicentre phase II efficacy trial. Lancet Oncol 2005; 5: 271–278.
110. Hines JF, Ghim SJ, Jenson AB. Prospects for human papillomavirus vaccine development: Emerging HPV vaccines. Curr Opin Obstet Gynecol 1998; 10: 15–19.
111. Mandel MJ, Lewis RJ. Molluscum contagiosum of the newborn. Br J Dermatol 1971; 84: 370–372.
112. Dohil MA, Lin P, Lee J, et al. The epidemiology of molluscum contagiosum in children J Am Acad Dermatol 2006; 54: 47–54.
113. Young WJ. Molluscum contagiosum with unusual distribution. Kentucky Med J 1926; 24: 467.
114. Wilkin JK. Molluscum contagiosum venereum in a women's outpatient clinic: A venereally transmitted disease. Am J Obstet Gynecol 1977; 128: 531–535.
115. Senkevich TG, Bugert JJ, Sisler JR, et al. Genome sequence of a human tumorigenic poxvirus: Prediction of specific host response-evasion genes. Science 1996; 273: 813–816.
116. Lewis EJ, Lam M, Crutchfield CE III. An update on molluscum contagiosum. Cutis 1997; 60: 29–34.
117. Castilla MT, Sanzo JM, Fuentes S. Molluscum contagiosum in children and its relationship to attendance at swimming-pools: An epidemiological study. Dermatology 1995; 191: 165.
118. Highet AS. Molluscum contagiosum. Arch Dis Child 1992; 67: 1248–1249.

14

Fungal Infections, Infestations and Parasitic Infections in Neonates

K. Robin Carder

FUNGAL INFECTIONS

Infections caused by fungi and yeasts are common in neonates and infants. Of these, the most frequent is *Candida* infection, presenting as thrush and diaper dermatitis. More extensive manifestations, such as congenital and systemic candidiasis, are less common. Significant fungal infections are being seen more often in very low-birthweight (VLBW), preterm infants. *Malassezia furfur* can colonize the skin or manifest as neonatal cephalic pustulosis, tinea versicolor, or fungemia. *Aspergillus* is second only to *Candida* as a cause of opportunistic fungal infections in these hosts. Zygomycosis and trichosporonosis are seen almost exclusively in premature infants. Dermatophyte infections include tinea capitis and tinea corporis.

Candidiasis

Epidemiology and Pathogenesis

Candida is the most common fungal pathogen in newborns.[1] Infection may be acquired vertically from the mother or horizontally by nosocomial transmission in the nursery.[1] *C. albicans* is responsible for approximately 75% of neonatal fungal infections.[2] Other *Candida* species associated with neonatal disease include *C. tropicalis*, *C. parapsilosis*, *C. lusitaniae*, and *C. glabrata* (*Torulopsis glabrata*). Normally these yeasts are saprophytes, inhabiting the skin or gastrointestinal tract without invasion unless host defenses are altered. *Candida* spp. may also colonize endotracheal tubes and catheters without causing systemic illness, but associated clinical illness is common in VLBW infants.[3] In extremely low-birthweight infants (<1000 g), invasive candidiasis is common. In one prospective study, 7% of 4379 infants had *Candida* isolated from blood or cerebrospinal fluid.[3a]

Virulence mechanisms associated with *Candida* infections include fungal proteinase, increased adherence of yeast to epithelial cells due to similarity to mammalian cell ligands, and resistance to neutrophil ingestion of hyphal forms.[4] Secretory IgA, functional T lymphocytes, and phagocytic cells are important in defense against *Candida* infections, hence the increased susceptibility to these infections in patients with secretory IgA deficiency, primary T-cell deficiency such as DiGeorge syndrome, severe combined immunodeficiency, chronic granulomatous disease, myeloperoxidase deficiency, and human immunodeficiency virus (HIV) infection. Recurrent or persistent yeast infections can be presenting symptoms of immunodeficiency. Host resistance to fungal infections also depends on activated macrophages, which in turn rely on T-lymphocyte release of interferon (IFN)-γ. Incomplete activation of macrophages by IFN in neonates[5] contributes to increased susceptibility to invasive fungal disease.

Predisposing factors for *Candida* (monilial) infections include excessive humidity, maceration, diabetes, and broad-spectrum antibiotics. Risk factors for systemic candidiasis in neonates include low birthweight, prematurity, broad-spectrum antibiotic therapy, indwelling catheters, prolonged endotracheal intubation, tracheostomy, prior fungal colonization, gastrointestinal pathology or abdominal surgery, enteral feeding, immunosuppression, defective neutrophil function or neutropenia, and steroid therapy.[2,6–11]

Various techniques in addition to culture are used to evaluate the epidemiology of fungal pathogens. They include polymerase chain reaction (PCR), restriction fragment endonuclease digestion of chromosomal DNA, electrophoretic karyotyping, and Southern blot hybridization analysis using DNA probes, β-glucan assay (β-D-glucan is a major component of the fungal cell wall) and gas chromatography mass spectrometry for D-arabitinol (a major metabolite of most *Candida* species).[1,15]

Clinical presentations of candidal infections are discussed in the next section, followed by diagnostic and treatment recommendations.

Congenital Candidiasis

Congenital candidiasis (CC) refers to *Candida* infection acquired in utero and presenting with symptoms in the first days of life.[12] Classic congenital candidiasis presents as a diffuse cutaneous infection, presumed to arise from an ascending intrauterine chorioamnionitis. The typical patient is an otherwise healthy term neonate who, within the first 12 hours of life, develops a monomorphous papulovesicular eruption that is intensely erythematous (Figs 14-1 and 14-2). The papular rash progresses to pustules, followed by late crusting and desquamation. Any area of the body surface, including the face, palms, and soles, can be involved, and widespread involvement is often evident (Fig. 14-3). *Candida* paronychia and onycho-

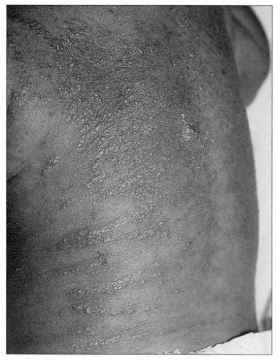

FIG. 14-1 Congenital candidiasis. Diffuse, erythematous, pustular eruption.

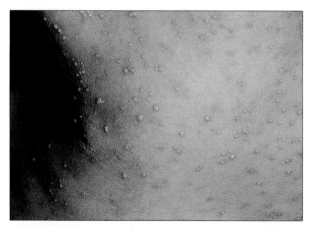

FIG. 14-2 Congenital candidiasis. Diffusely distributed, distinct pustules.

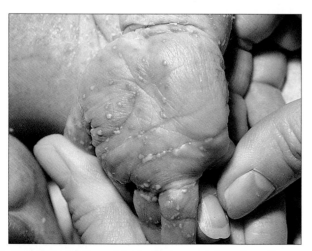

FIG. 14-3 Congenital candidiasis. Palmar pustules with erythema.

mycosis have been reported.[12–15] Congenital candidiasis is surprisingly uncommon given the 33% rate of vaginal colonization with *Candida* in pregnant women.[2] The presence of a foreign body in the maternal uterus or cervix is a risk factor for CC.[12] In the majority of term infants with CC systemic dissemination of yeast is rare, and the prognosis is excellent, with rapid clearance of the rash using topical treatment alone. Occasionally CC can present as pneumonia and sepsis without a rash.[16] CC with systemic involvement is more commonly seen in premature, low-birthweight infants (<1500 g).[12,17–19] Skin findings in these infants may be variable, with a burn-like dermatitis (similar to staphylococcal scalded skin syndrome) in addition to the usual red scaly or vesiculopustular eruption.[12] A widespread rash in a premature or ill-appearing infant, respiratory distress in the immediate postnatal period, leukocytosis, or hyperglycemia should alert the physician to the possibility of systemic candidiasis despite negative blood cultures.[12,19,20]

Systemic Candidiasis

Systemic candidiasis (SC), defined as *Candida* infection in an otherwise sterile body fluid such as blood, urine, or cerebrospinal fluid, affects 2–7% of VLBW newborns.[3a,6,21] Skin manifestations occur in up to 60% of these infants.[20] These infections can be acquired in utero (CC) or postnatally. Baley et al.[21] described skin manifestations of VLBW infants with SC. Included were an extensive burn-like dermatitis followed by desquamation, progressive diaper dermatitis involving papules and pustules, and isolated diaper rash with or without thrush (Fig. 14-4).[21] Cutaneous abscesses at the site of intravascular catheters may also be seen.[2] Systemic signs include apnea, bradycardia, abdominal distension, guaiac-positive stools, hyperglycemia, temperature instability, leukemoid reaction, and hypotension.[2,6,22]

Invasive Fungal Dermatitis

Invasive fungal dermatitis (IFD) is a clinicopathologic entity of erosive crusting lesions in VLBW infants. It is described by Rowen et al.[23] as a primary skin condition that leads to secondary dissemination and systemic disease. It is primarily due to *Candida albicans* or other *Candida* species. *Aspergillus*, *Trichosporon beigelii*, and *Curvularia* are also etiologic agents of invasive fungal dermatitis. Skin biopsy demonstrates fungal invasion beyond the stratum corneum, well into the epidermis, and at times extending into the dermis. Onset several days after birth, the presence of erosions and crusts, and typical histologic findings help to differentiate IFD from congenital candidiasis. Risk factors include extreme prematurity (<25 weeks' gestational age), vaginal birth, steroid administration, and hyperglycemia.[23]

Localized Neonatal Candidiasis
Oral Candidiasis (Thrush)

Acute oral candidiasis appears on the oropharyngeal mucosa as white adherent curd-like plaques resembling milk or formula (Fig. 14-5). Plaques can be scraped off only with difficulty, leaving a bright erythematous base (pseudomembranous and erythematous forms, respectively). Extensive infection can lead to feeding difficulties, particularly if the esophagus is involved.[2]

Candida Diaper Dermatitis

Candida infection of the diaper area may occur alone or in conjunction with thrush. Bright, erythematous plaques,

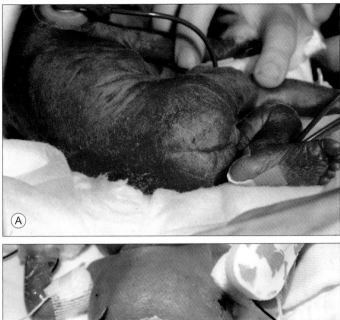
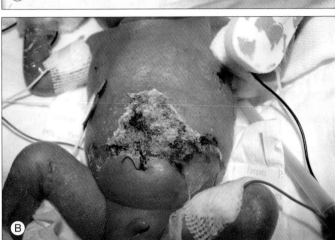

FIG. 14-4 (A) Congenital candidiasis in a premature infant presenting with diffuse erythema and a scald-like appearance (Courtesy of Robert Silverman, MD.) (B) Candidiasis with scald-like erythema with localized crusting and necrosis.

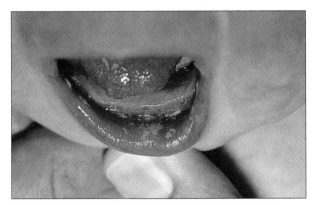

FIG. 14-5 White plaques of oral thrush.

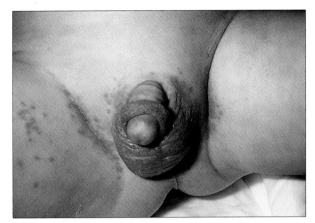

FIG. 14-6 Candidal diaper dermatitis. Red plaque with inguinal crease involvement and satellite pustules.

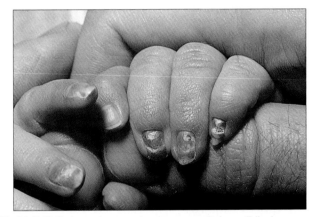

FIG. 14-7 Nail changes secondary to congenital candidiasis.

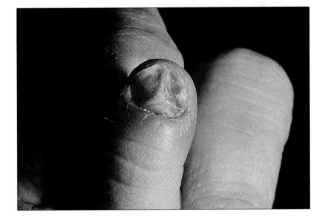

FIG. 14-8 Candidal paronychia.

papules, and pustules affect the moist intertriginous areas of the perineum, with a predilection for inguinal creases. White scale and satellite pustules are common along the periphery, often prominent at the border of involved and uninvolved skin (Fig. 14-6). Perianal involvement is common. Pustules may be very superficial and rupture easily. Candidal dermatitis may be seen in 4–6% of term newborns, with the incidence peaking at 3–4 months of age.[2] Similar bright erythema may be seen in napkin psoriasis. Further differential diagnoses include infectious and noninfectious entities outlined in Chapter 16.

Candida Infection of the Nail

Candidal infection of the nail may occur alone or in conjunction with systemic and congenital candidiasis. Finger sucking is a potential predisposing event. Erythema and swelling in proximal and lateral nail folds may resemble bacterial paronychia, and separation of the cuticle from the nail plate may be seen (Figs 14-7 and 14-8). The resultant onychodystrophy may lead to proximal-, distal-, and lateral-subungual, superficial white, or total dystrophic onychomycosis. The latter presents with a crumbling nail and an abnormally thickened nail bed. It is frequently seen in patients with chronic mucocutaneous candidiasis and other immunodeficiency states.[24] Tinea unguium, hereditary onychodystrophy, ectodermal dysplasia, epidermolysis bullosa, psoriasis, and acrodermatitis may present with similar nail findings.

Diagnosis of Candida Infections

Skin scrapings from pustules or peripheral scale should be examined using KOH solution or Giemsa, Gram, or calcofluor stains. Pseudohyphae and spores may be visualized with direct staining. Satellite pustules are most likely to yield positive results. Cultures from multiple sites, including skin, blood, cerebrospinal fluid, and urine, should be collected if systemic disease is suspected. Culture yield is inconsistent,[7] and negative cultures do not rule out systemic disease in the symptomatic infant.[2] Buffy coat smear microscopy, a rapid bedside test with 100% specificity, can confirm candidemia within 1–2 hours. Sensitivity is 62%, compared to 44% for peripheral blood smear examination.[25] In some centers, buffy coat culture may yield results faster than whole blood cultures.[25] A skin biopsy specimen may reveal a subcorneal pustule with neutrophils, and periodic acid–Schiff (PAS) staining will highlight the organisms. Invasive fungal dermatitis demonstrates invasion and inflammation of the epidermis, and possibly invasion of the dermis.

Treatment of Candida Infections

Localized forms of candidiasis can be treated topically in most infants. For thrush, nystatin solution (100 000 units/mL) is applied to the oral mucosa four times per day for at least 1 week. Resistant thrush may respond to once-daily oral fluconazole (2–3 mg/kg/day)[26] or itraconazole (2 mg/kg/day),[27] particularly in immunocompromised children. Oral amphotericin B has been studied for treatment of recurrent thrush.[28] Imidazole creams are useful for diaper dermatitis and nail infection. Nystatin, allylamines (including naftifine and terbinafine), or aqueous solutions of 1% gentian violet or 2% eosin are alternatives for localized disease. Inflamed or erosive monilial diaper dermatitis may require a combination of the above with a 1% hydrocortisone cream or ointment and barrier paste containing zinc oxide. Oral nystatin may also be a useful adjunct for the treatment of diaper dermatitis, especially for recurrent disease or concurrent oral candidiasis, thereby reducing the load of gastrointestinal Candida.

Congenital candidiasis in asymptomatic term infants can be treated with topical agents alone. However, for ill and VLBW preterm infants, systemic treatment is recommended.[12]

The drug of choice for systemic antifungal therapy is amphotericin B, a polyene macrolide antibiotic.[2] Intravenous doses of 0.5–1 mg/kg/day are recommended.[2,29,30] It should be diluted in dextrose water to 0.1 mg/mL and delivered over 4–6 hours to avoid infusion-related reactions. Treatment is usually continued for a minimum of 14–21 days, depending on the degree of systemic illness.[31] Associated nephrotoxicity is seen less commonly in neonates than in adults treated with amphotericin;[30] however, renal function should be monitored. Hepatotoxicity and bone marrow suppression are also potential side effects.[29] Lipid-associated amphotericin B formulations have been developed to deliver greater dosages, limit infusion

volume, and minimize toxicity.[32] Successful treatment of systemic fungal disease with these products has been reported in neonates.[33] Both the liposomal (5 mg/kg/day) and colloidal dispersion (3 mg/kg on day 1, then 5 mg/kg/day) forms of amphotericin B were shown to be safe and effective in extremely low-birthweight (ELBW) infants with candidemia and renal dysfunction.[30,34] Furthermore, high-dose (5–7 mg/kg/day) liposomal amphotericin B may add a therapeutic advantage with more rapid eradication of infection when used as first-line therapy.[35]

5-Fluorocytosine (5-FC) is a pyrimidine antimetabolite that acts synergistically with amphotericin B against fungal pathogens such as cryptococcus and Candida spp. 5-FC is given orally (50–150 mg/kg/day) and penetrates well into the CSF. For this reason, 5-FC is often added to amphotericin B therapy in the setting of candidal CSF infection.[30] Potential toxicity includes bone marrow suppression and gastrointestinal side effects. Bone marrow suppression is associated with serum 5-FC concentrations greater than 100 mg/L.[29]

Systemic fluconazole has been used successfully for treatment of systemic candidiasis in neonates.[36–38] The recommended daily dose is 6 mg/kg/day for infants over 4 weeks of age, with less-frequent dosing for infants with compromised renal function and for those less than 4 weeks old. It is a second-line therapy for infants in whom amphotericin B is ineffective or contraindicated.[30,36] Given in the first trimester of pregnancy, fluconazole has been reported to be teratogenic, leading to multiple malformations.[39] Resistance to fluconazole can be seen especially in nonalbicans Candida species, such as C. krusei, C. tropicalis, C. glabrata, C. parapsilosis strains, and some C. albicans[31], and susceptibility testing can be performed to document the utility of these agents.[31,40]

Oral itraconazole administered at 5 mg/kg/day has been safe and well tolerated in infants and children;[41,42] however, there are limited reports documenting its use in newborns with candidiasis.[43] Oral ketoconazole (3–6.5 mg/kg/day) has been largely supplanted by the newer triazoles for candidiasis, because of the risk of fulminant hepatitis.[44]

The echinocandins such as capsofungin, are a relatively new class of antifungal agent which irreversibly inhibit 1,3-β-D-glucan synthesis.[45] Capsofungin is fungicidal against Candida spp., including resistant strains. In one study of capsofungin use in neonates (one term and nine preterm) with invasive candidiasis unresponsive to amphotericin B, at a dose of 1 mg/kg/day for 2 days, then at 2 mg/kg/day there-after, all cultures cleared after 3–7 days of therapy, with no adverse events.[45]

Adjunctive therapy for systemic Candida infection includes changing or removing indwelling catheters when feasible.[30]

Because ELBW infants are most susceptible to and have a higher mortality from systemic Candida infections,[46] prevention of infection by means of fluconazole prophylaxis has become a topic of consideration. Potential concerns include unknown short- or long-term risks of fluconazole to the infant (the risk–benefit ratio); uncertainty regarding the group of infants that would benefit most and the optimum dose and duration of therapy; and the potential for increased fluconazole resistance.[47,48] Fluconazole has been shown to reduce rectal colonization with Candida.[49] Bertini et al.[50] gave fluconazole 6 mg/kg every 72 hours for week 1, then daily for weeks 2–4 in neonates<1500 g with central venous access and reduced the rate of candidemia from 7.6% to 0. Healy et al.[51] initiated fluconazole prophylaxis in all ELBW infants less than 5 days of age and reduced invasive candidiasis-related mortality from 12% to 0. As for dosing, twice-weekly fluconazole (3 mg/kg/dose) in ELBW infants with a central venous catheter or endotracheal tube was as effective as daily prophylaxis in decreasing *Candida* colonization and bloodstream infections.[48] Although these studies appear promising, larger multicenter studies looking closely at the morbidity and mortality from all causes, the emergence of resistant *Candida* strains, and unexpected consequences are needed before routine fluconazole prophylaxis for ELBW infants can be recommended.[48]

Malassezia Infections

Malassezia (previously *Pityrosporum* species) are saprophytic yeasts found on 90% of adults as normal skin flora. Skin colonization of newborns usually occurs in the first 1–3 months of life.[3,52–54] By means of genetic analysis, the species formerly called *M. furfur* alone has now been reclassified as *M. furfur* plus at least six other species.[55] Although *M. furfur* is the most commonly associated species, *M. pachydermatis*, *M. sympodialis*, and *M. globosa* have also been associated with neonatal infection.[54,56,57] Three clinical forms of *Malassezia* infection may present in neonates: tinea versicolor, cephalic pustulosis, and catheter-associated sepsis without cutaneous lesions.

Skin Colonization with Malassezia *Species*

Malassezia furfur is the main species responsible for human skin colonization and infection, but other *Malassezia* species, including *M. sympodialis*, *M. globosa*, and *M. pachydermatis*, have been implicated in human disease.[54,56,57] *Malassezia* colonizes the skin of adults who are usually asymptomatic. Skin colonization begins in infancy, and the prevalence of colonization increases with age.[53] The most common site of colonization in both infants (>78%) and neonates is the ear.[53] Ashbee et al.[53] showed that 97.6% of infants (>28 days of age) and 31.8% of neonates were colonized; the mean age of colonization was 14 days.[53] Risk factors for colonization include gestational age of <28 weeks and length of hospital stay >10 days.[53] Fungal growth from skin and catheter cultures is not always associated with clinical sepsis.[3]

Tinea Versicolor

Tinea versicolor (pityriasis versicolor) is less common in infants than in older children, adolescents, and young adults. Facial involvement is very typical in affected infants and young children, although lesions may also be seen on the neck and upper trunk.[58,59] Tinea versicolor presents with multiple, 0.3–1 cm oval macules or plaques with fine scaling (Fig. 14-9). Lesions may be hypopigmented, skin-colored, or hyperpigmented relative to normal skin. Wood's light examination highlights the pigmentary changes and may produce a golden fluorescence. Differential diagnoses include pityriasis alba, and postinflammatory hypopigmentation and hyperpigmentation.

Neonatal Cephalic Pustulosis

Neonatal cephalic pustulosis is a relatively new term, which may represent what has been previously called neonatal acne.[55,60] During the second or third week of life, multiple, tiny, monomorphous papulopustules on an erythematous base begin to cover the face, scalp, and neck. Contrary to classic acne, comedones are not a feature, and follicular accentuation is absent.[60] Both *M. globosa* and *M. sympodialis* have been reported in association with neonatal cephalic pustulosis.[54]

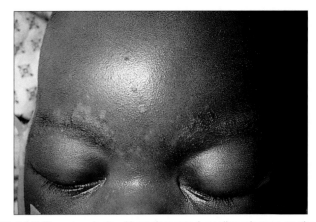

FIG. 14-9 Tinea versicolor. Hypopigmented, scaling plaques on the face in this premature infant revealed hyphae and spores on KOH preparation.

Higher rates of colonization were associated with increased severity of pustulosis.[54] Diagnosis is suggested by onset by 1 month of age, cephalic distribution, microscopic findings of yeast forms suggestive of *Malassezia*, exclusion of other pustular eruptions, and response to topical ketoconazole.[60] The differential diagnosis of this pustular eruption is discussed more extensively in Chapters 7 and 10.

Malassezia *Sepsis*

Malassezia fungemia is seen primarily in premature infants receiving intralipids through intravenous catheters. Skin colonization rates are much higher in premature infants than in full-term newborns, and the pathogenesis of disease probably involves organisms on the skin gaining venous access through indwelling catheters.[56,61] Although in one study of VLBW infants (<1250 g), skin colonization with *M. furfur* was not predictive of catheter infection or systemic illness, the skin colonization rate was 63%, and positive *M. furfur* blood cultures were common (9.6%) in infants with central venous catheters.[3] Clinical presentation ranges from asymptomatic colonization of the indwelling catheter to sepsis and death.[3,61] Fever, apnea, bradycardia, and thrombocytopenia in the presence of negative routine bacterial cultures suggest fungal disease. Clusters of cases of infantile bronchopneumonia in neonatal units have also been attributed to *M. furfur*.[61,62]

Diagnosis and Treatment of Malassezia *Infections*

Malassezia can be identified by KOH preparation or Giemsa stain examination of the fine scales or pus; this will reveal clusters of spherical yeast and associated filaments. *Malassezia* is differentiated from *Candida* and other yeasts by a broader budding base. *Malassezia furfur* is a lipophilic yeast that requires fatty acid supplementation for growth. Modified Dixon agar or an olive oil overlay on routine fungal media is used for isolation of these fungi from blood specimens.

Cutaneous infections can be treated with an imidazole cream.[44,60] A high level of suspicion for *Malassezia* sepsis is appropriate in premature infants with clinical signs of sepsis with negative bacterial and viral cultures, especially if intravenous lipid emulsions are being infused through venous catheters. Removal of the catheter and cessation of intravenous lipids, without systemic antifungal therapy, may be sufficient therapy for catheter-associated sepsis, although systemic antifungals may be considered if the infant does not show rapid clinical improvement.[61]

Trichosporonosis

Trichosporon asahii (formerly *T. beigelii*), a yeast found in soil and water, causes superficial mycoses in healthy persons (white piedra, onychomycosis, otomycosis).[63] Invasive disease is possible in immunocompromised hosts and has emerged as a cause of systemic fungal disease in very premature infants. Both *T. asahii* and *T. mucoides* have been associated with invasive infection in premature neonates.[63,64] Cutaneous manifestations of trichosporonosis are uncommon in neonates, but may include necrotic skin lesions or persistent generalized skin breakdown with serous or purulent drainage and white plaques;[63] neither erythema nor pustules are present. Unlike adults with trichosporonosis, neonates often have a normal absolute neutrophil count.[63] Both colonization of central venous lines without evidence of disease and sepsis associated with fungal dissemination are reported in VLBW infants.[63] Treatment is with a systemic antifungal agent. *Trichosporon* can exhibit tolerance to amphotericin B,[65,66] and lack of fungicidal activity has been associated with treatment failure and death.[65] Successful treatment of disseminated neonatal trichosporonosis with liposomal amphotericin B,[63] amphotericin plus flucytosine,[63] fluconazole,[64] and voriconazole (in a 10-week-old infant)[67] has been reported.

Aspergillosis

Aspergillus species are ubiquitous saprophytic fungi found in decaying vegetation and are infrequently pathogenic in healthy people.[68] The conidia can spread through the air, and there are reports of acquisition in immunosuppressed patients following hospital construction work.[69] *A. fumigatus* is the most common pathogen associated with neonatal infection, followed by *A. flavus*.[68–70] The pathogenesis of disease with systemic *Aspergillus* infection involves invasion of blood vessels with subsequent thrombosis and tissue necrosis. Macrophage and neutrophil function is an important immunologic defense mechanism against *Aspergillus* infection.[68–71] Risk factors for invasive aspergillosis include extreme prematurity, neutropenia or neutrophil incompetence, immunosuppression from severe disease such as malnutrition or bacterial sepsis, and induced immunosuppression with steroids.[68–71]

Aspergillosis in neonates presents with a spectrum of diseases, including primary cutaneous aspergillosis, single-system involvement such as pulmonary or gastrointestinal aspergillosis, and disseminated aspergillosis.[69] Mortality rates increase with more invasive disease. There can be overlap in clinical symptoms, and cutaneous lesions can be either primary or a manifestation of dissemination.

Primary Cutaneous Aspergillosis

Primary cutaneous aspergillosis (PCA) with infection limited to the skin is being reported more frequently in premature infants.[68,69,71] It is often associated with breaks in normal skin integrity, such as occur with intravenous catheter insertion, or skin erosion or maceration secondary to the use of adhesive tape, monitor leads, or prolonged armboard use.[68,70] Lesions are often confused with skin trauma or contact dermatitis, and diagnosis can be delayed unless a high level of suspicion is maintained. PCA may begin as a localized zone of erythema, evolving into a dark-red plaque with pustules, and finally a black eschar with a rim of erythema.[68] Clustered, erythematous papules or pustules, or a necrotic plaque or nodule with

an eschar, are characteristic (Fig. 14-10A, B). The differential diagnosis includes ecthyma gangrenosum, zygomycosis, noninfectious vasculitis, and pyoderma gangrenosum.[68] Histologic evaluation and culture of a biopsy specimen from the affected area can be diagnostic. Microscopically, vesicular surface erosion of a granuloma with infiltrating dichotomously branched septate hyphae is apparent. Growth of *Aspergillus* is supportive of a diagnosis, but lack of a positive culture does not rule out disease, especially if hyphal elements are seen on histologic examination.[69]

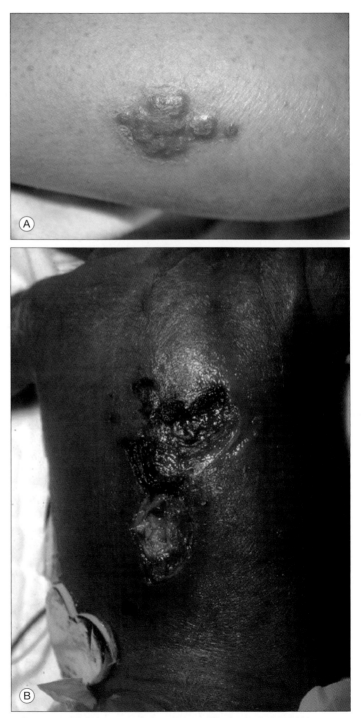

FIG. 14-10 (A) Primary cutaneous aspergillosis: an indurated, erythematous plaque. **(B)** Cutaneous aspergillosis with erosions and eschar in a premature neonate.

Systemic Aspergillosis

Isolated pulmonary, gastrointestinal, and central nervous system aspergillosis may not be associated with skin findings; however, disseminated aspergillosis can have cutaneous manifestations, and cutaneous aspergillosis may disseminate. A maculopapular eruption that may become pustular is described with systemic aspergillosis.[69] This often represents embolic phenomena from fungal dissemination. Mortality from systemic aspergillosis in neonates is high compared to that of primary cutaneous aspergillosis (up to 100% versus 27%, respectively).[69]

Systemic antifungal therapy is recommended for all forms of neonatal aspergillosis. Amphotericin B is the standard antimicrobial agent prescribed, either alone or in conjunction with flucytosine.[68–70] Lipid formulations of amphotericin B have been used in adults with aspergillosis,[68–71] but data in neonates are lacking. It is unclear whether complete surgical excision of cutaneous lesions is necessary for cure, but progression of the lesion during therapy may warrant surgical intervention.[68]

Cutaneous Zygomycosis (Mucormycosis, Phycomycosis)

Zygomycosis is the term for infection caused by fungi in the class Zygomycetes. There are six fungal genera that cause disease in humans: *Rhizopus, Cunninghamella, Mucor, Rhizomucor, Saksenea,* and *Absidia*.[72] These fungi are found in soil, decaying food, and other organic matter. Although infections may follow ingestion or inhalation of spores, direct inoculation into skin is the cause of primary cutaneous zygomycosis, which is seen predominantly in premature infants, as well as those who are immunocompromised from immunosuppressive drugs or underlying disease.[72,73] Similar to aspergillosis, zygomycosis can involve the skin alone (primary cutaneous) or may involve other organ systems, including the gastrointestinal, pulmonary, and central nervous systems. Skin lesions may represent dissemination, or primary cutaneous infection may disseminate. Zygomycosis in immunocompetent hosts includes cutaneous zygomycosis and sinusitis. The cutaneous lesions may present as pustules with or without discrete erythematous cellulitis, and may develop a sharply defined, black, necrotic plaque producing a pathognomonic black pus (Fig. 14-11).[73]

In a review of 31 cases of neonatal zygomycosis 22 were premature infants, and in 12 the skin was the initial site of

infection.[72] Reports include an association with contaminated dressings and tongue depressors used as splints for intravenous and arterial cannulation sites.[72–74] The Centers for Disease Control and Prevention (CDC) recommends that skin dressings be treated with cobalt irradiation as a preventive measure.[73]

Diagnosis is made by tissue biopsy and culture. Histologic examination shows large, nonseptate hyphae with right-angled branching.[75] The fungus invades downward into tissue and blood vessels, frequently leading to thrombosis with dermal edema and minimal inflammatory infiltrate.[75] Vascular invasion results in cutaneous ischemia and necrosis.[72,75]

Zygomycosis is treated with intravenous amphotericin B. As with aspergillosis, lipid formulations of amphotericin B can be used to deliver higher concentrations of drug, and other agents such as rifampin may be of use for antimicrobial synergy.[72,76] In vitro data reveal resistance to azoles (except for *Absidia*), flucytosine, and naftifine.[77] Although one successful case of medical treatment alone is reported,[73] surgical debridement is often imperative in the treatment of cutaneous zygomycosis, and wide excision with clean margins of involved tissue is recommended.[72,76]

Dermatophytosis

Dermatophytes are fungal pathogens responsible for the cutaneous infection known as tinea. Clinical conditions are named according to the affected anatomic location: tinea capitis (scalp), tinea faciei (face), tinea corporis (body), tinea diaper dermatitis (diaper area), and tinea unguium (nails); tinea cruris (groin) and tinea pedis (feet) are uncommon in infants.

Dermatophytosis in neonates may be acquired from infected caregivers or infected animals. Dermatophyte invasion of the stratum corneum is mediated by keratinase and other proteases.[78] Cell-mediated immunity and evidence of a delayed-type hypersensitivity response are important in host resistance.[78]

In North America, tinea faciei and corporis in infants are most often due to *Trichophyton tonsurans* and *Microsporum canis*.[79–82] In Europe, *M. canis* is the most common, followed by *T. mentagrophytes*.[82–85] In West African newborns *Microsporum landeronii* is a common cause.[84] The most common cause of tinea capitis in North America is *Trichophyton tonsurans*, which may also cause tinea faciei and corporis secondary to cutaneous spread. Fungal invasion in tinea capitis extends to the hair follicle, where infection may be either within the hair shaft (endothrix) or on the surface of the hair shaft (ectothrix). Neonatal tinea capitis has also been reported with other fungal species, including *T. rubrum, T. violaceum,* and *T. erinacei*.[82,86,87] Tinea diaper dermatitis is primarily due to *T. rubrum* and *Epidermophyton floccosum*.[88] Tinea unguium in childhood has been caused by *T. mentagrophytes* and *T. rubrum*.[89]

Tinea in babies occurs most commonly on the exposed scalp and face (Fig. 14-12)[3,79–81,83–87] Tinea capitis often presents as erythematous, scaling areas with partial alopecia.[82,85] Clinical manifestations vary from noninflammatory 'black dot' alopecia to a scaling, seborrheic dermatitis-like eruption without obvious hair loss.[82–84] Pustules may be present.[79] Kerions can be seen in conjunction with tinea capitis.[79] Kerions consist of pustules, nodules, and crusting, with underlying bogginess of scalp tissue. The inflammatory nature mimics bacterial infection and may lead to unsuccessful therapy with antibacterial agents. Tinea capitis associated with kerion formation has

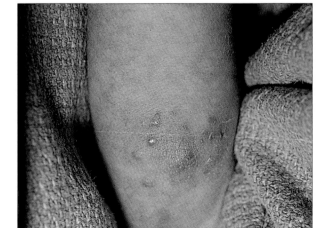

FIG. 14-11 Cutaneous rhizopus: pustules developed under tape adhesive.

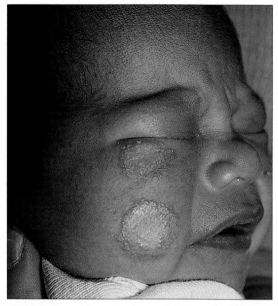

FIG. 14-12 Annular, scaling plaques on this 2-week-old infant due to *T. tonsurans* infection. The 4-year-old sibling was evaluated and had evidence of tinea capitis.

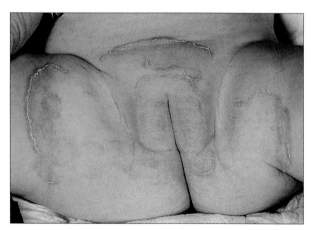

FIG. 14-13 Dermatophyte diaper dermatitis (note scaling edge).

been reported in a neonate.[79] Posterior cervical lymphadenopathy is usually present.

Tinea infection on other parts of the body usually presents as elevated, annular lesions with superficial scaling and/or tiny pustules.[81,86,87] These may be mistaken for dermatitis, and facial tinea may mimic neonatal lupus. Cases of tinea faciei and tinea corporis have been reported in neonates.[80,86,90] Cases of resistant diaper dermatitis in infants as a result of dermatophytes have been described.[88] In tinea diaper dermatitis, the presence of annular or arcuate plaques with a scaling peripheral border is a clue to the diagnosis (Fig. 14-13).

Onychomycosis is a fungal infection of the nail that may be caused by dermatophytes, nondermatophyte molds, and *Candida*. Tinea unguium, caused by dermatophytes, is uncommon in prepubertal children.[89] No cases of tinea unguium in neonates have been reported, but *Candida* onychomycosis is a relatively common finding in neonates with congenital cutaneous candidiasis.[14,15] Nails may have superficial white opaque patches, or yellowish discoloration with subungual hyperkera-

tosis. Hereditary onychodystrophy, acquired trachyonychia, psoriasis, lichen planus, and trauma may cause similar findings.

Diagnosis of dermatophytosis can be confirmed by several tests. A Wood's light examination may have limited usefulness in the diagnosis of tinea capitis; positive fluorescence is seen in ectothrix hair infections, but is absent in the more common endothrix infections such as those caused by *Trichophyton*. All suspected tinea infections should be confirmed by culture, or lesional scale or hair microscopically examined under 10% potassium hydroxide (KOH) solution or alternative stains (see Chapter 6). Although KOH preparations may demonstrate spores and hyphae, false-negative examinations are common. Scrapings of scales, brush or cotton-tipped applicator swabbings of the affected skin, or collections of hair are cultured on fungal media. Dermatophytes are slow growing and may take up to 1 month to grow in culture, although common pathogens generally grow within 2 weeks. Skin biopsy, although rarely necessary for diagnosis, may reveal hyperkeratosis with parakeratosis and a mixed inflammatory perivascular dermal infiltrate. Staining with periodic acid–Schiff (PAS) or Grocott–Gomori methenamine silver nitrate reveals fungal elements in the stratum corneum and possibly the hair follicle.[44]

Treatment of tinea capitis usually requires systemic antifungal therapy. Griseofulvin is the most commonly used agent, and successful treatment in neonates has been reported.[79,82,85] Griseofulvin doses of 15–20 mg/kg/day for 4–8 weeks may be needed.[79,82,85] Fluconazole (6 mg/kg/day) may also be effective.[91] Alternative medications include itraconazole and terbinafine, although experience with these in neonates is limited. Although topical therapy alone was successful in treatment five of six mostly preterm infants (four with tinea capitis) during a nursery outbreak of *M. canis*, and in three infants reported by Gilaberte et al.,[85] it is not generally recommended for scalp tinea infection.[80,85]

Tinea faciei and tinea corporis can be successfully treated with topical applications of azoles such as clotrimazole, econazole, and miconazole. Ciclopirox, as well as allylamines such as terbinafine or naftifine and amorfoline, may also be used.[92,93] If persistent, systemic griseofulvin or fluconazole for a period of 4–8 weeks may be required.[91,94]

It is important to identify the potential source of the fungal infection in family members. The prognosis for dermatophyte infections is excellent.

INFESTATIONS (ECTOPARASITIC INFESTATIONS)

Mites, flea larvae, protozoa, and helminth worms cause a variety of cutaneous lesions.[44] Mites are classified in the order Acari, class of arthropods Arachnida. The prototype is scabies, which is the most common parasitic infection in humans, including newborns. Flea larvae (myiasis) and other mites (demodicidosis) can occasionally cause disease in infants.

Scabies

Scabies is a common ectoparasitic infestation caused by the mite *Sarcoptes scabiei* ssp. *hominis*. Initial infestation by scabies may be asymptomatic, a carrier state being well recognized. A primary symptom of scabies is generalized pruritus, most intense at night. Infants, however, may not manifest symptoms despite extensive infection. Pruritus in a neonate unable to scratch may manifest as irritability, insomnia, and poor feeding. Congenital scabies is not seen, but infestation can develop in very young infants.[95,96]

Skin findings include a generalized erythematous vesiculo-papular eruption, with lesions commonly concentrated on the axillae, neck, palms, soles, and sometimes the head (Fig. 14-14). In older children and adults the head and neck are usually spared.[95,97] A burrow is the pathognomonic sign of scabies. Burrows appear as a small thin line with a tiny black dot at one end, indicating the location of the female mite.[95,98] They are found primarily on the hands, the flexural aspect of the wrists, and the medial or lateral aspects of the feet; visualization may be difficult because of secondary eczematous changes.[97]

In babies, vesicles and pustules are characteristically found on the palms and soles. Nodules may also appear during active infection, primarily in intertriginous areas, and these scabietic nodules may persist for some time after scabies has been successfully treated. Recurrent vesicular lesions similar to scabietic nodules may be manifestations of ongoing hypersensitivity response to the initial infestation.

A form of infantile scabies (scabies incognito) clinically resembling crusted (Norwegian) scabies is associated with prior topical corticosteroid therapy.[96] In addition to the generalized eruption, crusted and hyperkeratotic lesions on the palms and soles are described.[98] Unlike classic Norwegian scabies in adults, which is characterized by intense infestation by *Sarcoptes* mites, these infants lacked subungual hyperkeratosis and high mite counts.[98] There has also been a report in immunosuppressed children of a unique form of scabies consisting of fine scaling and minimal to absent pruritus, mimicking seborrheic dermatitis.[99]

The scabies mite is an obligate human ectoparasite unable to survive more than a few days without a host.[95] The microscopic adult female mite has eight legs and measures 400 µm. Throughout its life span of up to 30 days, the mite burrows into the stratum corneum, laying up to three eggs per day. Larvae hatch in 3–4 days, and mature into adult mites within 10–14 days.[95] Although only a few mites are present, hundreds of skin lesions may develop owing to hypersensitivity.[95]

Diagnosis is based on the clinical findings, as well as a history of contact with persons having a similar pruritic eruption. Definitive diagnosis is based on microscopic visualization of scrapings from a burrow or papule, demonstrating the mite, eggs, or scybala (feces) (see Chapter 6) (Fig. 14-15). Skin biopsy is rarely necessary. Histopathologic examination shows a mixed dermal inflammatory infiltrate with eosinophils and epidermal spongiosis. The mites, ova, and nymphs may also be seen.

The treatment of choice for neonatal scabies is permethrin 5% cream. It is approved for use in infants as young as 2 months old, with one report of safety and efficacy in a 23-day-old infant.[95] Permethrin is a neurotoxin that causes paralysis and death of ectoparasites; it has low potential for toxicity in humans, and there is no evidence of resistance to date.[95] Efficacy is superior to that of lindane, crotamiton, benzyl benzoate, and sulfur.[95] Permethrin applied to the entire body surface, including the scalp, and left on for 8–12 hours is 89–92% effective.[95] Reapplication 1 week later is advisable. Critical to success is the simultaneous treatment of all family members and close contacts, even if asymptomatic. Whereas adults are treated from the neck down, children under 2 years of age should have the head treated as well. In addition, bedding and clothing of patients and all contacts should be washed the following day in hot water for at least 5 minutes, or dry cleaned. Antihistamines such as hydroxyzine (2 mg/kg/day in divided doses every 6–8 hours) and a mild corticosteroid cream such as 1% hydrocortisone may help control the residual pruritus and eczematous dermatitis that can persist for several weeks following successful eradication of the parasite. Iver-

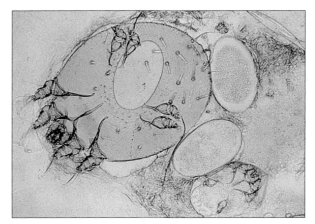

FIG. 14-15 Scabies. *Sarcoptes scabiei* mite and eggs.

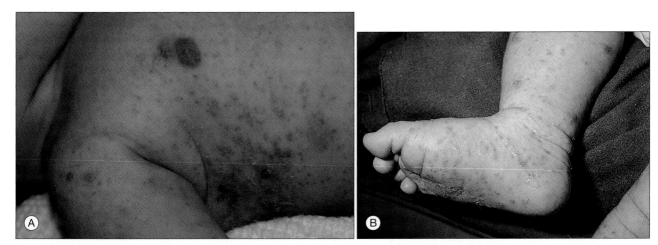

FIG. 14-14 (A) Scabies. Diffuse erythematous papules, pustules, crusted lesions, and scattered nodules. **(B)** Papules, vesicles, and pustules on the feet and legs, particularly on the instep, are characteristic in young infants.

mectin, an avermectin with antiparasitic and antinematode properties, has been used orally in cases of refractory scabies in adults,[100] but its use in neonates has not been studied.

Demodicidosis

Demodicidosis presents as perioral dermatitis, pustular folliculitis, and blepharitis.[101] Pruritic erythematous papules, pustules, nodules, and scaling occur primarily on the face, most commonly on the dorsum of the nose.[102] *Demodex folliculorum* and *D. brevis* are human ectoparasites that are normal inhabitants of the pilosebaceous ducts and glands. *D. canis* causes mange in animals. The role of the mite *Demodex* in human cutaneous disease is controversial,[101] and its specific role in neonatal disease has yet to be determined. To date, the youngest reported case is that of a 10-month-old infant.[102] Demodicidosis is found mainly in immunosuppressed children,[101,103] although disease in healthy hosts has been described.[102] Numerous mites are seen when skin scrapings are examined using KOH or when a skin biopsy is performed. A dramatic response may be seen within 2–3 weeks after the application of 5% permethrin cream.[101] Topical metronidazole and oral erythromycin help decrease the numbers of mites and may offer additional benefit.[101,102]

Myiasis

Myiasis is a parasitic infestation of dipterous larvae in mammals, found worldwide but primarily in the tropics and subtropics.[104] Cutaneous myiasis may occur in pre-existing wounds or present as a furuncle. Passage of maggots, discharge, a foul odor, and pain may be reported.[105,106] Myiasis is classified clinically according to the body site affected as cutaneous, nasopharyngeal, ocular, aural, intestinal, and genital. There have been reports of myiasis in neonates and infants chiefly in rural settings,[105] although cases have been reported in urban centers and neonatal intensive care units as well.[106] The diagnosis is made clinically and confirmed by identification of larvae, which can be preserved in 80% ethanol. Treatment involves extraction of the larvae by irrigation, manipulation, or ideally with surgery followed by debridement, cleansing, and possible primary suture closure.[104]

PARASITIC INFECTIONS

Parasitic infections with cutaneous manifestations are more commonly seen in developing countries and are infrequently reported in neonates. Table 14-1 presents summary of cutaneous diseases due to parasites. *Toxoplasma* are autonomous,

TABLE 14-1 Parasitic cutaneous infections in neonates

Parasite	Name	Source	Clinical findings	Therapy
Mite				
Sarcopies scabiei ssp. hominis	Scabies	Human	Classical burrow; vesicles on palms and soles; nodules, papules, and pustules on face and extensors	Permethrin 5% cream or lotion, including scalp, Tx contacts
Demodex folliculorum	Demodicidosis	Human saprophyte	Papules and pustules on face and extensors	Permethrin 5% cream or lotion
Protozoa				
Toxoplasma gondii	Toxoplasmosis	Cats	Acquired: variable. Congenital: chorioretinitis, hydrocephalus, intracranial calcifications, ± petechial rash	Pyrimethamine and sulfonamide, or spiramycin, or trimethoprim-sulfamethoxazole
Entamoeba histolytica	Amebiasis	Humans 10% worldwide GI tract colonized	Ulcer, draining sinus, vegetative plaque in the inguinal, perineal area, abdomen	Metronidazole and iodoquinol or paromomycin
L. major, L. tropica, L. ethiopica (Old World)	Cutaneous leishmaniasis	Female sandfly Mammal reservoir	Single or multiple papules and nodules ± ulcer resolving to leave scars	Sodium stibogluconate, Meglumine antimonite ± allopurinol, ketoconazole, itraconazole, amphotericin B, cryotherapy, heat
L. mexicana, L. braziliensis (New World)				
L. braziliensis	Mucocutaneous leishmaniasis		Destructive oral, nasopharyngeal lesions	
L. donovani	Visceral leishmaniasis (Kala-azar)		Gray skin color, nodules	
Myiasis: (fly larvae) order Diptera	Myiasis	Flies, gnats, mosquitos	Furuncle or infested ulcer	Surgical removal
Helminths:	Rare in newborns			
Platyhelminthes (tapeworms)				
Trematodes				
Cestodes				

single-cell organisms that are acquired in utero more frequently than postnatally in neonates. Cutaneous manifestations of helminth worms are discussed minimally here, but are treated in depth by Stein.[44] Toxoplasmosis and leishmaniasis are discussed in greater detail.

Toxoplasmosis

Toxoplasmosis is caused by the intracellular protozoon *Toxoplasma gondii*. Found worldwide in many animal species, cats are the only species in which the sexual stage (sporozoite) occurs.[107–109] Infection commonly occurs through consumption of undercooked meats containing *Toxoplasma* cysts or oocysts excreted by cats.[109,110] Toxoplasmosis may be acquired congenitally or postnatally. Congenital toxoplasmosis is a sequela of acute maternal infection or reactivation, with risk of transmission being 15% in the first trimester, 30% in the second, and 60% in the third.[108] Severity of fetal disease varies inversely with gestational age at the time of infection. Thus early infection more likely leads to fetal death or severe neurologic and ophthalmologic disease.[110] Most newborns infected in the second or third trimester have mild or subclinical manifestations. In at least 40% of cases the infection is discovered late, manifesting as chorioretinitis, visual impairment, and neurologic sequelae.[108,110] Risk of fetal infection is estimated to be <1–19.6 per 10 000 live births worldwide, varying with geographic location.[111]

Congenital toxoplasmosis has no specific cutaneous manifestations,[107–109] but in a report by Roizen et al.[112] petechial and nonpetechial rashes were seen in respectively 17% and 14% of affected infants. Deep blue-red papules and macules and nonspecific exanthems, both with involvement of the palms and soles, and a calcifying dermatitis have been described in affected neonates.[109] Neurologic sequelae such as seizures, hydrocephalus, microcephaly, and neuropsychomotor developmental delay are the main clinical manifestations.[110] Intracranial calcifications and increased CSF protein may be seen. Eye abnormalities include chorioretinitis (95%), microphthalmia, cataracts and retinal detachment. The most common clinical presentation of eye involvement is strabismus, seen in 49% of affected infants.[110] Neonatal disease may include systemic findings of hepatosplenomegaly, lymphadenopathy, hyperbilirubinemia, and thrombocytopenia. The prognosis of congenital toxoplasmosis has improved with therapy; however, many cases are not recognized in the newborn period.[107]

Postnatally acquired toxoplasmosis is asymptomatic in the majority of patients. However, in an immunocompromised host the disease can be serious. Symptomatic toxoplasmosis can involve the central nervous system and also disseminate to other organs.[108] Fever, malaise, and arthralgia are frequent symptoms, mimicking infectious mononucleosis.[108,109] Cutaneous manifestations are variable and include macular, papular, pustular, or vesiculobullous eruptions.[109] They may be hemorrhagic and may resemble roseola or erythema multiforme.[44] Lymphadenopathy and hepatosplenomegaly may accompany these eruptions.

The diagnosis of toxoplasmosis is based on isolation of the organism, characteristic histopathology of lymphadenitis, detection of *Toxoplasma* antigens in tissues and body fluids, and detection of *Toxoplasma* nucleic acid by PCR. The most commonly used diagnostic tool is serology. Early diagnosis may be difficult owing to delay in antibody response and the presence of maternal IgG. Both the enzyme-linked immunosorbent assay (ELISA) and immunosorbent agglutination assay (ISAGA) are useful tests.[108] The Sabin–Feldman dye test entails the uptake of methylene blue by *Toxoplasma* trophozoites lyzed in the presence of specific antibody and complement. It is very specific but only available through reference laboratories.[108] PCR testing of amniotic fluid has now replaced cordocentesis for the prenatal diagnosis of fetal infection.[113] Ultrasound abnormalities are found in up to 40% of congenitally infected infants, the most common being ventriculomegaly.[108]

Symptomatic acquired or congenital toxoplasmosis should be treated with pyrimethamine, sulfadiazine, and folinic acid.[108] Therapeutic abortion may be offered as an alternative. In some cases vertical transmission has been prevented by the administration of spiramycin to the mother.[113] Antibiotic therapy to reduce subsequent disease is recommended for symptomatic and asymptomatic neonates. Treatment should be continued for at least 1 year.

Leishmaniasis

Leishmaniasis is a parasitic infection due to *Leishmania* species (family Trypanosomatidae). There are 400 000 new cases each year in Asia, Africa, the Mediterranean, and the Americas. The flagellated, extracellular promastigote is transmitted by female phlebotomine sandflies to animal reservoirs, including rodents and dogs.[114] There it becomes an obligate intracellular amastigote. Recent reports of infants with leishmaniasis living in nonendemic areas emphasize the need to consider this diagnosis when unusual skin lesions are present.[114–117] Leishmaniasis is classified into the following categories: visceral (*L. donovani, L. infantum*), mucocutaneous (*L. braziliensis*), Old World cutaneous (*L. major, L. tropica, L. ethiopica*), and New World cutaneous (*L. mexicana, L. braziliensis*)[118] (see Table 14-1).

Visceral leishmaniasis due to *L. donovani* presents with fever, wasting of the face and extremities, hepatosplenomegaly, ascites, pancytopenia, and earth-gray skin pigmentation on the temples, perioral area, hands, and feet.[114] There may be a papular lesion seen early at the site of the sandfly bite.

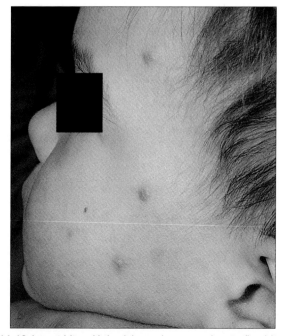

FIG. 14-16 Insect bites. Urticarial papules secondary to flea bites.

Mucocutaneous leishmaniasis due to *L. braziliensis* invades the midface, nose, and upper respiratory tract. A sporotrichoid lymphatic form has been described with *L. braziliensis* and *L. major*.

In countries where leishmaniasis is prevalent, infants and children are frequently affected by cutaneous leishmaniasis. The initial lesion is an erythematous papule derived from an insect bite that evolves to form a relatively painless crusted ulcer.[114] It is typically on an exposed site (primarily on the face and hands), paired or clustered, with a volcanic or iceberg appearance, and oriented to the skin creases. Satellite papules or nodules may be present with surrounding erythema.[117] Secondary bacterial infection is common. The lesions generally heal spontaneously in 3–12 months, although they may also evolve into chronic, treatment-resistant forms that are localized, lupoid, or disseminated.

Diagnosis is based on smears or skin biopsy specimens that permit visualization of the amastigote, culture, or animal inoculation that produces characteristic lesions.[114] The leishmanin skin test evaluates the degree of induration after an intradermal injection of antigen. Positive findings are seen 1–3 months after the initial lesion in cutaneous leishmaniasis. Serologic studies are most valuable in visceral leishmaniasis.[114]

Although visceral leishmaniasis is usually fatal if untreated, spontaneous resolution is the rule in cutaneous forms of the disease. Indications for treatment include lesions that are early, multiple, mucosal, or in cosmetically sensitive sites. Disseminated disease in an immunodeficient host also warrants treatment. If treatment is needed, there is no single ideal drug. Primary treatment is with pentavalent antimonials such as intramuscular or intravenous sodium stibogluconate

TABLE 14-2 Arthropod bites and stings

Class	Order	Source	Lesions	Treatment	Disease
Insecta (three pairs of legs)	Anoplura	Lice: Pediculus humanus, Phthirus pubis	Nits, pruritic bites, maculae caeruleae	5% permethrin; Tx fomites	
	Coleoptera	Beetles	'Kissing' or touching blisters and dermatitis	Topical corticosteroid, systemic antihistamine	Secondary bacterial infection
	Diptera	Mosquitos	Pruritic papules	Topical corticosteroid, systemic antihistamine	Vector for: Encephalitis Malaria Yellow fever Dengue fever Filariasis
		Flies (bloodsucking):	Pruritic, painful papules	Topical corticosteroid, systemic antihistamine	
		Tabanae: horseflies, deerflies, etc.	± angioedema	Topical corticosteroid, systemic antihistamine	Vector for: Tularemia
		Simulidae: black flies Midges: sand flies	± malaise		
	Hemiptera	Cimicidae (bedbugs)	Pruritic papules	Topical corticosteroid, systemic antihistamine	Vector for:
		Reduvidae (kissing bugs)	Painful bites	Topical corticosteroid, systemic antihistamine	Trypanosoma cruzi
	Hymenoptera	Apidea (bees) Vespidea (wasps, hornets) Formicoidea (ants)	Urticarial papule Angioedema	Quick removal of stinger, SQ epinephrine, corticosteroid, antihistamine	
	Lepidoptera	Caterpillars Moths	Urticarial linear papules	Topical corticosteroid, systemic antihistamine	
	Siphonoptera	Fleas: Pulicidae (human, cat, dog, bird)	Grouped papules	Topical corticosteroid, systemic antihistamine	Vector for: Plague Typhus
		Sarcopsyllidae (sand fleas)	Necrotic abscess	Topical corticosteroid, systemic antihistamine	
Arachnida (four pairs of legs)	Acari	Ticks: Argasidae Ixodidae	Papule, granuloma	Remove tick	Vector for: Lyme disease Rocky mountain spotted fever Colorado tick fever Tularemia
		Mites: Follicle, food, fowl, grain, harvest (chigger), murine, scabies	Pruritic papules	Topical corticosteroid, systemic antihistamine	Vector for: Rickettsialpox
	Araneae	Spiders	Painful bite ± necrosis ± systemic reaction	Ice, elevation, antihistamine, analgesic	
	Scorpiones	Scorpions	Bite and neurotoxin		
Chilopoda		Centipedes			
Diplopoda		Millipedes			

(10–20 mg/kg/day) or meglumine antimonate (not available in the United States).[119] Ketoconazole and amphotericin B may also be effective, and temperature-sensitive *Leishmania* may respond to cryotherapy or heat.[117]

ARTHROPOD BITES AND STINGS

Arthropod bites and stings may cause a variety of skin lesions, as well as be vectors for disease. Erythematous, urticarial papules and pustules with a central punctum can be seen, most commonly on exposed surfaces (Fig. 14-16). Vesicular lesions may be a manifestation of a hypersensitive response and not indicative of bacterial infection, particularly in infants.

These pink raised lesions are typically arranged in groups. Persistence of lesions for weeks to months (papular urticaria) is rarely seen in the first year of life.[120] Specific lesions and subsequent diseases are outlined in Table 14-2.

Skin lesions are caused by four of the nine classes of arthropod: Insecta, Chilopoda, Diplopoda, and Arachnida.[121] Although the terms bite and sting are often used interchangeably, in the strict sense, a 'bite' involves venom injected via structures of the mouth, such as fangs or mandibles, whereas a 'sting' connotes the injection of venom via a tapered posterior structure called the sting.[122] Secondary bacterial infection must be considered in infants with bites and stings. The presence of fever and wound drainage is suggestive of infection and may warrant antibiotic therapy.

REFERENCES

1. Ruiz-Diez B, Martinez V, Alvarez M, et al. Molecular tracking of *Candida albicans* in a neonatal intensive care unit: long-term colonizations versus catheter-related infections. J Clin Microbiol 1997; 35: 3032–3036.
2. Baley JE. Neonatal candidiasis: the current challenge. Clin.Perinatol 1991; 18: 263–80.
3. Shattuck KE, Cochran CK, Zabransky RJ, et al. Colonization and infection associated with *Malassezia* and *Candida* species in a neonatal unit. J Hosp Infect 1996; 34: 123–129.
3a. Benjamin DK, Jr, Stoll BJ, Fanaroff AA, et al., on behalf of the National Institute of Child Health and Human Development Neonatal Research Network. Neonatal candidiasis among extremely low birth weight infants: risk factors, mortality rates, and neurodevelopmental outcomes at 18 to 22 months. Pediatrics 2006; 117: 84–92.
4. Marodi L. Local and systemic host defense mechanisms against *Candida*: immunopathology of candidal infections. Pediatr Infect Dis J 1997; 16: 795–801.
5. Marodi L, Kaposzta R, Campbell DE, et al. Candidacidal mechanisms in the human neonate. Impaired IFN-gamma activation of macrophages in newborn infants. J Immunol 1994; 153: 5643–5649.
6. Baley JE, Kliegman RM, Fanaroff AA. Disseminated fungal infections in very low-birth-weight infants: clinical manifestations and epidemiology. Pediatrics 1984; 73: 144–152.
7. Stuart SM, Lane AT. *Candida* and *Malassezia* as nursery pathogens. Semin Dermatol 1992; 11: 19–23.
8. Shetty SS, Harrison LH, Hajjeh RA, et al. Determining risk factors for candidemia among newborn infants from population-based surveillance: Baltimore, Maryland, 1998–2000. Pediatr Infect Dis J 2005; 24: 601–604.
9. Benjamin DK, Jr, DeLong ER, Steinbach WJ, et al. Empirical therapy for neonatal candidemia in very low birthweight infants. Pediatrics 2003; 112: 543–547.
10. Saiman L, Ludington E, Pfaller M, et al. Risk factors for candidemia in neonatal intensive care unit patients. The National Epidemiology of Mycosis Survey study group. Pediatr Infect Dis J 2000; 19: 319–324.
11. Feja KN, Wu F, Roberts K, et al. Risk factors for candidemia in critically ill infants: a matched case-control study. J Pediatr 2005; 147: 156–161.
12. Darmstadt GL, Dinulos JG, Miller Z. Congenital cutaneous candidiasis: clinical presentation, pathogenesis, and management guidelines. Pediatrics 2000; 105: 438–444.
13. Raval DS, Barton LL, Hansen RC, Kling PJ. Congenital cutaneous candidiasis: case report and review. Pediatr Dermatol 1995; 12: 355–358.
14. Clegg HW, Prose NS, Greenberg DN. Nail dystrophy in congenital cutaneous candidiasis. Pediatr Dermatol 2003; 20: 342–344.
15. Kurgansky D, Sweren R. Onychomycosis in a 10-week-old infant. Arch Dermatol 1990; 126: 1371.
16. Gerberding KM, Eisenhut CC, Engle WA, Cohen MD. Congenital candida pneumonia and sepsis: a case report and review of the literature. J Perinatol 1989; 9: 159–161.
17. Johnson DE, Thompson TR, Ferrieri P. Congenital candidiasis. Am J Dis Child 1981; 135: 273–275.
18. Waguespack-LaBiche J, Chen SH, Yen A. Disseminated congenital candidiasis in a premature infant. Arch Dermatol 1999; 135: 510–512.
19. Cosgrove BF, Reeves K, Mullins D, et al. Congenital cutaneous candidiasis associated with respiratory distress and elevation of liver function tests: a case report and review of the literature. J Am Acad Dermatol 1997; 37: 817–823.
20. Santos LA, Beceiro J, Hernandez R, et al. Congenital cutaneous candidiasis: Report of four cases and review of the literature. Eur J Pediatr 1991; 150: 336–338.
21. Baley JE, Silverman RA. Systemic candidiasis: cutaneous manifestations in low birthweight infants. Pediatrics 1988; 82: 211–215.
22. Pradeepkumar VK, Rajadurai VS, Tan KW. Congenital candidiasis: varied presentations. J Perinatol 1998; 18: 311–316.
23. Rowen JL, Atkins JT, Levy ML, et al. Invasive fungal dermatitis in the < or = 1000-gram neonate. Pediatrics 1995; 95: 682–687.
24. Hay RJ, Baran R. Fungal (onychomycosis) and other infections of the nail apparatus. In: Dawber RPR, ed. Diseases of the nails and their management. Oxford: Blackwell Scientific, 1984; 121–156.
25. Reddy TC, Chakrabarti A, Singh M, Singhi S. Role of buffy coat examination in the diagnosis of neonatal candidemia. Pediatr Infect Dis J 1996; 15: 718–720.
26. Flynn PM, Cunningham CK, Kerkering T et al. Oropharyngeal candidiasis in immunocompromised children: a randomized, multicenter study of orally administered fluconazole suspension versus nystatin. The Multicenter Fluconazole Study Group. J Pediatr 1995; 127: 322–328.
27. Crutchfield CE, III, Lewis EJ The successful treatment of oral candidiasis (thrush) in a pediatric patient using itraconazole. Pediatr Dermatol 1997; 14: 246.
28. Stevens DA. Oral amphotericin B as an antifungal agent. J Mycol Med 1997; 7: 241–242.
29. van den Anker JN, van Popele NM, Sauer PJ. Antifungal agents in neonatal systemic candidiasis. Antimicrob Agents Chemother 1995; 39: 1391–1397.
30. Leibovitz E. Neonatal candidosis: clinical picture, management controversies and consensus, and new therapeutic options. J Antimicrob Chemother 2002; 49: 69–73.

31. Rowen JL, Tate JM. Management of neonatal candidiasis. Neonatal Candidiasis Study Group. Pediatr Infect Dis J 1998; 17: 1007–1011.

32. Friedlich PS, Steinberg I, Fujitani A, deLemos RA. Renal tolerance with the use of intralipid-amphotericin B in low-birth-weight neonates. Am J Perinatol 1997; 14: 377–383.

33. Scarcella A, Pasquariello MB, Giugliano B, et al. Liposomal amphotericin B treatment for neonatal fungal infections. Pediatr Infect Dis J 1998; 17: 146–148.

34. Linder N, Klinger G, Shalit I, et al. Treatment of candidaemia in premature infants: comparison of three amphotericin B preparations. J Antimicrob Chemother 2003; 52: 663–667.

35. Juster-Reicher A, Flidel-Rimon O, Amitay M, et al. High-dose liposomal amphotericin B in the therapy of systemic candidiasis in neonates. Eur J Clin Microbiol Infect Dis 2003; 22: 603–607.

36. Fasano C, O'Keeffe J, Gibbs D. Fluconazole treatment of neonates and infants with severe fungal infections not treatable with conventional agents. Eur J Clin Microbiol Infect Dis 1994; 13: 351–354.

37. Schwarze R, Penk A, Pittrow L. [Use of fluconazole in children less than 1 year old: review]. Mycoses 1998; 41: 61–70.

38. Melville C, Kempley ST. Treatment of invasive Candida infection in neonates with congenital cutaneous candidiasis. Pediatrics 2001; 108: 216.

39. Aleck KA, Bartley DL. Multiple malformation syndrome following fluconazole use in pregnancy: report of an additional patient. Am J Med Genet 1997; 72: 253–256.

40. Warren NG, Hazen KC. Candida, cryptococcus, and other yeasts of medical importance. Manual of clinical microbiology. Washington, DC: ASM Press, 2006; 723–737.

41. de Repentigny L, Ratelle J, Leclerc JM et al. Repeated-dose pharmacokinetics of an oral solution of itraconazole in infants and children. Antimicrob Agents Chemother 1998; 42: 404–408.

42. Tosti A, Piraccini BM, Vincenzi C, Cameli N. Itraconazole in the treatment of two young brothers with chronic mucocutaneous candidiasis. Pediatr Dermatol 1997; 14: 146–148.

43. Sciacca A, Betta P, Cilauro S, et al. [Oral administration of itraconazole in a case of neonatal hepatic candidiasis]. Pediatr Med Chir 1995; 17: 173–175.

44. Stein DH. Fungal, protozoan, and helminth infections. In: Schachner LAHRC, ed. Pediatric dermatology. New York: Churchill Livingstone, 1995; 1295–345.

45. Odio CM, Araya R, Pinto LE, et al. Caspofungin therapy of neonates with invasive candidiasis. Pediatr Infect Dis J 2004; 23: 1093–1097.

46. Colby CE, Drohan L, Benitz W, Hintz SR. Low yield of ancillary diagnostic studies in neonates infected with Candida. J Perinatol 2004; 24: 241–246.

47. Neely MN, Schreiber JR. Fluconazole prophylaxis in the very low birthweight infant: not ready for prime time. Pediatrics 2001; 107: 404–405.

48. Long SS, Stevenson DK. Reducing Candida infections during neonatal intensive care: management choices, infection control, and fluconazole prophylaxis. J Pediatr 2005; 147: 135–141.

49. Kicklighter SD, Springer SC, Cox T, et al. Fluconazole for prophylaxis against candidal rectal colonization in the very low birthweight infant. Pediatrics 2001; 107: 293–298.

50. Bertini G, Perugi S, Dani C, et al. Fluconazole prophylaxis prevents invasive fungal infection in high-risk, very low birthweight infants. J Pediatr 2005; 147: 162–165.

51. Healy CM, Baker CJ, Zaccaria E, Campbell JR. Impact of fluconazole prophylaxis on incidence and outcome of invasive candidiasis in a neonatal intensive care unit. J Pediatr 2005; 147: 166–171.

52. Leeming JP, Sutton TM, Fleming PJ. Neonatal skin as a reservoir of Malassezia species. Pediatr Infect Dis J 1995; 14: 719–721.

53. Ashbee HR, Leck AK, Puntis JW, et al. Skin colonization by Malassezia in neonates and infants. Infect Control Hosp Epidemiol 2002; 23: 212–216.

54. Bernier V, Weill FX, Hirigoyen V, et al. Skin colonization by Malassezia species in neonates: a prospective study and relationship with neonatal cephalic pustulosis. Arch Dermatol 2002; 138: 215–218.

55. Bergman JN, Eichenfield LF. Neonatal acne and cephalic pustulosis: is Malassezia the whole story? Arch Dermatol 2002; 138: 255–257.

56. Welbel SF, McNeil MM, Pramanik A, et al. Nosocomial Malassezia pachydermatis bloodstream infections in a neonatal intensive care unit. Pediatr Infect Dis J 1994; 13: 104–108.

57. Chang HJ, Miller HL, Watkins N, et al. An epidemic of Malassezia pachydermatis in an intensive care nursery associated with colonization of health care workers' pet dogs. N Engl J Med 1998; 338: 706–711.

58. Terragni L, Lasagni A, Oriani A, Gelmetti C. Pityriasis versicolor in the pediatric age. Pediatr Dermatol 1991; 8: 9–12.

59. Di Silverio A, Zeccara C, Serra F, et al. Pityriasis versicolor in a newborn. Mycoses 1995; 38: 227–228.

60. Rapelanoro R, Mortureux P, Couprie B, et al. Neonatal Malassezia furfur pustulosis. Arch Dermatol 1996; 132: 190–193.

61. Dankner WM, Spector SA, Fierer J, Davis CE. Malassezia fungemia in neonates and adults: complication of hyperalimentation. Rev Infect Dis 1987; 9: 743–753.

62. Marcon MJ, Powell DA. Human infections due to Malassezia spp. Clin Microbiol Rev 1992; 5: 101–119.

63. Salazar GE, Campbell JR. Trichosporonosis, an unusual fungal infection in neonates. Pediatr Infect Dis J 2002; 21: 161–165.

64. Gokahmetoglu S, Nedret KA, Gunes T, Cetin N. Case reports. Trichosporon mucoides infection in three premature newborns. Mycoses 2002; 45: 123–125.

65. Walsh TJ, Melcher GP, Rinaldi MG, et al. Trichosporon beigelii, an emerging pathogen resistant to amphotericin B. J Clin Microbiol 1990; 28: 1616–1622.

66. Perparim K, Nagai H, Hashimoto A, et al. In vitro susceptibility of Trichosporon beigelii to antifungal agents. J Chemother 1996; 8: 445–448.

67. Maples HD, Stowe CD, Saccente SL, Jacobs RF. Voriconazole serum concentrations in an infant treated for Trichosporon beigelii infection. Pediatr Infect Dis J 2003; 22: 1022–1024.

68. Woodruff CA, Hebert AA. Neonatal primary cutaneous aspergillosis: case report and review of the literature. Pediatr Dermatol 2002; 19: 439–444.

69. Groll AH, Jaeger G, Allendorf A, et al. Invasive pulmonary aspergillosis in a critically ill neonate: case report and review of invasive aspergillosis during the first 3 months of life. Clin Infect Dis 1998; 27: 437–452.

70. Steinbach WJ. Pediatric aspergillosis: disease and treatment differences in children. Pediatr Infect Dis J 2005; 24: 358–364.

71. Denning DW. Invasive aspergillosis. Clin Infect Dis 1998; 26: 781–803.

72. Robertson AF, Joshi VV, Ellison DA, Cedars JC. Zygomycosis in neonates. Pediatr Infect Dis J 1997; 16: 812–815.

73. Linder N, Keller N, Huri C, et al. Primary cutaneous mucormycosis in a premature infant: case report and review of the literature. Am J Perinatol 1998; 15: 35–38.

74. Holzel H, Macqueen S, MacDonald A, et al. Rhizopus microsporus in wooden tongue depressors: a major threat or minor inconvenience? J Hosp Infect 1998; 38: 113–118.

75. du Plessis PJ, Wentzel LF, Delport SD, van Damme E. Zygomycotic necrotizing cellulitis in a premature infant. Dermatology 1997; 195: 179–181.

76. Hughes C, Driver SJ, Alexander KA. Successful treatment of abdominal wall Rhizopus necrotizing cellulitis in a preterm infant. Pediatr Infect Dis J 1995; 14: 336.

77. Amin SB, Ryan RM, Metlay LA, Watson WJ Absidia corymbifera

infections in neonates. Clin Infect Dis 1998; 26: 990–992.

78. Weitzman I, Chin NX, Kunjukunju N, Della-Latta P. A survey of dermatophytes isolated from human patients in the United States from 1993 to 1995. J Am Acad Dermatol 1998; 39: 255–261.

79. Weston WL, Morelli JG. Neonatal tinea capitis. Pediatr Infect Dis J 1998; 17: 257–258.

80. Snider R, Landers S, Levy ML. The ringworm riddle: an outbreak of *Microsporum canis* in the nursery. Pediatr Infect Dis J 1993; 12: 145–148.

81. Johnson ML, Anderson LL. Papulosquamous plaques in a mother and newborn son. Pediatr Dermatol 1995; 12: 281–284.

82. Romano C, Gianni C, Papini M. Tinea capitis in infants less than 1 year of age. Pediatr Dermatol 2001; 18: 465–468.

83. Virgili A, Corazza M, Zampino MR. Atypical features of tinea in newborns. Pediatr Dermatol 1993; 10: 92.

84. Cabon N, Moulinier C, Taieb A, Maleville J Tinea capitis and faciei caused by *Microsporon langeronii* in two neonates. Pediatr Dermatol 1994; 11: 281.

85. Gilaberte Y, Rezusta A, Gil J, et al. Tinea capitis in infants in their first year of life. Br J Dermatol 2004; 151: 886–890.

86. Singal A, Baruah MC, Rawat S, Sharma SC. *Trichophyton rubrum* infection in a 3-day-old neonate. Pediatr Dermatol 1996; 13: 488–489.

87. Ghorpade A, Ramanan C, Durairaj P. *Trichophyton mentagrophytes* infection in a two-day-old infant. Int J Dermatol 1991; 30: 209–210.

88. Baudraz-Rosselet F, Ruffieux P, Mancarella A, et al. Diaper dermatitis due to *Trichophyton verrucosum*. Pediatr Dermatol 1993; 10: 368–369.

89. Ploysangam T, Lucky AW. Childhood white superficial onychomycosis caused by *Trichophyton rubrum*: report of seven cases and review of the literature. J Am Acad Dermatol 1997; 36: 29–32.

90. Alden ER, Chernila SA. Ringworm in an infant. Pediatrics 1969; 44: 261–262.

91. Mercurio MG, Silverman RA, Elewski BE. Tinea capitis: fluconazole in *Trichophyton tonsurans* infection. Pediatr Dermatol 1998; 15: 229–232.

92. Pierard GE, Arrese JE, Pierard-Franchimont C. Treatment and prophylaxis of tinea infections. Drugs 1996; 52: 209–224.

93. Rabinowitz LG, Esterly NB. Naftifine (Naftin) in pediatrics. Pediatrics 1992; 90: 652.

94. Friedlander SF, Suarez S. Pediatric antifungal therapy. Dermatol Clin 1998; 16: 527–537.

95. Peterson CM, Eichenfield LF. Scabies. Pediatr Ann 1996; 25: 97–100.

96. Haim A, Grunwald MH, Kapelushnik J, et al. Hypereosinophilia in red scaly infants with scabies. J Pediatr 2005; 146: 712.

97. Hurwitz S. Scabies in babies. Am J Dis Child 1973; 126: 226–228.

98. Camassa F, Fania M, Ditano G, et al. Neonatal scabies. Cutis 1995; 56: 210–212.

99. Duran C, Tamayo L, de la Luz OM, Ruiz-Maldonado R. Scabies of the scalp mimicking seborrheic dermatitis in immunocompromised patients. Pediatr Dermatol 1993; 10: 136–138.

100. Huffam SE, Currie BJ. Ivermectin for *Sarcoptes scabiei* hyperinfestation. Int J Infect Dis 1998; 2: 152–154.

101. Castanet J, Monpoux F, Mariani R, et al. Demodicidosis in an immunodeficient child. Pediatr Dermatol 1998; 14: 219–220.

102. Patrizi A, Neri I, Chieregato C, Misciali M. Demodicidosis in immunocompetent young children: report of eight cases. Dermatology 1997; 195: 239–242.

103. Sarro RA, Hong JJ, Elgart ML. An unusual demodicidosis manifestation in a patient with AIDS. J Am Acad Dermatol 1998; 38: 120–121.

104. Noutsis C, Millikan LE. Myiasis. Dermatol Clin 1994; 12: 729–736.

105. Bapat SS. Neonatal myiasis. Pediatrics 2000; 106: E6.

106. Koh TH. Neonatal myiasis: a case report and a role of the Internet. J Perinatol 1999; 19: 528–529.

107. Boyer KM. Diagnosis and treatment of congenital toxoplasmosis. Adv Pediatr Infect Dis 1996; 11: 449–467.

108. Lynfield R, Guerina NG. Toxoplasmosis. Pediatr Rev 1997; 18: 75–83.

109. Justus J Cutaneous manifestations of toxoplasmosis. Curr Probl Dermatol 1971; 4: 24–47.

110. Safadi MA, Berezin EN, Farhat CK, Carvalho ES. Clinical presentation and follow up of children with congenital toxoplasmosis in Brazil. Brazil J Infect Dis 2003; 7: 325–331.

111. Carvalheiro CG, Mussi-Pinhata MM, Yamamoto AY, et al. Incidence of congenital toxoplasmosis estimated by neonatal screening: relevance of diagnostic confirmation in asymptomatic newborn infants. Epidemiol Infect 2005; 133: 485–491.

112. Roizen N, Swisher CN, Stein MA, et al. Neurologic and developmental outcome in treated congenital toxoplasmosis. Pediatrics 1995; 95: 11–20.

113. Alger LS. Toxoplasmosis and parvovirus B19. Infect Dis Clin North Am 1997; 11: 55–75.

114. Kubba R, Al Gindan Y. Leishmaniasis. Dermatol Clin 1989; 7: 331–351.

115. Di rocco M, Vignola S, Borrone C, et al. Cutaneous leishmaniasis in a 6-month-old girl. J Pediatr 1998; 132: 748.

116. del Giudice P, Marty P, Lacour JP, et al. Cutaneous leishmaniasis due to *Leishmania infantum*. Case reports and literature review. Arch Dermatol 1998; 134: 193–198.

117. Reed BR, Orton PW, Marr JJ, et al. Cutaneous leishmaniasis in an infant. Pediatr Dermatol 1983; 1: 142–145.

118. Wittner M. Leishmaniasis. In: Feigin RD, Cherry JD, eds. Textbook of pediatric infectious diseases. Philadelphia: WB Saunders, 1998; 2452–2458.

119. Nelson JD, ed. 1998–1999 Pocket book of pediatric antimicrobial therapy. 13th edition Baltimore: Williams & Wilkins, 1998: p62.

120. Brimhall CL, Esterly NB. Summertime, and the critters are biting. Contemp Pediatr 1994; 11: 62–77.

121. Rees RS, King LE, Jr. Arthropod bites and stings. In: Fitzpatrick TB, ed. Dermatology in general medicine. New York: McGraw-Hill, 1987; 2495–2506.

122. Vetter RS, Visscher PK. Bites and stings of medically important venomous arthropods. Int J Dermatol 1998; 37: 481–496.

15

Eczematous and Papulosquamous Disorders

Laurie A. Bernard, Lawrence F. Eichenfield

Eczematous eruptions represent a significant portion of the skin disease seen in the neonate. The most common is atopic dermatitis (AD). Seborrheic dermatitis (SD) and irritant diaper dermatitis (IDD) are now seen less frequently. Allergic contact dermatitis is rare in infants, and many less common eczematous disorders that result from nutritional, metabolic, and immunologic diseases have clinical manifestations that may be difficult to differentiate from AD.

Dermatitis is an all-inclusive term for inflammation of the skin that appears clinically as erythema and scaling, or erythema and scaling with crusts. The term eczema (boiling over) refers either to the infantile form of AD or to the morphology of erythema, scaling, and crusts.

ATOPIC DERMATITIS

Atopic dermatitis was described by Besnier[1] in 1892 as prurigo diasthétique. In 1933 Wise and Sulzberger[2] coined the term atopic dermatitis, and in 1935 Hill and Sulzberger[3] characterized the clinical entity. The term atopy means 'without place' or 'a strange thing.' Atopic dermatitis is an inherited, chronic, relapsing, pruritic skin condition characterized clinically by xerosis, inflammation, spongiosis and lichenification, and a complex immunopathology. The disease imposes an enormous burden on the social, personal, emotional, and financial resources of patients and their families.[4] In the United States annual costs spent for AD care are estimated at $1.64 billion.[5]

There has been a great increase in prevalence of atopic dermatitis over the past 50 years, with prevalence rates of 10–20% in the United States, Europe, Japan, Australia, and other industrialized countries.[6–8] Although there are ethnic variations in prevalence, studies have shown that different countries with similar ethnic demographics have markedly different recorded prevalences, suggesting that environmental factors are important in disease expression.[8] Atopic dermatitis is slightly more common in girls, with a female-to-male ratio of 1.3:1, and in higher social classes.[9] There may also be an increased incidence associated with maternal smoking,[10] but a lower incidence in preterm infants.[11] Other potential risk factors that may be associated with a rise in atopic disease include small family size, migration from rural to urban environments, increased income and education, and the increased use of antibiotics.[12]

Clinical Findings
History
In approximately 60% of patients the onset of AD is during the first year of life, most commonly between 3 and 6 months of age; 90% will present by 5 years of age.[13,14] Often AD patients have an additional atopic disorder such as asthma or allergic rhinitis, and this phenomenon increases with advancing age. Atopic dermatitis is usually the first manifestation of the 'atopic triad,' which includes AD, asthma, and allergic rhinitis.[15]

Family history is often helpful in establishing a diagnosis of AD: approximately 70% of patients will have a family history of atopy. Additionally, studies have determined that children with one atopic parent develop allergy 50% of the time, with the percentage increasing to 75% if both parents are atopic. Absence of an atopic disorder in the family history makes the diagnosis less likely.

The predominant symptom in AD is pruritus, which often interferes with sleep patterns and quality of life and is a major cause of morbidity. Excoriation often leads to complications such as secondary infection. Parents should be questioned about the infant scratching and rubbing against objects such as bedding or carpeting.

Physical Examination
There are three distinct clinical age-related phases of atopic dermatitis: infantile, childhood, and adulthood. During each phase both the site and morphology of the lesions change, although the phases often overlap. The infantile phase generally lasts until 2–3 years of age, the childhood phase from 2 years until puberty, and the adult phase from puberty onward.

The eruption in infancy characteristically begins on the cheeks (Figs 15-1 and 15-2) and scalp (Fig. 15-3) and evolves over time to involve the lateral and extensor aspects of the legs and arms (Fig. 15-4). The periauricular areas are often involved. The trunk may be involved, although the diaper area is usually spared (Fig. 15-5). Lesions are generally symmetric, scaly, erythematous patches and plaques, within which crusting is common. Chronic findings such as lichenification and pigmentary changes are not seen as often in the infantile phase. During late infancy the childhood phase, the flexural surfaces of the extremities become the most commonly involved sites, particularly the antecubital and popliteal fossae (Fig. 15-6).

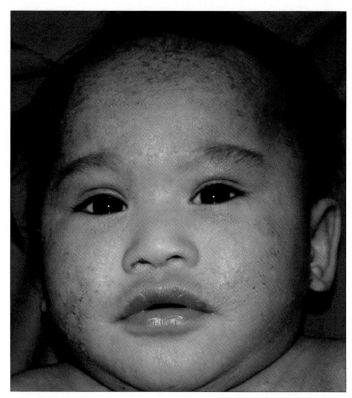

FIG. 15-1 Atopic dermatitis with typical early facial involvement.

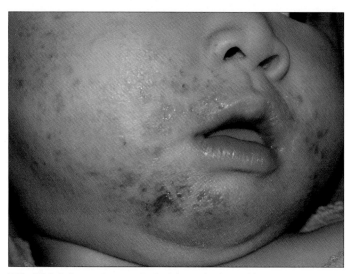

FIG. 15-2 Inflammatory acute facial atopic dermatitis.

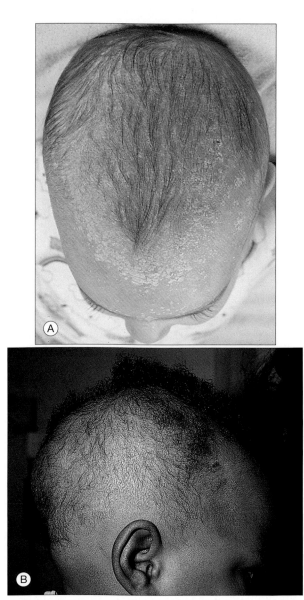

FIG. 15-3 (A) Typical 'cradle cap' may be the first manifestation of atopic dermatitis. (B) Temporary alopecia may result when an infant rubs the sides of the head against bedding to alleviate itching.

Other frequently involved sites include the neck, wrist and ankle flexures, and the creases between the thighs and buttocks. Lesions continue to be erythematous patches with crusting and excoriation. Lichenification and pigmentary changes also become prominent (Fig. 15-7). The pigment changes often evoke parental concerns about scarring, although lesions generally do not scar unless severely infected or excoriated.

There are a number of additional physical findings that, if present, aid in the diagnosis of atopic dermatitis. These are listed in Box 15-1. These findings are not specific to AD and may be seen in healthy patients as well.

Diagnosis

The diagnosis of AD is generally made clinically. It is often challenging to establish the diagnosis in early infancy, as AD can be difficult to distinguish from other infantile eczematous disorders. Clinical criteria have been formulated to assist in defining the disorder,[16–18] which is best viewed as a syndrome consisting of a number of clinical features:

A. Essential features (must be present)
  a. Pruritus
  b. Eczematous dermatitis (acute, subacute or chronic)
    i. Typical morphology and age-specific patterns
    ii. Chronic or relapsing history
B. Important features (seen in most cases, adding support to the diagnosis)
  a. Early age of onset
  b. Atopy
    i. Personal and/or family history
    ii. IgE reactivity
  c. Xerosis

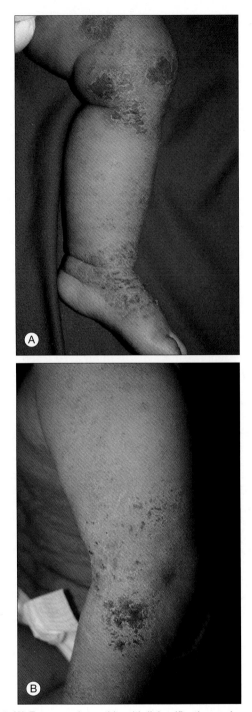

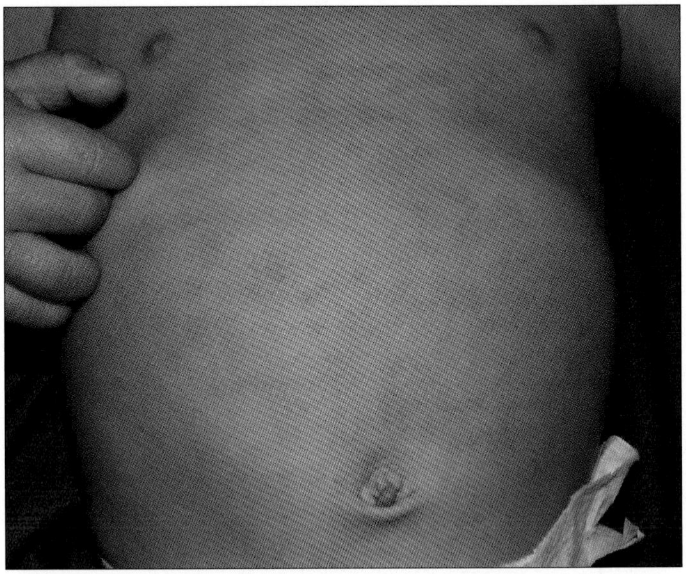

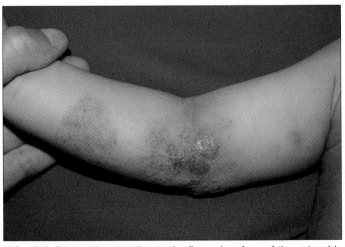

FIG. 15-5 Truncal atopic dermatitis with erythema, papules and scaling.

FIG. 15-6 Dermatitis extending to the flexural surface of the antecubital fossa.

FIG. 15-4 (A) Extensor dermatitis with lichenification and crusting of the leg. (B) Erythema and scale on the extensor surface of the arm.

C. Associated features (these clinical associations help to suggest the diagnosis of AD but are too nonspecific to be used to define or detect AD for research or epidemiologic studies)
   a. Atypical vascular responses (e.g. facial pallor, white dermatographism, delayed blanch response)
   b. Keratosis pilaris/hyperlinear palms/ichthyosis
   c. Ocular/periorbital changes
   d. Other regional findings (e.g. perioral changes/periauricular lesions)
   e. Perifollicular accentuation/lichenification/prurigo lesions.

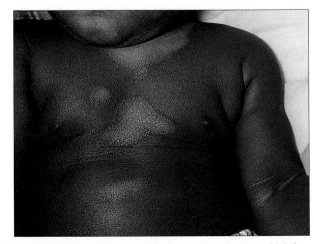

FIG. 15-7 Marked postinflammatory hypopigmentation, which is common in darkly pigmented infants.

Box 15-1 Features of atopic dermatitis

Major features
- Pruritus
- Rash on face and/or extensors in infants and young children
- Lichenification in flexural areas in older children
- Tendency toward chronic or chronically relapsing dermatitis
- Personal or family history of atopic disease: asthma, allergic rhinitis, atopic dermatitis

Other common findings
- Dryness
- Dennie–Morgan folds (accentuated lines or grooves below the margin of the lower eyelid)
- Allergic shiners (darkening beneath the eyes)
- Facial pallor
- Pityriasis alba
- Keratosis pilaris
- Ichthyosis vulgaris
- Hyperlinearity of palms and soles
- White dermatographism (white line appears on skin within 1 minute of being stroked with blunt instrument)
- Conjunctivitis
- Keratoconus
- Anterior subcapsular cataracts
- Elevated serum IgE
- Immediate skin test reactivity

Reproduced from Bernard LA, Eichenfield LF. How to identify atopic dermatitis vs. other eczemas. In: Leung DYM, Eichenfield LF, eds. Pediatric eczemas. New York: Summit Communications, 2004; 20.

Laboratory testing is not needed in the routine evaluation of uncomplicated AD. Serum IgE is elevated in approximately 70–80% of patients. The majority of patients also have peripheral blood eosinophilia.

Skin biopsies may be helpful in distinguishing AD from other inflammatory skin disorders, but biopsy findings alone are not diagnostic. The histology varies from an acute dermatitis with spongiosis and a lymphocytic infiltrate, to chronic changes in lichenified skin showing acanthosis, hyperkeratosis, parakeratosis, and a perivascular lymphocytic infiltrate around blood vessels and an accumulation of Langerhans' cells,[19] phagocytes, and mast cells.[20] The superficial venular plexus has endothelial cell hypertrophy, basement membrane thickening,[21] and increased numbers of immunoreactive nerve fibers.[22] Eosinophils are not commonly present in acute AD. Mast cells are found in normal numbers in different stages of degranulation.[23]

Etiology/Pathogenesis

Currently available data suggest that the etiology of AD is probably multifactorial. It appears that the disease results from genetic susceptibilities, including epidermal barrier dysfunction and an altered innate immune system, and a heightened response to allergens and microbial antigens.[24]

AD is genetically mediated with familial clustering; monozygotic twins are concordant, whereas dizygotic twins are discordant for AD;[25] and transfer of AD by bone marrow transplantation[26] has been reported. Genetic screening of families with AD has highlighted chromosome regions that are implicated in other inflammatory diseases,[27–30] and it is highly likely that many genes are involved in the immunologic abnormalities seen in AD, including high levels of IgE,[31] abnormal T-cell clones,[32] high levels of IL-4, and low levels of interferon-γ.[33] Loss-of-function mutations of the epidermal barrier protein filaggrin have been shown to be a major predisposing factor for AD, as well as ichthyosis vulgaris.[34,35]

Skin barrier dysfunction plays a major role in AD. It is markedly reduced owing to the downregulated cornified envelope genes (filaggrin and loricrin), reduced ceramide levels, increased levels of proteolytic enzymes, and enhanced transepidermal water loss.[34,35] Exogenous protease inhibitors, such as those produced by *Staphylococcus aureus* or dust mites, may also damage the epidermal barrier. Such epidermal changes may potentiate the absorption of allergens into the skin or lead to increased bacterial colonization. Keratinocytes play an important role in atopic skin inflammation, secreting chemokines and cytokines, influencing T-cell activation, and through innate immune responses, including toll-like receptor expression and antimicrobial peptides.[36]

Cytokine abnormalities are common in AD, and their interaction may represent another pathogenetic mechanism underlying the inflammation. It has been recognized that Th2 responses predominate in acute AD and lead to the overproduction of numerous cytokines, notably IL-4 and IL-13, which mediate switching of immunoglobulin isotypes to IgE synthesis.[37] IL-4 also stimulates mast cells to produce mediators such as histamine, which play a key role in the development of pruritus. IL-5 predominates in chronic AD and is involved in eosinophil development and survival.[37,38] Neuropeptides (substance P) stimulate release of histamine from skin mast cells and may link the central nervous system with cutaneous inflammation.[39] The repeated stimulation and abnormal biochemical responsiveness and mediator release by AD monocytes, mast cells, and eosinophils may sustain and initiate a vicious cycle, contributing to the inflammation.[40]

Antigens may trigger immune responses in AD. These include microbes, such as *S. aureus*, aeroallergens, and foods. The antigens may be presented to the allergen-specific IgE receptors on Langerhans' cells and inflammatory dendritic epidermal cells (IDEC), and these complexes may interact with allergen-specific T cells.[41] The impact of food exposure on the development of atopic dermatitis is controversial. Although it is known that food allergy and sensitization more commonly develop in children with atopic dermatitis, it is unclear how important food exposures are to the development of atopic dermatitis, nor how common food-induced eczematous dermatitis is during infancy.[42] Studies[43,44] have reported that prolonged breastfeeding protects against the development of AD, that maternal avoidance of allergens during early lactation reduces the incidence of AD,[43,44] and that the early introduction of solid food increases the incidence of AD.[43] The house dust mite *Dermatophagoides pteronyssinus* and the yeast *Pityrosporum ovale* have both been cited in the pathogenesis of AD.[45]

S. aureus colonization on the skin and nares is more common in AD than in other skin diseases (or in the normal population), and the further finding of *S. aureus* enterotoxin B producing superantigens suggests it may play a role in pathogenesis.[46]

Differential Diagnosis

The common disorders in the differential diagnosis of AD in neonates include SD, contact dermatitis, psoriasis, scabies, ichthyosis, tinea corporis, and keratosis pilaris (Box 15-2). Seborrheic dermatitis may be virtually indistinguishable from AD (Fig. 15-8), owing to the similarity in sites of involvement and morphology (see the following discussion). Contact dermatitis is rare in the newborn period, though irritant dermatitis is not uncommon. A configuration suggesting an external source of irritation may be evident and helpful in differentiating between the two.

Psoriasis is not commonly recognized in infants, although it may occur at birth or during the first year of life. Both psoriasis vulgaris and pustular psoriasis may occur in the neonate. The diaper area is most commonly affected in the former, where lesions are erythematous, well-demarcated plaques surmounted by scale, which is less silvery in the diaper area than in other areas (see the following discussion).

Scabies may be difficult to distinguish from AD because both diseases cause severe pruritus. Scabies is rarely considered in the newborn. The face is not usually involved in scabies, whereas the eczematous patches on the cheeks and xerosis are typical of AD. Moreover, the eruption of scabies is polymorphous, with burrows, papules, nodules, and eczema-tous and urticarial lesions, as well as typical pustules on the palms and soles. A recent onset of itching in family members is also helpful in differentiating the two conditions.

When the skin lesions are associated with failure to thrive, diarrhea, infection, and other systemic signs, it is important to consider rare disorders such as nutritional, metabolic, genetic, immunologic disorders and proliferative disorders, such as Langerhans' cell histiocytosis (Box 15-3).

Occasionally, AD may be so severe that the whole body becomes erythrodermic, causing confusion with other causes of erythroderma, particularly Netherton syndrome, and nutritional deficiencies (see Chapter 18).

Prognosis

Atopic dermatitis is a disease of exacerbations and remissions. Data from follow-up surveys show enormous variation in the prognosis, owing to differences in patient sampling techniques. The degree of severity of AD, its persistence into adolescence, and allergen sensitization, are predictors that the disease is more likely to continue into adult life.[47] Other reported risk factors for adult disease include the presence of other atopic diseases such as asthma and allergic rhinitis, a family history of AD in parents or siblings, early age of onset and high serum IgE levels, and null mutations in the filaggrin gene in early-onset AD.[48,49]

Vickers[48] reported that AD cleared by age 20 in 90% of patients, but the inclusion of patients with SD, which has an excellent prognosis and clears within weeks, biased his results. Nevertheless, there is a steady decline in AD, with the highest prevalence being in those under 2 years of age and a much

---

Box 15-2 Differential diagnosis of infantile atopic dermatitis: common disorders

Seborrheic dermatitis

Contact dermatitis (allergic and irritant)

Scabies

Psoriasis

Ichthyosis vulgaris

Keratosis pilaris

Box 15-3 Differential diagnosis of atopic dermatitis: rare disorders in infants

Metabolic/nutritional/genetic disorders

Acrodermatitis enteropathica

Zinc deficiency (prematurity; deficient breast milk zinc; cystic fibrosis)

Other nutritional deficiencies (biotin, essential fatty acids)

Netherton syndrome

Phenylketonuria

Omenn syndrome

Prolidase deficiency

Gluten-sensitive enteropathy

Eosinophilic gastroenteritis

Hurler syndrome

Immune disorders

Hyperimmunoglobulin-E syndrome

Severe combined immunodeficiency disorder

Wiskott–Aldrich syndrome

Agammaglobulinemia

Ataxia–telangiectasia

Neonatal lupus erythematosus

Proliferative disorders

Langerhans' cell histiocytosis

Adapted from Bernard LA, Eichenfield LF. How to identify atopic dermatitis vs. other eczemas. In: Leung DYM, Eichenfield LF, eds. Pediatric eczemas. New York: Summit Communications, 2004; 28.

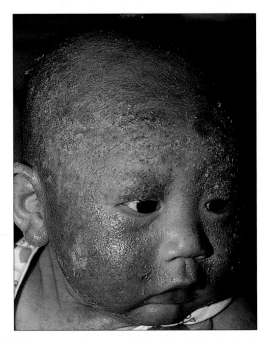

FIG. 15-8 This young infant was initially thought to have seborrheic dermatitis, but over time the diagnosis of atopic dermatitis became evident.

lower prevalence in adulthood.[48] Spontaneous resolution of AD has been reported to occur in 40–60% of patients affected during infancy, particularly in those with mild disease.

Figures on the incidence of asthma and hay fever following or associated with AD vary from 10% to 70%.[13,47] In one survey, 48% suffered from respiratory atopy, 36% from rhinitis, 28% from asthma, and 15% from both.[13] There is an added risk of developing either asthma or AD if there is a family history of either,[50] or if filaggrin gene null mutations are present.[51] Asthma can start at any time, but AD generally occurs earlier than other atopic diseases.[13]

Treatment

The management of atopic dermatitis should be directed at excellent skin care, avoidance of irritants and allergens, hydrating the skin, and treating pruritus, xerosis, and inflammation. It is extremely important to educate the parents on the nature of the disease and the goals of therapy. Understanding the chronic, relapsing nature of AD is important, as is counseling on the natural history and prognosis. Because parents are inundated with so much information, attention to detail, repetition of advice, and written handouts can improve treatment results.

Environmental Control

Dry skin, excessive sweating, changes in temperature and humidity and exogenous irritants and allergens are all triggers of eczema that are influenced by the environment.[52] Skin hyperreactivity in infants with atopic dermatitis is common, allowing factors that are not often discernible to induce pruritus and the 'itch–scratch' cycle that may cause eczema flares. Neonates with AD are irritated by coarse fibers, such as wool; 100% cotton clothing is traditionally recommended, although similar smooth-fibered clothing, such as commercially available silk fabrics, may also be useful. Bathing and moisturization can minimize skin dryness, which is more vulnerable to irritants, allergens and microbes. Avoidance of known triggers and irritants is an important cornerstone of therapy.

Pruritus

One of the major challenges of treatment is controlling the intense pruritus. Pruritus causes sleep deprivation in both patients and their families. Evidence for the effectiveness of antihistamines is contradictory,[53,54] and the impact of antihistamines on the itch of dermatitis is unclear. Sedating antihistamines, predominantly H_1, are commonly used, and effectiveness may be due to drowsiness from central nervous system (CNS) depression. Nonsedating antihistamines show variable results in controlling AD-associated pruritus. Effective control of skin inflammation and excellent hydration are the most effective interventions to reduce pruritus.

Xerosis (Dry Skin)

Xerosis is a significant component of AD, and hydrating the skin is a foundation of atopic dermatitis therapy. This is accomplished through frequent application of moisturizers and appropriate bathing techniques. The frequency of bathing is controversial. Evidence suggests that bathing, followed by the immediate application of an emollient while the skin is wet (the 'soak and seal' method), has an excellent hydrating effect, is steroid sparing, and is a tremendously useful treatment in AD patients.[55] The application of moisturizers independent of bathing can improve hydration status and improve

barrier function. Ideally, moisturizing agents should be safe, effective, inexpensive, and free of additives and other potential sensitizing agents. Products containing urea, lactic acid, and α-hydroxy acids may sting and their absorption in infants is unknown. Emollients should be applied all over the body when the skin is wet and after topical corticosteroids have been applied to lesional skin. Regular applications of emollients should be continued after the dermatitis has improved, to attempt to minimize disease flares and the need for anti-inflammatory agents.

Topical therapy to improve skin hydration, decrease skin barrier dysfunction, and to replace abnormal epidermal lipids may be useful. Studies with topical preparations having distinct compositions of lipids and ceramides, as well as a non-steroidal cream containing palmitamide MEA, an essential fatty acid, and a hydrolipidic cream with glycyrrhetinic acid (MAS063ADP),[56,57] have shown some benefit. Further clinical studies to define the benefits relative to traditional moisturizers and topical anti-inflammatory agents will be helpful.

Anti-Inflammatory Agents
Topical Corticosteroids

Topical corticosteroids were first introduced by Sulzberger and Witten[58] in 1952 and are the mainstay of treatment in AD because of their excellent anti-inflammatory effects. They are grouped according to their potency into seven classes, from very weak (VII) to superpotent (I). The early indiscriminate use of topical corticosteroids resulted in a number of local and systemic side effects, which has led to an unfounded fear and reluctance on the part of parents and physicians to use them appropriately, despite the extremely small number of reported side effects in those treated,[59,60] the majority of which occur in patients who have received inappropriate treatment.[61] Physicians should encourage the correct use of topical corticosteroid preparations on affected inflamed areas. Close monitoring and follow-up during treatment is appropriate. Precise information should be given to the parents regarding the manner of application, and written handouts are very useful.

There are many methods of prescribing topical corticosteroids and other anti-inflammatory therapies. Published algorithms may be used.[62] Mild cases or where facial or diaper areas are involved are generally treated with low-potency steroids, such as hydrocortisone 1% ointment, aclometasone, and desonide. For more significant flares, or if low-potency steroids are inadequate to control the eczema, stronger topical corticosteroids are used for truncal and body surfaces. Prescriptions should be given for sufficient medication for the area involved. Depending on the extent of the eruption and the size of the infant, 100 g will usually last for about a month. Areas should be treated two to three times a day until the inflammation disappears, with frequent use of emollients. Emollients should continue after corticosteroids are discontinued. In infants with persistent or frequently recurrent AD a maintenance regimen is essential which may use emollients, intermittent topical corticosteroids, newer barrier cream therapies, and topical calcineurin inhibitors (see below).

Systemic corticosteroids are not indicated for the treatment of AD in neonates.

Topical Calcineurin Inhibitors

Topical calcineurin inhibitors are a relatively new class of anti-inflammatory therapy for atopic dermatitis. Topical tacroli-

mus and pimecrolimus are approved for use in adults and children 2 years and older, and are not currently recommended for routine therapy of AD in infants.

Topical pimecrolimus has been studied in a large population of 1133 infants aged 3–23 months with mild to severe AD. The patients studied were treated intermittently for up to 2 years. The results of these studies demonstrated rapid symptom relief, prevention of progression to major flares, increased numbers of disease-free days, improved quality of life of patients and their parents, and good tolerability.[63–68] Pimecrolimus blood concentrations measured in 35 patients were low, irrespective of the disease severity and extent, and remained low during intermittent treatment for up to 1 year. The level of systemic exposure to pimecrolimus among infants was comparable to that observed for older children enrolled in the same studies and treated in the same way with pimecrolimus 1% cream, which indicated that infants are not at higher risk of significant percutaneous absorption of topically applied pimecrolimus.[69–71] In addition, no sign of immunosuppression was seen in infants treated during up to 2 years of intermittent therapy with topical pimecrolimus. These data suggest that pimecrolimus 1% cream may be a useful second-line therapy in infants with persistent AD despite intermittent corticosteroids.

Although long-term safety has not yet been established, current data indicate TCIs to be both safe and effective with proper use. Rare cases of skin malignancy have been reported with topical tacrolimus, though the level of data quality and applicability of the reports was judged to be low in the report of a scientific consensus conference.[72] The most common side effects are local reactions such as stinging and burning, and patients should be monitored for signs and symptoms of cutaneous viral infection, although ongoing surveillance and recent reports have not shown a trend for increased frequency of viral superinfections.[73]

Infections

S. aureus frequently colonizes the skin and nares of atopic individuals. Topical corticosteroids alone can reduce bacterial counts.[74] Oral antibiotics may be necessary to treat obvious secondary bacterial infection, presenting as pustules and honey-colored crusts. Antibiotics may also be used if the AD flares for no apparent reason. The usual first-line treatment is a first- or second-generation cephalosporin. Macrolides are of limited utility, with significant antibiotic resistance reported in most geographic areas. Methicillin-resistant *S. aureus* (MRSA) is another significant concern and, if suspected, clindamycin or trimethoprim-sulfamethoxazole are reasonable options. Bacterial culture and sensitivities may be needed to guide antibiotic therapy. Although prolonged oral antibiotic therapy is alleged to reduce the *S. aureus* superantigens,[46] resistant bacteria may develop. Because colonization is so common in this setting, antibiotics should only be used when signs of infection are present.

Mupirocin (pseudomonic acid) decreases the carrier rate of *S. aureus* on the skin,[75] but application in large areas is impractical. Antibacterial scrubs reduce the staphylococcal colony count, but irritation and potential toxicity limits their use in neonates. *S. aureus* colonization is difficult to eradicate from the nose and skin even with long-term antibiotic use, and all close contacts must be treated.[76] Bleach baths have been used to reduce staphylococcal colonization in children with AD, but have not been formally studied for use in infants.

Allergen Avoidance

General skin-care measures and topical anti-inflammatory agents are standard for atopic dermatitis. Allergies may develop in early life in a subset of infants. Sensitization to foods is uncommon in infants, though those with AD have a higher risk of developing food and dust mite allergies than infants or children without AD. Food exposures in allergic children may induce contact urticaria, urticaria, noncutaneous allergy symptoms such as gastrointestinal effects, wheezing and nasal congestion, or in a subset of individuals food-induced eczematous dermatitis. Egg, milk, wheat, soy, and peanut account for more than 90% of the foods allergies in children with AD. Food allergies usually are associated with positive immediate skin tests or elevated serum IgE specific to various foods, though positive tests do not necessarily correlate with clinically important allergy. Positive in-vitro tests should be confirmed with controlled food challenges and elimination diets. Extensive elimination diets are rarely, if ever, necessary because even in patients with multiple positive skin tests, the majority will react to three or fewer foods on controlled challenge.

Adjunctive and Alternative Therapies

Families of patients with atopic dermatitis often use alternative therapies. In one study, the second most common reason for patients to seek alternative medicine was for treatment of allergic conditions such as atopic dermatitis. In many cases, the safety and efficacy of these treatments has not been elucidated, although fortunately the number of published reports evaluating such therapies is increasing. Probiotics have recently emerged as a potentially useful therapy for atopic disease. A number of studies have appeared favorable, although to date these have mostly been small and short term.[77,78] Larger, long-term randomized trials are needed in order to determine safety, efficacy, optimal dosing, and treatment duration before such therapies can be recommended, particularly in infants. Chinese herbal therapy is the modality most extensively studied for the treatment of AD. A number of controlled trials have been conducted, but results have been mixed and inconclusive.[79] There are also significant safety concerns: a number of cases of serious hepatotoxicity have been reported with the use of Chinese herbals for AD. Some of these herbal medications have also been found to be contaminated with corticosteroids.

Essential fatty acid supplementation has also been studied for use in AD. It is theorized that the disturbed barrier function in the skin of these patients may be caused by altered metabolism of fatty acids. It is hypothesized that this disturbance could potentially be treated with agents high in certain fatty acids. Such agents include, among others, evening primrose oil, fish oil, and borage oil. The most extensively studied product is evening primrose oil, and results have been mixed. It has been difficult to compare trial results, as methodologies and dosing are quite variable. Currently, there is not sufficient evidence to support the use of evening primrose oil for treatment of AD, but further controlled trials are indicated. Other alternative therapies include acupuncture, massage therapy, hypnotherapy, transepidermal nerve stimulation, biofeedback, and other oral herbal supplements. Supportive data for their utility in infantile AD are scant.

SEBORRHEIC DERMATITIS

First described by Unna in 1887,[80] seborrheic dermatitis (SD) is a disease of unknown etiology that affects infants with a distinct inflammatory eruption that primarily involves the scalp and intertriginous areas. The disease affects both sexes and is most common within the first 4–6 weeks of life, but may occur up to 1 year of age. Many experts believe that severe SD is not seen as frequently as in the past, for uncertain reasons.[81]

Cutaneous Findings

The scalp is the first area to be involved, with 'cradle-cap,' a greasy, yellow scale on the vertex. Hair loss is uncommon, and erythema is variable (Fig. 15-9). The retroauricular creases are commonly affected. Lesions commonly involve the face, primarily the central forehead, glabella, eyebrows, malar eminences, nasolabial folds, and external ears with erythema and a yellow greasy scale (Fig. 15-10). Other commonly affected

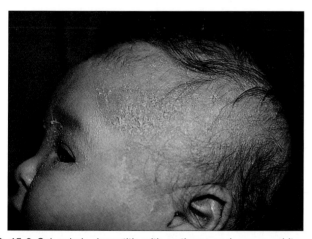

FIG. 15-9 Seborrheic dermatitis with erythema and greasy, white scalp scaling.

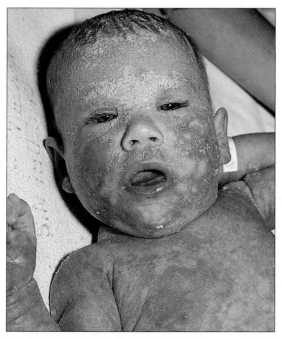

FIG. 15-10 Seborrheic dermatitis: this infant had unusually widespread disease.

areas include the diaper area, with well-demarcated, erythematous plaques and a variable degree of scale; the axillary area and other creases (Fig. 15-11); and the presternal and interscapular areas, where eczematous patches are common. After a few days, *Candida albicans* commonly invades the affected areas, causing maceration and crusting (see Chapter 14).

Secondary bacterial infection may rarely occur, with crusting and pustules on the existing lesions. Postinflammatory hypopigmentation is common in dark-skinned infants, but improves in the weeks after the dermatitis has resolved.

Etiology and Pathogenesis

The etiology and pathogenesis are unknown. Theories of increased sebaceous gland activity as a result of maternal hormones and nutritional factors are reasonable, but have not been validated.[81,82]

Studies have implicated the yeast-like organism *Pityrosporum ovale* (*Malassezia*) in the etiology of SD in infants.[83,84] The organism was detected in the majority of infants with SD, but in only a few of the controls.[84] In treatment studies of SD ketoconazole 2% and bifonazole shampoo resulted in rapid cure in most children treated.[85]

Diagnosis

The diagnosis is usually a clinical one. Histology of the lesions is not diagnostic and consists of a subacute dermatitis with elongation of the epidermal rete ridges. The presence of neutrophils is more suggestive of SD than other forms of dermatitis. There are no laboratory markers for diagnosing this condition.

Differential Diagnosis

Seborrheic dermatitis may be very difficult to distinguish from psoriasis. Psoriasis may occur in infants and often starts in the diaper area with persistent, well-demarcated, erythematous plaques surmounted by a scale (Fig. 15-12). The greasy scale in the scalp and creases that is typical of SD is not seen in psoriasis. Similarly, AD in newborns is easy to confuse with SD, particularly during the first few weeks of life.[86] The scalp is often involved in both. Cradle cap is caused by the retention of keratin and is often found in normal infants. It is also com-

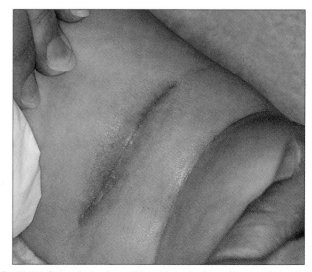

FIG. 15-11 Seborrheic dermatitis with typical involvement in body fold.

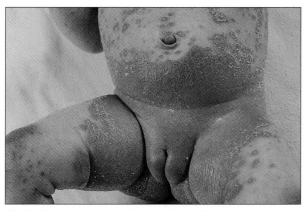

FIG. 15-12 Psoriasis: typical diaper-area involvement.

monly seen in AD, where the scale is dry rather than greasy, as is seen in SD. The term seboatopic is used for cases fitting both patterns, but the diagnosis usually becomes clear early on; the majority of cases represent AD. The morphology of the lesions and the presence or absence of pruritus and xerosis is helpful in differentiating between the two. The diagnosis of SD is more likely when the axillae are affected, and AD is more likely to be diagnosed when the shins and forearms are involved.

Persistent, hemorrhagic, atrophic, or ulcerative lesions should alert physicians to consider the diagnosis of Langerhans' cell histiocytosis (LCH; see Chapter 25), which in neonates and young infants can resemble SD, with a similar distribution in the scalp and the retroauricular and diaper areas. Well-demarcated, erythematous patches and crusts are evident, but the presence of petechiae and purpura is typical of LCH. Lesions of LCH may also involve other areas of the body with varying morphologies, including erythematous papules, vesicles, and nodules. Skin biopsy easily differentiates between the two conditions.

Other eczematous disorders, including immunodeficiency diseases, nutritional and metabolic disorders, may appear similar to SD.

Course, Management, Treatment, and Prognosis

Follow-up studies of patients with infantile SD have produced a variety of findings. Vickers[48] classified both AD and SD as one disease. Others[80,83] have concluded that many of the cases diagnosed as infantile SD evolved into AD. These reports may have based their diagnosis of SD on the finding of cradle cap, which was thought to be diagnostic of SD but is now known to frequently occur in AD. Reports of SD evolving into psoriasis may reflect the previous lack of recognition of psoriasis in infancy.[87]

Treatment consists of using a mild shampoo, such as selenium zinc for mild disease, and low-potency topical corticosteroid; these are usually effective in controlling the disease within several weeks. Antiyeast shampoos such as ketaconazole, and bifonazole are also highly effective as well. Recurrence of SD is rare. Salicylic acid preparations should not be used because absorption can cause salicylism and irritation.

PSORIASIS

Psoriasis is a common, chronic inflammatory skin disease characterized clinically by a typical, scaly eruption and pathogenetically by cutaneous inflammation and accelerated epidermal cell turnover. It affects 1–2% of the population[88,89] and while one-third of cases occur before the age of 20 it is uncommon in infants. Although rare, psoriasis may present at birth. Two per cent of cases present before age 2 years, and are often mistaken for SD. There is a slight female preponderance.[90] When psoriasis occurs in children, a family history is easier to ascertain.

Cutaneous Findings

Infantile psoriasis commonly presents in the diaper area (see Fig. 15-12) or on the scalp. It may, however, involve any area and, unlike the adult form, commonly affects the face. Lesions may be pruritic and consist of erythematous, well-demarcated plaques with a silvery scale, a feature that is often absent in the diaper area. In infancy the Koebner phenomenon (isomorphic response) is common. Nail changes are present in 10% of infants with psoriasis. The findings may include pitting, onycholysis, oil spots, and subungual hyperkeratosis. Severe, inflammatory nail changes (acrodermatitis continua of Hallopeau) may accompany pustular psoriasis.

Pustular psoriasis is a much rarer form of psoriasis in infancy. This may have its onset at birth or in the ensuing few weeks. The eruption often presents with fever and sheets of small pustules that may also be arranged in a circinate or annular pattern. In this instance, pustules are located at the peripheral edge of an erythematous scale. Associated findings in this pustular variety include geographic tongue, sterile osteomyelitis, and very rarely lung involvement with the capillary leak syndrome. Rarely, a diffuse psoriasiform Id-like eruption can be seen associated with severe candidiasis of the diaper area.

Etiology and Pathogenesis

The etiology of psoriasis is unknown. There is a strong family history, which is even more evident in the younger cases. This appears to be associated with certain HLA types, such as Cw6. The gene defect is not inherited in a simple autosomal dominant or recessive pattern. In older children, it is well recognized that guttate (teardrop) lesions may be related to infection with β-hemolytic streptococcus. Guttate psoriasis has been described after a perianal streptococcal infection. The ultimate pathogenesis of psoriasis is unknown and may represent a polygenic inheritance pattern that manifests after multifactorial environmental events.

Diagnosis

The diagnosis of 'napkin psoriasis' is often difficult and a biopsy may be necessary for confirmation. Characteristic histology includes parakeratosis, loss of the granular layer, Munro microabscesses, and spongiform pustules of Kogoj. A lymphocytic infiltrate is present within the dermis. A repeated sterile culture from the pustules should alert physicians to the diagnosis of pustular psoriasis, and a biopsy is helpful.

Differential Diagnosis

It is difficult to differentiate psoriasis in the diaper area and scalp from SD, but the absence of intertriginous involvement, a greasy yellow scale, and nail changes may be helpful. Other causes of eruptions in the diaper area, including LCH and Netherton syndrome, as well as nutritional and metabolic disorders, are relatively easy to exclude with the appearance of the lesions and the biopsy findings. It is important to rule out infectious etiologies in pustular psoriasis, particularly when osteomyelitis is present. Kawasaki disease may display psoriasis-like eruption in infants.[91] Erythrokeratodermas and ichthyosiform disorders may be considered in the differential diagnosis of infantile psoriasis.

Prognosis

The prognosis in infancy is variable. In a follow-up study[92] of nine patients, most were still affected but had mild disease and did not require constant follow-up. The more extensive the disease, the more likely lesions will persist.

Treatment

Many treatments are available for psoriasis in adults, most of which are inappropriate for neonates. A mild to mid-strength steroid preparation is often all that is required for the plaque variety. The pustular form is more difficult to treat. A conservative approach with the use of topical corticosteroid preparations is often the first line of treatment. If this is not successful, then alternative topical anti-inflammatory agents, vitamin D analogs, or systemic therapy such as methotrexate, retinoids, and cyclosporin may be considered.

Candidiasis with Psoriasiform Id

Candidiasis with psoriasiform id is rarely seen in the neonatal period. Lesions of *Candida* in the diaper area are treated with topical corticosteroids, and after days to weeks an explosive psoriasiform eruption occurs on the cheeks and trunk. Treatment of the candidal eruption with topical antifungal agents and mild to mid-strength corticosteroids to the psoriasiform areas results in remission in a few weeks. Whether the appearance of these lesions is associated with a psoriatic diathesis is not known.

CONTACT DERMATITIS

Contact dermatitis is an inflammatory process caused by the application of an irritating substance to the skin, or by a substance causing an allergic reaction. Although irritant contact dermatitis occurs in many individuals who are exposed to the irritating substance, allergic contact dermatitis (ACD) occurs only in a small number of individuals who become sensitized. Patients with AD are more predisposed to irritant contact dermatitis because of their disordered barrier function.

Both irritant dermatitis and ACD are rare in infants. Although infants are able to mount an immunologic response to a sensitizing substance, nickel is the only substance causing ACD seen with any frequency.

Cutaneous Findings

Nickel sensitivity in neonates is almost exclusively caused by wearing contact nickel snaps on clothing. The most commonly involved areas are on the center of the chest and upper abdomen, where there may be a pruritic, linear dermatitis corresponding to the areas where the nickel snaps are in contact with the skin. Id reactions are common, particularly in the antecubital fossae, but they can affect other areas as well. Infants with nickel sensitivity are often misdiagnosed as having AD; nickel sensitization may be more common in patients with AD, who may have both conditions. Another possible source of nickel allergy is ear-piercing, which in some cultures is performed in very young infants.

Allergic contact dermatitis may also occur in the diaper area. (See Chapter 16; Fig. 16-9).

Pathogenesis

The pathology is that of any acute dermatitis. Immunohistochemical stains show a predominance of helper cells with some suppressor cells, although only a small number of the T cells in the infiltrate have specificity for the antigen.

ACD is produced by a T-lymphocyte-mediated type IV immune response. There are two distinct phases in the development of ACD: the afferent or induction phase and the efferent or elicitation phase.[93] The sensitization following first exposure with an allergen takes 5–25 days. On repeat exposure the eruption develops within 24–48 hours.

Management of Nickel Dermatitis

Contact with metals containing nickel should be eliminated, including nickel zippers and underwear with nickel snaps. Topical corticosteroids are helpful until the inflammation has subsided.

KERATOSIS PILARIS

This very common condition is seen in patients with atopic dermatitis as well as otherwise healthy children. It is caused by perifollicular retention of scale, leading to plugging in the orifice of the hair follicle. Affected patients develop small papules on the lateral aspects of the upper arms and thighs; in infants the cheeks may be involved (Figs 15-13 A & B). The papules are generally flesh-colored and asymptomatic, but may become inflamed and erythematous. Treatment in infants is aimed at skin hydration with thick emollients.

SCABIES

This common infectious dermatosis is produced by infestation with the mite *Sarcoptes scabiei*. The rash is polymorphous and may appear papular, nodular, eczematous, or urticarial (Fig. 15-14). Burrows, if present, are diagnostic of scabies. The rash is profoundly pruritic, and if widespread can be difficult to distinguish from AD. In infants with scabies, tiny papules are often seen on the lateral surfaces of the hands and feet, which can help to distinguish the rash from AD. Additionally, facial involvement is more typical of AD. If the diagnosis is unclear, a parasite slide preparation may be performed in attempt to visualize the mite, eggs, or fecal material. The treatment for scabies is 5% permethrin cream applied from the neck down; infants should have the head treated as well. All family members must be treated simultaneously. See Chapter 14 for further discussion.

OTHER ETIOLOGIES OF ECZEMATOUS ERUPTIONS (See Boxes 15-2 and 15-3)

Many nutritional deficiencies, metabolic disorders, and conditions causing erythrodermas may appear eczematous (see Chapter 17). Zinc deficiency can result from inadequate intake, malabsorption, excessive loss, or a combination of these caused by inherited and acquired conditions.[94] The skin may have widespread involvement. Zinc is an essential nutrient involved in numerous biologic functions necessary for growth and development.[95]

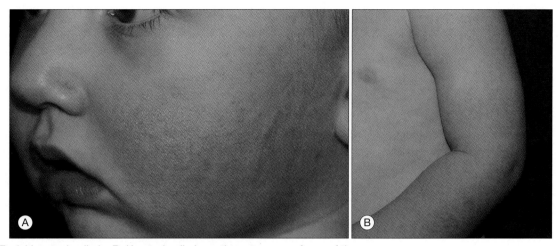

FIG. 15-13 A Facial keratosis pilaris. **B.** Keratosis pilaris on the extensor surfaces of the arms.

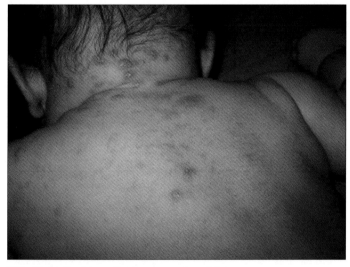

FIG. 15-14 Scabies with papules and nodules.

Acrodermatitis enteropathica is a rare, autosomal recessive disorder caused by an inborn error of metabolism that results in zinc malabsorption and deficiency. It typically presents when the child is weaned from breast to cow's milk or, in the case of formula-fed infants, after 4–10 weeks, when stores of zinc have been depleted. Both cow's and breast milk contain adequate amounts of zinc, but in acrodermatitis enteropathica the transport mechanism for absorbing zinc in the intestine is defective and the cow's milk lacks the ligand necessary for the transfer of zinc across the Paneth cells of the small intestine.[96]

Zinc deficiency can also result from inadequate intake of zinc. In the past, this condition was described in infants receiving parenteral alimentation without adequate zinc supplementation, but the routine addition of zinc to parenteral feeds has eliminated this problem. Zinc deficiency is still seen in premature infants who are exclusively breastfed. The most common cause is when the nutritional needs of premature infants increase in the first few months of life, at a time when the mother's breast milk zinc is decreasing. There is also increased secretion into the gut during the first few months, and poor zinc absorption.[95] It may also be rarely seen in term breastfed infants, resulting from low or completely absent zinc

in the mother's breast milk despite normal maternal plasma zinc levels. Thus the transfer of zinc from plasma to breast milk is defective.[95] The condition may be inherited, as there are reports of absence of breast milk zinc in numerous members of one family.[97]

The skin eruption is usually the first clinical sign of zinc deficiency. Lesions are present on the cheeks and chin in a horseshoe distribution with erythematous dermatitic erosions (Fig. 15-15A). Initially bullae may be present, but these rapidly erode. Over time, a more psoriasiform eruption develops. Periorbital involvement is common. The fingers and toes may have similar erosions and can be accompanied by nail dystrophy. They often become secondarily infected with *S. aureus* and *Candida*. A typical eruption occurs in the diaper area, consisting of a sharply demarcated area of erythema with accentuation of scale at the margin (Fig. 15-15B). Occasionally this may occur without facial involvement. Irritability, diarrhea, hair loss, and failure to thrive are additional features.

Low plasma zinc levels are the characteristic finding, and levels of zinc-dependent alkaline phosphatase may also be low. Care should be taken to use a plastic syringe when drawing zinc levels and to prevent zinc contamination from rubber stoppers on glass tubes. High levels of zinc are due to laboratory error, as the body excretes zinc and limits absorption when the levels get too high.[98]

Treatment with zinc sulfate 1–3 mg/kg/day (the latter being appropriate for acrodermatitis enteropathica) leads to rapid improvement, with irritability being the first symptom to respond.[99] The inherited condition (acrodermatitis enteropathica) may require long-term therapy. Occasionally zinc sulfate causes gastrointestinal symptoms and zinc gluconate may be substituted.[100]

Biotin deficiency (multiple carboxylase deficiency) is an autosomal recessive disorder that becomes apparent in the neonatal period or late infancy. Systemic signs and symptoms include vomiting, seizures, developmental delay, hypotonia, and later ataxia. Cutaneous lesions resemble those of zinc deficiency, affecting the area around the eyes, face, and perianal area. The lesions are eczematous or psoriasiform and are unresponsive to topical treatment with steroids. Secondary candidal infection is common and remains unresponsive to treatment until the biotin deficiency is corrected. The etiology of the condition in the neonate can be attributed to

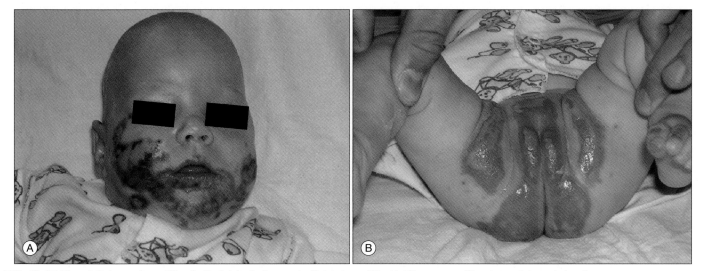

FIG. 15-15 Zinc deficiency dermatitis. **A.** Facial, including periorificial dermatitis. **B.** Diaper area (Courtesy of Joseph Lam).

the decreased activity of any or all of three carboxylases: 3-methylcrotonyl CoA carboxylase, propionyl CoA carboxylase, and pyruvate carboxylase. All are biotin-dependent enzymes in which biotin acts as a cofactor. The defect is in holocarboxylase synthetase. In the juvenile form of the disease biotinidase is absent.[101]

The absence of carboxylase enzymes leads to an accumulation of carboxyls in the urine, resulting in lactic acidosis or ketosis. Treatment consists of biotin 5–20 mg/day, leading to rapid improvement.[102] The biotin is well absorbed and does not accumulate in tissues. A dose of 10 mg is usually given empirically.[103]

Cystic fibrosis is an autosomal recessive disorder characterized by widespread dysfunction of the exocrine glands, resulting in chronic pulmonary disease, pancreatic insufficiency, and elevated sweat electrolytes. It can present in neonates or young infants with an erythematous, scaly rash with periorificial and/or perineal accentuation, closely resembling that of zinc deficiency.[104] Pedal edema is common. The usual presentation of failure to thrive, malabsorption, hepatosplenomegaly, and frequent pulmonary infections may be associated with the rash. The cause of the skin eruption is unknown, although essential fatty acid deficiency, low zinc levels, and protein deficiency may all be involved.[105]

Hartnup disease is an extremely rare heterogeneous autosomal recessive disorder characterized by a pellagra-like photosensitive eruption, cerebellar ataxia, emotional instability, encephalopathy, seizures, and aminoaciduria. The defect involves the disordered metabolism of tryptophan associated with the intestinal and renal transport of certain neutral α-amino acids. The disease is usually associated with consanguinity in the parents; it is extremely rare in the western hemisphere.[106]

Netherton syndrome is a rare disorder characterized by severe generalized erythroderma, scaling, and alopecia, caused by mutations in the *SPINK-5* gene (See Figure 17-4). Sparse eyebrows and hair are a hallmark of the disorder. Affected patients tend to have dramatic increases in metabolic demands due to their skin disease, often resulting in failure to thrive

and/or dehydration from increased insensible losses. Laboratory examination most often reveals elevated IgE levels. Definitive diagnosis may be made by genetic testing. Light microscopy of affected hair may reveal trichorrhexis invaginata or 'bamboo hair' (see Chapters 18 and 28).

Omenn syndrome is an autosomal recessive form of severe combined immunodeficiency (SCID) that presents in the neonatal period with an intensely pruritic generalized eczematous eruption that is difficult to distinguish from AD.[107] Failure to thrive, alopecia, eosinophilia, diarrhea, and repeated infections accompany the skin eruption. Hepatosplenomegaly and lymphadenopathy are common. Bone marrow transplantation is the first-line therapy for Omenn syndrome.[108]

Phenylketonuria[109] is a rare autosomal recessive disorder involving the metabolism of phenylalanine. Infants may appear normal at birth, although most have blond hair and blue eyes or, if African-American, are fairer than their parents. About 50% of patients develop dermatitis that is indistinguishable from AD. Neurological signs become evident later. At birth, all babies in the USA are screened for phenylketonuria, which is due to the absence of phenylalanine hydroxylase. This enzyme is required for the conversion of phenylalanine to tyrosine. To prevent the accumulation of phenylalanine in the blood, a low-phenylalanine diet is instituted as soon as possible after birth to prevent the resultant mental retardation.

Wiskott–Aldrich syndrome is an X-linked recessive disease affecting almost entirely males. It presents in the first few months of life with petechiae, ecchymoses, and an associated bloody diarrhea caused by both quantitative and qualitative abnormalities of platelets. The skin eruption, which usually develops after the bleeding diathesis, is characterized by an extremely pruritic, generalized eczematous eruption with bloody crusts. Apart from its hemorrhagic component, the eruption is indistinguishable from AD (Fig. 15-16). Skin abscesses from recurrent bacterial infections with pneumococci, meningococci, and *Haemophilus influenzae*, as well as molluscum contagiosum, verrucae, and herpes simplex, are common. There is a tendency to develop nephropathy and lymphoreticular malignancies later in life. The cell surface

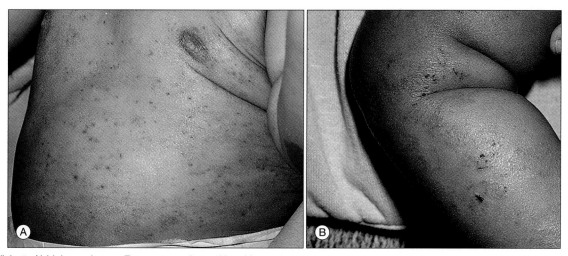

FIG. 15-16 Wiskott–Aldrich syndrome. Eczematous dermatitis with crusts.

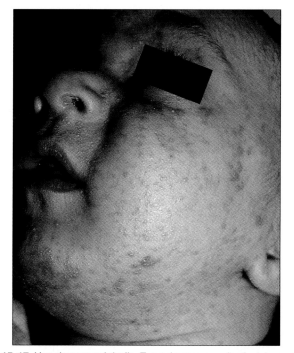

FIG. 15-17 Hypoimmunoglobulin-E syndrome: papular facial eruption.

Box 15-4 Characteristics distinguishing hyper-IgE syndrome from atopic dermatitis

Very high IgE levels, generally >2000 IU/mLl, or 10 times normal limit

Predominance of inflammatory facial papules in the context of an eczematous dermatitis

Recurrent infections in childhood (staphylococcal skin, pneumonias)

Skeletal abnormalities (repeated fractures, osteopenia)

Dental abnormalities (retained primary teeth)

Characteristic 'coarse' facial features (may not be distinctive until adolescence)

marker CD43 or sialophorin[110] is absent from most cells, but this does not account for the Wiskott–Aldrich phenotype. The Wiskott–Aldrich-associated gene and its gene product, the Wiskott–Aldrich-associated protein, have recently been identified.[111] This gene is present on Xp11.23. Bone marrow transplantation can be curative in patients with a histocompatible donor.

Hyper-IgE syndrome and Job syndrome are immunodeficiency diseases characterized by chronic dermatitis, skeletal and dental abnormalities. The rash has often been described as similar to AD, but inflammatory facial papules may predominate (Fig. 15-17), and the disease course usually allows differentiation (Box 15-4). The skeletal abnormalities consist of repeated fractures. The dental abnormalities include retained primary teeth. There are also recurrent infections with cold abscesses, eosinophilia, and extremely elevated levels of IgE. Coarse facies and cranial synostosis have been reported.[112] Job syndrome occurs mainly in females with red hair and fair skin and is a variant of the hyper-IgE syndrome. The inheritance pattern is not well established, with reports of both autosomal dominant and recessive forms. Mucocutaneous candidiasis has been reported in the hyper-IgE syndrome, although its significance remains unclear. Very high levels of IgE, associated with an IgA deficiency and cutaneous hypersensitivity reactions of *S. aureus* and *Candida albicans*, are noted. The cause may be related to a defect in granulocyte chemotaxis.[112]

OTHER PAPULOSQUAMOUS DISORDERS

Several papulosquamous disorders that are more common in later childhood may rarely present in infants. Pityriasis rosea has been reported in several infants 3 months of age and older.[113–115] Lichen planus has been recorded in an infant 3 weeks of age.[116] Keratosis lichenoides chronica, presenting with symmetric erythematous scaling, verrucous and lichenoid papules in a reticulate or linear pattern, usually presents in adults, and rarely is present in infancy.

REFERENCES

1. Besnier E. Premiere note et observations preliminaires pour servir d'introduction a l'étude diathesques. Ann Dermatol Syphiligr 1892; 4: 634.

2. Wise F, Sulzberger MB. Editorial remarks. In: Year book of dermatology and syphilology. Chicago: Year Book Medical Publishers, 1933; 59.

3. Hill LW, Sulzberger MR. Evolution of atopic dermatitis. Arch Derm Syphilol 1935; 32: 451–463.

4. Su JC, Kemp AS, Varigos GA, Nolan TM Atopic eczema: its impact on the family and financial cost. Arch Dis Child 1997; 76: 159–162.

5. Bickers DR, Lim HW, Margolis D, et al. The burden of skin diseases: 2004 a joint project of the American Academy of Dermatology Association and the Society for Investigative Dermatology. J Am Acad Dermatol 2006; 55: 490–500.

6. Walker RB, Warin RP. The incidence of eczema in early childhood. Br J Dermatol 1956; 68: 182.

7. Carroll CL, Balkrishnan R, Feldman SR, et al. The burden of atopic dermatitis: impact on the patient, family, and society. Pediatr Dermatol 2005; 22: 192–199.

8. Tay Y, Kong H, Koo L, et al. The prevalence and descriptive epidemiology of atopic dermatitis in Singapore school children. Br J Dermatol 2002; 146: 101–106.

9. Williams HC, Strachan DP, Hay RJ. Childhood eczema: disease of the advantaged? Br Med J 1994; 308: 1132–1135.

10. Schafer T, Dirschedl P, Kunz B, et al. Maternal smoking during pregnancy and lactation increases the risk for atopic eczema in the offspring. J Am Acad Dermatol 1997; 36: 550–556.

11. David TJ, Ewing CI. Atopic eczema and preterm birth. Arch Dis Child 1988; 63: 435–436.

12. Eichenfield LF, Hanifin JM, Beck LA, et al. Atopic dermatitis and asthma: parallels in the evolution of treatment. Pediatrics 2004: 111: 608–616.

13. Queille-Roussel C, Raynaud F, Saurat J-H. A prospective computerized study of 500 cases of atopic dermatitis in childhood. Acta Dermatol Venereol 1985; 114: 87–92.

14. Rajka G. Essential aspects of atopic dermatitis. Berlin: Springer-Verlag, 1989; 21.

15. Kuster W, Peterson M, Christophers E, et al. A family study of atopic dermatitis: Clinical and genetic characteristics of 188 patients and 2,151 family members. Arch Dermatol Res 1990; 282: 98–102.

16. Hanifin J, Rajka G. Diagnostic features of atopic dermatitis. Acta Dermatol Venereol 1980; 92: 44.

17. Williams HC, Burney PG, Hay RJ, et al. The UK Working Party's diagnostic criteria for atopic dermatitis. I. Derivation of a minimum set of discriminators for atopic dermatitis. Br J Dermatol 1994; 131: 383–396.

18. Eichenfield LF, Hanifin JM, Luger TA et al. Consensus conference on pediatric atopic dermatitis. J Am Acad Dermatol 2003; 49: 1088–1095.

19. Uno H, Hanifin JM. Ultrastructural and L-dopa histofluorescent observations of Langerhans' cells in atopic dermatitis. Clin Res 1979; 27: 538A.

20. Montgomery H. Dermatopathology. Vol. 1. New York: Harper & Row, 1967; 186–190.

21. Soter NA, Mihm MC Jr. Morphology of atopic eczema. Acta Dermatol Venereol 1980; 92: 11.

22. Tobin D, Nabarro G, Baart de la Faille H, et al. Increased number of immunoreactive nerve fibers in atopic dermatitis. J Allergy Clin Immunol 1992; 90: 613–622.

23. Mihm MC, Soter NA, Dvorak HF, Austen KF. The structure of normal skin and the morphology of atopic eczema. J Invest Dermatol 1976; 67: 305–312.

24. Leung D, Boguniewicz M, Howell M, et al. New insights into atopic dermatitis. J. Clin Invest 2004; 113: 651.

25. Schultz Larsen F. Atopic dermatitis: a genetic-epidemiologic study in a population-based twin sample. J Am Acad Dermatol 1993; 28: 719–723.

26. Bellou A, Kanny G, Fremont S, et al. Transfer of atopy following bone marrow transplantation. Ann Allergy Asthma Immunol 1997; 78: 513–516.

27. Cookson WOCM, Sharp PA, Faux JA, Hopkin JM. Linkage between immunoglobulin E responses underlying asthma and rhinitis and chromosome 11q. Lancet 1989; 10: 1292–1295.

28. Shirakawa T, Hashimoto T, Furuyama J, et al. Linkage between severe atopy and chromosome 11q13 in Japanese families. Clin Genet 1994; 46: 228–232.

29. Marsh DG, Meyers DA. A major gene for allergy – fact or fancy? Nature Genet 1992; 2: 252–254.

30. Coleman R, Trembath RC, Harper JI. Chromosome 11q13 and atopy underlying atopic eczema. Lancet 1993; 341: 1121–1122.

31. Blumenthal MN. The role of genetic factors in determining atopic conditions. Can J Allergy Clin Immunol 1997; 2: 69.

32. Juto P, Strannegard O. T lymphocytes and blood eosinophils in early infancy in relation to heredity for allergy and type of feeding. J Allergy Clin Immunol 1979; 64: 38–42.

33. Butler JM, Chan SC, Stevens S, Hanifin JM. Increased leukocyte histamine release with elevated cyclic AMP-phosphodiesterase activity in atopic dermatitis. J Allergy Clin Immunol 1983; 71: 490–497.

34. Cork MJ, Robinson DA, Vasilopoulos Y, et al. New perspectives on epidermal barrier dysfunction in atopic dermatitis: gene–environment interactions. J. Allergy Clin Immunol 2006; 118: 3–21.

35. Sugiura H, Ebise H, Tazawa T, et al. Large-scale DNA microarray analysis of atopic skin lesions shows overexpression of an epidermal differentiation gene cluster in the alternative pathway and lack of protective gene expression in the cornified envelope. Br J Dermatol 2005; 152: 146.

36. McGirt LY, Beck LA. Innate immune defects in atopic dermatitis. J Allergy Clin Immunol 2006; 118: 202–8. Epub 2006 Jun 6.

37. Hamid Q, Boguniewicz M, Leung D. Differential in in situ cytokine gene expression in acute vs chronic dermatitis. J Clin Invest 1994; 94: 870.

38. Homey B, Steinhoff M, Ruzicka T, Leung DY. Cytokines and chemokines orchestrate atopic skin inflammation. J Allergy Clin Immunol 2006; 118: 178–189.

39. Giannetti A, Fantini F, Cimitan A, Pincelli C. Vasoactive intestinal polypeptide and substance P in the pathogenesis of atopic dermatitis. Acta Dermatol Venereol 1992; 176: 90–92.

40. Cooper KD. Atopic dermatitis: Recent trends in pathogenesis and therapy. Prog Dermatol 1993; 27: 1–16.

41. Novak N, Bieber T. The role of dendritic cell subtypes in the pathophysiology of atopic dermatitis. J Am Acad Dermatol 2005; 53: S171–176.

42. Debra Rowlands D, Tofte SJ, Hanifin JM. Does food allergy cause atopic dermatitis? Food challenge testing to dissociate eczematous from immediate reactions. Dermatol Ther 2006; 19: 97–103.

43. Sigurs N, Hattevig G, Kjellman B. Maternal avoidance of eggs, cow's milk, and fish during lactation: effect on allergic manifestations, skin-prick tests, and specific IgE antibodies in children at age 4 years. Pediatrics 1992; 89: 735–739.

44. Sampson HA, Metcalfe DD. Food allergies. JAMA 1992; 268: 2840–2844.

45. Hanifin JM. Critical evaluation of food and mite allergy in the management of atopic dermatitis. J Dermatol 1997; 24: 495–503.

46. Leung DY, Harbeck R, Bina P, et al. Presence of IgE antibodies to staphylococcal exotoxins on the skin of patients with atopic dermatitis. J Clin Invest 1993; 92: 1374–1380.

47. Illi S, von Mutius E, Lau S et al. The natural course of atopic dermatitis from birth to age 7 years and the association with asthma. J Allergy Clin Immunol 2004; 113: 925–931.

48. Vickers CFH. The natural history of atopic eczema. Presented at International Symposium on Atopic Dermatitis 1979. Acta Dermatol Venereol 1980; 92: 113.

49. Barker JN, Palmer CN, Zhao Y, et al. Null mutations in the filaggrin gene (FLG) determine major susceptibility to early-onset atopic dermatitis that persists into adulthood. J Invest Dermatol 2006; [Epub ahead of print].

50. Lubs ML. Empiric risks for genetic counseling in families with allergy. J Pediatr 1972; 80: 26–31.

51. Palmer CN, Irvine AD, Terron-Kwiatkowski A, et al. Common loss-of-function variants of the epidermal barrier protein filaggrin are a major predisposing factor for atopic dermatitis. Nature Genet 2006; 38: 441–446.

52. Leung DYM, Boguniewicz M. Triggers of atopic dermatitis. In: Eichenfield LF, Leung DYM, eds. The eczemas. New York: Summit Communications, 2004; 55–63.

53. Hoare C, Li Wan Po A, Williams H. Systematic review of treatments for atopic eczema. Health Technol Assess 2000; 4: 1–191.

54. Berth-Jones J, Graham-Brown RA. Failure of terfenadine in relieving the pruritus of atopic dermatitis. Br J Dermatol 1989; 121: 635–637.

55. Lucky AW, Leach AD, Laskarzewski P, Wenck H. Use of an emollient as a steroid-sparing agent in the treatment of mild to moderate atopic dermatitis in children. Pediatr Dermatol 1997; 14: 321–324.

56. Chamlin SL, Kao J, Frieden IJ, et al. Ceramide-dominant barrier repair lipids alleviate childhood atopic dermatitis: changes in barrier function provide a sensitive indicator of disease activity. J Am Acad Dermatol 2002; 47: 198.

57. Abramovits, W, Boguniewicz, M: A multicenter, randomized, vehicle-controlled clinical study to examine the efficacy and safety of MAS063DP (Atopiclair) in the management of mild to moderate atopic dermatitis in adults. J Drugs Dermatol 2006; 5: 236.

58. Sulzberger MB, Witten VH. The effect of topically applied compound F in selected dermatoses. J Invest Dermatol 1952; 101–102.

59. Yamamoto K. How doctor's advice is followed by mothers of atopic children. Acta Dermatol Venereol 1989; 144: 31–34.

60. Charman CR, Morris AD, Williams HC. Topical corticosteroid phobia in patients with atopic eczema. Br J Dermatol 2000; 142: 931–936.

61. Callen J, Chamlin S, Eichenfield L, et al. A systematic review of the safety of topical therapies for atopic dermatitis. Br J Dermatol 2007; 156(2): 203–221.

62. Eichenfield LF. Consensus guidelines in diagnosis and treatment of atopic dermatitis. Allergy 2004; 59: 86–92.

63. Kapp A, Papp K, Bingham A, et al. Flare Reduction in Eczema with Elidel (infants) Multicentre Investigator Study Group: long-term management of atopic dermatitis in infants with topical pimecrolimus, a nonsteroid anti-inflammatory drug. J Allergy Clin Immunol 2002; 110: 277–284.

64. Whalley D, Huels J, McKenna SP, van Assche D. The benefit of pimecrolimus (Elidel, SDZ ASM 981) on parents' quality of life in the treatment of pediatric atopic dermatitis. Pediatrics 2002; 110: 1133–1136.

65. Ho VC, Gupta A, Kaufmann R, et al. Safety and efficacy of nonsteroid pimecrolimus cream 1% in the treatment of atopic dermatitis in infants. J Pediatr 2003; 142: 155–162.

66. Kaufmann R, Fölster-Holst R, Höger P, et al. Onset of action of pimecrolimus cream 1% in the treatment of atopic eczema in infants. J Allergy Clin Immunol 2004; 114: 1183–1188.

67. Papp KA, Werfel T, Fölster-Holst R, et al. Long-term control of atopic dermatitis with pimecrolimus cream 1% in infants and young children: a two-year study. J Am Acad Dermatol 2005; 52: 240–246.

68. Papp KA, Breuer K, Meurer M, et al. Long-term treatment of atopic dermatitis with pimecrolimus cream 1% in infants does not interfere with the development of protective antibodies after vaccination. J Am Acad Dermatol 2005; 52: 247–253.

69. Graham-Brown RAC, Grassberger M. Pimecrolimus: a review of pre-clinical and clinical data. Int J Clin Pract 2003; 57: 319–327.

70. Allen BR, Lakhanpaul M, Morris A, et al. Systemic exposure, tolerability, and efficacy of pimecrolimus cream 1% in atopic dermatitis patients. Arch Dis Child 2003; 88: 969–973.

71. Lakhanpaul M, Davies T, Allen B, et al. Pimecrolimus (SDZ ASM 981) cream 1%: minimal systemic absorption in infants with atopic dermatitis during long-term treatment [abstract]. Ann Dermatol Venereol 2002; 129: 415.

72. Berger TG, Duvic M, Van Voorhees AS, et al. The use of topical calcineurin inhibitors in dermatology: safety concerns. Report of the American Academy of Dermatology Association Task Force. J Am Acad Dermatol 2006; 54: 818.

73. Paul C, Cork M, Rossi AB, et al. Safety and tolerability of 1% pimecrolimus cream among infants: experience with 1133 patients treated for up to 2 years. Pediatrics 2006; 117: e118.

74. Nilsson EJ, Henning CG, Magnusson J. Topical corticosteroids and Staphylococcus aureus in atopic dermatitis. J Am Acad Dermatol 1992; 27: 29–34.

75. Lever R, Hadley K, Downey D, Mackie R. Staphylococcal colonization in atopic dermatitis and the effect of topical mupirocin therapy. Br J Dermatol 1988; 119: 189–198.

76. Dahl MV. Staphylococcus aureus and atopic dermatitis. Arch Dermatol 1983; 119: 840–846.

77. Kalliomaki M, Salminen S, Arvilommi H, et al. Probiotics in primary prevention of atopic disease: a randomised placebo-controlled trial. Lancet 2001; 357: 1076.

78. Kalliomaki M, Salminen S, Poussa T, et al. Probiotics and prevention of atopic disease: 4-year follow-up of a randomised placebo-controlled trial. Lancet 2003; 361: 1869.

79. Zhang W, Leonard T, Bath-Hextall F, et al. Chinese herbal medicine for atopic eczema. Cochrane Database System Review 2005; 2: CD002291.

80. Unna PG. Seborrhoeae eczema. J Cutan Dis 1887; 5: 499.

81. Krol A, Krafchik B. The differential diagnosis of atopic dermatitis in childhood. Dermatol Ther 2006; 19: 73–82.

82. Elish D, Silverberg NB. Infantile seborrheic dermatitis. Cutis 2006; 77: 297–300.

83. Ruiz-Maldonado R, Lopez-Matinez R, Perez Chavariea EL, et al. Pityrosporum ovale in infantile seborrheic dermatitis. Pediatr Dermatol 1989; 6: 16–20.

84. Broberg A, Faergemann J. Infantile seborrhoeic dermatitis and Pityrosporum ovale. Br J Dermatol 1989; 120: 359–362.

85. Zeharia A, Mimouni M, Fogel D. Treatment with bifonazole shampoo for scalp seborrhea in infants and young children. Pediatr Dermatol 1996; 13: 151–153.

86. Moises-Alfaro CB, Caceres-Rios HW, Rueda M et al. Are infantile seborrheic and atopic dermatitis clinical variants of the same disease? Int J Dermatol 2002; 41: 349–351.

87. Neville EA, Finn OA. Psoriasiform napkin dermatitis a follow-up study. Br J Dermatol 1975; 92: 279–285.

88. Nall L. Epidemiologic strategies in psoriasis research. Int J Dermatol 1994; 33: 313–319.

89. Elder JT, Nair RP, Guo SW, et al. The genetics of psoriasis. Arch Dermatol 1994; 130: 216–224.

90. Farber EM, Nall L. Epidemiology: Natural history and genetics. In: Roenigk HH Jr, Maibach HI, eds. Psoriasis, 3rd edn. New York: Marcel Dekker, 1998.

91. Menni S, Gualandri L, Boccardi D, et al. Association of psoriasis-like eruption and Kawasaki disease. J Dermatol 2006; 33: 571–573.

92. Farber EM, Mullen RH, Jacobs AH, Nall L. Infantile psoriasis: a follow-up study. Pediatr Dermatol 1986; 3: 237.

93. Mozzanica N. Pathogenetic aspects of allergic and irritant contact dermatitis. Clin Dermatol 1992; 10: 115–121.

94. Stevens J, Lubitz L. Symptomatic zinc deficiency in breast-fed term and premature infants. J Paediatr Child Health 1998; 34: 97–100.

95. Prasad AS. Zinc: an overview. Nutrition 1995; 11: 93–99.

96. Lonnerdal B, Stanislowski AG, Hurley LS. Isolation of a low molecular weight zinc binding ligand from human milk. J Inorg Biochem 1980; 12: 71–78.

97. Zimmerman AW, Hambidge KM, Lepow ML, et al. Acrodermatitis in breast-fed premature infants: Evidence for a defect of mammary zinc secretion. Pediatrics 1982; 69: 176–183.

98. Van Wouwe JP. Clinical and laboratory diagnosis of acrodermatitis enteropathica. Eur J Pediatr 1989; 149: 2–8.

99. Goskowicz M, Eichenfield LF. Cutaneous findings of nutritional deficiencies in children. Curr Opin Pediatr 1993; 5: 441–445.

100. Walsh CT, Sandstead HH, Prasad AS, et al. Zinc: health effects and research priorities for the 1990s. Environ Health Perspect 1994; 102: 5–46.

101. Wolf B, Heard GS. Screening for biotinidase deficiency in newborns: worldwide experience. Pediatrics 1990; 85: 512–517.

102. Nyhan WL. Inborn errors of biotin metabolism. Arch Dermatol 1987; 123: 1696–1698.

103. Zempleni J, Mock DM. Bioavailability of biotin given orally to humans in pharmacologic doses. Am J Clin Nutr 1999; 69: 504–508.

104. Darmstadt GL, Schmidt CP, Wechsler DS, et al. Dermatitis as a presenting sign of cystic fibrosis. Arch Dermatol 1992; 128: 1358–1364.

105. Schmidt CP, Tunnessen W. Cystic fibrosis presenting with periorificial dermatitis. J Am Acad Dermatol 1991; 25: 896–897.

106. Wilcken B, Yu JS, Brown DA. Natural history of Hartnup disease. Arch Dis Child 1977; 52: 38–40.

107. Omenn GS. Familial reticuloendotheliosis with eosinophilia. N Engl J Med 1965; 273: 427.

108. Gomez L, Le Deist F, Blanche S, et al. Treatment of Omenn syndrome by bone marrow transplantation. J Pediatr 1995; 127: 76–81.

109. Lee EB. Metabolic diseases and the skin. Pediatr Clin North Am 1983; 30: 597–608.

110. Remold-O'Donnell E, Kenney DM, Parkman R, et al. Characterization of a human lymphocyte surface sialoglycoprotein that is defective in Wiskott–Aldrich syndrome. J Exp Med 1984; 159: 1705–1723.

111. Ochs HD. The Wiskott–Aldrich syndrome. Semin Hematol 1998; 35: 332–345.

112. Grimbacher B, Holland SM, Gallin JI, et al. Hyper-IgE syndrome with recurrent infections – an autosomal dominant multisystem disorder. N Engl J Med 1999; 340: 692–702.

113. Rudunsky BM. PR in a 4 month old infant; an account of suggested contagiousness. J Pediatr 1963: 62; 159–160.

114. Hyatt HW. PR in a 3 month old infant. Arch Pediatr 1960: 77; 364–368.

115. Tay Y, Goh C. One year review of PR at the National Skin Centre, Singapore. Ann Acad Med Singapore 1999: 28; 829–831.

116. Paller AS, Mancini A. Hurwitz clinical pediatric dermatology, 3rd edn. Philadelphia: Elsevier Saunders, 2006; 101.

16

Diaper Area Eruptions

Alfons Krol, Bernice Krafchik

Eruptions in the diaper region have diverse origins. This chapter will review eruptions, both common and uncommon, that have major findings in the diaper area not only in neonates but also in young infants (Box 16-1). Many of the conditions listed in Chapter 10 (Vesicles, Pustules Bullae, Erosions, and Ulcerations) may be seen or arise in the diaper region. There are many diseases that may also involve other areas of the body and coincidentally affect the diaper area that are mentioned but not discussed in detail in this chapter. Table 16-1 describes the clinical setting, morphology, distribution, and best method for diagnosing the major conditions causing diaper area eruptions in neonates and infants.

The term 'diaper rash' refers to any eruption in the area covered by the diaper. There are eruptions that are directly related to the wearing of diapers; those aggravated by wearing diapers, and those that occur in the diaper region irrespective of whether diapers are worn or not. The majority of the severe eruptions, which have been a direct consequence of diapering itself, are more uncommon in countries where disposable diapers are used. Ethnic and cultural differences related to the practice of diapering newborn infants have evolved over hundreds of years, from swaddling in the middle ages and even later, to the high-technology, multilayered disposable diapers of the 21st century. These latter practices have lead to a marked reduction in the frequency of diaper eruptions, particularly irritant diaper dermatitis (IDD).

CARE OF THE DIAPER AREA IN THE NEWBORN

The diaper area in newborns is exposed to urine and feces and it is a combination of both that causes IDD. Normal care of the perineal area should be aimed at gentle removal of the excreta, frequent change of diapers, and use of a mild emollient (petrolatum) to prevent irritation. Normal infants should be bathed with a mild soap. In preterm infants or those with a tendency to develop irritant diaper dermatitis, a barrier product should be applied to the diaper area with each diaper change. A study integrating these practices into skin care routines for infants in a neonatal intensive care unit has led to significant improvements, with less dryness, redness, and skin surface damage.[1] Feces should be removed from the skin as soon as possible after soiling. Plain water alone or a very mild soap, with gentle use of a moist cotton washcloth, is sufficient to remove the feces and urine before the area is gently dried. Rubbing should be avoided. Fragrance- and alcohol-free baby

---

Box 16-1 Causes of diaper dermatitis

Inflammatory conditions
Irritant diaper dermatitis

Seborrheic dermatitis

Atopic dermatitis

Psoriasis

Psoriasiform diaper dermatitis with Id reaction

Erosive perianal eruption

Pseudoverrucous papules

Granuloma gluteale infantum

Allergic contact dermatitis due to diaper components

Diaper dye dermatitis and 'Lucky Luke' dermatitis

Infections
Candidiasis

Bullous impetigo/staphylococcal scalded skin syndrome

Perianal streptococcal dermatitis/streptococcal intertrigo

Pseudomonas/ecthyma gangrenosum

Diaper dermatophytosis

Herpes simplex

HPV infection (condylomata)

Molluscum contagiosum

Coxsackie viral infection (hand, foot, and butt exanthem)

Metabolic
Nutritional abnormalities

Zinc deficiency

Acrodermatitis enteropathica

Acrodermatitis enteropathica-like eruptions
  Methylmalonic acidemia
  Proprionic acidemia
  Glutaric aciduria (type1)
  Maple syrup urine disease
  Ornithine transcarbamylase deficiency
  Citrullinemia
  Biotin deficiency
  Holocarboxylase deficiency

Cystic fibrosis

Miscellaneous
Langerhans' cell histiocytosis

Kawasaki disease

Granular parakeratosis

Pyramidal perianal protrusion

Nascent hemangioma

Lichen sclerosis

Pyoderma gangrenosum

Chronic bullous disease of childhood

Bullous pemphigoid

245

wipes are another convenient option. Baby wipes are now universally alcohol free and contain 98% water.

The ideal or perfect barrier product has yet to be formulated. Traditionally both lipophilic and hydrophilic ointments and pastes have been used, often combined with zinc oxide. The more lipophilic products may be highly occlusive, whereas the hydrophilic products are more hydrating but function less effectively as a barrier. Pastes such as Zinc Oxide Paste USP (25% zinc oxide, 25% corn starch, 50% petrolatum) are a more effective barrier, but are more adherent and difficult to remove; parents may inadvertently irritate the infant's skin when trying to remove the residual feces and barrier cream. In general, water-in-oil formulations with a lipid content of 50% provide a better barrier than lighter oil-in-water products. Plain petrolatum is recommended for routine use. Soft zinc paste products such as Ihle's paste (Rougier Pharma Canada) or Triple Paste (Summers Labs, Collegeville, PA) contain a combination of ingredients such as zinc oxide, cornstarch, petrolatum and lanolin, and are excellent, affordable, nonsensitizing product for both prevention and treatment of IDD. Chapter 5 discusses many of the common ingredients in commercial diaper rash products. The use of talcum or baby powders and products containing boric acid is not recommended because of inherent or potential toxicities associated with their use.

Irritant Diaper Dermatitis

Jacquet[2] gave the first description of diaper dermatitis in 1905. Irritant diaper dermatitis (IDD) does not usually develop during the neonatal period, particularly in the first 3 weeks of life, and eruptions in the diaper area in this age group should be assumed to be due to causes other than irritation until proven otherwise. Onset of IDD is generally between 3 weeks and 2 years of age, with prevalence highest between 9 and 12 months.[3] The condition was previously common, affecting 25% of children seen in a clinic for dermatological diseases,[4] but the incidence has decreased remarkably in western cultures owing to the advent of disposable diapers. In certain societies, such as China, where diapering has not been a social convention, IDD has been distinctly uncommon until recently, with the adoption of western diapering practices.

Home laundering of diapers is now uncommon in western societies: most parents in developed countries diaper their infants with disposable or cloth diapers from a diaper service. Modern superabsorbable disposable diapers have been shown to be more effective than washable cloth diapers in reducing IDD,[3,5,6] yet it is estimated that 1–2% of the non-biodegradable waste in North American landfills is composed of disposable diapers.

The evolution of disposable diapers from paper to absorbable cellulose centers, to present-day disposable, which contain both an intricate wicking system that prevents backflow and an absorbable gel matrix that can hold 80 times its weight, has reduced the prevalence of IDD. The most recent advances include a slow-release petrolatum surface and a breathable outer sheet. The most important factor in preventing IDD is the frequency and number of diaper changes. Other factors causing IDD include episodes of diarrhea, antibiotic use, and anatomical problems such as short bowel syndrome. Whereas cloth diapers are less efficient at reducing skin wetness, friction and pH, there is a risk that the expense of superabsorbable

diapers may prevent parents from changing the diaper sufficiently often, thus contributing to the development of IDD.

Cutaneous Findings

IDD presents as erythema on the convex surfaces of the inner upper thigh, the lower abdomen, and buttock areas, the areas most in contact with the diaper. The creases and the suprapubic area in boys are spared (Fig. 16.1). The eruption may become more severe and inflammatory, with yeast colonization, and enlarging areas of involvement including the creases. In more severe cases the erythema may be accompanied by a glistening or glazed appearance and a wrinkled surface.

Jacquet's erosive dermatitis presents with well-demarcated punched-out ulcers and erosions (Fig. 16.2). It is seen less commonly with the use of disposable diapers, and has usually been associated with infrequent diaper changes and poor removal of chemicals used in home laundering. It may also be seen in infants who have short bowel syndrome or following surgery for Hirschsprung disease, which may result in chronic diarrhea.

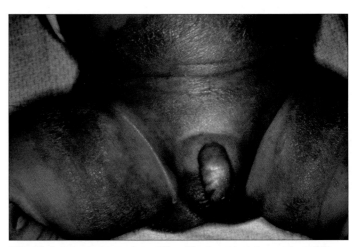

FIG. 16-1 Irritant diaper dermatitis with characteristic sparing of the folds.

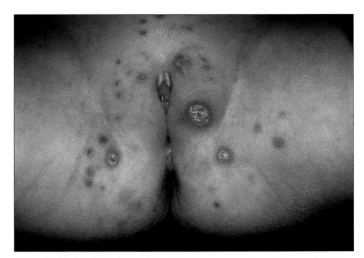

FIG. 16-2 Jacquet's dermatitis. Well-demarcated erosions, primarily on convex surfaces.

TABLE 16-1 The differential diagnosis of diaper area eruptions

Disease	Usual age	Skin: morphology	Skin: usual distribution	Clinical:other	Method of diagnosis/findings
Eruptions where the diaper/diaper environment is a central cause					
Irritant diaper dermatitis (IDD)	Between 3 weeks and 2 years. Peak ages 9–12 months	Erythema, with fine scaling and glazed skin surface. Erosions and ulcerations when severe	Convex surfaces of upper inner thigh, lower abdomen and buttock; spares intertriginous creases	Risk factors: cloth diapers, diarrhea	Clinical
Erosive perianal eruption	Usually infants 6 weeks to 3 months of age	Well demarcated erosions and superficial ulcerations 0.5–1.5 cm	Perianal skin, opposing areas of buttocks	Associated with frequent stooling of any etiology	Clinical
Pseudoverrucous papules	Usually infants rather than newborns	Well demarcated dome-shaped papules 2–10 mm, with shiny, smooth red or white surface	Perianal region, buttocks, vulvar, scrotal or around enterostomal openings	Severe, intractable diarrhea from any cause- short gut syndrome, following surgery for imperforate anus or pull through for Hirschsprung disease. May mimic condylomata clinically	Usually Clinical Biopsy shows reactive acanthosis or psoriasiform spongiotic dermatitis
Granuloma gluteale infantum	Usually infants rather than newborns	Oval red-brown to violaceous dermal papules or nodules 5 mm to 2–3 cm. Lesions run parallel to skin lines	Perianal, perivulvar or gluteal surfaces of the diaper region. Rarely inguinal folds, neck and axillae	Usually a history of chronic diaper eruption treated with multiple products, including fluorinated steroids	Clinical Biopsy shows dense superficial and deep inflammatory infiltrate composed of lymphocytes, histiocytes and plasma cells, proliferation of dermal blood vessels and extravasated red blood cells and hemosiderin
Granular parakeratosis	Usually 9–22 months of age	Asymptomatic, geometric, yellow brown, scaling plaques with underlying erythema	Areas of friction and pressure in diaper region. May involve axillae	None	Clinical Biopsy shows abnormal keratinization and retention hyperkeratosis
Infantile seborrheic dermatitis (ISD)	First 4–6 weeks of life, but any time in the first year	Erythematous, well demarcated patches involving the creases; may affect entire diaper region. Scale often minimal in diaper region	Multiple areas may be involved especially scalp, eyebrows, sides of nose, axillae, chest and diaper region	Generally happy babies, unlike infants with AD who have more pruritus	Clinical KOH to r/o associated Candidiasis
Psoriasis	Under 2 years	Brightly erythematous, well demarcated patches and plaques typically with absent or thin white scale	Often starts on convex surfaces, may affect entire diaper region including creases, gluteal cleft; may also involve face, scalp, trunk, and umbilicus	Eruption often asymptomatic and unresponsive to usual diaper dermatitis treatments	Clinical +/- Skin Biopsy Epidermal Acanthosis, parakeratosis dilated capillaries

TABLE 16-1 The differential diagnosis of diaper area eruptions—cont'd

Disease	Usual age	Skin: morphology	Skin: usual distribution	Clinical:other	Method of diagnosis/ findings
Candidal diaper dermatitis with psoriasiform Id	Usually infants 6–24 months but may occur earlier	Initial candidal diaper rash with erythematous patches and peripheral satellite papules or pustules with associated papules and scaly plaques elsewhere on body	Typical (usually severe) eruption diaper area followed by rapid onset of papules and plaques involving the torso, face, less prominent on extremities	Usually asymptomatic; occasionally pruritic	Clinical KOH + psuedohyphae and spores in diaper region early on
Allergic contact dermatitis	Usually after 6 months of age	Erythema and small vesicles leading to area of eczematous eruption of red papules and vesicles overlying areas of edema	Depends on contact allergen involved: diaper dye dermatitis at margins of diaper Entire diaper region if due to applied topical products	Associated pruritus	Clinical Biopsy shows spongiotic dermatitis with eosinophils
Infectious causes					
Candidiasis	Common after 2 months of age	Beefy-red eruption emanating from folds with satellite pustules or erythematous eruption extending over perineum with peripheral scale	Begins in inguinal folds, may involve entire perineum	Often history of preceding antibiotic use or diarrhea preceding eruption. May have associated oral thrush	Clinical KOH and Culture positive for Candida
Impetigo	Often in first few weeks of life in diaper region	Single or multiple flaccid bullae or moist superficial erosions	Often starts in umbilical stump; spreads to intertriginous areas of diaper region	Usually no other symptoms but neonates with hematogenous spread may develop septicemia, osteomyelitis or septic arthritis	Clinical Gram stain, Culture Biopsy rarely required but shows subcorneal pustule
Perianal/perineal streptococcal dermatitis	Usually after 6 months of age more common in toddlers	Moist, bright red erythema around perianal skin with yellowish sticky exudates at periphery. May have small pustules in surrounding skin	Perianal skin most common but can be in inguinal creases, other body folds	Local pain and tenderness common, fever rare. May have concomitant streptococcal pharyngitis. May be trigger for guttate psoriasis	Clinical Culture positive for B-Hemolytic Streptococci
Ecthyma gangrenosum	Usually seen in very premature or immunocompromised infants	Erythematous macule that rapidly evolves into grey nodule, necrotic bulla or ulceration with surrounding bright red areola	May occur anywhere but 50% occur in perineal/gluteal area	Associated neutropenia common. May rarely occur in diaper region in normal infants	Clinical gram stain and culture of lesions or + blood culture
Diaper dermatophytosis	Usually seen in toddlers	Erythematous scaling papules and plaques with border in diaper region. Deeper follicular papules and pustules in chronic cases	Buttocks, thighs and lower abdomen but may involve entire diaper area	Often family history of tinea pedis or other tinea infection	Clinical KOH and culture + For dermatophyte usually T. rubrum or T. Mentagrophytes
Herpes simplex	Presents 2–8 days after contact with infected individual	Grouped 2–3 mm umbilicated vesicles and erosions on erythematous base	Neonatal HSV may present on buttocks after breech delivery	Fever and regional adenopathy	Clinical + HSV culture or DFA or PCR. + tzanck smear of base of vesicle

TABLE 16-1 The differential diagnosis of diaper area eruptions—cont'd

Disease	Usual age	Skin: morphology	Skin: usual distribution	Clinical:other	Method of diagnosis/findings
Condylomata acuminata	Usually seen through vertical transmission from an infected mother; incidence in young infants from child abuse unknown but low	1–3 mm flesh-colored papules that may coalesce to form plaques. Verrucous to velvety surface	May occur on any part of the perineum	Usually asymptomatic	Clinical HPV serotyping available
Molluscum Contagiosum	Rare in neonates, increasingly common in toddlers and early childhood	Umbilicated flesh colored or pink papules, usually several, occasionally large numbers	Often in folds or areas of friction	May have associated molluscum dermatitis	Clinical or biopsy if diagnostic uncertainty
Coxsackie Viral Infection	1–4 yrs of age	Small red macules that rapidly evolve into superficial ovoid vesicles on hands and feet. Small papules and superficial erosions seen over buttocks and thighs	Hand, foot and 'butt' (diaper area) exanthem with erosions and vesicles of buccal area, tongue, gingiva and anterior tonsillar pillars	Fever and malaise Rarely, encephalitis, aseptic meningitis, myocarditis Enterovirus 71 cases pulmonary hemorrhage	Clinical Viral culture
Eruptions with accentuation in diaper area irrespective of presence of diapers/diaper environment					
Zinc deficiency/acrodermatitis enteropathica	True genetic AE occurs within 3 months after weaning; Zn deficiency common in breastfed premature infants within 1–2 months of age	Crusted, scaling, eczematous to psoriasiform dermatitis Face and diaper area	Periorificial, perineum, acral and periungual areas	Irritability, diarrhea, sparse hair, recurrent candidal infections especially paronychia, failure to thrive	Clinical Low serum Zinc Low Alkaline Phosphatase
Cystic fibrosis	Infancy	Periorificial and truncal dermatitis	Similar to AE	Significant edema, diarrhea, irritability, alopecia, failure to thrive	Clinical Sweat chloride test CFTR mutational analysis
Langerhans' cell histiocytosis	Birth to 4 years	Single, few or multiple lesions; Morphology may vary: yellow-brown papules, nodules, vesicles, erosions, ulcerations, atrophy, palpable petechial lesions, purpura, scale or crusting either alone or in combination	Folds of diaper region characteristic, also trunk scalp and retrauricular regions	Gums teeth and nails may be involved. Bony involvement in 50%; lymphadenopathy 14%; Liver or CNS in 10% (diabetes insipidus)	Clincal confirm with Skin biopsy showing infiltrate of CD1A + cells in epidermis and dermis
Pyramidal perianal protrusion	Usually 1–30 months of age	Pyramidal shaped soft tissue 'tag-like' protrusion – occasionally has a tongue-like lip	Seen in midline of perineum typically anterior to the anus but can be at other locations.	Often a history of constipation or diarrhea. May be associated with lichen sclerosus	Clinical Biopsy shows normal skin unless LS changes present (rarely required)
Nascent ulcerated infantile hemangioma	Birth to a few days of life	Oval to annular area of superficial to full thickness skin ulceration. Often surrounding telangiectasia or tiny vascular papules	Perianal, perivulvar and buttocks, may occur on lip or perioral region	Associated pain, occasionally secondary infection. Concern for spinal dysraphism/urogenital anomalies with very large lumbosacral lesions	Clinical- hemangioma becomes evident over next few days to weeks. Biopsy: Glut-1 + vessels

TABLE 16-1 The differential diagnosis of diaper area eruptions—cont'd

Disease	Usual age	Skin: morphology	Skin: usual distribution	Clinical:other	Method of diagnosis/findings
Lichen sclerosus	Usually in childhood 5–7 yrs, but may be seen in infancy	White, glistening, atrophic changes in the vulvar area and perianal skin. Associated purpura, and small hemorrhagic vesicles may be seen	Figure-of-eight distribution in perineum. Phimosis in boys; rarely extragenital lesions	Associated pain, itching, dysuria constipation and encopresis may be present	Clinical Biopsy confirms (rarely necessary)
Pyoderma gangrenosum	Uncommon in infancy but reported as young as 3 months	Tender papulopustule rapidly evolves into undermined ulcer with violaceous border. Rarely bullous and hemorrhagic	Head and anogenital sites most common in infants and children. Lower extremities in older children	Painful, usually associated with IBD, also seen in immunodeficiency, Leukocyte adhesion defect, leukemia, rheumatic disorders	Clinical Biopsy not specific but helpful to exclude other disorders ie infectious ulcers and vasculitis
Chronic bullous disease of childhood	Usually in early childhood Rare in infancy	Annular to polycyclic vesicles and bullae forming rosettes or 'string of pearls'	Diaper area, buttocks and inner thighs characteristic with spread to the trunk and scalp and face	May present initially with fever or other constitutional symptoms	Clinical Confirm with biopsy-subepidermal blister with polys and eosinophils Immunoflourescence + Linear IgA deposits
Bullous pemphigoid	Rare in infants and children but earliest reported case 2 months of age	Urticarial papules and plaques evolve into tense, often hemorrhagic bullae 0.25–2 cm in size. Blisters on normal or inflamed skin	Widespread distribution, often involves perineum, flexures of limbs and face mucosal involvement may occur in older children	Associated itching and pain	Clinical Confirm with biopsy-subepidermal Blister with eosinophils Immunoflourescence-deposits of C_3, And IgG at BMZ
Kawaski disease	Infancy to 5 yrs	Eruption may be polymorphous; often involves diaper region in young infants, with perineal erythema, small sterile pustules, urticarial lesions, early evidence of desquamation in perineal area	Accentuation perineal area but can be widespread macular erythema, urticarial, scarlatiniform, or maculopapular lesions	Persistent fever, irritability conjunctivitis, strawberry tongue, fissured lips, cervical adenopathy, peripheral edema, leukoocytosis, thrombocytosis, increased ESR, sterile pyuria, pericardial effusions and myocarditis	Diagnostic Clinical Criteria Echocardiogram

Extracutaneous Findings
None.

Etiology/Pathogenesis
At birth a newborn's skin undergoes a sudden transition accompanied by drying and cooling of the skin surface as it adapts to its new environment.[7] Visscher[8] has measured the changes in the newborn's epidermal barrier properties over the first 4 weeks of life, showing increased surface hydration, less transepidermal water movement under occlusion, and a decrease in surface pH. Diapered and nondiapered sites are indistinguishable at birth, but over the first 2 weeks of life diapered areas show consistently increased pH and hydration, thus setting the stage for IDD.

IDD results from the interaction of several factors associated with prolonged contact of the skin with a combination of both urine and feces (Table 16.1). The wearing of diapers causes a significant increase in skin wetness and pH.[9] Prolonged wetness leads to maceration of the stratum corneum due to disruption of the intercellular lipid lamellae.[10]

Weakening of the stratum corneum from excess hydration makes the skin more susceptible to damage by friction from the diaper. Fecal lipases and proteases are activated by the increased pH in the urine.[11] In addition, the acidic pH of the skin surface is essential for maintaining a normal cutaneous microflora, which protects against invasion by pathogenic bacteria and yeasts.[12] When diarrhea occurs, the fecal lipases and proteases increase in the diaper, leading to further damage to the stratum corneum. In the etiology of primary IDD, ammonia and *Candida* play less of a role than previously thought.

Differential Diagnosis

Ordinarily the diagnosis is straightforward and uncomplicated. Many of the disorders listed in Box 16.1 present with subtle differences from IDD, particularly psoriasis and allergic contact dermatitis. Atopic dermatitis (AD) classically spares the diaper region, but infants with widespread AD may have involvement of the skin just above the margin of the diaper. Strict attention to the morphology and location of lesions, the absence of pustules or vesicles, and the absence of lesions in the creases should lead the physician to the correct diagnosis.

Treatment and Care

Mild topical steroid therapy (1% hydrocortisone ointment) covered by a barrier product three times daily, will clear the majority of IDD that does not respond to barrier products alone. The use of potent fluorinated topical steroids in the diaper region is not recommended as the natural occlusion of this area will promote increased absorption and may cause atrophy, striae, and adrenal suppression. When the practitioner is faced with a severely inflamed recalcitrant dermatitis in the diaper area, it is safe to use a week-long course of a medium-potency topical steroid to bring the eruption under control. The role of topical immunomodulators in the management of diaper dermatitis is unclear and cannot be recommended until further data are available on their safety and use in infants under 2 years of age.

Erosive Perianal Eruption

This entity presents with erosions and ulcers in the perianal skin and occurs most commonly between 6 weeks and 3 months of age, but can be seen at other ages. The etiology is almost universally associated with frequent stooling, either in breastfed babies, children with diarrhea due to malabsorption, or infection in infants with short gut syndrome (Fig. 16-3). This condition may eventuate into pseudoverrucous perianal papules in infants who undergo enterostomal closure, or following pullthrough surgery for Hirschsprung disease.[13] In mild cases, frequent diaper changes and use of a barrier product such as zinc oxide or triple paste with a low- to medium-strength topical steroid ointment applied two to three times daily is helpful. In patients with short gut or other malabsorption syndromes the condition may be chronic, unremitting, and very difficult to treat.

Pseudoverrucous Papules

Pseudoverrucous papules (PVP; sometimes referred to as 'pseudoverrucous papules and nodules'), the more severe forms of Jacquet erosive diaper dermatitis, and granuloma gluteale infantum are probably best viewed as a reaction patterns fol-

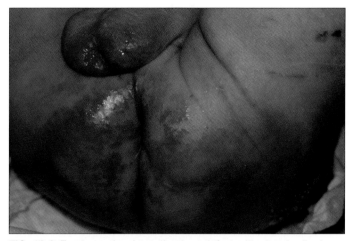

FIG. 16-3 Erosive perianal eruption in an infant with chronic diarrhea.

lowing chronic, unremitting irritation due to feces, urine, or a combination thereof. Pseudoverrucous papules were first described by Goldberg et al.[14,15] in the setting of chronic diaper dermatitis, encopresis or peristomal skin irritation.

Well documented precipitating factors leading to this condition include chronic diarrhea due to malabsorption or short-gut syndrome, postoperatively following repair of Hirschsprung disease or imperforate anus, around stomas (either urinary or fecal), and following chronic incontinence. Clinical features include dome-shaped papules, typically varying in size from 2 to 10 mm, often with a shiny, smooth, white or red surface (Fig. 16-4A, B). Biopsy specimens reveal reactive acanthosis or psoriasiform spongiotic dermatitis. The lesions regress when the irritating factor is removed. Recognition of this entity is important because pseudoverrucous papules and nodules may mimic other dermatoses, especially condyloma acuminatum, and unnecessary work-up for sexual abuse may be initiated.

Granuloma Gluteale Infantum

Granuloma gluteale infantum (GGI) was originally described by Tappeiner and Pfleger.[16] It is rarely seen today and there are only 30 cases reported in the literature. Infants present with oval red-brown to purple dermal nodules on the gluteal surface and diaper area[17,18] (Fig. 16-5). Rarely lesions may be present in the intertriginous areas, including the neck and axilla. The long axis of the lesions runs parallel to skin lines. In the majority of affected infants there is a history of a preceding eruption in the diaper region treated with fluorinated topical steroids. Similar granulomas in the diaper region have been noted in adults who are incontinent and confined to bed.[19] The etiology of GGI is unclear, but some have hypothesized that it is a skin response to the combined effects of inflammation, maceration, local infection with *Candida*, and use of fluorinated steroids. The sparing of deep folds suggests that occlusion by the diaper is necessary for its formation.

Treatment for these conditions should be directed at correcting the underlying cause of the chronic urine or fecal leakage whenever possible, as well as frequent use of a barrier product. Lesions generally resolve completely and spontaneously after a period of several months if the source of chronic irritation can be removed.

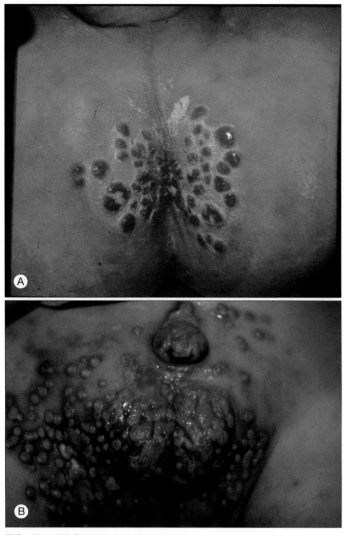

FIG. 16-4 (A) Extensive perianal pseudoverrucous papules. (B) Extensive pseudoverrucous papules in an infant with congenital genitourinary anomalies and chronic urinary leakage.

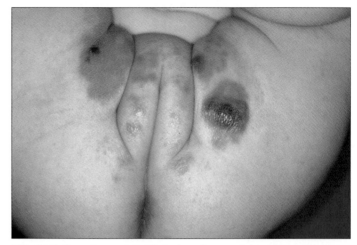

FIG. 16-5 Granuloma gluteal infantum. Larger violaceous nodules are evident.

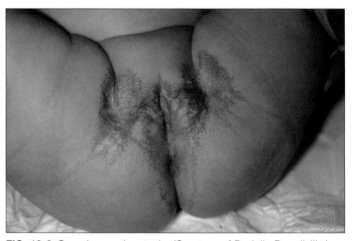

FIG. 16-6 Granular parakeratosis. (Courtesy of Dr Julie Prendiville.)

Granular Parakeratosis

Granular parakeratosis is a rare disorder of keratinization characterized by retention hyperkeratosis. Its precise etiology is unknown, but it is generally viewed as a reaction to chronic irritation or possibly as a reaction to certain topical products such as zinc oxide, which are commonly used in the diaper area. It was originally described in the axillary region of adults, but there have recently been several reports in infants from 9 to 22 months of age.

Infants usually present with asymptomatic, geometric yellow-brown, superficial scaling plaques with pronounced underlying erythema[20] in areas of friction and pressure in the diaper region. A second pattern of linear warty papules in the inguinal area has also been described[21] (Fig. 16-6).

The cause of this peculiar entity is obscure, but immuno-histochemical and electron microscopic studies suggest that there is a defect in processing of profillagrin to filaggrin which

results in failure of the normal degradation of keratohyalin and clumping of keratohyalin filaments during cornification.[22] These abnormal components result in the retention hyper-keratosis seen. Friction, moisture, and occlusion from diapers may trigger defective maturation of the stratum corneum at local sites in susceptible infants.

Treatment is empiric, with variable response to topical steroid, calcineurin inhibitors, keratolytics and emollients.[20] The majority of cases clear spontaneously after months, but occasional patients may have lesions for several years.

Infantile Seborrheic Dermatitis (ISD)
(See also Chapter 15)

First described by Unna in 1887,[23] ISD is a disease that affects infants usually in the first 2 years, with a distinct inflamma-tory eruption that primarily involves the scalp, retroauricular area, face, chest, diaper and intertriginous areas. A precise definition is lacking; some physicians confine the entity to the presence of scalp scaling called cradle cap, whereas others only use the term if there is inflammation of the scalp and in other seborrheic sites.

Cutaneous Features

The eruption usually begins under 6 weeks of age, but may occur up to a year or even later.[24] Both sexes are equally affected. The vast majority of infants develop cradle cap alone; this is a collection of asymptomatic, greasy keratin on the vertex of the scalp, without inflammation or involvement of other areas. A few patients develop multiple areas of involvement, including erythematous well-demarcated patches in the retroauricular area, eyebrows, along the sides of the nose, and involving the axillae, chest, and diaper area. The most commonly involved are the scalp and diaper area (Fig. 16-7A, B). Although there is often a yellow, greasy scale on the erythema, this is not invariably present and is usually absent in the diaper area, where lesions consist of erythematous, well-demarcated patches involving the creases, but sometimes affecting the whole region. Scale is unusual or minimal in the diaper area, unless there is invasion by *Candida albicans*, when crusting and scaling occur.[25]

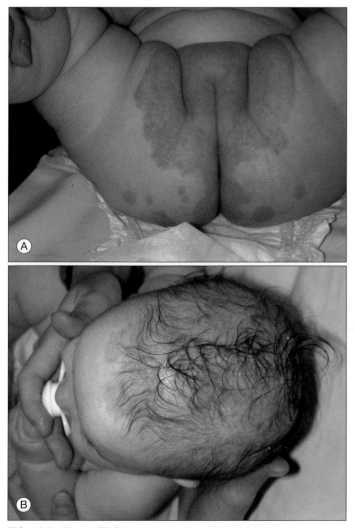

FIG. 16-7 (**A**) and (**B**) Seborrheic dermatitis involving the diaper area and scalp.

Extracutaneous Findings
None.

Differential Diagnosis

It is often difficult to differentiate ISD from atopic dermatitis (AD). The scalp is often involved in both conditions; the pruritus with AD may not be evident early in infancy, and occasionally ISD may be pruritic. The flexures are frequently involved in both conditions. Distinguishing features include xerosis of the skin and sparing of the diaper area in AD. Psoriasis in the diaper area is now more frequently recognized in infants, and is at times impossible to distinguish from ISD. The lesions are often confined to the diaper area as well-demarcated, erythematous and glistening plaques, with a thin, white scale. Infants seldom have the thick silvery scale that is normally seen with psoriasis in other areas.

Langerhans' cell histiocytosis (LCH) is a potentially lethal disease that can mimic ISD in the diaper area and scalp. Unlike ISD, LCH lesions are crusted, ulcerative, petechial and purpuric.

IDD usually spares the creases, and other eruptions in the diaper area have specific presentations that allow distinction from ISD.

Etiology/Pathogenesis

The etiology of ISD in infants is probably the result of colonization and proliferation of the yeast *Malassezia furfur (Pityrosporum ovale)*.[26] *Malassezia* organisms thrive in an oily environment and may proliferate more in those infants whose hair is only shampooed once or twice a week or who have emollients applied to the scalp. There is a marked decrease in the incidence of IDD in those infants whose hair is shampooed on a daily basis. A familial tendency may be relevant.[27] Other theories of causation, including biotin and essential fatty acid deficiency, have not been proved.[28]

Prognosis/Treatment

The majority of infants are cured within 2–4 weeks of treatment without recurrence;[29] the relationship to adult disease is not known.[27] Cradle cap can be treated with simple measures, including washing the scalp daily with a mild shampoo (Johnson's Baby Shampoo) following the application of oil (mineral oil, Aveeno oil) to loosen the scale. A topical steroid cream (either hydrocortisone or triamcinolone) three times a day may be necessary if there are any inflammatory lesions. In the intertriginous areas, hydrocortisone 1% cream can be applied three times a day. As the etiology of ISD is now thought to be an infection with a yeast organism, antifungal measures have proved to be as effective as topical steroids.[30] An antifungal shampoo (ketoconazole) daily, followed by the use of ketoconazole cream three times a day, is effective in treating the condition.

Psoriasis

Psoriasis is a common chronic inflammatory skin disease that affects both adults and children. It is characterized clinically by a typical scaly eruption, and pathogenetically by an accelerated epidermal cell turnover. The condition is being increasingly recognized in early infancy, and often affects the diaper area, particularly in those under 1 year.[31] Of the one-third of cases of psoriasis that occur before age 20, 2% occur before the age of 2.[32] There is often a family history of psoriasis in infants and children who develop the disease.[32]

Cutaneous Findings

Parents complain of an eruption in the diaper area that is asymptomatic and unresponsive to standard treatment. Lesions appear as erythematous, glistening, well-demarcated patches with a thin white scale, or they affect the whole diaper area including the creases[33] (Fig. 16-8A, B). Other areas are less frequently involved and include the face, scalp, trunk, and umbilical areas, with erythematous papules and plaques. The scale is often thin and lacks the characteristic silvery scale seen in older children and adults. Guttate lesions and nail changes are rare in infants.

Although pustular psoriasis does occur in infancy, it does not affect the diaper area specifically. Patients present with fever and malaise, associated with either small pustules on an erythematous base or annular erythema with peripheral pustules. Occasionally coalescence may lead to the formation of lakes of pus on the skin surface.

Extracutaneous Findings

It is increasingly recognized that psoriasis may be associated with internal organ involvement. Joints are affected in 10% of patients, although this is uncommon in infancy. Geographic tongue may be seen, particularly in pustular variants. There is a small but well recognized increase of psoriasis in patients with Crohn's disease. Patients with acute pustular psoriasis may develop a sterile osteomyelitis, and there have been a few reports of lung involvement in acute-onset psoriasis.

Differential Diagnosis

At times it may be impossible to distinguish between ISD and psoriasis. Many of the cases diagnosed as ISD who develop psoriasis later in life probably had psoriasis at the outset. Psoriasis is more chronic and more resistant to treatment, and usually spares the flexural areas, including the inguinal creases, which are commonly involved in ISD. The umbilical area is commonly involved in both conditions, but particularly in psoriasis. Resolution of psoriasis in infancy is often very rapid, unlike in older children, adding to the difficulty of distinction

from ISD. The lesions of atopic dermatitis are pruritic, poorly demarcated, and usually spare the diaper area.

IDD lesions have a typical pattern, spare the creases, and are not as well demarcated as those in psoriasis.

Etiology/Pathogenesis

There is a strong genetic component in patients with psoriasis, particularly in the younger age groups.[34] The pathogenesis is thought to involve an imbalance of T-helper cells resulting in a Th1-type cytokine reaction pattern. There is an increased cell turnover period of 4 days that is characteristic of psoriasis; in normal cells the turnover period is 28 days.

Prognosis/Treatment

The outcome of psoriasis in the younger age group is unknown. Many cases only have a single outbreak, others become chronic with frequent flares, and there are some patients who have a diagnosis of ISD or psoriasis in infancy who develop psoriasis many years later.

Daily bathing followed by the application of a mild topical steroid cream or ointment (hydrocortisone 1%) to the affected areas of the face and diaper area, and a moderate steroid ointment (triamcinolone) to the affected body areas three times a day, usually produces a rapid resolution of the lesions. If a mild steroid ointment is not sufficient to cause regression, a short trial of a medium-strength topical steroid in the diaper area may be given for a few weeks. It is important not to use anything stronger than this, as striae and atrophy and iatrogenic Cushing syndrome have resulted from the use of potent topical steroids under the occlusive environment of the diaper. If complete regression is not seen within 3–4 weeks, a refined tar product, liquor carbonis detergens (LCD), can be compounded with the steroid in a 5–10% concentration. Salicylic acid is not recommended in neonates and infants, as systemic absorption can lead to salicylism.

Candidal Diaper Dermatitis with Psoriasiform Id

This condition was first described in the 1960s as 'diaper dermatitis with psoriasiform ID.'[35] It consists of a candidal eruption in the diaper area, followed a few days to weeks later by

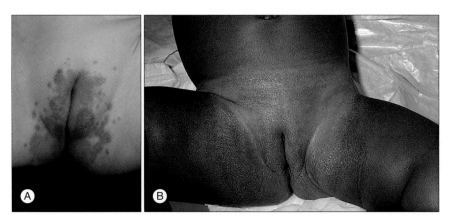

FIG. 16-8 (**A**) and (**B**) Psoriasis. Typical diaper involvement.

an explosive psoriasiform eruption on other areas of the body. It has been seen much less frequently in recent years.

Cutaneous Findings

The condition usually affects infants between 6 and 24 months, but may occur earlier. The sexes are equally affected. There is an initial infection with *Candida albicans* in the diaper area[36] that is severe, prolonged, or inadequately treated. The diaper lesions are erythematous patches with a peripheral scale, typical of *Candida albicans* infection. Days to weeks later, often soon after the initiation of effective therapy of the diaper rash, there is an acute explosion of lesions anywhere on the body and face that consist of well-demarcated psoriasiform plaques[37] (Fig. 16-9).

Extracutaneous Findings

None.

Etiology/Pathogenesis

The exact etiology of the psoriasiform Id reaction is unknown. Id (also known as auto-eczematization) reactions occur in conjunction with several other infectious and inflammatory diseases, including tinea capitis and pedis, but their pathogenesis remains obscure. Some infants may have a genetic predisposition to developing psoriasis, but this is not true in all cases.

Prognosis/Treatment

Lesions on the face are treated with a low-potency topical steroid cream 2–3 times a day, those on the body with a mid-potency topical corticosteroid cream 2–3 times a day, and those in the diaper area with an antifungal agent, usually a topical imidazole, 3–4 times a day. Cure occurs within 4–6 weeks and there is no recurrence, although there have been some reports of psoriasis developing some years later.[35]

Allergic Contact Dermatitis

Allergic contact dermatitis (ACD) may occur in the diaper region after exposure to fragrances, dyes, other components of the diaper itself, or to products applied by the parents to diapered skin.[38] Weston[39] has shown that ACD may account for up to 20% of all cases of childhood dermatitis, refuting the notion that ACD is rare in children. Sensitization may begin as early as 6 months of age.[40] Allergens that infants and children have become sensitized to include urushiol (poison ivy), nickel (in metal snaps on clothing), thimerosol, neomycin, chromates, Balsam of Peru, and formaldehyde and related preservatives.[41]

A specific form of ACD on the outer buttocks and hips was determined by patch testing to be due to rubber components in the elastic bands of the diapers. The authors termed this entity 'Lucky Luke Dermatitis' after the cartoon character who carries his gun holster in the same area[42] (Fig. 16-10). Recently Alberta et al.[43] reported several infants with ACD

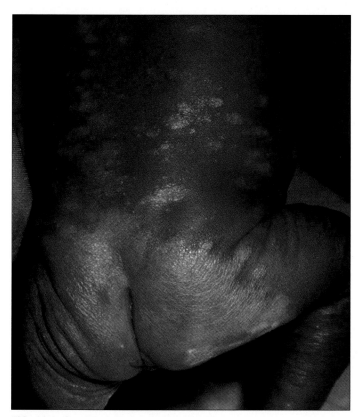

FIG. 16-9 *Candida* with psoriasiform Id. Note that lesions extend onto areas distant from the site of the diaper rash.

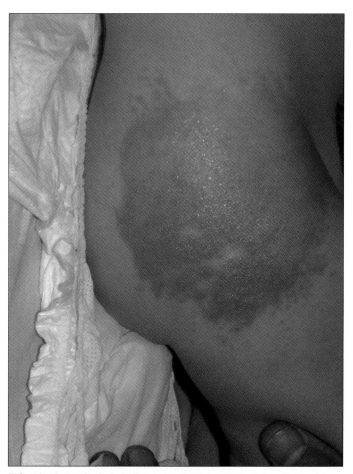

FIG. 16-10 'Lucky Luke' allergic contact dermatitis from disposable diaper components.

caused by the various blue, pink, and green dyes used in diapers. Changing to dye-free diapers quickly alleviated the rash.

ACD may be present in the same areas of the diaper as IDD, but the morphology of the lesions is different in ACD, beginning with erythema and small vesicles and leading to an eczematous eruption with red papules or vesicles overlying areas of edema.[38] Treatment with a medium-strength topical steroid provides rapid relief of symptoms, but removing the offending allergen is key to preventing recurrences.

INFECTIONS

Candidiasis (See Chapter 14)

Candidiasis, caused by the yeast *Candida albicans*, is the most common infection in newborns.[44] Three percent of infants are affected from the second to the fourth month of life.[45] Thrush (oral candidiasis) is common in early infancy, presumably owing to infection from the mother's vaginal canal. Candidiasis usually affects the skin and mucous membranes only, but in certain circumstances, such as low birthweight or with systemic infections around the birth period, invasive systemic disease may occur.

Clinical Picture

In congenital candidiasis lesions usually spare the diaper area but occur anywhere, including the hands and face. Candidal diaper dermatitis usually begins around 6 weeks of age and is seldom seen before this time. It is common to have a history of antibiotic use or diarrhea preceding the appearance of the eruption.

The entire perineal area, including the creases, may be affected. The morphology of the lesions takes two forms: a diffuse erythematous patch extending over the perineum with a peripheral scale, or small pink papules surmounted by a scale, and coalescence in some areas (Fig. 16-11A). The more classic picture of a beefy-red diaper area with satellite pustules (Fig. 16-11B) is less common, possibly because of earlier treatment with antifungal agents. Infants should be examined for evidence of oral candidiasis (thrush), which typically presents as small white patches on the buccal mucosa.

Differential Diagnosis

In IDD the creases are spared. Perianal streptococcus infection appears as painful, beefy-red lesions surrounding the anus. ISD presents with erythematous patches: it does not have the peripheral scale or the satellite papules or pustules seen in candidiasis.

Etiology/Pathogenesis

The lesions are formed when *Candida albicans* is excreted in excessive amounts in the feces. This is often preceded by the use of antibiotics and diarrhea of any cause. The significance of recovering *Candida albicans* from the diaper area is difficult to interpret, as the organism may be recovered in any irritant skin condition in the diaper area after 72 hours,[46] and may even be present in small amounts on normal skin. However, when candidal infection occurs, the organism is present in much larger numbers in the skin and feces.[47, 48] *Candida* has the ability to invade through the epidermal barrier by liberating keratinases.

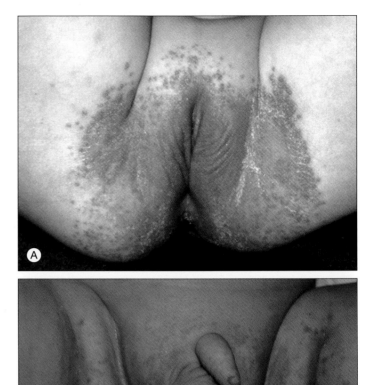

FIG. 16-11 (A) and **(B)** *Candida* diaper dermatitis. The skin folds are typically involved and satellite papules are a characteristic feature.

Prognosis/Treatment

Studies comparing the various treatment options for *Candida* diaper dermatitis are lacking.[49] Treatment with topical anticandidal therapy, either nystatin (cream or ointment) or one of the imidazoles (clotrimazole, miconazole, or ketoconazole), two or three times daily is generally effective in producing resolution in about 2 weeks. A formulation of miconazole 0.25% compounded in zinc oxide and petrolatum (Vusion, Barrier Therapeutics, Princeton, NJ) has recently been approved specifically for the treatment of documented *Candida* diaper dermatitis.[49a] The use of additional hydrocortisone 1% to one of the above agents provides an anti-inflammatory effect and may promote more rapid resolution of the rash, but this has not been studied in formal clinical trials. Potent topical corticosteroids should be avoided.

Burow's solution (5% aluminum subacetate) or normal saline compresses may be useful in inflammatory lesions. In a double-blind study, the oral use of nystatin (to eliminate *Candida* from the bowel), in conjunction with topical nystatin did not affect the outcome of the dermatitis more favorably than topical nystatin alone;[50] however, if oral candidiasis is present, oral nystatin suspension is required both to treat the thrush and to prevent recurrence of the diaper rash. Oral fluconazole (6 mg/kg as a loading dose and 3 mg/kg/day for 1–2 weeks is very effective in treating mucocutaneous *Candida* infection. However, if topical therapy is ineffective, an alternative diagnosis or the presence of a concomitant immunodeficiency should be considered.

Staphylococcal Infection: Impetigo/ Staphylococcus Scalded Skin Syndrome (SSSS) (See Chapter 12)

Impetigo is the most common bacterial skin infection seen in infants and children,[51] and the most common organism causing impetigo in infants is *Staphylococcus Aureus*, phage type 2. The diaper area is frequently affected with lesions, which appear as flaccid bullae. A generalized form of staphylococcal infection caused by a number of exotoxins of phage 2 is known as staphylococcal scalded skin syndrome (SSSS). Infants and young children are primarily affected, but the disease has been reported in adults, usually in immunocompromised patients, in whom there is a sizable mortality rate. The diaper area of the neonate is often affected by SSSS. Very occasionally a pseudomonas exotoxin may cause lesions that resemble SSSS. *Streptococcus pyogenes* is rarely the sole cause of impetigo in the neonate.

Cutaneous Findings

The infection can occur at any time and in any location, but often presents in the first 2 weeks of life in the diaper area. Constitutional signs are absent. The lesions may be single or multiple, and are either flaccid bullae or moist, superficial erythematous erosions (Fig. 16-12A) that have a thin peripheral collarette of scale after the bullae rupture. Initially pus is not present and one sees serous fluid in the bullae. After a few days the fluid becomes cloudy and pus is seen in the dependent area of the bulla. The lesions are superficial and there is no scarring once resolution occurs. A culture from the lesions or the umbilical stump usually yields a heavy growth of *S. aureus*.

SSSS presents with skin findings alone, but occasionally there may be a short prodrome of sore throat or conjunctivitis, followed by the release of toxin. The skin is sensitive to the touch and erythematous, with widespread exfoliation and fissuring around the mouth. Areas of involvement can be limited to the neck or diaper area (Fig. 16-12B). The mucous membranes are unaffected. The organisms are from the nose, pharynx and umbilicus, but not the skin. The Nikolsky sign is positive.

Extracutaneous Findings

None.

Etiology/Pathogenesis

The most common entry point in neonates is an infected umbilical stump. The eruption is caused by *S. aureus* phage type 2. Locally produced exfoliative or epidermolytic toxins A and B bind to desmoglein 1 in the desmosomes, with resultant proteolysis.[52,53] The toxins cleave the granular layer.[54] In bullous impetigo the exfoliating toxin is confined to the area of infection. In SSSS the exotoxin is spread hematogenously from a local source.

Differential Diagnosis

It is important to rule out other causes of blistering in the neonate. The most important are herpes simplex infection and

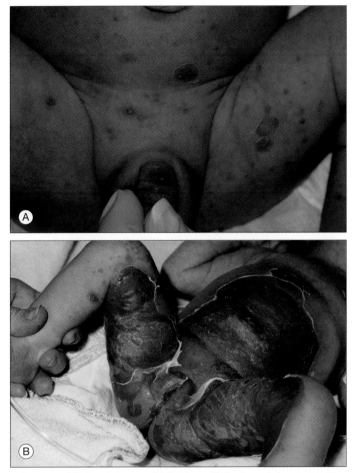

FIG. 16-12 **(A)** Staphylococcal infection with both pustules and bullae in an 11-day-old infant. **(B)** Staphylococcal scalded skin syndrome in a neonate involving the diaper region.

epidermolysis bullosa. In herpes simplex infection the vesicles are grouped and small, whereas in impetigo they tend to be larger bullae. Erythema toxicum presents with small pustules on an erythematous base, and small pustules are also seen with transient neonatal pustular melanosis, acropustulosis of infancy, and congenital candidiasis. Lesions are often smaller than those seen with impetigo and are pustular, whereas in impetigo the bullae are larger and flaccid or superficial erosions. Other rare causes of bullae in the neonate include pemphigus, pemphigoid, and incontinentia pigmenti, although these do not usually present with large flaccid bullae or erosions, and the diaper area is not specifically involved.

Prognosis/Treatment

Both bullous impetigo and SSSS have a good prognosis in infants and children. It is important to treat bullous impetigo immediately to prevent spread in the nursery. Oral antibiotics such as cloxacillin, cephalexin, and erythromycin are all effective as a 10-day course and lead to rapid cure in 5–7 days, with no scarring or recurrence. Some centers use IV antibiotics. In methicillin-resistant cases it may be feasible to use fucidic acid or mupirocin if the lesions are localized.[55]

Perianal and Perineal Streptococcal Dermatitis (See Chapter 12)

Infections with β-hemolytic streptococci may take several forms in this region, including perianal dermatitis, intertrigo, cellulitis, vulvovaginitis, and balanoposthitis.[56–60] Perianal streptococcal dermatitis[57] (PSD) is the most common presentation and is seen more frequently in males. Outbreaks have been recorded at daycare centers.[61] 'Streptococci love the folds,' and recently Honig et al.[60] published a cases series of infants less than 5 months of age with streptococcal intertrigo involving the inguinal, axillary, limb, and neck folds.

Cutaneous Findings

PSD presents as sharply circumscribed perianal erythema with occasional fissures, often with a sticky yellowish exudate that accumulates at the periphery (Fig. 16-13). Pustules may also be present at the border of the lesions. The surface is often tender to touch, and there are associated symptoms of itching, painful defecation, or blood-streaked stools.

Extracutaneous Findings

Infants may present with constipation, pain with defecation, or even encopresis. Fever is rare. Guttate psoriasis, which is typically associated with streptococcal pharyngitis, may be seen with PSD. Therefore any patient with new-onset guttate psoriasis should have an anogenital examination and appropriate cultures should be obtained.

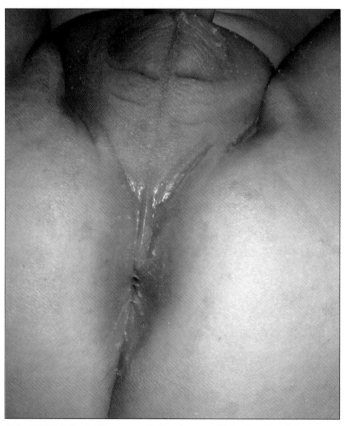

FIG. 16-13 Infant with group A streptococcal infection involving perinatal and inguinal creases. Moist erythema of the folds is characteristic.

Etiology/Pathogenesis

The mechanism of infection may be related to tropism of specific GABHS (group A β-hemolytic streptococcus) strains to this area, but colonization may occur through the passage of swallowed GABHS in the gastrointestinal tract, or orodigital contamination from a focus of GABHS pharyngitis.[58] Communal bathing has contributed to familial outbreaks.[62] Similar clinical presentations have been reported with cultures positive for *S. aureus* strains.

Diagnosis and Differential Diagnosis

The differential diagnosis includes psoriasis, seborrheic dermatitis, cutaneous candidiasis, pinworm infestation, Crohn's disease, and sexual abuse. The diagnosis is confirmed by bacterial culture of the affected area. Certain laboratories may use media selective for enteric pathogens when plating swabs from this area, so it is essential to specifically request isolation of GABS. If culture is negative but clinical suspicion is high, culture of the pharynx may provide additional evidence for GABHS.

Treatment and Care

Treatment with a 10-day course of oral penicillin V or amoxicillin, with or without adjunctive topical mupirocin ointment applied twice daily, is usually curative. Erythromycin may be used in penicillin-allergic patients. Recurrent disease may prompt the need for repeated or more prolonged oral therapy. Repeated recurrences are uncommon, but may require strategies similar to those used to eliminate streptococcal carriage from the pharynx.

Ecthyma Gangrenosum

Ecthyma gangrenosum (EG) is due to direct skin inoculation or more commonly to septicemia caused by infection with *Pseudomonas aeruginosa*. It may occur anywhere on the skin surface, but over 50% present in the perineal/gluteal area, particularly in immunocompromised infants.[63] Skin lesions begin as an erythematous macule that rapidly enlarges into a grey nodule, necrotic bulla, or ulceration with a bright red surrounding areola.[64] Differential diagnosis includes cutaneous anthrax[65] as well as opportunistic pathogens, including *Aeromonas*, *Aspergillus*, and *Mucor*. Treatment is with antipseudomonal systemic antibiotic therapy.

Diaper Dermatophytosis

Dermatophyte infections of the diaper region are rare but often misdiagnosed. Isolated organisms include *Trichophyton rubrum*, *T. mentagophytes*, and *T. verrucosum*, as well as *Epidermophyton floccosum*.[66, 67] Often other family members, particularly the patient's parent, have associated tinea pedis or cruris. Standard remedies for IDD or the use of topical nystatin (which is efficacious against *Candida* but not dermatophytes) will not alleviate the problem and may exacerbate it. Examination shows annular, erythematous, scaling papules and plaques in the diaper region. In chronic cases deeper follicular papules and pustules may be present (Fig. 16-14). Superficial infection responds well to topical antifungals, but when lesions are extensive or there is deeper follicular involvement, treatment with oral antifungals such as griseofulvin, fluconazole, or terbinafine may be required; experience with the use of terbinafine in neonates and very young infants is rather limited.

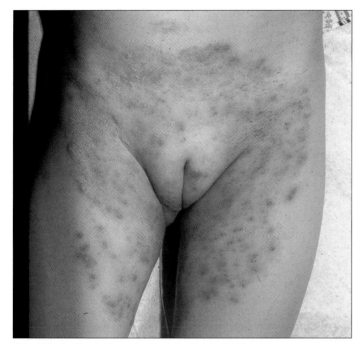

FIG. 16-14 Diaper dermatophytosis due to *Trichophyton mentagrophytes*.

Herpes Simplex infection (See Chapter 13)

Primary herpes infection presents with painful vesicles, clustered on an erythematous base, 2–8 days after contact with an infected individual. Neonatal herpes may present in the diaper region following breech delivery of an infant whose mother has genital HSV. The diagnosis of genital HSV in an older infant or child may raise the suspicion of sexual abuse, although innocent transmission from an infected caregiver or parent may occur. Maternofetal transmission of HSV resulting in neonatal HSV infection is discussed in Chapter 13.

Condyloma Acuminata and Mollusca Contagiosa (See Chapter 13)

Verrucae are caused by cutaneous infection with the human papilloma virus (HPV); such infection is very common in children. There are in excess of 130 HPV subtypes, most of which produce self-limited infection; a few lead to malignancies. When verrucae affect the genital area they are known as condyloma acuminata. At least 30–40 subtypes are implicated in causing condyloma acuminata.[68] Acquisition in infancy is usually through maternal transmission. The incubation period is unknown and may be anywhere between 1 and more than 24 months. They can occur on any part of the perineum, including the vaginal area and around and extending into the anus. Lesions appear as asymptomatic, flesh-colored papules that may coalesce to form plaques. They have a characteristic verrucous, velvety surface.

Although it is well recognized that condyloma may be the result of child abuse, most cases in young infants are either vertically acquired or from an unknown sources.[69] The exact percentage of cases acquired from sexual abuse in young infants is unknown and probably quite low, yet it is important to at least consider the possibility of abuse in all cases. There is a high rate of spontaneous resolution. Treatment regimens include imiquimod, podophyllin, and surgical removal (see Chapter 13).

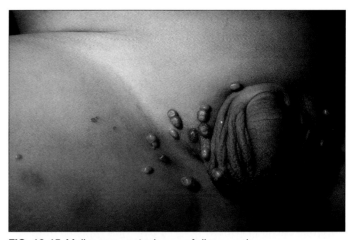

FIG. 16-15 Molluscum contagiosum of diaper region.

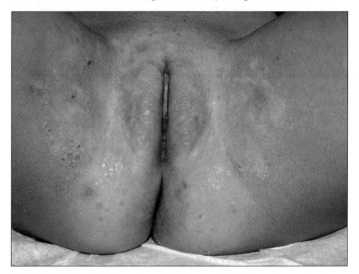

FIG. 16-16 Hand, foot and mouth disease. Vesicles and papules in the diaper area are a common manifestation.

Molluscum contagiosum (MC) is a poxviral infection of the skin characterized by discrete single or multiple, pink or flesh-colored, umbilicated papules.[70] There are four subtypes that are not area specific. It is rarely seen in the neonatal period, but increases in incidence in early childhood; 80% of patients are under 8 years old.[71] The lesions are thought to be spread by autoinoculation; they tend to cluster in creases such as the axillae, the antecubital and popiteal fossae, and the diaper area (Fig. 16-15). The latter often raises the specter of child abuse, but supportive evidence is usually lacking and genital involvement is common in childhood.[71] The disease is self-limited and often resolves with quite severe inflammation. Treatment includes curettage with topical anesthetics, liquid nitrogen (not an option in infants or young children), cantharidin and podophyllin.

Coxsackie Viral Exanthem (Hand, Foot and 'Butt' Exanthem) (See Chapter 13)

Hand, foot, and mouth disease is caused by various serotypes of Coxsackie virus, including A16, A5, A9, A10, B1, and B3. Infection with enterovirus 71 may cause a similar clinical presentation. The disease tends to be more severe in children under 5 years of age. Lesions consist of small red macules that rapidly evolve into ovoid vesicles. In the perineum vesicles are rarely seen[72] (Fig. 16-16). Thirty-one percent of affected children will have lesions in the buttocks or perineum, particularly those who are still wearing diapers[73] (see Chapter 13).

NUTRITIONAL AND METABOLIC DISORDERS
(See Chapter 17)

Zinc Deficiency

Zinc is an essential mineral element that is necessary for the normal function of humans. An acute deficiency of zinc, through various and different mechanisms, is associated with a specific clinical picture in the skin. The dermatitis affects the periorificial areas of the face, the diaper area, and acral sites. Acrodermatitis enteropathica (AE) is a rare, recessively inherited disorder caused by a lack of zinc transfer from the small intestine.[74] A similar and much more frequent clinical picture is seen with other causes of low zinc levels, such as in breastfed premature babies whose need for zinc outstrips the supply available in breast milk. In rare cases, a similar etiology can occur in term infants whose mothers' breast milk is deficient in zinc.[74] It can also occur in malabsorption states, particularly when associated with cystic fibrosis (see discussion below). Previously, zinc deficiency was reported in patients on parenteral alimentation, but it is rarely if ever seen nowadays, as zinc is routinely added to the feeds. A picture resembling zinc deficiency is also seen with other metabolic diseases, such methylmalonic acid deficiency, essential fatty acid deficiency, and vitamin A acid deficiency.

Clinical Presentation

The typical presentation is in a neonate who develops a crusted, scaling, erythematous dermatitis around the face and diaper area (Fig. 16-17A, B). Lesions on the face assume a characteristic horseshoe appearance around the mouth. The periorbital area may also be involved. In the diaper area lesions often affect the area around the anal cleft, with sharply demarcated erythema, superficial scale, and accentuated crusting at the periphery. Paronychia with candidal infection, maceration, and dermatitis are seen in the acral areas of the fingers and toes. Bullous lesions are rarely present on acral skin.

Extracutaneous Manifestations

It is common to have marked irritability, diarrhea, sparse hair or alopecia, and recurrent infections, particularly with *Candida albicans*, associated with the skin changes, but these may be absent early in the course of the disease, skin manifestations being the only finding. Nails may be dystrophic.

Etiology/Pathogenesis

The etiology of AE is thought to be an abnormality in the region of chromosome 8q24.3 affecting the zinc transporter system at the level of the small intestine.[75] Zinc is a cofactor in many enzymatic responses, hence the heterogeneity of the clinical signs in the disease. The serum zinc level is low; blood should be collected in a plastic container to avoid erroneously high laboratory levels. Alkaline phosphatase levels may also be low, as zinc is a cofactor in this enzyme.

Prognosis/Treatment

Oral zinc supplementation, given as zinc sulfate (3–5 mg/kg/day) or as zinc gluconate (which is better tolerated but more expensive), results in the rapid reversal of rash and associated symptoms. Patients with the genetic form of AE require treatment for life. Those infants with zinc deficiency due to a lack in breast milk require supplementation if breastfeeding is continued, but once formula or solid food is begun the supplemental zinc is no longer needed.[76]

Disorders that Resemble Acrodermatitis Enteropathica (See Chapter 17)

Biotin deficiency and certain organicacidurias[77] (see Chapter 17) may present with dermatitis of periorificial regions, including the diaper area, often in association with alopecia and changes in hair texture. The specific entities reported include deficiency of vitamin B_{12} or isoleucine from restrictive diets or methylmalonic acidemia, proprionic academia, glutaric aciduria (type 1),[78] maple syrup urine disease,[79] ornithine transcar-

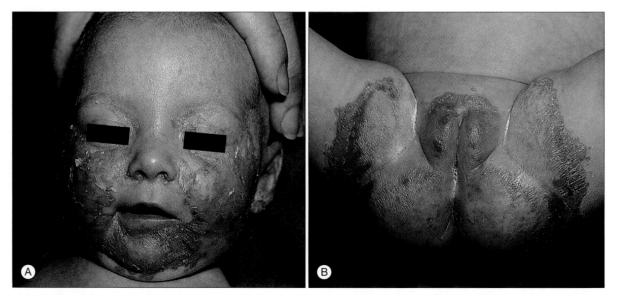

FIG. 16-17 Zinc deficiency (A) Periorificial eruption. **(B)** Diaper rash. The skin findings are typical of zinc deficiency, in this case caused by low levels of zinc in breast milk.

bamylase deficiency,[80] and citrullinemia.[81] Cystic fibrosis may present in infancy with failure to thrive and an AE-like eruption.[82] Edema is usually severe in cystic fibrosis because of marked hypoproteinemia, and the characteristic mucosal and paronychial lesions of AE are usually absent.

Biotin deficiency may be induced by a diet high in raw egg white, which contains avidin which prevents the absorption of biotin. It has also been reported during prolonged parenteral nutrition containing inadequate replacement of biotin. Several autosomal recessive disorders may present with AE-like eruptions because they require biotin as a cofactor, including methylmalonic academia, multiple carboxylase deficiency, and holocarboxylase deficiency.[83] Children undergoing long-term treatment with valproic acid for seizure disorders may have low biotin levels.[84]

MISCELLANEOUS

Langerhans' Cell Histiocytosis
(See also Chapter 25)

Langerhans' cell histiocytosis (LCH) is a disease of unknown origin that is caused by an accumulation of bone marrow-derived cells that originate from the granulocyte series. Cells divide into the macrophage and dendritic cell series. LHC is a

dendritic cell disorder and is the only histiocytic disease to affect neonates. The cells in this group of histiocytosis are all S100 and CD1a positive and have Birbeck granules on electron microscopy. The diaper area is often involved.

Clinical Presentation

LCH affects 2.6 per million child years,[85] with boys slightly more affected than girls. Spontaneous regression often occurs in limited forms, so the incidence may be higher than recorded. The age group most often affected is from 1 to 4 years, but the disease may occur at birth and can affect any age. The skin, including the gums, teeth, and nails, is the organ most commonly affected (40%) after bone.[86] Skin lesions may be single, few in number, or disseminated, and are the presenting sign in 50% of cases.[87] LCH in the newborn may involve the skin alone – the so-called congenital self-healing histiocytosis (Hashimoto–Pritzker disease) in which the majority of cases have nonspecific skin findings and are usually undiagnosed for a few months.[88] The most common sites affected in skin LCH are the trunk, scalp, and behind the ears, the diaper area, and the folds. Lesions are protean in their presentation: papules, nodules, vesicles, erosions, ulcerations, petechiae and purpura, scale and crusting can all be present either alone or together (Fig. 16-18A). The color varies from erythematous to yellow or brown. Lesions in the diaper area are erythematous with

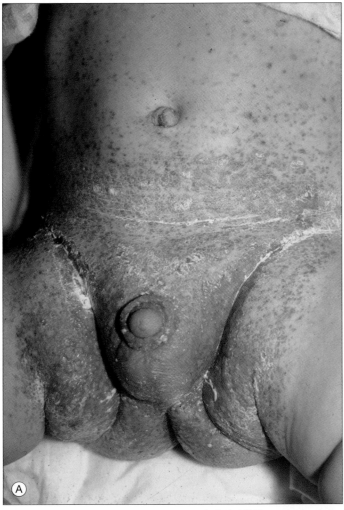

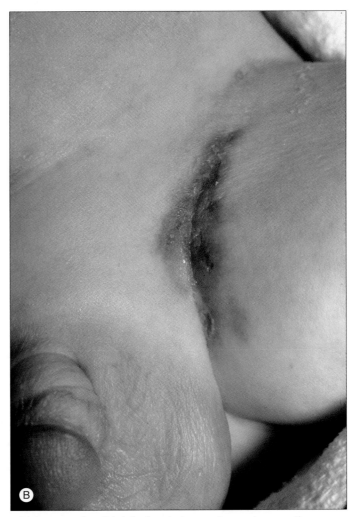

FIG. 16-18 Langerhans' cell histiocytosis (LCH). (**A**) Extensive eruption resembles severe *Candida* infection, but purpuric papules near the umbilicus are typical of LCH. (**B**) LCH with ulceration in the inguinal crease.

peripheral petechiae. Ulcerations or atrophy involving the inguinal creases may be present (Fig. 16-8B).

Extracutaneous Findings

Any organ may be affected in LCH, but it is unusual for the kidneys and gonads to be affected. In children under 2 with LCH the disease (Letterer–Siwe disease) is frequently disseminated, with skin and other organ involvement. The most common organ of involvement is bone (74%), followed by the skin (40%), lymph nodes (14%) and all other organs (<10%).[88]

Etiology/Pathogenesis

The precise etiology is unknown. Genetic factors have been implicated, as the disease is more common in monozygotic twins and in families. HLA studies have varied, but immune factors are thought to play a role. The theory of a reactive process invokes environmental factors, including malignancy.

Differential Diagnosis

Owing to the diversity of the symptoms and signs it is easy to miss the diagnosis. Nodular conditions such as neuroblastoma, congenital leukemia, mastocytosis, and hemangiomas all present with nodular lesions. Pustular lesions such as erythema toxicum, neonatal pustular melanosis, and acropustulosis of infancy can all mimic LCH. The dermatitic variant is easily confused with ISD. Petechiae are a helpful sign of differentiation. In any patient resistant to standard treatment for ISD should be evaluated for LCH; both conditions affect the scalp and diaper area, and both have erythema and scaling. There is more crusting in LCH, and petechiae are a valuable distinguishing sign.

Prognosis/Treatment

The diagnosis should be established based on biopsy and skin markers CD1a and S100 staining. The prognosis is not affected by the clinical appearance or the histology. In single system skin disease, or where few skin lesions are present, it is important to monitor carefully for signs of other organ progression and the appearance of diabetes insipidus. The prognosis in this group is good.[88] In the multinodular group of LCH called Hand–Schuller–Christian the disease is chronic and may be associated with the development of diabetes insipidus;[89] it has a better prognosis than the disseminated Letterer–Siwe disease, where mortality under the age of 2 years is 50%.[90] There are no good data on the definitive treatment of skin LCH. Treatment is geared toward the wellbeing of the patient, the number of organs involved, and the desire to minimize late effects. LCH involving multiple organs requires treatment[91] (see Chapter 25).

Infantile Perianal Pyramidal Protrusion

First described in 1996,[92] this entity consists of a protrusion around the anus that is often related to diarrhea, chronic constipation, or less commonly lichen sclerosus.[93] It has also been described in the literature as tags or skin folds.[94] The terminology has now been simplified to infantile perineal protrusion (IPP).[95]

Cutaneous Findings

IPP is fairly common, affecting up to 11% of prepubertal girls.[94] It has been reported in families,[93] and is almost exclusively

seen in females.[94] The age range is usually between 1 and 30 months, but it has been reported at birth.[94] Parents, when prompted, will often give a history of chronic constipation or diarrhea as the initial event, prior to the appearance of IPP. The lesion may be asymptomatic or there may be pain on defecation; it is sometimes associated with fissuring. IPP usually appears on the perianal mucous membrane in the midline just anterior to the anal opening; it may less commonly be seen on the posterior aspect of the anus.[96] It is a pyramidal soft tissue protrusion with a tongue-like lip[93] (Fig. 16-19). The surface is smooth. The pathology is unremarkable, those having lichen sclerosis changes showing evidence of the disease on biopsy.[95]

Extracutaneous Findings

There may be a history of diarrhea or constipation from various causes.

Etiology/Pathogenesis

The cause is unclear. IPP may be familial, functional (diarrhea or constipation), and lichen sclerosus-associated.[97] Weakness of the median raphe of the perineum, and perineal constitutional weakness have not been proved.

Differential Diagnosis

Other conditions affecting the anal area should all be considered. These include hemorrhoids, skin tags, sexual abuse condyloma acuminata, tag associated with anal fissure, granulomatous bowel disease, rectal prolapse, perineal midline malformation, and infantile hemangiomas.[93]

Prognosis/Treatment

Many cases resolve completely, whereas less commonly others persist.[96] Attending to either constipation, diarrhea or fissuring may be helpful in accelerating the resolution. Looking for other evidence of lichen sclerosus and treatment with high-potency corticosteroids is useful. Observation with petrolatum applied to the area is usually all that is needed until spontaneous resolution.

Nascent Hemangioma (See Chapter 20)

Infantile hemangiomas located in the perineum frequently become ulcerated, and this may actually be the presenting

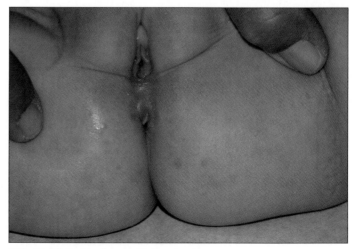

FIG. 16-19 Perianal pyramidal protrusion.

finding in a minority of patients. In these cases, an infant will be born with or develop an ulceration in the perineum in the first few days of life prior to a hemangioma being evident. Close inspection will often reveal telangiectasia or vascular papules at the margin of the ulceration, or occasionally in the surrounding skin (Fig. 16-20A). Days to several weeks later a superficial plaque-type hemangioma will develop in the region (Fig. 16-20B). Undiagnosed ulceration due to nascent hemangioma may be misdiagnosed as a rapidly expanding bacterial or viral infection, thermal burn, or child abuse.[98] The etiology of ulceration in nascent hemangiomas is unclear, but may be related to rapid apoptosis of endothelial cells in a portion of the evolving hemangioma.

Lichen Sclerosus (LS)

This disease of unknown origin affects the genital area of female children with a well-recognized clinical and histologic picture. Cases during infancy are uncommon, but the presence of histologic changes of LS in boys with congenital phimosis and a documented association with perineal pyramidal protrusion suggests than onset may occur quite early in infancy.[98a] The eruption may be symptomatic, but usually presents with pruritus in the genital area, or with constipation in girls and phimosis in boys.[99]

The latter is related to the fissuring of the perianal skin, with pain on defecation and subsequent holding of the stool. The classic clinical picture is of a white, glistening, atrophic vulval area, often with accentuation of the veins. The lesions may extend onto the anal area in a figure-of-eight distribution. Hemorrhagic areas and petechiae may be seen (Fig. 16-21). It is important to differentiate LS from child abuse and herpes simplex infection. If left untreated, adhesions and flattening of the clitoris and vaginal opening may occur. Response to potent topical steroids is excellent, but recurrence may occur.[100]

Pyoderma Gangrenosum (See also Chapter 10)

Pyoderma gangrenosum presents as papules that develop into pustules and then rapidly expand into painful deep ulcerations surrounded by a violaceous border. Pathergy often occurs. Although rare in infants, a case has been reported in a 3-week-old infant presenting with perineal lesions.[101] Crohn's disease should be considered when lesions of pyoderma gangrenosum develop in the perianal region, particularly with features of skin tags, perianal fissuring, and a history of diarrhea or constipation.[102]

Chronic Bullous Disease of Childhood (CBDC) (See also Chapter 10)

CBDC or linear IgA disease is an acquired blistering disorder that involved the skin and mucous membranes. The bullae are subepidermal. The etiology of CBDC is unknown; studies implicating infectious or autoimmune diseases have been inconclusive. Commonly, preschool children present with fever or other constitutional findings, followed by large tense bullae that are annular or polycyclic. The lesions are described as resembling a string of pearls. The underlying skin is normal. The diaper area is characteristically involved, with spread to the trunk and legs, although any site can be affected. Although not recognized initially, mucous membranes, particularly the oral mucosa, are frequently involved. Erosions and occasional intact bullae are seen. Conjunctival erosions are not uncommon. The prognosis for remission without treatment is

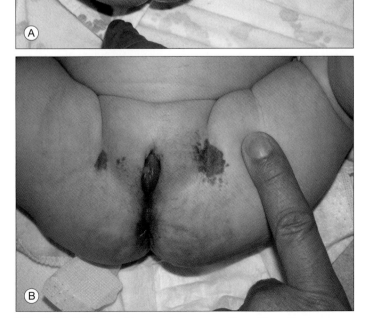

FIG. 16-20 (A) Nascent hemangioma presenting with perianal ulceration at birth. **(B)** Same patient at 6 weeks of age.

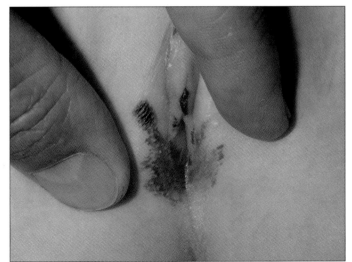

FIG. 16-21 Lichen sclerosus in a young infant; in addition to hypopigmentation and atrophy, hemorrhage is a relatively common finding.

between 3 and 5 years, although the disease may persist into adult life. Treatments, include dapsone, sulfapyridine, and prednisone, all have been utilized, with varying results.[103]

Bullous Pemphigoid (BP) (See Chapter 10)

A rare disease in childhood, BP is an acquired blistering disorder that overlaps with CBDC. It has been recorded in infants as young as 2–3 months. Tense bullae on a normal or erythematous base, with urticarial lesions, are typical. Common areas of involvement include the flexures, particularly the inner thighs, the forearms, the axillae, and the diaper area. Infants often present with hand and foot lesions. A variant of BP confined to the vulval area is known as localized vulval pemphigoid. Typically, BP antigens are designated BP 230 and 180. Immunofluorescence demonstrates IGG and C3 at the dermoepidermal junction. The prognosis is good, with remission within 1 year. Systemic or topical steroids have been used with good effect, as has a combination of tetracycline and nicotinamide.[104]

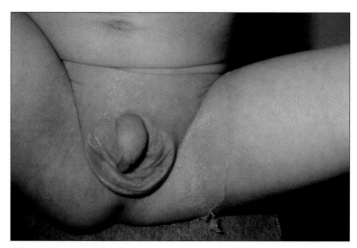

FIG. 16-22 Perineal erythema and scale in a young infant with Kawasaki syndrome.

Kawasaki Syndrome

Kawasaki syndrome is a well-characterized febrile illness with prominent cutaneous manifestations.[105] Approximately two-thirds of affected infants may have prominent erythema and early desquamation in the perineal area (Fig. 16-22). This finding which can be an important clue to diagnosis, as it often occurs early in the disease, before the presence of other diagnostic findings such as desquamation of the fingers and toes. The inguinal creases are often the most prominent area of involvement, but the entire perineal area may be involved. The initial bright-red erythema may persist or fade, resolving with prominent desquamation. Small sterile pustules are sometimes present.[106, 107]

REFERENCES

1. Lund CH, Kuller J, Lane AT, et al. Neonatal skin care: clinical outcomes of the AWHONN/NANN evidence-based clinical practice guideline. J Obstet Gynecol Neonat Nurs 2001; 30: 41–51.
2. Jaquet L. Traité des maladies de l'enfance. In: Grancher J, Comby J, Marfan AB, eds. Traité des maladies de l'enfance. Paris: Masson & Co, 1905; 714
3. Zahorsky J. The ammoniacal diaper in infants and young children. Am J Dis Child 1915; 10: 436.
4. Jordon WE, Lawson KD, Berg RW, et al. Diaper dermatitis: frequency and severity among a general infant population. Pediatr Dermatol 1986; 3: 198–207.
5. Ward DB, Fleischer AB Jr, Feldman SR, Krowchuk DP. Characterization of diaper dermatitis in the United States. Arch Pediatr Adolesc Med 2000; 154: 943–946.
6. Lane AT, Rehder PA, Helm K. Evaluations of diapers containing absorbent gelling material with conventional disposable diapers in newborn infants. Am J Dis Child 1990; 144: 315–318.
7. Visscher MO, Chatterjee R, Muinson KA, et al. Development of diaper rash in the newborn. Pediatr Dermatol 2000; 17: 52–57.
8. Visscher MO, Chatterjee R, Munson KA, et al. Changes in diapered and

non-diapered skin over the first month of life. Pediatr Dermatol 2000; 17: 45–51.
9. Berg RW, Milligan MC, Sarbaugh FC. Association of skin wetness and pH with diaper dermatitis. Pediatr Dermatol 1994; 11: 18–20.
10. Warner RR, Stone KJ, Boissy YL. Hydration disrupts stratum corneum ultrastructure. J Invest Dermatol 2003; 120: 275–284.
11. Berg RW, Buckingham KW, Stewart RL. Etiologic factors in diaper dermatitis: the role of urine. Pediatr Dermatol 1986; 3: 102–106.
12. Fluhr JW, Elias PM. Stratum corneum pH: formation and function of the 'acid mantle.' Exog Dermatol 2002; 1: 163–175.
13. Tokar B, Urer S. Factors determining the severity of perianal dermatitis after enterostoma closure of pediatric patients. Int J Dermatol 2005; 44: 168–169.
14. Goldberg NS, Esterly NB, Rothman KF, et al. Perianal pseudoverrucous papules and nodules in children. Arch Dermatol 1992 Feb; 128: 240–242.
15. Rodriguez-Poblador J, Gonzalez-Castro U, Herranz-Martinez S, Luelmo-Aguilar J. Jacquet erosive diaper dermatitis after surgery for Hirschsprung disease. Pediatr Dermatol 1998; 15: 46–47.

16. Tappeiner J, Pfleger L. Granuloma gluteale infantum. Hautartzt 1971; 22: 383–388.
17. Delacretaz J, Grigoriu D, De Crousaz H, et al. Candidose nodulaire de la région inguinogénitale et des fesses. Dermatologica 1972; 144: 144.
18. Ortonne J, Perrot H, Thivolet J. Granuloma gluteale infantile (GGI): Etude ultrastructurale. Ann Dermatol Venereol (Paris) 1980; 107: 631–634.
19. Dytoc M, Fiorillo L, Liao J, Krol AL. Granuloma gluteale adultorum associated with use of topical benzocaine preparations: Case report and literature review. J Cutan Med Surg 2002; 6: 221–225.
20. Chang MW, Kaufmann JM, Orlow SJ, et al. Infantile granular parakeratosis: Recognition of two clinical patterns. J Am Acad Dermatol 2004; 50: S93–96.
21. Patrizi A, Neri I, Misciali C, et al. Granular parakeratosis: four pediatric cases. Br J Dermatol 2002; 147: 1003–1006.
22. Metze D, Rutten A. Granular parakeratosis – a unique aaquired disorder of keratinization. J Cutan Pathol 1999; 26: 339–352.
23. Unna PG. Seborrhoeic eczema. J Cutan Dis 1887; 5: 499.
24. Williams JV, Eichenfield LF, Burke BL, et al. Prevalence of scalp scaling in prepubertal children. Pediatrics 2005; 115: e1–e6.

25. Gupta AK, Bluhm R. Seborrheic dermatitis. J Eur Acad Dermatol Venereol 2004; 18: 13–26.

26. Wananukul S, Chindamporn A, Yumyourn P, et al. Malassezia furfur in infantile seborrheic dermatitis. Asia Pacific J Allergy Immunol 2005; 23: 101–105.

27. Mimouni K, Mukamel M, Zaheria A, et al. Prognosis of infantile seborrheic dermatitis. J Pediatr 1995; 127: 744–746.

28. Erlichman M, Goldstein R, Levi E, et al. Infantile flexural seborrheic dermatitis. Neither biotin nor essential fatty acid deficiency. Arch Dis Childhood 1981; 56: 560–562.

29. Wannanukul S, Chiabunkana J. Comparative study of 2% ketoconazole cream and 1% hydrocortisone cream in the treatment of infantile seborrheic dermatitis. J Med Assoc Thai 2004; 87: S68–S71.

30. Cohen S. Should we treat infantile seborrheic dermatitis with topical antifungals or topical steroids? Arch Dis Childhood 2000; 89: 288–289.

31. Farber EA, Jacobs AH. Infantile psoriasis. Am J Dis Child 1977; 131: 1266.

32. Farber EM, Nall L. Epidemiology: Natural history and genetics. In: Roenigk HH Jr, Maibach HI, eds. Psoriasis, 3rd edn. New York: Marcel Dekker, 1998; 107–158.

33. Farber EM. Juvenile psoriasis. Early interventions can reduce risk for problems later. Postgrad Med 1998; 103: 89–100.

34. Morris A, Rogers M, Fischer G, Williams K. Childhood psoriasis: a clinical review of 1262 cases. Pediatr Dermatol 2001; 18: 188–198.

35. Fergusson AG, Fraser ND, Grant PW. Napkin dermatitis with psoriasiform 'id.' Br J Dermatol 1966; 78: 289–296.

36. Rattet JP, Headley JL, Barr RJ. Diaper dermatitis with psoriasiform ID eruption. Int J Dermatol 1981; 20: 122–125.

37. Nevill EA, Finn OA. Psoriasiform napkin dermatitis: a follow-up study. Br J Dermatol 1975; 92: 279.

38. Friedlander SF. Contact dermatitis. Pediatr Rev 1998; 19: 166–171.

39. Weston WL, Weston JA. Allergic contact dermatitis in children. Am J Dis Child 1984; 138: 932–936.

40. Bruckner AL, Weston WL, Morelli JG. Does sensitization to contact allergens begin in infancy? Pediatrics 1986; 78: 1070–1074.

41. Barros MA, Baptista A, Correia M, Azevedo F. Patch testing in children: a study of 562 school children. Contact Dermatitis 1991; 25: 156–159.

42. Roul S, Ducombs G, Leaute-Labreze C, Taieb A. 'Lucky Luke' contact dermatitis due to rubber components of diapers. Contact Dermatitis 1998; 38: 363–364.

43. Alberta L, Sweeney SM, Wiss K. Diaper dye dermatitis. Pediatrics 2005; 116: e450–e452.

44. Ruiz-Diez B, Martinez V. Molecular tracking of Candida albicans in a neonatal intensive care unit: long-term colonizations versus catheter-related infections. J Clin Microbiol 1997; 35: 3032–3036.

45. Bound JP. Thrush napkin rashes. Br Med J 1956; 1: 782.

46. Beare JM, Cheeseman EA, MacKenzie DWR. The association between Candida albicans and lesions of seborrheic eczema. Br J Dermatol 1968; 80: 675–681.

47. Leyden J. The role of microorganisms in diaper dermatitis. Arch Dermatol 1978; 114: 56–59.

48. Rebora A, Leyden J. Napkin (diaper) dermatitis and gastrointestinal carriage of Candida albicans. Br J Dermatol 1981; 105: 551–555.

49. Hoppe JE. Treatment of oropharyngeal candidiasis and candidal diaper dermatitis in neonates and infants: review and reappraisal. Pediatr Infect Dis J 1997; 16: 885–894.

49A. Spraker MK, Gisoldi EM, Siegfried EC, et al. Topical miconazole nitrate ointment in the treatment of diaper dermatitis complicated by candidiasis. Cutis 2006; 77: 113–120.

50. Munz D, Powell KR, Pai CH. Treatment of candidal diaper dermatitis: a double-blind placebo-controlled comparison of topical nystatin with topical plus oral nystatin. J Pediatr 1982; 101: 1022–1025.

51. Darmstadt G, Lane AT. Impetigo. An overview. Pediatr Dermatol 1994; 11: 293–303.

52. Elias P, Fritsch P, Dahl MS. Staphyloccocal toxic epidermal necrolysis. Pathogenesis and studies on the subcellular site of action of exfoliatin. J Invest Dermatol 1975; 65: 501–512.

53. Yamasaki O, Yamaguchi T, Sugai M, et al. Clinical manifestations of staphylococcal scalded skin syndrome depend on T serotypes of exfoliatin organisms. J Clin Microbiol 2005; 43: 1890–1893.

54. Amagai M, Yamaguchi T, Hanakawa Y, et al. Staphylococcal exfoliative toxin B specifically cleaves desmoglein 1. J Invest Dermatol 2002; 118: 845–850.

55. Johnston GA. Treatment of bullous impetigo and staphylococcal skin syndrome in infants. Exp Rev Anti Infect Ther 2004; 2: 439–446.

56. Amren DP, Anderson AS, Wannamaker LW. Perianal cellulites associated with group A streptococci. Am J Dis Child 1966; 112: 546–552.

57. Krol AL. Perianal streptococcal dermatitis. Pediatr Dermatol 1990; 7: 97–100.

58. Kokx NP, Comstock JA, Facklam RR. Streptococcal perianal disease in children. Pediatrics 1987; 80: 659–663.

59. Rehder PA, Eliezer ET, Lane AT. Perianal cellulites. Cutaneous group A streptococcal disease. Arch Dermatol 1988; 124: 702–704.

60. Honig P, Frieden I, Kim H, Yan A. Streptococcal intertrigo: an underrrecognized condition in children. Pediatrics 2003; 112: 1427–1429.

61. Muotiala A, Saxen H, Vuopio-Varkila J. Group A streptococcal outbreak of perianal infection in a day care center. Adv Exp Med Biol 1997; 418: 211–215.

62. Mogielnicki NP, Schwartzman JD, Elliott JA. Perineal group A streptococcal disease in a pediatric practice. Pediatrics 2000; 106: 276–281.

63. Guclear H, Ergun T, Demircay Z. Ecthyma gangrenosum. Int J Dermatol 1999; 38: 298–305.

64. Taieb A, Boisseau AM, Sarlangue J, et al. Gangrenous ecthyma of the diaper area in infants. Ann Pediatr (Paris) 1992; 39: 443–446.

65. Tutrone WD, Scheinfield NS, Weinberg JM. Cutaneous anthrax: a concise review. Cutis 2002; 69: 27–33.

66. Parry EL, Foshee WS, Marks JG. Diaper dermatophytosis. Am J Dis Child 1982; 136: 273–274.

67. Baudraz-Rosselet F, Ruffieux PH, Mancarella A, et al. Diaper dermatitis due to Trichophyton verrucosum. Pediatr Dermatol 1993; 10: 368–369.

68. Sinclair KA, Woods CR, Kirse DJ, Sinal SH. Anogenital and respiratory tract human papillomavirus infections among children: age, gender, and potential transmission through sexual abuse. Pediatrics 2005; 116: 815–825.

69. Handley J, Hanks E, Armstrong K, et al. Common association of HPV2 in anogenital warts in prepubertal children. Pediatr Dermatol 1997; 14: 339–343.

70. Gottlieb SL, Myskowski PL. Molluscum contagiosum. Int J Dermatol. 1994; 33: 45.

71. Dohil MA, Lin P, Lee J, et al. The epidemiology of molluscum contagiosum in children. J Am Acad Dermatol 2006; 54: 47–54.

72. Slavin KA, Frieden IJ. Picture of the month: Hand, foot and mouth disease. Arch Pediatr Adolesc Med 1998; 152: 505–506.

73. Richardson HB Jr, Leibovitz A. Hand, foot, and mouth disease in children. J Pediatr 1965; 67: 6–12.

74. Aggett PJ, Harries JT. The current staus of zinc in health and disease states. Arch Dis Child 1979; 54: 909–917.

75. Wang K, Pugh EW, Griffen S, et al. Homozygosity mapping places the acrodermatitis enteropathica gene on chromosome region 8q24.3. Am J Hum Genet 2001; 68: 1055–60 Epub 2001.

76. Perafan-Riveros C, Sayago-Franca LF, Fortes-Alves AC, et al. Acrodermatitis enteropathica: Case report and review of the literature. Pediatr Dermatol 2002; 19: 426–431.

77. De Raeve L, De Meirleir L, Ramet J, et al. Acrodermatitis enteropathica-like cutaneous lesions in organic aciduria. J Pediatr 1994; 124: 416–420.
78. Niyama S, Koelker S, Degen I, et al. Acrodermatitis academia secondary to malnutrition in glutaric aciduria type 1. Eur J Dermatol 2001; 11: 244–246.
79. Koch SE, Pachman S, Koch TK, Williams ML. Dermatitis in treated maple syrup urine disease. J Am Acad Dermatol 1993; 28: 289–292.
80. Lee JY, Chang SE, Suh CW, et al. A case of acrodermatitis enteropathica-like dermatosis caused by ornithine transcarbamylase deficiency. J Am Acad Dermatol 2002; 46: 965–967.
81. Goldblum OM, Brusilow SW, Maldonado YA, Farmer ER. Neonatal citrullinemia associated with cutaneous manifestations and arginine deficiency. J Am Acad Dermatol 1986; 14: 321–326.
82. Crone J, Huber WD, Eichler I, et al. Acrodermatitis enteropathica-like eruption as the presenting sign of cystic fibrosis. Case report and review of the literature. Eur J Pediatr 2002; 161: 475–478.
83. Seymons K, De Moor A, De Raeve H, et al. Dermatologic signs of biotin deficiency leading to the diagnosis of multiple carboxylase deficiency. Pediatr Dermatol 2004; 21: 231–235.
84. Schulpis KH, Karikas GA Tjamouranis J, et al. Low serum biotinidase activity in children with valproic acid monotherapy. Epilepsia 2001; 42: 1359–1362.
85. Alston RD, Tatevossian RG, McNally RJ, et al. Incidence and survival of childhood Langerhans' cell histiocytosis in Northwest England from 1954 to 1998. Pediatr Blood Cancer 2006; [Epub ahead of print].
86. The French Langerhans' Cell Histiocytosis Study Group. A multicenter retrospective survey of LCH. 348 cases observed between 1983–93 Arch Dis Child 1996; 75: 17–12.
87. Munn S, Chu AC. Langerhans' cell histiocytosis of the skin. Hematol Oncol Clin North Am 1998; 12: 269–228.
88. Stein SL, Paller AS, Haut PR, et al. Langerhans' cell histiocytosis presenting in the neonatal period: a retrospective case series. Arch Pediatr Adolesc Med 2001; 155: 778–783.
89. Yu RC, Chu AC. Lack of T-cell rearrangement in cells involved in Langerhans' cell histiocytosis. Cancer 1995; 75: 1162–1166.
90. Rivera-Luna R, Alter-Molxhadsky N, Cardens-Cardos R, et al. Langerhans' cell histiocytosis in children under 2 years of age. Med Pediatr Oncol 1996; 26: 70–74.
91. Ladisch S, Gadner H. Treatment of Langerhans' cell histiocytosis: evolution and current approaches. Br J Cancer 1994; 70: S41–S46.
92. Kayashima K, Kitoh M, Ono T. Infantile perianal pyramidal protrusion. Arch Dermatol 1996; 132: 1481–1484.
93. Amor Khachemoune CWS, Kjetil KG, Ehrsam E. Infantile perineal protrusion. J Am Acad Dermatol 2006; 54: 1046–1049.
94. CrucesMJ, De La Torre C, Losada A, et al. Infantile pyramidal protrusion as a manifestation of lichen sclerosus et atrophicus. Arch Dermatol 1998; 134: 1118–1120.
95. Merigou D, Labreze C, Lamireau T, et al. Infantile perinanal pyramidal protrusion: a marker of constipation. Dermatol 1998; 15: 143–144.
96. Patrizi A, Baone B, Neri I, D'Antuono A. Infantile perianal protrusion: 13 new cases. Pediatr Dermatol 2002; 19: 15–18.
97. McCann J, Voris J, Simon M, Wells R. Infantile perineal findings in prepubertal children selected for nonabuse: a descriptive study. Child Abuse Neglect 1989; 13: 1799.
98. Liang MG, Frieden IJ. Perineal and lip ulcerations as the presenting manifestations of hemangioma of infancy. Pediatrics 1997; 99: 256–259.
98A. Fischer G, Rogers M. Vulvar disease in children: a clinical audit of 130 cases. Pediatr Dermatol 2000; 17: 1–6.
99. Maronn ML, Esterly NB. Constipation as a feature of anogenital lichen sclerosis in children. Pediatrics 2005; 115: e230–232.
100. Smith YR, Haefner HK. Vulval lichen sclerosus: Pathophysiology and treatment. Am J Clin Dermatol 2004; 5: 105–125.
101. Graham JA, Hansen KK, Rabinowitz LG, Esterly NB. Pyoderma gangrenosum in infants and children. Pediatr Dermatol 1994; 11: 10–17.
102. Dinulos JGH, Darmstadt GL, Len MK, et al. Infantile Crohn disease presenting with diarrhea and pyoderma gangrenosum. Pediatr Dermatol 2006; 23: 43–48.
103. Kanwar AJ, Sandhu K, Handa S. Chronic bullous disease of childhood in north India. Pediatr Dermatol 2004; 21: 610–612.
104. Walsh SR, Hogg D, Mydlarski R. Bullous pemphigoid: from bench to bedside. Drugs 2005; 65: 905–926.
105. Falcini F. Kawasaki disease. Curr Opin Rheumatol 2006; 18: 33–38.
106. Friter BS, Lucky AW. The perineal eruption of Kawasaki syndrome. Arch Dermatol 1988; 124: 1805–1810.
107. Krowchuk DP, Bass J, Elgart GW. Kawasaki disease with an exanthem limited to the diaper area. Am J Dis Child 1988; 142: 1136–1137.

17

Erythrodermas, Immunodeficiency, and Metabolic Disorders

Brandie J. Metz, Moise L. Levy

ERYTHRODERMAS

The term erythroderma is used in dermatology to describe a skin eruption characterized by diffuse erythema, usually in association with scaling. Infantile erythroderma is caused by or associated with a large number of disorders (Box 17-1). The differential diagnosis includes inflammatory, infectious, inherited, and immunologic diseases, many of which have a hereditary basis. Some of these diseases are potentially life-threatening, and erythroderma itself can cause serious medical complications, such as electrolyte imbalance, sepsis, and temperature instability resulting from heat loss. It is therefore important for the physician to accurately diagnose and treat the problem.

INFLAMMATORY DISEASES

Atopic Dermatitis

Severe generalized atopic dermatitis is unusual in neonates, but because atopic dermatitis is such a common problem it is the most common cause of acquired or noncongenital erythroderma in infants (see Chapter 15). Classic infantile atopic dermatitis involves the scalp, cheeks, and extensor surfaces of the extremities and may not appear until the infant is several months of age.[1] When the distribution is generalized and the onset is early, diagnosis can be more difficult.

The presence of pruritus, an almost invariable feature of this condition, is not always apparent in neonates and young infants.[2] Typically, the diaper region is spared even in cases of widespread atopic dermatitis, as a result of the moist, occlusive environment of diapered skin. In contrast to infants with severe metabolic or immunologic disease, infants with atopic dermatitis usually grow normally and thrive, assuming the disease is recognized and treated promptly. There is often a family history of atopy. Atopic dermatitis generally responds rapidly to appropriate therapy with topical corticosteroids and emollients. Skin biopsy in atopic dermatitis demonstrates acanthosis (thickening of the epidermis) and varying degrees of spongiosis (epidermal edema), as well as lymphohistiocytic inflammatory infiltrates, often with scattered eosinophils and plasma cells.

Seborrheic Dermatitis

Seborrheic dermatitis is a common problem during the neonatal period and is generally easily recognized (see also Chapter 15). Typically there is scaling and erythema involving seborrheic areas such as the scalp and body folds.[3] The yellow, greasy, scalp scale may encompass the entire forehead, including the eyebrows, and erythema and maceration can involve body folds such as the retroauricular areas, neck, axillae, and groin. When the disease is mild, only the scalp is affected and body fold involvement is either focal or absent entirely. Occasionally, however, a more diffuse pattern of seborrheic dermatitis can occur, which must be distinguished from atopic dermatitis, neonatal candidiasis, psoriasis, and other causes of infantile erythroderma (Fig. 17-1) (see Box 17-1).

The distribution of the dermatitis is more helpful than any other criterion in differentiating between atopic and seborrheic dermatitis,[2] but it can be difficult and sometimes impossible to differentiate the two conditions accurately early in their course. Although the scalp can be red and scaly in both conditions, seborrheic dermatitis tends to involve the groin and other body folds, which are generally spared in atopic dermatitis because they are better hydrated. As treatment for both conditions in infancy is similar, from a practical standpoint accurate differentiation can be an academic exercise. However, the course of this disease differs: seborrheic dermatitis usually resolves over several months, whereas atopic dermatitis often persists for several years. Skin biopsy findings in seborrheic dermatitis are similar to those in atopic dermatitis. There is mild acanthosis, spongiosis, and a mild lymphohistiocytic inflammatory infiltrate; parakeratotic scale may be present.

If clinical features suggest widespread seborrheic dermatitis in an infant who is otherwise well and thriving, and the skin readily clears after the application of low- to mid-potency topical corticosteroids without chronic rebound when therapy is tapered, the diagnosis of seborrheic dermatitis is probably accurate. Otherwise, alternative diagnoses should be considered.

Psoriasis

Less than 1% of all cases of psoriasis are said to occur in infants under 1 year of age.[3] Infantile psoriasis can be a diffi-

Box 17-1 Erythrodermas: red scaly baby – differential diagnosis

Inflammatory diseases
Atopic dermatitis

Seborrheic dermatitis

Psoriasis

Boric acid poisoning

Diffuse mastocytosis

Infectious disease
Staphylococcal scalded skin syndrome

Candida/other fungal infections

Herpes simplex virus

Syphilis

Inherited diseases
Ichthyosis

    Netherton's syndrome

    Nonbullous ichthyosiform erythroderma

    Bullous ichthyosis (epidermolytic hyperkeratosis)

    Sjögren-Larsson syndrome

    Chondrodysplasia punctata

Ectodermal dysplasia

Cobalamin deficiency

Maple syrup urine disease

Carbamoyl phosphate synthetase deficiency

Argininosuccinicaciduria

Methylmalonic aciduria

Propionic acidemia

Cystic fibrosis

Essential fatty acid deficiency

Biotinidase deficiency

Immunologic diseases
Leiner's phenotype

Omenn's syndrome

DiGeorge Anomaly

Graft versus host disease

Severe combined immunodeficiency

Bruton's hypogammaglobulinemia

Common variable hypogammaglobulinemia

Eosinophilic gastroenteritis

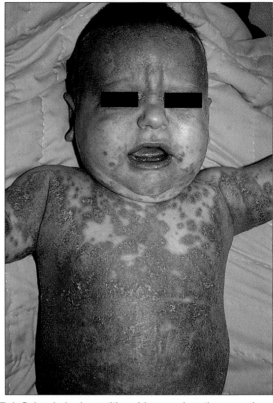

FIG. 17-1 Seborrheic dermatitis: widespread erythema and scale.

Rarely, infantile psoriasis is generalized, a presentation that has been reported in young infants, and can even be present at birth.[5] Erythroderma can evolve into and even alternate with pustulosis. Infantile generalized pustular psoriasis can be associated with lytic bone lesions,[6] and be complicated by the acute respiratory distress syndrome (pulmonary capillary leak syndrome) that can also be seen in adults with acute generalized pustular psoriasis (personal communication, B. Krafchik).[7] Skin biopsy can be helpful in diagnosis and in some cases is diagnostic. Biopsy usually shows psoriasiform hyperplasia with elongated rete ridges and parakeratotic scale, often containing neutrophils. Occasionally, the diagnostic finding of a spongiform micropustule or microabscess in the upper epidermis is seen. Skin biopsies of erythrodermic psoriasis are often indistinguishable from those of chronic dermatitis, and it may take several biopsies and close observation over time to confirm the diagnosis.

Localized psoriasis may be treated with emollients and low-potency topical corticosteroids, but often clears only partially or recurs. Cases of infantile psoriasis may prove to be mild and occasionally even clear completely as the child gets older.[8] The prognosis of generalized erythrodermic or pustular psoriasis in infancy is more guarded, and treatment usually requires systemic retinoid therapy, as well as supportive care.

Boric Acid Poisoning

Boric acid poisoning is now very rare, but was seen in the past as a result of the frequent use of boric acid-containing powders and lotions for the treatment of diaper dermatitis. It presents with a maculopapular eruption that can evolve into a generalized erythroderma, the appearance of which has been likened to a boiled lobster. A positive Nikolsky sign and desquamation are additional features.[9] Like staphylococcal scalded skin syn-

cult disorder to diagnose because of its clinical similarity to both seborrheic dermatitis and atopic dermatitis. Infantile psoriasis can look like that seen in older individuals, with discrete oval erythematous plaques with white scale involving the trunk, extremities, and face. Psoriatic plaques in infants usually have less white scale than the typical hyperkeratotic plaque seen in adults. Facial involvement is more common in the infant, and the scalp, palms, and soles may have diffuse erythema and scaling. A periumbilical distribution may be helpful in distinguishing psoriasis from either seborrheic or atopic dermatitis. Pustular psoriasis, either in a diffuse distribution or limited to the palms and soles, may be seen rarely. In contrast to atopic dermatitis, psoriasis in young infants often involves the diaper area because it develops in areas of injured skin (the Koebner phenomenon), e.g. after a prior irritant or *Candida* diaper dermatitis (see Chapter 15).[4]

drome, the condition may be accentuated in periorificial and intertriginous areas. Alopecia may also develop. Affected infants are usually ill, with fever, irritability, vomiting, and diarrhea, which can progress to shock and even death.

Diffuse Mastocytosis

The various forms of cutaneous mastocytosis are discussed fully in Chapter 25. Only the rare diffuse form of the disease is associated with neonatal erythroderma.[10] The affected infant usually has generalized thickening of the skin, which can be subtle. The thickening is due to infiltration of the dermis by mast cells. Because these mast cells release histamine and other vasoactive substances, they cause the skin to be very reactive, with a tendency to develop erythema, flushing, and wheals. Urtication with minor trauma (Darier's sign), and blisters, which develop either spontaneously or superimposed upon wheals, may be seen. The absence of scale and the presence of the above findings differentiate mastocytosis from other causes of erythroderma.

Skin biopsy is diagnostic: there is a dense, band-like infiltrate of mast cells in the upper dermis, which can be confirmed with Giemsa stain.

INFECTIOUS DISEASES

Staphylococcal Scalded Skin Syndrome

Staphylococcal scalded skin syndrome (SSSS) is an uncommon cause of neonatal erythroderma (see Chapter 12). It is characterized by the abrupt onset of diffuse erythema, which rapidly evolves to erosive desquamation involving most skin surfaces. Although there is often periorificial accentuation, the staphylococcal toxin requires keratinizing epithelium and therefore spares mucous membrane surfaces. Epidermal sloughing, occurring with minor trauma, helps distinguish SSSS from the other causes of infantile erythroderma, with the exception of toxic epidermal necrolysis (TEN)[11] (see Chapter 12) and boric acid poisoning (see the previous discussion). Rarely, a widespread form of staphylococcal pustulosis can occur acutely in an otherwise healthy infant (personal observations, MK Spraker 1997, WL Weston 1997). The pustules develop on an erythematous macular base and are small and superficial. They subsequently desquamate, thereby mimicking a true erythroderma.

Candidiasis

Candidal infection can cause neonatal erythroderma in two clinical settings: intrauterine acquisition with the development of congenital candidiasis, and postnatal onset in very premature infants. Congenital candidiasis typically presents either at birth or within the first few days of life with generalized erythema, vesicles, pustules, papules, and scaling. The pustules can be subtle at first, with erythroderma predominating. The palms and soles are often involved, which may be a helpful clue to diagnosis. The condition can occur in either term or preterm infants. *Candida albicans* can also cause a diffuse burn-like erythema within the first 2 weeks of life in premature infants (See Fig. 14-4A);[12] the authors have seen a number of cases in which the diffuse scaling and erythema were most pronounced over the back.[13] The diagnosis is made by examination of skin scrapings (KOH preparation) and/or surface culture for *Candida*, or by skin biopsy. The latter will show fungal elements within the epidermis and/or dermis, mixed inflammatory infiltrates, and occasional areas of necrosis and hemorrhage.

The risk of extracutaneous disease and the prognosis depend on the gestational age of the infant. In term infants the prognosis is excellent, and topical antiyeast therapies are usually curative. In infants weighing less than 1500 g with either congenital or acquired generalized cutaneous candidiasis, there is a significant risk of disseminated disease, and parenteral antifungal agents are recommended. Skin biopsies of affected areas in such infants may be used to predict the ultimate dissemination of disease. In one series, the finding of subcorneal invasion of *Candida* on skin biopsy was associated with a 69% risk for disseminated disease.[13] Both conditions are discussed in more detail in Chapter 14.

Herpes Simplex

Although most cases of herpes simplex (HSV) infection have characteristic lesions localized on the presenting part, the so-called intrauterine variant of HSV can present at birth with either isolated or diffuse erythema, and scaling or crusted erosions on an erythematous base (see Chapter 13). It may be difficult to recognize clinically because vesicles may not be present.[14,15] This type of widespread involvement is generally associated with very severe neurologic disease. Multinucleated giant cells should be demonstrable on Tzanck smears of vesicular lesions. A skin biopsy, scrapings for direct fluorescent antibody staining, and viral cultures will help confirm the diagnosis.

Syphilis

Congenital syphilis may cause diffuse erythema and scaling (see Chapter 12). This presentation is most typically seen in infants at 6–8 weeks of age, in whom exposure to syphilis occurred either very late in pregnancy or at the time of delivery.[16] Superficial erosions or bullae over the hands or feet of a newborn, together with a diffuse scaling dermatitis (Fig. 17-2), should alert the practitioner to the possibility of syphilis. Infiltrated mucosal papules and plaques (condyloma lata) may be seen in a perianal location and are similar to the mucous patches seen on other mucous membrane sites in older patients with secondary syphilis. Periosteal changes of long bones, such

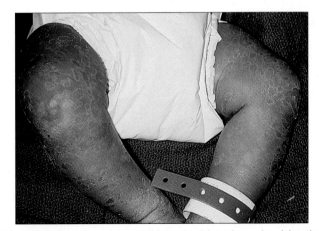

FIG. 17-2 Diffuse superficial scaling and mild erythema involving the skin of an infant with congenital syphilis.

as the clavicles, as well as hepatosplenomegaly, are additional features. Appropriate serologies are generally diagnostic, and darkfield examination of mucous membranes lesions should reveal spirochetes.

INHERITED DISEASES

Ichthyosis

The ichthyoses are a group of genetic disorders characterized by generalized skin scaling; generalized erythroderma is a common presentation for some types of ichthyosis (see Chapter 18). Many infants with this presentation have the congenital ichthyosiform erythroderma (CIE) phenotype,[17] which is notable for the diffuse erythematous appearance of the skin and overlying fine white scale (Fig. 17-3). Ectropion can occur

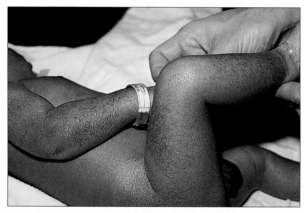

FIG. 17-3 Diffuse erythema with fine scale in an infant with nonbullous congenital ichthyosiform erythroderma.

but is less common, and when present is less severe than in patients with classic lamellar ichthyosis. In these patients there is less erythema and thicker, darker, more plate-like scale. Infants with autosomal dominant bullous ichthyosis (bullous CIE; epidermolytic hyperkeratosis) typically present with diffusely erythematous skin and mild hyperkeratosis, often in association with areas of denuded skin. The lack of mucous membrane involvement in bullous CIE helps distinguish it from epidermolysis bullosa. Over subsequent weeks and months the blistering subsides and is replaced by varying degrees of an ichthyosiform erythroderma. Ultimately, marked hyperkeratosis is evident diffusely, with accentuation on flexural surfaces. The characteristic histopathologic findings of epidermal cytolysis of the upper spinous and granular layers help confirm the diagnosis of bullous ichthyosis.

The ichthyosis most likely to be confused with other causes of erythroderma is Netherton syndrome, a rare disorder caused by mutations in *SPINK5*, which encodes a serine protease inhibitor.[18] Netherton syndrome is marked by severe diffuse erythroderma, scaling, and varying degrees of alopecia, including sparse eyebrows (Fig. 17-4).[19,20] Affected infants often fail to thrive as a result of the extreme metabolic demands presented by their skin disease, and they can also develop hypernatremic dehydration. Most have a markedly elevated IgE level. The diagnosis of Netherton syndrome is often delayed because of the late presentation of the diagnostic hair shaft abnormality, trichorrhexis invaginata (bamboo hair). Such hairs, when examined by routine light microscopy, will appear to have telescoped into themselves along the length of the shaft. Small bulbous areas of thickening at the site of the telescoping correspond to the areas of increased fragility and ultimate breakage of affected hairs. Plucking of eyebrow hairs and evaluation of multiple areas of the scalp over time may be

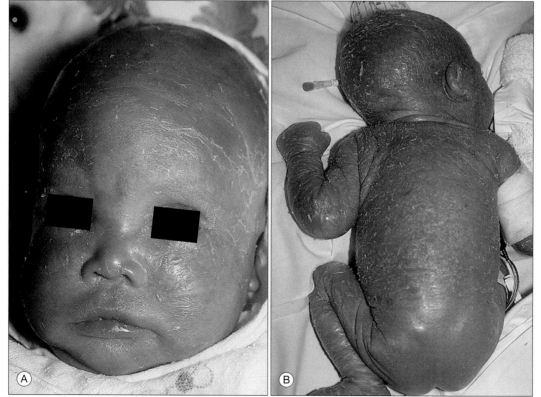

FIG. 17-4 Netherton's syndrome. Diffuse erythema, scale, and alopecia.

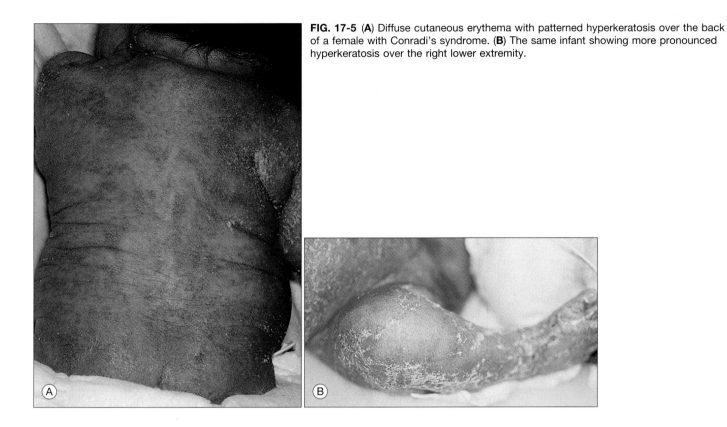

FIG. 17-5 (**A**) Diffuse cutaneous erythema with patterned hyperkeratosis over the back of a female with Conradi's syndrome. (**B**) The same infant showing more pronounced hyperkeratosis over the right lower extremity.

required to visualize the characteristic hair changes. Later in the course, patients may show a distinctive skin finding, ichthyosis linearis circumflexa. This is an erythematous scaling eruption with polycyclic and/or serpiginous morphology and elevated borders.

Sjögren–Larsson syndrome is due to a deficiency of fatty acid aldehyde dehydrogenase and can present with varying degrees of erythroderma.[21,22] A collodion membrane at birth is unusual. Affected infants may have a phenotype consistent with either CIE or lamellar ichthyosis. Nonprogressive spasticity and mental retardation become apparent during the early years of life. After the first year many affected patients have distinctive glistening dots seen on careful retinal examination.

Chondrodysplasia punctata (Conradi–Hünermann syndrome) presents with either diffuse erythroderma or bands of erythema, and a patterned ichthyosis occurring along Blaschko's lines (Fig. 17-5).[23,24] These areas of ichthyosis typically resolve and may be replaced by a follicular atrophoderma. This syndrome is also marked by skeletal defects (dwarfism), cataracts, and other features. Plain radiographs at the time of birth may show stippling of the epiphyseal areas of bones. Some cases have been found to be caused by a peroxisomal deficiency.

Infantile erythroderma can also be seen in keratosis–ichthyosis–deafness (KID) syndrome,[25,26] neutral lipid storage disease with ichthyosis (Chanarin–Dorfman syndrome),[27] and in newborns with trichothiodystrophy (Tay syndrome).[28]

Occasionally, males affected with X-linked hypohidrotic ectodermal dysplasia may present at birth with a mild diffuse erythroderma and fine superficial scaling (Fig. 17-6).[29] Such

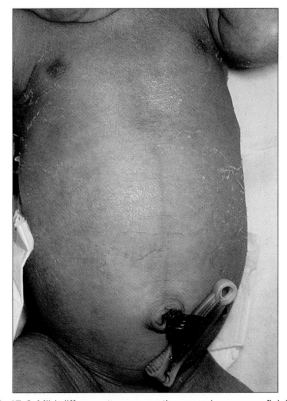

FIG. 17-6 Mild diffuse cutaneous erythema and very superficial scaling on a child with X-linked hypohidrotic ectodermal dysplasia. These findings were present at birth.

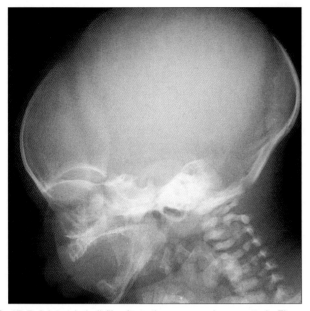

FIG. 17-7 A lateral skull film from the same male neonate in Figure 17-6, showing the absence of tooth buds.

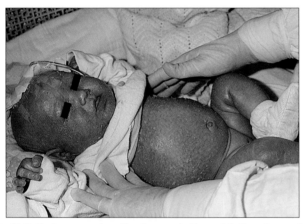

FIG. 17-8 Erythema and scaling is seen in the exfoliative phase of GVHD.

infants have the typical facial features of ED and sparse hair, lashes, and eyebrows. Periorbital hyperpigmentation and fine wrinkling can be seen at birth, and lateral plain films of the skull will demonstrate no or few tooth buds (Fig. 17-7).

IMMUNOLOGIC DISEASES

Graft-versus-host Disease

Graft-versus-host disease (GVHD) is caused by the interaction between immunocompetent lymphoid cells and immunodeficient host cells.[30] Nearly all cases in neonates and young infants are caused by severe T-cell immunodeficiency states (such as severe combined immunodeficiency) with maternal engraftment either in utero or at the time of delivery.[31] Clinically, affected infants typically present with a scaly erythematous rash that often begins on the scalp and face and moves downward. Fine erythematous papules may also occur. The findings may be patchy or diffuse, in some cases progressing to frank erythroderma (Fig. 17-8).[31,32] The most severe cuta-

neous manifestation of GVHD is toxic epidermal necrolysis, a finding that may rarely be evident at the time of delivery. Diffuse alopecia is a common finding and often involves the eyebrows as well as scalp hair. Although milder forms of GVHD sometimes respond (at least partially) to emollients or topical corticosteroids, recurrences are the rule. If unrecognized and untreated, GVHD progresses and may affect a variety of organ systems.

The diagnosis should be suspected in any young infant with erythroderma and frequent infections, chronic diarrhea, and/or failure to thrive. If present, a family history of prior early infant deaths is helpful because many forms of immunodeficiency are familial. Skin biopsy can be very useful in confirming the diagnosis. The histopathologic changes of GVHD are usually graded by severity (from I to IV).[33] Most authors agree that minimum criteria for the histopathologic diagnosis of GVHD include the presence of epidermal lymphocytes, dyskeratosis, and satellite cell necrosis. The latter refers to the finding of a lymphocyte apposed to an eosinophilic keratinocyte (dyskeratotic epidermal cell) within the epidermis. Similar changes may also result from the conditioning therapy utilized for some patients before bone marrow transplantation, as well as from the effect of certain viruses.[34,35] In some cases of GVHD caused by maternal engraftment, a spongiotic dermatitis may predominate.[31,36] Multiple skin biopsies obtained over days or weeks may be necessary if the diagnosis is strongly suspected, but without confirmatory histopathology. Immunophenotyping of skin biopsies has been used to complement the characteristic findings on routine histopathology described previously.[37] The finding of strong staining for HLA-DR within the epidermis is strongly suggestive of GVHD. It should be emphasized, however, that immunophenotyping alone should not be considered diagnostic of GVHD, and that the lack of such features should not discount the presence of compatible clinical and histopathologic findings of this condition.

Because the diagnosis of GVHD in the absence of a known organ or bone marrow transplant implies a severe immunodeficiency, a complete evaluation of the immune system should be undertaken. Although lymphopenia is characteristic of severe T-cell or severe combined immunodeficiency, the lymphocyte count in the blood may be normal or even elevated because of the presence of circulating maternal lymphocytes. Eosinophilia is often present. Although small numbers of circulating maternal cells are considered a normal finding in the first few weeks of life, the presence of large numbers of maternal lymphocytes is highly suggestive of an underlying immunodeficiency, and in the setting of erythroderma strongly suggests the diagnosis of GVHD. Maternal engraftment can be documented by demonstrating extra circulating HLA haplotypes, or by demonstrating an XX genotype in the blood of a male infant.[36,38]

The differential diagnosis is generally confined to other more common conditions, such as seborrheic dermatitis, infantile eczema, or the unusual viral or drug eruptions.

The course of this condition can be variable and depends on the degree of organ involvement, as well as the severity of the immunodeficiency. In most instances the skin can be treated with bland emollients, as well as low- or mid-potency topical corticosteroid preparations. More severe reactions, particularly those with systemic manifestations, may require systemic corticosteroid therapy, cytotoxic drugs, or monoclonal antibodies.[30] For subacute or chronic skin disease, in the absence of systemic involvement, phototherapy, either PUVA or narrowband UVB, has proved useful both as a primary therapy and as a means to decrease or discontinue altogether the use of systemic therapies.[39-41] Such therapy is reserved for older patients.

The skin manifestations of GVHD occurring after transplantation, or rarely resulting from transfusions, have been well characterized and include an acute phase with a morbilliform erythema, a papular dermatitis, diffuse erythroderma, or in severe cases, diffuse bullae or frank necrosis, such as are seen in toxic epidermal necrolysis. Often, such skin changes begin on the head and neck and extend in a caudal fashion. The palms and soles are usually predominantly involved. Chronic changes (more than 100 days post transplantation) may include oral mucous membrane changes, nail dystrophy, and localized or diffuse lichenoid (flat-topped) papules. Extracutaneous features of the disease are primarily gastrointestinal. A hepatitis may be found, as well as varying degrees of diarrhea. Skin biopsies of representative lesions will generally reveal features of GVHD, such as vacuolization of the basal cell layer and dyskeratosis within the epidermis.

Eosinophilic Gastroenteritis

Eosinophilic gastroenteritis was first reported by Waldman et al.,[42,43] who called the condition allergic gastroenteropathy. Cutaneous features included edema, particularly over the face, as well as generalized atopic dermatitis. The extracutaneous manifestations are striking and include growth retardation, extreme hypoalbuminemia, hypogammaglobulinemia, anemia, and eosinophilia, as well as mild gastrointestinal symptoms consisting of intermittent diarrhea or vomiting after the ingestion of certain foods, and excessive loss of protein into the gastrointestinal tract. Asthma and allergic rhinitis may also be present. Diagnosis is confirmed with intestinal biopsies, which reveal mucosal eosinophilia. The disease is now subclassified into protein-sensitive and idiopathic forms.[44] The protein-sensitive form is more common, responds to dietary restriction of cow's milk or soy protein, and ultimately resolves with time. The idiopathic form requires steroid therapy to control symptoms. The dermatitis improves rapidly and dramatically with resolution of the other symptoms when the dermatitis is aggressively treated.

Leiner's Phenotype

A chapter on infantile erythroderma would not be complete without a discussion of Leiner's disease, or what we prefer to call Leiner's phenotype. Leiner's disease or syndrome was initially described in 1908 by Dr Carl Leiner,[45,46] who reported a distinctive dermatitis he had seen in 43 children at a children's hospital in Vienna over 5 years. These infants developed a generalized erythematous desquamative dermatitis that appeared during the first few weeks of life but which was not present at birth. Most had diarrhea and weight loss, and the disease did not respond to any known topical or oral medication. Many improved when their diet was changed to rice water and cow's milk, but one-third died from their illness. Because all but two of these infants had been breastfed, he hypothesized that breastfeeding was causative. Similar patients were seen in Prague and Belgrade during and after World War II in a time of serious food shortages.[47] Many of these infants improved when fed cow's milk, so it was postu-

lated that the disease was caused by a deficiency of biotin, as the biotin content in cow's milk was higher than that of human milk.

Subsequently, the term Leiner's disease was often used to describe any infant with widespread dermatitis in association with diarrhea and/or failure to thrive. In 1968 two sibling infants with erythroderma, diarrhea, and failure to thrive, who also had an increased susceptibility to infection, were shown to have a yeast opsonization defect;[48] the dermatitis cleared in one of the children after an infusion of fresh frozen plasma. It was hypothesized that a yeast opsonization defect resulting from a dysfunction of the fifth component of complement was the cause of Leiner's disease. Additional patients were then studied, but most did not have this opsonization defect, which was subsequently shown to be quite common in the general population. Moreover, not all improved with fresh frozen plasma.[49]

In 1988 Glover et al.[50] reported a group of five infants with erythroderma, diarrhea, and failure to thrive. None had a yeast opsonization defect, but instead a variety of other immunologic abnormalities, including elevated IgE levels and hypogammaglobulinemia, were found. Some were subsequently diagnosed as having Netherton or Omenn syndromes.[50] This paper established the need to consider the diagnosis of immunodeficiency when evaluating erythrodermic infants, and established the multiple etiologies of what had formerly been called Leiner's disease.

Leiner's disease, if the term is used today, should be used to describe a clinical phenotype defined as an infant with (1) noncongenital or acquired erythroderma (Fig. 17-9); (2) diar-

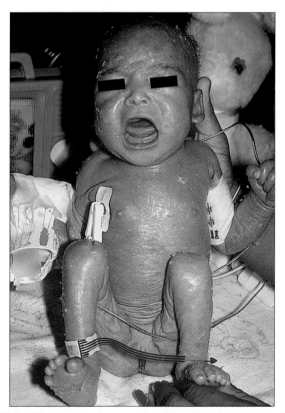

FIG. 17-9 Diffuse erythroderma and scaling with failure to thrive in an infant with hypogammaglobulinemia.

rhea; and (3) failure to thrive, without associating it with a specific immunologic defect. Infants with these findings need thorough investigations searching for the underlying cause of their disorder. Most of the diseases listed in Box 17-1 need to be considered, especially immunodeficiencies, Netherton syndrome, Omenn syndrome, and eosinophilic gastroenteritis (see the following discussion). Baseline immune studies of such infants should include chest radiograph, full blood count, quantitative immunoglobulins, and skin testing before or after specific immunizations. More detailed testing should be pursued as indicated.

The prognosis and treatment of this condition are entirely dependent on the specific diagnosis. The associated diarrhea and failure to thrive must be treated aggressively with adequate nutritional support up to and including parental hyperalimentation, as indicated.

EVALUATION AND MANAGEMENT OF THE RED SCALY BABY

The history and physical examination may provide important diagnostic clues to the etiology of erythroderma. Specific parameters that may be of value in determining an underlying cause include congenital onset; skin induration; and the presence of large scaling plaques, alopecia with or without hair dysplasia, evolution, response to corticosteroid therapy, presence of infections, and failure to thrive.[51] If the infant appears to have atopic or seborrheic dermatitis, then appropriate therapy can be instituted. If there is no response to therapy, or if the infant appears to be systemically ill, fails to thrive, or shows other evidence of a more generalized disease, a more comprehensive evaluation should be undertaken (Boxes 17-1 and 17-2). Laboratory tests useful in evaluating erythroderma in neonates and infants are outlined in Box 17-2. The selection of which tests to perform depends on which disease(s) are most suspected. Appropriate smears and cultures for fungal, bacterial, or viral disease should be performed if infection is suspected. A chest radiograph may be useful to evaluate the thymic shadow, which may be absent in neonates with SCID. IgG levels, if obtained during the first months of life, are reflective of maternal values. These may, however, be useful in infants over 6 months of age. Liver function tests may be indicated in primary or secondary nutritional disease, such as cystic fibrosis. In the latter, one would expect elevations of the transaminases and severely decreased serum albumin. Serum amino and urine organic acids are necessary to screen for suspected cases of primary metabolic diseases, such as the aminoacidurias or biotin deficiencies. A biotinidase level can be obtained if biotin deficiency is suspected. Lastly, skin biopsy can be useful for direct histopathologic examination of representative lesions, and fibroblast culture can help in definitive diagnosis of several metabolic diseases.

When an infant presents with erythroderma, immediate attention to fluid and electrolytes is paramount. For example, infants with ichthyosis can develop life-threatening hypernatremic dehydration. Infectious complications, primarily bacterial or fungal, must also be considered. These infants need a warm, humid environment to minimize their metabolic demands. Topical therapy consisting of bland emollients such as petrolatum or Aquaphor is helpful in minimizing transepidermal water loss and may decrease potential infectious complications.[52]

A summary of the evaluation and management of many of the disorders is found in Table 17-1.

IMMUNODEFICIENCY

Several types of immunodeficiency may produce similar initial clinical signs, with an eczematous dermatitis, diarrhea and failure to thrive. Children with a persistent eczematous eruption accompanied by failure to thrive may warrant an immunologic evaluation. The following discussion encompasses immunodeficiency syndromes with either erythroderma or other cutaneous manifestations in the neonatal period. These are outined in Table 17-2.

Severe Combined Immunodeficiency

Severe combined immunodeficiency (SCID) is a heterogeneous group of inherited disorders with similar clinical manifestations and immunologic deficiencies, with a profound deficiency of T lymphocytes and defects in both cellular and humoral immunity. Subtypes are classified by the abnormal development of other lymphocyte lineages, predominantly B lymphocytes and natural killer (NK) cells. Most cases are inherited in an autosomal recessive manner, although approximately 40% are X-linked recessive. About 20% of SCID is caused by adenosine deaminase (ADA) deficiency.[53]

The immunologic deficiency results in an increased susceptibility to bacterial, viral, fungal and protozoan infections. Recurrent infections, diarrhea, and failure to thrive are evident by 3–6 months of age.[54] Among the most common mucocutaneous infections are those due to *C. albicans*, *Staphylococcus aureus*, and *Streptococcus pyogenes*. In addition to infectious cutaneous manifestations, all reported forms SCID can present with a diffuse skin involvement, either erythroderma (see Fig. 17-8) or morbilliform or seborrheic dermatitis-like eruptions. Patients with SCID may develop

---

Box 17-2 Red scaly baby—laboratory evaluation

Gram stain (if infection suspected)

Fungal smear (if infection suspected)

Tzanck smear (if infection suspected)

Appropriate cultures (e.g. nasopharynx/rectum for viruses or staph)

Chest radiograph (may reveal absence thymic shadow in neonate with SCID)

CBC, platelets

Quantitative immunoglobulins

Isohemagglutinins

Liver function tests

Electrolytes

Plasma zinc

Biotinidase

RPR

HIV

Sweat chloride

Serum amino/urine organic acids

Trichogram

Skin biopsy

T/B cell functional/quantitative assays (by immunologist)

TABLE 17-1 Evaluation and management of disorders

Diagnosis	Usual onset	Clinical features	Associated features	Management
Inflammatory disorders				
Atopic dermatitis	Birth-6 months	Pruritus, xerosis, scaling, and erythema	Skin biopsy: acanthosis, spongiosis	Emollients Topical corticosteroids
Seborrheic dermatitis	Birth-1 month	Greasy scale: Scalp, face, body Erythema of body folds and diaper region	Skin biopsy shows features of mild dermatitis and is generally nonspecific	Routine cleansing; occasionally mild topical corticosteroids for short courses
Psoriasis	Birth-adulthood	Mild or thick scale over the scalp and, diaper areas as well as the abdomen. Periumbilical involvement is typical	Skin biopsy often shows features of chronic dermatitis; spongiotic pustules may rarely be seen	Emollients, low potency, corticosteroids, coal tar/petrolatum
Diffuse mastocytosis	Birth-2 months	Absence of scale Flushing Positive Darier's sign	Skin biopsy: dense dermal infiltrate of mast cells. Some infants may show severe syncope, diarrhea, or shock	Prevention of degranulation is important Counseling regarding direct mast cell degranulators should be offered Oral antihistamines (both H1 and H2)
Infectious diseases				
Staphylococcal scalded skin syndrome	Anytime	Diffuse cutaneous erythema followed by superficial desquamation. Mucous membranes are spared	Skin culture of nasopharynx, rectum, or pustule should grow S. aureus Skin biopsy shows superficial epidermal split	Appropriate antibiotics Superficial wound care
Candida	Birth or neonatal	Generalized erythema, papules, scaling, pustules, diffuse erythema	KOH examinations of scraping should be positive Cervical culture for yeast Skin biopsy should show typical fungal elements	Topical therapy for limited disease Systemic antifungal therapy for invasive/ disseminated disease
Herpes simplex	Birth or later	Grouped vesicles on erythematosus base over presenting part: erosions, scaling, erythema (intrauterine variant)	Tzanck smears showing multiple nucleated giant cells; skin biopsy will show intra-epidermal vesicles with ballooning degeneration of keratinocytes Viral culture should be diagnostic Direct fluorescent antibody of scrapings may also be done	Appropriate antiviral therapy
Congenital syphilis	Birth or 6–8 weeks	Bullae, erythema, scaling, eroded papules and plaques over anogenital areas	Dark field examination of mucous membrane lesions: spirochetes specific serology positive	Appropriate antibiotic therapy
Inherited diseases				
Ichthyosis	Birth or later	Diffuse scale, bullae with hyperkeratosis, patterned hyperkeratosis (depending on particular disorder)	Skin biopsy showing epidermolysis with (EHK); retinal changes (Sjögren-Larsson Syndrome);bone radiographs showing epiphyseal stipling (chondrodysplasia punctata)	Supportive, emollients, hydration
Immunologic diseases				
Leiner's phenotype	Weeks to months	Erythematous scaling, desquamative dermatitis, diarrhea, failure to thrive, alopecia	Immunoglobulin abnormalities, hair shaft abnormalities (Netherton's), T cell abnormalities	Definitive therapy depends on ultimate diagnosis; attention to fluid and electrolytes

graft-versus-host disease from nonirradiated blood products or engraftment of maternal lymphocytes (Fig. 17-10). Cutaneous manifestations vary from a morbilliform rash or exfoliative dermatitis in acute GVHD, to a lichenoid or sclerodermoid rash in chronic GVHD.[55] Early extracutaneous infections may also include viral-induced chronic diarrhea, otitis media, and pneumonia due to bacteria, viruses or *Pseudomonas carinii*.

The prognosis of SCID is poor, and without intervention most patients die from overwhelming infection by 1 year of

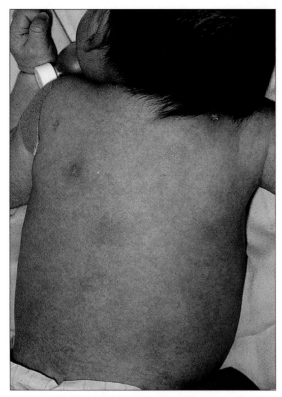

FIG. 17-10 A male child diagnosed with SCID. He manifested a diffusely distributed blanching erythema. The skin eruption was caused by post bone-marrow transplant GVHD.

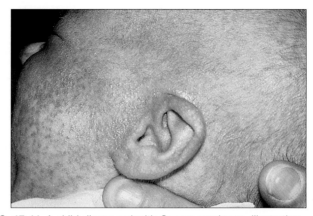

FIG. 17-11 A child diagnosed with Omenn syndrome, illustrating diffusely distributed scaling, erythematous papules. These findings were present over the entire skin surface.

age. Management includes protective isolation and vigorous treatment of infections. All blood products should be irradiated to prevent GVHD. HLA-identical bone marrow transplantation is the treatment of choice. Enzyme replacement with ADA coupled to polyethylene glycol (PEG-ADA) has helped several infants with ADA deficiency, and ADA is a target for gene therapy protocols.[53]

Omenn Syndrome

Omenn syndrome is a rare autosomal recessive form of SCID with reticuloendothelial cell proliferation caused by recombinase-activating gene (RAG1 or RAG2) deficiency in most patients. This syndrome was originally described as familial reticuloendotheliosis with eosinophilia. This T cell-deficient state is marked by abnormal histiocytic cells and extreme elevations of eosinophils in affected tissues and in the peripheral blood. During early infancy these patients develop a generalized exfoliative erythroderma (Fig. 17-11), lymphadenopathy, hepatosplenomegaly, recurrent infections, and failure to thrive.[56] Diffuse alopecia may be seen as well. Although the condition is primarily one of T-cell dysregulation, both humoral and cellular immune defects are seen.[57] Abnormal antibody production and elevated IgE levels occur. There is usually a marked leukocytosis with eosinophilia, anemia, hypogammaglobulinemia, and depressed T cell-mediated immunity. A gene defect has been identified that maps to chromosome 11, though some authors believe there is genetic heterogeneity.[58,59] The disorder is often difficult to distinguish from GVHD. The only known effective treatment is bone marrow transplantation.

DiGeorge Anomaly

The DiGeorge anomaly (DGA) is one of a group of disorders that have in common a chromosomal deletion resulting in monosomy 22q11, known as the DiGeorge syndrome chromosome region, or DGCR. A small fraction of patients with clinical features of DGA have deletions of chromosome 10p14.[60] Autosomal dominant, autosomal recessive and X-linked inheritance have all been reported. All forms are associated with a T-cell defect and normal humoral immunity. The compromise in T-cell production is a result of thymic hypoplasia or aplasia, which is in turn part of a larger developmental anomaly of the third and fourth pharyngeal pouches. In addition to the thymus defect, conotruncal cardiac anomalies, hypoparathyroidism, dysmorphism, and cleft palate are prominent features. Characteristic facial features include a short philtrum, low-set ears and hypertelorism.[61] Neonatal tetany may occur with hypocalcemia due to aplastic parathyroid glands.

Infants with DiGeorge syndrome can have a maculopapular or eczematous dermatitis that may become generalized.[62,63] Many patients have recurrent mucocutaneous candidal infections as neonates, as well as increased susceptibility to viral, Pneumocystis carinii and other fungal infections. GVHD may occur in patients who are given nonirradiated blood products. Noninfectious granulomas have also been described. Patients with DGA may have erythroderma, similar to that seen in Omenn syndrome, which occurs in association with a dramatic oligoclonal expansion of a few founding T cells, often of an exclusively memory type.[60]

Management of the immunodeficiency in DGA includes prophylactic trimethoprim/sulfamethoxazole. No live vaccines should be given and blood products should be irradiated. Patents with dramatically low levels of T cells should be considered for a HLA-identical bone marrow transplant or a thymus transplant.[60]

Wiskott–Aldrich Syndrome

Wiskott–Aldrich sydrome (WAS) is a rare X-linked recessive disorder characterized by recurrent pyogenic infections, bleeding due to thrombocytopenia, and recalcitrant eczematous dermatitis. The gene for WAS has been mapped to chromosome Xp11[20] and encodes for WAS protein (WASP), a cytoplasmic protein constitutively expressed in all hematopoietic stem cell-derived lineages.[64]

The most consistent finding in WAS is thrombocytopenia with small platelets. Because it is present from birth, initial presenting signs in the majority of patients are related complications such as petechiae, purpura, epistaxis, gastrointestinal bleeding, or intracranial hemorrhage.[65] Recurrent bacterial infections begin in infancy and include otitis media, pneumonia, infectious diarrhea, sinusitis, meningitis, and septicemia. There is also increased susceptibility to viruses and *Pneumocystis carinii*. There is also an increased risk of autoimmune disease and malignancy, mainly lymphoreticular malignancies.[66] Laboratory examination may also reveal characteristic elevated IgA and IgE and decreased IgM.[64]

Dermatitis usually develops during the first few months of life and meets the criteria for atopic dermatitis (See Fig. 15-14). The face, scalp, and flexural areas are usually the most severely involved, although involvement can be widespread. Excoriated areas often have associated petechiae or purpura, and secondary infection of eczematous lesions is common, as are eczema herpeticum and molluscum.[66] Other infections of the skin may be present independently, and may include impetigo, cellulites, and abscesses.

Treatment is largely symptomatic and includes antibiotics and intravenous immunoglobulin in selected cases. Splenectomy may be used to treat thrombocytopenia, although there is an increased risk of postsplenectomy sepsis. Platelet transfusion is reserved for cases of life-threatening hemorrhage.[66] Blood products should be irradiated. At present, BMT or cord blood stem cell transplant is the only curative therapy for WAS.[65]

Hyperimmunoglobulin E Syndrome

Hyperimmunoglobulin E (hyper-IgE) syndrome, formerly also known as Job syndrome, consists of a severe dermatitis with recurrent abscess formation and recurrent sinopulmonary infections associated with markedly elevated serum IgE levels.[67] Inheritance follows an autosomal dominant pattern with variable penetrance.

The severe dermatitis may be present from birth or early childhood, and as in atopic dermatitis the rash is typically pruritic and often lichenified, although its distribution may be atypical for true atopic dermatitis (See Figs 10-8 and 15-17). A distinct papulopustular eruption of the face and scalp has been reported in the first year of life.[68]

Cutaneous infections are frequent and start in infancy. They may take the form of crusted plaques, pustules, furuncles, cellulitis, lymphangitis, or abscesses. The abscesses may be erythematous and tender, or may be fluctuant masses which are neither hot nor tender and are not associated with systemic symptoms ('cold abscesses'). They are filled with pus that grows *Staphylococcus aureus*. This diagnosis should be considered in children with recurrent abscesses complicating chronic eczema. Skin biopsy reveals an eosinophilic infiltrate similar to that seen in eosinophilic pustular folliculitis. Infection with nonbacterial pathogens may also occur, especially *Candida* infections of the mouth, nails, and skin.[69]

In addition to skin infections, sinopulmonary and bone infections are common. *S. aureus* is also the most common organism for these infections. Skeletal abnormalities are seen in hyper-IgE syndrome, particularly long bone fractures, which occur with minimal trauma.[69] Coarse facial features manifested by a prominent forehead and a broad nasal bridge are typically not seen at birth but appear later in childhood.

The management of hyper-IgE syndrome includes prophylactic antibiotics to prevent *S. aureus* infections. The eczematous dermatitis may require treatment with topical corticosteroids to reduce inflammation and antihistamines to control pruritus. Incision and drainage may be required for abscesses.[70]

Chronic Granulomatous Disease

Chronic granulomatous disease (CGD) represents a group of genetic disorders in which impaired intracellular microbial killing by phagocytes leads to recurrent bacterial and fungal infections and granuloma formation. Defects in the nicotinamide dinucleotide phosphate (NADPH) oxidase complex result in failure to generate superoxide radicals during the respiratory burst, leading to an inability of phagocytic lymphocytes to kill intracellular bacteria and fungi, especially *Aspergillus* spp. CGD can be caused by mutations in any of the four structural genes of the NADPH oxidase. The most common type is X-linked recessive, and the remainder are autosomal recessive.[71]

The earliest lesions are usually staphylococcal infections of the skin around the nose and mouth, which may be present at birth. Skin abscesses, usually caused by *S. aureus*, occur in 42% of patients. Purulent inflammatory reactions may occur at sites of minor cutaneous trauma or sites of regional lymph node drainage with suppurative lymphadenitis.[72] There are also reports of cutaneous granulomas containing the typical pigmented macrophages also seen in visceral granulomas.[73]

The extracutaneous organs most frequently involved are the lymph nodes, lungs, and liver. Bronchopneumonia is the most prevalent infection, with abscess formation and empyema as frequent complications. These patients have hepatosplenomegaly, and granulomas of the liver and spleen are common. Hepatic abscesses are usually caused by *S. aureus* and may require surgical drainage.

The screening test for CGD is the nitroblue tetrazolium (NBT) reduction assay. Management includes antibacterial and antifungal prophylaxis. Patients with all forms of CGD have shown clinical improvement after administration of subcutaneous recombinant IFN-γ.[74] HLA-matched BMT has also been performed successfully in CGD.

METABOLIC DISORDERS

Disorders of metabolism often present during the neonatal period and may exhibit skin manifestations. Rarely, metabolic diseases are associated with erythroderma, either shortly after birth, or later resulting from subsequent therapeutic dietary restrictions. Although cutaneous manifestations may be seen with such diseases, many metabolic disorders manifest themselves with feeding or neurological abnormalities, or through biochemical abnormalities alone.[75,76] Lysosomal storage diseases may present with coarse facial features as well as organomegaly.

Many metabolic conditions have been well described over the last several decades and are now associated with docu-

TABLE 17-2 Immunodeficiency syndromes with cutaneous manifestations in the neonatal period

Immunodeficiency	Cause/gene	Infectious organisms	Cutaneous findings	Associated findings
Severe combined immunodeficiency	T-cell deficiency (20% ADA deficiency)	Bacterial (*S. aureus, S. pyogenes*) Viral Fungal (*C. albicans*) Protozoan	Erythroderma Morbilliform Seborrheic dermatitis-like GVHD	Diarrhea Failure to thrive Pneumonia
Omenn's syndrome	RAG gene mutation	Same as SCID	Erythroderma Alopecia	Lymphadenopathy Hepatosplenomegaly Failure to thrive Elevated IgE, eosinophilia
DiGeorge anomaly	Monosomy 22q11 Deletion 10p14	Fungal Viral *Pneumocystis carinii*	Eczematous dermatitis Erythroderma GVHD	Thymic aplasia/hypoplasia Cardiac anomalies Hypoparathyroidism Cleft palate
Wiskott-Aldrich syndrome	WAS gene	Bacterial Viral *Pneumocystis carinii*	Eczematous dermatitis Petechiae, purpura	Thrombocytopenia Autoimmune disease Lymphoreticular malignancy
Hyperimmunoglobulin E syndrome	STAT3 mutations (some patients)	*S. aureus* *Candida*	Severe dermatitis Abscesses	Sinopulmonary infections Elevated IgE Bone fractures
Chronic granulomatous disease	Impaired phagocyte killing NADPH oxidase genes	Bacterial Fungal (*Aspergillus*)	Granulomas	Pulmonary infections Hepatic abscesses Hepatosplenomegaly

mented molecular bases. Evidence of this is the increase in size of major texts devoted to this group of diseases, such as *The Metabolic Basis of Inherited Diseases*, which was published in one volume in 1960 and which now as *The Metabolic and Molecular Basis of Inherited Diseases* consists of four volumes.

Case Report

A male infant born to unrelated parents was seen at 5 months of age for an erythematous dermatitis involving intertriginous areas. This was treated with topical steroids and dietary management for presumed atopic dermatitis, seborrheic dermatitis, and candidiasis. At 11 months the dermatitis had worsened and the child then manifested fever, feeding problems, and irritability. He was also tachypneic and hypotonic. He demonstrated psychomotor delay. Laboratory studies showed a severe metabolic acidosis with elevated serum lactate and ketonuria. Serum amino acids showed elevated alanine, and urinary organic acid investigation suggested multiple carboxylase deficiency (typically, elevated 3-hydroxyisovalerate, 3-methylcrotonylglycine, methylcitrate, and 3-hydroxypropionate). This was confirmed by enzymatic assay on cultured fibroblasts. Biotinidase was normal. The child was supplemented with biotin and responded well.[77] Other such cases may not respond well to biotin supplementation, perhaps because of a variety of mutations in the affected gene(s).[77,78] This case illustrates the varied presentation of children with inherited metabolic disease.

Metabolic diseases can be bewildering to consider for any clinician. An appreciation of a classification system is helpful when considering this group of diseases, in addition to a clinical basis for their presentation. Such conditions can be considered under headings of organic acid disorders, fatty acid oxidation disorders, disorders of amino acid metabolism, and others such as biotinidase deficiency, galactosemia, and cystic fibrosis.[79] A few of these diseases with erythroderma as a manifestation are highlighted below; the others are summarized in Tables 17–3 and 17–4.

TABLE 17-3 Classification of inherited metabolic disorders

Organic acid disorders	Fatty acid disorders	Amino acid disorders	Others
BKT	MCAD	PKU	BIOT
GA 1	VLCAD	MSUD	GALT
HMG	LCHAD	HCY	CF
MCD	CUD	CIT	LSD
IVA			
MUT			
3MCC			
Cb1 A, B			
PROP			

BKT: β-ketothiolase deficiency; GA-1: glutaric academia, type 1; HMG: 3-OH 3-CH3 glutaric aciduria; MCD: multiple carboxylase deficiency; IVA: isovaleric academia; MUT: methylmalonic acidemia (mutase deficiency); 3MCC: 3-methylcrotonyl-CoA carboxylase deficiency; Cb 1 A, B: methylmalonic acidemia (cobalamin 1 A, B); PROP: propionic academia; MCAD: medium-chain acyl-CoA dehydrogenase deficiency; VLCAD: very long-chain acyl-CoA dehydrogenase deficiency; LCHAD: long-chain L-3-OH acyl-CoA dehydrogenase deficiency; CUD: carnitine uptake defect; PKU: phenylketonuria; MSUD: maple syrup urine disease; HCY: homocystinuria; CIT: citrullinemia; ASA: argininosuccinyl-CoA lyase deficiency (argininosuccinic aciduria); BIOT: biotinidase deficiency; GALT: classical galactosemia; CF: cystic fibrosis; LSD: lysosomal storage disease
Modified from Seashore and Seashore[79] p 183

TABLE 17-4 Clinical clues to metabolic disorders

Clinical sign/Lab finding	Differential diagnosis	Suggested testing
Metabolic acidosis without lactic acidosis or ketonuria	Pyroglutamic aciduria	Urine organic acids
Metabolic acidosis without lactic acidosis, with ketonuria	Organic acidemias	Urine organic acids Plasma acylcarnitine profile
Lactic acidosis with ketonuria	Pyruvate carboxylase deficiency (severe) Glycogen storage disease I	Urine organic acids Plasma amino acids
Lactic acidosis, no ketonuria	Pyruvate carboxylase deficiency (mild) Pyruvate dehydrogenase deficiency Mitochondrial dysfunction Hypoxia or hypoperfusion	Urine organic acid analysis
Hyperammonemia, moderate-severe	Urea cycle disorders Organic acidemias Transient hyperammonemia of newborn HHH syndrome Lysinuric protein intolerance	Plasma amino acids Plasma acylcarnitine profile Urine organic acids
Hyperammonemia, mild-moderate	Organic acidemias Severe pyruvate carboxylase deficiency Fatty acid oxidation disorders Carnitine disorders Non-fasting sample	Urine organic acids Plasma amino acids Plasma acylcarnitine profile Plasma carnitine, free & total
Hypoglycemia	Fatty acid oxidation disorders Carnitine disorders Glycogen storage diseases Hyperinsulinism	Urine organic acids Plasma acylcarnitine profile Plasma carnitine, free & total
Seizures	Non-ketotic hyperglycinemia Sulfite oxidase deficiency Molybdenum cofactor deficiency Pyridoxal phosphate sensitive encephalopathy Serine deficiency disorder GLUT-1 deficiency	Plasma amino acids CSF amino acids Urine sulfite (dipstick) Blood and CSF glucose
Liver disease	Galactosemia Disorders of bile acid synthesis	Galactose-1-phosphate (RBC) GALT enzyme assay (RBC)
Cataracts	Galactosemia, mitochondrial dysfunction	Galactose and galactose-1-phosphate. GALT enzyme assay, urine organic acids
Neutropenia	Bath syndrome, glycogen storage disease 1b, organic acidemias, abnormalities of folate and B12 metabolism	Urine organic acids, plasma total homocysteine, plasma amino acids
Cardiomyopathy, arrhythmia	Long chain fatty acid oxidation disorders, carnitine disorders, Barth syndrome, mitochondrial dysfunction	Plasma acylcarnitine profile Plasma carnitine, free & total Urine organic acids

ORGANIC ACID DISORDERS

Methylmalonic Acidemia

Methylmalonic acidemia (MMA) is an inborn error of metabolism inherited in an autosomal recessive manner.[80,81] It is a group of diseases caused by a defect in the metabolism of branched-chain amino acids, which results in the accumulation of methylmalonic acid. Although some cases of methylmalonic acidemia, especially those caused by a cobalamin F and cobalamin C type of defect, have presented with a dermatitis similar to that seen in acrodermatitis enteropathica,[80,81] more commonly the dermatitis begins after the institution of dietary restrictions.[82] In either case the appearance is similar and in a primarily periorificial location. There are erythema and ulceration in the corners of the mouth and genital areas. A more diffuse dermatitis resembling SSSS has also been described. Extracutaneous manifestations can include poor feeding, vomiting, hypotonia, and acidosis, often leading to coma and death.

Assays for serum amino acid and metabolic analysis of cultured skin fibroblasts from affected patients confirm the diagnosis. Urinary organic acids should also be examined for elevations of methyl malonate and homocystine. Skin biopsy shows vacuolar dermatitis with dyskeratotic keratinocytes, mild psoriasiform changes, and epidermal pallor as seen in acrodermatitis enteropathica. There is a lymphocytic perivascular infiltrate within the dermis, as well as areas of orthokeratosis and parakeratosis, with spongiosis of the epidermis. The differential diagnosis of this disease includes other metabolic and nutritional deficiency states, such as acrodermatitis enteropathica, other aminoacidurias, and biotinidase deficiency. Management consists of dietary restrictions of branched-chain amino acids, specifically isoleucine and valine, and in those cases marked by cobalamin deficiency, supplementation with cobalamin. The prognosis of MMA is guarded, with many patients remaining severely impaired neurologically in spite of aggressive dietary support.

FATTY ACID DISORDERS

Essential Fatty Acid Deficiency

Essential fatty acid (EFA) deficiency was seen more frequently before 1975, in patients on parenteral hyperalimentation, before the need for EFA supplementation was recognized.[83] It is now an extremely unusual condition. It presents with a diffuse fine desquamation and mild or even absent erythema. The condition sometimes occurs in patients with severe fat malabsorption and may be one of the causes of the dermatitis of cystic fibrosis.

AMINO ACID DISORDERS

Maple Syrup Urine Disease and Other Inborn Errors of Metabolism

In maple syrup urine disease (MSUD)[84–88] diffuse exfoliative erythroderma has been well described. MSUD is another inborn error of metabolism in which the metabolism of branched-chain amino acids is defective. There is an abnormality in the degradation of the branched-chain amino acids causing diagnostic elevations of isoleucine, leucine, and valine in the serum, as well as in urine and cultured tissue fibroblasts. An erythematous scaling eruption that becomes erosive begins in a primarily periorificial distribution within days after initiating dietary therapy. The eruption is similar to that seen in acrodermatitis enteropathica. It can generalize, however. Such infants may also present with poor feeding, vomiting, lethargy, and seizures. Death may occur if the disorder is not promptly recognized. The problem may be caused by low isoleucine levels due to the dietary restrictions required for the disease. A similar, albeit milder dermatitis has been induced in infants fed diets deficient in isoleucine,[89] and similar eruptions have also been noted in citrullinemia,[90] carbamoyl phosphate synthetase deficiency, and argininosuccinicaciduria.[91] The cause of the dermatitis in each of these cases is also presumed to be caused by an abnormality of branched-chain amino acids, such as isoleucine. Histopathology of skin biopsies may show a very superficial perivascular lymphohistiocytic infiltrate with erosion of the outer epidermis, again as

may be seen in skin biopsies from patients with other inborn errors of metabolism. The differential diagnosis includes other inborn errors of metabolism in which periorificial dermatitis may occur after initiation of dietary therapy, such as propionic acidemia and methylmalonic acidemia[92] (Fig. 17-12). Treatment requires diligent attention to dietary restrictions. The diet must be liberalized so that sufficient branched-chain amino acids are delivered to raise plasma concentrations above the subnormal range.

OTHER DISORDERS

Cystic Fibrosis

Infants with cystic fibrosis (CF) can develop widespread, scaly erythematous lesions as a manifestation of global malnutrition during the first 3 or 4 months of life, and these are occasionally the initial presentation of CF.[93–95] The dermatitis is variable. A diffuse erythematous papular dermatitis, diffuse desquamating erythema or erythroderma, or a distinctly periorificial erythema and scaling may be seen (Fig. 17-13). However, in the author's experience most infants present with impressive generalized desquamative erythroderma. The der-

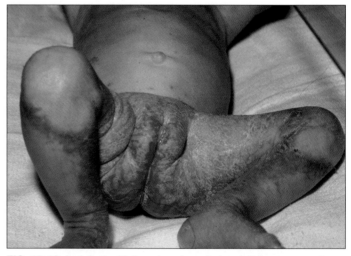

FIG. 17-12 An infant with tyrosinemia and zinc deficiency presents with perineal scaly plaques similar to the eruption seen in acrodermatitis enteropathica.

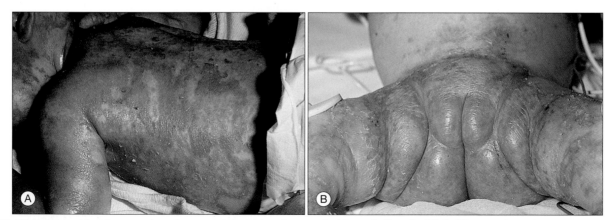

FIG. 17-13 (A) Diffuse erythroderma and scaling on an infant later diagnosed with cystic fibrosis. **(B)** A different infant with periorificial erythema and scale. This child was later diagnosed with cystic fibrosis.

matitis does not respond to treatment with topical corticosteroids or antifungals. In contrast to infants affected with classic acrodermatitis enteropathica, infants with cystic fibrosis typically lack paronychial involvement. Affected infants often have mild depressions of zinc levels, increased liver transaminases, and normal or slightly depressed levels of alkaline phosphatase. The dermatitis of CF occasionally clears with zinc therapy, but does so more reliably with appropriate enzyme replacement and nutritional supplements.

In spite of the abundance of diagnostic testing for metabolic diseases, most are not currently included in mandated state newborn screening programs.[79] Newborn screening began with testing for phenylketonuria (PKU) in 1940 and – in addition to hypothyroidism – might include only galactosemia routinely. Testing availability varies by locality.[96] The American College of Medical Genetics established a task force which has suggested that 30 conditions be screened in newborn infants in the whole of the United States.[97] The importance of such screening is intervention at a time in advance of the often devastating consequences of these disorders. Many of these disorders will present during the first week of life with metabolic acidosis and/or hyperammonemia, as well as altered neurologic status or emesis. Such findings are nonspecific and may be initially diagnosed as sepsis. Severe mental status alteration, however, should be a clue to a primary metabolic disease. Extreme elevations in the anion gap will suggest organic acidemias, such as propionic acidemia, methylmalonic academia, isovaleric acidemia, or multiple carboxylase deficiency. Elevations in serum ammonia levels may be a sign of the organic acid disorders, as well as urea cycle abnormalities, mitochondrial diseases, or disorders of fatty acid β-oxidation. Table 17-4 lists diseases to be considered when a clinical or laboratory finding is present, along with suggested testing.

Many of these disorders now have well-described molecular diagnoses. Most are inherited in either autosomal recessive or X-linked recessive fashion. Basic screening tests include plasma amino acid levels and urine organic acids. Screening for acylcarnitine levels can provide clues to both organic acidurias and fatty acid oxidation disorders, such as medium-chain acyl-CoA dehydrogenase deficiency (MCAD). Serum amino acid studies will diagnose disorders such as maple syrup urine disease and homocystinuria. More specific testing is required for disorders such as biotinidase deficiency, galactosemia, cystic fibrosis, peroxisomal, or lysosomal storage diseases. Clinicians caring for infants should be aware of the often broad and nonspecific presentation of metabolic disorders and work closely with genetic/metabolic consultants. The goal of prompt diagnosis and treatment is to attempt to avoid the severe long-term sequelae of neurologic deficits or death.

REFERENCES

1. Bonifazi E, Meneghini CL. Atopic dermatitis in the first six months of life. Acta Dermatol Venereol 1989; 144: 20–22.
2. Yates VM, Kerr R, Frier K, et al. Early diagnosis of infantile seborrheic dermatitis and atopic dermatitis – total and specific IgE levels. Br J Dermatol 1983; 108: 639–645.
3. Puissant A. Psoriasis in children under the age of ten: A study of 100 observations. Gazetta Sanitaria 1970; 19: 191.
4. Janniger CK, Schwartz RA, Musumeci ML, et al. Infantile psoriasis. Cutis 2005; 76: 173–177.
5. Beylot C, Puissant A, Bioulac P, et al. Particular clinical features of psoriasis in infants and children. Acta Dermatol Venereol 1979; 87: 95–97.
6. Ivker RA, Grim-Jorgensen CM, Vega VK, et al. Infantile generalized pustular psoriasis associated with lytic lesions of the bone. Pediatr Dermatol 1993; 10: 277–282.
7. Abou-Samra T, Constantin J-M, Amarger S, et al. Generalized pustular psoriasis complicated by acute respiratory distress syndrome. Br J Dermatol 2004; 150, 353–356.
8. Farber EM, Mullen RH, Jacobs AH, et al. Infantile psoriasis: A follow-up study. Pediatr Dermatol 1986; 3: 237–243.
9. Valdes-Dapena MA, Arey JB. Boric acid poisoning. J Pediatr 1962; 61: 521.
10. Has C, Misery L, David L, et al. Recurring staphylococcal scalded skin syndrome-like bullous mastocytosis: the utility of cytodiagnosis and the rapid regression with steroids. Pediatr Dermatol 2002; 19: 220–223.
11. Lohmeier K, Megahed M, Schulte, KW, et al. Toxic epidermal necrolysis in a premature infant of 27 weeks' gestational age. Br J Dermatol 2005; 152: 150–151.
12. Smolinski KN, Shah SS, Honig PJ, et al. Neonatal cutaneous fungal infections. Curr Opin Pediatr 2005; 17: 486–493.
13. Rowan JL, Atkins JT, Levy ML, et al. Invasive fungal dermatitis in the < or 1000 gm neonate. Pediatrics 1995; 95: 682.
14. Hutto C, Arvin A, Jacobs R, et al. Intrauterine herpes simplex infections. J Pediatr 1987; 110: 97–101.
15. Honig PJ, Brown D. Congenital herpes simplex infection initially resembling epidermolysis bullosa. J Pediatr 1982; 101: 958–960.
16. Chawla V, Pandit PB, Nkrumah FK. Congenital syphilis in the newborn. Arch Dis Child 1988; 63: 1393–1394.
17. Williams ML, Elias PM. Heterogeneity in autosomal recessive ichthyosis: Clinical and biochemical differentiation of lamellar ichthyosis and non-bullous congenital ichthyosiform erythroderma. Arch Dermatol 1985; 121: 477–488.
18. Chavanas S, Bodemer C, Rochat A, et al. Mutations in SPINK5, encoding a serine protease inhibitor, cause Netherton syndrome. Nature Genet 2000; 25: 141–142.
19. Fartasch M, Williams ML, Elias PM. Altered lamellar body secretion and stratum corneum membrane structure in Netherton syndrome: differentiation from other infantile erythrodermas and pathogenic implications. Arch Dermatol 1999; 135: 823–832.
20. Judge MR, Morgan G, Harper JI. A clinical and immunological study of Netherton's syndrome. Br J Dermatol 1994; 131: 615–621.
21. Williams ML, Shwayder TA. Ichthyosis and disorders of cornification. In: Schachner LA, Hansen RC, eds. Pediatric dermatology. New York: Churchill Livingstone, 1995; 413–418.
22. Alio AM, Bird LM, McClellan SD, et al. Sjogren–Larsson syndrome: a case report and literature review. Cutis 2006; 78: 61–65.
23. Kalter DC, Atherton DJ, Clayton PT. X-linked dominant Conradi–Hunermann syndrome presenting as congenital erythroderma. J Am Acad Dermatol 1989; 21: 248–256.
24. Corbi MR, Conejo-Mir JS, Linares M, et al. Conradi–Hunermann syndrome with unilateral distribution. Pediatr Dermatol 1998; 15: 299–303.
25. Nazzaro V, Blanchet-Burdon C, Lorette G, et al. Familial occurrence of KID (keratosis, ichthyosis, deafness) syndrome. Case reports of a mother and daughter. J Am Acad Dermatol 1990; 23: 385–388.
26. Lenane P, Cammisuli S, Chitayat D, et al. What syndrome is this? KID syndrome (keratitis, ichthyosis, deafness). Pediatr Dermatol 2006; 23: 81–81.
27. Srebrnik A, Tur E, Perluk C, et al. Dorfman–Chanarin syndrome: A case report and a review. J Am Acad Dermatol 1987; 17: 801–808.

28. Happle R, Traupe H, Grobe H, et al. The Tay syndromes (congenital ichthyosis with trichothiodystrophy). Eur J Pediatr 1984; 147–152.

29. Executive and SCIENTIFIC ADVISORY BOARDS of the National Foundation for Ectodermal Dysplasia. Scaling skin in the neonate: A clue to the early diagnosis of X-linked hypohidrotic ectodermal dysplasia (Christ–Siemens–Touraine syndrome). J Pediatr 1989; 114: 600–602.

30. Dinulos JG, Levy ML. Graft-versus-host disease in children. Semin Dermatol 1995; 14: 66–69.

31. Denianke KS, Frieden IJ, Cowan MJ. Cutaneous manifestations of maternal engraftment in patients with severe combined immunodeficiency: a clinicopathologic study. Bone Marrow Transplant 2001; 28: 227–233.

32. Farrell A. Scerri L, Stevens A, et al. Acute graft-versus-host disease with unusual cutaneous intracellular vacuolation in an infant with severe combined immunodeficiency. Pediatr Dermatol 1995; 12: 311–313.

33. Lerner KG, Kao GF, Storb R, et al. Histopathology of graft-vs-host reaction (GVHR) in human recipients of marrow from HLA matched sibling donors. Transplant Proc 1974; 6: 367–371.

34. Sale GE, Lerner KG, Barker EA, et al. The skin biopsy in the diagnosis of acute graft-versus-host disease in man. Am J Pathol 1977; 89: 621–635.

35. Fujinami RS, Nelson JA, Walker L, et al. Sequence homology and immunologic cross-reactivity of human cytomegalovirus with HLA-DR chain: A means for graft rejection and immunosupression. J Virol 1988; 62: 100–105.

36. Appleton AL, Curtis A, Wilkes J, et al. Differentiation of materno-fetal GVHD from Omenn's syndrome in pre-BMT patients with severe combined immunodeficiency. Bone Marrow Transplant 1994; 14: 157–159.

37. Paller AS, Nelson A, Steffan L. T-lymphocyte subsets in the lesional skin of allogeneic and autologous bone marrow transplant patients. Arch Dermatol 1988; 124: 1795–1801.

38. Katz F, Malcolm S, Strobel S, et al. The use of locus-specific minisatellite probes to check engraftment following allogenic bone marrow transplantation for severe combined immunodeficiency disease. Bone Marrow Transplant 1990; 5: 199–204.

39. Hymes SR, Morison WL, Farmer ER, et al. Methoxsalen and ultraviolet A radiation in treatment of chronic cutaneous graft-vs-host reaction. J Am Acad Dermatol 1985; 12: 30–70.

40. Vogelsa GB, Wolff D, Altomonte V, et al. Treatment of chronic graft-versus-host disease with ultraviolet irradiation and psoralen (PUVA). Bone Marrow Transplant 1996; 17: 1061–1067.

41. Grundmann-Kollmann M, Martin H, Ludwig R, et al. Narrowband UV-B phototherapy in the treatment of cutaneous graft versus host disease. Transplantation 2002; 75: 1631–1634.

42. Waldman TA, Wochner RD, Laster L, et al. Allergic gastroenteropathy – a cause of excessive gastrointestinal protein loss. N Engl J Med 1967; 276: 761–769.

43. Jenkins HR, Walker-Smith JA, Atherton DO. Protein-losing enteropathy in atopic dermatitis. Pediatr Dermatol; 1986; 3: 125–129.

44. Katz AJ, Twarog FJ, Zeiger RS, et al. Milk sensitive and eosinophilic gastroenteropathy: Similar clinical features with contrasting mechanisms and clinical course. J Allergy Clin Immunol 1984; 74: 72–78.

45. Leiner C. Über erythrodermia disquamativa, eine eingenartige universalle dermatose der brustlkinder. Arch Dermatol Syphilol 1908; 89: 163–189.

46. Leiner C. Erythodermia desquamation (universal dermatitis of children at the breast). Br J Child Dis 1908; 5: 244–251.

47. Vujasin J, Petrovic D. Biotin in some erythemato-squamous dermatoses of babies. Dermatologica 1952; 105: 180–183.

48. Miller ME, Seals J, Kaye R, et al. A familial, plasma-associated defect of phagocytosis. Lancet 1968; ii: 60–63.

49. Weston WL, Humber JR. Failure of fresh plasma in Leiner disease. Arch Dermatol 1977; 113: 233–234.

50. Glover MT, Atherton DJ, Levinsky RJ. Syndrome of erythroderma, failure to thrive and diarrhea in infancy: A manifestation of immunodeficiency. Pediatrics 1988; 81: 66–72.

51. Pruszkowski A, Bodemer C, Fraitag S, et al. Neonatal and infantile erythrodermas. Arch Dermatol 2000; 136: 875–880.

52. Nopper AJ, Horii KA, Sokdeo-Drost S, et al. Topical ointment therapy benefits premature infants. J Pediatr 1996; 128: 660–669.

53. Fischer A. Severe combined immunodeficiencies (SCID). Clin Exp Immunol 2000; 122: 143–149.

54. Hague RA, Rassam S, Morgan G, et al. Early diagnosis of severe combined immunodeficiency syndrome. Arch Dis Child 1999; 70: 260–263.

55. De Raeve L, Song M, Levy J, et al. Cutaneous lesions as a clue to severe combined immunodeficiency. Pediatr Dermatol 1992; 9: 49–51.

56. Pupo RA, Tyring SK, Raimer SS, et al. Omenn's syndrome and related combined immunodeficiency syndromes: Diagnostic considerations in infants with persistent erythroderma and failure to thrive. J Am Acad Dermatol 1991; 25: 442–446.

57. Omenn GS. Familial reticuloendothiliosis with eosinophilia. N Engl J Med 1965; 273: 427.

58. Villa A, Sautagata S, Bozzi F, et al. Partial V(D) J recombination activity leads to Omenn syndrome. Cell 1998; 93: 885–896.

59. Giliani S, Bonfim C, de Saint Basile G, et al. Omenn syndrome in an infant with IL7RA gene mutation. J Pediatr 2006; 148: 272–274.

60. Sullivan KE. The clinical, immunological, and molecular spectrum of chromosome 22q11.2 deletion syndrome and DiGeorge syndrome. Curr Opin Allergy Clin Immunol 2004; 4: 505–512.

61. Hong R. The DiGeorge Anomaly (Catch 22, DiGeorge/velocardiofacial syndrome). Semin Hematol. 1998; 35: 282–290.

62. Conley ME, Beckwith JB, Mancer JFK, et al. The spectrum of the DiGeorge syndrome. J Pediatr 1979; 94: 883–890.

63. Archer E, Chuan T-Y, Hong R. Severe eczema in a patient with DiGeorge syndrome. Cutis 1990; 45: 455–459.

64. Ochs HD. The Wiskott–Aldrich syndrome. Semin Hematol. 1998; 35: 332–345.

65. Thrasher AJ, Kinnon C. The Wiskott–Aldrich syndrome. Clin Exp Immunol 2000; 120: 2.

66. Sullivan KE, Mullen CA, Blaese RM, et al. A multiinstitutional survey of the Wiskott–Aldrich syndrome. J Pediatr 1994; 125: 876–885.

67. Grimbacher B, Holland SM, Gallin JI, et al. Hyper-IgE syndrome with recurrent infections – an autosomal dominant multisystem disorder. N Engl J Med 1999; 340: 692–702.

68. Chamlin SL, McCalmont TH, Cunningham BB, et al. Cutaneous manifestations of hyper-IgE syndrome in infants and children. J Pediatr 2002; 141: 572–575.

69. Erlewyn-Lajeunesse M. Hyperimmunoglobulin-E syndrome with recurrent infection: a review of current opinion and treatment. Pediatr Allergy Immunol 2000; 11: 133–141.

70. Leung DY, Geha RS. Clinical and immunologic aspects of the hyperimmunogobulin E syndrome. Hematol Oncol Clin North Am 1988; 2: 81–100.

71. Rosenzweig SD, Holland SM. Phagocyte immunodeficiencies and their infections. J Allergy Clin Immunol 2004; 113: 620–626.

72. Windhorst DB, Good RA. Dermatologic manifestations of fatal granulomatous disease of childhood. Arch Dermatol 1971; 103: 351–357.

73. Dohil M, Prendiville JS, Crawford RI, Speert DP. Cutaneous manifestations of chronic granulomatous disease: A report of four cases and review of the literature. J Am Acad Dermatol 1997; 36: 899–907.

74. International Chronic Granulomatous Disease Cooperative Study Group. A controlled trial of interferon-gamma to prevent infection in chronic granulomatous disease. N Engl J Med 1991; 324: 509–516.

75. Garganta CL, Smith WE. Metabolic evaluation of the sick neonate. Semin Perinatol 2005; 29: 164–172.

76. Ellaway CJ, Wilcken B, Christodoulou J. Clinical approach to inborn errors of

metabolism presenting in the newborn period. J Paediatr Child Health 2002; 38: 511–517.

77. Morrone A, Malvagia S, Donati MA, et al. Clinical findings and biochemical and molecular analysis of four patients with holocarboxylase synthetase deficiency. Am J Med Genet 2002; 111: 10–18.

78. Wilson DJ, Myer M, Darlow BA, et al. Severe holocarboxylase synthetase deficiency with incomplete biotin responsiveness resulting in antenatal insults in Samoan neonates. J Pediatr 2005; 147: 115–118.

79. Seashore MR, Seashore CJ. Newborn screening and the pediatric practioner. Semin Perinatol 2005; 29: 182–188.

80. Shih VE, Axel SM, Tewksbury JC, et al. Defective lysosomal release of vitamin B12 (cbIF): A hereditary cobalamin metabolic disorder associated with sudden death. Am J Med Genet 1989; 33: 555–563.

81. Howard R, Frieden IJ, Crawford D, et al. Methylmalonic aciduria, cobalamin c type, presenting with cutaneous manifestations. Arch Dermatol 1997; 133: 1563–1566.

82. Koopman RJ, Happle R. Cutaneous manifestations of methylmalonic aciduria. Arch Dermatol Res 1990; 282: 272–273.

83. Hansen AE, Wiese HF, Boelsche AR, et al. Role of linoleic acid in infant nutrition. Pediatrics 1963; 31: 171–192.

84. DiLiberti JH, DiGeorge AM, Ayerback VH. Abnormal leucine/isoleucine ratio and acrodermatitis enteropathica-like rash in maple syrup urine disease (MSUD). Pediatr Res 1973; 7: 382.

85. Spraker MK, Helminski MA, Elsas LJ. Periorificial dermatitis secondary to dietary deficiency of isoleucine in treated infants with maple syrup urine disease [abstract]. J Invest Dermatol 1986; 86: 508.

86. Koch SE, Packman S, Koch TK, et al. Dermatitis in treated maple syrup urine disease. J Am Acad Dermatol 1993; 28: 289–292.

87. Northrup H, Sigman ES, Hebert AA. Exfoliative erythroderma resulting from inadequate intake of branched-chain amino acids in infants with maple syrup urine disease. Arch Dermatol 1993; 129: 384–385.

88. Giacoia GP, Berry GT. Acrodermatitis enteropathica-like syndrome secondary to isoleucine deficiency during treatment of maple syrup urine disease. Am J Dis Child 1993; 147: 954–956.

89. Snyderman SE, Boyer A, Norton PM, et al. The essential aminoacid requirements of infants: isoleucine. Am J Clin Nutr 1964; 15: 313.

90. Theone J, Batshaw M, Spector E. Neonatal citrullinemia: Treatment with ketoanalogues of essential aminoacids. J Pediatr 1977; 90: 218–224.

91. Kline JJ, Hug G, Schubert WK, et al. Arginine deficiency syndrome: Its occurrence in carbamoyl phosphate synthetase deficiency. Am J Dis Child 1981; 135: 437–442.

92. DeRaeve L, DeMeirlier L, Ramet J, et al. Acrodermatitis enteropathica-like cutaneous lesions in organic aciduria. J Pediatr 1994; 124: 416–420.

93. Hansen RC, Lemen R, Rersin B. Cystic fibrosis manifesting with acrodermatitis enteropathica-like eruption: Associated with essential fatty acid and zinc deficiencies. Arch Dermatol 1983; 119: 51–55.

94. Darmstadt GL, Schmidt CP, Wechsler DS, et al. Dermatitis as a presenting sign of cystic fibrosis. Arch Dermatol 1992; 128: 1358–1364.

95. Hansen RC. Dermatitis and nutritional deficiency: Diagnostic and therapeutic considerations [editorial]. Arch Dermatol 1992; 128; 1389–1390.

96. National Newborn Screening Status Report, 11.14.05. *http://genes-r-us.uthscsa.edu/nbsdisorders.pdf*

97. Genome News Network. Panel urges states to screen newborns for 30 disorders. *http://www.genomenewsnetwork.org/articles/2004/10/01/screening*

18

Disorders of Cornification (Ichthyosis)

Alan D. Irvine, Amy S. Paller

The term 'inherited disorders of cornification' covers a wide range of genetic conditions with molecular defects that preclude the formation of a normal epidermis. The term is usually considered to include entities divided on morphological grounds into ichthyoses, follicular keratoses, and palmoplantar keratodermas (Table 18-1). In addition, many inherited disorders usually considered as ectodermal dysplasias have significant defects in epidermal development or differentiation. Several ichthyotic conditions first manifest in the neonatal period, usually as either collodion baby or scaling erythroderma, or more rarely as a harlequin fetus. In some situations, such as harlequin ichthyosis or Netherton syndrome, associated complications are life-threatening. For most of these conditions, therapy during the neonatal and early infantile periods is supportive (Box 18-1), involving frequent application of bland emollients and monitoring for evidence of infection or fluid and electrolyte imbalance. The use of topical medications with keratolytic agents neonatally and during the first 6 months of life is usually unnecessary and risks significant absorption of potentially toxic substances (e.g. lactic acid, salicylic acid). In the past 15 years the molecular bases of the great majority of these disorders have been elucidated, thereby laying the groundwork for confirmatory molecular diagnosis and opening up the possibility of DNA-based prenatal diagnosis for several of the devastating conditions (Table 18-1). A wonderful support group is available for all families with a disorder of cornification, the Foundation for Ichthyosis and Related Skin Types (FIRST; www.scalyskin.org).

Box 18-1 Principles of care of the collodion baby

Intervention	Reason
Careful fluid and electrolyte balance	Increased TEWL
Humidity controlled environment	Increased TEWL
Temperature controlled environment	Diminished ability to control temperature
Regular bland emollients	Diminished barrier function
Avoid potentially toxic topicals (e.g. steroids, TIMs, urea, lactic acid)	Diminished barrier function
Prevent infection	Diminished barrier function
Good eye care	Keratitis from prolonged ectropion

TEWL = transepidermal water loss

COLLODION BABY

Cutaneous Features

The collodion baby (Figs 18-1 and 18-2) is the phenotype at birth of several ichthyotic disorders, but autosomal recessive congenital ichthyosiform erythroderma or lamellar ichthyosis of variable severity are the eventual phenotype in most

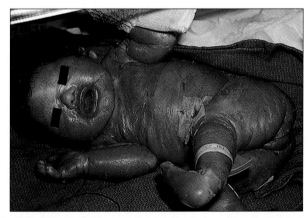

FIG. 18-1 Shiny collodion membrane of a 1-day-old collodion baby. Note the eclabion and tightened skin of the hands.

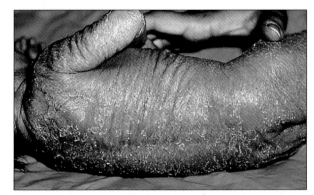

FIG. 18-2 One week after birth this collodion baby with congenital ichthyosiform erythroderma is showing desquamation of scale. Despite the severity of the early phenotype, this infant had very mild congenital ichthyosiform erythroderma at 6 months of age. (From Paller AS. Ichthyosis in the neonate. In: Dyall-Smith D, Marks R, eds. Dermatology at the millennium: Overview of past achievements, current knowledge and future trends. London: Parthenon Publishing Group, 1998, with permission.)

TABLE 18-1 Genetic disorders of cornification

Disorder	OMIM #	Inh	Cutaneous findings	Extracutaneous findings	Gene defect (s)	Protein (s)	Class of protein/ function
Ichthyoses							
Bullous congenital ichthyosiform erythroderma (epidermolytic hyperkeratosis)	113800	AD	Warty hyperkeratosis	None	*KRT1* and *KRT10*	Keratins 1 and 10	Cytoskeleton structural protein
Chanarin–Dorfman syndrome (neutral lipid storage disease; also termed NClE2)	275630	AR	Fine scales with occasional background erythema	Myopathy Hepatosplenomegaly	*CGI58*	CGI-58	Enzyme, a member of the esterase/lipase/ thioesterase subfamily
CHILD syndrome	308050	XD	Unilateral ichthyosiform erythroderma	Chondrodysplasia punctata Cataracts Limb reduction defects Asymmetric organ hypoplasia	*NSDHL*	3-beta-hydroxysteroid-delta(8),delta(7)-isomerase	Enzyme involved cholesterol biosynetesis
CHIME syndrome	280000	AR	Ichthyotic erythema Occasionally migratory plaques	Colobomas Conductive hearing loss Mental retardation	NK	NK	NK
Collodion baby (self-healing)	242300	AR	Collodion baby at birth, not subsequent ichthyotic phenotype	None	*TGM1*	Keratinocyte transglutaminase 1	Enzyme involved in crosslinking of stratum corneum
Congenital ichthyosiform erythroderma	242100	AR	Fine white scales, background erythema	None	*TGM1* *ALOX12B* *ALOXE3* *Also mapped to loci on 4q23 and 12p11.2-q13*	Keratinocyte transglutaminase 1 Arachidonate 12-lipoxygenase, r type Arachidonate lipoxygenase 3 NK	Transglutaminase, cornified envelope cross linking Lipoxygenase Epoxy alcohol synthase Function unknown
Congenital ichthyosiform erythroderma	None assigned	AR	Fine white scales, background erythema Mild PPK White nails	None	*ICHTHYIN*	Ichthyin, member of DUF803 protein family	Uncertain, probably a membrane–bound receptor
Cyclic ichthyosis with epidermolytic hyperkeratosis	607602	AD	Cyclical occurrence of polycyclic hyperkeratotic plaques	None	*KRT1*	Keratin 1	Cytoskeleton structural protein
Ectodermal dysplasia/ skin fragility syndrome	604536	AR	Skin fragility Keratotic plaques on limbs Palmoplantar keratoderma Alopecia	Diminished sweating	*PKP1*	Plakophilin-1	Desmosomal component
Familial peeling skin syndrome	270300	AR	Superficial acral peeling	None	*TGM5*	Keratinocyte tramnsglutaminase 5	Enzyme

Disease	OMIM	Inheritance	Cutaneous features	Extracutaneous features	Gene	Protein	Function
Gaucher syndrome, type 2	230900	AR	Collodion baby, mild scaling later	Hepatosplenomegaly retroflexion of the head, strabismus, dysphagia, choking spells, hypertonicity Death usually occurs in the first year	GBA	Acid beta-glucosidase	Enzyme
Harlequin ichthyosis	242500	AR	Rigid plates	Ectropion Eclabion	ABCA12	ATP-binding cassette, subfamily a, member 12	ABC transporter
Ichthyosis bullosa of Siemens	146800	AD	Mild flexural hyperkeratosis	None	KRT2E	Keratin 2 e	Cytoskeletal structural protein in suprabasal layer
Ichthyosis hystrix (Curth–Macklin)	146590 146600	AD	Spiky hyperkeratosis	None	KRT1	Keratin 1	Cytoskeletal structural protein
Ichthyosis vulgaris	146700	AD	Fine, white scale	None	FLG	Filaggrin	Structural component of stratum corneum
IFAP syndrome (ichthyosis follicularis)	398205	XR	Spiny follicular ichthyosis Nail dystrophy Alopecia	Photophobia Psychomotor delay Short stature	NK	NK	NK
Keratitis–ichthyosis–deafness syndrome (KID; includes HID syndrome)	242150 602540	AD	Verrucous plaques Stippled pattern of keratoderma	Keratitis Sensorineural deafness	GJB2	Connexin 26	Gap junction protein
Lamellar ichthyosis type 1	242300	AR	Large adherent plates	None	TGM1	Keratinocyte transglutaminase 1	Enzyme involved in crosslinking of stratum corneum
Lamellar ichthyosis type 2	601277	AR	Large adherent plates	None	ABCA12	ATP-binding cassette, subfamily a, member 12	ABC transporter
Lamellar ichthyosis type 3	604777	AR	Large adherent plates	None	Mapped to 19p12-q12	NK	NK
Lamellar ichthyosis (autosomal dominant form)	146750	AD	Large adherent plates	None	NK	NK	NK
Multiple sulfatase deficiency	272200	AR	Mild scale	Mental retardation Mucopolysaccharidosis Metachromatic leukodystrophy	SUMF1	Sulfatase-modifying factor-1	Modifier of sulphatase enzyme activity
Netherton syndrome	256500	AR	Erythroderma in infancy Ichthyosis linearis circumflexa	Atopic diathesis, food allergies Structural hair defects (trichorrhexis nodosa) Growth delay	SPINK5	LETKI	Serine protease inhibitor

TABLE 18-1 Genetic disorders of cornification—cont'd

Disorder	OMIM #	Inh	Cutaneous findings	Extracutaneous findings	Gene defect(s)	Protein(s)	Class of protein/function
Neu–Laxova syndrome	256520	AR	Variable: mild scaling to harlequin ichthyosis appearance	Intrauterine growth retardation, Microcephaly, Sensorineural hearing loss, Subcapsular cataracts, Nystagmus, strabismus, Mental retardation	NK	NK	NK
Nonlamellar, nonerythodermic ichthyosis phenotype	604781	AR	Fine, nonerythematous scaling more prominent in the knees, ankles, and ears	None	Mapped to 19p13.1-p13.2	NK	NK
Refsum disease	266500	AR	Late onset, fine scale	Retinitis pigmentosa, Cardiac failure	PAHX or PHYH, PEX7	Phytanoyl-CoA hydroxylase, Peroxin-7	Enzymes involved in phytanic acid metabolism
Sjögren–Larsson syndrome	270200	AR	Fine lamellar scale	Di- or tetraplegia, Retinal glistening white dots			
Trichothiodystrophy syndromes	601675	AR	May have collodion membrane, Can vary from mild scaling to marked adherent plaques	Photosensitivity, Brittle hair with 'tiger tail' pattern, Decreased fertility, Short stature, Susceptibility to infection	XPD, or ERCC2, XPB, or ERCC3	Xeropigmentosum group D protein, Xeropigmentosum group B protein	DNA repair enzymes also involved in regulation of transcription
X-linked chondrodysplasia punctata (Conradi–Hünerman syndrome)	302960	XD	Striated ichthyosiform hyperkeratosis, Follicular atrophoderma, Alopecia	Cataracts, Frontal bossing, Short proximal limbs	EBP	Emopamil-binding protein	Enzyme involved cholesterol biosynthesis
X-linked ichthyosis	308100	XR	Large, dark scales	Prolongation of labor, Cryptorchidism, Corneal opacities	STS	Steroid sulfatase	Enzyme
Follicular keratoses							
Darier–White disease (including acral hemorrhagic variant)	124200	AD	Yellow-brown, greasy papules	Neuropsychiatric features, Frequent HSV infections	ATP2A2	SERCA2 Ca(2+)-ATPase	Ca^{2+} ion pump protein
Keratosis pilaris	604093	AD	Follicular hyperkeratosis	None	NK	NK	NK
Keratosis pilaris spinulosa decalvans	308800	XD	Follicular hyperkeratosis	Corneal degeneration, Alopecia, Loss of eyebrows	Mapped to Xp22.1, some evidence that mutations in SAT may be relevant	SAT encodes Spermidine/spermine N(1)-acetyltransferase	Enzyme (N(1)-acetylation)
Erythrokeratodermas							
Erythrokeratoderma variabilis	133200	AD	Hyperkeratotic patches, Figurate erythema	None	GJB3, GJB4	Connexin 31, Connexin 30.3	Gap junction protein
Erythrokeratoderma variabilis with erythema gyratem repens	133200	AD	Hyperkeratotic patches, Migratory annular morphology	None	GJB4	Connexin 30.3	Gap junction protein

Disease	OMIM	Inheritance	Hyperkeratotic patches		*LOR*	Loricrin	Cornified cell envelope protein
Erythrokeratoderma progressiva symmetrica	602036	AD	None	None	*LOR*	Loricrin	Cornified cell envelope protein

Palmoplantar keratodermas

Disease	OMIM	Inheritance	Hyperkeratotic patches	Associated features	Gene/Locus	Protein	Function
Acrokeratoelastoidalis	101850	AD	Punctate PPK	None	NK	NK	NK
Bart–Pumphrey syndrome	149200	AD	Diffuse PPK; Knuckle pads; Leukonychia	Sensorineural deafness	*GJB2*	Connexin 26	Gap junction protein
Corneodermatosseous syndrome	122440	AD	Diffuse PPK	Photophobia; Corneal dystrophy; Distal onycholysis; Brachydactyly; Short stature; Medullary narrowing of the digits; Dental decay	NK	NK	NK
Haim–Munk syndrome	245010	AR	Focal PPK; Onychogryphosis	Severe periodontosis; Arachnodactyly; Acroosteolysis	*CTSC*	Cathepsin C	Enzyme
Hidrotic ectodermal dysplasia (Clouston syndrome)	129500	AD	Diffuse PPK; Nail dystrophy; Recurrent paronychia; Alopecia; Oral leukokeratoses	Sensorineural deafness	GJB6	Connexin 30	Gap junction protein
Howel-Evans syndrome	148500	AD	Focal PPK	Esophageal carcinoma; Oral leukokeratosis; Oral carcinoma	*Mapped to 17q25*	NK	NK
Keratolytic winter keratoderma (Outsthoorn syndrome)	148370	AD	Diffuse PPK; Centrifugal peeling of palms, soles and occasionally buttocks and trunk	None	*Mapped to 8p23-p22*	NK	NK
Mal de Meleda	248300	AR	Diffuse PPK; Knuckle pads; Koilonychia; Subungual hyperkeratosis	Digital autoamputation	*AMS*	SLURP1	Secreted protein, function not entirely understood
Naegeli–Franceschetti–Jadassohn syndrome	161000	AD	Diffuse PPK; Reticulate pigmentation; Nail dystrophy; Absent dermatoglyphics	Dental dystrophy	*Mapped to 17q11.2-q21*	NK	NK
Naxos disease	148500	AR	Focal PPK; Woolly hair	Arrhythmogenic right ventricular dysplasia/cardiomyopathy	*JUP*	Plakoglobin	Desmosomal component
Olmsted syndrome	None assigned	AD	Focal/Diffuse PPK; Hypotrichosis; Periorifacial plaques	None	NK	NK	NK
Pachyonychia congenita type I (Jadassohn–Lewandowsky syndrome)	167200	AD	Focal PPK; Symmetric subungual hyperkeratosis; Follicular hyperkeratosis	Natal teeth (rare); Oral leukokeratoses	*KRT6A and KRT16*	Keratins 6A and 16	Cytoskeletal structural proteins

TABLE 18-1 Genetic disorders of cornification—cont'd

Disorder	OMIM #	Inh	Cutaneous findings	Extracutaneous findings	Gene defect (s)	Protein (s)	Class of protein/ function
Pachyonychia congenita type II (Jackson–Lawler syndrome)	167210	AD	Focal PPK, Symmetric subungual hyperkeratosis, Follicular hyperkeratosis, Steatocysts	Oral leukokeratoses, Natal teeth (more common than PC-1)	*KRT6B and KRT 17*	Keratins 6B and 17	Cytoskeletal structural proteins
Papillon–Lefèvre syndrome	245000	AR	Focal PPK, Hypotrichosis, Nail fragility, Eyelid cysts	Periodontitis, Premature loss of dentition, Calcification of dura mater	*CTSC*	Cathepsin C	Enzyme
Porokeratosis punctata palmaris et plantaris	175860	AD	Punctate PPK	None	NK	NK	NK
PPK of Sybert	None	AD	Diffuse PPK	Pseudoainhum, Digital autoamputation	NK	NK	NK
Punctate PPK (Buschke–Fischer–Brauer)	148600	AD	Punctate PPK	Lynch type II malignancies in some families	NK	NK	NK
Richner–Hanhart syndrome (Tyrosinemia II)	276600	AR	Focal PPK	Photophobia, Corneal erosions, Mental retardation	*TAT*	Tyrosine transaminase	
Sclerotylosis (Huriez syndrome)	181600	AD	PPK, Atrophic fibrosis of the skin of the limbs, Hypoplasia of nails, Skin cancer	Bowel cancer	*Mapped to 4q23*	NK	NK
Schöpf–Schultz–Passarge syndrome	224750	AR	Diffuse PPK, Hypotrichosis, Eyelid cysts, Facial telangiectasia, Multiple squamous cell carcinomas	Hypodontia	NK	NK	NK
Striate PPK	148700	AD	Focal/Striate PPK	None	*DSP DSG1 KRT1*	Desmoplakin 1, Desmoglein 1, Keratin 1	Desmosomal structural component, Cytoskeletal structural protein
Striate PPK with dilated cardiomyopathy and woolly hair	605676	AR	Focal/striate PPK	Dilated cardiomyopathy, Woolly hair	*DSP*	Desmoplakin 1	Desmosomal structural component
Vohwinkel syndrome (classic variant)	124500	AD	Diffuse PPK	Sensorineural deafness, Pseudoainhum, Digital autoamputation	*GJB2*	Connexin 26	Gap junction protein
Vohwinkel syndrome (ichthyotic/camisa variant)	604117	AD	Diffuse PPK, Diffuse ichthyosis	None	*LOR*	Loricrin	Cornified cell envelope protein
Vörner syndrome (EPPK)	144200	AD	Diffuse PPK	None	*KRT9*	Keratin 9	Cytoskeletal structural protein

patients.[1] Others include autosomal dominant lamellar ichthyosis, Sjögren–Larsson syndrome, Conradi–Hunermann syndrome, trichothiodystrophy, and neonatal Gaucher's disease.[2] In 5–6% of collodion babies normal-appearing skin replaces the collodion membrane, an autosomal recessive disorder called lamellar ichthyosis of the newborn or spontaneously healing collodion baby.[3] Collodion babies are encased in thickened, shiny, variably erythematous skin that resembles cellophane (Fig. 18-1).

Extracutaneous Features

Despite the thickening of the stratum corneum, the collodion membrane is actually a poor barrier, which can result in excessive transcutaneous fluid and electrolyte loss with resultant hypernatremic dehydration,[4,5] increased metabolic requirements, and temperature instability owing to increased evaporative cooling. Collodion babies are often premature, and the combined skin disorder and prematurity further increase the risk of complications. In addition, numerous cutaneous fissures may be present which, together with the poor skin barrier, increase the risk of the skin being a site of entry for bacteria and subsequent sepsis. Infection may be also be difficult to diagnose owing to the intrinsic temperature instability and fluid imbalances associated with the underlying skin condition. Aspiration of squamous material in the amniotic fluid may lead to neonatal pneumonia.[6] In addition, the thickening of the skin may restrict movement, making sucking, eye closure, and rarely respiration, difficult.

Etiology/Pathogenesis

Although most cases are due to persistent forms of ichthyosis (discussed in more detail below), approximately 5% are self-healing. The self-healing collodion baby phenotype has been shown in one kindred to be due to mutations in *TGM1*.[7] In two affected siblings, increased hydrostatic pressure significantly reduced the activity of the mutant enzyme, suggesting that this pressure both traps water molecules and locks the mutated enzyme in an inactive *trans* conformation in utero. After birth these water molecules are removed and the enzyme is predicted to isomerize back to a partially active *cis* form, explaining the dramatic improvement of this skin condition.[7]

Differential Diagnosis

Several conditions can result in the collodion baby phenotype (Box 18-2). Occasionally severe cases can be confused with harlequin ichthyosis.

Treatment and Care (see Box 18-1)

Collodion babies should be placed in high-humidity environments to increase hydration, and bland emollients should be applied. Electrolytes should be monitored,[4] as should fluid intake and output. The membrane usually sloughs during the first month of life (Fig. 18-2). The use of topical keratolytic agents should be avoided in view of the increased potential for toxicity resulting from absorption through the compromised permeability barrier.[4]

HARLEQUIN ICHTHYOSIS

Cutaneous Features

Harlequin ichthyosis (HI) is a rare autosomal recessive disorder in which the neonate is born with a thick covering of

---

> **Box 18.2 Eventual outcomes of neonatal collodion baby phenotype**
>
> **Common**
> NCIE
> Lamellar ichthyosis
> Self-healing collodion baby
>
> **Uncommon**
> Chanarin–Dorfman syndrome
> Loricrin keratoderma
> Gaucher disease, type II
> Trichothiodystrophy syndromes
> Sjögren–Larsson syndrome
> Conradi–Hünermann
> Neu–Laxova syndrome

armor-like scales, severe ectropion and eclabium, and underdeveloped nose and ears (Fig. 18-3). Occasionally infants with HI present with a thick vernix-like coating.

Extracutaneous Features

There is high neonatal mortality due to respiratory complications, infections through the defective skin barrier, and dehydration.

Differential Diagnosis

Severe forms of collodion baby may cause confusion but the diagnosis of harlequin ichthyosis is usually straightforward.

Etiology/Pathogenesis

All patients have hyperkeratosis, lipid accumulation within corneocytes, and absence of normal lamellar granules.[8] Recently mutations have been identified in the lipid transporter *ABCA12* in several families,[9,10] firmly establishing a defect in lipid transport as the primary defect in harlequin ichthyosis. Less deleterious missense mutations in this same gene have been shown to underlie lamellar ichthyosis in some families[11] (see Table 18-1 and below). These data also now allow the possibility of DNA-based prenatal diagnosis of this devastating disorder. The recovery of lipid secretion after gene correction[9] raises hope for future therapeutic approaches. The integrity of the stratum corneum barrier is largely due to corneocytes embedded in intracellular lipid lamellae. These extracellular lipid lamellae are in turn formed from intracellular granules. Absence of *ABCA12* prevents the transfer of lipids into lamellar granules, explaining the previously described ultrastructural abnormalities.[12] It is likely that the dysmorphic features observed in harlequin ichthyosis are at least in part secondary to restricted fetal movement; this condition has been termed 'fetal deformation sequence' (FADS).[13]

Treatment and Care

In general, harlequin babies require vigorous supportive therapy, including a humid environment, the aggressive use of emollients, and careful monitoring of fluid and electrolyte needs. Survival past the neonatal period is uncommon, but reported. Most affected infants have complications, such as systemic infection through fissured skin, difficulties with feeding and respiration, and distal gangrene. Therapy with

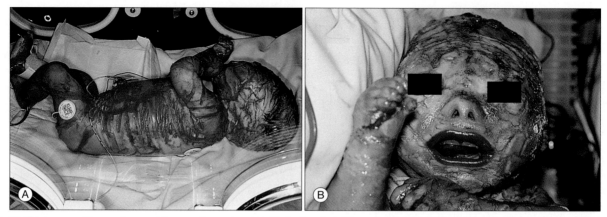

FIG. 18-3 (A) Thick armor-like scaling and fissures in a neonate with harlequin ichthyosis. (B) Note the severe ectropion, eclabion, and digital contractures. (Courtesy of Dr. Sylvia Suarez, Alexandria, VA.)

retinoids may improve the clinical appearance, but the condition at best evolves into a severe generalized ichthyosiform erythroderma phenotype.[14–18] Harlequin ichthyosis is the only ichthyotic condition in the neonate that may justify the use of systemic retinoid therapy during the newborn period. Treatment with retinoids was first undertaken in 1985.[19] Infants can survive, and the oldest known survivor is now in her early 20s.[14, 20] The administration of systemic retinoids should generally be considered in infants who have survived the first few weeks with intensive nursing support, in the knowledge that the persistent resultant ichthyotic condition is severe and associated with a poor quality of life. A possible exception is infants with particularly thick areas of plate-like scale causing digital constriction, where early use of retinoids may cause more prompt desquamation, potentially helping to avoid digital gangrene.

ICHTHYOSIS VULGARIS

Cutaneous Features

Ichthyosis vulgaris is one of the most common genetic disorders of skin, occurring in approximately 1 in 250 individuals, based on a survey of healthy English schoolchildren.[21] In contrast to other forms of ichthyosis, ichthyosis vulgaris does not manifest during the neonatal period. The condition usually appears after 3 months of age as fine, light-colored scales that are larger and coarser on the lower extremities. Palmoplantar markings are accentuated (hyperlinearity).

Extracutaneous Features

There is an association in some cases with atopic asthma and rhinitis in later life.

Etiology/Pathogenesis

Several lines of evidence point to a genetic defect in the filaggrin gene (FLG) in ichthyosis vulgaris (IV). Immunoblotting studies show that filaggrin protein and/or keratinocytes are absent or markedly reduced in the skin of IV patients.[22] In addition, reduced filaggrin mRNA has been demonstrated in some individuals with IV.[23] A recessive mouse mutant, flaky tail (ft), bears the histological and ultrastructural hallmarks of human IV[24] and strong genetic linkage to the murine filaggrin locus (Flg) has been obtained. Importantly, genetic linkage in an American family was identified between IV associated with a histologically absent granular layer and markers in the epidermal differentiation complex (EDC) on chromosome 1q21.[25] Recently homozygous or compound heterozygous stop mutations predicting stop codons were identified in the filaggrin gene as the cause of moderate or severe IV in 15 kindreds.[26] In addition, these mutations were semidominant; heterozygotes exhibit a very mild phenotype with incomplete penetrance. The mutations show a combined allele frequency of ~4% in caucasian populations, explaining the high incidence of IV.

Differential Diagnosis

In affected boys, ichthyosis vulgaris in the young infant may need to be distinguished from X-linked recessive ichthyosis (see below).

Treatment and Care

In the neonatal period no specific care is necessary. Good skin care with regular emollients and the avoidance of irritants such as detergents is advisable, as these infants tend to have lifelong dry skin and a high incidence of atopic dermatitis.[21]

X-LINKED RECESSIVE ICHTHYOSIS

Cutaneous Features

X-linked recessive ichthyosis (RXLI), a disorder that affects 1 : 6000–1 : 2000 males, is present by 3 months of age in 84% of patients, although only 17% show evidence of exaggerated neonatal desquamation and peeling at birth. Extensor surfaces, the preauricular areas, and the sides of the neck are most severely affected by the large, dark, adherent scales (Fig. 18-4).

Extracutaneous Features

The absence of steroid sulfatase activity during fetal life also leads to increased fetal production of DHEAS (dehydroepiandrosterone sulfate) and decreased placental estrogen production, which may delay the progression of parturition. Occasionally, affected boys have hypogonadism with undescended testes, hypoplasia of the penis and scrotum, and failure of normal sexual maturation. The development of testicular cancer has been described in one patient without undescended testes. Approximately 10% of affected boys have a contiguous gene deletion syndrome, a larger deletion which encompasses genes that are contiguous with the steroid sulfatase gene on the terminal short arm of the X chromosome.

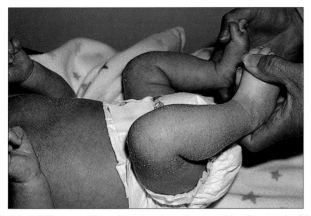

FIG. 18-4 Diffuse scaling of the trunk and extremities is seen in this 2-week-old infant with X-linked ichthyosis.

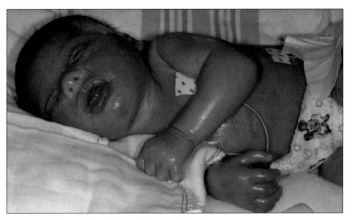

FIG. 18-5 Lamellar ichthyosis in an infant.

Deletion of surrounding genes results in mental retardation, hypogonadism, and anosmia (Kallmann syndrome), or a bone dysplasia characterized radiographically by stippled epiphyses (X-linked recessive chondrodysplasia punctata).

Etiology/Pathogenesis

X-linked ichthyosis results from mutations of the gene for steroid sulfatase (arylsulfatase C), particularly deletions (90% of patients). In a study assessing the clinical and molecular features in 28 patients with Kallmann syndrome 1, submicroscopic deletions were found at Xp22.3 involving four genes, including VCXA, STS, KAL1, and OA1, in three familial cases and one sporadic male case affected by a contiguous gene syndrome.[27]

Differential Diagnosis

X-linked recessive ichthyosis (XLRI) in the neonate is not associated with collodion membrane and is therefore distinguishable from other ichthyotic disorders associated with collodion membranes and early skin thickening. IV is an important differential diagnosis in older male infants and can be distinguished by measurements of cholesterol sulfate levels in plasma. Babies with the rare autosomal recessive disorder multiple sulfatase deficiency manifest with scaling typical of XLRI and decreased steroid sulfatase because of a global deficiency of sulfatases. Affected patients also show neurologic abnormalities characteristic of metachromatic leukodystrophy, and features of storage diseases because of the deficiency of several additional sulfatases.

Treatment and Care

In the neonatal period no specific care is necessary, but patients will generally need lifelong skin care advice and appropriate emollients. XLRI may be detected prenatally. The most common scenario for this is in pregnancies not known to be at risk with an abnormal 'triple screen' test that detects decreased maternal estriol levels. XLRI may then be confirmed by FISH (fluorescent in situ hybridization); STS (steroid sulphatase); and DHEAS for deletions and/or the demonstration of decreased placental sulfatase activity in amniotic fluid cells and increased DHEAS levels in amniotic fluid. Corrective gene therapy has been performed in an animal model by transplantation to mouse skin of grafts of XLRI keratinocytes that have been stably transfected with the normal steroid sulfatase gene.[28]

LAMELLAR ICHTHYOSIS

Cutaneous Features

Lamellar ichthyosis (LI) is usually inherited as an autosomal recessive disorder, although an autosomal dominant form has been described.[29] Babies with lamellar ichthyosis are usually born with collodion membranes (see the previous discussion). After shedding of the collodion membrane the scales are large and plate-like (Fig. 18-5) and are hyperpigmented, particularly in patients with darker skin.[30] Underlying erythroderma is minimal, but ectropion and alopecia may be severe. Biopsies from patients with LI have massive thickening of the stratum corneum, mild acanthosis, and a normal granular layer. The epidermis in LI may show papillomatosis with regular psoriasiform blunting and broadening of the rete ridges.

Extracutaneous Features

Exposure keratitis can result from prolonged ectropion.

Etiology/Pathogenesis

The molecular basis for many patients with LI is mutations in keratinocyte transglutaminase I,[31] an enzyme that is involved in cornified envelope formation by cross-linking precursor proteins such as involucrin. Prenatal diagnosis by molecular analysis of fetal DNA, obtained by chorionic villus sampling, is a preferred method of prenatal diagnosis, but is only possible in families in which the molecular defect is known.[32] Based on the discovery of the underlying gene defect in some families with LI, gene therapy has been performed in mouse models of LI, generated by transplantation of cultured LI keratinocytes that have been transfected with the normal transglutaminase I gene onto immunodeficient mice. Although the expression of the normal transglutaminase I is transient in vivo, it restores not only the transglutaminase but also normal involucrin cross-linking and involucrin expression.[33] However, the genetic basis for lamellar ichthyosis is heterogeneous, and several families have been described with normal keratinocyte transglutaminase.[34] Recent work has identified mutations in the lipid transporter *ABCA12* in several families[11] (see Harlequin ichthyosis). In three consanguineous Moroccan families the transglutaminase I gene locus was excluded and the mutant gene was instead strongly linked to 2q33-35.[35] A third genetic locus for LI has been identified on 19p12-q12.[36]

Differential Diagnosis

Lamellar ichthyosis can be difficult to distinguish from nonbullous congenital ichthyosiform erythroderma in the neonatal period.

Treatment and Care

In the neonatal period general supportive measures are appropriate (see Box 18-1). In older children and adults more potent topical keratolytic preparations and oral retinoids may be appropriate, but these should be avoided in infancy.

NONBULLOUS CONGENITAL ICHTHYOSIFORM ERYTHRODERMA

Cutaneous Features

Patients with nonbullous congenital ichthyosiform erythroderma (NCIE) also usually present as collodion babies. Underlying erythroderma is common, and the scales tend to be finer and lighter in color than those of infants with lamellar ichthyosis. Alopecia and ectropion may be associated.[30]

Extracutaneous Features

Not uncommonly patients with NCIE have associated neurologic abnormalities, and the NCIE phenotype may be part of other multisystem conditions, such as neutral lipid storage disease (Chanarin–Dorfman syndrome).

Etiology/Pathogenesis

Histopathology shows marked acanthosis of the epidermis with a moderately thickened stratum corneum and variable focal parakeratosis.[30] NCIE is a genetically heterogeneous condition. The CIE phenotype can be caused by less deleterious mutations in the *TGM1* gene,[37] in which more mutations with more profound functional consequences cause lamellar ichthyosis. In addition to the causative gene for Chanarin–Dorfman syndrome, an NCIE phenotype has been attributed to mutations in four further genes, and two additional genetic loci have been mapped in ethnic kindreds. Thus at least six distinct genes can underscore this cutaneous phenotype (Table 18-1).

Differential Diagnosis

Because of the associated neurological abnormalities and the potential to respond to dietary tailoring, it is important to exclude Chanarin–Dorfman syndrome (see below). However, this is a very uncommon cause of the CIE phenotype.

Treatment and Care

See Box 18-1 for general principles of care in the neonatal period.

ICHTHYOSIS PREMATURITY SYNDROME

Cutaneous Features

Ichthyosis prematurity syndrome (IPS) is a distinct form of ichthyosis that is reported almost exclusively in the Norwegian population.[38] To date, the only exceptions are two Finnish families and one north Italian family. At birth, the skin, particularly on the head and peripheral extremities, is covered by a thick, caseous, desquamating epidermis. Within 2 weeks this improves to a simple dryness of the skin. Later, the phenotype is mild, with persisting dryness and white scaling. The skin shows a cobblestone-like surface, particularly on distal extremities, and a leather-like thickening on the lower back. Hypereosinophilia is common.[38]

Extracutaneous Features

Pregnancies are complicated by polyhydramnios, and ultrasound shows opaque amniotic fluid. The birth is premature, and delivery usually takes place at around weeks 30–32. Affected children may suffer from postnatal asphyxia, possibly related to aspiration of amnionic debris.

Etiology/Pathogenesis

The pattern on electron microscopy is characterized by membrane aggregations in the upper epidermal cells.

Although the aetiology and pathogenesis are not understood, ichthyosis prematurity syndrome segregates independently of the known ichthyosis loci and is more prevalent in a defined region in the adjacent middle parts of Norway and Sweden. The condition has recently been linked to chromosome 9q33.3-34.13.[38]

Differential Diagnosis

The differential diagnosis in the neonatal period includes collodion membrane and harlequin ichthyosis.

Treatment and Care

For general neonatal management principles see Box 18-1.

EPIDERMOLYTIC HYPERKERATOSIS (BULLOUS CONGENITAL ICHTHYOSIFORM ERYTHRODERMA, BCIE)

Cutaneous Features

This autosomal dominant disorder manifests in the neonate as widespread areas of denuded skin with only subtle skin thickening and/or scaling (Fig. 18-6). Confusion with other blistering disorders in the neonate is common, particularly epidermolysis bullosa, and secondary cutaneous bacterial infection caused by *Staphylococcus aureus* often occurs. As patients age the scaling becomes more verrucous, with large dark scales, particularly at intertriginous sites, and the propensity towards blistering tends to decrease.

Extracutaneous Features

In the neonatal period infants with BCIE risk dehydration, electrolyte imbalance, and infection; however, most babies do well and death rarely occurs in neonates.

Etiology/Pathogenesis

The gene defects of BCIE involve abnormalities of keratins 1 or 10,[39,40] the major differentiation-specific keratins of the upper epidermis. These mutations cause the formation of

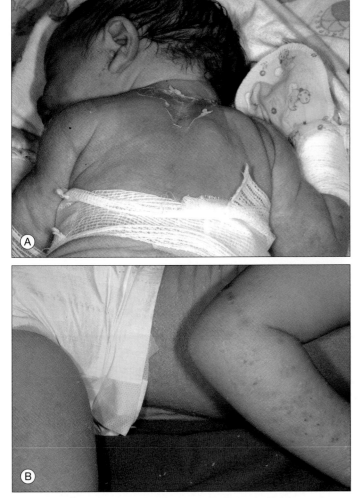

FIG. 18-6 Epidermolytic hyperkeratosis. **(A)** Blistering in a neonate often occurs at site of trauma. **(B)** In this 18-month-old infant, erythema and fine scale are more prominent. Scaling becomes more verrucous as the patient becomes older, especially in intertriginous areas and overlying joints.

defective keratin filaments, which are functionally responsible for the tonofilament clumping and blistering of this disorder. Prenatal diagnosis has been performed at 20–24 weeks of gestation by fetal skin biopsy, based on the abnormal clumping of keratin filaments,[41] but also by molecular analysis of keratin 10 in an affected family.[42]

Differential Diagnosis

Distinction from epidermolysis bullosa is important in the neonatal period. The principles of care at this stage remain the same, but accurate diagnosis is important in order to properly inform and counsel parents. The histologic appearance of lesional skin confirms the diagnosis, showing vacuolization of the granular and upper spinous layers. Hyperkeratosis, acanthosis, and papillomatosis are variable, but the granular layer is thickened. On electron microscopy the tonofilaments are seen to be clumped in the lower epidermal layers and form perinuclear shells in the granular cell and upper spinous layers.

Treatment and Care

The neonate should be managed according to the same broad principles as outlined in Box 18-1, but with additional specific precautions on skin handling of neonates with fragile skin directed by a detailed nursing protocol.

ICHTHYOSIS HYSTRIX

Cutaneous Features

Ichthyosis hystrix (Curth–Macklin) is a rare autosomal dominant ichthyotic disorder characterized by plaques of spiny hyperkeratosis. The extent of involvement varies from patchy to generalized and severe. In patients with patchy involvement, the distribution is not along the lines of Blaschko. Usually the face, palms, and soles are not affected, but involvement of the penis and scrotum has been described. Affected infants tend to show cutaneous changes within the first weeks of life, with subsequent progression of involvement, although onset during childhood has been described in some patients. Erythroderma may be present at birth, but disappears with time.

Extracutaneous Features

None.

Etiology/Pathogenesis

Microscopic examination of skin biopsy specimens shows orthokeratosis, papillomatosis, and acanthosis of the granular and upper spinous layers, with perinuclear vacuolization. Keratinocytes may have two nuclei. Ultrastructural examination shows concentric shells of tonofibrils that encase the nuclei with perinuclear vacuoles, lamellar body abnormalities, and binuclear keratinocytes.[43] In two families the ichthyosis hystrix phenotype has been attributed to mutations in keratin 1.[44,45] The condition is genetically heterogeneous; in other families linkage to the keratin gene clusters has been excluded.[46]

Differential Diagnosis

Ichthyosis hystrix can be confused with epidermolytic hyperkeratosis. The lack of erythroderma, blistering, and typical ultrastructural characteristics distinguish these conditions. Epidermal nevi, although they may resemble ichthyosis hystrix both clinically and histologically, are distinguishable by their distribution along the lines of Blaschko.

Treatment and Care

Neonatal care is as in outlined in Box 18-1. In older children keratolytics and oral retinoids may be of value.

FAMILIAL PEELING SKIN SYNDROME

Cutaneous Features

This rare autosomal recessive condition is characterized by spontaneous superficial peeling of skin, sometimes accompanied by pruritus and occasionally by erythema or vesiculation. Skin involvement is usually generalized, but the palms, soles, face, and scalp may be unaffected. The Nikolsky sign tends to be positive, and a skin biopsy often shows psoriasiform epidermal changes and shedding of the stratum corneum just above the granular layer. Two subgroups have been noted, based on the ultrastructural level of cleavage. Type A, which begins either at birth or at 3–6 years of age, shows a split through the corneocyte cytoplasm. Type B, which always begins at birth, shows cleavage along the intercellular spaces.[47] In a further variant, peeling is limited to acral areas.[48]

Extracutaneous Features

Transient eosinophilia and elevation of IgE levels may be associated with both types.

Etiology/Pathogenesis

The genetic defect in types A and B remains unknown, but the acral variant has been shown to be caused by homozygous mutations in keratinocyte transglutaminase 5.[48] Some cases with *SPINK5* mutations have also been demonstrated, suggesting that this may be a heterogeneous, rather than a singular distinct disease.[49]

Differential Diagnosis

The clinical appearance of types A and B may be confused with staphylococcal scalded skin syndrome but the duration and distribution should make the distinction.

Treatment and Care

General principles of care apply (see Box 18-1).

SJÖGREN–LARSSON SYNDROME

Cutaneous Features

This autosomal recessive disorder usually manifests in the neonatal period with slight or moderate widespread ichthyosis,[50-52] although rarely features may not occur until the infant is older than 6 months. Mild erythema is occasionally present at birth, which clears within months. Only one baby with Sjögren–Larsson syndrome has been reported to have had a collodion membrane at birth. Affected babies usually show thickening of the skin, especially at the umbilicus, neck, and flexural areas, that resembles lichenification. Scaling, if present, is fine and lamellar, so that some neonates have been misdiagnosed as being postmature. Some neonates with Sjögren–Larsson syndrome have had taut, shiny fingers and toes. By 1 year of age the ichthyosis is fully developed, with generalized thickening, lamellar scaling, and relative sparing of the central face, and often the palms and soles. The ichthyosis of Sjögren–Larsson is less scaly and more lichenified in appearance, reminiscent of a mild generalized acanthosis nigricans, and pruritus is typically more prominent than in other forms of ichthyosis. Hair and nails are normal. Histopathologic examination of biopsied skin shows significant hyperkeratosis and papillomatosis, with abnormal lamellar or membranous inclusions.[53]

Extracutaneous Features

Most infants with SLS are born preterm.[54] Mental and developmental retardation and spastic diplegia or tetraplegia are the most common extracutaneous features. Many patients have speech abnormalities, seizures, short stature, and kyphosis. Pathognomonic retinal 'glistening dots' are not present in all patients. The neurologic disease usually becomes apparent by 3 months of age, with failure to reach normal developmental milestones and the onset of spasticity. Phenotypic variability may be seen: in one family three of four siblings had skin findings but none were typical of SLS, and one lacked skin lesions entirely.[55]

Etiology/Pathogenesis

Sjögren–Larsson syndrome results from mutations in fatty aldehyde dehydrogenase, a component of fatty alcohol: nicotinamide adenine dinucleotide oxidoreductase (FAO), which converts fatty alcohol to fatty acid.[52,56] Fatty alcohol is used for the biosynthesis of wax esters, which are largely produced in skin, and of glycerol ether lipids, which are prominent in myelin. There appears to be no genotype–phenotype correlation.[54] Prenatal diagnosis of Sjögren–Larsson syndrome is possible by measurement of FAO activity in cultured amniocytes or chorionic cells, histologic analysis, and/or analysis of fetal DNA if the gene defect is known.[57]

Differential Diagnosis

The differential diagnosis includes all of the CIE phenotypes (Table 18-1). The development of neurological manifestations distinguishes SLS. The ethnic background also provides a useful clue as to the possible diagnosis, the incidence being much higher in northern Sweden, where inbreeding has led to a high prevalence of 8.3 in 100 000 persons; elsewhere in Sweden and worldwide the incidence is 0.4 per 100 000.[54]

Treatment and Care

There are no well established specific treatments, but there have been some encouraging data on 5-lipoxygenase inhibitors, the use of which for 5 weeks was reported to improve behavior and pruritus.[58]

NEUTRAL LIPID STORAGE DISEASE (CHANARIN–DORFMAN SYNDROME)

Cutaneous Features

This autosomal recessive disorder is characterized by the multisystemic accumulation of neutral lipids (triglycerides).[59] Approximately 65% of affected patients have associated ichthyosis, which is always present at birth as nonbullous congenital ichthyosiform erythroderma, or occasionally as a collodion baby.

Extracutaneous Features

Hepatomegaly occurs in 46% of patients, although fatty liver may be universal. Liver levels of transaminases are often elevated.[60,61] Almost 70% of patients have either elevated serum creatine kinase activity or muscle weakness, or both, usually mild and first symptomatic in adulthood. Other features may include ataxia, mental retardation, neurosensory hearing loss, and cataracts.

Etiology/Pathogenesis

Sections of skin show accumulation of neutral lipids, and these nonmembrane-bound cytosolic triacylglycerol droplets are also found in liver, muscle, intestinal mucosa, and neutrophils. Vacuolated neutrophils are considered the most consistent marker for neutral lipid storage disease. Mutations in the *CGI-58* gene have been found in several families.[62] The gene product belongs to a large series of proteins most of which are enzymes in the esterase/lipase/thioesterase subfamily. It is widely expressed in skin, lymphocytes, liver, skeletal muscle, and brain.

Differential Diagnosis

In the neonate, the ichthyosis may be impossible to distinguish from other NCIE phenotypes and possible causes of collodion baby. Diagnosis is usually made by a peripheral blood smear, which shows lipid droplets in granulocytes.[63]

Treatment and Care

Preliminary observations suggest that a low-fat diet, including medium-chain triglycerides, may improve liver function and the skin, especially if begun in early childhood.[64]

NETHERTON SYNDROME

Cutaneous Features

Netherton syndrome should be suspected in the neonate with generalized scaling erythroderma, especially if there is failure to thrive (Fig. 18-7).[65] Affected infants are often born prematurely and develop the typical ichthyosiform erythroderma in utero or during the first weeks of life. A collodion baby phenotype is not associated. The classic hair shaft abnormality, trichorrhexis invaginata ('bamboo hairs,' 'ball-and-socket deformity'), is thought to result from a defect in keratinization of the internal root sheath. Multiple hairs from different areas should be examined, as only 20–50% of hairs may be affected. Although trichorrhexis invaginata may be present in the neonatal period, delayed and sparse hair growth at this time, as well as the easy breakage of these hairs, makes demonstration of the hair defect in the neonatal period difficult. Ichthyosis linearis circumflexa, the characteristic skin change associated with Netherton syndrome, is not seen before 2 years of age, but occurs eventually in 70% of patients. It manifests episodically, often lasting for a few weeks and then clearing for weeks or months. The ichthyosiform erythroderma, however, frequently improves with age. The atopic diathesis becomes problematic in two-thirds of patients, with the development of pruritic atopic dermatitis, multiple food allergies, and often accompanying, urticaria, angioedema, asthma, and/or anaphylaxis.

Extracutaneous Features

The failure to thrive is often profound, requiring hospitalization for nutritional support and correction of the hypernatremic dehydration that may be associated. Patients may have diarrhea, and occasionally demonstrate villus atrophy if intestinal biopsy is performed. Most patients have increased levels of IgE, but other laboratory and clinical evidence of immune dysfunction may be present as well. The increased risk of sepsis occurs as a result of both the abnormal skin barrier and the associated immune defects that are only in part owing to malnutrition.

Etiology/Pathogenesis

The underlying molecular basis for Netherton syndrome is mutations in *SPINK5*, a serine protease inhibitor.[66,67] Lymphoepithelial Kazal-type-related inhibitor (LEKTI), a putative serine protease inhibitor, is strongly expressed in differentiated keratinocytes in normal skin. The lamellar granule system transports and secretes LEKTI earlier than its potential serine protease targets kallikrein 5 and kallikrein 7, thus preventing degradation of desmoglein 1 and premature loss of stratum corneum integrity/cohesion.[68,69] Deficiency of LETKI also leads to excessive cleavage of profilaggrin to filaggrin, further affecting differentiation.

Differential Diagnosis

Netherton syndrome in the neonatal period must be distinguished from several other disorders with extensive scaling erythroderma, failure to thrive, and increased risk of infection, particularly several immunodeficiency disorders, other ichthyoses, and atopic or psoriasiform erythroderma (see also Chapter 17). Skin biopsy sections show subacute or chronic seborrheic or psoriasiform dermatitis with spongiosis.[70] The stratum corneum is thin and focally parakeratotic, and the granular layer is reduced. Electron microscopic studies have revealed features in skin biopsy specimens that are specific to Netherton syndrome, particularly the premature secretion of lamellar body contents, foci of electron-dense material separating lipid membranes, and disturbed maturation of lamellar membrane structures. Immunohistochemical staining to LETKI, the protein product of *SPINK5*, is also possible and with increasing availability will become a highly useful diagnostic investigation,[71] but is currently not widely available.

Treatment and Care

Treatment of Netherton syndrome is extremely difficult. Despite their pruritic, erythematous skin, patients tend to respond poorly to topical steroids, although some have improved after topical application of calcineurin inhibitors or calcipotriol. The poor cutaneous barrier of patients with Netherton syndrome may result in significant absorption of topically applied agents. For example, high blood levels of tacrolimus have been found following topical application for the associated dermatitis.[72] The application of keratolytic agents or administration of systemic retinoids often worsens the severity of the disorder, and their use is inappropriate during the neonatal period. Most patients prefer to use bland, thick emollients as the only therapy throughout life.

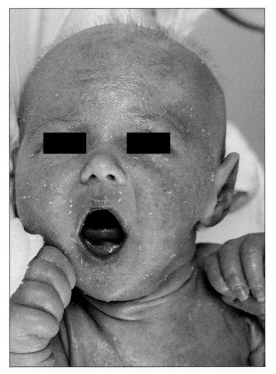

FIG. 18-7 A 32-day-old infant with failure to thrive, hypernatremic dehydration, and ichthyosiform erythroderma was diagnosed with Netherton syndrome by microscopic examination of one of just a few sparse hairs. Note the sparse hair secondary to trichorrhexis invaginata. The infant died of sepsis at 3 months of age. (Courtesy of Dr. Bernice Krafchik, Toronto, Canada.)

TRICHOTHIODYSTROPHY (TAY SYNDROME, IBIDS SYNDROME, PIBIDS SYNDROME, SIBIDS SYNDROME)

Cutaneous Features

Three autosomal recessive subsets of trichothiodystrophy (TTD) are associated with ichthyosis: IBIDS (ichthyosis with brittle hair, intellectual impairment, decreased fertility, and short stature), PIBIDS (IBIDS with photosensitivity; Tay syndrome), and SIBIDS (IBIDS with osteosclerosis). Of these, PIBIDS is the most common, comprising approximately 50% of cases of TTD. Neonates with TTD and ichthyosis are usually born with a collodion membrane. The severity of the ichthyosis after the membrane is shed is variable, ranging from a mild to a severe lamellar ichthyosis phenotype. In trichothiodystrophy the hair has a 10–50% reduction in sulfur content, leading to brittle hair that shows transverse fractures (trichoschisis), a decreased cuticular layer with twisting, and a nodular appearance that mimics trichorrhexis nodosa. Polarizing microscopy shows a 'tiger-tail' pattern of alternating light and dark bands consistent with the alternating content of sulfur in the hair. Examination of hairs at birth by polarizing microscopy may not reveal the tiger-tail pattern, and repeated examinations may be necessary later in the first months of life.[73]

Extracutaneous Features

Several other clinical features may be associated, including low birthweight, nail dystrophy, increased susceptibility to infection, neutropenia, hypothyroidism, nystagmus, optic atrophy, cataracts, and hypertonia.[74] Not uncommonly, patients die of sepsis during childhood.

Etiology/Pathogenesis

Cells from patients with PIBIDS show decreased DNA repair levels similar to those of patients with xeroderma pigmentosum (XP), but the development of skin cancer has not been described. The variable and multiple clinical features of PIBIDS may be due in part to the many genes that can result in this phenotype. TTD syndromes have been shown to be due to phenotype-specific mutations in either XPB or XPD. These genes encode the helicase subunits of TFIIH, a DNA repair factor that is also required for transcription of class II genes,[75] so that the brittle hair of PIBIDS syndrome may result from decreased transcription of the genes that encode the sulfur-rich matrix of hair and nails. TFIIH is a complex factor that includes the XPD and XPB gene products.[76] Recently a 75 amino-acid protein, designated p8 or GTF2H5, was identified as the tenth protein in this complex. This peptide appears to be critical in maintaining TFIIH base levels, which are known to be diminished in TTD-A.[77] Inactivating mutations in this gene have been shown to cause TTD-A.[78]

Differential Diagnosis

In the neonatal period other causes of collodion membrane need to be excluded. The development of extracutaneous features facilitates the diagnosis.

Treatment and Care

Management of the ichthyosis is as usual (see Box 18-1). Prenatal diagnosis of PIBIDS has been performed by DNA repair measurements in amniotic fluid cells, with confirmation by polarizing microscopic analysis of fetal hair.[79]

KERATITIS–ICHTHYOSIS–DEAFNESS (KID) SYNDROME

Cutaneous Features

The constellation of vascularizing keratitis, ichthyosiform hyperkeratosis, and sensorineural deafness is the characteristic feature of KID syndrome. Patients are usually born with erythematous or erythrokeratodermatous skin that is mildly scaling, although in some the presence of excessive vernix-like material is the presenting finding. Occasionally skin abnormalities are not noted until a few weeks of age.[80] The characteristic thick, leathery skin with tiny stippled papules develops during the first year of life, particularly during the first 3 months (Fig. 18-8). Well-defined verrucous hyperkeratotic plaques develop in 90% of patients, often localized to the face and limbs. Diffuse palmoplantar hyperkeratosis with a stippled or leathery pattern also occurs in almost all patients. Alopecia occurs overall in 80% of patients, ranging from minimal loss of eyebrows or eyelashes to total scalp alopecia; in 25% of patients the alopecia is congenital. An additional 17% of patients have sparse, fine hair without frank alopecia. The scalp may be markedly thickened in the affected neonate. Nails are dystrophic in the majority of patients. Sweating may be decreased or absent. Biopsy of skin shows nonspecific acanthosis with papillomatosis and basket-weave hyperkeratosis. Hair follicles may be atrophic. Squamous cell carcinoma of the skin and tongue has been described in more than 10% of patients, and may occur during childhood.

Extracutaneous Features

The hearing loss is sensorineural, congenital, and can be progressive. It can be detected in the neonate by brainstem-evoked auditory potential testing. Unlike the auditory changes, ophthalmologic features are progressive and most commonly develop in childhood or early adolescence, although photophobia from birth has been described. The keratoconjunctivitis sicca with corneal vascularization leads to pannus formation and markedly decreased visual acuity.[81] Approximately 45% of patients have recurrent infections, especially bacterial and candidal infections of the skin, auditory canals, and eyes. Some patients have shown evidence of immunodeficiency, with moderate increases in IgE levels, defective chemotaxis, and absent lymphocyte proliferative responses to Candida albicans.[82] Death from infection during infancy or early childhood has been reported.[83]

Etiology/Pathogenesis

Mutations in the GJB2 gene encoding the gap junction protein connexin 26 are now known to be the cause of KID syndrome in a majority of cases.[84] There does appear to be genetic heterogeneity, however, with mutations also identified in GJB6, which encodes connexin 30.[85] Gap junctions facilitate efficient cell–cell communication between all cells in multicellular organisms. This system facilitates a synchronized cellular response to a variety of intercellular signals by regulating the direct passage of low-molecular-weight metabolites (<1 kDa) and ions between the cytoplasm of adjacent cells.[86] The skin and inner ear have a high number of gap junctions, and in the skin they appear to have a role in the coordination of keratinocyte growth and differentiation.[87] Connexins are the major proteins of gap junctions and may be classified into three major groups, based on sequence homology: gap junction α (GJA), gap junction β (GJB), gap junction γ (GJC). Mutations

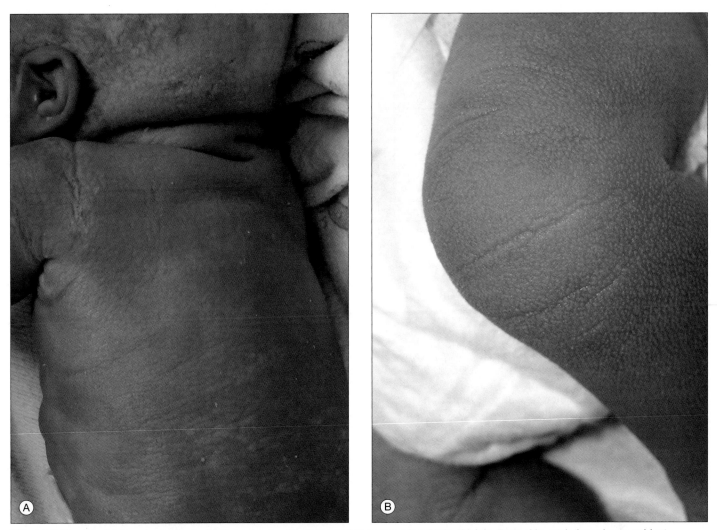

FIG. 18-8 Keratitis–ichthyosis–deafness (KID) syndrome. (**A**) Characterististic hyperkeratosis, thick leathery skin, and alopecia are evident. (**B**) Close-up of the leg demonstrates skin furrows and tiny stippled papules commonly seen in KID syndrome. (Courtesy of Marcos Antezana MD.)

in the β connexins have been shown to underlie epidermal disease, sensorineural hearing loss, and peripheral neuropathy. For detailed reviews of connexin biology see Richard[88] and Kelsell.[89] The relationship between epidermal disease and deafness is complex, and three out of the four autosomal dominant connexin mutations that are associated with epidermal disease are also associated with hearing loss.

Differential Diagnosis

Distinction from Clouston syndrome (see below) can be difficult and, as noted above, mutations in connexin 30 can underlie both phenotypes.[85] In both conditions the associated keratoderma has a characteristic 'stippled' quality that is quite distinctive. Erythrokeratoderma variabilis (EKV) can also closely resemble KID syndrome. Detection of deafness is indicative of KID syndrome. Molecular diagnosis is now relatively straightforward, as connexin genes are small and easily screened for mutations.

Treatment and Care

Therapy is supportive, but corneal and cochlear implants[90] have been successfully performed to treat corneal vasculariza-

tion and the hearing loss, respectively. Oral fluconazole therapy of recalcitrant fungating candidiasis can result in complete resolution and remission for at least a year.[91]

ERYTHROKERATODERMA VARIABILIS

Cutaneous Features

This autosomal dominant disorder manifests as two types of skin change. Some patients have migratory patches of erythema, which are often targetoid or circinate and last for days to months. With time, the lesions become more fixed, erythematous, and hyperkeratotic (Fig. 18–9). In other patients the disorder manifests as sharply demarcated, fixed hyperkeratotic plaques. Both types of lesion may be seen in the same patient. The typical areas of involvement are the extensor surfaces of the extremities, trunk, buttocks, and face. The palms and soles are not usually involved. Lesions are present at birth in up to one-third of patients.[92] Most begin to show evidence of involvement during the first year of life, with progression during childhood and stabilization at puberty. Later improvement has been described, including clearing with fevers.

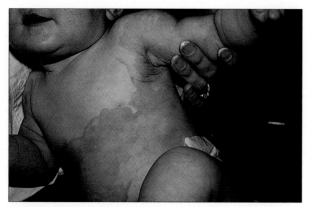

FIG. 18-9 Erythrokeratoderma variabilis. Sharply demarcated erythematous hyperkeratotic plaques on the trunk of an affected child.

Extracutaneous Features

There are usually no extracutaneous features, although ataxia has been described.[93]

Etiology/Pathogenesis

Mutations in the *GJB3* gene which encodes for connexin 31,[94] and the *GJB4* gene which encodes for connexin 30.3,[95,96] have been shown to cause erythrokeratoderma variabilis. There is likely to be further genetic heterogeneity as mutations in these two genes do not account for all cases of EKV.[96]

Differential Diagnosis

KID syndrome and Clouston syndrome can cause diagnostic confusion, but palmoplantar keratoderma is not usually a feature of EKV.

Treatment and Care

Treatment with systemic retinoids has resulted in improvement or clearing.

CLOUSTON SYNDROME (HIDROTIC ECTODERMAL DYSPLASIA)

Cutaneous Features

This autosomal dominant genodermatosis was first described in a very extensive family of French Canadian extraction who subsequently migrated to Scotland and the United States.[97–99] The characteristic features are total alopecia, severe nail dystrophy, hyperpigmentation over the joints, strabismus, bulbous fingertips, and a distinctive palmoplantar keratoderma. In contrast to hypohidrotic ectodermal dysplasia, sweating is unimpaired and the facies, teeth, and breast development are normal.[100] The original kindred has been followed extensively for years, and multiple cutaneous carcinomas of the nail bed and palmar tissue have been observed in several affected individuals.[101–103]

Extracutaneous Features

There are none.

Etiology/Pathogenesis

In 1996, Clouston syndrome was linked to chromosome 13q11-q12.1,[104] and subsequent studies have shown genetic homogeneity to this locus.[105–109] Recently mutations in the *GJB6* gene encoding the β connexin 30 were identified in all available kindreds. Interestingly, only two mutations in *GJB6* (G11R and A88V) accounted for all the families tested.[110] Mutations in *GJB6* had previously been identified in a small family with dominant nonsyndromic hearing loss,[111] emphasizing the complexity and diversity of phenotypes caused by dominant-acting connexin mutations.

Differential Diagnosis

Distinction from other connexin disorders such as KID syndrome and EKV is important and not always obvious. Alopecia is most commonly associated with Clouston syndrome. The stippled palmoplantar keratoderma is seen in both KID and Clouston syndrome.

Treatment and Care

No specific treatment is needed in the neonatal period. In the older child the nail dystrophy can be severe and require podiatric attention. In some individuals the alopecia is a major issue: psychological support and wigs may be required.

ERYTHROKERATODERMA PROGRESSIVA SYMMETRICA

Cutaneous Features

This autosomal dominant disorder is characterized by symmetric erythematous scaling plaques that may spare the trunk but which are commonly found on the knees, buttocks, and groin. The palms and soles are affected in approximately 50% of patients, and the face is occasionally involved. Features are usually present during the first few years of life.

Extracutaneous Features

There are usually no extracutaneous features.

Etiology/Pathogenesis

Skin biopsies show acanthosis with perinuclear vacuolization of granular cells. Ultrastructural studies show lipid vacuoles in the stratum corneum, and increased numbers of swollen mitochondria in granular cells.[112] Mutations in loricrin have been shown in some patients with this condition.[113, 114] Patients with these mutations may show features of Vohwinkel syndrome (VS), progressive symmetric erythrokeratoderma, or congenital ichthyosiform erythroderma with a collodion baby phenotype at birth.[115] Common clinical features include hyperkeratosis of the palms and soles, with digital constriction. Histologic characteristics common to all of these conditions include parakeratotic hyperkeratosis with hypergranulosis, and nuclear accumulation of mutant loricrin. The term 'loricrin keratoderma' has been proposed to encompass all these phenotypes.[116] The molecular basis in individuals with no palmoplantar involvement is not clear.

Differential Diagnosis

EKV can be distinguished by absence of palmoplantar involvement and transient migratory plaques (Table 18-1).

Treatment and Care

The use of oral retinoids has been reported to be effective. Topical keratolytics, retinoids, and glucocorticoids have also been used with more variable effects.[117]

CHILD SYNDROME

Cutaneous Features

The term CHILD syndrome is an acronym for congenital hemidysplasia with ichthyosiform nevus and limb defects. The condition occurs almost exclusively in girls, and is presumed to be lethal in affected males. The only case in a boy is thought to represent early postzygotic mosaicism.[118] The inflammatory ichthyosiform skin lesion of CHILD syndrome may be present at birth or develop during the first few months of life.[118,119] It is characterized by yellow, waxy scaling and is strikingly unilateral, generally with a sharp demarcation at the ventral and dorsal midline regions (Fig. 18-10). Streaks of inflammation and scaling can also follow Blaschko's lines, with involvement of the apparently unaffected side of the body. Similarly, streaks of normal skin may be interspersed within the area of the CHILD nevus. With increasing age, the skin lesions may improve or clear spontaneously, but thickened erythematous plaques in intertriginous areas tend to persist and be the most severely affected sites (ptychotropism).[120] The skin lesions of CHILD syndrome nevus can occur without any other abnormalities, but the occurrence of all features of CHILD syndrome in a sibling of a patient with only the CHILD nevus suggests variable expressivity within the spectrum of CHILD syndrome.[121]

Extracutaneous Features

A variable degree of ipsilateral skeletal hypoplasia is an important feature of CHILD syndrome. As with the skin changes, unilaterality is not absolute and slight changes may be present on the contralateral side. Punctate epiphyseal calcifications may be demonstrable by X-ray, but tend to disappear after the first few years of life. Cardiovascular and renal abnormalities are the major visceral problems in CHILD syndrome, although anomalies of other viscera have been described.[119]

Etiology/Pathogenesis

Biopsy of skin lesions shows epidermal acanthosis with marked parakeratosis alternating with orthokeratosis. Basophilic ghost cells of the granular layer are common. The papillary dermis is often filled with histiocytes showing foamy cytoplasm, resulting in the characteristic histopathologic pattern of verrucous xanthoma. Patients with CHILD syndrome have mutations in 3β-hydroxysteroid dehydrogenase.[122]

Differential Diagnosis

The nevus of CHILD syndrome needs to be distinguished from inflammatory linear verrucous epidermal nevus and linear psoriasis by the histopathologic features and the constellation of other clinical manifestations, if present. CHILD syndrome shares features with Conradi–Hünermann syndrome (see the following discussion), including the prevalence in girls with a presumed X-linked dominant inheritance pattern, ichthyosiform erythroderma, limb reduction defects, stippled epiphyses, and peroxisomal defects. The unilateral nature of the nevus and limb deformities helps to distinguish these conditions.

Treatment and Care

Multisystem care will include cardiology and renal workup. The limb hypoplasia requires orthopedic follow-up.

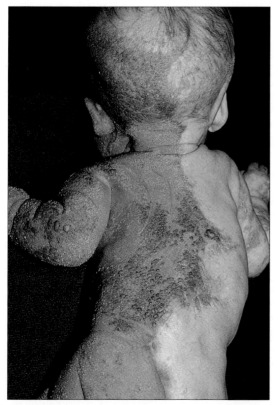

FIG. 18-10 CHILD syndrome. Sharply demarcated, erythematous ichthyosiform lesions with mostly unilateral distribution and hemidysplasia are characteristic findings. Thickened, yellow-brown scale in a whorled pattern is seen within areas of the CHILD nevus.

CONRADI–HÜNERMANN SYNDROME (X-LINKED CHONDRODYSPLASIA PUNCTATA)

Cutaneous Features

Most cases of chondrodysplasia punctata seen by dermatologists are the X-linked dominant Conradi–Hünermann form. Affected neonates are usually female, because the disorder is considered lethal to male fetuses. However, Conradi syndrome has been described in a few male patients with and without Kleinfelter syndrome.[123] At birth, patients most commonly have patterned erythroderma with overlying thin to thick psoriasiform scale (Fig. 18-11). In severe cases generalized ichthyosiform erythroderma occurs,[124] and later evolves into the typical patterning along Blaschko's lines. Involvement may be predominantly unilateral. With advancing age the ichthyosiform erythroderma and stippling improve, leaving finer scaling without underlying erythema and follicular atrophoderma. Cicatricial alopecia occurs as scalp scaling resolves. Ptychotropism may be seen (see CHILD syndrome).

Extracutaneous Features

Extracutaneous features include limb reduction, typically asymmetric, and facies with frontal bossing, saddle nose, and malar hypoplasia. Asymmetric, focal stippled calcifications of the epiphyseal regions are common. Cataracts usually develop later during childhood, but may be present at birth.[123]

Etiology/Pathogenesis

The underlying molecular basis is mutations in emopamil binding protein (3β-hydroxysteroid-Δ8, Δ7-isomerase), which

301

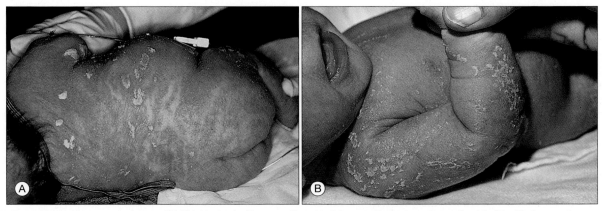

FIG. 18-11 Conradi–Hünermann syndrome. (**A**) Thick, psoriasiform scaling overlying erythema in a 1-month-old girl with the syndrome and chondrodysplasia punctata.. As the scaling desquamated, the underlying erythema along Blaschko's lines became more apparent. (**B**) The pattern of scale along Blaschko's lines is more evident in this neonate with Conradi–Hünermann syndrome. (From Paller AS. Ichthyosis in the neonate. In: Dyall-Smith D, Marks R, eds. Dermatology at the millennium: Overview of past achievements, current knowledge and future trends. London: Parthenon Publishing Group, 1998, with permission.)

is involved in plasmalogen synthesis.[125] Chondrodysplasia punctata can be inherited in both autosomal and X-linked fashion, and may also be the result of an environmental insult, particularly fetal exposure to warfarin.[124]

Differential Diagnosis

The differential diagnosis usually includes two other forms of chondrodysplasia punctata: autosomal recessive rhizomelic chondrodysplasia punctata,[124] and X-linked recessive chondrodysplasia punctata with steroid sulfatase deficiency.[126] The rhizomelic form is also associated with multiple peroxisomal defects. The ichthyosis occurs in approximately one-third of patients and is poorly described. Affected patients have developmental retardation and tend to die as infants. The X-linked recessive form occurs as a contiguous gene deletion syndrome of Xp, not at the site of Conradi syndrome. The ichthyosis is consistent with recessive X-linked ichthyosis, but stippled epiphyses are associated. Affected infants are deficient in steroid sulfatase activity, and have no peroxisome defects.

Treatment and Care

There is no specific care for the neonate with Conradi's syndrome.

ICHTHYOSIS FOLLICULARIS (IFAP SYNDROME)

Cutaneous Features

Patients are born with thickening of the skin, including the palms and soles, with generalized prominent follicular keratoses and mild erythema.[127,128] The clinical findings have been described as a 'nutmeg grater'.[129] The scalp is hairless, and severe photophobia is noted from birth. The nails may be dystrophic, and follicular pustules may be present. Biopsies show a hyperkeratotic stratum corneum with a thinned dermis. The hair follicles are atrophic and shortened, with abnormal localization of the bulbs to the deep portion of the dermis, rather than a subcutaneous location. There are no normal hair shafts, and sebaceous glands are absent. It is possible that at least two other forms exist in addition to this classic form.[130,131]

Extracutaneous Features

Some patients have had short stature, psychomotor delay, and/or seizures. Ocular changes including corneal ulceration, greatly reduced visual acuity,[132] and cataract[133] have been reported.

Etiology/Pathogenesis

The underlying gene defect in patients with IFAP is unknown. The predominance of the classic form of the disorder in male patients suggests an X-linked recessive disorder, and female carriers of this form may have linear involvement.[134] An autosomal recessive form has also been described.

Differential Diagnosis

The constellation of clinical signs should make the diagnosis apparent.

Treatment and Care

Systemic retinoids have been used in children as young as 3 years, with reported improvement.[135]

CHIME SYNDROME

Cutaneous Features

The acronym CHIME derives from coloboma, heart defects, ichthyosiform dermatosis, mental retardation, and ear anomalies, including conductive hearing loss. The skin is thick and dry at birth. Some patients show pruritic ichthyotic erythema during the first month of life. Lesions in the neonate may be sharply marginated and migratory (Fig. 18-12). Examination of biopsied skin specimens shows nonspecific changes.[136] The hair may be fine and sparse, with trichorrhexis nodosa seen on light microscopy.

Extracutaneous Features

The colobomas are most commonly retinal, although choroidal colobomas have been described.[137] A variety of heart defects have been associated, including tetralogy of Fallot, transposition of the great vessels, pulmonic stenosis, and ventricular septal defect.[136] Typical facial features include hypertelorism with a broad, flat nasal root, upslanting palpebral fissures, epicanthal folds and ptosis, macrostomia with a long colu-

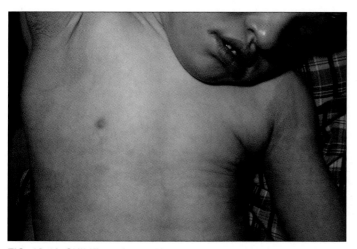

FIG. 18-12 CHIME syndrome. Note the migratory erythema in both axillae, and the characteristic thick lips seen in this syndrome.

mella but a short philtrum, and full lips. The ears tend to be cupped, with rolled helices. Brachydactyly is a constant feature. Other frequent characteristics include seizures and a wide-based gait. Cleft palate and renal or urologic anomalies have been described.

Etiology/Pathogenesis
The underlying defect is unknown.

Differential Diagnosis
CHIME syndrome must be distinguished from other ichthyotic disorders of infancy with developmental delay and seizures, particularly Sjögren–Larsson syndrome, Netherton syndrome, KID syndrome, and IBIDS syndrome. The characteristic ocular, cardiac, ear, and dysmorphic features help confirm the diagnosis.

GAUCHER DISEASE

Cutaneous Features
Gaucher disease (β-glucocerebrosidase deficiency) is an autosomal recessive disorder that results from the deficient activity of lysosomal glucocerebrosidase. Several infants with the type II (acute infantile cerebral or acute neuronopathic) form of Gaucher have been born with a collodion membrane.[2,138,139] The enzyme deficiency with resultant abnormalities in glucocerebrosidase degradation appears directly responsible for the abnormal skin of these infants. Glucosylceramide and ceramide are components of the intercellular bilayers in the stratum corneum that participate in skin permeability barrier function, so that the absence of glucocerebrosidase (which increases glucosylceramide and reduces the generation of ceramide) leads to abnormal skin thickening and increased transepidermal water loss.

Extracutaneous Features
Extracutaneous features of type II Gaucher disease include enlargement of the abdomen due to hepatosplenomegaly, and neurologic signs such as retroflexion of the head, strabismus, dysphagia, choking spells, and hypertonicity are features. Death usually occurs before the age of 1 year. Although patients with type II typically have acute neurologic progression and those with type III have slow progression, some children have been reported with an intermediate phenotype of delayed age of onset, rapid progression of neurologic disease with refractory seizures, and oculomotor abnormalities.[140] Based on the clinical presentation, along with the detected genotypic heterogeneity found by identification of all 18 alleles, it has been suggested that neuronopathic Gaucher disease is more likely to be a continuum of phenotypes, from the severe perinatal cases to mild involvement with oculomotor problems.[140] A subset of patients with this form of disease have intrauterine onset of symptoms and early perinatal death.[141]

Etiology/Pathogenesis
Gaucher disease type II is caused by mutation in the gene encoding acid β-glucosidase (GBA). Mutations in this gene also cause Gaucher disease type I and type IIII. Type II is the least common form.[142]

Treatment and Care
Management of Gaucher disease type II is palliative, as most children die in the first year.[143] Knowledge of genotype–phenotype correlation and assessment of biomarkers[144] may be helpful in delineating severity and counseling parents.

PALMOPLANTAR KERATODERMAS

The keratoderma of many forms of hereditary palmoplantar keratoderma (PPK) is first apparent during the first months of life, whereas in others (e.g. punctate keratoderma, keratoderma striata, Howell–Evans) it is not seen until early to late childhood.[145] In the neonatal period the affected areas may appear hyperhydrated (Fig. 18-13). The majority of types of palmoplantar keratoderma are autosomal dominant. Table 18-1 provides a comprehensive summary of the recognized PPK phenotypes and their genetic cause. Some of the more common conditions are discussed briefly below.

In the Unna form of palmoplantar keratoderma (nonepidermolytic), the palms and soles are usually red at birth or soon thereafter. The skin progressively thickens on the palms and soles, starting at the margins and extending centrally, with red borders that usually disappear after several years. Keratotic lesions may occasionally be found on the dorsum of the hands and feet, the volar wrists, and the knees and elbows. The overall extent of involvement is variable. Palmoplantar hyperhidrosis is commonly associated with the nonepidermolytic form. A mild defect of keratin 1 and defects in keratins 6a and 16 have been described in families with nonepidermolytic palmoplantar keratoderma.[146] In Greither syndrome (transgrediens form), the onset of thickening tends to be later, but the diffuse palmoplantar keratoderma extends onto the dorsum of the hands and feet. The knees, elbows, shins, and forearms are often involved. This syndrome is now known to be caused by mutations in keratin 1.[147–149]

Vorner palmoplantar keratoderma (epidermolytic palmoplantar keratoderma) can also begin at an early age, and is clinically indistinguishable from the nonepidermolytic form during the first years of life, when the keratoderma is confined to the palms and soles. Epidermolytic palmoplantar keratoderma results from mutations in keratin 9, a gene that is only expressed in the skin of the palms and soles, limiting its distribution of expression. It should be noted that descendants of the family described by Thost[150] as having nonepidermolytic

303

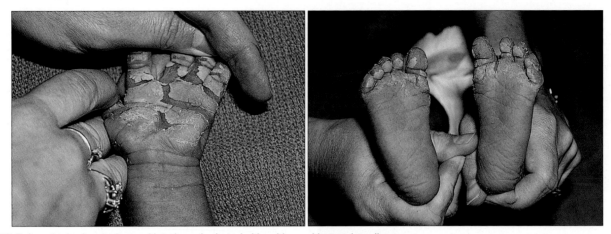

FIG. 18-13 Palmoplantar keratoderma. Note hyperhydrated skin with cracking and peeling.

palmoplantar keratoderma actually have keratin 9 mutations, demonstrating that the epidermolytic hyperkeratosis found in biopsy sections is an inconstant feature that may require several biopsies for detection.

The keratoses of Vohwinkel syndrome also are first noted shortly after birth, and gradually develop into the typical honeycombed diffuse palmoplantar hyperkeratoses with starfish-like keratoses on the backs of the hands, fingers, and toes. The constricting bands of the digits (pseudoainhum) first develop at 5 years of age or later, and can lead to autoamputation, as well as decreased motility of the hands. Some patients with Vohwinkel syndrome have alopecia, and an erythrokeratoderma has been described as well. The gene defect involves mutations in the gene that codes for loricrin.[151] Patients with deafness and the palmoplantar changes of Vohwinkel have connexin 26 mutations, not loricrin gene mutations.

Mal de Meleda, an autosomal recessive form of palmoplantar keratoderma, is not congenital but is present during the first 6 months of life as a diffuse palmoplantar keratoderma. The dorsal surfaces of the hands and feet are involved, and keratotic plaques tend to be present on the knees and elbows as well.[152] Koilonychia, nail thickening, and subungual hyperkeratosis are usually associated. Mild perioral erythema and hyperkeratosis may be present. Mal de Maleda is known to be caused by mutations in the secreted protein SLURP1.[153,154]

OLMSTED SYNDROME

Cutaneous Features
This extremely rare disorder usually presents with progressive thickening of the palms and soles during the first few years of life.[155] Typically, lesions are absent during the neonatal period, but begin as discrete lesions that become more confluent with time. The borders of keratoderma are erythematous. Contractures of the palms and soles, and autoamputation from progressive digital constriction are common. Lesions, particularly on the feet, tend to be exquisitely painful. After the onset of palmoplantar keratoderma the periorificial areas become hyperkeratotic, with fissured plaques. This involvement of periorificial areas, particularly perioral, perianal, perinasal, pericrural, and periumbilical, distinguishes this condition from other forms of palmoplantar keratoderma. Oral leukokeratosis, alopecia, and nail dystrophy have been described in association.

Extracutaneous Features
There are no extracutaneous features.

Etiology/Pathogenesis
The cause of this disorder is unknown.

Differential Diagnosis
Olmsted syndrome is usually easily distinguished from other mutilating keratodermas (Table 18-1).

Treatment and Care
In the neonatal period no specific care is necessary, and indeed keratolytics are best avoided as they do not tend to be helpful. In the older child regular paring and sometimes grafting is needed to preserve good hand function and the ability to walk.

TYROSINEMIA II

Cutaneous Features
Tryosinemia II (Richner–Hanhart syndrome) is an autosomal recessive disorder comprising a triad of ocular manifestations, cutaneous hyperkeratoses, and mental retardation. The early cutaneous lesions may be seen during the first year of life as sharply demarcated, yellowish keratotic papules of the palmar and plantar surfaces, but more commonly appear later, sometimes as late as the second decade. The lesions become more erythematous, erosive, and painful with time. In one case the clinical phenotype was of a diffuse PPK.[156] Nail dystrophy may also be associated.

Extracutaneous Features
The ocular manifestations of the disorder appear soon after birth.[157] Photophobia and bilateral tearing commonly occur within the first 3 months of life, and progress to corneal erosions. Ocular lesions are typically transitory, and are subject to intermittent relapses. The corneal lesions are frequently misdiagnosed as herpetic keratitis, and remissions may be misinterpreted as a response to antiviral therapy. The eye changes occasionally develop after the skin manifestations. Varying degrees of intellectual impairment have been described in less than half of affected patients.

Etiology/Pathogenesis

Tyrosinemia type II is caused by a deficiency of hepatic tyrosine aminotransferase (TAT)[158] that results in elevated tyrosine levels in the plasma and urine.

Differential Diagnosis

Diagnosis is occasionally delayed until adulthood. Early diagnosis is important, as appropriate dietary advice can help diminish the severity of neurological and ocular manifestations. In the neonate the corneal erosions can be mistaken for herpetic infections. The focal PPK that occurs later in life can resemble that associated with keratin 6A, 6B, 16, and 17 mutations, but may be more erosive.

Treatment and Care

The treatment of choice is dietary restriction of tyrosine with a low-phenylalanine, low-tyrosine diet.

RESTRICTIVE DERMOPATHY

Cutaneous Features

Neonates with this lethal autosomal recessive condition are born with rigid skin, attributed to fetal akinesia or hypokinesia deformation sequence.[159–161] Polyhydramnios with reduced fetal movements usually results in premature delivery at approximately 31 weeks' gestational age. Premature rupture of the membranes and an enlarged placenta with a short umbilical cord are often associated. The skin typically is thin, shiny, and red, with prominent vessels. Scaling and erosions are frequently seen (Fig. 18-14).

Extracutaneous Features

The facies are characterized by micrognathia, a small open mouth (O-shaped), pinched nares with choanal atresia or stenosis, and flattened or low-set pinnae. The constraint of movement in utero also leads to flexion contractures of the joints, and bony changes such as poor ossification of the clavicle; over-tubulation of the radius, ulna, and distal phalanges; and widened sutures and large fontanelles. Natal teeth have been described in 25–50% of patients with restrictive dermopathy. Most patients die of pulmonary hypoplasia with respiratory insufficiency or sepsis.

Etiology/Pathogenesis

Restrictive dermopathy may be caused by dominant de novo *LMNA* (encoding lamin A) mutations,[162] or, more frequently,

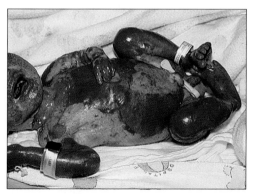

FIG. 18-14 Eroded, shiny skin is seen in this neonate with restrictive dermopathy.

by recessive null *ZMPSTE24* mutations, most of which lie in a mutational hotspot within exon 9.[163] This gene encodes a metalloproteinase specifically involved in the post-translational processing of lamin A. It is likely that many of the dysmorphic features observed in restrictive dermopathy are secondary to restricted fetal movement; this condition has been termed fetal akinesia deformation sequence (FADS).[13]

Differential Diagnosis

Skin biopsy at 20 weeks' gestational age may be normal,[164] and DNA-based prenatal diagnosis is best if the familial gene defect is known. The onset of intrauterine growth retardation, restricted fetal movement, and polyhydramnios that raise suspicion of the diagnosis may occur late in gestation, precluding prenatal testing. Histopathologic examination of skin biopsy sections shows a thick epidermis, and a thin dermis with a paucity and hypoplasia of cutaneous appendages. Collagen bundles are abnormally arranged, and elastic fibers are almost absent.

Treatment and Care

Most patients die during the neonatal period; the longest survivor with restrictive dermopathy died at 4 months of age.

NEU–LAXOVA SYNDROME

Cutaneous Features

Neu–Laxova syndrome is a rare, lethal, autosomal recessive trait characterized by severe intrauterine growth retardation, microcephaly with abnormal brain development, edema, and ichthyosis.[165,166] The ichthyosis is present at birth, but varies from mildly scaling skin to a harlequin fetus appearance. Histologic findings are nonspecific and show the acanthosis and orthokeratosis of lamellar ichthyosis. Excessive subcutaneous adipose tissue and myxomatous connective tissue may contribute to the characteristic edema.

Extracutaneous Features

The lack of brain development is characterized by lissencephaly and agenesis of the corpus callosum. Characteristic facial features include a slanted forehead, protuberant eyes, a flattened nose, deformed ears, micrognathia, and a short neck. Microphthalmia and cleft palate are occasionally associated. The limbs, fingers, and toes are abnormal, with syndactyly, hypoplasia, and contractures. Skeletal X-rays often show poor mineralization. The craniofacial and limb abnormalities are related to the reduced intrauterine movement, and are therefore defined as fetal akinesia/hypokinesis sequence, as has been described in other syndromes.

Etiology/Pathogenesis

The etiology of this rare and devastating disorder is unknown, but is the condition is likely to cover an number of heterogeneous disorders.[167]

Differential Diagnosis

The constellation of features usually makes the diagnosis clear.

Treatment and Care

Treatment is palliative.

NEONATAL SCALING OF HYPOHIDROTIC ECTODERMAL DYSPLASIA

The ectodermal dysplasias encompass a complex and highly diverse group of heritable disorders that share in common developmental abnormalities of ectodermal appendages (see Chapter 26). The most common form is hypohidrotic ectodermal dysplasia, which can be X-linked, autosomal dominant, or autosomal recessive. Scaling of the skin during the newborn period has been described in 70% of patients with X-linked hypohidrotic ectodermal dysplasia.[168] The skin has been described as 'like plastic,' peeling off in sheets, and 'like a snake peeling.' Some infants have been described as very dry at birth, and others as collodion membrane-like. Later in infancy the typical facial features, sparsity of hair, decreased ability to sweat, and eventually dental abnormalities allow the diagnosis to be confirmed. Patients tend to have an increased risk of upper respiratory tract infections and atopy, particularly manifesting as asthma and atopic dermatitis. The genetic defects underlying both X-linked and autosomal forms of hypohidrotic ectodermal dysplasia encode proteins of the ectodyplasin/NFκB signalling pathways.[169]

REFERENCES

1. Larregue M, Gharbi R, Daniel J, et al. [Collodion baby. Clinical course based on 29 cases]. Ann Dermatol Syphiligr (Paris) 1976; 103: 31–56.
2. Lui K, Commens C, Choong R, Jaworski R. Collodion babies with Gaucher's disease. Arch Dis Child 1988; 63: 854–856.
3. Frenk E, de Techtermann F. Self-healing collodion baby: evidence for autosomal recessive inheritance. Pediatr Dermatol 1992; 9: 95–97.
4. Buyse L, Graves C, Marks R, et al. Collodion baby dehydration: the danger of high transepidermal water loss. Br J Dermatol 1993; 129: 86–88.
5. Garty BZ, Wiseman Y, Metzker A, et al. Hypernatremic dehydration and hypothermia in congenital lamellar ichthyosis. Pediatr Dermatol 1985; 3: 65–68.
6. Perlman M, Bar-Ziv J. Congenital ichthyosis and neonatal pulmonary disease. Pediatrics 1974; 53: 573–575.
7. Raghunath M, Hennies H-C, Ahvazi B, et al. Self-healing collodion baby: a dynamic phenotype explained by a particular transglutaminase-1 mutation. J Invest Dermatol 2003; 120: 224–228.
8. Dale BA, Holbrook KA, Fleckman P, et al. Heterogeneity in harlequin ichthyosis, an inborn error of epidermal keratinization: variable morphology and structural protein expression and a defect in lamellar granules. J Invest Dermatol 1990; 94: 6–18.
9. Akiyama M, Sugiyama-Nakagiri Y, Sakai K, et al. Mutations in lipid transporter ABCA12 in harlequin ichthyosis and functional recovery by corrective gene transfer. J Clin Invest 2005; 115: 1777–1784.
10. Kelsell DP, Norgett EE, Unsworth H, et al. Mutations in ABCA12 underlie the severe congenital skin disease harlequin ichthyosis. Am J Hum Genet 2005; 76: 794–803.
11. Lefevre C, Audebert S, Jobard F et al. Mutations in the transporter ABCA12 are associated with lamellar ichthyosis type 2. Hum Mol Genet 2003; 12: 2369–2378.
12. Hovnanian A. Harlequin ichthyosis unmasked: a defect of lipid transport. J Clin Invest 2005; 115: 1708–1710.
13. Witters I, Moerman P, Fryns JP. Fetal akinesia deformation sequence: a study of 30 consecutive in utero diagnoses. Am J Med Genet 2002; 113: 23–28.
14. Haftek M, Cambazard F, Dhouailly D, et al. A longitudinal study of a harlequin infant presenting clinically as non-bullous congenital ichthyosiform erythroderma. Br J Dermatol 1996; 135: 448–453.
15. Prasad RS, Pejaver RK, Hassan A, et al. Management and follow-up of harlequin siblings. Br J Dermatol 1994; 130: 650–653.
16. Roberts LJ. Long-term survival of a harlequin fetus. J Am Acad Dermatol 1989; 21: 335–339.
17. Rogers M, Scraf C. Harlequin baby treated with etretinate. Pediatr Dermatol 1989; 6: 216–221.
18. Ward PS, Jones RD. Successful treatment of a harlequin fetus. Arch Dis Child 1989; 64: 1309–1311.
19. Lawlor F, Peiris S. Harlequin fetus successfully treated with etretinate. Br J Dermatol 1985; 112: 585–590.
20. Akiyama M, Yoneda K, Kim SY, et al. Cornified cell envelope proteins and keratins are normally distributed in harlequin ichthyosis. J Cutan Pathol 1996; 23: 571–575.
21. Wells RS, Kerr CS. Clinical features of autosomal dominant and sex-linked ichthyosis in an English Population. Br Med J 1966; 1: 947–950.
22. Penabad P, Arellano PE, Becker E, et al. Differential patterns of filaggrin expression in lamellar ichthyosis. Br J Dermatol 1998; 139: 958–964.
23. Nirunsuksiri W, Zhang S-H, Fleckman P. Reduced stability and biallelic, coequal expression of profilaggrin mRNA in keratinocytes cultured from subjects with ichthyosis vulgaris. J Invest Dermatol 1998; 110: 854–861.
24. Presland RB, Boggess D, Lewis SP, et al. Loss of normal profilaggrin and filaggrin in flaky tail (ft/ft) mice: an animal model for the filaggrin-deficient skin disease ichthyosis vulgaris. J Invest Dermatol 2000; 115: 1072–1081.
25. Compton JG, DiGiovanna JJ, Johnston KA, et al. Mapping of the associated phenotype of an absent granular layer in ichthyosis vulgaris to the epidermal differentiation complex on chromosome 1. Exp Dermatol 2002; 11: 518–526.
26. Smith FJ, Irvine AD, Terron-Kwiatkowski A, et al. Loss-of-function mutations in the gene encoding filaggrin cause ichthyosis vulgaris. Nature Genet 2006; 38: 337–342.
27. Sato N, Katsumata N, Kagami M, et al. Clinical assessment and mutation analysis of Kallmann syndrome 1 (KAL1) and fibroblast growth factor receptor 1 (FGFR1, or KAL2) in five families and 18 sporadic patients. J Clin Endocrinol Metab 2004; 89: 1079–1088.
28. Freiberg RA, Choate KA, Deng H, et al. A model of corrective gene transfer in X-linked ichthyosis. Hum Mol Genet 1997; 6: 927–933.
29. Traupe H, Kolde G, Happle R. Autosomal dominant lamellar ichthyosis: a new skin disorder. Clin Genet 1984; 26: 457–461.
30. Williams ML, Elias PM. Heterogeneity in autosomal recessive ichthyosis. Clinical and biochemical differentiation of lamellar ichthyosis and nonbullous congenital ichthyosiform erythroderma. Arch Dermatol 1985; 121: 477–488.
31. Huber M, Rettler I, Bernasconi K, et al. Mutations of keratinocyte transglutaminase in lamellar ichthyosis. Science 1995; 267: 525–528.
32. Schorderet DF, Huber M, Laurini RN, et al. Prenatal diagnosis of lamellar ichthyosis by direct mutational analysis of the keratinocyte transglutaminase gene. Prenat Diagn 1997; 17: 483–486.
33. Choate KA, Medalie DA, Morgan JR, Khavari PA. Corrective gene transfer in the human skin disorder lamellar ichthyosis. Nature Med 1996; 2: 1263–1267.
34. Huber M, Rettler I, Bernasconi K, et al. Lamellar ichthyosis is genetically heterogeneous–cases with normal keratinocyte transglutaminase. J Invest Dermatol 1995; 105: 653–654.
35. Parmentier L, Lakhdar H, Blanchet-Bardon C, et al. Mapping of a second

locus for lamellar ichthyosis to chromosome 2q33–35. Hum Mol Genet 1996; 5: 555–559.

36. Fischer J, Faure A, Bouadjar B, et al. Two new loci for autosomal recessive ichthyosis on chromosomes 3p21 and 19p12-q12 and evidence for further genetic heterogeneity. Am J Hum Genet 2000; 66: 904–913.

37. Pigg M, Gedde-Dahl T, Jr, Cox D, et al. Strong founder effect for a transglutaminase 1 gene mutation in lamellar ichthyosis and congenital ichthyosiform erythroderma from Norway. Eur J Hum Genet 1998; 6: 589–596.

38. Klar J, Gedde-Dahl T, Jr, Larsson M, et al. Assignment of the locus for ichthyosis prematurity syndrome to chromosome 9q33.3–34.13. J Med Genet 2004; 41: 208–212.

39. Paller AS. Lessons from skin blistering: molecular mechanisms and unusual patterns of inheritance? Am J Pathol 1996; 148: 1727–1731.

40. Irvine AD, McLean WH. Human keratin diseases: the increasing spectrum of disease and subtlety of the phenotype–genotype correlation. Br J Dermatol 1999; 140: 815–828.

41. Golbus MS, Sagebiel RW, Filly RA, et al. Prenatal diagnosis of congenital bullous ichthyosiform erythroderma (epidermolytic hyperkeratosis) by fetal skin biopsy. N Engl J Med 1980; 302: 93–95.

42. Rothnagel JA, Longley MA, Holder RA, et al. Prenatal diagnosis of epidermolytic hyperkeratosis by direct gene sequencing. J Invest Dermatol 1994; 102: 13–16.

43. Kanerva L, Karvonen J, Oikarinen A, et al. Ichthyosis hystrix (Curth–Macklin). Light and electron microscopic studies performed before and after etretinate treatment. Arch Dermatol 1984; 120: 1218–1223.

44. Sprecher E, Ishida-Yamamoto A, Becker OM, et al. Evidence for novel functions of the keratin tail emerging from a mutation causing ichthyosis hystrix. J Invest Dermatol 2001; 116: 511–519.

45. Richardson ES, Lee JB, Hyde PH, Richard G. A novel mutation and large size polymorphism affecting the V2 domain of keratin 1 in an African-American family with severe, diffuse palmoplantar keratoderma of the ichthyosis hystrix Curth–Macklin type. J Invest Dermatol 2006; 126: 79–84.

46. Bonifas JM, Bare JW, Chen MA, et al. Evidence against keratin gene mutations in a family with ichthyosis hystrix Curth–Macklin. J Invest Dermatol 1993; 101: 890–891.

47. Janin A, Copin MC, Dubos JP, et al. Familial peeling skin syndrome with eosinophilia: clinical, histologic, and ultrastructural study of three cases. Arch Pathol Lab Med 1996; 120: 662–665.

48. Cassidy AJ, van Steensel MA, Steijlen PM, et al. A homozygous missense mutation in TGM5 abolishes epidermal transglutaminase 5 activity and causes acral peeling skin syndrome. Am J Hum Genet 2005; 77: 909–917.

49. Geyer AS, Ratajczak P, Pol-Rodriguez M, et al. Netherton syndrome with extensive skin peeling and failure to thrive due to a homozygous frameshift mutation in SPINK5. Dermatology 2005; 210: 308–314.

50. Jagell S, Liden S. Ichthyosis in the Sjögren–Larsson syndrome. Clin Genet 1982; 21: 243–252.

51. Lacour M. Update on Sjögren–Larsson syndrome. Dermatology 1996; 193: 77–82.

52. Rizzo WB. Sjögren–Larsson syndrome. Semin Dermatol 1993; 12: 210–218.

53. Ito M, Oguro K, Sato Y. Ultrastructural study of the skin in Sjögren–Larsson syndrome. Arch Dermatol Res 1991; 283: 141–148.

54. Willemsen MAAP, Ijlst L, Steijlen PM, et al. Clinical, biochemical and molecular genetic characteristics of 19 patients with the Sjögren–Larsson syndrome. Brain 2001; 124: 1426–1437.

55. Nigro JF, Rizzo WB, Esterly NB. Redefining the Sjögren–Larsson syndrome: atypical findings in three siblings and implications regarding diagnosis. J Am Acad Dermatol 1996; 35: 678–684.

56. De Laurenzi V, Rogers GR, Hamrock DJ, et al. Sjögren–Larsson syndrome is caused by mutations in the fatty aldehyde dehydrogenase gene. Nature Genet 1996; 12: 52–57.

57. Sillen A, Jagell S, Wadelius C. A missense mutation in the FALDH gene identified in Sjögren–Larsson syndrome patients originating from the northern part of Sweden. Hum Genet 1997; 100: 201–203.

58. Willemsen MA, Rotteveel JJ, Steijlen PM, et al. 5-Lipoxygenase inhibition: a new treatment strategy for Sjögren–Larsson syndrome. Neuropediatrics 2000; 31: 1–3.

59. Igal RA, Rhoads JM, Coleman RA. Neutral lipid storage disease with fatty liver and cholestasis. J Pediatr Gastroenterol Nutr 1997; 25: 541–547.

60. Chanarin I, Patel A, Slavin G, et al. Neutral-lipid storage disease: a new disorder of lipid metabolism. Br Med J 1975; 1: 553–555.

61. Dorfman ML, Hershko C, Eisenberg S, Sagher F. Ichthyosiform dermatosis with systemic lipidosis. Arch Dermatol 1974; 110: 261–266.

62. Lefevre C, Jobard F, Caux F, et al. Mutations in CGI-58, the gene encoding a new protein of the esterase/lipase/thioesterase subfamily, in Chanarin–Dorfman syndrome. Am J Hum Genet 2001; 69: 1002–1012.

63. Jordans GH. The familial occurrence of fat containing vacuoles in the leukocytes diagnosed in two brothers suffering from dystrophia musculorum progressiva (ERB). Acta Med Scand 1953; 145: 419–423.

64. Kakourou T, Drogari E, Christomanou H, et al. Neutral lipid storage disease – response to dietary intervention. Arch Dis Child 1997; 77: 184.

65. Judge MR, Morgan G, Harper JI. A clinical and immunological study of Netherton's syndrome. Br J Dermatol 1994; 131: 615–621.

66. Chavanas S, Bodemer C, Rochat A, et al. Mutations in SPINK5, encoding a serine protease inhibitor, cause Netherton syndrome. Nature Genet 2000; 25: 141–142.

67. Bitoun E, Chavanas S, Irvine AD, et al. Netherton syndrome: disease expression and spectrum of SPINK5 mutations in 21 families. J Invest Dermatol 2002; 118: 352–361.

68. Ishida-Yamamoto A, Deraison C, Bonnart C, et al. LEKTI is localized in lamellar granules, separated from KLK5 and KLK7, and is secreted in the extracellular spaces of the superficial stratum granulosum. J Invest Dermatol 2005; 124: 360–366.

69. Descargues P, Deraison C, Bonnart C, et al. Spink5-deficient mice mimic Netherton syndrome through degradation of desmoglein 1 by epidermal protease hyperactivity. Nature Genet 2005; 37: 56–65.

70. Scheimberg I, Hoeger PH, Harper JI, et al. Omenn's syndrome: differential diagnosis in infants with erythroderma and immunodeficiency. Pediatr Dev Pathol 2001; 4: 237–245.

71. Ong C, O'Toole EA, Ghali L, et al. LEKTI demonstrable by immunohistochemistry of the skin: a potential diagnostic skin test for Netherton syndrome. Br J Dermatol 2004; 151: 1253–1257.

72. Allen A, Siegfried E, Silverman R, et al. Significant absorption of topical tacrolimus in 3 patients with Netherton syndrome. Arch Dermatol 2001; 137: 747–750.

73. Brusasco A, Restano L. The typical 'tiger tail' pattern of the hair shaft in trichothiodystrophy may not be evident at birth. Arch Dermatol 1997; 133: 249.

74. Hersh JH, Klein LR, Joyce MR, et al. Trichothiodystrophy and associated anomalies: a variant of SIBIDS or new symptom complex? Pediatr Dermatol 1993; 10: 117–122.

75. Bergmann E, Egly JM. Trichothiodystrophy, a transcription syndrome. Trends Genet 2001; 17: 279–286.

76. Cleaver JE. Splitting hairs – discovery of a new DNA repair and transcription factor for the human disease trichothiodystrophy. DNA Repair (Amsterdam) 2005; 4: 285–287.

77. Vermeulen W, Bergmann E, Auriol J, et al. Sublimiting concentration of TFIIH transcription/DNA repair factor causes TTD-A trichothiodystrophy disorder. Nature Genet 2000; 26: 307–313.

78. Giglia-Mari G, Coin F, Ranish JA, et al. A new, tenth subunit of TFIIH is responsible for the DNA repair syndrome trichothiodystrophy group A. Nature Genet 2004; 36: 714–719.

79. Sarasin A, Blanchet-Bardon C, Renault G, et al. Prenatal diagnosis in a subset of trichothiodystrophy patients defective in DNA repair. Br J Dermatol 1992; 127: 485–491.

80. Caceres-Rios H, Tamayo-Sanchez L, Duran-Mckinster C, et al. Keratitis, ichthyosis, and deafness (KID syndrome): review of the literature and proposal of a new terminology. Pediatr Dermatol 1996; 13: 105–113.

81. Sonoda S, Uchino E, Sonoda KH, et al. Two patients with severe corneal disease in KID syndrome. Am J Ophthalmol 2004; 137: 181–183.

82. Harms M, Gilardi S, Levy PM, Saurat JH. KID syndrome (keratitis, ichthyosis, and deafness) and chronic mucocutaneous candidiasis: case report and review of the literature. Pediatr Dermatol 1984; 2: 1–7.

83. Janecke AR, Hennies HC, Gunther B, et al. GJB2 mutations in keratitis–ichthyosis–deafness syndrome including its fatal form. Am J Med Genet A 2005; 133: 128–131.

84. Richard G, Rouan F, Willoughby CE, et al. Missense mutations in GJB2 encoding connexin-26 cause the ectodermal dysplasia keratitis–ichthyosis–deafness syndrome. Am J Hum Genet 2002; 70: 1341–1348.

85. Jan AY, Amin S, Ratajczak P, et al. Genetic heterogeneity of KID syndrome: identification of a Cx30 gene (GJB6) mutation in a patient with KID syndrome and congenital atrichia. J Invest Dermatol 2004; 122: 1108–1113.

86. Pitts JD. The discovery of metabolic co-operation. Bioessays 1998; 20: 1047–1051.

87. Choudhry R, Pitts JD, Hodgins MB. Changing patterns of gap junctional intercellular communication and connexin distribution in mouse epidermis and hair follicles during embryonic development. Dev Dyn 1997; 210: 417–430.

88. Richard G. Connexins: a connection with the skin. Exp Dermatol 2000; 9: 77–96.

89. Kelsell DP, Di WL, Houseman MJ. Connexin mutations in skin disease and hearing loss. Am J Hum Genet 2001; 68: 559–568.

90. Hampton SM, Toner JG, Small J. Cochlear implant extrusion in a child with keratitis, ichthyosis and deafness syndrome. J Laryngol Otol 1997; 111: 465–467.

91. Shiraishi S, Murakami S, Miki Y. Oral fluconazole treatment of fungating candidiasis in the keratitis, ichthyosis and deafness (KID) syndrome. Br J Dermatol 1994; 131: 904–907.

92. Knipe RC, Flowers FP, Johnson FR, Jr, et al. Erythrokeratoderma variabilis: case report and review of the literature. Pediatr Dermatol 1995; 12: 21–23.

93. Giroux JM, Barbeau A. Erythrokeratodermia with ataxia. Arch Dermatol 1972; 106: 183–188.

94. Richard G, Smith LE, Bailey RA, et al. Mutations in the human connexin gene GJB3 cause erythrokeratodermia variabilis. Nature Genet 1998; 20: 366–369.

95. Macari F, Landau M, Cousin P, et al. Mutation in the gene for connexin 30.3 in a family with erythrokeratodermia variabilis. Am J Hum Genet 2000; 67: 1296–1301.

96. Common JEA, O'Toole EA, Leigh IM, et al. Clinical and genetic heterogeneity of erythrokeratoderma variabilis. J Invest Dermatol 2005; 125: 920–927.

97. Clouston HR. A hereditary ectodermal dystrophy. Can Med Assoc J 1929; 21: 18–31.

98. MacKay H, Davidson AM. Congenital ectodermal dysplasia. Br J Dermatol 1929; 41: 1–5.

99. Joachim H. Hereditary dystrophy of the hair and nails in six generations. Ann Intern Med 1936; 10: 400–402.

100. Hassed SJ, Kincannon JM, Arnold GL. Clouston syndrome: an ectodermal dysplasia without significant dental findings. Am J Med Genet 1996; 61: 274–276.

101. Campbell CJ, Keokarn T. Squamous-cell carcinoma of the nail bed in epidermal dysplasia. J Bone Joint Surg Am 1966; 48: 92–99.

102. Mauro JA, Maslyn R, Stein AA. Squamous-cell carcinoma of nail bed in hereditary ectodermal dysplasia. NY State J Med 1972; 72: 1065–1066.

103. Williams M, Fraser FC. Hydrotic ectodermal dysplasia – Clouston's family revisited. Can Med Assoc J 1967; 96: 36–38.

104. Kibar Z, Der Kaloustian VM, Brais B, et al. The gene responsible for Clouston hidrotic ectodermal dysplasia maps to the pericentromeric region of chromosome 13q. Hum Mol Genet 1996; 5: 543–547.

105. Kibar Z, Dube MP, Powell J, et al. Clouston hidrotic ectodermal dysplasia (HED): genetic homogeneity, presence of a founder effect in the French Canadian population and fine genetic mapping. Eur J Hum Genet 2000; 8: 372–380.

106. Lamartine J, Laoudj D, Blanchet-Bardon C, et al. Refined localization of the gene for Clouston syndrome (hidrotic ectodermal dysplasia) in a large French family. Br J Dermatol 2000; 142: 248–252.

107. Radhakrishna U, Blouin JL, Mehenni H, et al. The gene for autosomal dominant hidrotic ectodermal dysplasia (Clouston syndrome) in a large Indian family maps to the 13q11-q12.1 pericentromeric region. Am J Med Genet 1997; 71: 80–86.

108. Stevens HP, Choon SE, Hennies HC, Kelsell DP. Evidence for a single genetic locus in Clouston's hidrotic ectodermal dysplasia. Br J Dermatol 1999; 140: 963–964.

109. Taylor TD, Hayflick SJ, McKinnon W, et al. Confirmation of linkage of Clouston syndrome (hidrotic ectodermal dysplasia) to 13q11-q12.1 with evidence for multiple independent mutations. J Invest Dermatol 1998; 111: 83–85.

110. Lamartine J, Munhoz Essenfelder G, Kibar Z, et al. Mutations in GJB6 cause hidrotic ectodermal dysplasia. Nature Genet 2000; 26: 142–144.

111. Grifa A, Wagner CA, D'Ambrosio L, et al. Mutations in GJB6 cause nonsyndromic autosomal dominant deafness at DFNA3 locus. Nature Genet 1999; 23: 16–18.

112. Nazzaro V, Blanchet-Bardon C. Progressive symmetric erythrokeratoderma. Histological and ultrastructural study of patient before and after treatment with etretinate. Arch Dermatol 1986; 122: 434–440.

113. Ishida-Yamamoto A, McGrath JA, Lam H, et al. The molecular pathology of progressive symmetric erythrokeratoderma: a frameshift mutation in the loricrin gene and perturbations in the cornified cell envelope. Am J Hum Genet 1997; 61: 581–589.

114. Suga Y, Jarnik M, Attar PS, et al. Transgenic mice expressing a mutant form of loricrin reveal the molecular basis of the skin diseases, Vohwinkel syndrome and progressive symmetric erythrokeratoderma. J Cell Biol 2000; 151: 401–412.

115. Matsumoto K, Muto M, Seki S, et al. Loricrin keratoderma: a cause of congenital ichthyosiform erythroderma and collodion baby. Br J Dermatol 2001; 145: 657–660.

116. Ishida-Yamamoto A. Loricrin keratoderma: a novel disease entity characterized by nuclear accumulation of mutant loricrin. J Dermatol Sci 2003; 31: 3–8.

117. Gray LC, Davis LS, Guill MA. Progressive symmetric erythrokeratodermia. J Am Acad Dermatol 1996; 34: 858–859.

118. Happle R, Effendy I, Megahed M, et al. CHILD syndrome in a boy. Am J Med Genet 1996; 62: 192–194.

119. Hebert AA, Esterly NB, Holbrook KA, Hall JC. The CHILD syndrome. Histologic and ultrastructural studies. Arch Dermatol 1987; 123: 503–509.

120. Happle R. Ptychotropism as a cutaneous feature of the CHILD syndrome. J Am Acad Dermatol 1990; 23: 763–766.

121. Baptista AP, Cortesao JM. [Inflammatory variable epidermal naevus (atypical ILVEN? A new entity?) (author's transl)]. Ann Dermatol Venereol 1979; 106: 443–450.

122. Konig A, Happle R, Bornholdt D, et al. Mutations in the NSDHL gene, encoding a 3beta-hydroxysteroid

dehydrogenase, cause CHILD syndrome. Am J Med Genet 2000; 90: 339–346.

123. Happle R. X-linked dominant chondrodysplasia punctata/ichthyosis/cataract syndrome in males. Am J Med Genet 1995; 57: 493.

124. Kalter DC, Atherton DJ, Clayton PT. X-linked dominant Conradi–Hünermann syndrome presenting as congenital erythroderma. J Am Acad Dermatol 1989; 21: 248–256.

125. Has C, Bruckner-Tuderman L, Muller D, et al. The Conradi–Hünermann–Happle syndrome (CDPX2) and emopamil binding protein: novel mutations, and somatic and gonadal mosaicism. Hum Mol Genet 2000; 9: 1951–1955.

126. Bick D, Curry CJ, McGill JR, et al. Male infant with ichthyosis, Kallmann syndrome, chondrodysplasia punctata, and an Xp chromosome deletion. Am J Med Genet 1989; 33: 100–107.

127. Hamm H, Meinecke P, Traupe H. Further delineation of the ichthyosis follicularis, atrichia, and photophobia syndrome. Eur J Pediatr 1991; 150: 627–629.

128. Eramo LR, Esterly NB, Zieserl EJ, et al. Ichthyosis follicularis with alopecia and photophobia. Arch Dermatol 1985; 121: 1167–1174.

129. Zeligman I, Fleisher TL. Ichthyosis follicularis. Arch Dermatol 1959; 80: 413–420.

130. Happle R. What is IFAP syndrome? Am J Med Genet A 2004; 124: 328.

131. Megarbane H, Zablit C, Waked N, et al. Ichthyosis follicularis, alopecia, and photophobia (IFAP) syndrome: report of a new family with additional features and review. Am J Med Genet A 2004; 124: 323–327.

132. Traboulsi E, Waked N, Megarbane H, Megarbane A. Ocular findings in ichthyosis follicularis–alopecia–photophobia (IFAP) syndrome. Ophthalm Genet 2004; 25: 153–156.

133. Tsolia M, Aroni K, Konstantopoulou I, et al. Ichthyosis follicularis with alopecia and photophobia in a girl with cataract: histological and electron microscopy findings. Acta Dermatol Venereol 2005; 85: 51–55.

134. Konig A, Happle R. Linear lesions reflecting lyonization in women heterozygous for IFAP syndrome (ichthyosis follicularis with atrichia and photophobia). Am J Med Genet 1999; 85: 365–368.

135. Khandpur S, Bhat R, Ramam M. Ichthyosis follicularis, alopecia and photophobia (IFAP) syndrome treated with acitretin. J Eur Acad Dermatol Venereol 2005; 19: 759–762.

136. Tinschert S, Anton-Lamprecht I, Albrecht-Nebe H, Audring H. Zunich neuroectodermal syndrome: migratory ichthyosiform dermatosis, colobomas, and other abnormalities. Pediatr Dermatol 1996; 13: 363–371.

137. Shashi V, Zunich J, Kelly TE, Fryburg JS. Neuroectodermal (CHIME) syndrome: an additional case with long term follow up of all reported cases. J Med Genet 1995; 32: 465–469.

138. Fujimoto A, Tayebi N, Sidransky E. Congenital ichthyosis preceding neurologic symptoms in two sibs with type 2 Gaucher disease. Am J Med Genet 1995; 59: 356–358.

139. Sidransky E, Sherer DM, Ginns EI. Gaucher disease in the neonate: a distinct Gaucher phenotype is analogous to a mouse model created by targeted disruption of the glucocerebrosidase gene. Pediatr Res 1992; 32: 494–498.

140. Goker-Alpan O, Schiffmann R, Park JK, et al. Phenotypic continuum in neuronopathic Gaucher disease: an intermediate phenotype between type 2 and type 3. J Pediatr 2003; 143: 273–276.

141. Felderhoff-Mueser U, Uhl J, Penzel R, et al. Intrauterine onset of acute neuropathic type 2 Gaucher disease: identification of a novel insertion sequence. Am J Med Genet A 2004; 128: 138–143.

142. Charrow J, Andersson HC, Kaplan P, et al. The Gaucher Registry: Demographics and disease characteristics of 1698 patients with Gaucher disease. Arch Intern Med 2000; 160: 2835–2843.

143. Grabowski GA. Recent clinical progress in Gaucher disease. Curr Opin Pediatr 2005; 17: 519–524.

144. Deegan PB, Moran MT, McFarlane I, et al. Clinical evaluation of chemokine and enzymatic biomarkers of Gaucher disease. Blood Cells Mol Dis 2005; 35: 259–267.

145. Irvine AD, Paller AS. Molecular genetics of the inherited disorders of cornification: an update. Adv Dermatol 2002; 18: 111–149.

146. Irvine AD, McLean WH. Human keratin diseases: the increasing spectrum of disease and subtlety of the phenotype–genotype correlation. Br J Dermatol 1999; 140: 815–828.

147. Terron-Kwiatkowski A, Paller AS, Compton J, et al. Two cases of primarily palmoplantar keratoderma associated with novel mutations in keratin 1. J Invest Dermatol 2002; 119: 966–971.

148. Terron-Kwiatkowski A, Terrinoni A, Didona B, et al. Atypical epidermolytic palmoplantar keratoderma presentation associated with a mutation in the keratin 1 gene. Br J Dermatol 2004; 150: 1096–1103.

149. Gach JE, Munro CS, Lane EB, et al. Two families with Greither's syndrome caused by a keratin 1 mutation. J Am Acad Dermatol 2005; 53: S225–230.

150. Kuster W, Zehender D, Mensing H, et al. [Vorner keratosis palmoplantaris diffusa. Clinical, formal genetic and molecular biology studies of 22 families]. Hautarzt 1995; 46: 705–710.

151. Maestrini E, Monaco AP, McGrath JA, et al. A molecular defect in loricrin, the major component of the cornified cell envelope, underlies Vohwinkel's syndrome. Nature Genet 1996; 13: 70–77.

152. Lestringant GG, Frossard PM, Adeghate E, Qayed KI. Mal de Meleda: a report of four cases from the United Arab Emirates. Pediatr Dermatol 1997; 14: 186–191.

153. Chimienti F, Hogg RC, Plantard L, et al. Identification of SLURP-1 as an epidermal neuromodulator explains the clinical phenotype of Mal de Meleda. Hum Mol Genet 2003; 12: 3017–3024.

154. Fischer J, Bouadjar B, Heilig R, et al. Mutations in the gene encoding SLURP-1 in Mal de Meleda. Hum Mol Genet 2001; 10: 875–880.

155. Perry HO, Su WP. Olmsted syndrome. Semin Dermatol 1995; 14: 145–151.

156. Madan V, Gupta U. Tyrosinaemia type II with diffuse plantar keratoderma and self-mutilation. Clin Exp Dermatol 2006; 31: 54–56.

157. Benoldi D, Orsoni JB, Allegra F. Tyrosinemia type II: a challenge for ophthalmologists and dermatologists. Pediatr Dermatol 1997; 14: 110–112.

158. Natt E, Kida K, Odievre M, et al. Point mutations in the tyrosine aminotransferase gene in tyrosinemia type II. Proc Natl Acad Sci USA 1992; 89: 9297–9301.

159. Mau U, Kendziorra H, Kaiser P, Enders H. Restrictive dermopathy: report and review. Am J Med Genet 1997; 71: 179–185.

160. Smitt JH, van Asperen CJ, Niessen CM, et al. Restrictive dermopathy. Report of 12 cases. Dutch Task Force on Genodermatology. Arch Dermatol 1998; 134: 577–579.

161. Welsh KM, Smoller BR, Holbrook KA, Johnston K. Restrictive dermopathy. Report of two affected siblings and a review of the literature. Arch Dermatol 1992; 128: 228–231.

162. Navarro CL, De Sandre-Giovannoli A, Bernard R, et al. Lamin A and ZMPSTE24 (FACE-1) defects cause nuclear disorganization and identify restrictive dermopathy as a lethal neonatal laminopathy. Hum Mol Genet 2004; 13: 2493–2503.

163. Navarro CL, Cadinanos J, Sandre-Giovannoli AD, et al. Loss of ZMPSTE24 (FACE-1) causes autosomal recessive restrictive dermopathy and accumulation of Lamin A precursors. Hum Mol Genet 2005; 14: 1503–1513.

164. Hamel BC, Happle R, Steylen PM, et al. False-negative prenatal diagnosis of restrictive dermopathy. Am J Med Genet 1992; 44: 824–826.

165. Naveed, Manjunath CS, Sreenivas V. New manifestations of Neu–Laxova syndrome. Am J Med Genet 1990; 35: 55–59.

309

166. Abdel Meguid N, Temtamy SA. Neu–Laxova syndrome in two Egyptian families. Am J Med Genet 1991; 41: 30–31.
167. Manning MA, Cunniff CM, Colby CE, et al. Neu–Laxova syndrome: detailed prenatal diagnostic and post-mortem findings and literature review. Am J Med Genet A 2004; 125: 240–249.
168. Executive and Scientific Advisory Boards of the National Foundation for Ectodermal Dysplasias. Scaling skin in the neonate: a clue to the early diagnosis of X-linked hypohidrotic ectodermal dysplasia (Christ–Siemens–Touraine syndrome). J Pediatr 1989; 114: 600–602.
169. Courtois G. The NF-kB signaling pathway in human genetic diseases. Cellular and Molecular Life Sciences (CMLS) 2005; 62: 1682–1691.

19

Inflammatory and Purpuric Eruptions

Eulalia Baselga, Antonio Torrelo

This group of eruptions is composed of lesions of variable morphology and diverse etiology. However, all have erythema as a common feature, a reflection of their inflammatory nature. Several disorders appear to represent hypersensitivity reactions, but for most the etiologic agents are unknown. The differential diagnosis of purpura is extensive in neonates, and includes hematological disorders, infections, trauma, and iatrogenic disorders.

ANNULAR ERYTHEMAS

Annular erythema is a descriptive term that encompasses several entities of unknown etiology characterized by circinate polycyclic lesions that extend peripherally from a central focus.[1,2] Because of subtle differences in clinical features, age of onset, duration of individual lesions, and total duration of the eruptions, a variety of descriptive terms have been coined for these disorders (Table 19-1). For prognostic reasons, it is useful to subdivide annular erythemas into transient and persistent forms.[3] Transient forms include annular erythema of infancy and the less well-established entity erythema gyratum atrophicans transient neonatale. Persistent annular erythemas include erythema annulare centrifugum, familial annular erythema, and erythema gyratum perstans. Other annular erythemas known to be a manifestation of well-defined diseases (e.g. neonatal lupus) or with distinctive clinical or histologic features (e.g. erythema multiforme, erythema chronicum migrans, erythema marginatum rheumaticum, and erythema gyratum repens) are not considered under this heading.

Annular Erythema of Infancy

Annular erythema of infancy is a benign disease of early infancy characterized by urticarial papules that enlarge peripherally, forming 2–3 cm rings or arcs with firm, raised, cord-like or urticarial borders.[4–6] Adjacent lesions become confluent, forming arcuate and polycyclic lesions (Fig. 19-1). Neither vesiculation nor scaling is present at the border. The eruption is asymptomatic. Individual lesions resolve spontaneously without a trace within several days, but new lesions continue to appear in a cyclical fashion until complete resolution within the first year of life. A few cases lasting for years have been described.[7–9]

The cause of annular erythema is unknown, and there are no associated systemic findings. Histologic studies reveal a superficial and deep, dense, perivascular infiltrate of mononuclear cells and eosinophils. No flame figures are observed. The epidermis is normal or mildly spongiotic.

Laboratory studies are normal. Peripheral eosinophilia does not accompany tissue eosinophilia. Immunoglobulin levels, including IgE levels, are normal. The differential diagnosis should include other annular lesions of infancy (see the following discussion). No treatment is warranted because of the self-limited nature of the eruption.

Erythema gyratum atrophicans transiens neonatale is a less well-defined entity,[10] characterized clinically by annular plaques with an erythematous border and an atrophic center. The lesions appear in the newborn period and resolve within the first year of life. Histologic findings include epidermal atrophy and a mild perivascular mononuclear infiltrate. Immunofluorescence studies reveal granular deposits of IgG, C3, and C4 at the dermoepidermal junction and around capillaries. Erythema gyratum atrophicans transiens neonatale possibly represents a variant of neonatal lupus erythematosus.[11]

Erythema Annulare Centrifugum

Erythema annulare centrifugum is a more persistent type of annular erythema that usually affects adults,[12] but may also occur in children and rarely in newborns.[3,13–16] The lesions are clinically somewhat similar to those of annular erythema of infancy, but scaling or vesiculation is seen at the border. The scales lag behind the advancing border, which, in contrast to annular erythema of infancy, is not indurated. Individual lesions resolve spontaneously after a few weeks, but new plaques continue to develop for years, or may be a lifelong condition. There is no associated pruritus.

Erythema gyratum perstans falls within the spectrum of erythema annulare centrifugum.[16–18] Some authors defend the distinctness of erythema gyratum perstans and consider distinctive features of this disorder to be its early onset, a duration of more than 15 years, the presence of slight to severe pruritus, and especially the presence of vesiculation.[16]

Erythema annulare centrifugum is thought to represent a hypersensitivity reaction to several trigger factors, including infectious agents (*Candida*,[19,20] Epstein–Barr virus,[14] and *Ascaris*[21]), drugs or foods,[22,23] and neoplasia, especially in adults. Intradermal injection of candidin or trichophytin may reproduce the clinical lesions.[13,24]

TABLE 19-1 Annular erythemas

	Age of onset	Clinical features	Duration of individual lesions	Duration of eruption	Healing	Histopathology
Transient Forms						
Annular erythema of infancy[4]	Early infancy	Annular plaques No scaling or vesiculation	Days	Transient (5–6 wk; cyclic course)	No residual lesions	Perivascular infiltrate of eosinophils
Persistent Forms						
Erythema annulare centrifugum[11]	Adulthood, newborn period possible	Mild scaling may be seen at borders	Weeks	Persistent (months or years, with new lesions developing continuously)	Residual hyperpigmentation	Superficial and deep perivascular cuff of lymphocytes
Familial annular erythema[22]	Early infancy to puberty Autosomal dominant	Possible vesiculation or scaling Geographic tongue may be associated Pruritus	Days	Persistent (lifelong, short remissions)	Transient hyperpigmentation	Superficial perivascular cuff of lymphocytes Spongiosis and parakeratosis
Erythema gyratum perstans[12]	Early infancy	Scaling, constant Vesiculation possible Central atrophy	Weeks	Persistent (lifelong)	Transient hyperpigmentation	Perivascular cuff of lymphocytes Spongiosis and parakeratosis

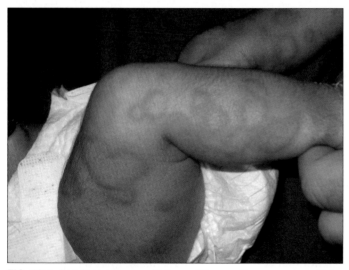

FIG. 19-1 Annular erythema of infancy: The eruption was congenital.

Histologic features consist of a dense, superficial, perivascular mononuclear infiltrate. Parakeratosis or epidermal spongiosis may be present. No therapy has been successful in all cases. Treatment agents include oral nystatin,[20] oral amphotericin B,[19] topical antifungals, antihistamines, disodium cromoglycate, and interferon-α.[13]

Familial Annular Erythema

Familial cases of annular erythema with autosomal dominant inheritance have been described.[25,26] The onset is in early infancy. Scaling, vesiculation, and pruritus may be more common than in erythema annular centrifugum. Lesions resolve with residual hyperpigmentation. Chronicity is the rule. Geographic tongue may be associated.[26]

Differential Diagnosis of Annular Erythemas

Differential diagnosis includes other eruptions with ringlike lesions, such as neonatal lupus, erythema multiforme, urticaria, urticarial lesions of pemphigoid, fungal infections, erythema chronicum migrans, and congenital Lyme disease.[7,27,28] Serum antibody determinations (antinuclear, SS-A, and SS-B) are recommended to exclude neonatal lupus.

NEONATAL LUPUS ERYTHEMATOSUS[29–36]

Neonatal lupus erythematosus (NLE) is a disease of newborns caused by maternally transmitted autoantibodies. The major manifestations are dermatologic and cardiac. Skin findings are transient. Cardiac disease, which is responsible for the morbidity and mortality of NLE, begins in utero and affects the cardiac conduction system permanently. Other findings include hepatic and hematologic abnormalities. Mothers of infants with neonatal lupus have anti-Ro/SS-A autoantibodies in 95% of cases. Anti-La/SS-B and anti-U1RNP autoantibodies have also been implicated in the pathogenesis of NLE in a minority of patients.[37,38]

Cutaneous Findings

Fifty per cent of infants with NLE have skin lesions, and congenital heart block is present in about 10%.[29,36] Lesions commonly develop at a few weeks of age but may be apparent at birth, which suggests that ultraviolet (UV) radiation is not essential for the development of skin lesions in NLE.[39] Clinically, skin lesions are analogous to those of subacute cutaneous lupus in its two variants: papulosquamous and annular. Papulosquamous lesions are more common and are

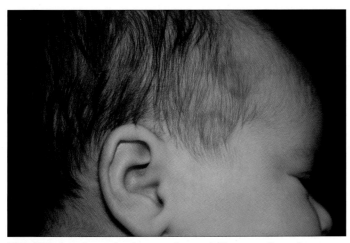

FIG. 19-2 Annular scaly plaques of neonatal lupus erythematosus resembling tinea corporis.

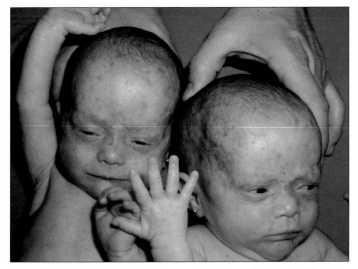

FIG. 19-3 Atrophic plaques and raccoon eyes on the faces of twins with neonatal lupus.

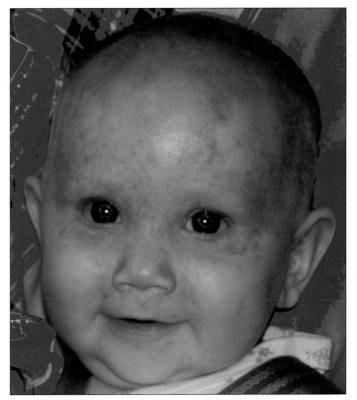

FIG. 19-4 'Raccoon eyes' and prominent facial erytnema in an infant with neonatal lupus (courtesy of Dr. Joseph Lam).

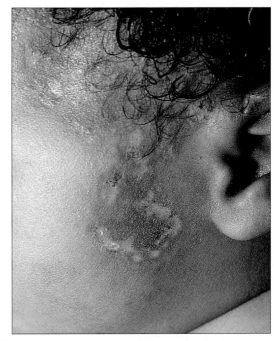

FIG. 19-5 Atrophy and pigmentary changes in an infant with neonatal lupus erythematosus. This boy also had congenital A-V block.

characterized by erythematous, nonindurated scaly plaques (Fig. 19-2). Sometimes the skin lesions have an atrophic appearance (Fig. 19-3). Ulcerations may be present.[40] In contrast to discoid lupus, scarring and follicular plugging are absent. The annular variant, which occurs almost exclusively in Japan, consists of annular, more inflammatory plaques.[41] Lupus profundus and generalized poikiloderma with erosions and patchy alopecia are rare manifestations.[42,43]

NLE lesions may be widespread but are most common on the face and scalp, predominantly affecting the periorbital and malar areas and often causing a 'raccoon eyes' appearance (Figs 19-3 and 19-4). The eruption is frequently precipitated or aggravated by sun exposure. Sun exposure is not strictly required, however, as the lesions may occur in sun-protected areas such as the diaper region, palms, and soles.[39,44,45] Skin lesions are transient and cease to appear around the age of 6 months, after the disappearance of maternal antibodies. Transient hypopigmentation and epidermal atrophy may result (Fig. 19-5).[36] Telangiectasia is a more permanent sequela. Telangiectasia also may be an initial sign of NLE, occurring without preceding identifiable inflammatory lesions; features of cutis marmorata telangiectatica congenita have been observed.[35,46] A case of NLE with a serological profile consis-

tent with drug-induced lupus has been described in a newborn whose mother was treated with α-interferon during pregnancy.[47]

Extracutaneous Findings

The most significant manifestation is isolated complete congenital heart block. More than 90% of such cases are due to

NLE. Most patients have third-degree block, but progression from a second-degree block has been reported.[48] Heart block can often be detected as early as 20 weeks of gestation.

Transient liver disease, manifesting as hepatomegaly (with a picture of cholestasis) or elevation of liver enzymes,[35,49–51] and thrombocytopenia or other isolated cytopenias, may occur.[52] Petechiae and purpura have been described as presenting signs of NLE.[53] Less common findings include thrombosis associated with anticardiolipin antibodies, hypocalcemia, spastic paraparesis, pneumonitis, and transient myasthenia gravis.[54–56] Central nervous system (CNS) involvement has been reported in 10 of 11 consecutive infants with NLE, in the form of ultrasound and CT scan abnormalities which did not result in clinical neurological manifestations.[57] Such CNS involvement in NLE is probably a transient phenomenon.

Between 30% and 50% of mothers of infants with NLE have a connective tissue disease, most commonly SLE or Sjögren syndrome. Most, however, are asymptomatic. The risk for developing overt connective tissue disease in these mothers is highly debated, with estimates ranging from 2% to more than 70%.[36,58–63]

Etiology and Pathogenesis

It is universally agreed that placentally transmitted maternal IgG autoantibodies are necessary for the pathogenesis of NLE, but not sufficient.[64] The most commonly implicated autoantibodies have been anti-Ro/SS-A and anti-La/SS-B. More than 95% of NLE infants have anti-Ro antibody, and 60–80% have anti-La antibodies. A small subset of affected infants do not have detectable anti-Ro or anti-La antibodies, but instead have anti-U1RNP.[37,38] Mothers with high titers of anti-Ro and anti-La antibodies are at greater risk of delivering an infant with NLE. Despite initial observations based on immunoblot or ELISA testing that anti-52 kDa Ro antibodies conferred a higher risk of NLE than anti-60 kDa Ro antibodies, more precise testing with line immunoassay has revealed that antibodies to 60 kDa Ro are significantly more sensitive than antibodies to 52 kDa Ro and 48 kDa La.[65] Furthermore, comparing mothers of children with NLE with rash alone or with congenital heart block, there is no significant difference in the prevalence of any of the three antibodies between the two groups.[65] However, significantly more symptomatic mothers of children with congenital heart block have anti-La antibodies than do disease-matched mothers with unaffected children.[65] Moreover, the mean level of anti-La seems to be higher in mothers of infants with congenital heart block than in mothers of children with cutaneous NLE.[66]

It is not clear why only less than 5% of mothers with anti-Ro and anti-La antibodies give birth to affected children and why mothers of affected infants are often asymptomatic despite having the same antibodies. Furthermore, fraternal twins are often discordant for NLE, and NLE does not occur in every pregnancy. Genetic factors may be important for the development of NLE in children with maternal lupus antibodies. A link has been suggested between NLE rash and the allele HLA-DRB1*03, as well as a -308A polymorphism in the TNF-α gene.[34] Alternatively, maternal and/or sibling microchimerism may play an additional role, as levels of microchimerism have been reported to correlate with NLE disease activity.[67]

Laboratory Tests and Histopathology

Serologic studies for autoantibodies in the mother and infant demonstrate anti-Ro, anti-La, and/or anti-U1RNP antibodies.

Anti-nDNA, anticardiolipin antibodies, antinuclear antibody, and rheumatoid factor may also be present. Anti-Sm antibody, highly specific for systemic lupus erythematosus, is not found in NLE. The maternal antibody titer is usually higher than the infant titer, which may even be negative if only immunodiffusion techniques are used. More sensitive methods, such as ELISA, immunoblotting, or line immunoassay, should be used in such instances. Skin biopsy, which is usually not necessary for diagnosis, shows changes characteristic of lupus erythematosus, that is, epidermal atrophy and vacuolization of the basal layer with a sparse lymphohistiocytic infiltrate at the dermoepidermal junction and in a periappendageal distribution. In many instances, histopathological features in children with NLE rash are subtle. Direct immunofluorescence is positive in 50% of cases, demonstrating granular deposits of IgG, C3, and IgM at the dermoepidermal junction. Histopathologic examination of the heart shows replacement of the atrioventricular node by fibrosis or fatty tissue. Endomyocardial fibroelastosis and patent ductus arteriosus may also be seen,[68,69] as well as deposits of IgG and complement.[70]

Differential Diagnosis

The differential diagnosis includes congenital rubella, cytomegalovirus infection, annular erythema of infancy, tinea corporis, and seborrheic dermatitis. Congenital syphilis should also be considered, but mucosal lesions are not a feature of NLE. False positive serologic tests for syphilis may occur in NLE. Telangiectasia and photosensitivity may suggest Bloom syndrome or Rothmund–Thomson syndrome. Serologic studies for autoantibodies in both infant and mother help to confirm the diagnosis. Skin biopsy for histologic and direct immunofluorescence studies is seldom necessary.

Course, Management, Treatment, and Prognosis

Neonates with suspected NLE should receive a complete physical examination, electrocardiogram, complete blood count with platelet count, and liver function tests (Box 19-1).

Skin lesions are transient. Treatment of skin disease consists of sun protection and the application of topical steroids. Pulsed dye laser therapy may be considered for residual telangiectasia. Congenital heart block is permanent. Half of newborns with complete congenital heart block require implantation of a pacemaker in the neonatal period.[32,61,71] The average

---

Box 19-1 Recommended evaluation of children with neonatal lupus erythematosus

- Clinical skin examination
- Complete clinical examination
- Skin biopsy (if clinical diagnosis not achieved)
- Full blood count (including platelets)
- Coagulation screen (including lupus anticoagulant and antiphospholipid antibodies)
- Serum chemistry (including liver function test)
- Autoantibody screening: antinuclear antibodies, anti-Ro, anti-La, anti-RNP
- Electrocardiogram and echocardiogram. Referral to pediatric cardiologist
- CNS ultrasound. Consider brain CT scan or MRI if clinical examination abnormal

mortality from complete congenital heart block in the neonatal period is 15%; another 10–20% die of pacemaker complications.[27,32] Late-onset cardiomyopathy may develop in a few infants.[72–74]

For mothers with anti-Ro or anti-La antibodies, the risk of delivering an infant with NLE is 1–20%, depending on whether they have asymptomatic or symptomatic SLE.[29,32] The risk of recurrence of congenital heart block in subsequent pregnancies may be as high as 25%.[61] Such pregnancies should be closely monitored, with repeated fetal echocardiograms.[75] If signs of intrauterine congestive heart failure are detected dexamethasone or plasmapheresis, or both, have been given.[32,76–79]

Although NLE is usually self-limited, SLE or other rheumatologic/autoimmune diseases may develop later in life in a small subset of patients.[62,80,81] The exact risk is unknown.

DRUG ERUPTIONS[82–85]

Cutaneous drug reactions are extremely rare in the neonatal period because the ability to generate a drug-induced immune response appears to be lower in infants.[86–88] Furthermore, most drug reactions require time for sensitization, which may range from 1 to 4 weeks or more, as well as re-exposure to the causative drug. Finally, newborns and young infants are less exposed to drugs than adults. Cutaneous adverse reactions to drugs may be classified according to the clinical characteristics of the eruption (Box 19-2). Whenever a suspect eruption is observed, a detailed history of medications should be obtained, including drugs administered to the mother, which may be present in breast milk. Morbilliform (Fig. 19-6) or maculopapular eruptions (Fig. 19-7) are the most frequent type of drug reaction in neonates, and antibiotics are commonly implicated (Fig. 19-8). Distinguishing a drug eruption from a viral exanthem is often difficult.

EMLA cream, a local anesthetic that may be used with great frequency in neonatal units, has been noted to produce a localized purpuric eruption.[89,90] This type of reaction is seen preferentially in neonates, and subsequent applications of the cream do not always reproduce the purpuric lesions. Methemoglobinemia is another complication of EMLA use in this age group.[90] EMLA cream should therefore be used with caution in infants who are taking methemoglobin-inducing medications such as sulfonamides, acetaminophen, nitroglycerin, nitroprusside, and phenytoin, and particularly in those with a history of methemoglobinemia.

Vancomycin, an antibiotic frequently administered to premature newborn infants for *Staphylococcus epidermidis* nosocomial infections, may produce shock and rash in newborns

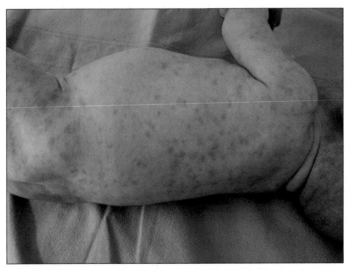

FIG. 19-7 Maculopapular eruption caused by diazoxide.

Box 19-2 Clinical patterns of cutaneous drug reactions

Maculopapular

Urticarial

Serum sickness–like

Hypersensitivity syndrome

Erythema multiforme

Toxic epidermal necrolysis

Fixed drug

Purpuric

Vasculitic

Lichenoid

Photo induced

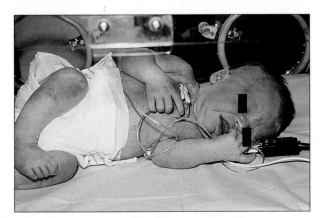

FIG. 19-6 Drug eruption resulting from procainamide.

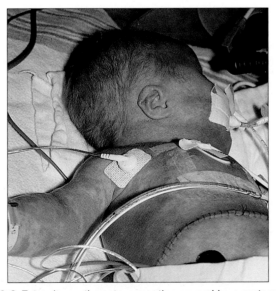

FIG. 19-8 Extensive erythematous eruption caused by a systemic antibiotic.

(red-baby syndrome).[91–93] This reaction is characterized by the appearance of an intense, macular, erythematous eruption on the neck, face, and upper trunk shortly after the infusion is completed. It may be accompanied by hypotension and shock. The reaction resolves rapidly in a matter of hours. It is frequently associated with rapid infusion; however, lengthening the infusion to more than 1 hour does not completely eliminate the risk.[92]

Newborns with AIDS have an increased susceptibility to drug reactions.[94,95] Reactions to trimethroprim/sulfamethoxazole in patients with HIV infections can be severe and life-threatening.[96]

Fixed drug reactions of the scrotum and penis, with erythema and edema resulting from hydroxyzine hydrochloride, have been described in early infancy.[97] However, hydroxyzine hydrochloride is administered infrequently in the neonatal period because of the risk of antimuscarinic effects, such as restlessness and excitation.

Serum sickness-like reaction is a type of drug reaction that occurs predominantly in children and has been reported in infants 5 months of age.[98] It is characterized by fever, an urticarial eruption, and arthralgias. Lymphadenopathy may be present. In contrast to true serum sickness, there are no immune complexes, vasculitis, or renal impairment. The most commonly implicated drug has been cefaclor.[98–100] This type of reaction may be seen in infants with an unknown or presumably viral etiology (Fig. 19-9)

Hypersensitivity syndrome reaction is a serious drug reaction characterized by fever, skin rash, lymphadenopathy, and internal organ involvement, especially of the liver.[101,102] The most commonly implicated drugs are anticonvulsants, and therefore it is not rare in children. A fatal case in a 3-month-old infant has been reported, as well as a case in a premature infant.[103,104]

Toxic epidermal necrolysis (TEN) is extremely rare in newborns. Cases of TEN in newborns have been related to antibiotics and phenobarbital.[105] All cases described so far proved fatal.

Vegetant bromoderma is a reaction to bromides characterized by coalescing papules and pustules which form vegetant inflammatory or pseudotumoral lesions. It usually affects the scalp, face, and legs. Most cases of vegetant bromoderma have

been described in infants after the ingestion of syrups and solutions containing bromide, which has sedative and expectorant properties, or the spasmolytic agent scopolamine bromide.[106] The eruption ceases after withdrawal of bromide. The risk of systemic intoxication, known as bromism, makes it advisable to avoid bromide use in newborns and infants.

Other anectodal reports of toxicoderma in very young infants or newborns have been described, such as a papular eruption from G-CSF for collection of stem cells (Fig. 19-10),[107] a lichenoid reaction to ursodeoxycholic acid for neonatal hepatitis,[108] and a maculopapular rash from diazoxide used for neonatal hyperglycemia (see Fig. 19-7).

URTICARIA

Urticaria (hives) occurs frequently in childhood but is uncommon in children younger than 6 months and even rarer in the neonatal period.[82,109–117] Urticaria is usually sporadic; however, familial forms with autosomal dominant inheritance have been described for many of the physical urticarias, such as dermographism, heat urticaria, cold urticaria, and vibratory urticaria.

Urticaria can be divided into acute (lasting less than 6 weeks) and chronic (lasting more than 6 weeks) types. Nevertheless, this arbitrary division has prognostic and etiopathogenic significance. In infants, chronic urticaria is very rare.[111,118] Physical urticarias represent a special subgroup of urticaria in which wheals are elicited by different types of physical stimuli.[119] These include dermographism, cold, pressure, cholinergic, aquagenic, vibratory, and solar urticaria.

Cutaneous Findings

Urticaria is characterized by transient edematous pruritic wheals (Fig. 19-11). By definition, individual lesions last less than 24 hours. Hives may occur on the skin and mucous membranes. Angioedema or giant urticaria is a closely related entity in which there is swelling of the deep subcutaneous tissues and diffuse swelling of the eyelids, genitalia, lips, and tongue. It may be seen alone, or more often in association with 'common' urticaria. Urticaria in children has certain characteristic features. The hives tend to coalesce, forming bizarre polycyclic, serpiginous, or annular shapes (figurative urticaria, Fig. 19-12; or annular urticaria, Fig. 19-13), and may become hemorrhagic.[109,112] Edema is often pronounced

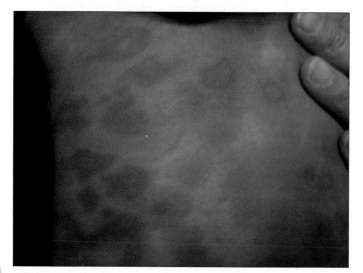

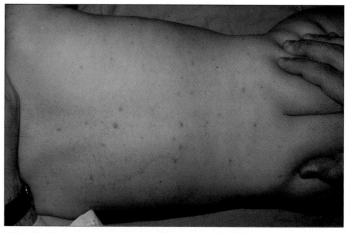

FIG. 19-9 Infant with serum sickness-like eruption.

FIG. 19-10 Papulopustular eruption due to G-CSF.

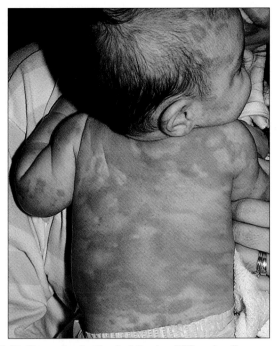

FIG. 19-11 Generalized urticaria following DPT and polio immunizations.

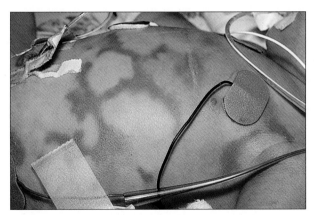

FIG. 19-12 Polycyclic lesions of urticaria associated with prostaglandin E₂ infusion.

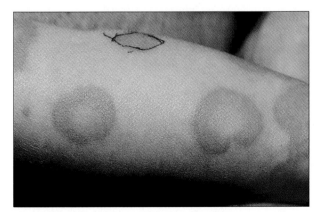

FIG. 19-13 Annular urticaria of unknown etiology.

and painful. These features confer a dramatic appearance to the eruption. in children the itching may be absent. Urticaria may be more common and recurrent in atopic patients.[112,115]

Extracutaneous Findings

Acute urticaria may be accompanied by signs of anaphylactic shock. In cases of angioedema, abdominal pain, diarrhea, vomiting, respiratory compromise, and joint pain may occur.

Etiology and Pathogenesis[82,113]

Urticaria develops as a result of an increased permeability of capillaries and small venules, which leads to leakage of fluid into the extravascular space. Mast cell activation and subsequent mediator release are responsible for these changes. Histamine is the best-known mediator. Many triggers (secretagogues) initiate mast cell degranulation through receptors on mast cell membranes, either via an IgE-dependent mechanism or through complement activation (immunologic secretagogues) or by acting directly without the need for receptors (nonimmunologic secretagogues).

The most common provocative agents in children are drugs, foods, and infections, which account for 40% of the cases of acute urticaria.[112,115,117] Antipyretics (primarily aspirin) and antibiotics (amoxicillin, macrolides, and oral cephalosporins) are the most frequently incriminated drugs. Food-related urticaria is associated with atopy.[112] Cow's milk allergy is one of the main causes of urticaria in infants, being present in 6–35% of cases of cow's milk intolerance.[116,120,121]

Diagnosis

The diagnosis of urticaria is made on clinical grounds. Histopathologic examination of a skin biopsy specimen shows vascular dilation, edema, and a perivascular inflammatory infiltrate composed of lymphohistiocytic cells, polymorphonuclear cells, and more specifically eosinophils. Neutrophils may predominate.

Laboratory tests are not usually necessary for the evaluation of acute urticaria. IgE levels can be elevated in some patients. An exhaustive search for an underlying cause not elicited by history alone is not warranted. An erythrocyte sedimentation rate may suffice as a screening test in cases of chronic urticaria because it is usually elevated in diseases associated with chronic urticaria (e.g. collagen vascular diseases). In 10–15% of patients no cause is identified. Intradermal skin tests to discover suspected allergens are not reliable.

Differential Diagnosis

Urticaria in infants is often misdiagnosed as erythema multiforme, acute hemorrhagic edema, annular erythema of infancy, or Kawasaki disease. In an infant with urticaria and dermographism the possibility of diffuse cutaneous mastocytosis without visible cutaneous lesions should also be considered.[122] NOMID/CINCA (see below) should be considered in young infant with urticaria. The predominance of neutrophils in skin biopsies of children with NOMID may help in the differential diagnosis, although it is not 100% specific. In case of doubt, genetic testic for NOMID is now available.

Course, Management, Treatment, and Prognosis

Despite its alarming symptoms, urticaria in early infancy is usually benign. Exceptions are chronic infantile neurological cutaneous and articular syndrome (CINCA) (see below) and the inherited physical urticarias, which may have a lifelong course. If medication is required, antihistamines such as diphenhydramine or hydroxyzine are the mainstay of therapy. However, newborns have an increased susceptibility to antimuscarinic side effects, such as central nervous system (CNS) excitation causing convulsions. Systemic corticosteroids should be reserved for cases of intractable urticaria.

Familial Physical Urticarias

Autosomal dominant variants have been described for many of the physical urticarias. Although rare, these familial cases begin early in life, even immediately after birth, and have a lifelong course, usually with increased severity. The exact pathogenic mechanism for many of the physical urticarias is unknown.

Familial cold urticaria (FCU) is an autosomal dominant disorder characterized by the development of burning wheals, and frequently pain and swelling of joints, stiffness, chills, and even fever after exposure to cold, especially in combination with damp and windy weather.[123-126] The skin lesions appear on exposed areas and generalize afterwards. Leukocytosis may be present during the attacks. The reaction may be delayed for up to 6 hours after cold challenge. In contrast to acquired cold urticaria, the reaction cannot be elicited by an ice cube test: rather, the patient must be subjected to cold environmental temperatures or cold water immersion. On skin biopsy a neutrophilic infiltrate predominates. The symptoms tend to improve with age. Responses to H_1 and H_2 blockers and ketotifen are poor. Stanozolol has been of limited benefit.[127] FCU has also been described along with amyloidosis and deafness as Muckle–Wells syndrome (MWS).[128] It has been recently demonstrated that both FCU and MWS are due to mutations in the *CIAS1* (cryopyrin) gene: in fact they are the same disorder and may share exactly the same genetic mutation.[129] FCU and MWS are also allelic diseases with CINCA syndrome (see below), which is also due to *CIAS1* gene mutations.[130]

Familial dermographism (autosomal dominant) has been described in a single large family.[131] In neonates dermographism can also be a manifestation of 'silent' diffuse cutaneous mastocytosis.[122,132] Vibratory urticaria is an autosomal dominant physical urticaria in which wheals develop after repetitive vibratory stimulation or stretching.[133,134] The need for repetitive trauma differentiates it from dermographism. Familial aquagenic urticaria and familial heat urticaria usually have onset in childhood.[135-137]

CHRONIC INFANTILE NEUROLOGICAL CUTANEOUS AND ARTICULAR SYNDROME (CINCA)[138-141]

CINCA syndrome, also known as neonatal onset multisystemic inflammatory disease (NOMID), is a chronic systemic inflammatory disease of neonatal onset characterized by skin rash, arthropathy, and CNS manifestations. Cutaneous findings are the presenting signs. The disease follows a chronic course with acute febrile exacerbations, lymph node enlargement, and hepatosplenomegaly. Two-thirds of patients are born prematurely.

Cutaneous Findings

A skin eruption is usually the first manifestation of the disease and is present at birth or develops during the first 6 months of life. It is characterized by generalized, evanescent, urticarial macules and papules that migrate over the course of a single day and wax and wane in intensity (Fig. 19-14). The rash is persistent, although recrudescence of the skin lesions is noted at flare-ups. The lesions may be pruritic, especially after sun exposure, but are usually asymptomatic.[140,141] Geographic tongue and oral ulcers have been noted in a single patient.[141]

Extracutaneous Findings

Symmetric or asymmetric arthropathy is another constant finding and is severe in half of patients. It is often absent in the first few weeks of life, but usually develops during the first year.[140,142] The severity of the arthropathy correlates with an early onset of joint symptoms. The knees are most frequently affected, followed by the ankles and feet, elbows, wrists, and hands. Joint swelling and pain are more severe during febrile flare-ups. On palpation, a bony consistency is characteristic as a result of epiphyseal and growth cartilage involvement and overgrowth of the patellae. Joint contractures and severe deformities result.

Neurologic signs and symptoms such as headache, vomiting, and seizures develop at a variable age. Intellectual impairment is also common. Both spasticity and hypotonia have been described. Eye involvement is an inconstant finding. Papilledema with or without optic nerve atrophy is the most common feature. Other ocular manifestations include uveitis, keratitis, conjunctivitis, and chorioretinitis.[143] These changes may lead to complete blindness in adulthood. Progressive sensorineural hearing loss and hoarseness are also common.

Affected children have a characteristic phenotype. There is progressive growth retardation and increased head circumference with frontal bossing. Fontanel closure is retarded. Icterus may be present in the neonatal period, especially in patients with severe arthropathy.[140]

Etiology and Pathogenesis

Mutations in the *CIAS1* gene have been identified in 60% of patients with CINCA syndrome.[144,145] *CIAS1* encodes a protein called cryopyrin, which is involved in the regulation of apoptosis and the inflammatory signaling pathway.[145] It is proposed that familial cold urticaria and CINCA represent extreme groups of the same disease, defined by the magnitude of phenotypic expression.[145] Considerable clinical overlapping exists between these disorders.

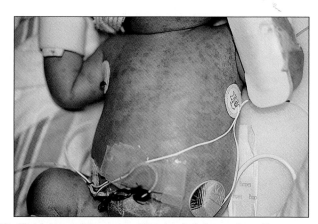

FIG. 19-14 Neonatal onset multisystemic inflammatory disease.

Laboratory Tests, Radiologic Findings, and Histopathology

Nonspecific findings typical of a chronic inflammatory process include microcytic anemia; leukocytosis with high neutrophil and eosinophil counts, elevated platelet counts, sedimentation rates, and acute-phase reactants; and polyclonal hyperglobulinemia G, A, or M. Rheumatoid factor and antinuclear antibodies are usually absent. Liver enzymes may be mildly elevated. CSF examination shows pleocytosis and high protein levels.

Radiologic studies of the affected joints show irregularly enlarged, bizarre, spiculated epiphyses with a grossly coarsened trabecular appearance.[140,142] There is periosteal new bone formation, and growth cartilage abnormalities are frequent. With time, there is bowing deformity of long bones and shortening of diaphyseal length. CT scans of the head have demonstrated hydrocephalus and cerebral atrophy.

Histopathologic examination of the skin reveals interstitial and perivascular neutrophilia.[141,142] Neutrophilic eccrine hidradenitis has been described.[141] Biopsies of lymph nodes, liver, and synovium show nonspecific signs of chronic inflammation.

Differential Diagnosis

NOMID must be differentiated from systemic onset juvenile arthritis. The main differences are its neonatal onset, persistent rash, the short duration of bouts of fever, absence of morning stiffness, and central nervous system involvement. The arthropathy is more deforming, and the radiographic findings of enlarged and disorganized epiphyses are distinctive. In addition, the response to NSAIDs is poor. Urticaria should also be considered and the predominance of eosinophils in skin biopsy may be a relative clue.

Course, Management, Treatment, and Prognosis

The disease follows a chronic course with acute febrile exacerbations. Occasionally it causes death in the first or second decade. Nonsteroidal anti-inflammatory drugs may be effective for pain relief but do not alter the course of the disease. Prednisone has been palliative in doses ranging from 0.5 to 2.0 mg/kg/day.[142] Chlorambucil and penicillamine have been tried, with limited success.[146,147] Thalidomide has shown beneficial effects in a single patient.[148] Other choices include methotrexate, the recombinant human IL-1 receptor antagonist anakinra,[149–152] and the anti-TNF-α agent etanercept.[153]

ERYTHEMA MULTIFORME

Erythema multiforme (EM) is an acute, self-limited disorder of skin and mucous membranes.[154–156] It has been considered a spectrum of disorders, designated EM minor, consisting of skin involvement only or of both the skin and the mouth, and as EM major (Stevens–Johnson syndrome; SJS), which involves at least two mucous membranes with variable cutaneous lesions. Some authors include toxic epidermal necrolysis within this spectrum as a severe form of SJS. Recent evidence suggests that EM and SJS have distinct clinical features and different precipitating factors, so perhaps the terms EM major and EM minor are best avoided.[157,158] EM is a common disease in children[155] but extremely unusual in the neonatal period.[94,155,159–162] Toxic epidermal necrolysis is discussed in Chapter 10.

Cutaneous Findings

The prototypic lesion of EM is a 1–3 cm erythematous, edematous papule that develops a dusky vesicular, purpuric, or necrotic center. A raised edematous ring of pallor surrounded by an erythematous outer ring is often present. These concentric color changes produce the typical target, or iris, lesion. In many cases only two zones are seen, with a single ring around the central papule (atypical target lesions). The lesions are distributed symmetrically and acrally on the extensor surface of the extremities. They may extend to the trunk, flexural surfaces, palms, and soles. In children, lesions on the face and ears are common, but are rare on the scalp[163] (Fig. 19-15).

In SJS, the lesions are more centrally located, predominating on the trunk. The targets are atypical and are usually flat. Individual lesions tend to coalesce in large patches. Areas of epidermal detachment may occur, but usually affect less than 10% of the body surface area. Mucosal lesions occur frequently in EM and are requisite for a diagnosis of SJS. Mucous membrane involvement is characterized by erythema or blisters that rapidly evolve to confluent erosions with pseudomembrane formation. The oral mucosa and conjunctiva are most commonly involved, but genital, anal, pharyngeal, and upper respiratory tract involvement may be seen. The number of mucous membranes involved has been considered one of the main distinguishing features of EM and SJS.

Extracutaneous Findings

Mild, nonspecific, prodromal symptoms of cough, rhinitis, and low-grade fever are occasionally present in EM. Fever, arthralgias, and prostration are common in SJS.

Etiology and Pathogenesis

EM has been considered a hypersensitivity phenomenon to multiple precipitating factors such as infectious agents or drugs. Three etiologic factors have been well documented: herpes simplex for erythema multiforme, and *Mycoplasma* infections and drugs for SJS. Herpes simplex (HSV-1 or HSV-2) is considered to be responsible for more than 80% of EM in children, even if clinical infection is inapparent.[164] HSV-associated EM follows the lesions of herpes by 1–3 weeks and is often recurrent. However, not every episode of recurrent herpes is followed by EM. HSV-specific DNA has been detected by polymerase chain reaction and in situ hybridization in lesional skin from a large number of children with EM, whether 'idiopathic' or clearly HSV related.[164]

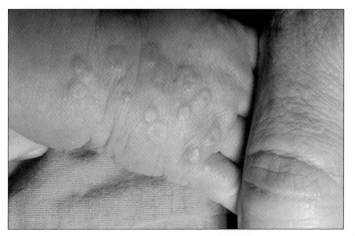

FIG. 19-15 Target lesions of erythema multiforme in a newborn.

Cow's milk intolerance has been described as a cause of erythema multiforme in a neonate.[159] Drugs are the most common cause of SJS. Sulfonamides, phenylbutazone, diphenylhydantoin, and penicillin derivatives are most frequently implicated.[163] Vaccinations were the only known possible causative agents in a newborn and two infants with erythema multiforme.[162,165]

Laboratory Tests and Histopathology

In cases of extensive involvement an elevated sedimentation rate, leukocytosis, and mild elevation of transaminases may be seen. Electrolyte imbalance and hypoproteinemia may be encountered in SJS. Eosinophilia may be seen in drug-related cases.

Histopathologic examination of early lesions reveals a lymphocytic band-like infiltrate at the dermoepidermal junction, with exocytosis and individual necrotic keratinocytes in close proximity to lymphocytes ('satellite cell necrosis'). There is vacuolization of the basal layer with focal cleft formation at the dermoepidermal junction. The upper dermis is edematous. Over time, more extensive confluent necrosis of the epidermis supervenes, resulting in subepidermal blister formation. In EM a lichenoid infiltrate predominates, whereas in SJS epidermal necrosis predominates.

Differential Diagnosis

In typical cases EM or SJS is rarely confused with other entities. Urticarial vasculitis may be considered in some cases. Kawasaki disease may produce target-like lesions; however, associated findings should allow differentiation. Serum sickness-like reactions often associated with the use of Cefaclor or other antibiotics, or even without any known etiology, can also produce targetoid lesions (see Fig. 19-9).

Course, Management, Treatment, and Prognosis

Erythema multiforme is usually self-limited. Individual lesions heal in 1–2 weeks, with residual hyperpigmentation. Conservative supportive care is the preferred form of treatment. Possible underlying causes should be sought. Treatment of underlying infection and discontinuation of nonessential drugs are indicated. Corticosteroids are unnecessary and may even worsen a concurrent infection.[166,167] In HSV-associated EM, early intervention or even prophylactic treatment with oral aciclovir may be beneficial.[168]

SJS has a less favorable prognosis, with a mortality rate of 5–15% if left untreated. The use of corticosteroids in SJS is more controversial.[166,167,169,170] No controlled study has proved their efficacy, and in some studies patients treated with corticosteroids have had a worse prognosis.[171] Corticosteroids may predispose to secondary infection while suppressing the signs of sepsis. Supportive care is extremely important.

SWEET SYNDROME

Sweet syndrome, or acute febrile neutrophilic dermatosis, is a benign disease characterized by tender, raised erythematous plaques, fever, peripheral leukocytosis, histologic findings of a dense dermal infiltrate of polymorphonuclear leukocytes, and a rapid response to systemic corticosteroids.[172–176] Only a few pediatric cases have been reported,[177–190] the youngest being 5 weeks of age.[180] Two brothers with Sweet syndrome starting at 2 weeks of life have been reported.[188]

Cutaneous Findings

The lesions of Sweet syndrome have an acute, explosive onset and are characterized by indurated, tender, erythematous plaques or nodules that vary in size from 0.5 to 4 cm (Fig. 19-16). Tiny pustules may appear at a later stage. The borders may be raised, mammillated, or even vesicular. Some of the lesions may show central clearing, forming annular or gyrate plaques (Fig. 19-17). The lesions are usually multiple and distributed over the face and extremities or, more rarely, the trunk. Without treatment, they tend to heal spontaneously

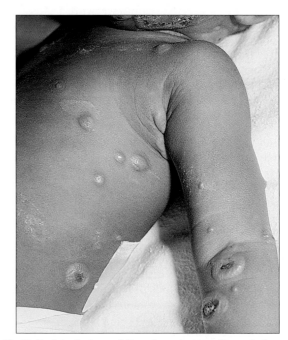

FIG. 19-16 Nodular lesions of Sweet syndrome with central crusting.

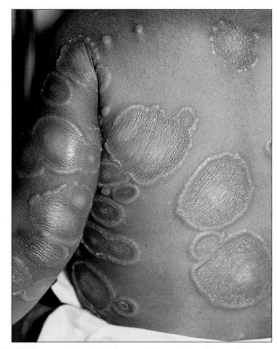

FIG. 19-17 Progression of lesions of Sweet syndrome in the same patient as in Figure 19-16. Plaques and nodules have flattened and are clearing centrally.

within a few months. In some patients, especially children, the lesions heal with areas of secondary cutis laxa, also known as Marshall syndrome.[179,189,191]

Extracutaneous Findings

A high, spiking fever is characteristic but may be absent in up to 50% of patients.[176] Arthralgias or asymmetric arthritis may be associated, and conjunctivitis or iridocyclitis may be seen in one-third of patients.[176] Renal involvement manifesting as proteinuria or hematuria, as well as lung involvement with infiltrates visible on chest radiographs, has also been described. Central nervous system involvement may occur in rare instances and manifest as headaches, convulsions, or disturbance of consciousness. Cerebrospinal fluid pleocytosis with lymphocyte predominance is usually found in such cases.[192]

Etiology and Pathogenesis

The pathogenesis is unknown. Many of the patients reported have had a preceding respiratory tract infection or elevated antistreptolysin O titers.[176] Ten per cent of the cases have been seen in the setting of a variety of hematologic malignancies, particularly acute myeloid and myelomonocytic leukemias.[193] Sweet syndrome has also been associated with solid tumors, inflammatory bowel disease, connective tissue diseases, and chronic granulomatous disease, or it may occur as an adverse reaction to drugs,[194–196] particularly granulocyte colony-stimulating factor[197] or after vaccination.[198] Because of these associations and the rapid response to systemic corticosteroids, Sweet syndrome is thought to represent a hypersensitivity reaction to infectious agents or tumoral antigens.

Laboratory Tests and Histopathology

An elevated erythrocyte sedimentation rate and peripheral leukocytosis are frequent accompanying abnormalities. Eosinophilia, microcytic anemia, mild elevation of liver enzymes, and urinalysis abnormalities may be present occasionally. Antineutrophil cytoplasmic antibodies have been detected in some cases.[176] α_1-Antitrypsin deficiency has been documented in one case of Marshall syndrome.[191]

The histopathologic findings are diagnostic.[173] There is a dense perivascular infiltrate composed almost entirely of neutrophils. The dermis appears edematous, and subepidermal blisters may form. Spongiosis, exocytosis, and intraepidermal vesiculation may be seen. There is endothelial swelling and nuclear dust, but true vasculitis is characteristically absent.

Differential Diagnosis

The lesions of Sweet syndrome may initially resemble those of EM or acute hemorrhagic edema. Lesions on the lower extremities may resemble those of erythema nodosum, but lesions more characteristic of Sweet syndrome are usually present in other locations.

Course, Management, Treatment, and Prognosis

Sweet syndrome is a benign disease but may be a marker of malignancy. If left untreated it resolves spontaneously over weeks to months. Recurrences are common. Marshall syndrome may have a poorer prognosis, with the development of elastolysis in the lungs or cardiovascular involvement.

Oral corticosteroids are the treatment of choice and usually elicit a prompt response.[199] Potassium iodide administration has been successful in a few cases,[200] as have colchicine,[201] dapsone,[202] clofazimine,[189] and intravenous immunoglobulin.[184]

KAWASAKI DISEASE

Kawasaki disease is an acute systemic vasculitis involving small and medium-sized muscular arteries, especially the coronary arteries, of young children. In the past, many cases were called infantile polyarteritis nodosa. The disease is characterized by fever lasting at least 5 days, nonpurulent conjunctivitis, a polymorphous exanthem, erythema and swelling of the hands and feet, inflammatory changes of the lips and oral cavity, and acute nonpurulent cervical adenopathy.[203–206] Coronary artery aneurysms or ectasia develop in 15–25% of untreated children and may lead to ischemic heart disease or sudden death.

Kawasaki disease occurs predominantly in children under 5 and has a peak incidence between 9 and 11 months.[207–209] It is infrequent before 6 months of age, although it has been reported in patients less than 2 weeks of age.[210–212] Boys are affected 1.5 times as often as girls. Kawasaki disease is an endemic disease with epidemic and geographic clustering. There is seasonal predominance in late winter and spring, although this may differ in different countries.[213,214] It is most common in Japan, with an annual incidence of 112 cases per 100 000 children under 5, and is steadily increasing.[215,216] Familial cases in household contacts have been described.[217] The recurrence rate is 3%, with some patients having two or more recurrences.

Cutaneous Findings[205,218]

The skin is involved in 99% of patients. The first sign often consists of diffuse erythema and painful induration of the hands and feet. Between 1 and 3 weeks after disease onset the eruption characteristically begins to desquamate beneath the distal nail plates, and peeling may extend to involve the entire palm and sole. Horizontal depressions in the nail plates (Beau's lines) usually result.

A polymorphous exanthem on the trunk and proximal extremities usually appears within 5 days of onset of fever (Fig. 19-18). It is a nonspecific, diffuse maculopapular or

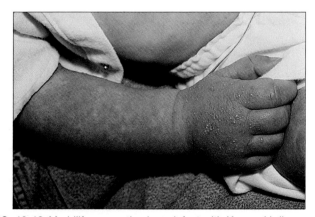

FIG. 19-18 Morbiliform eruption in an infant with Kawasaki disease.

morbilliform eruption, but may be urticarial, scarlatiniform, targetoid, or even pustular. Bullous or vesicular eruptions have not been described. The rash is usually in the perineum, which is a distinctive feature at this early stage, and it desquamates within 48 hours, preceding finger-tip and toe-tip desquamation[219] (Fig. 19-19). Plaque-type, guttate, and pustular psoriasis have been described, either during the acute or the convalescent phase of the disease, which supports a superantigen-mediated etiology.[220–223]

Changes in the lips and oral mucosa include erythema, swelling and fissuring of the lips, strawberry tongue, and erythema of the oropharynx. Oral ulcerations and pharyngeal exudates are not seen.

Intermittent acrocyanosis has been observed in infants younger than 6 months of age,[209] as well as peripheral gangrene.[224] Inflammatory changes with necrosis at the site of a previous BCG inoculation have been reported.[225–228]

Extracutaneous Findings[205,206,218,229]

Prolonged fever for at least 5 days is the cardinal and initial feature of the disease. It begins abruptly and is high, with peak temperatures generally >39°C (102°F) and in many cases >40°C (104°F), with several spikes each day (remittent fever). In the absence of appropriate therapy, fever persists for a mean of 11 days, but it may continue for 3–4 weeks and, rarely, even longer.

Bilateral nonexudative conjunctival injection, involving mainly the bulbar conjunctivae, begins shortly after disease onset and may already be resolved at time of first consultation. Anterior uveitis is frequently noted on slit-lamp examination but is rarely symptomatic.

Cervical lymphadenopathy is the least common diagnostic sign, with a prevalence of approximately 65%. It is usually unilateral, and confined to the anterior cervical triangle. The lymph nodes are often firm, nonfluctuant, and only slightly tender.

Cardiac conditions are the main cause of long-term morbidity and mortality. The pericardium, myocardium, endocardium, and coronary arteries may all be involved. Myocarditis may manifest in the acute phase, and arrhythmias due to ischemia, congestive heart failure, and valvular involvement, usually mitral, may occur. Occasionally there may low cardiac output syndrome or shock. Cardiac auscultation of the infant or child with Kawasaki disease in the acute phase often reveals a hyperdynamic precordium, tachycardia, a gallop rhythm, and an innocent flow murmur. A pansystolic regurgitant murmur may be heard in children with significant mitral regurgitation. Electrocardiography may show arrhythmia, prolonged PR interval, or nonspecific ST and T-wave changes. Pericardial effusion may be detected by an echocardiogram in 30% of patients. Without treatment, coronary artery aneurysms develop in 20% and are most commonly detected 10 days to 4 weeks after onset. Risk factors for the development of coronary aneurysms include age younger than 1 year, male gender, fever for more than 2 weeks, recurrent fever, and delayed treatment. Aneurysms may also develop in systemic medium-sized arteries and result in peripheral gangrene.[224]

Polyarticular arthritis and arthralgias may occur in the first weeks of the illness. It affects small as well as large joints. Irritability is usually prominent. Lethargy and other signs of aseptic meningitis may be present. Abdominal symptoms such as vomiting, diarrhea, and pain are common. In rare instances acute abdominal pain, mimicking a surgical abdomen, may herald the onset of the disease. Mild hepatitis occurs frequently, as does acute distension of the gallbladder (hydrops).

Transient unilateral peripheral facial nerve palsy occurs rarely. Respiratory symptoms due to pulmonary nodules, infiltrates, or pleural effusion may also be observed.[230–232] Rare findings include testicular swelling, hemophagocytic syndrome,[233] and transient high-frequency sensorineural hearing loss (20–35 dB).[234]

Etiology and Pathogenesis[235–237]

Epidemiologic and clinical data suggest that Kawasaki disease has features of infectious disease in an immunologically susceptible host and of an immune-mediated vasculitis. Many etiologic agents, ranging from bacteria such as *Propionibacterium*, *Staphylococcus*, *Streptococcus*, *Chlamydia* and *Yersinia* to viruses such as Epstein–Barr, parvovirus, adenoviruses, retroviruses, and a novel human coronavirus, have been linked to Kawasaki disease in different geographic outbreaks, but none has been consistently demonstrated.[235] Much of the continuing debate in the literature concerns whether Kawasaki disease is caused by a superantigen or a conventional antigen.[235,237] Evidence of a superantigen-mediated disease process includes the identification of superantigen-producing organisms, isolation of bacterial superantigens, or finding the hallmark of superantigen activation in affected children, such as selective expansion of Vβ2 and Vβ8 T-cell receptor families. However, the immune response in Kawasaki disease is oligoclonal (antigen driven, i.e. similar to a response to a conventional antigen) rather than polyclonal (as found typically in superantigen-driven responses), and immunoglobulin A (IgA) plasma cells play a central role.[235,237]

Regardless of the cause, evidence points to a generalized immune activation with production of various proinflammatory cytokines and endothelial cell activation which lead to coronary artery alteration.[238–241] The most studied cytokine has been TNF-α, which is usually elevated in children with Kawasaki disease. Enzymes, including matrix metalloproteinases that are capable of damaging arterial wall integrity, may also be important in the development of aneurysmal dilatation. Various chemotactins that attract neutrophils and monocytes to coronary arteries may also play an important role.[242]

Host genetic determinants play a role in both susceptibility and coronary artery outcome in Kawasaki disease.[243] The

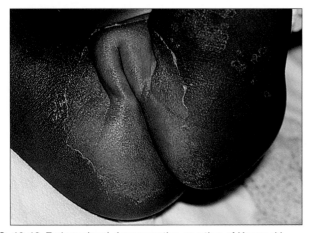

FIG. 19-19 Early perineal desquamative eruption of Kawasaki disease.

incidence rate in siblings is 10 times the population incidence.[217,244,245] The risk of occurrence in twins is higher than in ordinary siblings. Parents who had Kawasaki disease in childhood are more likely to have affected children, and children with recurrent disease.[246]

Laboratory Tests and Histopathology

In the acute phase, laboratory studies show leukocytosis ($>15 000/mm^3$) with a left shift, normochromic normocytic anemia, increased sedimentation rate and other acute-phase reactants, depressed albumin, and elevated IgM and IgE levels. The degree of elevation of ESR and C-reactive protein may show discrepancy, and both should be measured. Furthermore, elevation of ESR can be caused by IVIG therapy and therefore can not be the sole determinant of the degree of inflammatory activity.[218] Plasma lipids are altered in the acute stage, with depressed plasma cholesterol and HDL.[247,248] There may be mild elevation of transaminases and polyclonal hypergammaglobulinemia. In the subacute stage, in the second and third weeks of illness, there is a marked and almost universal thrombocytosis, which returns to normal in 4–8 weeks. Thrombocytopenia is rarely seen in the acute stage and may be a sign of disseminated intravascular coagulation. Antineutrophil cytoplasmic antibodies may be detectable as a nonspecific epiphenomenon. There may be sterile pyuria with mild proteinuria. Cerebrospinal fluid shows a mononuclear pleocytosis with normal protein and glucose levels. Skin biopsy findings are not specific. There is edema in the papillary dermis, with a mild perivascular mononuclear cell infiltrate. Vasculitis of medium and large arteries is observed.

Diagnosis[218]

There is no single diagnostic test for Kawasaki disease and therefore clinical criteria have been established to guide treatment decisions (Box 19-3). The classic diagnosis has been based on the presence of 5 days of fever and four of the five principal clinical features. Clinical features usually appear sequentially and are not all present at a single point in time, therefore watchful waiting is sometimes necessary before a diagnosis can be made. To avoid holding treatment until more than four clinical criteria are met, and the recognition that many patients with 'incomplete' Kawasaki still develop coronary artery disease, one may diagnose and treat Kawasaki on day 4 of illness in the presence of four principal criteria.[230,249] Also, the diagnosis can be made in patients with fever for 5 days and fewer than four principal features when coronary artery disease is detected by two-dimensional echocardiography (2DE) or coronary angiography. Kawasaki disease should be considered in the differential diagnosis of a young child, specially under 1 year of age, with unexplained fever for 5 days that is associated with any of the principal clinical features of this disease, or even in the presence of other clinical and laboratory findings that are not classic criteria but which are commonly encountered in this disease (Box 19-3).[218] For example, an elevated CRP or ESR and elevated platelet count after 7 days of illness are uncommon in viral infections but are universally seen in children with Kawasaki disease. Echocardiography may be useful in evaluating 'incomplete Kawasaki disease' and should be considered in any infant under 6 months with fever of more than 7 days' duration, laboratory evidence of systemic inflammation, and no other explanation for the febrile illness.[218] Although aneurysms rarely form before day 10 of illness there may be signs of coronary arteritis, decreased

contractility, mitral regurgitation, and pericardial effusion. With all these considerations a new algorithm has been proposed to help in deciding which patient with incomplete Kawasaki disease should undergo echocardiography or receive IVIG treatment (Fig. 19-20).[218]

Box 19-3 Classic diagnostic criteria for Kawasaki disease*

1. Fever of 5 days' duration and at least four of the following:**
2. Changes in the extremities: Erythema of palms, soles; edema of hands, feet; periungual peeling of fingers, toes.
3. Polymorphous exanthem
4. Bilateral conjunctival injection without exudation
5. Changes in the lips and oral cavity: fissuring, strawberry tongue, difuse injection of the oral or pharyngeal mucosa
6. Cervical lymphadenopathy of at least 1.5 cm in diameter.
7. Exclusion of other diseases with similar findings

*Patients with fever of at least 5 days and < four principal criteria can be diagnosed with Kawasaki disease when coronary artery abnormalities are detected by 2DE or angiography.
**Patients with four principal criteria can be diagnosed on day 4 of fever.

Other clinical/laboratory findings in Kawasaki disease

Other clinical and laboratory findings
  Cardiovascular findings
    Congestive heart failure, myocarditis, pericarditis, valvular regurgitation
    Coronary artery abnormalities
    Aneurysms of medium-sized noncoronary arteries
    Raynaud's phenomenon
    Peripheral gangrene
  Musculoskeletal system
    Arthritis, arthralgia
  Gastrointestinal tract
    Diarrhea, vomiting, abdominal pain
    Hepatic dysfunction
    Hydrops of gallbladder
  Central nervous system
    Extreme irritability
    Aseptic meningitis
    Sensorineural hearing loss
  Genitourinary system
    Urethritis/meatitis
  Other findings
    Erythema, induration at BCG inoculation site
    Anterior uveitis (mild)
    Desquamating rash in groin

Laboratory findings in acute Kawasaki disease
  Leukocytosis with neutrophilia and immature forms
  Elevated ESR
  Elevated CRP
  Anemia
  Abnormal plasma lipids
  Hypoalbuminemia
  Hyponatremia
  Thrombocytosis after week 1§
  Sterile pyuria
  Elevated serum transaminases
  Elevated serum gamma glutamyl transpeptidase
  Pleocytosis of cerebrospinal fluid
  Leukocytosis in synovial fluid

Modified from Pediatrics 2004; 114: 1708–1133.

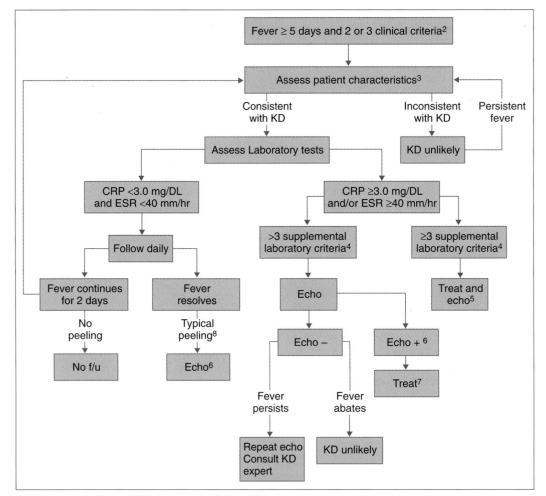

FIG. 19-20 Evaluation of suspected incomplete Kawasaki disease. (1) In the absence of gold standard for diagnosis, this algorithm cannot be evidence based but rather represents the informed opinion of the expert committee. Consultation with an expert should be sought anytime assistance is needed. (2) Infants ≤6 months old on day ≥7 of fever without other explanation should undergo laboratory testing and, if evidence of systemic inflammation is found, an echocardiogram, even if the infants have no clinical criteria. (3) Patient characteristics suggesting Kawasaki disease are listed in Box 19-3. Characteristics suggesting disease other than Kawasaki disease include exudative conjunctivitis, exudative pharyngitis, discrete intraoral lesions, bullous or vesicular rash, or generalized adenopathy. Consider alternative diagnoses. (4) Supplemental laboratory criteria include albumin ≤3.0 g/dL, anemia for age, elevation of alanine aminotransferase, platelets after 7 days ≥450 000/mm³, white blood cell count ≥15 000/mm³, and urine ≥10 white blood cells/high-power field. (5) Can treat before performing echocardiogram. (6) Echocardiogram is considered positive for purposes of this algorithm if any of 3 conditions are met: z score of LAD or RCA ≥2.5, coronary arteries meet Japanese Ministry of Health criteria for aneurysms, or ≥3 other suggestive features exist, including perivascular brightness, lack of tapering, decreased LV function, mitral regurgitation, pericardial effusion, or z scores in LAD or RCA of 2–2.5. (7) If the echocardiogram is positive, treatment should be given to children within 10 days of fever onset and those beyond day 10 with clinical and laboratory sings (CRP, ESR) of ongoing inflammation. (8) Typical peeling begins under nail bed of fingers and then toes.

Sometimes Kawasaki disease may be 'atypical,' presenting at onset with clinical features that are not generally seen, such as acute abdominal pain, renal impairment, meningeal irritation, pneumonia, or retropharyngeal abscess.

Differential Diagnosis

Many diseases mimic Kawasaki disease, including viral infections, streptococcal infection, juvenile rheumatoid arthritis, erythema multiforme, staphylococcal scalded skin syndrome, toxic shock syndrome, drug hypersensitivity reactions, Rocky Mountain spotted fever, leptospirosis, mercury hypersensitivity reaction (acrodynia), and bacterial cervical adenitis. Low white blood cell count, lymphocytosis and low platelet count may be useful in suggesting a viral infection instead of Kawasaki disease.

Course, Management, Treatment, and Prognosis

The morbidity and mortality of Kawasaki disease depend primarily on coronary artery lesions.[250–254] Coronary artery aneurysms or ectasia develop in 15–25% of untreated children and may lead to ischemic heart disease or sudden death. With early treatment the risk is reduced to around 5–12%.[215,216] Small aneurysms resolve completely within the first 2 years after disease onset in 30–60% of these patients.[255] However, coronary aneurysms, especially if giant (>8 mm), may persist and be complicated by thrombotic occlusion or the development of stenosis at the outlet of the aneurysm. Stenotic lesions as well as early coronary atherosclerosis may develop gradually over several years, so long-term follow-up is warranted.[252,253,256,257]

Several scoring systems have been developed to predict risk for coronary artery aneurysms.[258] The Harada score is one that is used in Japan.[259]

Because the major sequelae of Kawasaki disease are related to coronary artery systems, cardiac imaging is critical in the evaluation of all patients with suspected Kawasaki disease, and serial echocardiograms are recommended. Echocardiography should focus on coronary artery visualization and measurement, but also on left ventricle contractibility, valve function, the presence of pericardial effusion, and measurement of the aortic root.[260] An initial examination should be performed as soon as the diagnosis is suspected and is useful as a baseline for follow-up. Thereafter, for uncomplicated cases it should be repeated at 2 weeks and at 6–8 weeks after disease onset.[218] For those who develop coronary artery aneurysms or other cardiac abnormalities more frequent evaluation is recommended. Other noninvasive imaging modalities, such as MRI, MRA, and ultrafast CT, as well as cardiac stress testing, are being evaluated in the management of Kawasaki disease. Until the aneurysm resolves a stress test may be needed to guide recommendations for physical activity and the need for angiography.

Treatment in the acute phase of the disease is directed to reducing inflammation in the coronary artery wall and preventing coronary thrombosis, whereas long-term therapy in individuals who develop coronary aneurysms is aimed at preventing myocardial ischemia or infarction. Intravenous γ-globulin (IVIG) combined with high-dose aspirin is the treatment of choice in the acute phase of the disease.[229] Aspirin alone does not appear to reduce the frequency of the development of coronary abnormalities, but together with IVIG it has an additive anti-inflammatory effect. In the acute stage aspirin is given in doses of 80–100 mg/kg divided into four. The duration of high-dose aspirin varies in different centers. In many institutions the dose is reduced after the child has been afebrile for 48–72 hours. Others continue until day 14 of illness and >48–72 hours after fever cessation. Following this acute phase low-dose aspirin (3–5 mg/kg) is given as an antiplatelet agent until there is no evidence of coronary changes at 6–8 weeks from disease onset. For patients who develop coronary abnormalities, low-dose aspirin is continued until regression of coronary artery aneurysms, but some clinicians continue indefinitely. Ibuprofen should be avoided in children taking aspirin for its antiplatelet effect because it antagonizes platelet inhibition.

IVIG has been shown to reduce the incidence of coronary artery aneurisms from 20% to 3–4%.[261–264] A single dose of 2 mg/kg has been shown to be superior than lower doses for 4 consecutive days.[261,262] IVIG should be started early, within 10 days of disease onset and preferably within 7 days. Treatment before day 5 does not appear to prevent cardiac sequelae and may be associated with an increased need for IVIG retreatment.[265,266] Treatment after day 10 should be considered if there are still signs of ongoing inflammation (elevated ESR or CRP) or persistent fever.[267] Not all patients respond to a single dose of IVIG and may have persistent or recrudescent fever 36 hours after completion of the initial treatment, and require a second dose. It has been observed that those children who received IVIG very early in the illness are more prone to require a second infusion. Vaccination with live or other vaccines should be deferred for at least 11 months after high-dose IVIG treatment, both to ensure correct immunization and to avoid flares of Kawasaki disease.[268]

The usefulness of steroids in combination with IVIG in the initial therapy of Kawasaki disease is not well established. Steroids shorten the duration of fever and lower ESR and CRP,

but do not seem to influence the coronary outcome.[269,270] Steroids have also been used for IVIG treatment failures, but their role in preventing or reversing coronary anomalies is uncertain. It has been recommended to restrict their use in children who have persistent fever after two infusions of IVIG.[218] The most common regimen is intravenous pulse methylprednisolone, 30 mg/kg for 1–3 days.

Because of its inhibition of TNF-α messenger RNA transcription, pentoxifylline may have a theoretical benefit in the initial treatment of Kawasaki disease, although there are only small clinical trials reported.[271] The role of TNF-α antagonists such as infliximab; abciximab, a platelet glycoprotein IIb/IIa receptor inhibitor; plasma exchange; and cytotoxic agents for patients with refractory Kawasaki disease, remains uncertain.[218,272]

ACUTE HEMORRHAGIC EDEMA

Acute hemorrhagic edema (AHE), purpura en cockade, or Finkelstein disease, is an acute, benign leukocytoclastic vasculitis of limited skin involvement occurring in children under 2 years of age.[273–280] AHE has been considered an infantile variant of Henoch–Schönlein purpura; however, because of clinical and prognostic differences it is sometimes regarded as a separate entity.

Cutaneous Findings

The disease is characterized by the abrupt onset of fever; tender edema of the face, eyelids, ears, scrotum, and acral extremities; and ecchymotic purpura on the face and extremities. The trunk is usually spared. Individual lesions often have a darker center and expand centrifugally, giving them a cockade or target-like configuration. Lesions range in size from 0.5 to 4.0 cm and may become confluent, forming polycyclic, annular plaques (Fig. 19-21). Necrotic[279,281] and bullous lesions may be seen.[279,282] Petechiae in the mucous membranes have also been described.[283]

Extracutaneous Findings

Except for fever, there are no associated manifestations. In many patients there is a preceding upper respiratory tract infection. The dramatic cutaneous findings contrast with the general wellbeing of the patient.

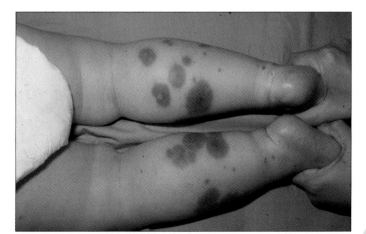

FIG. 19-21 Acute hemorrhagic edema.

Etiology and Pathogenesis

The cause of AHE is unknown. It is thought to represent an immune complex-mediated disease precipitated by a preceding infection, particularly an upper respiratory tract infection, drug intake, or immunization. Staphylococci and *Streptococcus* spp. and viruses (adenoviruses, rotavirus) have been implicated most commonly.

Laboratory Tests and Histopathology

Leukocytosis (both lymphocytic and granulocytic), thrombocytosis, eosinophilia, and an elevated ESR may be present. Urinalysis, tests for occult blood in the stool, immunoglobulin, and complement levels are usually normal or negative. Circulating immunocomplexes may occasionally be found.[282]

Histopathologic examination of skin biopsy specimens demonstrates a small vessel leukocytoclastic vasculitis. Direct immunofluorescence shows deposition of C3 and fibrinogen in the vessel wall. IgM, IgG, IgA, and IgE deposition has also been noted in up to one-third of cases.[282,284-286]

Differential Diagnosis

The differential diagnosis includes Henoch–Schönlein purpura, child abuse, meningococcemia and other infectious purpuras, erythema multiforme, Kawasaki disease, and Sweet syndrome.[273,283] Distinction from Henoch–Schönlein purpura may be impossible[280] (Table 19-2). Perivascular deposits of IgA are not useful for differentiation because they may be present in both entities.

Course, Management, and Prognosis

The prognosis is excellent. The eruption resolves spontaneously without sequelae in 1–3 weeks. Treatment with corticosteroids is not necessary and may lead to complications and worsen the prognosis.[284] Exacerbations may be observed during the clinical evolution, with new crops of lesions and fever,[281,285] but true recurrences weeks or months after the first episode are rare.[280,283] There has been a single report of a fatal ileoileal intussusception in an infant with cutaneous lesions otherwise typical for AHE.[281]

TABLE 19-2 Differential diagnosis between acute hemorrhagic edema and Henoch–Schönlein purpura

	Acute hemorrhagic edema	Henoch–Schönlein purpura
Onset	Acute and dramatic	Less dramatic
Age	2 m–2 years	>2 years
Sex	Male predominance	Male predominance
Location	Face, ears, extremities	Lower extremities, buttocks
Morphology	Large medallion-like purpura Facial edema	Palpable purpura Edema of lower extremities
Course	No recurrences	Frequent relapses
Histopathology	Leukocytoclastic vasculitis	Leukocytoclastic vasculitis
Immunodeposits	Variable IgA, IgM, C3	IgA
Systemic involvement	No	Renal, gastrointestinal, joint, CNS

THE PORPHYRIAS[287-295]

The porphyrias are a group of diseases characterized by abnormalities of porphyrin–heme metabolism. Each type results from deficient activity of one of the enzymes of the heme biosynthetic pathway, which leads to an accumulation of heme precursors within plasma, red blood cells, urine, and feces.[295] The genes for these enzymes have been characterized.[287,289,295] Porphyrias are mainly inherited in an autosomal dominant manner with incomplete penetrance, but autosomal recessive and more complex patterns of inheritance are also possible. Porphyrias are classified as hepatic or erythropoietic, according to the organ site in which the underlying defect of heme synthesis is predominantly expressed (see Table 19-3). Cutaneous manifestations in porphyrias may be classified as acute photosensitivity with burning pain, edema, and erythema shortly after sun exposure, or delayed photosensitivity manifesting as skin fragility, subepidermal blisters, milia, disorders of pigmentation, and sclerodermoid signs. Hepatic porphyrias usually manifest acute neurovisceral attacks and delayed photosensitivity, and rarely present before puberty except from the homozygous variants. Elevated porphyrins may be detected in the stool or urine. Erythropoietic porphyrias are characterized by acute cutaneous photosensitivity from early childhood. The more delayed photosensitivity, although less characteristic of this type of porphyria, may be also present.[293] Erythrocyte and plasma porphyrin levels are elevated in erythropoietic porphyrias.

Photosensitivity in porphyrias is maximum for ultraviolet wavelengths between 400 and 410 nm ('Soret band'), the spectrum of maximum absorption of porphyrins.

The pathophysiologic mechanisms involved in the cutaneous manifestations of the porphyrias are multiple and involve the creation of reactive oxygen specimens.[296-298]

Childhood porphyrias are relative uncommon and their exact incidence is unknown. Only those porphyrias manifesting early in infancy are reviewed here.

Congenital Erythropoietic Porphyria

Congenital erythropoietic porphyria (CEP), also called Günther disease, is a rare autosomal recessive disorder caused by deficient activity of uroporphyrinogen III (UROGEN III) synthase which leads to nonenzymatic conversion of hydroxymethylbilane to uroporphyrinogen I, a nonphysiologic substrate that is converted to coproporphyrinogen I; these porphyrinogen I isomers are then oxidized to uroporphyrin I (URO-I) and coproporphyrin I (COPRO-I), which are phototoxic compounds. Elevated levels of URO-I and COPRO-I in erythrocytes result in massive hemolysis, and the released porphyrins accumulate in peripheral blood, skin, bone, and teeth and are excreted in large amounts in the urine and feces.

Cutaneous Findings[292,299,300]

CEP presents with severe photosensitivity from birth or early infancy with formation of vesicles and bullae on areas exposed to sun, phototherapy devices, or even ambient lighting.[301] There is also marked skin fragility. As a result of the phototoxic injury and the increased skin fragility, there are severe mutilations, mainly of the fingers, hands, and face, particularly the nose and ears, but also in sun-protected areas. Hypertrichosis of the face and extremities, scarring alopecia of the scalp and eyebrows, and pigmentary changes (hyperpig-

TABLE 19-3 Classification of the porphyrias, enzymatic defect, porphyrin profile, and age of onset

Tissue origin	Type	Enzyme deficiency	Porphyrin profile				Age of onset
			Erythrocyte	Plasma	Urine	Stool	
Erythropoietic	Congenital erythropoietic porphyria (CEP)	Uroporphyrinogen III synthase	URO-I, COPRO-I, PROTO	URO-I, COPRO-I, PROTO	URO-I > COPRO-I	COPRO-I	Birth, infancy
	Erythropoietic protoporphyria (EPP)	Ferrochelatase	PROTO	PROTO	Normal	PROTO	Infancy, early childhood
Hepatic	Acute intermittent porphyria (AIP)	Porphobilinogen deaminase	Normal	Normal	ALA, PBG	Normal	After puberty, no cutaneous manifestations
	Variegate porphyria (VP)	Protoporphyrinogen oxidase	Normal	COPRO, PROTO	COPRO > URO	PROTO > COPRO	Second decade, homozygous variant at birth, infancy, or early childhood
	Hereditary coproporphyria (HCP)	Coproporphyrinogen oxidase	Normal	COPRO	COPRO	COPRO	After puberty, homozygous variant (hardero-porphyria) at birth, infancy, or early childhood
	Porphyria cutanea tarda (PCT)	Uroporphyrinogen decarboxylase	Normal	URO	URO-I > III	ISOCOPRO	Third of fourth decade
	ALA dehydratase porphyria	ALA dehydratase	PROTO	ALA, COPRO, PROTO	ALA, COPRO, URO	COPRO, PROTO	Any age, no cutaneous manifestations
Hepatoerythropoietic	Hepatoerythropoietic porphyria (HEP)	Uroporphyrinogen decarboxylase	Zn-PROTO	URO	URO-(I and III)	ISOCOPRO	Early infancy

ALA, *5-aminolevulinate;* COPRO, *coproporphyrin;* ISOCOPRO, *isocoproporphyrin;* PBG, *porphobilinogen;* PROTO, *protoporphyrin;* URO, *uroporphyrin.*

mentation and hypopigmentation) are also common. Over time, severe facial mutilation results, with destruction of nasal and auricular cartilages, ectropion, and eclabium, as well as shortening and contraction of the fingers. Milder phenotypes may have onset later in childhood.[302]

Extracutaneous Findings
The accumulation of porphyrins in deciduous and permanent teeth produces red discoloration (erythrodontia) and reddish fluorescence on Wood's light examination, which is pathognomonic. The urine is also reddish, which causes pink discoloration of the diapers that fluoresces – an early bed-side diagnostic sign. Porphyrins accumulate in the amniotic fluid and brownish amniotic fluid may be observed. Severe hemolytic anemia and secondary splenomegaly occur. Anemia may be so severe as to lead to hydrops fetalis and death in utero. Patients with late-onset disease may not develop hemolytic anemia but only thrombocytopenia and myelodysplasia. Ocular changes include ectropion, photophobia, and keratoconjunctivitis.[303] Other manifestations include osteodystrophy with increased bone fragility, and porphyrin-rich gallstones.

Genetics
The gene for UROGEN III synthase is localized on chromosome 10. Several mutations have been identified,[304] and different mutations correlate with the level of residual enzyme activity and hence with disease severity and genotypes.[302,305,306]

Laboratory Tests and Histopathology
Histologic examination of skin biopsy specimens from blisters reveals subepidermal cleavage (within the lamina lucida) and minimal inflammatory infiltrate. Perivascular accumulation of PAS-positive, diastase-resistant, homogeneous hyaline material (porphyrins) may be seen, which is best viewed with fluorescence microscopy. See Table 19-3 for porphyrin excretion profile. Measurement of URO III synthase activity is available. Prenatal diagnosis from amniotic fluid is possible by either measurement of uroproporphyrin I or direct gene mutation analysis.[307–310]

Differential Diagnosis
Other photosensitivity diseases presenting early in life (Box 19-4) or diseases manifesting with blisters, such as epidermolysis bullosa and bullous pemphigoid, should be considered. Determination of porphyrins is diagnostic and allows differentiation from other porphyrias presenting early in life with photosensitivity.

Prognosis
The clinical severity of CEP is highly variable, ranging from hydrops fetalis, hepatosplenomegaly, and severe anemia in utero to adult-onset disease with only cutaneous manifestations.[311] In most cases, however, patients survive well into adulthood, albeit with severe mutilations or major disfigurement.

Box 19-4 Causes of photosensitivity in neonates

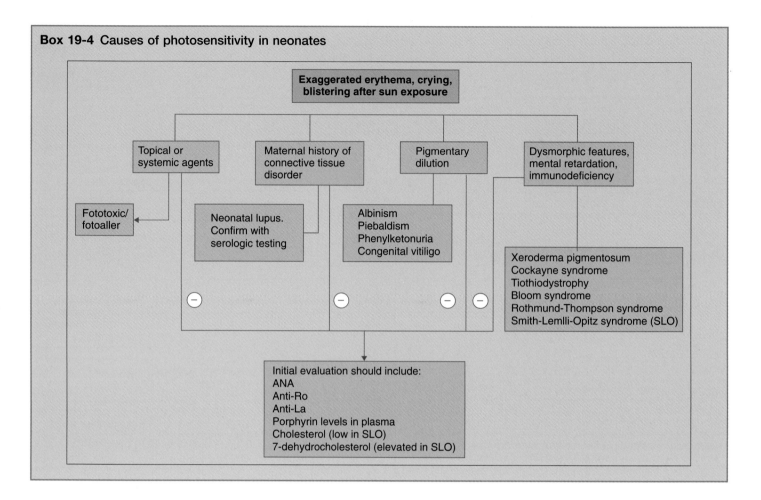

Treatment[312]

Protection from sun exposure is essential. Chemical sunscreens do not achieve good protection against Soret band radiation, so protective clothing and physical sunblocks are necessary. Long-wavelength, UV-absorbing films are encouraged on car windows and windows at home. Children with the severe phenotypes and severe hemolysis benefit from repeated erythrocyte transfusions and hydroxyurea to suppress erythropoiesis. Hematocrits should be maintained above 32%, with appropriate iron chelation. The efficacy or repeated erythrocyte transfusion may decrease at puberty. Subsequent splenectomy is often needed to control hemolytic anemia.[313,314] Activated charcoal,[315–318] and β-carotene[319,320] have been used, with inconsistent results. Bone marrow transplantation or stem cells from cord blood offer the possibility of correcting enzyme activity.[321–325] Replacement gene therapy has been accomplished in vitro.[326,327]

Erythropoietic Protoporphyria[287,298,328]

Erythropoietic protoporphyria (EPP) is the most common form of cutaneous porphyria apart from porphyria cutanea tarda (PCT). EPP is caused by deficient activity of ferrochelatase, leading to the accumulation of protoporphyrin in erythrocytes, plasma, and feces. Clinical symptoms typically begin in infancy or early childhood, with a peak incidence between 2 and 4 years of age. EPP is usually inherited as an autosomal dominant condition, but most individuals who are heterozygous for the inherited mutations are asymptomatic, because of half-normal ferrochelatase activity[329] For protoporphyrin to accumulate sufficiently to cause photosensitivity, a reduction of enzymatic activity to below a critical threshold of about 35% of normal is required. Some families may have autosomal recessive inheritance.[329–331]

Cutaneous Manifestations

Clinical manifestations are those of an acute phototoxic reaction, which triggers an episode of crying within minutes of sunlight exposure due to burning pain or stinging sensations on exposed areas (the face and the dorsal aspect of hands). Some patients are photosensitive to fluorescent lighting.[328] Erythema, edema, and urticarial lesions occur, but vesicles and bullae are rare (Fig. 19-22). Fine petechiae may occur on sun-exposed areas after prolonged exposure. Some patients have only subjective symptoms.[328] With chronic exposure there is characteristic thickening and wrinkling of the knuckle pads, furrowing around the mouth (pseudorhagades), and shallow elliptical scars on the nose, cheeks, and forehead.

Hemolytic anemia is absent, but in some patients a mild hypochromic, microcytic anemia may occur. Protoporphyrin-rich gallstones may develop in childhood. Fatal liver failure resulting from the progressive accumulation of protoporphyrin in hepatocytes is a possible outcome in about 2.5% of patients, altering the prognosis for an otherwise clinically benign disorder. Recessive inheritance may predispose to severe liver disease.[329,332]

Genetics

The gene for ferrochelatase is localized on chromosome 18. Over 70 mutations in this gene have been identified in EPP

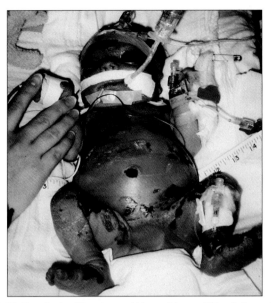

FIG. 19-22 Porphyria. (Courtesy of Henry Lim and Tor Schwayder.)

families.[329,333] In most symptomatic patients inheritance of a second mutation is needed in order to reduce the enzymatic activity to a critical threshold where clinical symptoms are caused. Autosomal recessive inheritance has been demonstrated in 3% of patients with EPP.[329]

Laboratory tests and Histopathology

Histopathologic examination of skin biopsy specimens of sun-exposed areas shows marked concentric deposits of a hyaline material around dermal blood vessels. This material is PAS positive and diastase resistant.

Patients with EPP should undergo frequent liver function tests, and those with persistent abnormalities should have a liver biopsy. Children with high erythrocyte protoporphyrins should have periodic determination of blood, urinary, and fecal porphyrins because increased excretion of copropophyrins, high erythrocyte protoporphyrins and reduced excretion of faecal protoporhyrins can predict liver failure.[334]

Diagnosis

The diagnosis of EPP is established by detecting elevated levels of protoporphyrin in erythrocytes, plasma, and feces. In addition, fecal and erythrocyte coproporphyrins may be increased. A rapid microfluorometric assay for free erythrocyte protoporphyrins and examination of a blood smear for fluorescent erythrocytes may also be used as screening tests.[335] The differential diagnosis includes other types of porphyria, but causes of immediate photosensitivity such as PMLE or solar urticaria do not occur in infants.

Treatment

The mainstay of treatment for erythropoietic protoporphyria is sun avoidance and the use of physical sunscreens.[336,337] Topical dihydroxyacetone may be helpful in some patients by producing brown pigment.[287] Oral administration of β-carotene (30–90 mg/day for children) has been shown in uncontrolled studies to increase tolerance to sun exposure because it quenches the formation of free radicals.[334,338,339] Narrowband ultraviolet B phototherapy has been proposed, as

this wavelength does not cause photosensitivity.[340] Desensitization with PUVA therapy has also been used. Oral iron, intravenous hematin, transfusion therapy, and a high-carbohydrate diet have been used to prevent protoporphyrin accumulation in the liver by reducing protoporphyrin production, but their efficacy is unproven.[334] Cholestyramine or activated charcoal have been used to interrupt the enterohepatic circulation of protoporphirins.[341] Avoidance of alcohol and drugs that interfere with hepatic excretory function is also essential. Liver transplantation has been performed in a few patients with liver failure, although the enzymatic defect is not thereby corrected and hence the long-term outcome is poor.[342–345] Modification of the lighting in the operating room is necessary to avoid photoxicity to exposed organs.

Hepatoerythropoietic Porphyria

Hepatoerythropoietic porphyria (HEP) is an extremely rare disorder caused by a marked deficiency of uroporphyrinogen decarboxylase due to a homozygous state.[346–349] Clinical manifestations begin in infancy, or more commonly in early childhood, and resemble both porphyria cutanea tarda and Günter disease. The disease usually presents with darkening of the urine and delayed-type cutaneous photosensitivity, with vesicles, skin fragility, milia, and scarring. With time, hypertrichosis, sclerodermoid changes, and mutilation similar to the manifestations of Günter disease become apparent. Anemia, hepatosplenomegaly, and abnormalities of liver function of varying degrees may also occur, but are less common than in congenital erythropoietic porphyria. The porphyrin excretion pattern resembles that of porphyria cutanea tarda (PCT), with elevated urinary uroporphyrins and 7-carboxylated porphyrins, and a smaller elevation of coproporphyrins, 6- and 5-carboxylated porphyrins. Increased isocoproporphyrins in feces are characteristic. Unlike in PCT, erythrocyte proto is increased.

Treatment is directed to sun protection. Hypertrichosis in hepatoerythropoietic porphyria has been treated successfully with high-intensity pulses of noncoherent light.[350]

Other Porphyrias

Homozygous Porphyrias

Other porphyrias with onset of symptoms in infancy or early childhood include homozygous variants of aminolevulinate dehydratase (ALAD) deficiency, homozygous coproporphyria (harderoporphyria), homozygous variegate porphyria, and homozygous acute intermittent porphyria.[351]

ALAD deficiency porphyria is rare (fewer than 10 patients reported) and usually manifests later in childhood or adulthood, but neonatal onset has been reported.[352] Clinical manifestations from birth are recurrent attacks of pain, vomiting, hyponatremia, and symptoms of polyneuropathy affecting motor functions, including respiration. Raised levels of 5-aminolevulinic acid and coproporphyrin in urine are found. Very low erythrocyte aminolevulinate dehydratase activity is diagnostic. Liver transplantation in patients with neonatal onset has little effect.[353]

In harderoporphyria, neonatal jaundice, hemolytic anemia, and hepatosplenomegaly dominate the clinical picture.[354–357] Blisters may occur during phototherapy for neonatal jaundice. Diagnosis depends on detecting very low coproporphyrinogen oxidase activity, elevated coproporphyrin in urine, markedly elevated harderoporphyrin and coproporphyrin in feces, and zinc protoporphyrin in erythrocytes.

Homozygous variegate porphyria may present shortly after birth with marked photosensitivity or, more commonly, with erosions, blisters, and milia following minor trauma in sun-exposed areas.[358–360] Acute attacks are absent, but mental and growth retardation, seizures, nystagmus, and clinodactyly have been described.

Homozygous variant of acute intermittent porphyria may present early in life with ataxia, mental retardation, convulsions, cataracts, and hepatosplenomegaly, but acute attacks typical of acute intermittent porphyria do not occur in these children.[361–364] There are no cutaneous manifestations. Markedly increased porphobilinogen and ALAD in urine are found and are responsible for the orange urine.

TRANSIENT PORPHYRINEMIAS[365–368]

Transient increases in porphyrin levels have been described in neonates with hemolytic disease of the newborn and in a neonate with severe liver failure due to tyrosinemia type 1.[368] These infants develop erythema, violaceous discoloration, purpura, erosions, and blisters in areas exposed to phototherapy, with sharp demarcation at photoprotected sites. Sensitivity to sunlight may occur.

Elevated levels of plasma/urine porphyrins (mainly coproporphyrin) and/or erythrocyte protoporphyrin are found, which normalize spontaneously during the first few months. The cause of transient porphyrinemia is unclear but is probably due to cholestasis. Other factors likely to be involved include blood transfusions and drug use.

PURPURA IN THE NEWBORN

Purpura in the neonate is almost always an emergency and should prompt an immediate search for an underlying disorder. Apart from trauma, purpura in the newborn may be due to coagulation defects, platelet abnormalities, or infections (see Box 19-5). Extramedullary erythropoiesis also causes purpuric lesions by a different mechanism.

In the evaluation of a neonate with purpura it is important to obtain a maternal and familial history of bleeding diathesis and thromboembolic phenomena, drug intake, and symptoms of infectious diseases. A general physical examination and workup for sepsis is warranted. Laboratory studies should include hemoglobin and hematocrit values, platelet count, white blood count, coagulation studies, and TORCH serologies.

DERMAL ERYTHROPOIESIS (BLUEBERRY MUFFIN BABY)

Persistence of the erythropoietic activity of fetal dermal mesenchyme into the newborn period produces a characteristic purpuric eruption for which the term blueberry muffin baby was coined. The eruption, first observed in newborns with congenital rubella (Fig. 19-23), may be the result of other intrauterine infections (Fig. 19-24) and hematologic dyscrasias.[369–371] A blueberry muffin-like eruption may also represent metastatic infiltration of the dermis by congenital malignancies, without true extramedullary erythropoiesis (Fig. 19-25).

Cutaneous Findings

The cutaneous lesions of blueberry muffin babies consist of dark blue or magenta, nonblanchable, round to oval papules

---

Box 19-5 Differential diagnosis of neonatal purpura

1. Extramedullary erythropoiesis (blueberry muffin baby)
2. Coagulation defects
   Protein C and S deficiency (neonatal purpura fulminans)
   Hemorrhagic disease of the newborn
   Hereditary clotting factor deficiencies
3. Platelet abnormalities
   a. Immune platelet destruction
      Alloimmune neonatal thrombocytopenia
      Maternal autoimmune thrombocytopenia (ITP, lupus)
      Drug-related immune thrombocytopenia
   b. Primary platelet production/function defects
      Thrombocytopenia with absent radii syndrome
      Wiskott-Aldrich syndrome
      Fanconi anemia
      Congenital megakaryocytic thrombocytopenia
      X-linked recessive thrombocytopenia
      Other hereditary thrombocytopenias
      Giant platelet syndromes (Bernard-Soulier, May-Hegglin)
      Trisomy 13 or 18
      Alport syndrome variants
      Gray platelet syndrome
      Glanzmann thrombasthenia
   c. Kasabach-Merritt syndrome*
4. Infections†
   Congenital (TORCH)
   Sepsis
   HIV
   Parvovirus B19
5. Trauma
6. Purpuric phototherapy-induced eruption

Modified from Baselga E, Drolet BA, Esterly NB. J Am Acad Dermatol 1997;37:673–705.
*Both thrombocytopenia and consumption coagulopathy are involved in the pathogenesis.
†Infection may cause purpura by several mechanisms.

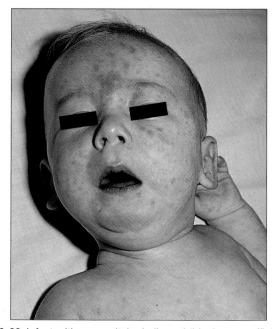

FIG. 19-23 Infant with congenital rubella and 'blueberry muffin' lesions.

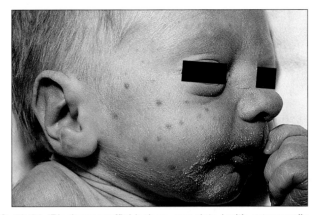

FIG. 19-24 'Blueberry muffin' lesions associated with cytomegalic inclusion disease.

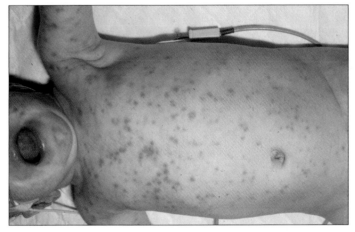

FIG. 19-25 Infiltration of the skin by leukemia cutis producing a blueberry muffin appearance.

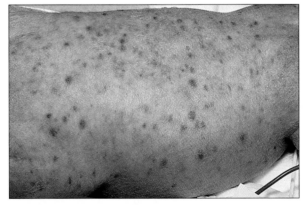

FIG. 19-26 Lesions of dermal erythropoiesis in an infant with Rh incompatibility due to RhoGAM failure.

ranging in size from 1 to 7 mm and have a generalized distribution, with emphasis on the head, neck, and trunk (Fig. 19-26). The papules are firm to palpation, with an infiltrative quality that distinguishes them from petechiae and purpura, which often coexist in the same patient. These lesions evolve into dark purple to brown macules and involute spontaneously within 2–6 weeks.[273] Blueberry muffin lesions caused by infiltrative processes are usually larger, more nodular, less hemorrhagic, fewer in number, and firmer to palpation.

Extracutaneous Findings
Accompanying abnormalities vary with the underlying cause.

Etiology and Pathogenesis
In the prevaccination era rubella was the most common cause of dermal erythropoiesis, but now congenital cytomegalovirus (CMV) infection is the major cause.[369,370] Dermal erythropoiesis has been associated with other intrauterine infections, such as Coxsackie B2[369] and parvovirus B19,[372] as well as hematologic dyscrasias such as Rh incompatibility (Fig. 19-24),[373,374] maternofetal ABO incompatibility,[369] spherocytosis,[375] and the twin transfusion syndrome[210,216] (Box 19-6). In rare instances it may occur in otherwise healthy newborns.[369,376]

Laboratory Tests and Histopathology
Histopathologic examination demonstrates poorly circumscribed collections of nucleated and nonnucleated red blood cells, predominantly confined to the reticular dermis and extending to the subcutaneous tissue.[369–371] Occasionally a few myeloid precursors may be interspersed.

Laboratory findings depend on the underlying cause. In the evaluation of a blueberry muffin baby the following tests are indicated: peripheral blood count, hemoglobin level, TORCH serologies, viral cultures, and a Coombs' test. Skin biopsy is not always necessary for diagnosis, but may be helpful if an infiltrative process is suspected.

Differential Diagnosis
The differential diagnosis includes other causes of neonatal purpura, such as coagulation defects, platelet abnormalities, and infections.[273] Neoplastic diseases that produce infiltrative metastases in the neonatal period, such as neuroblastomas,[377–379] rhabdomyosarcomas,[380] myelogenous leukemias,[381–383] and Langerhans' cell histiocytosis, especially the congenital self-healing reticulohistiocytosis variant (Hashimoto–Pritzker),[384,385] should be considered.

Course, Management, Treatment, and Prognosis
The lesions of true dermal erythropoiesis fade and resolve spontaneously 3–6 weeks after birth. Treatment is directed at the underlying condition.

PROTEINS C AND S DEFICIENCIES (NEONATAL PURPURA FULMINANS)

Neonatal purpura fulminans is a rare condition characterized by massive and progressive hemorrhagic necrosis of the skin accompanied by thrombosis of the cutaneous vasculature in the neonatal period.[386–391] Occasionally larger vessels and other organs are involved. The primary pathologic event is widespread thrombosis, which is responsible for a hematologic picture of disseminated intravascular coagulation (DIC). In neonates, purpura fulminans is usually the result of inherited thrombophilic disorders that are attributable to protein C deficiency, protein S deficiency, or resistance to activated protein C due to factor V mutations.

Cutaneous Findings
Neonatal purpura fulminans manifests 2–12 hours after birth. In rare instances, delayed onset of up to 6–10 months of age has been described.[392] Cutaneous lesions consist of extensive

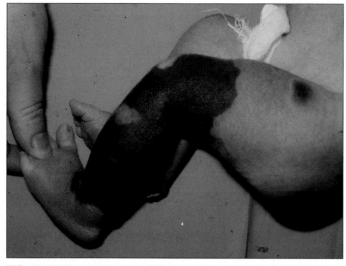

FIG. 19-27 Neonatal purpura fulminans due to protein C deficiency.

ecchymoses in a diffuse and often symmetric distribution that rapidly evolve into hemorrhagic bullae and purple-black necrotic skin lesions, which ultimately form a thick eschar (Fig. 19-27). The initial ecchymotic areas are sharply defined from the surrounding skin and usually have a red, advancing inflammatory rim. They are most common at sites of trauma or pressure, the buttocks, extremities, trunk, and scalp. Mucous membranes may rarely be involved.[393] If treatment is instituted in the first 1–3 hours, before necrosis ensues, the initial lesions may be reversible.[390]

Extracutaneous Findings

Other organs may be affected by the microvascular thrombosis, most commonly the CNS and eye, but also the kidney and gastrointestinal tract. Cavernous sinus involvement, which may occur in utero, can result in hydrocephalus, seizures, intracerebral hemorrhage, and mental retardation.[388,394,395] Microphthalmia, cataracts, and blindness due to vitreous or retinal hemorrhage may be seen.[388,389] Deep venous thrombosis and pulmonary embolism have also been described.[394]

Etiology and Pathogenesis

Purpura fulminans in the neonatal period is almost always caused by inherited thrombophilic states such as homozygous protein C and S deficiency or resistance to activated protein C. Severe bacterial infection associated with DIC can also induce purpura fulminans in the neonate, although it is more common in infancy or early childhood.[396,397] Proteins C and S are vitamin K-dependent glycoproteins with antithrombotic properties.[398,399]

Protein C deficiency is an autosomal dominant disease with incomplete penetrance.[399] Homozygous or compound heterozygous patients have a severe clinical phenotype and usually present with neonatal purpura fulminans, although they may be asymptomatic or present later in life with recurrent thrombosis.[400,401]

Protein S deficiency is also transmitted as an autosomal dominant trait with incomplete penetrance.[399] Homozygous patients may develop neonatal purpura fulminans, although the risk is lower than in patients with homozygous protein C deficiency.[387,402]

Neonatal purpura fulminans may also be caused by activated protein C resistance due to a mutation in the factor V gene.[393,403] Resistance to activated protein C may coexist with protein S and protein C deficiencies, becoming an additional genetic risk factor for purpura fulminans or thromboembolic complications, and explaining in part the incomplete clinical penetrance of inherited thrombophilic disorders.[404]

Laboratory Tests and Histopathology

Blood coagulation studies demonstrate evidence of DIC, including prolonged prothrombin and partial thromboplastin times, increased fibrin split products, reduced fibrinogen, and reduced platelets. Microangiopathic hemolytic anemia may occur.

Biopsy of the early skin lesions demonstrates occlusion of dermal blood vessels by microthrombi. Hemorrhage and dermal necrosis are present in the more advanced stages. Necrosis of the overlying epidermis with subepidermal hemorrhagic bullae occurs in later phases. Secondary fibrinoid necrosis of dermal vessel walls may be present in the necrotic areas, but primary vasculitis is absent.[390,405]

A definitive diagnosis of protein C and S deficiency is established by measurements of protein C and S levels.[399] Protein C deficiencies can be identified by immunoenzymatic assays measuring the actual concentration of the protein in plasma, and two functional assays measuring the enzymatic activity and the anticoagulant activity. These tests distinguish two types of protein C deficiency. In type I, which is the most common, reduced synthesis of the normal protein leads to a low plasma concentration in all three assays. In type II, a qualitative deficiency, levels are normal but functional assays are abnormal. For protein S deficiency, functional and immunoenzymatic assays are available, and both the free form and the inactive form that circulates bound to C4b-binding protein have to be measured.[399] Type I deficiency is characterized by low total and free protein S, type II by normal free protein S and low activity, and type III by low free protein levels with normal total levels.

Interpreting the results of the assays may be difficult because protein C and S levels are physiologically reduced in the neonatal period, and may be undetectable in sick newborns with liver disease, respiratory distress syndrome, DIC, or sepsis.[389,390,396,397,406] A complete sepsis workup is therefore recommended in any case of neonatal purpura fulminans. Serial determination of protein levels in patients and other family members is necessary to exclude a transient deficiency and confirm true congenital deficiency.

Differential Diagnosis

The cutaneous lesions of purpura fulminans are very characteristic and rarely mistaken for any other condition. Other causes of purpuric eruptions in the newborn may be considered (see Box 19-6).

Course, Management, Treatment, and Prognosis

Without treatment, neonatal purpura fulminans is often fatal. If the diagnosis is suspected, therapy should be initiated immediately without waiting for the results of protein C and S measurements. Prompt treatment may completely reverse early skin lesions. Initial therapy consists of the administration of fresh frozen plasma (10–15 mL/kg/12 h) or prothrombin complex concentrate, sources of protein C, protein S, and activated protein C.[389,390] A protein C concentrate has been developed that has the advantage of avoiding blood volume overload and does not carry the risk of transmission of viral

ment therapy to avoid coumarin-induced skin necrosis. Experience with long-term treatment using protein C infusions is limited. There are few case reports of a successful liver transplant for homozygous protein C deficiency.[409,410]

PURPURIC PHOTOTHERAPY-INDUCED ERUPTION

This benign, transient purpura in transfused neonates who undergo phototherapy is characterized by raspberry-colored, nonblanching lesions at exposed sites, sparing sites that are protected from lights (e.g. leads and temperature probes).[206,208] The eruption develops after 1–4 days of phototherapy and clears spontaneously after discontinuation of light therapy. Histologically there is extravasation of red blood cells in the dermis without epidermal damage. The pathogenesis of this disease is unknown, although transient porphyrinemia has been detected in some patients.[367,411] The purpuric nature of the eruption and the absence of 'sunburn cells' differentiate this eruption from 'sunburn' caused by exposure to UVA from fluorescent lamps.[412] Congenital erythropoietic porphyria and transient elevated porphyrin levels in neonates with hemolytic disease may also cause photosensitivity.[411] Drug-induced phototoxicity in neonates who have received photosensitizing chemicals such as fluorescein dye, furosemide or methylene-blue must be considered.[413-416]

diseases.[407,408] Protein S concentrate is not yet available for clinical use. Replacement therapy should be continued until all lesions have healed, usually after 4–8 weeks. Long-term treatment involves careful administration of oral anticoagulants, starting at very low doses and with protective replace-

REFERENCES

1. Bressler GS, Jones RE, Jr. Erythema annulare centrifugum. J Am Acad Dermatol 1981; 4: 597–602.
2. Harrison P, V. The annular erythemas. Int J Dermatol 1979; 18: 282–290.
3. Toonstra J, de Wit RF. 'Persistent' annular erythema of infancy. Arch Dermatol 1984; 120: 1069–1072.
4. Cox NH, McQueen A, Evans TJ, Morley WN. An annular erythema of infancy. Arch Dermatol 1987; 123: 510–513.
5. Hebert AA, Esterly NB. Annular erythema of infancy. J Am Acad Dermatol 1986; 14: 339–343.
6. Peterson AO, Jr, Jarratt M. Annular erythema of infancy. Arch Dermatol 1981; 117: 145–148.
7. Wong LC, Kakakios A, Rogers M. Congenital annular erythema persisting in a 15-year-old girl. Australas J Dermatol 2002; 43: 55–61.
8. Helm TN, Bass J, Chang LW, Bergfeld WF. Persistent annular erythema of infancy. Pediatr Dermatol 1993; 10: 46–48.
9. Bottoni U, Innocenzi D, Bonaccorsi P, et al. Erythema annulare centrifugum: report of a case with neonatal onset. J Eur Acad Dermatol Venereol 2002; 16: 500–503.
10. Gianotti F, Ermacora E. Erythema gyratum atrophicans transiens neonatale. Arch Dermatol 1975; 111: 615–616.
11. Puig L, Moreno A, Alomar A, de Moragas JM. Erythema gyratum atrophicans transiens neonatale: a

variant of cutaneous neonatal lupus erythematosus. Pediatr Dermatol 1988; 5: 112–116.
12. Tyring SK. Reactive erythemas: erythema annulare centrifugum and erythema gyratum repens. Clin Dermatol 1993; 11: 135–139.
13. Guillet MH, Dorval JC, Larregue M, Guillet G. Erytheme annulaire centrifuge de Darier à debut neonatal avec 15 ans de suivi. Efficacité de l'interféron et role de cytokines. Ann Dermatol Venereol 1995; 122: 422–426.
14. Hammar H. Erythema annulare centrifugum coincident with Epstein–Barr virus infection in an infant. Acta Paediatr Scand 1974; 63: 788–792.
15. Fried R, Litt JZ, Schonberg IL. Erythema annulare centrifugum (Darier) in a newborn infant. J Pediatr 1957; 50: 66–67.
16. Klaber R. Erythema gyratum perstans (Colcott Fox): a case report, with discussion on relations with erythema centrifugum annulare (Darier) and dermatitis herpetiformis. Br J Dermatol 1946; 58: 111–121.
17. Larregue M, Beuve-Mery M, Dupuy JM, et al. Érythème annulaire centrifuge type Colcott–Fox (erythema gyratum perstans). Ann Dermatol Venereol 1977; 104: 217–223.
18. Woederman MJ. Erythema gyratum repens. Dermatologica 1964; 128: 391–392.
19. Schmid MH, Wollenberg A, Sander CA, Bieber T. Erythema annulare centrifugum and intestinal Candida

albicans infection – coincidence or connection? Acta Dermatol Venereol 1997; 77: 93–94.
20. Shelley WB. Erythema annulare centrifugum due to candida albicans. Br J Dermatol 1965; 77: 383–384.
21. Hendricks AA, Lu C, Elfenbein GJ, Hussain R. Erythema annulare centrifugum associated with ascariasis. Arch Dermatol 1981; 117: 582–585.
22. Ashurst PJ. Erythema annulare centrifugum due to hydroxychloroquine sulfate and chloroquine sulfate. Arch Dermatol 1967; 95: 37–39.
23. Shelley WB. Erythema annulare centrifugum. A case due to hypersensitivity to blue cheese penicillium. Arch Dermatol 1964; 90: 54–58.
24. Jillson OF, Hoekelman RA. Further amplification of the concept of dermatophytid. I. Erythema annulare centrifugum as a dermatophytid. AMA Arch Derm Syphilol 1952; 66: 738–745.
25. Watsky KL, Hansen T. Annular erythema in identical twins. Cutis 1989; 44: 139–140.
26. Beare JM, Froggatt P, Jones JH, Neill DW. Familial annular erythema. An apparently new dominant mutation. Br J Dermatol 1966; 78: 59–68.
27. Kikuchi I, Ogata K, Inoue S. Pityrosporum infection in an infant with lesions resembling erythema annulare centrifugum. Arch Dermatol 1984; 120: 380–382.
28. Trevisan G, Stinco G, Cinco M.

Neonatal skin lesions due to a spirochetal infection: a case of congenital Lyme borreliosis? Int J Dermatol 1997; 36: 677–680.

29. Lee LA. Neonatal lupus erythematosus. J Invest Dermatol 1993; 100: 9S–13S.

30. Lee LA. Neonatal lupus: clinical features, therapy, and pathogenesis. Curr Rheumatol Rep 2001; 3: 391–395.

31. Lee LA. Neonatal lupus erythematosus: clinical findings and pathogenesis. J Invest Dermatol Symp Proc 2004; 9: 52–56.

32. Silverman ED, Laxer RM. Neonatal lupus erythematosus. Rheum Dis Clin North Am 1997; 23: 599–618.

33. Watson RM, Lane AT, Barnett NK, et al. Neonatal lupus erythematosus. A clinical, serological and immunogenetic study with review of the literature. Medicine (Baltimore) 1984; 63: 362–378.

34. Buyon JP, Clancy RM. Neonatal lupus: basic research and clinical perspectives. Rheum Dis Clin North Am 2005; 31: 299–313.

35. Weston WL, Morelli JG, Lee LA. The clinical spectrum of anti-Ro-positive cutaneous neonatal lupus erythematosus. [Abstract] J Am Acad Dermatol 1999; 40: 675–681

36. Neiman AR, Lee LA, Weston WL, Buyon JP. Cutaneous manifestations of neonatal lupus without heart block: Characteristics of mothers and children enrolled in a national registry. [Abstract] J Pediatr 2000; 137: 674–680.

37. Sheth AP, Esterly NB, Ratoosh SL, et al. U1RNP positive neonatal lupus erythematosus: association with anti-La antibodies? Br J Dermatol 1995; 132: 520–526.

38. Provost TT, Watson R, Gammon WR, et al. The neonatal lupus syndrome associated with U1RNP (nRNP) antibodies. N Engl J Med 1987; 316: 1135–1138.

39. Diociaiuti A, Paone C, Giraldi L, et al. Congenital lupus erythematosus: case report and review of the literature. Pediatr Dermatol 2005; 22: 240–242.

40. Elish D, Silverberg NB. Neonatal lupus erythematosus. Cutis 2006; 77: 82–86.

41. Miyagawa S. Neonatal lupus erythematosus: a review of the racial differences and similarities in clinical, serological and immunogenetic features of Japanese versus Caucasian patients. J Dermatol 2005; 32: 514–522.

42. Nitta Y. Lupus erythematosus profundus associated with neonatal lupus erythematosus. Br J Dermatol 1997; 136: 112–114.

43. Crowley E, Frieden IJ. Neonatal lupus erythematosus: an unusual congenital presentation with cutaneous atrophy, erosions, alopecia, and pancytopenia. Pediatr Dermatol 1998; 15: 38–42.

44. Cimaz R, Biggioggero M, Catelli L, et al. Ultraviolet light exposure is not a requirement for the development of cutaneous neonatal lupus. Lupus 2002; 11: 257–260.

45. See A, Wargon O, Lim A, et al. Neonatal lupus erythematosus presenting as papules on the feet. Australas J Dermatol 2005; 46: 172–176.

46. Thornton CM, Eichenfield LF, Shinall EA, et al. Cutaneous telangiectases in neonatal lupus erythematosus. J Am Acad Dermatol 1995; 33: 19–25.

47. Fritz M, Vats K, Goyal RK. Neonatal lupus and IUGR following alpha-interferon therapy during pregnancy. J Perinatol 2005; 25: 552–554.

48. Geggel RL, Tucker L, Szer I. Postnatal progression from second- to third-degree heart block in neonatal lupus syndrome. J Pediatr 1988; 113: 1049–1052.

49. Lee LA, Sokol RJ, Buyon JP. Hepatobiliary disease in neonatal lupus: prevalence and clinical characteristics in cases enrolled in a national registry. Pediatrics 2002; 109: E11.

50. Cimaz R, Spence DL, Hornberger L, Silverman ED. Incidence and spectrum of neonatal lupus erythematosus: a prospective study of infants born to mothers with anti-Ro autoantibodies. J Pediatr 2003; 142: 678–683.

51. Scheker LE, Kasteler JS, Callen JP. Neonatal lupus erythematosus mimicking Langerhans' cell histiocytosis. Pediatr Dermatol 2003; 20: 164–166.

52. Kanagasegar S, Cimaz R, Kurien BT, et al. Neonatal lupus manifests as isolated neutropenia and mildly abnormal liver functions. J Rheumatol 2002; 29: 187–191.

53. Watson R, Kang JE, May M, et al. Thrombocytopenia in the neonatal lupus syndrome. Arch Dermatol 1988; 124: 560–563.

54. Bourke JF, Burns DA. Neonatal lupus erythematosus with persistent telangiectasia and spastic paraparesis. Clin Exp Dermatol 1993; 18: 271–273.

55. Rider LG, Sherry DD, Glass ST. Neonatal lupus erythematosus simulating transient myasthenia gravis at presentation. J Pediatr 1991; 118: 417–419.

56. Contractor S, Hiatt M, Kosmin M, Kim HC. Neonatal thrombosis with anticardiolipin antibody in baby and mother. Am J Perinatol 1992; 9: 409–410.

57. Prendiville JS, Cabral DA, Poskitt KJ, et al. Central nervous system involvement in neonatal lupus erythematosus. Pediatr Dermatol 2003; 20: 60–67.

58. Lawrence S, Luy L, Laxer R, et al. The health of mothers of children with cutaneous neonatal lupus erythematosus differs from that of mothers of children with congenital heart block. Am J Med 2000; 108: 705–709.

59. Julkunen H, Eronen M. Long-term outcome of mothers of children with isolated heart block in Finland. Arthritis Rheum 2001; 44: 647–652.

60. Brucato A, Franceschini F, Gasparini M, et al. Isolated congenital complete heart block: longterm outcome of mothers, maternal antibody specificity and immunogenetic background. J Rheumatol 1995; 22: 533–540.

61. McCune AB, Weston WL, Lee LA. Maternal and fetal outcome in neonatal lupus erythematosus. Ann Intern Med 1987; 106: 518–523.

62. Brucato A, Franceschini F, Buyon JP. Neonatal lupus: long-term outcomes of mothers and children and recurrence rate. Clin Exp Rheumatol 1997; 15: 467–473.

63. Press J, Uziel Y, Laxer RM, et al. Long-term outcome of mothers of children with complete congenital heart block. Am J Med 1996; 100: 328–332.

64. Buyon JP, Kim MY, Copel JA, Friedman DM. Anti-Ro/SSA antibodies and congenital heart block: necessary but not sufficient. Arthritis Rheum 2001; 44: 1723–1727.

65. Gordon P, Khamashta MA, Rosenthal E, et al. Anti-52 kDa Ro, anti-60 kDa Ro, and anti-La antibody profiles in neonatal lupus. J Rheumatol 2004; 31: 2480–2487.

66. Silverman ED, Buyon J, Laxer RM, et al. Autoantibody response to the Ro/La particle may predict outcome in neonatal lupus erythematosus. Clin Exp Immunol 1995; 100: 499–505.

67. Stevens AM, Hermes HM, Lambert NC, et al. Maternal and sibling microchimerism in twins and triplets discordant for neonatal lupus syndrome-congenital heart block. Rheumatology (Oxford) 2005; 44: 187–191.

68. Costedoat-Chalumeau N, Amoura Z, Villain E, et al. Anti-SSA/Ro antibodies and the heart: more than complete congenital heart block? A review of electrocardiographic and myocardial abnormalities and of treatment options. Arthritis Res Ther 2005; 7: 69–73.

69. Nield LE, Silverman ED, Smallhorn JF, et al. Endocardial fibroelastosis associated with maternal anti-Ro and anti-La antibodies in the absence of atrioventricular block. J Am Coll Cardiol 2002; 40: 796–802.

70. Lee LA, Coulter S, Erner S, Chu H. Cardiac immunoglobulin deposition in congenital heart block associated with maternal anti-Ro autoantibodies. Am J Med 1987; 83: 793–796.

71. Cruz RB, Viana VS, Nishioka SA, et al. Is isolated congenital heart block associated to neonatal lupus requiring pacemaker a distinct cardiac syndrome? Pacing Clin Electrophysiol 2004; 27: 615–620.

72. Costedoat-Chalumeau N, Amoura Z, Lupoglazoff JM, et al. Outcome of pregnancies in patients with anti-SSA/Ro antibodies: a study of 165

pregnancies, with special focus on electrocardiographic variations in the children and comparison with a control group. Arthritis Rheum 2004; 50: 3187–3194.

73. Taylor-Albert E, Reichlin M, Toews WH, et al. Delayed dilated cardiomyopathy as a manifestation of neonatal lupus: case reports, autoantibody analysis, and management. Pediatrics 1997; 99: 733–735.

74. Moak JP, Barron KS, Hougen TJ, et al. Congenital heart block: development of late-onset cardiomyopathy, a previously underappreciated sequela. J Am Coll Cardiol 2001; 37: 238–242.

75. Eronen M, Heikkila P, Teramo K. Congenital complete heart block in the fetus: hemodynamic features, antenatal treatment, and outcome in six cases. Pediatr Cardiol 2001; 22: 385–392.

76. Saleeb S, Copel J, Friedman D, Buyon JP. Comparison of treatment with fluorinated glucocorticoids to the natural history of autoantibody-associated congenital heart block: retrospective review of the research registry for neonatal lupus. Arthritis Rheum 1999; 42: 2335–2345.

77. Yang CH, Chen JY, Lee SC, Luo SF. Successful preventive treatment of congenital heart block during pregnancy in a woman with systemic lupus erythematosus and anti-Sjögren's syndrome A/Ro antibody. J Microbiol Immunol Infect 2005; 38: 365–369.

78. Buyon JP, Swersky SH, Fox HE, et al. Intrauterine therapy for presumptive fetal myocarditis with acquired heart block due to systemic lupus erythematosus. Experience in a mother with a predominance of SS-B (La) antibodies. Arthritis Rheum 1987; 30: 44–49.

79. Ishimaru S, Izaki S, Kitamura K, Morita Y. Neonatal lupus erythematosus: dissolution of atrioventricular block after administration of corticosteroid to the pregnant mother. Dermatology 1994; 189: 92–94.

80. Martin V, Lee LA, Askanase AD, et al. Long-term followup of children with neonatal lupus and their unaffected siblings. Arthritis Rheum 2002; 46: 2377–2383.

81. Buyon JP, Clancy RM. Neonatal lupus: review of proposed pathogenesis and clinical data from the US-based Research Registry for Neonatal Lupus. Autoimmunity 2003; 36: 41–50.

82. Carder KR. Hypersensitivity reactions in neonates and infants. Dermatol Ther 2005; 18: 160–175.

83. Wintroub BU, Stern R. Cutaneous drug reactions: pathogenesis and clinical classification. J Am Acad Dermatol 1985; 13: 167–179.

84. Bonnetblanc JM. Réactions cutanées aux médicaments chez l'enfant. Ann Dermatol Venereol 1997; 124: 339–345.

85. Knowles S, Shapiro L, Shear NH. Drug eruptions in children. Adv Dermatol 1999; 14: 399–415; discussion 416.

86. Knowles S, Shapiro L, Shear NH. Serious dermatologic reactions in children. Curr Opin Pediatr 1997; 9: 388–395.

87. Kramer MS, Hutchinson TA, Flegel KM, et al. Adverse drug reactions in general pediatric outpatients. J Pediatr 1985; 106: 305–310.

88. Sharma VK, Dhar S. Clinical pattern of cutaneous drug eruption among children and adolescents in north India. Pediatr Dermatol 1995; 12: 178–183.

89. Calobrisi SD, Drolet BA, Esterly NB. Petechial eruption after the application of EMLA cream. Pediatrics 1998; 101: 471–473.

90. Gourrier E, Karoubi P, el HA, Merbouche S, et al. Use of EMLA cream in a department of neonatology. Pain 1996; 68: 431–434.

91. Lacouture PG, Epstein MF, Mitchell AA. Vancomycin-associated shock and rash in newborn infants. J Pediatr 1987; 111: 615–616.

92. Odio C, Mohs E, Sklar FH, et al. Adverse reactions to vancomycin used as prophylaxis for CSF shunt procedures. Am J Dis Child 1984; 138: 17–19.

93. Schaad UB, McCracken GH, Jr, Nelson JD. Clinical pharmacology and efficacy of vancomycin in pediatric patients. J Pediatr 1980; 96: 119–126.

94. Salomon D, Saurat JH. Erythema multiforme major in a 2-month-old child with human immunodeficiency virus (HIV) infection. Br J Dermatol 1990; 123: 797–800.

95. Prose NS. Cutaneous manifestations of pediatric HIV infection. Pediatr Dermatol 1992; 9: 326–328.

96. Chanock SJ, Luginbuhl LM, McIntosh K, Lipshultz SE. Life-threatening reaction to trimethoprim/sulfamethoxazole in pediatric human immunodeficiency virus infection. Pediatrics 1994; 93: 519–521.

97. Cohen HA, Cohen Z, Frydman M. Fixed drug eruption of the scrotum due to hydroxyzine hydrochloride (Atarax). Cutis 1996; 57: 431–432.

98. King BA, Geelhoed GC. Adverse skin and joint reactions associated with oral antibiotics in children: The role of cefaclor in serum sickness-like reactions. J Paediatr Child Health 2003; 39: 677–681.

99. Vial T, Pont J, Pham E, et al. Cefaclor-associated serum sickness-like disease: eight cases and review of the literature. Ann Pharmacother 1992; 26: 910–914.

100. Hebert AA, Sigman ES, Levy ML. Serum sickness-like reactions from cefaclor in children. J Am Acad Dermatol 1991; 25: 805–808.

101. Carroll MC, Yueng-Yue KA, Esterly NB, Drolet BA. Drug-induced hypersensitivity syndrome in pediatric patients. Pediatrics 2001; 108: 485–492.

102. Bessmertny O, Hatton RC, Gonzalez-Peralta RP. Antiepileptic hypersensitivity syndrome in children. Ann Pharmacother 2001; 35: 533–538.

103. Yigit S, Korkmaz A, Sekerel B. Drug-induced hypersensitivity syndrome in a premature infant. Pediatr Dermatol 2005; 22: 71–74.

104. Chen CJ, Huang YC, Wang CY, Lin TY. Fatal anticonvulsant hypersensitivity syndrome in an infant. Eur J Pediatr 2003; 162: 893–894.

105. Lohmeier K, Megahed M, Schulte KW, et al. Toxic epidermal necrolysis in a premature infant of 27 weeks' gestational age. Br J Dermatol 2005; 152: 150–151.

106. Bel S, Bartralot R, Garcia D, et al. Vegetant bromoderma in an infant. Pediatr Dermatol 2001; 18: 336–338.

107. Torrelo A, Madero L, Mediero IG, Zambrano A. A cutaneous eruption from G-CSF in a healthy donor. Pediatr Dermatol 2000; 17: 205–207.

108. Buyukgebiz B, Arslan N, Ozturk Y, et al. Drug reaction to ursodeoxycholic acid: lichenoid drug eruption in an infant using ursodeoxycholic acid for neonatal hepatitis. J Pediatr Gastroenterol Nutr 2002; 35: 384–386.

109. Tamayo-Sanchez L, Ruiz-Maldonado R, Laterza A. Acute annular urticaria in infants and children. Pediatr Dermatol 1997; 14: 231–234.

110. Haas N, Birkle-Berlinger W, Henz BM. Prognosis of acute urticaria in children. Acta Dermatol Venereol 2005; 85: 74–75.

111. Sackesen C, Sekerel BE, Orhan F, et al. The etiology of different forms of urticaria in childhood. Pediatr Dermatol 2004; 21: 102–108.

112. Mortureux P, Leaute-Labreze C, Legrain-Lifermann V, et al. Acute urticaria in infancy and early childhood: a prospective study. Arch Dermatol 1998; 134: 319–323.

113. Beltrani VS. Urticaria: reassessed. Allergy Asthma Proc 2004; 25: 143–149.

114. Ghosh S, Kanwar AJ, Kaur S. Urticaria in children. Pediatr Dermatol 1993; 10: 107–110.

115. Legrain V, Taieb A, Sage T, Maleville J. Urticaria in infants: a study of forty patients. Pediatr Dermatol 1990; 7: 101–107.

116. Kauppinen K, Juntunen K, Lanki H. Urticaria in children. Retrospective evaluation and follow-up. Allergy 1984; 39: 469–472.

117. Carter EL, Garzon MC. Neonatal urticaria due to prostaglandin E1. Pediatr Dermatol 2000; 17: 58–61.

118. Hamel-Teillac D. Les urticaires chroniques de l'enfant. Ann Dermatol Venereol 2003; 130: 1S69–1S72.

119. Dice JP. Physical urticaria. Immunol Allergy Clin North Am 2004; 24: 225–246.

120. Heine RG, Elsayed S, Hosking CS, Hill DJ. Cow's milk allergy in infancy. Curr Opin Allergy Clin Immunol 2002; 2: 217–225.

121. Guillet MH, Guillet G. L'urticaire alimentaire de l'enfant. Revue de 51 observations. Allerg Immunol (Paris) 1993; 25: 333–338.

122. Ruiz-Maldonado R, Tamayo L, Ridaura C. Diffuse dermographic mastocytosis without visible skin lesions. Int J Dermatol 1975; 14: 126–128.

123. Wanderer AA, Hoffman HM. The spectrum of acquired and familial cold-induced urticaria/urticaria-like syndromes. Immunol Allergy Clin North Am 2004; 24: 259–286.

124. Zip CM, Ross JB, Greaves MW, et al. Familial cold urticaria. Clin Exp Dermatol 1993; 18: 338–341.

125. Tindall JP, Beeker SK, Rosse WF. Familial cold urticaria. A generalized reaction involving leukocytosis. Arch Intern Med 1969; 124: 129–134.

126. Doeglas HM, Bleumink E. Familial cold urticaria. Clinical findings. Arch Dermatol 1974; 110: 382–388.

127. Ormerod AD, Smart L, Reid TM, Milford-Ward A. Familial cold urticaria. Investigation of a family and response to stanozolol. Arch Dermatol 1993; 129: 343–346.

128. Haas N, Kuster W, Zuberbier T, Henz BM. Muckle–Wells syndrome: clinical and histological skin findings compatible with cold air urticaria in a large kindred. Br J Dermatol 2004; 151: 99–104.

129. Dode C, Le DN, Cuisset L, et al. New mutations of CIAS1 that are responsible for Muckle–Wells syndrome and familial cold urticaria: a novel mutation underlies both syndromes. Am J Hum Genet 2002; 70: 1498–1506.

130. Pradalier A, Cauvain A, Oukachbi Z. Inherited autoinflammatory recurrent fevers. Allerg Immunol (Paris) 2006; 38: 5–9.

131. Jedele KB, Michels VV. Familial dermographism. Am J Med Genet 1991; 39: 201–203.

132. Sahihi T, Esterly NB. Atypical diffuse cutaneous mastocytosis. Am J Dis Child 1972; 124: 133–135.

133. Epstein PA, Kidd KK. Dermo-distortive urticaria: an autosomal dominant dermatologic disorder. Am J Med Genet 1981; 9: 307–315.

134. Patterson R, Mellies CJ, Blankenship ML, Pruzansky JJ. Vibratory angioedema: a hereditary type of physical hypersensitivity. J Allergy Clin Immunol 1972; 50: 174–182.

135. Pitarch G, Torrijos A, Martinez-Menchon T, et al. Familial aquagenic urticaria and Bernard–Soulier syndrome. Dermatology 2006; 212: 96–97.

136. Bonnetblanc JM, Andrieu-Pfahl F, Meraud JP, Roux J. Familial aquagenic urticaria. Dermatologica 1979; 158: 468–470.

137. Michaelsson G, Ros AM. Familial localized heat urticaria of delayed type. Acta Dermatol Venereol 1971; 51: 279–283.

138. Kilcline C, Shinkai K, Bree A, et al. Neonatal-onset multisystem inflammatory disorder: the emerging role of pyrin genes in autoinflammatory diseases. Arch Dermatol 2005; 141: 248–253.

139. Hull KM, Shoham N, Chae JJ, et al. The expanding spectrum of systemic autoinflammatory disorders and their rheumatic manifestations. Curr Opin Rheumatol 2003; 15: 61–69.

140. Prieur AM. A recently recognised chronic inflammatory disease of early onset characterised by the triad of rash, central nervous system involvement and arthropathy. Clin Exp Rheumatol 2001; 19: 103–106.

141. Huttenlocher A, Frieden IJ, Emery H. Neonatal onset multisystem inflammatory disease. J Rheumatol 1995; 22: 1171–1173.

142. Torbiak RP, Dent PB, Cockshott WP. NOMID – a neonatal syndrome of multisystem inflammation. Skeletal Radiol 1989; 18: 359–364.

143. Dollfus H, Hafner R, Hofmann HM, et al. Chronic infantile neurological cutaneous and articular/neonatal onset multisystem inflammatory disease syndrome: ocular manifestations in a recently recognized chronic inflammatory disease of childhood. Arch Ophthalmol 2000; 118: 1386–1392.

144. Feldmann J, Prieur AM, Quartier P, et al. Chronic infantile neurological cutaneous and articular syndrome is caused by mutations in CIAS1, a gene highly expressed in polymorphonuclear cells and chondrocytes. Am J Hum Genet 2002; 71: 198–203.

145. Neven B, Callebaut I, Prieur AM, et al. Molecular basis of the spectral expression of CIAS1 mutations associated with phagocytic cell-mediated autoinflammatory disorders CINCA/NOMID, MWS, and FCU. Blood 2004; 103: 2809–2815.

146. Miura M, Okabe T, Tsubata S, et al. Chronic infantile neurological cutaneous articular syndrome in a patient from Japan. Eur J Pediatr 1997; 156: 624–626.

147. Hassink SG, Goldsmith DP. Neonatal onset multisystem inflammatory disease. Arthritis Rheum 1983; 26: 668–673.

148. Kallinich T, Hoffman HM, Roth J, Keitzer R. The clinical course of a child with CINCA/NOMID syndrome improved during and after treatment with thalidomide. Scand J Rheumatol 2005; 34: 246–249.

149. Hawkins PN, Lachmann HJ, Aganna E, McDermott MF. Spectrum of clinical features in Muckle–Wells syndrome and response to anakinra. Arthritis Rheum 2004; 50: 607–612.

150. Boschan C, Witt O, Lohse P, et al. Neonatal-onset multisystem inflammatory disease (NOMID) due to a novel S331R mutation of the CIAS1 gene and response to interleukin-1 receptor antagonist treatment. Am J Med Genet A 2006; 140: 883–886.

151. Lovell DJ, Bowyer SL, Solinger AM. Interleukin-1 blockade by anakinra improves clinical symptoms in patients with neonatal-onset multisystem inflammatory disease. Arthritis Rheum 2005; 52: 1283–1286.

152. Matsubayashi T, Sugiura H, Arai T, et al. Anakinra therapy for CINCA syndrome with a novel mutation in exon 4 of the CIAS1 gene. Acta Paediatr 2006; 95: 246–249.

153. Federico G, Rigante D, Pugliese AL, et al. Etanercept induces improvement of arthropathy in chronic infantile neurological cutaneous articular (CINCA) syndrome. Scand J Rheumatol 2003; 32: 312–314.

154. Brice SL, Huff JC, Weston WL. Erythema multiforme minor in children. Pediatrician 1991; 18: 188–194.

155. Dikland WJ, Oranje AP, Stolz E, van JT. Erythema multiforme in childhood and early infancy. Pediatr Dermatol 1986; 3: 135–139.

156. Hurwitz S. Erythema multiforme: a review of its characteristics, diagnostic criteria, and management. Pediatr Rev 1990; 11: 217–222.

157. Roujeau JC. Stevens–Johnson syndrome and toxic epidermal necrolysis are severity variants of the same disease which differs from erythema multiforme. J Dermatol 1997; 24: 726–729.

158. Bastuji-Garin S, Rzany B, Stern RS, et al. Clinical classification of cases of toxic epidermal necrolysis, Stevens–Johnson syndrome, and erythema multiforme. Arch Dermatol 1993; 129: 92–96.

159. Ashkenazi S, Metzker A, Rachmel A, Nitzan M. Erythema multiforme as a single manifestation of cow's milk intolerance. Acta Paediatr 1992; 81: 729–730.

160. Johnston GA, Ghura HS, Carter E, Graham-Brown RA. Neonatal erythema multiforme major. Clin Exp Dermatol 2002; 27: 661–664.

161. Nanda S, Pandhi D, Reddy BS. Erythema multiforme in a 9-day-old neonate. Pediatr Dermatol 2003; 20: 454–455.

162. Torrelo A, Moreno M, de P, I, Celma ML, Zambrano A. Erythema multiforme in a neonate. J Am Acad Dermatol 2003; 48: S78–S79.

163. Sakurai M. Erythema multiforme in children: unusual clinical features with seasonal occurrence. J Dermatol 1989; 16: 361–368.

164. Weston WL, Brice SL, Jester JD, et al. Herpes simplex virus in childhood erythema multiforme. Pediatrics 1992; 89: 32–34.

165. Frederiksen MS, Brenoe E, Trier J. Erythema multiforme minor following vaccination with paediatric vaccines. Scand J Infect Dis 2004; 36: 154–155.

166. Renfro L, Grant-Kels JM, Feder HM, Jr, Daman LA. Controversy: are systemic steroids indicated in the treatment of erythema multiforme? Pediatr Dermatol 1989; 6: 43–50.

167. Yeung AK, Goldman RD. Use of steroids for erythema multiforme in children. Can Fam Phys 2005; 51: 1481–1483.

168. Tatnall FM, Schofield JK, Leigh IM. A double-blind, placebo-controlled trial of continuous acyclovir therapy in recurrent erythema multiforme. Br J Dermatol 1995; 132: 267–270.

169. Samimi SS, Siegfried E. Stevens-Johnson syndrome developing in a girl with systemic lupus erythematosus on high-dose corticosteroid therapy. Pediatr Dermatol 2002; 19: 52–55.

170. Kakourou T, Klontza D, Soteropoulou F, Kattamis C. Corticosteroid treatment of erythema multiforme major (Stevens–Johnson syndrome) in children. Eur J Pediatr 1997; 156: 90–93.

171. Halebian PH, Corder VJ, Madden MR, Finklestein JL, Shires GT. Improved burn center survival of patients with toxic epidermal necrolysis managed without corticosteroids. Ann Surg 1986; 204: 503–512.

172. Cohen PR, Kurzrock R. Sweet's syndrome revisited: a review of disease concepts. Int J Dermatol 2003; 42: 761–778.

173. Callen JP. Neutrophilic dermatoses. Dermatol Clin 2002; 20: 409–419.

174. Fitzgerald RL, McBurney EI, Nesbitt LT, Jr. Sweet's syndrome. Int J Dermatol 1996; 35: 9–15.

175. von den DP. Sweet's syndrome (acute febrile neutrophilic dermatosis). J Am Acad Dermatol 1994; 31: 535–556.

176. Kemmett D, Hunter JA. Sweet's syndrome: a clinicopathologic review of twenty-nine cases. J Am Acad Dermatol 1990; 23: 503–507.

177. Dunn TR, Saperstein HW, Biederman A, Kaplan RP. Sweet syndrome in a neonate with aseptic meningitis. Pediatr Dermatol 1992; 9: 288–292.

178. Hassouna L, Nabulsi-Khalil M, Mroueh SM, et al. Multiple erythematous tender papules and nodules in an 11-month-old boy. Sweet syndrome (SS) (acute febrile neutrophilic dermatosis). Arch Dermatol 1996; 132: 1507, 1510.

179. Levin DL, Esterly NB, Herman JJ, Boxall LB. The Sweet syndrome in children. J Pediatr 1981; 99: 73–78.

180. Prasad PV, Ambujam S, Priya K, et al. Sweet's syndrome in an infant – report of a rare case. Int J Dermatol 2002; 41: 928–930.

181. Sedel D, Huguet P, Lebbe C, et al. Sweet syndrome as the presenting manifestation of chronic granulomatous disease in an infant. Pediatr Dermatol 1994; 11: 237–240.

182. Brady RC, Morris J, Connelly BL, Boiko S. Sweet's syndrome as an initial manifestation of pediatric human immunodeficiency virus infection. Pediatrics 1999; 104: 1142–1144.

183. Collins P, Rogers S, Keenan P, McCabe M. Acute febrile neutrophilic dermatosis in childhood (Sweet's syndrome). Br J Dermatol 1991; 124: 203–206.

184. Haliasos E, Soder B, Rubenstein DS, et al. Pediatric Sweet syndrome and immunodeficiency successfully treated with intravenous immunoglobulin. Pediatr Dermatol 2005; 22: 530–535.

185. Hazen PG, Kark EC, Davis BR, et al. Acute febrile neutrophilic dermatosis in children. Report of two cases in male infants. Arch Dermatol 1983; 119: 998–1002.

186. Itami S, Nishioka K. Sweet's syndrome in infancy. Br J Dermatol 1980; 103: 449–451.

187. Lipp KE, Shenefelt PD, Nelson RP, Jr, et al. Persistent Sweet's syndrome occurring in a child with a primary immunodeficiency. J Am Acad Dermatol 1999; 40: 838–841.

188. Parsapour K, Reep MD, Gohar K, et al. Familial Sweet's syndrome in 2 brothers, both seen in the first 2 weeks of life. J Am Acad Dermatol 2003; 49: 132–138.

189. Saxe N, Gordon W. Acute febrile neutrophilic dermatosis (Sweet's syndrome). Four case reports. S Afr Med J 1978; 53: 253–256.

190. Tuerlinckx D, Bodart E, Despontin K, et al. Sweet's syndrome with arthritis in an 8-month-old boy. J Rheumatol 1999; 26: 440–442.

191. Hwang ST, Williams ML, McCalmont TH, Frieden IJ. Sweet's syndrome leading to acquired cutis laxa (Marshall's syndrome) in an infant with alpha 1-antitrypsin deficiency. Arch Dermatol 1995; 131: 1175–1177.

192. Nobeyama Y, Kamide R. Sweet's syndrome with neurologic manifestation: case report and literature review. Int J Dermatol 2003; 42: 438–443.

193. Cohen PR, Kurzrock R. Sweet's syndrome and cancer. Clin Dermatol 1993; 11: 149–157.

194. Walker DC, Cohen PR. Trimethoprim-sulfamethoxazole-associated acute febrile neutrophilic dermatosis: case report and review of drug-induced Sweet's syndrome. J Am Acad Dermatol 1996; 34: 918–923.

195. Govindarajan G, Bashir Q, Kuppuswamy S, Brooks C. Sweet syndrome associated with furosemide. South Med J 2005; 98: 570–572.

196. Khan DB, Jappe U. Drug-induced Sweet's syndrome in acne caused by different tetracyclines: case report and review of the literature. Br J Dermatol 2002; 147: 558–562.

197. Jain KK. Sweet's syndrome associated with granulocyte colony-stimulating factor. Cutis 1996; 57: 107–110.

198. Jovanovic M, Poljacki M, Vujanovic L, Duran V. Acute febrile neutrophilic dermatosis (Sweet's syndrome) after influenza vaccination. J Am Acad Dermatol 2005; 52: 367–369.

199. Cohen PR, Kurzrock R. Sweet's syndrome: a review of current treatment options. Am J Clin Dermatol 2002; 3: 117–131.

200. Myatt AE, Baker DJ, Byfield DM. Sweet's syndrome: a report on the use of potassium iodide. Clin Exp Dermatol 1987; 12: 345–349.

201. Suehisa S, Tagami H, Inoue F, et al. Colchicine in the treatment of acute febrile neutrophilic dermatosis (Sweet's syndrome). Br J Dermatol 1983; 108: 99–101.

202. Aram H. Acute febrile neutrophilic dermatosis (Sweet's syndrome). Response to dapsone. Arch Dermatol 1984; 120: 245–247.

203. Kawasaki T, Kosaki F, Okawa S, et al. A new infantile acute febrile mucocutaneous lymph node syndrome (MLNS) prevailing in Japan. Pediatrics 1974; 54: 271–276.

204. Burns JC, Glode MP. Kawasaki syndrome. Lancet 2004; 364: 533–544.

205. Newburger JW, Fulton DR. Kawasaki disease. Curr Opin Pediatr 2004; 16: 508–514.

206. Falcini F. Kawasaki disease. Curr Opin Rheumatol 2006; 18: 33–38.

207. Levin M, Tizard EJ, Dillon MJ. Kawasaki disease: recent advances. Arch Dis Child 1991; 66: 1369–1372.

208. Rosenfeld EA, Corydon KE, Shulman ST. Kawasaki disease in infants less than one year of age. J Pediatr 1995; 126: 524–529.

209. Burns JC, Wiggins JW, Jr, Toews WH, et al. Clinical spectrum of Kawasaki disease in infants younger than 6 months of age. J Pediatr 1986; 109: 759–763.

210. Stanley TV, Grimwood K. Classical Kawasaki disease in a neonate. Arch Dis Child Fetal Neonatal Ed 2002; 86: F135–F136.

211. Krapf R, Zimmermann A, Stocker F. Lethal vasculitis of coronary arteries in a neonate and two infants: possible neonatal variant of the MLNS/IPN complex? Helv Paediatr Acta 1981; 36: 589–598.

212. Bolz D, Arbenz U, Fanconi S, Bauersfeld U. Myocarditis and coronary dilatation in the 1st week of life: neonatal incomplete Kawasaki disease? Eur J Pediatr 1998; 157: 589–591.

213. Burgner D, Harnden A. Kawasaki disease: what is the epidemiology telling us about the etiology? Int J Infect Dis 2005; 9: 185–194.

214. Bell DM, Morens DM, Holman RC, et al. Kawasaki syndrome in the United States 1976 to 1980. Am J Dis Child 1960; 1983; 137: 211–214.

215. Yanagawa H, Nakamura Y, Yashiro M, et al. Incidence survey of Kawasaki disease in 1997 and 1998 in Japan. Pediatrics 2001; 107: E33.

216. Yanagawa H, Nakamura Y, Yashiro M, et al. Results of the nationwide epidemiologic survey of Kawasaki disease in 1995 and 1996 in Japan. Pediatrics 1998; 102: E65.

217. Fujita Y, Nakamura Y, Sakata K, et al. Kawasaki disease in families. Pediatrics 1989; 84: 666–669.

218. Newburger JW, Takahashi M, Gerber MA, et al. Diagnosis, treatment, and long-term management of Kawasaki disease: a statement for health professionals from the Committee on Rheumatic Fever, Endocarditis, and Kawasaki Disease, Council on Cardiovascular Disease in the Young, American Heart Association. Pediatrics 2004; 114: 1708–1733.

219. Friter BS, Lucky AW. The perineal eruption of Kawasaki syndrome. Arch Dermatol 1988; 124: 1805–1810.

220. Eberhard BA, Sundel RP, Newburger JW, et al. Psoriatic eruption in Kawasaki disease. J Pediatr 2000; 137: 578–580.

221. Zvulunov A, Greenberg D, Cagnano E, Einhorn M. Development of psoriatic lesions during acute and convalescent phases of Kawasaki disease. J Paediatr Child Health 2003; 39: 229–231.

222. Garty B, Mosseri R, Finkelstein Y. Guttate psoriasis following Kawasaki disease. Pediatr Dermatol 2001; 18: 507–508.

223. Tsai HJ, Wu WM, Chang YC, et al. Annular pustules in Kawasaki disease: a further case indicating the association with psoriasis? Cutis 2003; 72: 354–356.

224. Tomita S, Chung K, Mas M, et al. Peripheral gangrene associated with Kawasaki disease. Clin Infect Dis 1992; 14: 121–126.

225. Hsu YH, Wang YH, Hsu WY, Lee YP. Kawasaki disease characterized by erythema and induration at the Bacillus Calmette–Guérin and purified protein derivate inoculation sites. Pediatr Infect Dis J 1987; 6: 576–578.

226. Bellet JS, Prose NS. Skin complications of Bacillus Calmette–Guérin immunization. Curr Opin Infect Dis 2005; 18: 97–100.

227. Sinha R, Balakumar T. BCG reactivation: a useful diagnostic tool even for incomplete Kawasaki disease. Arch Dis Child 2005; 90: 891.

228. Weinstein M. Inflammation at a previous inoculation site: an unusual presentation of Kawasaki disease. CMAJ 2006; 174: 459–460.

229. Dajani AS, Taubert KA, Gerber MA, et al. Diagnosis and therapy of Kawasaki disease in children. Circulation 1993; 87: 1776–1780.

230. Witt MT, Minich LL, Bohnsack JF, Young PC. Kawasaki disease: more patients are being diagnosed who do not meet American Heart Association criteria. Pediatrics 1999; 104: e10.

231. Alexandra FF. Inflammatory pulmonary nodules in Kawasaki disease. Pediatr Pulmonol 2003; 36: 102–106.

232. Palmer AL, Walker T, Smith JC. Acute respiratory distress syndrome in a child with Kawasaki disease. South Med J 2005; 98: 1031–1033.

233. Palazzi DL, McClain KL, Kaplan SL. Hemophagocytic syndrome after Kawasaki disease. Pediatr Infect Dis J 2003; 22: 663–666.

234. Knott PD, Orloff LA, Harris JP, et al. Sensorineural hearing loss and Kawasaki disease: A prospective study. Am J Otolaryngol 2001; 22: 343–348.

235. Yeung RS. Pathogenesis and treatment of Kawasaki's disease. Curr Opin Rheumatol 2005; 17: 617–623.

236. Wang CL, Wu YT, Liu CA, et al. Kawasaki disease: infection, immunity and genetics. Pediatr Infect Dis J 2005; 24: 998–1004.

237. Burgner D, Harnden A. Kawasaki disease: what is the epidemiology telling us about the etiology? Int J Infect Dis 2005; 9: 185–194.

238. Hirao J, Nagayoshi I. Development of coronary artery lesions in Kawasaki disease patients in relation to plasma interferon-gamma and interleukin-4 levels in the acute phase. Acta Paediatr Jpn 1997; 39: 293–295.

239. Hirao J, Yamashita T. Circulating soluble CD23 levels in Kawasaki disease with coronary artery lesions. Acta Paediatr Jpn 1997; 39: 397–399.

240. Hirao J, Hibi S, Andoh T, Ichimura T. High levels of circulating interleukin-4 and interleukin-10 in Kawasaki disease. Int Arch Allergy Immunol 1997; 112: 152–156.

241. Sato N, Sagawa K, Sasaguri Y, et al. Immunopathology and cytokine detection in the skin lesions of patients with Kawasaki disease. J Pediatr 1993; 122: 198–203.

242. Hirao J, Yamashita T. Circulating soluble L-selectin levels in Kawasaki disease with coronary artery lesions. Acta Paediatr Jpn 1997; 39: 290–292.

243. Burns JC, Shimizu C, Gonzalez E, et al. Genetic variations in the receptor-ligand pair CCR5 and CCL3L1 are important determinants of susceptibility to Kawasaki disease. J Infect Dis 2005; 192: 344–349.

244. Hewitt M, Smith LJ, Joffe HS, Chambers TL. Kawasaki disease in siblings. Arch Dis Child 1989; 64: 398–399.

245. Dergun M, Kao A, Hauger SB, et al. Familial occurrence of Kawasaki syndrome in North America. Arch Pediatr Adolesc Med 2005; 159: 876–881.

246. Uehara R, Yashiro M, Nakamura Y, Yanagawa H. Clinical features of patients with Kawasaki disease whose parents had the same disease. Arch Pediatr Adolesc Med 2004; 158: 1166–1169.

247. Salo E, Pesonen E, Viikari J. Serum cholesterol levels during and after Kawasaki disease. J Pediatr 1991; 119: 557–561.

248. Newburger JW, Burns JC, Beiser AS, Loscalzo J. Altered lipid profile after Kawasaki syndrome. Circulation 1991; 84: 625–631.

249. Simonini G, Rose CD, Vierucci A, et al. Diagnosing Kawasaki syndrome: the need for a new clinical tool. Rheumatology 2005; 44: 959–961.

250. Singh-Grewal D, Wong M, Isaacs D. Diagnosis, treatment and outcome of Kawasaki disease in an Australian tertiary setting: a review of three years experience. J Paediatr Child Health 2005; 41: 495–499.

251. Tsuda E, Kitamura S. National survey of coronary artery bypass grafting for coronary stenosis caused by Kawasaki disease in Japan. Circulation 2004; 110: II61–II66.

252. Nakamura Y, Aso E, Yashiro M, et al. Mortality among persons with a history of Kawasaki disease in Japan: can paediatricians safely discontinue follow-up of children with a history of the disease but without cardiac sequelae? Acta Paediatr 2005; 94: 429–434.

253. Nakamura Y, Yanagawa H, Harada K, et al. Mortality among persons with a history of Kawasaki disease in Japan: the fifth look. Arch Pediatr Adolesc Med 2002; 156: 162–165.

254. Levy DM, Silverman ED, Massicotte MP, et al. Longterm outcomes in patients with giant aneurysms secondary to Kawasaki disease. J Rheumatol 2005; 32: 928–934.

255. Kato H, Sugimura T, Akagi T, et al. Long-term consequences of Kawasaki disease. A 10- to 21-year follow-up study of 594 patients. Circulation 1996; 94: 1379–1385.

256. Dajani AS, Taubert KA, Takahashi M, et al. Guidelines for long-term management of patients with Kawasaki disease. Report from the Committee on Rheumatic Fever, Endocarditis, and Kawasaki Disease, Council on Cardiovascular Disease in the Young, American Heart Association. Circulation 1994; 89: 916–922.

257. Nakamura Y, Yanagawa H, Harada K, et al. Mortality among persons with a history of Kawasaki disease in Japan: existence of cardiac sequelae elevated the mortality. J Epidemiol 2000; 10: 372–375.

258. Nakamura Y, Yashiro M, Uehara R, et al. Use of laboratory data to identify risk factors of giant coronary aneurysms due to Kawasaki disease. Pediatr Int 2004; 46: 33–38.

259. Harada K. Intravenous gamma-globulin treatment in Kawasaki disease. Acta Paediatr Jpn 1991; 33: 805–810.

260. de ZA, Colan SD, Gauvreau K, Baker AL, et al. Coronary artery dimensions may be misclassified as normal in Kawasaki disease. J Pediatr 1998; 133: 254–258.

261. Terai M, Shulman ST. Prevalence of coronary artery abnormalities in

Kawasaki disease is highly dependent on gamma globulin dose but independent of salicylate dose. J Pediatr 1997; 131: 888–893.

262. Durongpisitkul K, Gururaj VJ, Park JM, Martin CF. The prevention of coronary artery aneurysm in Kawasaki disease: a meta- analysis on the efficacy of aspirin and immunoglobulin treatment. Pediatrics 1995; 96: 1057–1061.

263. Newburger JW, Takahashi M, Burns JC, et al. The treatment of Kawasaki syndrome with intravenous gamma globulin. N Engl J Med 1986; 315: 341–347.

264. Furusho K, Kamiya T, Nakano H, et al. High-dose intravenous gammaglobulin for Kawasaki disease. Lancet 1984; 2: 1055–1058.

265. Fong NC, Hui YW, Li CK, Chiu MC. Evaluation of the efficacy of treatment of Kawasaki disease before day 5 of illness. Pediatr Cardiol 2004; 25: 31–34.

266. Muta H, Ishii M, Egami K, et al. Early intravenous gamma-globulin treatment for Kawasaki disease: The nationwide surveys in Japan. J Pediatr 2004; 144: 496–499.

267. Marasini M, Pongiglione G, Gazzolo D, et al. Late intravenous gamma globulin treatment in infants and children with Kawasaki disease and coronary artery abnormalities. Am J Cardiol 1991; 68: 796–797.

268. Brogan PA, Bose A, Burgner D, et al. Kawasaki disease: an evidence based approach to diagnosis, treatment, and proposals for future research. Arch Dis Child 2002; 86: 286–290.

269. Sundel RP, Baker AL, Fulton DR, Newburger JW. Corticosteroids in the initial treatment of Kawasaki disease: Report of a randomized trial. J Pediatr 2003; 142: 611–616.

270. Okada Y, Shinohara M, Kobayashi T, et al. Effect of corticosteroids in addition to intravenous gamma globulin therapy on serum cytokine levels in the acute phase of Kawasaki disease in children. J Pediatr 2003; 143: 363–367.

271. Furukawa S, Matsubara T, Umezawa Y, et al. Pentoxifylline and intravenous gamma globulin combination therapy for acute Kawasaki disease. Eur J Pediatr 1994; 153: 663–667.

272. Burns JC, Mason WH, Hauger SB, et al. Infliximab treatment for refractory Kawasaki syndrome. J Pediatr 2005; 146: 662–667.

273. Baselga E, Drolet BA, Esterly NB. Purpura in infants and children. J Am Acad Dermatol 1997; 37: 673–705.

274. Caksen H, Odabas D, Kosem M, et al. Report of eight infants with acute infantile hemorrhagic edema and review of the literature. J Dermatol 2002; 29: 290–295.

275. Cox NH. Seidlmayer's syndrome: postinfectious cockade purpura of early

childhood. J Am Acad Dermatol 1992; 26: 275.

276. Cunningham BB, Caro WA, Eramo LR. Neonatal acute hemorrhagic edema of childhood: case report and review of the English-language literature. Pediatr Dermatol 1996; 13: 39–44.

277. Cunningham BB, Eramo L, Caro W. Acute hemorrhagic edema of childhood present at birth. Pediatr Dermatol 1999; 16: 68.

278. Gonggryp LA, Todd G. Acute hemorrhagic edema of childhood (AHE). Pediatr Dermatol 1998; 15: 91–96.

279. Ince E, Mumcu Y, Suskan E, et al. Infantile acute hemorrhagic edema: a variant of leukocytoclastic vasculitis. Pediatr Dermatol 1995; 12: 224–227.

280. Legrain V, Lejean S, Taieb A, et al. Infantile acute hemorrhagic edema of the skin: study of ten cases. J Am Acad Dermatol 1991; 24: 17–22.

281. Larregue M, Lorette G, Prigent F, Canuel C. Oedème aigu hémorragique du nourrisson avec complication léthale digestive. Ann Dermatol Venereol 1980; 107: 901–905.

282. Saraclar Y, Tinaztepe K, Adalioglu G, Tuncer A. Acute hemorrhagic edema of infancy (AHEI) – a variant of Henoch–Schonlein purpura or a distinct clinical entity? J Allergy Clin Immunol 1990; 86: 473–483.

283. Dubin BA, Bronson DM, Eng AM. Acute hemorrhagic edema of childhood: an unusual variant of leukocytoclastic vasculitis. J Am Acad Dermatol 1990; 23: 347–350.

284. Amitai Y, Gillis D, Wasserman D, Kochman RH. Henoch–Schonlein purpura in infants. Pediatrics 1993; 92: 865–867.

285. Lambert D, Laurent R, Bouilly D, et al. Cedeme aigu hémorragique du nourrisson. Données immunologiques et ultrastructurales. Ann Dermatol Venereol 1979; 106: 975–987.

286. Saraclar Y, Tinaztepe K. Infantile acute hemorrhagic edema of the skin. J Am Acad Dermatol 1992; 26: 275–276.

287. Ahmed I. Childhood porphyrias. Mayo Clin Proc 2002; 77: 825–836.

288. Gross U, Hoffmann GF, Doss MO. Erythropoietic and hepatic porphyrias. J Inherit Metab Dis 2000; 23: 641–661.

289. Kauppinen R. Porphyrias. Lancet 2005; 365: 241–252.

290. Mascaro JM. Porphyrias in children. Pediatr Dermatol 1992; 9: 371–372.

291. Lim HW. Porphyria update. Pediatr Dermatol 2000; 17: 75–83.

292. Lim HW, Cohen JL. The cutaneous porphyrias. Semin Cutan Med Surg 1999; 18: 285–292.

293. Jensen JD, Resnick SD. Porphyria in childhood. Semin Dermatol 1995; 14: 33–39.

294. Murphy GM. The cutaneous porphyrias: a review. British

Photodermatology Group. Br J Dermatol 1999; 140: 573–581.

295. Elder GH. Update on enzyme and molecular defects in porphyria. Photodermatol Photoimmunol Photomed 1998; 14: 66–69.

296. Lim HW. Pathogenesis of photosensitivity in the cutaneous porphyrias. J Invest Dermatol 2005; 124: xvi–xvii.

297. Poh-Fitzpatrick MB. Molecular and cellular mechanisms of porphyrin photosensitization. Photo-Dermatology 1986; 3: 148–157.

298. Poh-Fitzpatrick MB. Clinical features of the porphyrias. Clin Dermatol 1998; 16: 251–264.

299. Lim HW, Murphy GM. The porphyrias. Clin Dermatol 1996; 14: 375–387.

300. Fritsch C, Bolsen K, Ruzicka T, Goerz G. Congenital erythropoietic porphyria. J Am Acad Dermatol 1997; 36: 594–610.

301. Huang JL, Zaider E, Roth P, et al. Congenital erythropoietic porphyria: clinical, biochemical, and enzymatic profile of a severely affected infant. J Am Acad Dermatol 1996; 34: 924–927.

302. Berry AA, Desnick RJ, Astrin KH, et al. Two brothers with mild congenital erythropoietic porphyria due to a novel genotype. Arch Dermatol 2005; 141: 1575–1579.

303. Venkatesh P, Garg SP, Kumaran E, Tewari HK. Congenital porphyria with necrotizing scleritis in a 9-year-old child. Clin Exp Ophthalmol 2000; 28: 314–318.

304. Fontanellas A, Bensidhoum M, Enriquez de SR, et al. A systematic analysis of the mutations of the uroporphyrinogen III synthase gene in congenital erythropoietic porphyria. Eur J Hum Genet 1996; 4: 274–282.

305. Desnick RJ, Astrin KH. Congenital erythropoietic porphyria: advances in pathogenesis and treatment. Br J Haematol 2002; 117: 779–795.

306. Xu W, Astrin KH, Desnick RJ. Molecular basis of congenital erythropoietic porphyria: mutations in the human uroporphyrinogen III synthase gene. Hum Mutat 1996; 7: 187–192.

307. Kaiser IH. Brown amniotic fluid in congenital erythropoietic porphyria. Obstet Gynecol 1980; 56: 383–384.

308. Lazebnik N, Lazebnik RS. The prenatal presentation of congenital erythropoietic porphyria: report of two siblings with elevated maternal serum alpha-fetoprotein. Prenat Diagn 2004; 24: 282–286.

309. Ikha-Dahmane F, Dommergues M, Narcy F, et al. Congenital erythropoietic porphyria: prenatal diagnosis and autopsy findings in two sibling fetuses. Pediatr Dev Pathol 2001; 4: 180–184.

310. Ged C, Moreau-Gaudry F, Taine L, et al. Prenatal diagnosis in congenital

erythropoietic porphyria by metabolic measurement and DNA mutation analysis. Prenat Diagn 1996; 16: 83–86.

311. Horiguchi Y, Horio T, Yamamoto M, et al. Late onset erythropoietic porphyria. Br J Dermatol 1989; 121: 255–262.

312. Dawe SA, Peters TJ, Du VA, Creamer JD. Congenital erythropoietic porphyria: dilemmas in present day management. Clin Exp Dermatol 2002; 27: 680–683.

313. Guarini L, Piomelli S, Poh-Fitzpatrick MB. Hydroxyurea in congenital erythropoietic porphyria. N Engl J Med 1994; 330: 1091–1092.

314. Piomelli S, Poh-Fitzpatrick MB, Seaman C, et al. Complete suppression of the symptoms of congenital erythropoietic porphyria by long-term treatment with high-level transfusions. N Engl J Med 1986; 314: 1029–1031.

315. Gorchein A, Guo R, Lim CK, et al. Porphyrins in urine, plasma, erythrocytes, bile and faeces in a case of congenital erythropoietic porphyria (Gunther's disease) treated with blood transfusion and iron chelation: lack of benefit from oral charcoal. Biomed Chromatogr 1998; 12: 350–356.

316. Minder EI, Schneider-Yin X, Moll F. Lack of effect of oral charcoal in congenital erythropoietic porphyria. N Engl J Med 1994; 330: 1092–1094.

317. Hift RJ, Meissner PN, Kirsch RE. The effect of oral activated charcoal on the course of congenital erythropoietic porphyria. Br J Dermatol 1993; 129: 14–17.

318. Pimstone NR, Gandhi SN, Mukerji SK. Therapeutic efficacy of oral charcoal in congenital erythropoietic porphyria. N Engl J Med 1987; 316: 390–393.

319. Maleville J, Babin JP, Mollard S, et al. Porphyrie erythropoietique congenitale de Gunther et carotenoides. Essai therapeutique de 4 ans. Ann Dermatol Venereol 1982; 109: 883–887.

320. Seip M, Thune PO, Eriksen L. Treatment of photosensitivity in congenital erythropoietic porphyria (CEP) with beta-carotene. Acta Dermatol Venereol 1974; 54: 239–240.

321. Tezcan I, Xu W, Gurgey A, et al. Congenital erythropoietic porphyria successfully treated by allogeneic bone marrow transplantation. Blood 1998; 92: 4053–4058.

322. Thomas C, Ged C, Nordmann Y, et al. Correction of congenital erythropoietic porphyria by bone marrow transplantation. J Pediatr 1996; 129: 453–456.

323. Shaw PH, Mancini AJ, McConnell JP, et al. Treatment of congenital erythropoietic porphyria in children by allogeneic stem cell transplantation: a case report and review of the literature. Bone Marrow Transplant 2001; 27: 101–105.

324. Harada FA, Shwayder TA, Desnick RJ, Lim HW. Treatment of severe congenital erythropoietic porphyria by bone marrow transplantation. J Am Acad Dermatol 2001; 45: 279–282.

325. Dupuis-Girod S, Akkari V, Ged C, et al. Successful match-unrelated donor bone marrow transplantation for congenital erythropoietic porphyria (Gunther disease). Eur J Pediatr 2005; 164: 104–107.

326. Geronimi F, Richard E, Lamrissi-Garcia I, et al. Lentivirus-mediated gene transfer of uroporphyrinogen III synthase fully corrects the porphyric phenotype in human cells. J Mol Med 2003; 81: 310–320.

327. Kauppinen R, Glass IA, Aizencang G, et al. Congenital erythropoietic porphyria: prolonged high-level expression and correction of the heme biosynthetic defect by retroviral-mediated gene transfer into porphyric and erythroid cells. Mol Genet Metab 1998; 65: 10–17.

328. DeLeo VA, Poh-Fitzpatrick M, Mathews-Roth M, Harber LC. Erythropoietic protoporphyria. 10 years experience. Am J Med 1976; 60: 8–22.

329. Whatley SD, Mason NG, Khan M, et al. Autosomal recessive erythropoietic protoporphyria in the United Kingdom: prevalence and relationship to liver disease. J Med Genet 2004; 41: e105.

330. Goerz G, Bunselmeyer S, Bolsen K, Schurer NY. Ferrochelatase activities in patients with erythropoietic protoporphyria and their families. Br J Dermatol 1996; 134: 880–885.

331. Norris PG, Nunn AV, Hawk JL, Cox TM. Genetic heterogeneity in erythropoietic protoporphyria: a study of the enzymatic defect in nine affected families. J Invest Dermatol 1990; 95: 260–263.

332. Sarkany RP, Alexander GJ, Cox TM. Recessive inheritance of erythropoietic protoporphyria with liver failure. Lancet 1994; 344: 958–959.

333. Frank J, Nelson J, Wang X, et al. Erythropoietic protoporphyria: identification of novel mutations in the ferrochelatase gene and comparison of biochemical markers versus molecular analysis as diagnostic strategies. J Invest Med 1999; 47: 278–284.

334. Murphy GM. Diagnosis and management of the erythropoietic porphyrias. Dermatol Ther 2003; 16: 57–64.

335. Poh-Fitzpatrick MB, Piomelli S, Young P, et al. Rapid quantitative assay for erythrocyte porphyrins. Arch Dermatol 1974; 110: 225–230.

336. Mathews-Roth MM. The treatment of erythropoietic protoporphyria. Semin Liver Dis 1998; 18: 425–426.

337. Todd DJ. Therapeutic options for erythropoietic protoporphyria. Br J Dermatol 2000; 142: 826–827.

338. Miao LL, Mathews-Roth MM, Poh-Fitzpatrick MB. Beta carotene treatment and erythrocytic protoporphyrin levels. Arch Dermatol 1979; 115: 818.

339. Mathews-Roth MM. Erythropoietic protoporphyria: treatment with antioxidants and potential cure with gene therapy. Meth Enzymol 2000; 319: 479–484.

340. Warren LJ, George S. Erythropoietic protoporphyria treated with narrow-band (TL-01) UVB phototherapy. Australas J Dermatol 1998; 39: 179–182.

341. Gorchein A, Foster GR. Liver failure in protoporphyria: long-term treatment with oral charcoal. Hepatology 1999; 29: 995–996.

342. Leone N, Marzano A, Cerutti E, et al. Liver transplantation for erythropoietic protoporphyria: report of a case with medium-term follow-up. Dig Liver Dis 2000; 32: 799–802.

343. McGuire BM, Bonkovsky HL, Carithers RL, Jr, et al. Liver transplantation for erythropoietic protoporphyria liver disease. Liver Transpl 2005; 11: 1590–1596.

344. Meerman L, Haagsma EB, Gouw AS, et al. Long-term follow-up after liver transplantation for erythropoietic protoporphyria. Eur J Gastroenterol Hepatol 1999; 11: 431–438.

345. Pimstone NR. Roles and pitfalls of transplantation in human porphyria. Liver Transpl 2005; 11: 1460–1462.

346. Elder GH, Smith SG, Herrero C, et al. Hepatoerythropoietic porphyria: a new uroporphyrinogen decarboxylase defect or homozygous porphyria cutanea tarda? Lancet 1981; 1: 916–919.

347. Lim HW, Poh-Fitzpatrick MB. Hepatoerythropoietic porphyria: a variant of childhood-onset porphyria cutanea tarda. Porphyrin profiles and enzymatic studies of two cases in a family. J Am Acad Dermatol 1984; 11: 1103–1111.

348. Piñol-Aguade J, Herrero C, Almeida J, et al. Porphyrie hepato-erythroctaire, une nouvelle forme de porphyrie. Ann Dermatol Syphiligr 1975; 102: 129–136.

349. Toback AC, Sassa S, Poh-Fitzpatrick MB, et al. Hepatoerythropoietic porphyria: clinical, biochemical, and enzymatic studies in a three-generation family lineage. N Engl J Med 1987; 316: 645–650.

350. Garcia-Bravo M, Lopez-Gomez S, Segurado-Rodriguez MA, et al. Successful and safe treatment of hypertrichosis by high-intensity pulses of noncoherent light in a patient with hepatoerythropoietic porphyria. Arch Dermatol Res 2004; 296: 139–140.

351. Elder GH. Hepatic porphyrias in children. J Inherit Metab Dis 1997; 20: 237–246.

352. Thunell S, Holmberg L, Lundgren J. Aminolaevulinate dehydratase porphyria in infancy. A clinical and biochemical study. J Clin Chem Clin Biochem 1987; 25: 5–14.

353. Thunell S, Henrichson A, Floderus Y, et al. Liver transplantation in a boy with acute porphyria due to aminolaevulinate dehydratase deficiency. Eur J Clin Chem Clin Biochem 1992; 30: 599–606.

354. Lee DS, Flachsova E, Bodnarova M, et al. Structural basis of hereditary coproporphyria. Proc Natl Acad Sci USA 2005; 102: 14232–14237.

355. Lamoril J, Puy H, Whatley SD, et al. Characterization of mutations in the CPO gene in British patients demonstrates absence of genotype–phenotype correlation and identifies relationship between hereditary coproporphyria and harderoporphyria. Am J Hum Genet 2001; 68: 1130–1138.

356. Lamoril J, Martasek P, Deybach JC, et al. A molecular defect in coproporphyrinogen oxidase gene causing harderoporphyria, a variant form of hereditary coproporphyria. Hum Mol Genet 1995; 4: 275–278.

357. Nordmann Y, Grandchamp B, de VH, et al. Harderoporphyria: a variant hereditary coproporphyria. J Clin Invest 1983; 72: 1139–1149.

358. Palmer RA, Elder GH, Barrett D, Keohane SG. Homozygous variegate porphyria: a compound heterozygote with novel mutations in the protoporphyrinogen oxidase gene. Br J Dermatol 2001; 144: 866–869.

359. Kauppinen R, Timonen K, von M, et al. Homozygous variegate porphyria: 20 year follow-up and characterization of molecular defect. J Invest Dermatol 2001; 116: 610–613.

360. Roberts AG, Puy H, Dailey TA, et al. Molecular characterization of homozygous variegate porphyria. Hum Mol Genet 1998; 7: 1921–1925.

361. Beukeveld GJ, Wolthers BG, Nordmann Y, et al. A retrospective study of a patient with homozygous form of acute intermittent porphyria. J Inherit Metab Dis 1990; 13: 673–683.

362. Picat C, Delfau MH, de Rooij FW, et al. Identification of the mutations in the parents of a patient with a putative compound heterozygosity for acute intermittent porphyria. J Inherit Metab Dis 1990; 13: 684–686.

363. Llewellyn DH, Smyth SJ, Elder GH, et al. Homozygous acute intermittent porphyria: compound heterozygosity for adjacent base transitions in the same codon of the porphobilinogen deaminase gene. Hum Genet 1992; 89: 97–98.

364. Solis C, Martinez-Bermejo A, Naidich TP, et al. Acute intermittent porphyria: studies of the severe homozygous dominant disease provides insights into the neurologic attacks in acute porphyrias. Arch Neurol 2004; 61: 1764–1770.

365. Crawford GH, Kim S, James WD. Skin signs of systemic disease: an update. Adv Dermatol 2002; 18: 1–27.

366. Mallon E, Wojnarowska F, Hope P, Elder G. Neonatal bullous eruption as a result of transient porphyrinemia in a premature infant with hemolytic disease of the newborn. J Am Acad Dermatol 1995; 33: 333–336.

367. Paller AS, Eramo LR, Farrell EE, et al. Purpuric phototherapy-induced eruption in transfused neonates: relation to transient porphyrinemia. Pediatrics 1997; 100: 360–364.

368. Vanden Eijnden S, Blum D, Clercx A, et al. Cutaneous porphyria in a neonate with tyrosinaemia type 1. Eur J Pediatr 2000; 159: 503–506.

369. Bowden JB, Hebert AA, Rapini RP. Dermal hematopoiesis in neonates: report of five cases. J Am Acad Dermatol 1989; 20: 1104–1110.

370. Brough AJ, Jones D, Page RH, et al. Dermal erythropoiesis in neonatal infants: a manifestation of intrauterine viral disease. Pediatrics 1967; 40: 627–635.

371. Klein HZ, Markarian M. Dermal erythropoiesis in congenital rubella. Description of an infected newborn who had purpura associated with marked extramedullary erythropoiesis in the skin and elsewhere. Clin Pediatr (Phila) 1969; 8: 604–607.

372. Silver MM, Hellmann J, Zielenska M, et al. Anemia, blueberry-muffin rash, and hepatomegaly in a newborn infant. J Pediatr 1996; 128: 579–586.

373. Hebert AA, Esterly NB, Gardner TH. Dermal erythropoiesis in Rh hemolytic disease of the newborn. J Pediatr 1985; 107: 799–801.

374. Pizarro A, Elorza D, Gamallo C, et al. Neonatal dermal erythropoiesis associated with severe rhesus immunization: amelioration by high-dose intravenous immunoglobulin. Br J Dermatol 1995; 133: 334–336.

375. Argyle JC, Zone JJ. Dermal erythropoiesis in a neonate. Arch Dermatol 1981; 117: 492–494.

376. Hendricks WM, Hu CH. Blueberry muffin syndrome: cutaneous erythropoiesis and possible intrauterine viral infection. Cutis 1984; 34: 549–551.

377. Hawthorne HC, Jr, Nelson JS, Witzleben CL, Giangiacomo J. Blanching subcutaneous nodules in neonatal neuroblastoma. J Pediatr 1970; 77: 297–300.

378. Shown TE, Durfee MF. Blueberry muffin baby: neonatal neuroblastoma with subcutaneous metastases. J Urol 1970; 104: 193–195.

379. van E, I. Cutaneous metastases in neuroblastoma. Dermatologica 1968; 136: 265–269.

380. Kitagawa N, Arata J, Ohtsuki Y, et al. Congenital alveolar rhabdomyosarcoma presenting as a blueberry muffin baby. J Dermatol 1989; 16: 409–411.

381. Gottesfeld E, Silverman RA, Coccia PF, et al. Transient blueberry muffin appearance of a newborn with congenital monoblastic leukemia. J Am Acad Dermatol 1989; 21: 347–351.

382. Meuleman V, Degreef H. Acute myelomonocytic leukemia with skin localizations. Dermatology 1995; 190: 346–348.

383. Resnik KS, Brod BB. Leukemia cutis in congenital leukemia. Analysis and review of the world literature with report of an additional case. Arch Dermatol 1993; 129: 1301–1306.

384. Enjolras O, Leibowitch M, Guillemette J, et al. 'Blueberry muffin baby': hematopoiese extramedullaire neonatale? Leucemie monoblastique congenitale involutive? Ou histiocytose congenitale involutive? Ann Dermatol Venereol 1990; 117: 810–812.

385. Enjolras O, Leibowitch M, Bonacini F, et al. Histiocytoses langerhansiennes congenitales cutanees. A propos de 7 cas. Ann Dermatol Venereol 1992; 119: 111–117.

386. Auletta MJ, Headington JT. Purpura fulminans. A cutaneous manifestation of severe protein C deficiency. Arch Dermatol 1988; 124: 1387–1391.

387. Mahasandana C, Suvatte V, Chuansumrit A, et al. Homozygous protein S deficiency in an infant with purpura fulminans. J Pediatr 1990; 117: 750–753.

388. Marciniak E, Wilson HD, Marlar RA. Neonatal purpura fulminans: a genetic disorder related to the absence of protein C in blood. Blood 1985; 65: 15–20.

389. Marlar RA, Montgomery RR, Broekmans AW. Diagnosis and treatment of homozygous protein C deficiency. Report of the Working Party on Homozygous Protein C Deficiency of the Subcommittee on Protein C and Protein S, International Committee on Thrombosis and Haemostasis. J Pediatr 1989; 114: 528–534.

390. Marlar RA, Neumann A. Neonatal purpura fulminans due to homozygous protein C or protein S deficiencies. Semin Thromb Hemost 1990; 16: 299–309.

391. van der Horst RL. Purpura fulminans in a newborn baby. Arch Dis Child 1962; 37: 436–441.

392. Tuddenham EG, Takase T, Thomas AE, et al. Homozygous protein C deficiency with delayed onset of symptoms at 7 to 10 months. Thromb Res 1989; 53: 475–484.

393. Pipe SW, Schmaier AH, Nichols WC, et al. Neonatal purpura fulminans in association with factor V R506Q mutation. J Pediatr 1996; 128: 706–709.

394. Seligsohn U, Berger A, Abend M, et al. Homozygous protein C deficiency manifested by massive venous thrombosis in the newborn. N Engl J Med 1984; 310: 559–562.

395. Sills RH, Marlar RA, Montgomery RR, et al. Severe homozygous protein C deficiency. J Pediatr 1984; 105: 409–413.

396. Chuansumrit A, Hotrakitya S, Kruavit A. Severe acquired neonatal purpura

fulminans. Clin Pediatr (Phila) 1996; 35: 373–376.

397. Gurses N, Islek I. Causes of purpura fulminans. Pediatr Infect Dis J 1995; 14: 552–553.

398. Petaja J, Manco-Johnson MJ. Protein C pathway in infants and children. Semin Thromb Hemost 2003; 29: 349–362.

399. Aiach M, Borgel D, Gaussem P, et al. Protein C and protein S deficiencies. Semin Hematol 1997; 34: 205–216.

400. Grundy CB, Melissari E, Lindo V, et al. Late-onset homozygous protein C deficiency. Lancet 1991; 338: 575–576.

401. Tripodi A, Franchi F, Krachmalnicoff A, Mannucci PM. Asymptomatic homozygous protein C deficiency. Acta Haematol 1990; 83: 152–155.

402. Gomez E, Ledford MR, Pegelow CH, et al. Homozygous protein S deficiency due to a one base pair deletion that leads to a stop codon in exon III of the protein S gene. Thromb Haemost 1994; 71: 723–726.

403. Dahlback B. The discovery of activated protein C resistance. J Thromb Haemost 2003; 1: 3–9.

404. Dahlback B. Blood coagulation and its regulation by anticoagulant pathways: genetic pathogenesis of bleeding and thrombotic diseases. J Intern Med 2005; 257: 209–223.

405. Adcock DM, Hicks MJ. Dermato-pathology of skin necrosis associated with purpura fulminans. Semin Thromb Hemost 1990; 16: 283–292.

406. Minutillo C, Pemberton PJ, Willoughby ML, et al. Neonatal purpura fulminans and transient protein C deficiency. Arch Dis Child 1990; 65: 561–562.

407. Baliga V, Thwaites R, Tillyer ML, et al. Homozygous protein C deficiency – management with protein C concentrate. Eur J Pediatr 1995; 154: 534–538.

408. Dreyfus M, Masterson M, David M, et al. Replacement therapy with a monoclonal antibody purified protein C concentrate in newborns with severe congenital protein C deficiency. Semin Thromb Hemost 1995; 21: 371–381.

409. Angelis M, Pegelow CH, Khan FA, et al. En bloc heterotopic auxiliary liver and bilateral renal transplant in a patient with homozygous protein C deficiency. J Pediatr 2001; 138: 120–122.

410. Casella JF, Lewis JH, Bontempo FA, et al. Successful treatment of homozygous protein C deficiency by hepatic transplantation. Lancet 1988; 1: 435–438.

411. Crawford RI, Lawlor ER, Wadsworth LD, Prendiville JS. Transient erythroporphyria of infancy. J Am Acad Dermatol 1996; 35: 833–834.

412. Siegfried EC, Stone MS, Madison KC. Ultraviolet light burn: a cutaneous complication of visible light phototherapy of neonatal jaundice. Pediatr Dermatol 1992; 9: 278–282.

413. George M. Methylene-blue-induced hyperbilirubinemia and phototoxicity in a neonate. Clin Pediatr (Phila) 2000; 39: 659–661.

414. Porat R, Gilbert S, Magilner D. Methylene blue-induced phototoxicity: an unrecognized complication. Pediatrics 1996; 97: 717–721.

415. Kearns GL, Williams BJ, Timmons OD. Fluorescein phototoxicity in a premature infant. J Pediatr 1985; 107: 796–798.

416. Burry JN, Lawrence JR. Phototoxic blisters from high frusemide dosage. Br J Dermatol 1976; 94: 495–499.

20

Vascular Stains, Malformations, and Tumors

Odile Enjolras, Maria C. Garzon

CLASSIFICATION OF VASCULAR BIRTHMARKS

In 1982, Mulliken and Glowacki[1] proposed a biologic classification of vascular birthmarks that has become widely accepted. It was modified slightly in 1996 by the International Society for the Study of Vascular Anomalies.[2] Two major groups of vascular birthmarks are recognized: vascular malformations, which are composed of dysplastic, malformed vessels; and vascular tumors, which demonstrate cellular hyperplasia. The distinction between malformations and tumors is emphasized by their varying histologic appearance, cellular markers, and natural history[3,4] (Table 20.1). This classification also helps avoid confusing terminology such as 'cavernous hemangioma,' which had been previously used to describe both tumors and malformations[3]. It has endured for more than two decades, has international acceptance, and is a clinically useful framework for understanding vascular birthmarks. In rare instances, however, overlap between malformations and tumors can occur.

Vascular malformations are subcategorized according to flow characteristics and predominant anomalous channels: slow flow (capillary, C; venous, V; lymphatic, L) or fast flow (arteriovenous malformation, AVM; and arteriovenous fistula, AVF). A number of complex combined vascular malformations (M) exist: CVM, CLVM, LVM, AVM, CAVM, CLAVM, and so forth, with some of them known by eponyms. Infantile hemangioma is the most common vascular tumor of infancy, others being less common or rare, and some having only recently been characterized.

VASCULAR MALFORMATIONS

Capillary, venous, lymphatic, arterial, and arteriovenous malformations occur either alone or in combination. They are often localized and circumscribed lesions, but can also present in a segmental, systematized pattern or in a diffuse, disseminated form. Some are part of a more complex syndromic pathology (Table 20.2). Vascular malformations are often erroneously referred to in articles and texts as 'hemangioma' or 'hemangiomatosis,' and this complicates analysis of the literature. The majority of vascular malformations occur as sporadic anomalies. However, some are familial. Identification of gene mutations responsible for some forms of vascular malformations has helped in understanding the pathogenesis of some types of vascular malformation.

Capillary Malformations
Salmon Patch (Nevus Simplex)
A salmon patch is a capillary malformation (CM), also known as an 'angel kiss' when it is located on the forehead or eyelids, and 'stork bite' when located on the nape. It is present in nearly half of all newborns and affects males and females equally. It has a characteristic predilection for the midline, with the most common locations being the nape, upper glabella, nose, and upper lip (Fig. 20-1). The occiput and lower back may also be affected[5]. If a salmon patch involves an upper eyelid and does not occur concomitantly with a V-shaped patch in the middle of the forehead, it may be difficult to differentiate from a partial V1 port wine stain or a hemangioma precursor.

Salmon patches usually disappear within 1 or 2 years, but some persist, particularly those at the nape.[6] Persistent involvement of the glabella is sometimes referred to as medial telangiectatic nevus. Although most salmon patches have no associations, rarely they are a manifestation of another condition, such as Beckwith–Wiedemann, macrocephaly–CMTC, or Nova syndromes (see discussion below).

Butterfly-Shaped Mark and Sacral Medial Telangiectatic Vascular Nevus
Localized in the midline sacral region, the 'butterfly-shaped mark' has been described as a variant of the salmon patch. Involvement at this site is most often seen in infants with multiple salmon patches elsewhere. Some authors have asserted that evaluation of the spine seems unnecessary in these infants unless other signs are present,[7] but controversy still exists regarding the need for evaluation. Like salmon patches on the nape, this sacral stain may persist. A condition known as 'sacral medial telangiectatic vascular nevus' is closely related; it is localized to the sacral midline or extends to the entire back or the buttocks, often in infants with salmon patches elsewhere. Whereas some authors have reported a lack of associated spinal dysraphism,[8] prospective studies with MR imaging are lacking, so it is not possible to definitively exclude this risk completely.

TABLE 20-1 Major differences between hemangiomas and vascular malformations

	Infentile Hemangiomas	Vascular malformations
Clinical	Variably visible at birth Subsequent rapid growth Slow, spontaneous involution	Usually visible at birth (AVMs may be quiescent) Growth proportionate to the skin's growth (or slow progression); present lifelong
Sex ratio (f:m)	3:1 to 5:1 and 9:1 in severe cases	1:1
Pathology	Proliferating stage: hyperplasia of endothelial cells and SMC-actin+ cells Multilaminated basement membrane Higher mast cell content in involution	Flat endothelium Thin basement membrane Often irregularly attenuated walls (VM, LM)
Radiology	Fast-flow lesion on Doppler sonography Tumoral mass with flow voids on MR Lobular tumor on arteriogram	Slow flow (CM, LM, VM) or fast flow (AVM) on Doppler sonography MR: Hypersignal on T2 when slow flow (LM, VM); flow voids on T1 and T2 when fast flow (AVM) Arteriography of AVM demonstrates AV shunting
Bone changes	Rarely mass effect with distortion but no invasion	*Slow-flow VM*: distortion of bones, thinning, underdevelopment *Slow-flow CM*: hypertrophy *Slow-flow LM*: distortion, hypertrophy, and invasion *High-flow AVM*: destruction, rarely extensive lytic lesions *Combined malformations* (e.g., slow-flow [CVLM = Klippel-Trenaunay syndrome] or fast-flow [CAVM = Parkes-Weber syndrome]): overgrowth of limb bones, gigantism
Immunohistochemistry on tissue samples	*Proliferating hemangioma*: high expression of PCNA, type IV collagenase, VEGF, urokinase, and bFGF *Involuting hemangioma*: high TIMP-1, high bFGF (at all growth stages) Express GLUT-1, merosin, FcγRII and Lewis Y antigen	Lack expression of PCNA, type IV collagenase, urokinase, VEGF, and bFGF Lack expression of GLUT-1, merosin, FcγRII and Lewis Y antigen One familial (rare) form of VM linked to a mutated gene on 9p (VMCM1)
Hematology	No coagulopathy (Kasabach-Merritt syndrome is a complication of other vascular tumors of infancy, e.g., kaposiform hemangioendothelioma and tufted angioma, with a LM component)	Slow-flow VM or LM or LVM may have an associated LIC with risk of bleeding (DIC).

AVM, Arteriovenous malformation; *SMC*, smooth muscle cell; *VM*, venous malformation; *LM*, lymphatic malformation; *MR*, magnetic resonance imaging; *CM*, capillary malformation/port wine stain; *CLVM*, capillary lymphatic venous malformation; *CAVM*, capillary arteriovenous malformation; *PCNA*, proliferating cell nuclear antigen; *VEGF*, vascular endothelial growth factor; *bFGF*, basic fibroblast growth factor; *TIMP*, tissue inhibitor of metalloproteinase; *LIC*, localized intravascular coagulopathy; *DIC*, disseminated intravascular coagulation. *GLUT-1*, glucose transporter protein-1.

TABLE 20-2 Vascular anomalies with associated extracutaneous findings – selected syndromes

Syndrome	Cutaneous	Extracutaneous
Sturge-Weber	CM	Glaucoma, seizures
Klippel-Trenaunay	CVM, CLVM	Limb hypertrophy
Parkes Weber	CAVM, CLAVM	Limb hypertrophy
Proteus	CM, LM, CLVM Epidermal nevi, thickened palms and soles	Hemihypertrophy, visceral lipomas, visceral vascular malformations, endocrine tumors
Servelle-Martorell	CVM	Limb undergrowth
Bannayan-Riley-Ruvalcaba	CM, LM, VM Lipomas, pigmented macules (genitalia)	Macrocephaly, mental retardation, visceral lipomas, intestinal polyposis
Beckwith-Wiedemann	CM	Macroglossia, macrosomia, renal disorders, embryonal tumors
Adams-Oliver	CMTC Aplasia cutis congenita	Cranium defects, limb anomalies
Blue rubber bleb nevus (Bean)	VM, LVM	Gastrointestinal, CNS vascular malformations
Wyburn-Mason	AVM	CNS AVM
Cobb	AVM	Spinal AVM
PHACE	Hemangioma	Posterior fossa, arterial, cardiac, ocular anomalies
Kasabach-Merritt	KHE, tufted angioma	Thrombocytopenic coagulopathy

CM, Capillary malformation/port wine stain; *CVM*, capillary venous malformation; *CLVM*, capillary lymphatic venous malformation; *CAVM*, capillary arteriovenous malformation; *CLAVM*, capillary lymphatic arteriovenous malformation; *LM*, lymphatic malformation; *VM*, venous malformation; *CMTC*, cutis marmorata telangiectatica congenita; *AVM*, arteriovenous malformation; *KHE*, kaposiform hemangioendothelioma.

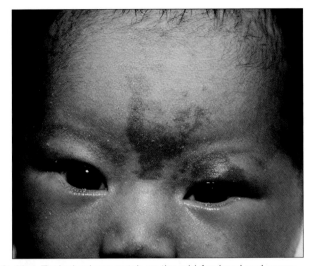

FIG. 20-1 Typical salmon patch on the mid-forehead and upper eyelid.

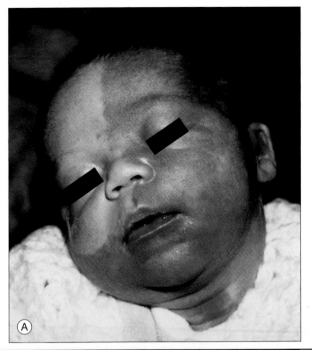

Port Wine Stains

Port wine stains (PWS) are capillary malformations that are almost always evident at birth. They usually occur as sporadic lesions, but families with multiple PWS scattered over the body have demonstrated a possible autosomal dominant pattern of inheritance.

Cutaneous Findings

PWS are pink or red patches that arise at birth. They typically grow proportionately with the child's somatic growth, and, if left untreated, persist throughout the patient's life. They consist of ectatic dermal capillaries and may occur anywhere on the body (Fig. 20-2A, B). PWS may appear to lighten over the first 3–6 months of life, but this should not be taken as a sign of resolution. Rather it is most likely due to the decrease in blood hemoglobin concentration (typically 15–17 g/dL at birth to a nadir of 8–10 g/dL by age 3 months). The natural history of port wine stains over a lifetime is often one of gradual darkening from pink-red to a crimson or deep purple hue. Skin thickening and soft tissue hypertrophy may also occur, particularly in stains on the medial cheek and upper lip area. Eczematous changes can occur in PWS and salmon patches, either with or without treatment. Nodular vascular lesions may appear within PWS during childhood or adult life and may require surgical intervention.[9] PWS are sometimes contiguous with a nevus anemicus. The association of PWS ('nevus flammeus') with pigmentary anomalies such as extensive mongolian spots, nevus spilus, or nevoid hyperpigmentation is a feature of phakomatosis pigmentovascularis (Fig. 20-3) (see Chapter 22).

Extracutaneous Findings

Progressive soft tissue and bony overgrowth may occur during childhood, especially with V2 PWS, and subtle changes are sometimes noted even in the neonatal period.[10] Asymmetric maxillary hypertrophy associated with distortion of the facial features will require orthodontic follow-up and treatment. Some patients require procedures to correct skeletal overgrowth in late childhood. Gum hypertrophy may also develop. Syndromic PWS are discussed later in this chapter.

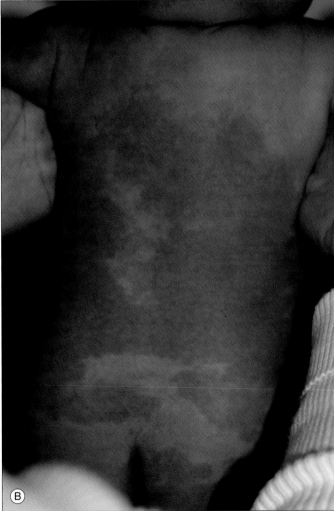

FIG. 20-2 (A) Port wine stain involving left facial V1 + V2 + V3 and right V3 areas. The V1 involvement indicates a risk of Sturge–Weber syndrome, which this infant had. **(B)** Extensive port wine stain on the back of a young infant.

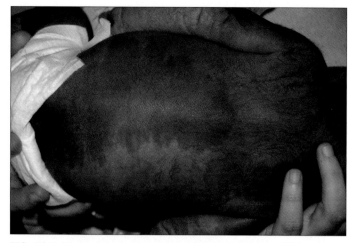

FIG. 20-3 Phakomatosis pigmentovascularis (courtesy of H.P. Makkar).

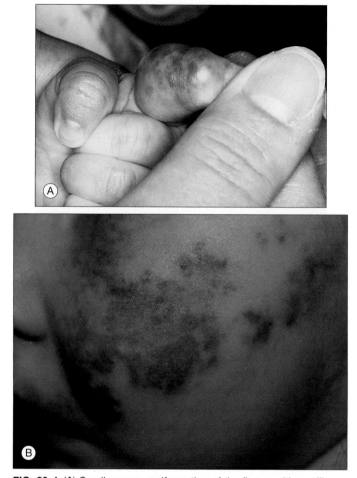

FIG. 20-4 (A) Small venous malformation of the finger, with swelling and blue nodularity. **(B)** More extensive venous malformation on the face.

Management and Treatment

The gradual thickening and nodularity of PWS provide a medical rationale for treatment during infancy and childhood.[9] The flashlamp-pumped pulsed dye laser (FPDL) is a now well-established treatment for PWS and poses a very low risk of scarring, even in young infants. Although only 15–20% of PWS clear completely with FPDL, the majority of treated lesions lighten significantly.[11,12] Response to laser treatment varies by region: outcomes are better on the face and neck, albeit with less improvement in V2 than other facial sites.[12] The extremities do not respond so well.[11–13] Recent developments in laser technology (such as built-in epidermal cooling devices) have led to more effective treatments for darker-skinned individuals and some previously resistant lesions, but in large and confluent PWS, improvement rather than complete clearing is the expected outcome. Other light sources can also be effective, but are generally not recommended for young infants. Controversy exists regarding the age at which treatment should begin. Some authors have noted a better therapeutic response with fewer treatments when treatment was begun in early infancy,[14] but others have found no difference.[15] Initiating treatment in infancy or early childhood can be helpful in reducing stigmatization and to help prevent skin thickening.

Telangiectasia

A variety of telangiectatic skin lesions have been described. They are usually composed of small, punctate telangiectasias distributed in either a segmental, unilateral nevoid, or diffuse pattern. Most are absent at birth, often developing before or at puberty. A pale halo of vasoconstriction may surround small telangiectasia. Toddlers and young children sometimes develop so-called spider angiomas. Risk factors include fair skin and a history of minor skin injury at the site. These may disappear spontaneously or persist. Fine telangiectasias are occasionally present on the cheeks of normal young children, but extensive telangiectasias in the photo-distribution should prompt consideration of conditions with photosensitivity such as Rothmund–Thomson syndrome. Persistent telangiectasias can also be seen as a sequela of neonatal lupus (see Chapter 19). The facial telangiectasias associated with hereditary hemorrhagic telangiectasia (HHT) and ataxia–telangiectasia usually present later in life.

Venous Malformations

Venous malformations (VM) are slow-flow vascular malformations that are usually evident at birth. They may involve skin, mucosa, subcutaneous tissues, and deeper structures. They are composed of ill-defined venous channels with irregularly attenuated walls, focally lacking smooth muscle cells, permeating the skin and adnexal structures.

Cutaneous Findings

At birth, the majority of VM are subtle, bluish, ill-defined, compressible birthmarks, but a bulky venous mass develops in some patients during intrauterine life (Fig. 20-4). VMs may be diffuse or localized. Affected skin and mucous membranes are typically blue with normal skin temperature, without a thrill or bruit. Lesions swell when dependent or with crying. Local venous thromboses can lead to the formation of phleboliths, which can be tender when palpated and are visible on radiographs as round calcifications. They can be present at

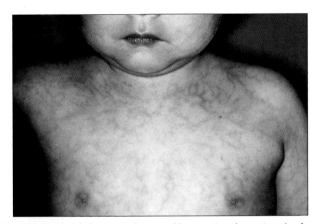

FIG. 20-5 Bockenheimer syndrome with an extensive network of dilated veins.

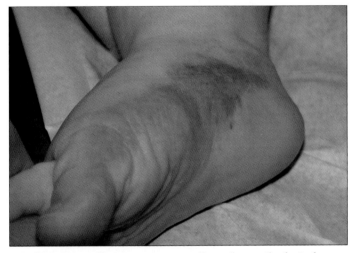

FIG. 20-6 Plaque-like glomuvenous malformation on the foot of a young infant. (Courtesy of Susan B. Mallory.)

birth in rare cases. Cutaneous and mucosal VM (VMCM) is a familial form of VM, inherited in an autosomal dominant fashion. Multifocal disease with skin, mucosal and intramuscular VMs may be present.[16,17] Diffuse congenital genuine phlebectasia of Bockenheimer is a rare type of VM with dilated blue linear veins visible on the entire skin surface (Fig. 20-5). Glomuvenous malformations (GVM; formerly called 'glomangioma') are a distinct type of venous malformation. They may be solitary or multiple, and may be localized or involve a larger territory of skin (Fig. 20-6). When present at birth, they are nodular or plaque-like, poorly demarcated pink or bluish (or both) lesions. During childhood they typically acquire a deeper blue hue and thicken, and become tender when palpated. Congenital plaque-like GVMs are usually pink at birth, with noticeable thickening and change in color to blue-purple during childhood. These plaque-like GVMs may arise sporadically, or occur as a manifestation of autosomal dominant GVM. Other family members may have smaller, blue vascular lesions scattered over the skin, increasing in number with age.[18]

Extracutaneous Findings

In addition to skin and mucosal involvement VM can also involve deeper soft tissues, muscles, joints, and in severe cases visceral sites such as the abdomen and pelvis. A majority of

patients with extensive VMs have a chronic localized intravascular coagulopathy (LIC), which can manifest in newborns and be erroneously diagnosed as the Kasabach–Merritt syndrome (KMS). This coagulopathy, which can result in either thrombosis (with pain and phlebolith formation) or bleeding, can persist throughout life. It differs from KMS because the primary process is one of ongoing clotting, with consumption of clotting factors, low fibrinogen and elevated D-dimers, but without the marked thrombocytopenia of KMS.[16,17] The 'blue rubber bleb nevus' syndrome, the association of multiple cutaneous venous malformations with gastrointestinal and other internal lesions, is discussed later in this chapter. In contrast to VMs, GVMs are typically localized to the skin and soft tissues without intramuscular involvement.

Pathogenesis

VMs are sporadic in the majority of cases, but, as noted, familial cases of both VM and GVM occur. Molecular biology has now permitted a clear distinction between VM (sometimes referred to as VMCM) and GVM. The mutated gene *VMCM1* maps to chromosome 9p17; this is an activating mutation in the kinase domain of the receptor tyrosine kinase Tie2.[19] GVM can be either a sporadic or an autosomal dominant condition, linked to mutations in the glomulin gene (mapping to 1p21-p22). Unlike VMs, far more cases of GVM are familial (approximately 64%).[18,20] Unlike VM and VMCM, individuals with GVM have venous-like channels which, rather than lacking smooth muscle cells in their walls, instead have several rows of actin-positive cells in their thick walls.

Diagnosis

The diagnosis is usually established on the basis of clinical features, but ultrasound, Doppler, MRI, and CT scans are useful for evaluating the extent of involvement.[21] Apart from diagnosis, the decision to image early in infancy depends on whether functional problems are present or early treatments are planned. Many VMs, however, especially larger ones, eventually do require imaging studies, MRI with contrast being the single best study to delineate disease. In individuals with craniofacial VMs it is advisable to image the brain: developmental venous anomalies (DVA) in the brain are more common in patients with craniofacial VMs than in the general population (25% vs 0.5%).[22] DVAs are uncommon trajectories of the brain's venous drainage and pose little risk of cerebral hemorrhage, but documenting their presence can help avoid misdiagnosis of a more worrisome condition later in life.

Differential Diagnosis

Extensive blue VMs in a leg or an arm and adjacent trunk must be differentiated from Klippel–Trenaunay syndrome (see later discussion). Sinus pericranii should be considered in the differential diagnosis of a VM located on the central forehead. This presents as a bluish, nonpulsating mass that is usually congenital and quickly expands when the patient puts their head in a dependent position or with crying. Sinus pericranii represents a direct communication between superficial veins and intracranial venous sinuses through a bony defect. It is best imaged using CT bone windows.

Course

The clinical course and complications of venous malformations depend on anatomic location, with differing problems in the craniofacial area, trunk, and limbs.[17] The cheek and lip are common locations for superficial craniofacial VMs, and there is sometimes extension to the temporal and orbital areas. Swelling is noted with changes in position and activity. As the child grows older, the VM may progressively distort the facial features and mold the underlying developing bones, which can result in deformities such as an open bite or enlargement of the orbit. Extensive retropharyngeal involvement can result in obstructive sleep apnea, occasionally even in young children. VMs located on the trunk and limbs may involve skin, skeletal muscles, joints, and bones. During infancy and early childhood, the skin component of the VM expands and becomes deep blue. However, the deeper component may remain undiagnosed until it causes pain. Swelling, functional impairment, and limited joint motion occur when the child becomes older and more active, especially if playing sports. The chronic coagulopathy often associated with diffuse limb VM can manifest as early as the neonatal period.

Treatment

Treatment of craniofacial VM should be considered if there is significant functional impairment or disfigurement, but is rarely initiated in the first year of life. Therapy is aimed at preventing distortion of facial features, limiting bone deformity, gaping, shift of the dental midline, lip expansion, and displacement of the lip commissures.[23,24] Small lesions can be treated using percutaneous sclerotherapy or excisional surgery alone. MRI features may be especially helpful in determining optimal management.[24] Larger VMs are usually treated with percutaneous sclerotherapy, either alone or combined with surgical excision.[25] Multiple treatments are often required over the years. Laser surgery or radiofrequency ablation is occasionally helpful. Extensive pure VMs of the limb are usually managed in a conservative manner. Elastic stockings are encouraged from infancy in extensive cases. Compression increases comfort, limits swelling, and improves coagulopathy. Indications for sclerotherapy and surgery of limb VMs are limited in infancy, but well-localized lesions are sometimes excised. Evaluation of large VMs includes assessment for coagulopathy. Complex VMs is best managed at a center with a multidisciplinary vascular anomalies group.

Lymphatic Malformations

Lymphatic malformations (LMs) (known in much of the literature as 'lymphangioma') can be macrocystic, microcystic, or combined.

Cutaneous Findings

Macrocystic LMs are usually visible at birth and are commonly diagnosed by prenatal ultrasound investigation. They occur more commonly in the neck and axilla, where they are often referred to as cystic hygroma (Fig. 20-7).[26] The detection in utero of some huge LMs of the neck, axilla, and thoracic area may lead to a discussion about terminating the pregnancy, as the prognosis is poor. Microcystic LMs can infiltrate diffusely throughout the dermis. Clear or hemorrhagic vesicles (so-called lymphangioma circumscriptum), which may intermittently leak lymphatic fluid, may be visible on the surface of the lesion. This type of LM is rarely evident during the neonatal period and becomes apparent on skin and mucous membranes later in childhood. Severe combined LMs may also occur on the trunk and limbs.[27]

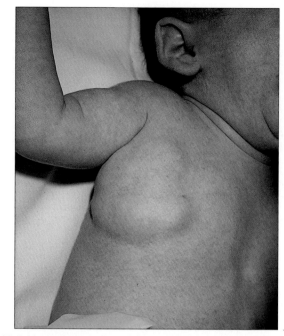

FIG. 20-7 Large thoracic lymphatic malformation ('cystic hygroma') present at birth.

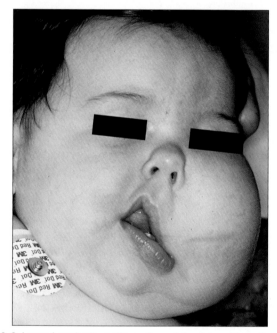

FIG. 20-8 Large lymphatic malformation of the face with both microcystic and macrocystic elements involving the skin and mucosa.

Extracutaneous Findings

Cervicofacial LMs involving the tongue and floor of the mouth will interfere with normal development of the jaw and create an open bite deformity. The most severe forms of combined micro-/macrocystic LMs, which are more common in the head region, particularly the cheek and mouth, can cause life-threatening airway disease and other functional problems in the neonate (Fig. 20-8). Intraoral involvement also causes halitosis, aggressive caries, and loss of teeth, and involvement of the mandible is present in 41% of these patients.[28,29] Extra- and intraconal orbital LM occurs in association with eyelid LM; this uncommon location causes severe complications including disfigurement, bleeding, infection, proptosis, and visual loss.[30] Severe cervicofacial LMs, usually the combined micro-/macrocystic type, involving the hypopharynx and larynx, the tongue and the floor of the mouth, can cause airway and esophageal obstruction requiring nasogastric tube feeding and emergency tracheotomy in the newborn.[31] Of 31 cases with such severe involvement, 58% required tracheostomy in infancy and one-third could not be decannulated.[29] Visceral LMs, intrathoracic or abdominal, are less common, representing about one-tenth of cases. A chronic coagulopathy may be associated with extensive visceral LMs and may manifest even in infancy with intralesional bleeding. LMs are more susceptible to bacterial infections, and infection itself can worsen the malformation.

Pathogenesis

Severe hydrops fetalis and multiple cystic hygromas are the major cause of spontaneous abortion of fetuses with the 45, X genotype of Turner syndrome.[32] Controversy remains regarding the diagnostic and nosologic boundaries between microcystic and macrocystic LMs, diffuse lymphangiomatosis (both superficial and visceral), congenital diffuse lymphangioma of the leg, transient localized lymphedema with puffiness of the dorsum of the feet (as seen in Turner and Noonan syndromes), and primary congenital lymphedema of limbs (Milroy–Meige–Nonne disease) (Fig. 20-9). Two genotypes of congenital

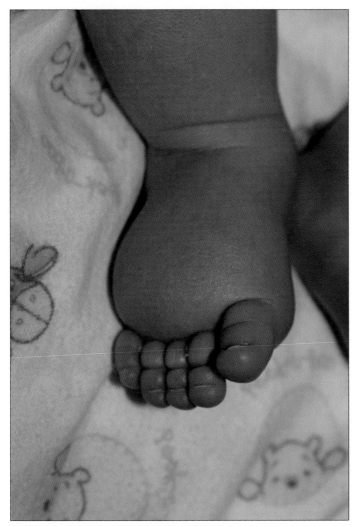

FIG. 20-9 Lymphedema of the foot in a 3-week-old infant with Milroy's disease.

lymphedema are identified: Milroy syndrome is linked to *VEGFR3* mutation, and lymphedema–distichiasis syndrome is linked to *FOXC2* mutation.

Diagnosis

The diagnosis is established either clinically or using CT, MRI, or ultrasound. Fluid aspiration and analysis may be helpful because a number of neonatal growths, including some malignant tumors, can present with large cyst-like swellings.[33] Histologically, lymphatic vessels or cysts have thin walls and lumina appear empty. Several positive markers of lymphatic vessels have been used, including LYVE-1, VEGFR-3 and D2-40.

Treatment

Congenital macrocystic LMs can be treated after birth using sclerotherapy. A variety of sclerosing agents have been used, including ethanol, OK-432, and doxycycline. Surgical resection is another therapeutic option for macrocystic LMs, as well as for microcystic and combined types, but recurrences and complications such as seroma or chronic lymphatic leakage may occur.[28–30,34,35] A multidisciplinary approach is required for complex LMs.[29]

Arteriovenous Malformations

Arteriovenous malformations (AVMs) are fast-flow anomalies that most commonly arise in the head and neck area. A significant percentage are visible at birth,[36,37] but they may be quite subtle in appearance, mimicking a port wine stain or involuting hemangioma (Fig. 20-10). Macular erythema with increased local warmth, a typical pattern of skin distribution, and subtle skin thickening can be clues to the diagnosis. An actual vascular mass with tense draining veins, a thrill, and a bruit is a rare presentation of an AVM in the newborn, and when present more likely represents a congenital hemangioma (see discussion below). Color Doppler ultrasound examination as well as MR with MR angiography may also be helpful in diagnosis, as well as delineating the extent of disease. Arteriography, the gold-standard for diagnosis, is not indicated in young infants with quiescent AVMs.

AVMs are dangerous lesions and may severely worsen over time. In some adults, an uncontrolled course may lead to disfigurement, pain, hemorrhage, and even death. Among the main factors triggering this devastating evolution are puberty and trauma, which may be accidental or the result of ill-advised and partial treatment. Superficial AVMs in infants are rarely amenable to a satisfactory treatment. Laser treatments, cryosurgery, or partial excision may initiate expansion and trigger the growth of an AVM. Severe congenital AVM with associated high-output heart failure at birth is a rare occurrence that requires endovascular embolization if pharmacologic treatment does not control cardiac complications. AVMs can be sporadic, familial, and seen in association with certain syndromes.

Syndromes Associated with Vascular Malformations

Vascular malformations may be a feature of several well-characterized syndromes, many of which have attached eponyms. Many are apparent at birth, with cutaneous lesions as a cardinal feature.[38] Some are familial, but the majority are sporadic (Table 20-2).

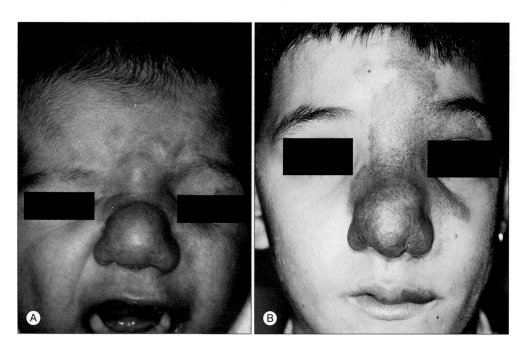

FIG. 20-10 (A) Five-day-old neonate with a midfacial quiescent arteriovenous malformation that subsequently worsened and proved to be part of a Bonnet–Dechaume–Blanc syndrome. (B) The same child at 8 years of age.

Rendu–Osler–Weber Syndrome

Also known as hereditary hemorrhagic telangiectasia (HHT), this familial autosomal dominant disorder with various phenotypes corresponds to at least three distinct genotypes.[39] DNA testing makes early diagnosis available to relatives in a given affected family. HHT is characterized by skin and mucosal telangiectasia, and a risk of arteriovenous malformations in lungs, brain, and liver.[40] Telangiectasia of the skin, lips, and mouth are not visible during infancy, and mucosal and visceral hemorrhages do not occur until later in life.

Ataxia–Telangiectasia (AT)

This is a rare autosomal recessive disease characterized by progressive cerebellar ataxia, telangiectasia, elevated α-fetoprotein levels, B- and T-cell immunodeficiency with sinopulmonary infections, cancer susceptibility (in particular breast cancer), sensitivity to ionizing radiation and radiomimetic drugs, and premature aging.[41] The onset of telangiectasia in the newborn period is rare. In a group of 48 patients, the median age of onset of gait abnormalities was 15 months, and 72 months for telangiectasias. The median age of diagnosis was 78 months, shortly after the appearance of telangiectasia in two-thirds of patients.[42] The mutated gene (*ATM*) maps to 11q22-23; it was isolated in 1995, and more than 100 mutations have been documented in affected individuals.

Cutis Marmorata Telangiectatica Congenita

Cutis marmorata telangiectatica congenita (CMTC) is a form of vascular malformation with a distinctive reticulated pattern. Most cases are sporadic. A female predominance is reported.[43] CMTC can be confined to a small area, have a regional distribution, or more diffuse skin involvement. At birth, a reticulated purple network is noted. The skin is streaked with linear and patchy vascular lesions intermingled with telangiectasia. In areas of involvement there are often focal areas of atrophy and/or ulceration, even during the neonatal period (Fig. 20-11). These changes are often most prominent over the limb joints. This conspicuous atrophic reticulate pattern differs from phys-

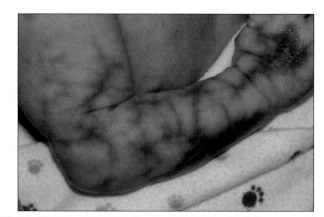

FIG. 20-11 Neonate with cutis marmorata telangiectatica congenita (CMTC) on arm.

iologic cutis marmorata, a normal finding in newborns, in that the pattern is coarse and less regular. CMTC may be associated with port wine stains, which can become more apparent after 1 year of age as the reticulate lesions fade. CMTC may improve with age, but rarely disappears completely. Ulcerations continue to arise during infancy and childhood, particularly in areas overlying the joints, resulting in scaly areas of scarring.

In our experience, regional CMTC with involvement of one or two areas of skin (most often the extremities) is far more common than the diffuse type, but it is less frequently reported in the literature. A difference in limb girth is common, and the affected limb may have a thinner, pseudo-'athletic' appearance compared to the normal extremity as a result of having less fat or diminished muscles and bones. Subsequent growth is usually proportional to the original degree of limb asymmetry.[44]

Associated developmental defects are far more common in children affected with widespread CMTC than with more localized disease. Multiple associated abnormalities have been reported, including musculoskeletal anomalies, vascular abnormalities (arterial stenosis), cardiac defects, and the Adams–Oliver syndrome (see below). Less frequently reported anomalies include brain and spinal cord defects, glaucoma and other ocular anomalies, imperforate anus, abnormal genitalia, dystrophic teeth, congenital hypothyroidism, stenosing tendonitis, and others.[43–48] We observed an infant with CMTC intermingled with mongolian spots on the trunk and one lower extremity (a very rare type of phakomatosis pigmentovascularis).

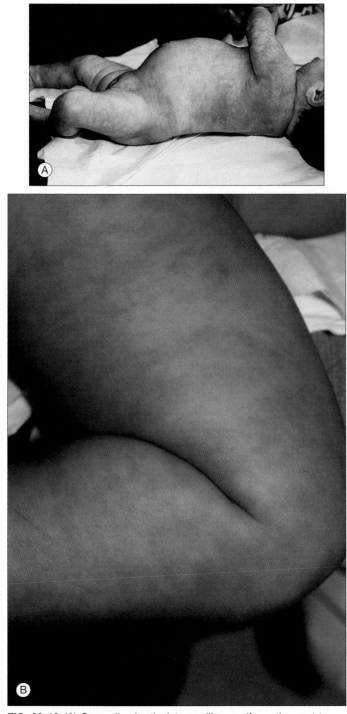

FIG. 20-12 **(A)** Generalized reticulate capillary malformation, not true CMTC. This child had multisystem disease with renal vascular anomalies, blindness, and brain ischemic attacks early in life. **(B)** Blotchy port wine stains such as this one are sometimes mistaken for CMTC.

CMTC can be confused with a generalized reticulate capillary malformation, but the latter lacks the patchy or linear atrophy and telangiectasia (Fig. 20-12A). Reticulate CM is a rare, diffuse type of CM that in our experience is often associated with multiple visceral vascular anomalies (eye, kidney, and lungs) and may be associated with a risk of developing early ischemic brain symptoms.[44] The syndrome known as macrocephaly–CMTC, also as megalencephaly–CMTC (OMIM 602501), includes various abnormalities such as asymmetric growth, developmental delay, 2–3 syndactyly of the toes, high forehead and frontal bossing, joint laxity, and a distinctive facies. The vascular lesions in this condition are *not* classic CMTC and most closely resemble reticulated capillary malformations. Most affected individuals also have prominent salmon patch-like lesions of the forehead and upper lip.[49] The differential diagnosis of CMTC also includes neonatal lupus: cases beginning during intrauterine life can result in extensive livedo, telangiectasia, and atrophic striae.[50] Less generalized PWS with a blotchy reticulated quality are also sometimes mistaken for CMTC (Fig. 20-12B).

The residual, persistent, reticulate vascular lesions of CMTC respond poorly to pulsed dye laser treatments and are associated with a greater risk of scarring than is usually associated with this mode of therapy. Associated port wine stains, however, may be more amenable to therapy. Management of extracutaneous associated abnormalities is directed at specific signs or symptoms. Infants with CMTC located in a distri-bution similar to the port wine stain of Sturge–Weber syndrome are at higher risk for CNS and ophthalmologic complications.

Sturge–Weber Syndrome
The classic triad in Sturge–Weber syndrome (SWS) includes the association of a facial port wine stain, invariably involving V1 (although it may be more extensive) (see Fig. 20-2A), ipsilateral eye abnormalities (choroidal vascular anomalies, increased ocular pressure, buphthalmos, and glaucoma in about 30%), and leptomeningeal and brain abnormalities (leptomeningeal vascular malformation, calcifications, cerebral atrophy, enlarged choroid plexus, and developmental venous anomalies in the brain). The risk of SWS with V1 PWS alone is approximately 10%, but with either bilateral V1 or concurrent V1, V2, V3 this rises to 25% or higher. Patients with V2 or V3 PWS alone without involvement of the V1 skin are not at risk for SWS. However, individual anatomic variations in the distribution of V1 and V2 at the internal or external canthus of the eye may pose difficulties in determining whether a port wine stain involves V1, with its associated risk of SWS (Fig. 20-13).

SWS can cause significant medical and ophthalmologic problems. Consequences of intracranial vascular anomalies include seizures, brain hypoxia, neuronal loss, disturbed regional cerebral blood flow, and a risk of contralateral hemiplegia. Developmental delay of cognitive skills may occur to varying degrees. Migraine headache is also common. Potential visual loss via acute or chronic glaucoma requires ongoing ophthalmologic follow-up.

The three mesectodermal tissues involved (the nasofrontal skin known as V1 skin, the ocular choroid, and the leptomeninges) have a common origin in the anterior neural primordium. A somatic mutation arising during development has been hypothesized. The possibility of SWS should be considered in any infant with a PWS that includes the V1 distribution.[51]

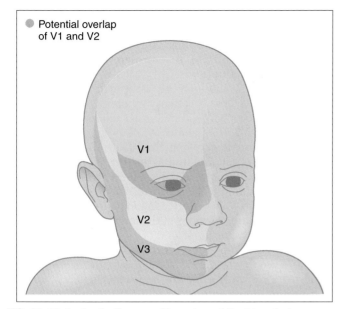

● Potential overlap of V1 and V2

V1

V2

V3

FIG. 20-13 Anatomic diagram of branches of the trigeminal nerve. The pink area denotes the potential overlap of V1 and V2. Adapted from Enjolras O, Riche MC, Merland JJ. Facial port-wine stains and Sturge–Weber Syndrome. Pediatrics 1985; 76: 48–51.

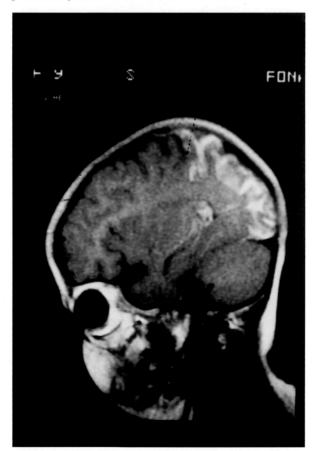

FIG. 20-14 Leptomeningeal lesion in Sturge–Weber syndrome well evidenced on T$_1$-weighted MRI sequence with gadolinium enhancement.

Neuroimaging consisting of MRI with gadolinium enhancement may be helpful in making an early diagnosis, but can be normal in some cases. Early subtle changes can include an enlarged choroid plexus or a pattern of local accelerated myelination. Typical neuroimaging changes include visualiza-

Box 20-1 Management of Sturge–Weber syndrome
- Regular ophthalmologic evaluation
- Treatment of glaucoma (surgical and/or medical)
- Neurologic evaluation
- Optimal control of seizures
- Laser treatment of PWS (after seizure disorder is controlled or prophylactically treated)
- Management of maxilla overgrowth, open bite deformity, and gingival hyperplasia when present

Patient/Family Support:

Contact information for The Sturge–Weber Foundation in the United Kingdom and Germany can be found at www.sturge-weber.com

The Sturge-Weber Foundation
Contact Information
International:
PO Box 418
Mount Freedom, NJ 07970, USA
Phone: 800-627-5482
URL: www.sturge-weber.com
E-mail:swf@sturge-weber.com
Canada:
1960 Prairie Avenue
Port Coquitlam, BC
V3B 1V4, Canada
Phone/Fax: 604-942-9209
E-mail: sturge-weber@shaw.com

tion of the pial vascular malformation, cerebral atrophy, and calcifications of the leptomeninges, the abnormal cortex and the underlying white matter (Fig. 20-14).[52] In most patients the first seizures in SWS occur before 2 years of age. The progressive nature of SWS has been demonstrated using functional neuroimaging tools, with hyperperfusion noted prior to the development of seizures, followed by hypoperfusion with decreased glucose utilization after the onset of seizures.[53,54]

Careful clinical follow-up is recommended in newborns with an at-risk V1 PWS. Although controversial, some pediatric neurologists believe that prophylactic anti-seizure medications are worth considering for at-risk infants.[55] Therapeutic management of SWS is often characterized by a lifelong struggle to preserve vision, motor and psychomotor development, and to ameliorate disfigurement (Box 20-1).

Klippel–Trenaunay, Parkes–Weber, and Servelle–Martorell Syndromes

These three syndromes are distinctive complex-combined vascular malformation syndromes that characteristically involve the limbs, are evident at birth, and have the potential for subsequent worsening, including interference with normal limb growth.[56] They are different vascular anomalies and are not synonymous. Klippel–Trenaunay syndrome (KTS) is a slow-flow vascular anomaly characterized by a vascular stain (usually a capillary malformation or mixed capillary–lymphatic malformation), varicose veins including persistent embryonic veins, and overgrowth of the soft tissue and/or bone of the affected limb. The presence at birth of a sharply demarcated geographic

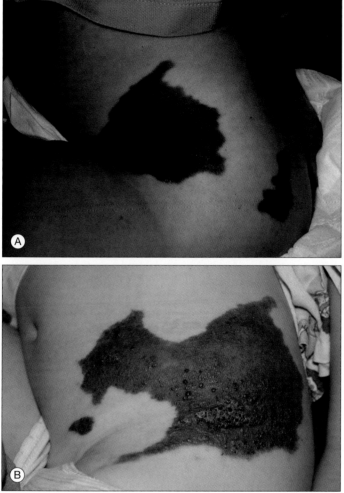

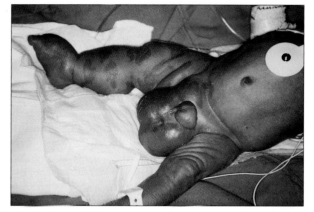

FIG. 20-16 Parkes–Weber syndrome in a newborn with evidence of a capillary lymphatic malformation, limb overgrowth, and arteriovenous fistulae (and cardiac failure) at birth.

FIG. 20-15 Klippel–Trenaunay syndrome with a prominent geographic stain on the abdomen, thigh, and buttock. Initially the stain is flat (**A**), but over time numerous 'blebs' develop on the surface due to increased lymphatic and venous pressure (**B**).

stain on the external lateral aspect of the affected extremity, mainly the thigh, is predictive of associated lymphatic anomalies and a poorer prognosis. If there is an associated lymphatic anomaly, small hemorrhagic 'blebs' which are actually lymphatic vesicles are often visible from birth or develop during early infancy[57] (Fig. 20-15). Bony hypertrophy can increase progressively, resulting in a limb length discrepancy. Some infants have a milder form of KT, with a large PWS involving a limb, soft tissue hypertrophy, but minimal to absent venous or lymphatic venous disease. These patients often have proportionate limb growth and a less morbid course than more severe cases of KTS. Parkes–Weber syndrome (PaWS) is the association of vascular stain, limb overgrowth (length and girth), and a fast-flow vascular anomaly with multiple arteriovenous shunts (Fig. 20-16). Severe cases in newborns have also had lymphedema at birth. In rare instances PaWS is complicated at birth by high-output cardiac failure. In the neonatal period noninvasive assessment of PaWS is best done using ultrasound/color Doppler and MR angiography. Arteriography is not performed in the neonatal period, unless endovascular arterial embolization of the AVFs is mandatory to reduce the arterial overload accountable for congestive heart failure. Thus KTS is a slow-flow CVLM, whereas PaWS is a fast-flow

CAVM, but both can result in gigantism of the affected limb. KTS may occur in association with SWS but not PaWS. Servelle–Martorell syndrome, also a slow-flow vascular syndrome, combining capillary stains and dysplastic veins, unlike KTS, leads to a progressive *undergrowth* of the affected limb.

Diagnosis

These diagnoses are usually made clinically, but modern vascular imaging techniques help delineate the vascular defects. The differential diagnosis of KTS, especially severe cases, includes Proteus syndrome (see discussion later in this chapter). Doppler ultrasound evaluation is helpful. MRI and MRA are helpful in more severe cases. Arteriography, phlebography, or lymphography are rarely needed during infancy and childhood. Routine screening for Wilms' tumor, as advised in infants with congenital hemihypertrophy, is not necessary for KTS,[58] with the exception of patients having true generalized hemihypertrophy and KTS.[59]

Treatment

Therapeutic management includes close orthopedic follow-up of limb growth.[56] If limb length discrepancy is significant after 1 year of age, radiographic studies may be appropriate, and a shoe lift or other orthopedic appliance may be used. Ultimately, surgical approaches to equalize limb lengths may be necessary, but this is not done during infancy. If capillary stains are extensive the use of a laser may be impractical, and responses on the extremities are poorer than at other sites.[13] Varicosities worsen over time, and later in life varicose veins in KTS, and AV fistulae in PaWS in selected patients, may require treatment. Ideally, patients should use compressive stockings, but proper fitting is difficult in infants and young children who are undergoing rapid somatic growth. Low-grade clotting and consumption coagulopathy similar to that seen in venous malformations can be seen in KTS (see previous discussion). Deep vein thrombosis is rare and pulmonary embolism is an exceptional but life-threatening event.[60] Long-term iatrogenic complications and a bad cosmetic outcome can result from overenthusiastic aggressive treatments early in life. Parents need educational information and support, both in the newborn period and over time. The Klippel–Trenaunay Association has a web site providing information to families:

www.k-t.org. A multidisciplinary approach is important, especially in more severe cases.

Capillary Malformation–Arteriovenous Malformation Syndrome

The Capillary Malformation–Arteriovenous Malformation (CM-AVM) syndrome[61] combines an AVM (either localized, more widespread such as Parkes–Weber syndrome, or visceral) and multiple small cutaneous red stains of a few millimeters or centimeters in diameter. It is inherited as an autosomal dominant trait, with wide expressivity – some affected family members may have symptomatic AVMs, whereas other exhibit only small, harmless skin stains. The disease has been linked to mutations of *RASA1*.

Wyburn–Mason, Bonnet–Dechaume–Blanc, and Brégeat Syndromes

These rare syndromes are characterized by arteriovenous malformations in the craniofacial area with fast-flow vascular anomalies in the skin (midline or hemifacial), orbit, retina, and brain. These eponyms are now considered to be synonymous. In infancy, the cutaneous AVM commonly mimics a facial port wine stain, although it is usually fainter and less well demarcated than PWS (see Fig. 20-10). It is warm on palpation and is sometimes associated with an abnormally increased skin thickness at birth. MR and CT angiography are helpful noninvasive tools that may be used in infants for the detection of the enlarged tortuous vessels and AV shunting. These findings are more clearly delineated later in life with conventional arteriography. Lesions slowly enlarge over years and may cause distortion of facial features, visual loss, and cerebral hemorrhage.

Cobb Syndrome

Cobb syndrome is the association of a dermatomal skin vascular malformation (trunk and arm or leg), a fast-flow intramedullary spinal AVM, and a vertebral vascular anomaly in the same segment. This metameric angiomatosis is the truncal counterpart of the syndromic cephalic AVMs. In infancy this syndrome may be undiagnosed because the cutaneous vascular signs are subtle or are misdiagnosed as skin capillary malformation. The diagnosis is often established later, when an abnormal vertebra is incidentally imaged or if neurologic symptoms of spinal cord compression occur. There is one report of a 5-month-old who, after developing paraparesis, was diagnosed as having Cobb syndrome documented with MRI and arteriography.

Maffucci Syndrome

Maffucci syndrome (MS) is a very rare sporadic syndrome, without sex prevalence, that begins in childhood and worsens during the patient's life. Congenital forms occur in only 17% of cases. MS is characterized by enchondromas of bones, and skin lesions which clinically resemble venous malformations. These blue skin lesions are nodular, develop slowly, and are rare in infancy. Although they have features of slow-flow venous anomalies – phleboliths, hypersignal on signal-enhanced T_2 sequences with MRI, histologic examination may reveal a spindle cell hemangioendothelioma, in addition to malformed venous channels.[4] Enchondromas, identical to those present in Ollier disease, involve both the metaphyses and the diaphyses, and may cause bony distortion and fragility, and shortening of an affected limb. The hands and feet are involved in 90% of patients. Cranial enchondromas result in severe neuro-ophthalmologic consequences. Over time, enchondromas may develop malignant transformation.

Blue Rubber Bleb Nevus Syndrome (Bean Syndrome)

The vascular anomalies associated with blue rubber bleb nevus syndrome (BRBNS) are small black-blue papules and nodular colorless 'nipples' which are venous malformations often involving the palms and soles. Lesions occasionally develop during infancy or later, increasing in number over time. Larger VM or LVM lesions, often congenital, can coexist with smaller ones and may occur in the skin or extend to muscles and retroperitoneum. On MRI they show well-defined, often septate, pouches that are strongly hyperintense on T_2-weighted images.[62] BRBNS can be sporadic or inherited as an autosomal dominant trait, but many previously reported familial cases probably correspond to the familial VMCM (though the latter does not include gastrointestinal bleeding). Gastrointestinal bleeding is uncommon early in life. Evaluation depends on whether extracutaneous symptoms are present. A coagulation disorder that sometimes develops soon after birth may manifest with bleeding, and can be treated with low molecular weight heparin. The differential diagnosis of BRBNS in the newborn period includes multifocal lymphangioendotheliomatosis (see discussion below).

Gorham Syndrome

This sporadic syndrome of bony destruction is associated with a vascular lesion that is usually a lymphatic or capillary–venous–lymphatic malformation. The cause of the extensive bone destruction is not clearly understood. Lesions usually become obvious in childhood. Visceral life-threatening lymphatic anomalies, including pleural effusions and abdominal macrocystic LM, may develop in association with the bone destructive process.

Hennekam Syndrome

An autosomal recessive disorder, Hennekam syndrome is the association of intestinal lymphangiectasia resulting in protein-losing enteropathy, lymphedema of the four limbs, abnormal facies, and mental retardation. The expansion of the phenotype raises the question of more than one gene defect.

Aagenaes Syndrome (Hereditary Cholestasis with Lymphedema)

Aagenaes syndrome is an autosomal recessive disease that occurs mostly in infants of Norwegian ancestry. Significant leg lymphedema due to lymph vessel hypoplasia that is congenital or develops later in life requires lifelong treatment. Cholestasis and obstructive jaundice are present at birth and may improve in adulthood, but in childhood they may be lethal. Children have severe bleeding if vitamin K supplementation is not provided. They also complain of itching, and have growth retardation.

Beckwith–Wiedemann Syndrome

Beckwith–Wiedemann syndrome is associated with a capillary stain of the mid-forehead that is clinically identical to salmon patch but has a greater likelihood of persistence. Other common abnormalities include macroglossia and umbilical anomalies, usually omphalocele, and overgrowth of tissues and organs (liver, spleen, and kidney). There is a high risk of malignant embryonal tumors in infancy, and of nonmalignant renal diseases. Other reported findings are a high birthweight, hemihypertrophy, and neonatal hypoglycemia. Intelligence is usually not impaired. Prenatal ultrasound diagnosis is possible because of visceromegaly.

Proteus Syndrome

This sporadic syndrome, first described by Wiedemann,[63] is discussed in more detail in Chapter 26. It is characterized by asymmetric localized overgrowth of various body parts, affecting soft tissues and bones. The syndrome may be evident at birth, but a progressive course and mosaic distribution of the lesions are characteristic and necessary for diagnosis.[64,65] The most characteristic features are the asymmetric, disproportionate growth with regional gigantism and cutaneous manifestations, including connective tissue nevus (cerebriform dermal thickening of soles and palms), epidermal nevi, lipomas, café au lait spots, and vascular malformations of the slow-flow type, such as extensive capillary, venous and lymphatic malformations.[64,65] Visceral benign tumors, mainly lipomas, but also tumors in the endocrine glands or CNS, and visceral vascular malformations are observed as well. Intelligence is normal in most patients, but learning disabilities are present in one-third. Ophthalmologic and neurologic alterations or seizures have been reported. Surgical reconstruction is the primary method of rehabilitation for these children. Orthopedic management is essential because of discrepancies in limb and foot growth. Excision of lipomas or laser treatment of vascular lesions is sometimes indicated. In addition to Klippel–Trenaunay syndrome, a major differential diagnosis of Proteus syndrome is a condition which has been called hemihyperplasia–lipomatosis syndrome, in which there is body asymmetry, soft tissue lipomas and both superficial and deep vascular malformations as associated findings. The major differences between this condition and Proteus syndrome appear to be the more aggressive disproportionate growth, more marked bony overgrowth, and cerebriform connective tissue nevi of the feet that characterize Proteus syndrome.[66]

Riley–Smith, Bannayan–Zonana, and Ruvalcaba–Myhre–Smith Syndromes

These familial autosomal dominant disorders are now considered together because they share overlapping clinical features and may represent a continuum, the Bannayan–Riley–Ruvalcaba syndrome (BRRS). BRRS is characterized by vascular and multiple other anomalies. The vascular lesions, many of which have not been well characterized, appear to represent several types of vascular anomaly, including capillary stains, venous malformations, and lymphatic malformations, but are often referred to in the medical literature as 'hemangiomas.' Other features include macrocephaly with normal ventricular size, pseudopapilledema, localized superficial soft tissue and visceral overgrowths, mainly lipomas, mild to severe mental retardation, juvenile intestinal polyposis, and pigmented macules arising on the genitalia. The common feature of juvenile intestinal polyps in BRRS and Cowden disease is explained by a shared mutation in a tumor suppressor gene, *PTEN*, which is localized on chromosome 10q23.

'Hemangiomatous' Branchial Clefts, Lip Pseudoclefts, Unusual Facies

Facial midline capillary malformation may occur in association with bony and facial abnormalities, including pseudocleft lip, cleft lip, cleft palate, unusual facies (hypoplastic nares, micrognathia, malformed ears, hypertelorism), and limb defects (hypomelia/phocomelia). When these features occur together, it is known as Roberts syndrome, pseudothalidomide syndrome, or SC phocomelia syndrome. Marked growth retardation and sparse, silvery hair are also reported. The branchiooculofacial syndrome has a distinctive phenotype of ear, eye, mouth, and craniofacial anomalies and may include 'hemangiomatous' aplastic skin overlying branchial or supraauricular defects.[66a,67]

Adams–Oliver Syndrome

Adams–Oliver syndrome is characterized by CMTC occurring in association with scalp aplasia cutis congenita, cranium defects, and distal limb-reduction abnormalities, ranging from hypoplastic nails, partial absence of toes or fingers, to total absence of a limb. When the cranial bone defect exposes the dura mater, necrosis, infection, and bleeding may be fatal. Additional features, in a series of nine families, were cryptorchidism and cardiac abnormalities. The clinical spectrum, may also include palate and auricular malformations, microphthalmia, spina bifida, and intracranial calcifications, without proven infection.[68–71] Most cases are transmitted as an autosomal dominant trait.

Nova Syndrome

Nova syndrome is a familial disorder in which a congenital glabellar capillary stain occurs in association with neurologic malformations, including Dandy–Walker malformation, hydrocephalus, cerebellar vermis agenesis, and mega cisterna magna.

VASCULAR TUMORS IN THE NEONATE

Traditionally, both fully formed hemangiomas in young infants and those that are either absent or barely noticeable at birth, with rapid postnatal growth, were considered to be variants of hemangiomas. An increased understanding of clinical and immunohistochemical differences has helped clarify the classification of these tumors and helped delineate them from one another.

Congenital Hemangiomas

Hemangiomas that are fully formed tumors at the time of birth and do not proliferate in postnatal life are referred to as 'congenital hemangioma' or 'congenital nonprogressive hemangioma'.[72,73] Two subtypes of congenital hemangioma are described based on their natural history: the rapidly involuting congenital hemangioma (RICH), and noninvoluting congenital hemangioma (NICH). Although some investigators hypothesize that these rare forms of congenital hemangioma and common infantile hemangioma may be variations of a single disorder, they have many clinical, histologic, and immunohistochemical features that help distinguish them from true infantile hemangiomas.[74,75] Both types are more common on the extremities, close to a joint, or on the head and neck close to an ear. The proliferating phase of both RICH and NICH occurs in utero, and no further growth occurs after birth. Three clinical morphologies of RICH are: 1) a raised, violaceous tumor with large, radiating veins; 2) a hemispheric tumor with overlying telangiectasia, often with a halo of pallor; and 3) a pink tumor with central red nodules (Fig. 20-17). Rarely the

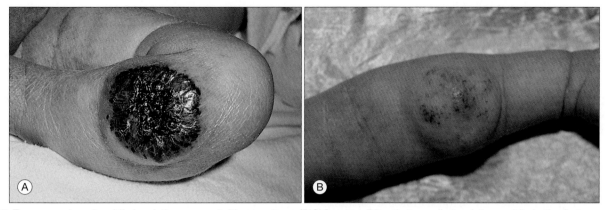

FIG. 20-17 Two examples of rapidly-involuting congenital hemangioma (RICH), a condition that usually involutes rapidly in the first year of life.

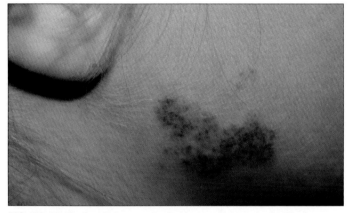

FIG. 20-18 Noninvoluting congenital hemangioma on cheek of a young child. The pallor admixed with vascular papules and telangiectasias is typical of the condition, which can mimic the early stages of an infantile hemangioma.

overlying skin may show hypertrichosis or milia that resolves in the first month of life. Linear ulceration, a central black necrotic crust and ulceration, and hemorrhage may complicate congenital hemangiomas. Occasionally, congenital hemangiomas are noted on routine prenatal ultrasound evaluation and may be mistaken for vascular malformations or other forms of neoplasia. Those that are detected usually reveal prominent vascularity and high flow. The majority of reported cases of RICH demonstrated accelerated spontaneous involution,[2,72,73] with regression by 14 months of age, potentially leaving areas of skin atrophy.

Noninvoluting congenital hemangioma (NICH) occurs slightly more frequently in males and is also present at birth. The lesions are usually flatter and less impressive in appearance than in RICH. They often present as a well-circumscribed round to oval, slightly indurated or raised soft tissue mass with a blue-purple color, or with coarse superficial telangiectasias and a rim of pallor (Fig. 20-18). They grow proportionately with the child and do not regress spontaneously. Some of these lesions clearly show arteriovenous micro-fistulas on Doppler, and these may develop increasing equatorial draining veins after years. They are often misdiagnosed in infancy as 'involuting hemangioma,' and the diagnosis may then be delayed until adolescence or adulthood, when they are excised, after having failed to involute. Some cases of RICH involute only partially,

and the residual tumor resembles NICH, supporting the concept that RICH and NICH may be variants of each other.[75]

Indications for treatment of RICH include ulceration and bleeding, functional impairment (depending upon location), congestive heart failure, and prominent residual skin changes. Early excision may be particularly important in infants with ulceration or when a necrotic area is present, as there are often large, fast-flow vessels close to the surface, conferring a risk of life-threatening hemorrhage.[76] Indications for treatment of NICH (typically surgical excision) depend on whether their appearance is bothersome, or whether bleeding or other symptoms are present.

Congenital hemangiomas are usually diagnosed based on clinical characteristics, but Doppler ultrasound and MRI can assist in the diagnosis. MRI is mandatory in the newborn whose tumor has a central crust or wound at birth, in order to evaluate the risk for hemorrhage: strikingly, some RICH are highly vascularized, with large tortuous flow voids on MRI, and others are relatively poorly vascularized, with MRI demonstrating a tumor of intermediate signal on T_1-weighted signal-enhanced sequences. The main differential diagnosis of both RICH and NICH is common infantile hemangioma, but in atypical cases other soft tissue tumors, including malignancies, must be considered. Transient thrombocytopenia can lead to consideration of other vascular tumors and Kasabach–Merritt phenomenon (see below), but the drop in platelet count is usually brief, rather than progressive. A biopsy may occasionally be required to differentiate RICH or NICH from other neoplasms, including fibrosarcoma and infantile myofibromatosis (see subsequent discussion).[72] Both RICH and NICH demonstrate the histologic features of both proliferative elements and dysplastic vessels more typical of those seen in vascular malformations. They are GLUT-1 negative, which helps distinguish them from infantile hemangiomas.[73,74]

Infantile Hemangioma

The infantile hemangioma is the most common vascular tumor encountered during early infancy (Table 20-1). It is a benign proliferation of endothelial cells that undergoes a phase of rapid growth followed by spontaneous involution. Although this chapter often uses the word 'hemangioma' rather than 'infantile hemangioma,' whenever this tumor is discussed in the context of other vascular tumors, the adjective 'infantile'

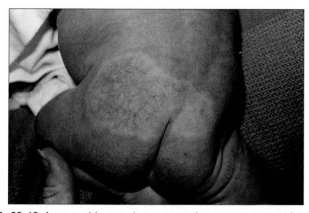

FIG. 20-19 A nascent hemangioma presenting as a vasoconstricted macule.

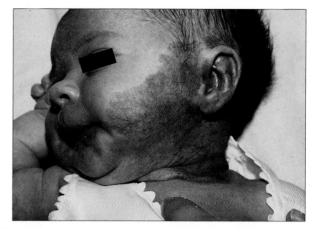

FIG. 20-20 Telangiectatic nascent hemangioma involving the 'beard' area, neck, and extending intraorally, a distribution that carries a high risk of airway hemangioma. Despite high-dose corticosteroid therapy, this patient developed respiratory distress 2 weeks later and was found to have an extensive laryngeal hemangioma, which required excision and laryngoplasty using an ear cartilage graft.

should be added to distinguish it from other vascular tumors or malformations.

Infantile hemangiomas are noted in 1–2.6% of healthy infants in the immediate newborn period,[77] but more often they become evident slightly later, most typically in the first few days to weeks of life. Although good population-based studies of their incidence are lacking, their reported overall incidence may be as high as 5–10%. The incidence may also vary by race, with the highest rates being reported in Caucasian infants, and lower rates in black and Asian infants.[78–80] All studies show an increased rate in females, with ratios varying from 2 : 1 to 9 : 1.[38,81,82] Severe complicated hemangiomas have an even higher incidence in females, with a reported ratio of 7 : 1.[83] Infantile hemangiomas are also more common in premature infants, occurring in 22–30% of infants weighing less than 1000 g and in 15% of infants with birthweight between 1000 and 1500 g.[79,84] Infants weighing more than 1500 g show no significant increase compared to term infants. A threefold increased incidence of hemangiomas has been noted in infants born to mothers who undergo chorionic villus sampling, compared to those whose mothers undergo amniocentesis.[85] A prospective study of over 1000 children with infantile hemangiomas confirmed previously known demographic risk factors, including Caucasian race, female gender, prematurity, and low birthweight, and also found an increased incidence in twins or higher-order multiples.[82,86] The majority of hemangiomas arise sporadically; however, a family history can be elicited in some patients, and autosomal dominant transmission has been reported.[87]

Clinical Characteristics of Infantile Hemangiomas

Hemangioma Precursors Although the medical literature frequently states that hemangiomas are rarely evident at birth, rather developing within the first few weeks, a large series reported evidence at birth in 50–60%. This is probably due to recognition of the subtle skin changes of hemangioma precursors (or so-called premonitory marks). Findings most commonly are fine telangiectasias superimposed on an area of pallor, a faint erythematous patch, or a bruise-like area.[80,88] It may be difficult initially to differentiate an erythematous precursor of hemangioma from a capillary malformation, but clues include a more ill-defined border, fine telangiectasias, and, if present, skin ulceration (Figs 20-19 and 20-20). Serial examinations may be necessary to establish the correct diag-

nosis. Rarely a hemangioma on the perineum or lip may present in the neonate with ulceration without an obvious hemangioma, mimicking bacterial or herpetic infection. In these cases the hemangioma becomes evident over the subsequent days to weeks. Biopsies obtained from the border of the ulcers in these patients demonstrate increased vascularity in the dermis, but are not clearly diagnostic of hemangioma.[89] Special stains demonstrating small and scanty capillaries with GLUT1 can help confirm the diagnosis.

Clinical Variants of Infantile Hemangiomas Hemangiomas can be classified into three morphologic subtypes based on their location within the skin: superficial, combined (superficial and deep), and deep. Superficial hemangiomas are the most common type, occurring in approximately 50–60% of cases. Combined hemangiomas are estimated to occur in 25–35% of cases, and deep hemangiomas in 15%.[38] The superficial hemangioma is characterized by its bright red color and finely lobulated surface.[90] These characteristics have led to the use of the term strawberry hemangioma (Fig. 20-21). Deep hemangiomas are not commonly noted in the neonatal period, often appearing at 1–3 months of life as a warm, subcutaneous mass caused by proliferation of the tumor in the deeper portion of the dermis or subcutis. The overlying skin may appear normal or have relatively inconspicuous superficial changes, such as telangiectasia or dilated veins, making it more difficult to diagnose. Larger, deep hemangiomas may be highly vascularized, with 'high-flow' arterial blood supply during the proliferating phase. In rare cases this may be detected on physical examination by the presence of a bruit, but it is important to consider arteriovenous malformations in the differential diagnosis. Many hemangiomas exhibit characteristics of both deep and superficial hemangiomas and are called combined, or mixed, hemangiomas. At the end of the proliferating phase these lesions frequently exhibit a configuration resembling a poached-egg, with a well-circumscribed superficial portion overlying a less well-defined deeper component.[90]

Although the majority of hemangiomas are small, a significant minority are large. Thus, in addition to characterizing hemangiomas according to their depth and location within the

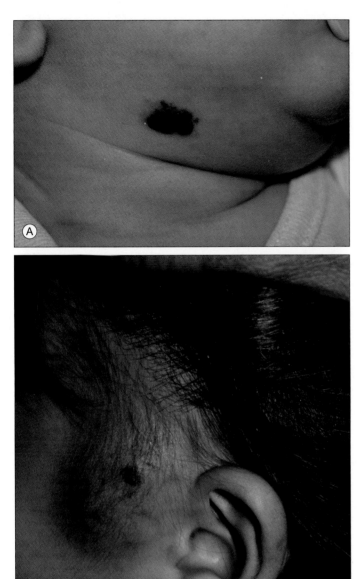

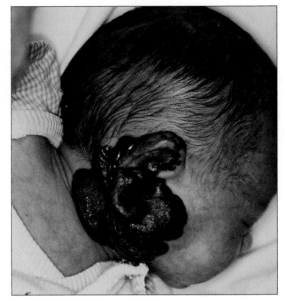

FIG. 20-22 Segmental hemangioma. Note the aggressive growth, which is more common in segmental hemangiomas than in localized ones.

FIG. 20-21 Two examples of localized hemangioma. (A) Superficial hemangioma on the neck. (B) Mainly deep hemangioma of the preauricular skin.

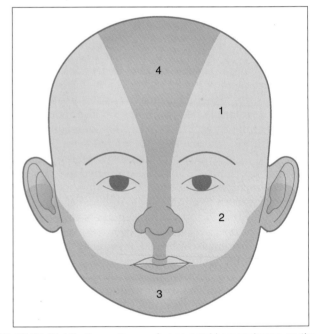

FIG. 20-23 Distribution patterns of segmental hemangiomas on the face. 1: frontotemporal, 2: maxillary, 3: mandibular, 4: frontonasal. (From Haggstrom AN, Lammer EJ, Schneider RA et al. Patterns of infantile hemangioma: new clues to hemangioma pathogenesis and embryonic facial development. Pediatrics 2006; 117:698–703. With permission.)

skin, recent studies have emphasized the pattern of involvement as a predictor of prognosis and risk for associated complications.[91,92] Described patterns include focal lesions that appear to arise from a central focus (Fig. 20-21), and segmental lesions which demonstrate a more diffuse area of involvement, appearing to arise from a broad area or developmental subunit (Fig. 20-22).

Some lesions are difficult to classify as either focal or segmental and are thus designated indeterminate. Segmental lesions are more often associated with extracutaneous anomalies, including spinal dysraphism, genitourinary anomalies, and PHACE syndrome.[92] The observation that hemangiomas demonstrate a predilection for the head and neck area[93] suggests that they are not randomly distributed. The patterns of segmental hemangiomas correspond to known embryologic prominences, suggesting a neuroectodermal derivation for their distribution[94] (Fig. 20-23).

Extracutaneous Hemangiomas Whereas most infants (75–90%) have only a single hemangioma, those with multiple hemangiomas, large segmental hemangiomas, or hemangiomas localized to certain anatomic sites have an increased risk of extracutaneous hemangiomas. The liver and airway are among the most common extracutaneous sites causing symptoms.[95–98]

Multiple Hemangiomas Approximately 10–25% of infants with hemangiomas have multiple hemangiomas. Numerous, small, superficial hemangiomas may herald visceral hemangiomatosis (Fig. 20-24). The term 'benign neonatal hemangiomatosis' has been used to describe infants with numerous cutaneous hemangiomas without clinically evident visceral lesions,[99] whereas 'diffuse neonatal hemangiomatosis' has been used to describe infants with both cutaneous and visceral hemangiomas.[100] Multiple hemangiomas appear early in the neonatal period, and girls are more commonly affected. Hepatic and cutaneous hemangiomas have been reported on prenatal ultrasound evaluation at 32 weeks.[101] The cutaneous lesions may range in size from a few millimeters to more than several centimeters in diameter. There is no consensus regarding the number of cutaneous lesions required to suspect visceral involvement, but 83% of infants with multiple liver hemangiomas have five or more, suggesting that this might be a useful threshold number for screening ultrasound. In particularly widespread disseminated cases, many other organs, including the gastrointestinal tract, lungs, CNS, oral mucosa, and eyes may be affected.[95,99,100,102] Additional complications of diffuse neonatal hemangiomatosis include high-output congestive heart failure, visceral hemorrhage, hydrocephalus, thyroid abnormalities (see below), and ocular abnormalities.[97] Untreated patients have a high mortality rate, with estimates as high as 29–81% with various treatment regimens.[95,97,103] Infants with segmental hemangiomas are also at increased risk for extracutaneous hemangiomas, especially of the liver, gastrointestinal tract, and CNS, but the scope of this risk is not completely understood.[98] Occasionally visceral involvement occurs in the setting of only a few seemingly innocuous cutaneous lesions. Newborns with multiple cutaneous hemangiomas need to be monitored closely with serial physical examinations to assess for visceral involvement. Evaluation for visceral involvement is typically suggested for young infants with five or more skin lesions. Serial radiologic evaluation of the liver, especially screening abdominal ultrasound, with further evaluation with CT or MRI, may be necessary to follow progression of visceral lesions.

Not all patients with hepatic involvement require therapy, but serial evaluation is essential, particularly in very young infants, as symptoms may develop in the first few months of life. Thereafter the risk of symptomatic liver disease decreases considerably. Kassarjian et al.[104] have recently proposed a clinical classification of liver hemangiomas into three groups based on the pattern of involvement within the liver and imaging characteristics. Solitary hepatic lesions in the absence of cutaneous hemangiomas must be differentiated from hepatic vascular malformations. These focal single lesions are usually GLUT1 negative, regress rapidly, and most likely represent a form of vascular tumor in the liver similar to RICH in skin, rather than true infantile hemangioma. If large vascular shunts are present, they may need embolization to treat their hemodynamic effects. Multifocal lesions usually occur in the setting of multiple small skin hemangiomas. They may be completely asymptomatic without the need for treatment, but if they have arteriovenous shunts, they may require liver embolization and/or medical therapy to manage congestive heart failure, as well as hemangioma-specific therapy (such as corticosteroids). Hepatic hemangiomatosis associated with an arteriovenous or arterioportal shunt or portovenous fistula is associated with greater morbidity.[104] Diffuse liver hemangiomas cause massive hepatomegaly, abdominal compartment syndrome, and are associated with hypothyroidism (see discussion below). They have a high rate of mortality and require aggressive medical therapy, and even consideration of liver transplantation.[86,105]

Airway Hemangiomas Segmental hemangiomas in a 'beard distribution,' involving the skin overlying the mandible, chin, and neck, have a high risk of concomitant upper airway or subglottic area involvement. There is a striking female predilection of 6–7:1 for 'beard' and severe complicated hemangiomas.[83,106] Affected infants typically present within the first few weeks of life with an increasing degree of noisy breathing, stridor, hoarse cry, or other signs of airway obstruction.

Hemangiomas and Structural Malformations

Hemangiomas, particularly when segmental, may have associated structural malformations.[83,92,107–113] There is a striking female predilection, exceeding the 3:1 ratio reported for hemangiomas overall, especially for hemangiomas occurring on the upper body (Box 20-2). The term PHACE syndrome refers to the association of posterior fossa brain malformations, hemangiomas, arterial anomalies, coarctation of the aorta and cardiac defects, and eye abnormalities (e.g. microphthalmia, optic nerve hypoplasia, cataracts, and increased retinal vascu-

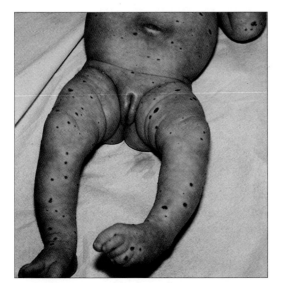

FIG. 20-24 Disseminated cutaneous (and liver) neonatal hemangiomatosis.

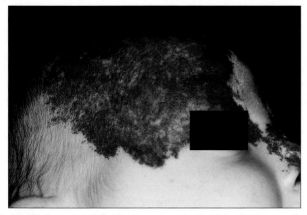

FIG. 20-25 Segmental distribution of a very flat infantile hemangioma mimicking a capillary malformation. Although the location resembles a V1 distribution, there is no risk of Sturge–Weber syndrome. However, the patient did have intra-cranial arterial defects (PHACE syndrome).

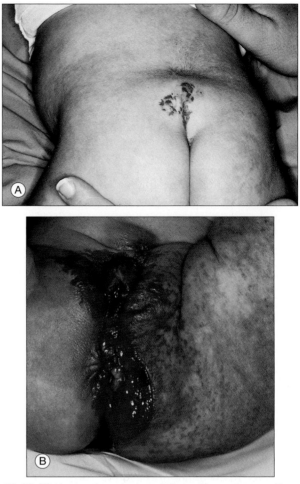

FIG. 20-26 (A) Hemangioma in association with a cutaneous lipoma and spinal dysraphism. **(B)** This infant had perineal hemangioma as well as a telangiectatic hemangioma of the entire lower limb in association with abnormal external genitalia, exstrophy of the bladder, and umbilical malposition. Note the large ulceration, which is a common complication of perineal hemangiomas.

larity). The term PHACE(s) is sometimes used when associated sternal anomalies or a supra-umbilical raphe are present.[110,114] A recent prospective study noted that 20% of infants with facial segmental hemangiomas had PHACE syndrome, and that PHACE was as commonly seen as Sturge–Weber syndrome during the period of the study.[115] Most affected infants have only one or two of the extracutaneous features, rather than all of the elements of the syndrome. Structural CNS malformations include the Dandy–Walker malformation and other posterior fossa anomalies, such as arachnoid cyst, enlarged fourth ventricle, enlarged cisterna magna, and cerebellar or vermian hypo-plasia.[111,113,116] Other CNS anomalies have been reported, including cerebral atrophy, gray matter heterotopia, pituitary abnormalities, and absent corpus callosum. Macrocephaly, ophthalmologic abnormalities, hypotonia, seizures, and psychomotor retardation may be a presenting sign of an underlying structural malformation. Both extra- and intracranial arterial anomalies have been reported involving the brachio-cephalic arteries, persistent embryonic arteries, such as the trigeminal artery, and cerebro-vascular abnormalities (e.g. hypoplastic arteries, aneurysms, aberrant internal carotid artery, stenosis, occlusion of the internal carotid, posterior or anterior cerebral artery, vertebral circulation and others) (Fig. 20-25).[108,110,111,117] Patients with intracranial anomalous vessels may demonstrate progressive occlusive arterial changes and cerebral infarction.[112] Cardiac abnormalities include abnormalities of the aortic arch, coarctation of the aorta, and cor tritriatum with partial anomalous pulmonary venous return, tricuspid and aortic atresia, patent ductus arteriosus, and ventricular septal defects.[108–111] Partial or complete sternal agenesis and supraumbilical raphe may also occur in patients with large facial hemangiomas or multiple hemangiomas.[109,112,118,119] Hemangiomas arising over the lumbosacral area may be associated with malformations of the genitourinary, gastrointes-tinal, neurologic, and skeletal systems (Fig. 20-26A, B). Imperforate anus, rectoscrotal fistula, renal anomalies, abnormal external genitalia, lipomyelomeningocele, tethered cord, and bony deformities of the sacrum have been reported.[99,120,121]

Thyroid Function Abnormalities

Hypothyroidism may complicate the course of infants with large and or visceral hemangiomas. A few infants with PHACE have been noted to have absent or lingual thyroid glands. Another mechanism of hypothyroidism has been found to be the deactivation of thyroxine by a type 3 iodothyronine deiodinase produced by the hemangioma tissue.[122–124] In addition, production of a TSH-like hormone has been described in an infant with severe hypothyroidism and multiple hepatic hemangiomas.[124] This form of hypothyroidism occurs during the phase of active hemangioma proliferation, and can be detected by the presence of markedly elevated TSH and low T_3. T_4 levels may be normal or low. Neonatal screening for hypothyroidism is inadequate to assess for this complication, as the most active phase of hemangioma proliferation typically occurs after this period. This consumptive form of hypothyroidism may be extremely difficult to correct, requiring large doses of thyroid hormone replacement, initially given intravenously. The hypothyroidism typically resolves as the hemangioma regresses, but may have already caused significant morbidity if not detected promptly. This complication is most commonly reported in association with hepatic hemangiomatosis; however, type 3 iodothyronine deiodinase activity has been found in cutaneous hemangiomas. Therefore it is recommended that children with very large cutaneous or hepatic hemangiomas have thyroid function tests performed.[122]

Pathogenesis

The pathogenesis of hemangioma has not been clearly elucidated, and remains poorly understood.[107,125] Hemangiomas are believed to represent localized areas of abnormal angiogenesis, and several hypotheses have been proposed.

Some studies have demonstrated clonality in hemangioma endothelial cells, with mutations in regions having genes that play a significant role in vascular growth or vascular regulatory pathways, including mutations in several genes involved in the VEGF signaling pathway (VEGF receptors), and Tie2.[126] However, it remains unclear whether these mutations are the direct cause of the hemangioma phenotype.[127,128] Initial analysis of several pedigrees of familial hemangiomas revealed a linkage to chromosome 5q.[129] Subsequent analysis of sporadic hemangiomas demonstrated loss of heterozygosity of 5q, supporting the possibility that somatic mutations play a role in hemangioma formation.[130] Several hypotheses regarding the nature of hemangioma growth (hemangiogenesis) have been postulated.[131] They may represent a clonal expansion of human endothelial cell progenitors in which a somatic mutation has occurred, leading to differences in both immunophenotype and behavior compared to normal endothelium. Another hypothesis is that extrinsic factors such as abnormalities in other surrounding cells induce the microvasculature to undergo aberrant proliferation and lead to hemangioma formation.[132]

Infantile hemangiomas express unique immunohistochemical markers which are not present in normal cutaneous vasculature, and these markers are shared with the human placenta microvasculature. North and co-workers[133] reported that glucose transporter protein-1 (GLUT-1) is expressed by infantile hemangiomas during all phases of their development (proliferating, involuting, and involuted), thereby distinguishing infantile hemangiomas from vascular malformations and other vascular tumors. Other placenta-associated vascular antigens, including merosin, FcγRII and Lewis Y antigen, are also present in hemangiomas.[134] Recent studies using DNA microarray techniques have revealed that the gene expression profiles of hemangiomas and placenta vascular endothelium are remarkably similar.[135] The shared immunohistochemical phenotype and gene expression profiles with placental microvasculature, and the observation that hemangiomas are significantly more common in infants whose mothers underwent chorionic villus sampling, has led to speculation that hemangioma endothelial cells may originate from placental vascular endothelium. Local factors and loss of mechanisms controlling intrauterine angiogenesis might contribute to their postnatal growth. Alternatively, these similarities may be due to their sharing a similar immature vascular phenotype, rather than direct implantation from placenta to fetus.[125,136]

The mechanisms that govern the growth and involution of hemangiomas are not completely understood. During proliferation, hemangiomas demonstrate proliferating cell nuclear antigen (PCNA), as well as increased levels of vascular endothelial growth factor (VEGF) and basic fibroblast growth factor (bFGF).[3,137,138] Angiogenesis mediators, including monocyte chemoattractant protein-1 and the adhesion molecules E-selectin and ICAM-3, are expressed at high levels.[139–142] Myeloid cell markers such as CD-83, -32, -14 and -15 co-label with hemangioma endothelial cells, particularly during the proliferative phase.[143] Proteins involved in extracellular matrix remodeling are also expressed during the proliferating phase.[3,131,144] Increased levels of urinary matrix metalloproteinase (MMP) proteins, specifically high molecular weight MMP, are noted in proliferating infantile hemangiomas, suggesting a role in extracellular matrix remodeling.[145] The expression of lymphatic endothelial hyaluronan receptor-1 (LYVE-1) in proliferating hemangiomas, with loss during the involuting phase, has led authors to propose that proliferating hemangiomas are arrested in an early developmental stage of vascular differentiation, which might help explain the rapid growth seen in the proliferating phase.[146] Local factors are also believed to play a significant role in hemangioma proliferation. Investigators have noted that hemangioma growth correlates with hyperplasia of the overlying epidermis, with these tissues elaborating angiogenic factors (e.g. VEGF, bFGF). Moreover, these tissues lacked expression of the angiogenesis inhibitor interferon (IFN)-β.[147]

The factors involved in hemangioma involution are being actively investigated, but no single integrated explanation has yet emerged. The levels of angiogenic factors found during proliferation decrease,[3,141,142] whereas levels of the angiogenesis inhibitor TIMP-1 (tissue inhibitor of metalloproteinase-1) increase. Interferon-regulated genes are upregulated during involution, suggesting a role for these genes in involution.[3,148] Apoptosis increases during involution and is believed to be the primary cellular mechanism of involution,[149,150] whereas inhibitors of apoptosis are upregulated during proliferation.[149,151]

Diagnosis

Most hemangiomas can be diagnosed on the basis of their history and clinical appearance. The differential diagnosis includes other vascular and nonvascular tumors that are discussed in this chapter. Where history and physical examination are not helpful, further studies may be necessary to confirm the diagnosis. Doppler ultrasound and MRI are most helpful in confirming the diagnosis of hemangioma. Doppler studies demonstrate the presence of a vascular lesion, but it may be difficult to differentiate a proliferating hemangioma from an arteriovenous malformation because both are high-flow lesions. Doppler ultrasonography is less helpful than MRI in delineating the extent of the hemangioma and its relationship to surrounding structures.[152] T_1-weighted MRI sequences demonstrate flow voids as a result of high-flow vessels, but also delineate the solid tissue mass with an intermediate signal that enhances on T_2-weighted sequences. The presence of a solid tissue mass differentiates a hemangioma from an arteriovenous malformation. CT is less helpful than MRI for distinguishing a hemangioma from a vascular malformation, but may define tissue involvement.[153] Angiography is no longer needed to establish the diagnosis, and is performed only for embolization therapy. Measurement of urinary bFGF levels may be helpful for differentiating a proliferating hemangioma from a vascular malformation, and for following response to therapy.[154–156]

A careful history and thorough physical examination should be performed in every infant with hemangioma, and particularly in those with multiple cutaneous hemangiomas, to assess for visceral hemangiomatosis. Further evaluation should be performed as indicated by the physical symptoms and location of hemangiomas.

Histopathology

If there is significant diagnostic uncertainty, a biopsy may be necessary to exclude other soft tissue tumors or vascular malformations. Early in the proliferating stage the tumor consists predominantly of a mass of endothelial cells. Lumina, lined by normal-appearing endothelial cells, become evident somewhat later in the late proliferative phase. PAS stains reveal a thickened basement membrane. Mast cells are increased within proliferating hemangiomas compared to normal tissue. As hemangiomas mature, they show lobules of endothelial channels separated by fibrous septa. Actin-positive smooth muscle cells are deposited around the vessels. Fat cells may be prominent in some involuted hemangiomas. Immunohistochemical analysis may be used to confirm the diagnosis of infantile hemangioma. GLUT-1 immunoreactivity and other placenta-associated vascular proteins, including FcγRII, merosin, and Lewis Y antigen, are present in the endothelial cells within infantile hemangiomas at all phases of development, but are lacking in normal vessels of the skin and subcutis, other types of vascular tumors and vascular malformations.[74,133,134]

Differential Diagnosis

Deep hemangiomas may be particularly difficult to differentiate from other tumors and malformations. Infantile myofibromatosis may mimic vascular tumors but is firmer to palpation and has distinct histopathologic features. Infantile fibrosarcoma, a rare tumor that is sometimes congenital, may resemble a deep hemangioma or lymphatic malformation.[33] Rhabdomyosarcoma is the most common sarcoma of early childhood and may present in newborns as a rapidly enlarging red cutaneous mass, usually involving the head and neck, that may be difficult to differentiate from a deep hemangioma. Other benign and malignant tumors that may resemble hemangiomas include adrenal carcinoma, spindle and epithelioid nevi, hemangiopericytoma, dermatofibrosarcoma protuberans, lipoblastoma, neuroblastoma, and nasal glioma. Congenital Langerhans' cell histiocytosis may mimic diffuse neonatal hemangiomatosis. Developmental anomalies such as encephaloceles, dermoid cysts, meningoceles, and teratomas may all be mistaken for deep hemangiomas.

Clinical Course

Several early studies have documented the natural history of hemangiomas. Three clinical phases are generally noted: proliferation, involution, and completion of involution. Onset of proliferation is almost invariably in the first weeks to months of life, and lasts for variable periods from weeks to months, in rare cases continuing beyond age 1. Some studies indicate that superficial and combined hemangiomas have a shorter duration of proliferation than deep ones. Most hemangiomas establish the boundaries of their anatomic territory relatively early, growing only in volume thereafter. Superficial hemangiomas have a characteristic bright red color during this phase. Both combined and deep hemangiomas may feel tense, and fluctuations in size and volume may be noted with crying or activity. The proliferating phase is followed by an involuting phase that may begin as early as within the first year of life. Change in the surface color and texture of a superficial hemangioma is often the earliest sign of spontaneous regression. The color changes from a bright crimson to a violaceous gray, and is often accompanied by flattening of the surface texture. The superficial portion ultimately breaks up into smaller areas and then resolves. The deeper portion also regresses, but this is often not as apparent clinically. Parents may note less fluctuation in size during crying, and the tumor is less firm to touch.[79,90] Increased warmth slowly diminishes to normal temperature. Prominent radiating veins are often noted as the hemangioma involutes and may mimic a venous malformation. Doppler studies indicate persistent high flow, and this can help in differentiating the two conditions. During the later phases of involution, the surface becomes wrinkled, and the mass may develop a fibrofatty consistency. Some resolve leaving normal or nearly normal skin, whereas others resolve with residua of variable cosmetic significance. Involuted hemangiomas often show residual telangiectasia, pallor or a yellowish color, fibrofatty tissue deposition, and atrophy (Fig. 20-27A, B). Several studies have shown that completion of involution occurs at a rate of approximately 10% per year, with 30% completing involution at 3 years, 50% at 5 years, etc.[79,82,90] Although not specifically mentioned in these studies, our experience is that small hemangiomas generally involute sooner than very large, bulky ones.

Ulceration is the most common complication of infantile hemangioma, occurring in approximately 10–15%, most often during the rapid growth phase. It is more common on the lip and perineum. Superimposed bacterial infection may develop, and virtually always resolves leaving textural change or scarring.[82] Bleeding can also occur, but profuse bleeding is surprisingly rare, occurring mainly with deeply ulcerated hemangiomas or those located on the scalp. Recurrent ulceration and infection may complicate hemangiomas located in the perineum, and conservative treatments routinely used to manage ulcer-

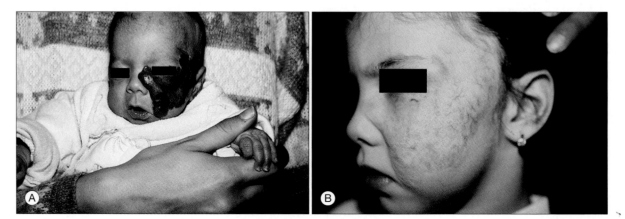

FIG. 20-27 (A) This segmental hemangioma grew rapidly with focal ulcerations in a premature infant girl. She had a dramatic response to corticosteroid treatment but did have some atrophic skin changes after involution **(B)**.

ated hemangiomas may be ineffective. Lesions in this area need to be monitored closely for this potential complication.

In addition to perineal and lip hemangiomas, certain lesions arising on the head and neck require closer follow-up or intervention because of a greater likelihood of complications. Segmental facial hemangiomas may be associated with PHACE syndrome and airway hemangiomas. Hemangiomas on the pinna may ulcerate and become secondarily infected, contributing to structural deformity. Hemangiomas obstructing the external auditory canal may cause conductive hearing loss.[79] Destruction of portions of the ear may result from hemangioma invasion and ulceration of the helix and/or pinna.

Growth of periorbital and lid hemangiomas may cause visual impairment by obstructing the visual axis, leading to amblyopia or deformation of the cornea, creating refractory errors. Large and/or segmental hemangiomas in the periocular area have the greatest risk of these complications, but even small lesions may pose a threat to normal visual development, with astigmatism being the most common sight-threatening ocular complication.[157,158] Proliferation of retrobulbar lesions may lead to proptosis, strabismus, and visual compromise.[159] Strabismus may be associated. Mixed hemangiomas located on the nasal tip distort the underlying cartilage. Plastic surgical repair is often necessary to correct the 'Cyrano-nose' deformity. Ulceration involving the columella can lead to destruction of the nasal septum.

Large cervicofacial hemangiomas may impair vital functions, distort normal anatomy, or lead to congestive heart failure as they proliferate. Retrospective review of 'alarming,' life-threatening, or function-threatening hemangiomas (excluding vascular tumors complicated by Kasabach–Merritt syndrome) reveals several distinct characteristics. These problematic hemangiomas are more common in females than males and frequently arise on the head and neck. Alarming hemangiomas are more often identified at birth (with precursor lesions), most are segmental, and rapid growth and proliferation are noted in the neonatal period in 80% of cases. They can have associated extracutaneous hemangiomas including subglottic and gastrointestinal hemangiomas.[98,160] Patients with large facial hemangiomas and visceral involvement have an increased incidence of congestive heart failure, though this complication is rare.[161] PHACE syndrome and other congenital malformations also occur more commonly in these infants.[115,162] The Kasabach–Merritt phenomenon (KMP) was originally believed to be a complication of large hemangiomas, but studies have proved that KMP is a complication of other vascular tumors, including Kaposiform hemangioendothelioma and tufted angioma, rather than infantile hemangiomas (see subsequent discussion).

Management

Before it was recognized that the majority of hemangiomas resolved spontaneously with few complications, X-ray therapy and surgery were mainstays of treatment. Subsequently it was appreciated that allowing hemangiomas to regress spontaneously resulted in better cosmetic outcomes and fewer complications. In addition, long-term cutaneous morbidity and thyroid cancer, as well as an increased risk of intracranial tumors, were reported after ionizing radiation treatment of hemangiomas in infants. More diverse management options[107] are currently available, but none is without potential side effects.[105,154]

Perhaps the greatest challenge in managing hemangiomas in infancy is the identification of those lesions that need treatment. Because of widely divergent sizes, location(s), and the rapid changes that can occur in early infancy, it may be difficult to predict prognosis at the time of initial evaluation. Frequent assessments during the first few weeks to months of life may be needed, particularly if high-risk features are present. The indications for treatment are controversial. The major goals of management are prevention and treatment of life-threatening or function-threatening complications caused by the growth of the hemangioma, prevention of permanent disfigurement, avoidance of overly aggressive, potentially toxic or scarring procedures for hemangiomas that are likely to have a very good prognosis without active intervention, attention to the psychosocial needs of the patient and family, and treatment of ulcerated hemangiomas that may result in pain, infection, or permanent scarring. The indications for considering treatment are summarized in Box 20-3.[105,162,163]

Despite these recommended guidelines, it may still be difficult to determine which hemangiomas should be treated, and how. The potential benefits of any form of treatment should be carefully weighed against the associated risks. The long-term effects of newer treatment methods may not be known. It is important to consider not only anatomic location, but also the size, type, and pattern of the hemangioma (superficial, deep, or combined, focal or segmental). It is also extremely important to assess the phase: is it actively proliferating, is it stable, or is involution predominating? It is essential to have a candid discussion with the parents regarding the possible outcomes with and without therapy, and the morbidity associated with treatment. There is no single 'recipe' for hemangioma treatment, and reassessment over time is needed to determine whether treatment, even if not initially recommended, becomes indicated. The following sections describe some of the treatment methods that have been employed.

Active Nonintervention The term 'active non-intervention' refers to the active observation and anticipatory guidance that can be given to parents, even if no specific therapy is instituted. Parents may feel significant distress as they await spontaneous involution and may react with disbelief, fear, and mourning. Some feel a degree of social stigmatization and many are accused of child abuse, either jokingly or in earnest. Parent–child interactions may be adversely affected.[164] A careful discussion of the natural history of hemangiomas, with photographic examples to demonstrate natural involution, as

> **Box 20-3 Indications for considering early hemangioma treatment**
> - Life-threatening or function-threatening hemangiomas, including those causing impairment of vision, respiratory compromise, or congestive heart failure
> - Hemangiomas in certain anatomic locations (nose, lip, glabellar area, and ear) that may cause permanent deformity or scars
> - Large facial hemangiomas, particularly those with a large dermal component
> - Ulcerated hemangiomas
> - Pedunculated hemangiomas which are virtually certain to leave fibrofatty residua

well as a frank discussion of therapeutic options, can help allay parental fears in most cases. Frequent visits, measurements, and photographs during the proliferating phase are recommended, and as the hemangioma begins to involute visits can become less frequent. If the hemangioma is small or innocuous, an explanation of why those seen on the internet may be more severe can also be reassuring. Acknowledgement of the intrusive questions and advice parents may receive can also be helpful.

Treatment of Ulceration Ulceration is the most common complication of infantile hemangioma and should be treated promptly. All ulcerations leave some degree of scarring. Ulceration can also cause pain, which can be severe, particularly in perioral and perineal locations. Topical antibiotics and occlusive dressings are usually the initial mode of therapy,[165] but medications to control pain, oral antibiotics, and other modalities may be necessary. Pulsed dye laser has been reported to accelerate healing in some cases. There have also been reports of improvement after the application of 0.01% becaplermin (recombinant platelet-derived growth factor),[165,166] but becaplermin is approved for the treatment of diabetic ulcers in adults and not approved for use in children. Its mechanism of action includes the promotion of angiogenesis, which raises questions about its potential for stimulating growth and worsening of hemangiomas. Further studies would be useful to determine the effectiveness and long- term safety of treatment. Corticosteroid therapy may be indicated in some patients with ulcerated hemangiomas, and excisional surgery may need to be considered when medical therapy fails. An approach to the management of ulceration is summarized in Box 20-4.

Corticosteroid Therapy Systemic corticosteroids have remained the mainstay of treatment for problematic hemangiomas since initial reports of their efficacy in the 1960s. The mechanism of action is unknown. Prednisone or prednisolone at a dosage of 2–3 mg/kg/day is used during the proliferating phase to slow or halt the growth of the hemangioma, and some authors advocate even higher doses.[107] A meta-analysis of systemic corticosteroids used during the proliferating phase of infantile hemangioma[167] found that most infants responded to treatment with cessation of growth. A mean dose of 2.9 mg/kg/day was used over a mean period of 1.8 months before tapering, with a response rate of 84%. Doses exceeding 3 mg/kg/day resulted in a response rate of 94%, but a greater incidence of adverse effects was noted. Overall, few major adverse effects were reported.

Most patients receive 2–3 mg/kg/day as a single morning dose. If a response is noted, patients are often maintained on this regimen for 4–6 weeks. Thereafter the dose is slowly tapered over the following months. The duration of treatment depends on response to therapy and the amount of time the hemangioma remains in the proliferating period. Approximately 30% of patients respond to treatment within 2–3 weeks, as evidenced by a cessation of growth and shrinkage of the mass (Fig. 20-28A, B). Another 40% demonstrate cessation

---

Box 20-4 Management of hemangioma ulceration

- Topical wound care. May include one or more of the following:
  - Sparing application of topical antibiotic, such as polymyxinB/bacitracin ointment or metronidazole gel
  - Liberal use of petrolatum or Aquaphor to create an occlusive environment
  - Polyurethane film or ultrathin hydrocolloid dressing if able to adhere to surrounding skin
- Pain control including acetaminophen with or without codeine as needed
- Judicious application of topical lidocaine periodically if pain is severe
- Bacterial culture if malodorous, purulent exudate, or other signs of infection
- Consider other modalities (pulsed dye laser, becaplermin gel, systemic corticosteroids, excisional surgery) as indicated by the clinical situation

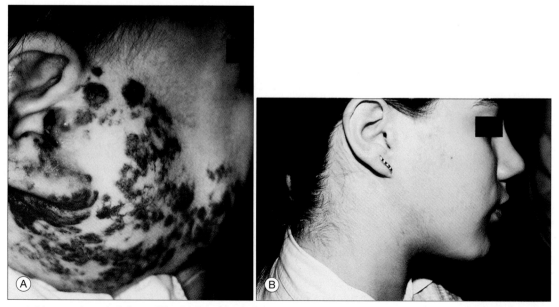

FIG. 20-28 Segmental hemangioma in infancy (**A**), which responded to corticosteroid therapy, leaving virtually normal skin at 14 years (**B**).

of growth without shrinkage in the size of the hemangioma, a finding that may be the result of either a corticosteroid effect or of spontaneous leveling-off in the growth of the lesion. Approximately 30% may fail to respond to therapy, even if prednisone dosages are increased.[83,161]

Before corticosteroid therapy is started, parents should be counseled about the potential side effects (Box 20-5). Although the adverse effects of corticosteroids have been well documented in the literature for other systemic diseases, there is limited information regarding side effects associated with the treatment of hemangiomas. A review of 62 children treated with prednisone or prednisolone at an initial dose of 2–3 mg/kg/day tapered over a mean of 7.9 months showed a low incidence of serious side effects.[168] Cushingoid facies, 'personality changes,' gastric irritation, and perineal and oral candidiasis are the most frequently reported short-term side effects. Retardation of growth, including both height and weight, is also noted, with infants experiencing catch-up growth after cessation of therapy. Hypothalamopituitary–adrenal axis suppression is common, and the need to taper steroid doses prior to discontinuation is emphasized. Steroid myopathy is rare. Hypertension is a potential complication of higher-dose therapy.[169] In addition, patients should be cautioned about the risk of immunocompromise and susceptibility to infection, and live-virus vaccines should be avoided during corticosteroid treatment. Pneumocystis carinii pneumonia has been reported in an infant receiving corticosteroid therapy for infantile hemangioma.[170] There are recent reports of neurotoxicity occurring in very premature infants receiving corticosteroid therapy within the first few weeks of life (in an attempt to prevent chronic lung disease).[171] This type of neurotoxicity has not been reported to date in term infants receiving systemic corticosteroids; however, further studies would be helpful to determine optimal treatment protocols and to assess for short- and long-term side effects.

Intralesional corticosteroid treatment may be useful in the treatment of small, localized hemangiomas in problematic locations such as the lips, tip of the nose, ear, or face. Long-acting triamcinolone acetonide, alone or in combination with the shorter-acting dexamethasone sodium phosphate, is the most frequently used agent.[152,172,173] No treatment protocols have been established and the frequency of injections is governed by clinical response: generally one to three treatments at 4–6-week intervals are needed. The dose of triamcinolone should not exceed 1–3 mg/kg per treatment session. Intralesional injection of hemangiomas on the eyelid with long-acting corticosteroid preparations may be complicated by occlusion of the central retinal or ophthalmic arteries, which may cause blindness.[174] Other complications associated with intralesional treatment in this area include intraocular deposits, eyelid necrosis, and scleroderma-like linear atrophy of the skin. Therefore caution is advised when using intralesional steroids in this location.[175] HPA axis suppression is reported in infants receiving large doses intralesionally.[176]

Topical use of ultrapotent (class I) corticosteroids can be variably effective. A few case series have been published, with the largest noting some degree of improvement in the majority of patients and no major adverse effects, but not all patient responded. Topical corticosteroid treatment should not be a substitute for more aggressive systemic corticosteroid therapy when indicated. Further studies are needed to assess efficacy and identify which subset of hemangiomas may respond most favorably.[177–179]

Other Therapies

- Interferon-α. Recombinant interferon-α has been successful in the treatment of life-threatening hemangiomas that have failed to respond to corticosteroid therapy.[180–183] Both interferon-α2a and -α2b have been used. The most common treatment regimen consists of a daily injection of 3 million U/m² as needed.[181] The response to therapy is variable, with some patients responding rapidly over the course of 3–6 months and others needing longer periods of treatment. Side effects associated with treatment include fever, neutropenia, altered hepatic function chemistries, flu-like complaints, and agitation. Spastic diplegia, a side effect reported in five of 26 infants receiving interferon-α_{2a} for hemangiomas, is a particularly worrisome potential complication.[185,185a] Although this has led some to recommend the use of the α2b preparation, neurotoxicity has also been reported with this preparation. However, use of α interferon may still be useful particularly for aggressive hemangiomas in infants over 1 year of age with ongoing proliferation, as the risk of neurotoxicity after this age may be lower.[185] Neuro-developmental status should be assessed at baseline, and monthly during and after treatment with interferon-α.[185,186]

- There are a few case reports of treating infantile hemangioma with the topical immunomodulator 5% imiquimod cream.[187–190] This cream is approved for the treatment of genital warts, actinic keratoses and superficial BCC in adults. Further studies are needed to determine the safety and efficacy of this therapy in infants.

- Vincristine has been used to treat corticosteroid-resistant hemangiomas and 'vascular tumors' as well as Kasabach–Merritt syndrome.[191] This chemotherapeutic agent is a vinca alkaloid that interferes with microtubule formation during mitosis by inhibiting tubulin. In vitro, it induces apoptosis of tumor and endothelial cells.[192] Peripheral neuropathy, constipation, jaw pain, anemia, and leukopenia are potential toxicities. Administration through a central venous catheter may be necessary, and the participation of a pediatric oncologist/hematologist is advised. It is usually effective, but studies are needed to determine the indications for its use, the incidence of adverse reactions, and the optimal dosage regimen.[192–197]

Surgical Therapies

The flashlamp-pumped pulsed dye laser (PDL) has been used to treat hemangiomas. Superficial lesions appear to respond

---

Box 20-5 Potential adverse effects of systemic corticosteroids used for treating hemangiomas

Common side effects Irritability, spitting up, trouble sleeping, gastrointestinal discomfort, Cushingoid facies, adrenal suppression, decrease or increase of weight, decreased height, increased blood pressure

Uncommon side effects Increased susceptibility to infections, especially chickenpox, certain bacterial infections, Candida albicans infections

Rare side effects Pneumocystis carinii pneumonia, myopathy, pseudotumor cerebri, premature thelarche, decreased head circumference growth

best to this treatment.[198–200] Hemangiomas with a deeper dermal component may show lightening of the superficial erythematous portion, but treatment does not affect the deeper portion. Early laser treatment does not necessarily prevent the growth of a deeper component. Multiple treatment sessions over several months may be needed to treat superficial hemangiomas. Treatment appears to be relatively well tolerated, but the risk of scarring appears to be higher than when treating similarly aged infants with port wine stains, particularly for large hemangiomas in a rapidly proliferative state. A randomized controlled study of PDL for early hemangiomas failed to show substantial benefits at 1 year of age, but this study has been criticized by some because it used a type of PDL without more recent improvements, such as a cooling spray to spare epidermal injury.[201] Side effects include transient pigmentary alteration and atrophic scarring.[201] Severe ulceration and scarring have been reported, especially when treating segmental hemangiomas in the proliferative phase.[202]

The pulsed dye laser is an effective treatment for residual telangiectasia in involuted hemangiomas, and may also be effective for ulcerated hemangiomas. Patients who failed to respond to treatment with topical agents respond with healing of the ulceration, and subjective reduction of pain may be noted after two or three treatments.[203,204] Other laser light sources, including the argon and Nd:YAG lasers, were used to treat hemangiomas in earlier series, but may cause more significant scarring. Percutaneous treatment with a bare fiber Nd:YAG laser has been used to treat deep hemangiomas.[205] Experience with this technique is limited and is probably operator dependent. Contact cryotherapy has been used to treat small, early-proliferating hemangiomas.[206] Surgical excision is usually reserved for involuted hemangiomas to remove residual fibrofatty tissue and redundant skin. Early excision is indicated for a small subset of hemangiomas. These include periorbital hemangioma that fail to respond to pharmacologic therapy, or in which medical therapy is believed to pose a greater risk, painful chronically ulcerated hemangiomas that have failed more conservative treatment, some large nasal tip hemangiomas, and some pedunculated hemangiomas that will inevitably result in prominent fibrofatty residual tissue even after involution is complete. Arterial embolization has been employed to treat life-threatening hemangiomas with high output that have failed medical therapy, to improve the cardiovascular status by reducing the tumor volume and flow.

Other Vascular Tumors

The diagnosis of the rare vascular tumors discussed in the sections that follow requires a skilled pathologist who is familiar with vascular lesions, as the criteria for their recognition are based primarily on histopathologic features and the immunohistochemical markers that are used to help delineate one vascular growth from another are absent. Moreover, many of these entities have been described only recently, so they may be unfamiliar to some pathologists.[4]

Tufted Angioma

Tufted angioma (TA) was described by Wilson-Jones and Orkin.[207] It was long known in the Japanese literature as angioblastoma of Nakagawa. The pathologic features are diagnostic. Most cases are acquired early in childhood and have a protracted course. Rare congenital forms also exist.[208] Congenital TAs display various patterns at birth, either as a large,

plaque-like, infiltrated, red or dusky blue-purple lesion or as a large, exophytic, firm, violaceous, cutaneous nodule (Fig. 20-29A). Not all TAs are present at birth, but may develop as papules, plaques, or nodules in the first few weeks to months of life. Increased hair overlying the tumor is a relatively common finding (Fig. 20-29B). A diagnostic biopsy is advised to rule out a congenital sarcoma. Histologically, both acquired and congenital TAs demonstrate vascular tufts of tightly packed capillaries, randomly dispersed throughout the dermis in a typical cannonball distribution, semilunar empty vascular spaces around the vascular tufts, and lymphatic-like spaces.[208] TAs must be differentiated from infantile hemangiomas as well as other vascular tumors. They are often somewhat firmer and may be tender. TAs may regress completely within a few years,[209,210] shrink leaving a residuum, or persist unchanged, requiring further treatment. A small number of congenital TAs develop Kasabach–Merritt phenomenon (see below). After resolution of the coagulopathy they may leave minor lesions

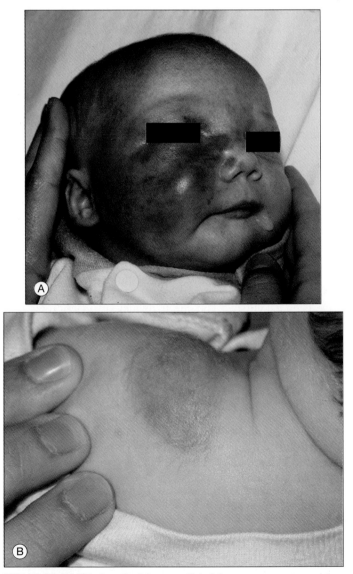

FIG. 20-29 (A) This hemifacial congenital violaceous mass proved to be a tufted angioma, which involuted with corticosteroid treatment. **(B)** Tufted angioma on the shoulder of a young infant. Hypertrichosis is a common feature. (Courtesy of Denise Metry.)

with a fibrotic texture or an extensive red stain with coalescent papules and tenderness.[211]

Kaposiform Hemangioendothelioma

Kaposiform hemangioendothelioma (KHE) is a rare vascular tumor that has been reported in association with Kasabach–Merritt phenomenon (see following section) and with lymphangiomatosis.[212] Histologic and clinical overlap with tufted angioma is sometimes seen. This tumor is distinct from typical infantile hemangioma and behaves more aggressively. It may present as a brown-red stain-like area at birth which begins to thicken and become purpuric, or as a plaque or nodule similar to tufted angioma. In a large pathologic study of 33 cases, lymph node involvement was present in two patients, but no patient developed distant metastases.[213] Histologic examination reveals densely infiltrating nodules composed of spindled cells with minimal atypia and infrequent mitoses, lining slit-like or crescentic vessels containing hemosiderin. The tumor is GLUT-1 negative.[133,213] Some histologic features are similar to those of tufted angioma, and some investigators feel that these two entities lie within a single spectrum.[214] The proliferation is associated with lymphatic spaces. It is rarely recognized in neonates, when, occurring without thrombocytopenia, it is probably misdiagnosed as 'congenital hemangioma.' Spontaneous involution is rare. Most reported cases have had associated Kasabach–Merritt phenomenon, but KHE can occur in the absence of a coagulopathy.[215]

Kasabach–Merritt Phenomenon

Since the first case report in 1940, the label Kasabach–Merritt phenomenon (KMP) has been used to describe infants with vascular anomalies and thrombocytopenia or other coagulopathy, and the syndrome was long considered to be a complication of 'hemangioma.'[216] Several publications have now documented that this biologic phenomenon is not associated with a 'true' hemangioma of infancy, but rather with other vascular tumors, especially kaposiform hemangioendothelioma (KHE) or tufted angioma (TA), which may occur in association with a lymphatic malformation.[217–221]

Cutaneous Findings

KMP is a rare and distinctive condition. Affected infants have a congenital tumor or a lesion soon after birth, with subsequent development of an inflammatory, bruising, reddish or purple mass, and purpura (Fig. 20-30A, B). Before the development of thrombocytopenia and platelet trapping, the clinical appearance may be quite variable. Infants may have a red-brown stain, a yellowish, bluish, or red plaque-like lesion, often congenital, or no lesion at all. Conversely, they may have a history of a congenital bulky tumor detected by prenatal ultrasound requiring a diagnostic biopsy as a neonate.[222]

Extracutaneous Findings

Severe thrombocytopenia is the hallmark of KMP. Consumption of fibrinogen, elevated D-dimers, and decreased coagulation factors occur to varying degrees, depending on the severity and phases of the disease. KMP has no anatomic site of predilection. Although more cases are within the skin and musculature, KMP can involve deeper visceral structures. Visceral KMP – cervicothoracic, abdominal, pelvic, or intracranial – is always life threatening.

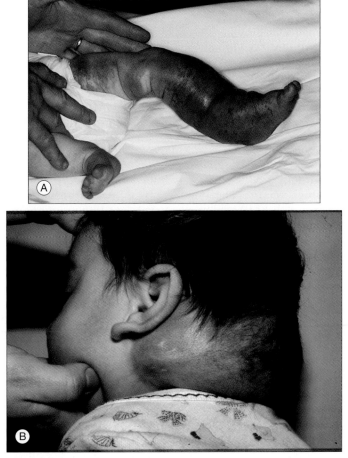

FIG. 20-30 Kasabach–Merritt phenomenon involving the leg. Note both the ecchymotic and the inflammatory patterns of the skin. Kasabach–Merrit phenomenon involving (**A**) the leg and (**B**) the neck.

Course

Thrombocytopenia may persist for a few years, but more commonly resolves with treatment by 12–18 months or sooner. Hemorrhage, infection, or iatrogenic complications may cause death. When the hematologic phenomenon is cured, the tumor shrinks but the patient has residual changes that are clearly different from those of an involuted hemangioma. These residua are more or less prominent, painful, persistent vascular tumors in a dormant stage. Their appearance varies from that of a pseudo-port wine stain, with infiltrated areas and papules, stain-like areas with haloes, and nodular residua, to a poorly delineated, fibrotic-feeling plaque. In some cases muscle and joint fibrosis remains.[223]

Diagnosis

The diagnosis can be suspected in a newborn or young infant with a rapidly growing soft tissue mass, often with tenderness and surrounding purpura. Skin biopsy may be necessary to distinguish the condition from other soft tissue tumors or even infection, but in typical cases, especially those with characteristic MR findings, the diagnosis can be made clinically, as biopsy of a highly vascular mass in a profoundly thrombocytopenic infant can be difficult.

Differential Diagnosis

Newborns or young infants with malignant soft tissue tumors will occasionally present with a large soft tissue mass and thrombocytopenia. Moderate thrombocytopenia can also be present in congenital hemangiomas or large lymphatic malformations, but it does not become as severe or as persistent as in KMP. KMP is virtually always due to solitary tumors. As previously discussed, large vascular malformations can have an associated coagulopathy, but elevated D-dimers and consumption of clotting factors, rather than platelet trapping, is the primary pathologic process involved. Multifocal vascular growths with associated thrombocytopenia are more likely to be due to 'multifocal lymphangioendotheliomatosis with thrombocytopenia' than to KMP.

Treatment

Kasabach–Merritt phenomenon is a medical emergency. Infants with KMP exhibit an inconsistent response to many therapeutic regimens. The choice of treatment is empiric. Both success and failure have been documented with various drugs prescribed either alone or in combination, which increases the risk of toxicity. Currently the best therapeutic options appear to be corticosteroids, vincristine, interferon-α, and ticlopidine plus aspirin. Surgical excision, arterial embolization, and radiotherapy may also benefit some patients.[224]

Multifocal Lymphangioendotheliomatosis with Thrombocytopenia (also known as Cutaneovisceral Angiomatosis with Thrombocytopenia)

This rare condition is characterized by multiple cutaneous vascular papules and plaques which are often present at birth or develop during the neonatal period. More skin lesions may develop over time. Affected infants typically have chronic fluctuating thrombocytopenia and gastrointestinal bleeding due to identical lesions within the GI tract.[225] Other reported sites of involvement include bones, synovium, lungs, liver, and spleen. Skin biopsy specimens demonstrated thin-walled vessels, some hobnailed endothelial cells, and intraluminal papillary projections. North et al.[225] demonstrated vessels staining for lymphatic markers (LYVE-1) suggesting a lymphatic origin for these lesions, but Prasad et al.[226] disagree, as they found only one of 10 cases with immunopositivity for the lymphatic marker D2-40.

Infantile Hemangiopericytoma (versus Infantile Myofibromatosis)

Infantile hemangiopericytoma is considered a rare tumor and different from the more common adult type because of its benign prognosis.[227] The congenital form, more common in boys, is a red, partially necrotic tumor, with a branching vasculature, a multilobular pattern, a collagenous matrix, and mitotic figures. This is a controversial lesion, considered by some to be part of a continuum with solitary infantile myofibromatosis.[227] However, more recent classification places this lesion in the category of solitary fibrous tumors.[228] Infantile myofibromatosis presents as a congenital rubbery red or pink nodule, corresponding to a richly vascularized tumor and

dense infiltration of plump, spindle-shaped cells. Solitary infantile myofibromatosis has a good outcome and involutes by massive apoptosis. A multinodular multisystemic form may be present in a neonate; this generalized form may have a bad outcome, being lethal soon after birth, although spontaneous resolution has also been reported.

Spindle Cell Hemangioendothelioma

Spindle cell hemangioendothelioma (SCHE) occurs at any age and site but seems more common in the limbs. It has a protracted course. Lesions are solitary or multiple. The nodular, dense, spindle cell proliferation is associated with 'cavernous' vessels of attenuated, irregularly thickened walls. Lesions tend to multiply locally and to recur when excised. Among 78 cases, four had Maffucci syndrome. No metastases were reported in this large series of SCHE, thereafter renamed SC-hemangioma (for a solitary lesion) or SC-hemangiomatosis (for multiple skin lesions).[229]

Congenital Eccrine Angiomatous Hamartoma (Sudoriparous Angioma)

Congenital forms of this tumor present as a nodule or as a large, ill-defined angiomatous plaque with lanugo and sweating at the site of the lesion.[230] The lesions are usually located on the extremities or abdomen and may involute. It is not clear whether the rarely reported congenital cases[231,232] are identical to the slowly growing, persistent forms that are characterized by an acquired bluish or flesh-colored nodule or a bossed erythematous and pigmented firm nodule or plaque with excess hair, hyperhidrosis, and pain overlying a slow-flow vascular malformation. Diagnosis is established on the basis of the presence of characteristic histologic findings. Closely packed eccrine sweat glands are associated with dilated capillaries, a few dysplastic venous channels, and a dense collagenous matrix.

Pyogenic Granuloma (Lobular Capillary Hemangioma)

Pyogenic granuloma (PG) – also known by its correct histopathologic description 'lobular capillary hemangioma' rather than its historic misnomer – is a common vascular tumor of infants and children, albeit relatively rare in the newborn period. PGs usually present as a solitary, red, rapidly growing papule or nodule, often located on the malar area or forehead. They often develop an eroded surface, bleeding easily and relatively profusely, prompting their nickname 'the Bandaid disease.' When a PG occurs in a very young infant, it may be mistaken for an infantile hemangioma.[233] Rare multifocal forms have been observed in newborns, but before specific immunohistochemical identification of infantile hemangiomas was possible they were often mistaken for infantile hemangiomas.[234,235] PGs do not involute spontaneously, but simple curettage with electrocautery is usually curative.[236,237]

REFERENCES

1. Mulliken JB, Glowacki J. Hemangiomas and vascular malformations in infants and children: a classification based on endothelial characteristics. Plast Reconstr Surg 1982; 69: 412–420.

2. Enjolras O, Mulliken J. Vascular tumors and vascular malformations, new issues. Adv Dermatol 1998; 13: 375–423.

3. Takahashi K, Mulliken JB, Kozakewich H, et al. Cellular markers

that distinguish the phases of hemangioma during infancy and childhood. J Clin Invest 1994; 93: 2357–2364.

4. Requena L, Sangueza OP. Cutaneous vascular proliferations. II. Hyperplasias

and benign neoplasms. J Am Acad Dermatol 1997; 37: 887–920.

5. Leung AKC, Telmesani AMA. Salmon patches in Caucasian children. Pediatr Dermatol 1989; 6: 185–187.

6. Maniscalco M, Guareschi E, Noto G, Patrizi A. Midline telangiectatic nevus (salmon patch) of the nape of the neck. Eur J Pediatr Dermatol 2003; 13: 81–84.

7. Metzker A, Shamir R. Butterfly-shaped mark: a variant form of nevus flammeus simplex. Pediatrics 1990; 85: 1069–1071.

8. Patrizi A, Neri I, Orlandi C, et al. Sacral medial telangiectatic vascular nevus: a study of 43 children. Dermatology 1996; 192: 301–306.

9. McClean K, Hanke CW. The medical necessity for treatment of port-wine stains. Dermatol Surg 1997; 23: 663–667.

10. Boyd JB, Mulliken JB, Kaban LB, et al. Skeletal changes associated with vascular malformations. Plast Reconstr Surg 1984; 74: 789–795.

11. Lanigan SW, Taibjee SM. Recent advances in laser treatment of port-wine stains. Br J Dermatol 2004; 151: 527–533.

12. Renfro L, Geronemus RG. Anatomical differences of port-wine stains in response to treatment with the pulsed dye laser. Arch Dermatol. 1993; 129: 182–188.

13. Sommer S, Seukeran DC, Sheehan-Dare RA. Efficacy of pulsed dye laser treatment of port-wine stain malformations of the lower limb. Br J Dermatology 2003; 149: 770–775.

14. Ashinoff R, Geronemus RG. Flashlamp-pumped pulsed dye laser for port-wine stains in infancy: earlier versus later treatment. J Am Acad Dermatol 1991; 24: 467–472.

15. Van Der Horst C, Koster P, De Borgie C, et al. Effect of the timing on the treatment of port-wine stains with the flash-lamp-pumped pulsed-dye laser. N Engl J Med 1998; 338: 1028–1033.

16. Enjolras O, Ciabrini D, Mazoyer E, et al. Extensive pure venous malformations in the upper and lower limbs: a review of 27 cases. J Am Acad Dermatol 1997; 36: 219–225.

17. Mazoyer E, Enjolras O, Laurian C, et al. Coagulation abnormalities associated with extensive venous malformations of the limbs: differentiation from Kasabach–Merritt syndrome. Clin Lab Haematol. 2002; 24: 243–251.

18. Boon LM, Mulliken JB, Enjolras O, Vikkula M. Glomuvenous malformation (glomangioma) and venous malformation. Arch Dermatol 2004; 140: 971–976.

19. Vikkula M, Boon LM, Carraway KL, et al. Vascular dysmorphogenesis caused by an activating mutation in the receptor tyrosine kinase TIE2. Cell 1996; 87: 1181–1190.

20. Brouillard P, Ghassibe M, Penington A, et al. Four common glomulin mutations cause two thirds of glomuvenous malformations ('familial glomangiomas'): evidence for a founder effect. J Med Genet 2005; 42: e 13.

21. Burrows PE, Mason KP. Percutaneous treatment of low flow vascular malformations. J Vasc Intervent Radiol 2004; 15: 431–445.

22. Boukobza M, Enjolras O, Guichard JP, et al. Cerebral developmental venous anomaly associated with head and neck venous malformations. Am J NeuroRadiol 1996; 17: 987–994.

23. Gelbert F, Enjolras O, Deffrenne D, et al. Percutaneous sclerotherapy for venous malformation of the lips: a retrospective study in 23 patients. Neuroradiology 2000; 42: 692–696.

24. Fayad L, Hazirolan T, Bluemke D, Mitchell S. Vascular malformations in the extremities: emphasis of MR imaging features that guide treatment options. Skeletal Radiol 2006; 35: 127–137.

25. Burrows PE, Fellows KE. Techniques for management of pediatric vascular anomalies. Current techniques in interventional radiology. Curr Med 1995; 2: 12–27.

26. Tanriverdi HA, Hendrick HJ, Ertan AK, et al. Hygroma colli cysticum: prenatal diagnosis and prognosis. Am J Perinatol 2001; 18: 415–420.

27. Davies D, Rogers M. Morphology of lymphatic malformations: a pictorial review. Aust J Dermatol 2000; 41: 1–7.

28. Padwa BL, Hayward PG, Ferrero NF, et al. Cervicofacial lymphatic malformation, clinical course, surgical intervention, and pathogenesis of skeletal hypertrophy. Plast Reconstr Surg 1995; 95: 951–960.

29. Edwards PD, Rahbar R, Ferraro NF, et al. Lymphatic malformation of the lingual base and oral floor. Plast Reconstr Surg 2005; 115: 1906–1015.

30. Greene AK, Burrows PE, Smith L, Mulliken JB. Periorbital lymphatic malformation: clinical course and management in 42 patients. Plast Reconstr Surg 2005; 115: 22–30.

31. Orvidas LJ, Kasperbauer JL. Pediatric lymphangiomas of the head and neck. Ann Otol Rhinol Laryngol 2000; 109: 411–421.

32. Loewenstein EJ, Kim KH, Glick SA. Turner's syndrome in dermatology. J Am Acad Dermatol 2004; 50: 767–776.

33. Hayward PG, Orgill DP, Mulliken JB, Perez-Atayde AR. Congenital fibrosarcoma masquerading as lymphatic malformation: report of two cases. J Pediatr Surg 1995; 30: 84–88.

34. Enjolras O, Deffrennes D, Borsik M, et al. Les 'tumeurs' vasculaires. Règles de prise en charge chirurgicale. Ann Chir Plast Esthet 1998; 43: 455–490.

35. Luzzato C, Midrio P, Tchaprassian Z, Guglielmi M. Sclerosing treatment of lymphangiomas with OK-432. Arch Dis Child 2000; 82: 316–318.

36. Enjolras O, Logeart I, Gelbert F, et al. Malformations artérioveineuses: à propos de 200 cas. Ann Dermatol Venereol 1999; 127: 17–22.

37. Wu JK, Bisdorff A, Gelbert F, et al. Auricular arteriovenous malformation: evaluation, management, and outcome. Plast Reconstr Surg 2005; 115: 985–995.

38. Esterly NB. Cutaneous hemangiomas, vascular stains and malformations, and associated syndromes. Curr Probl Dermatol 1995; 3: 69–107.

39. Cole SG, Begbie ME, Wallace GM, Shovlin CL. A new locus for hereditary haemorrhagic telangiectasia (HHT3) maps to chromosome 5. J Med Genet 2005; 42: 577–582.

40. Begbie ME, Wallace GMF, Shovlin CL. Hereditary haemorrhagic telangiectasia (Osler–Weber–Rendu syndrome): a view from the 21st century. Postgrad Med J 2003; 79: 18–24.

41. Taylor AM, Byrd PJ. Molecular pathology of ataxia telangiectasia. J Clin Pathol 2005; 58: 1009–1015.

42. Cabana M, Crawford TO, Winkelstein JA, et al. Consequences of the delayed diagnosis of ataxia–telangiectasia. Pediatrics 1998; 102: 98–100.

43. Picascia DD, Esterly NB. Cutis marmorata telangiectatica congenita: report of 22 cases. J Am Acad Dermatol 1989; 20: 1098–1104.

44. Enjolras O. Cutis marmorata telangiectatica congenita. Ann Dermatol Venereol. 2001; 128: 161–166.

45. Moroz PK. Cutis marmorata telangiectatica congenita: long-term follow-up, review of the literature, and report of a case in conjunction with congenital hypothyroidism. Pediatr Dermatol 1993; 10: 6–11.

46. Devillers ACA, de Waard-Van der Spek FB, Oranje AP. Cutis marmorata telangiectatica congenita: clinical features in 35 cases. Arch Dermatol 1999; 135: 34–38.

47. Gelmetti C, Schianchi R, Ermacora E. Cutis marmorata telangiectatica congenita: quatre nouveaux cas et revue de la littérature. Ann Dermatol Venereol 1987; 114: 1517–1528.

48. Fujita M, Darmstadt GL, Dinulos JG. Cutis marmorata telangiectatica congenita with hemangiomatous histopathologic features. J Am Acad Dermatol 2003; 48: 950–954.

49. Garavelli L, Leask K, Zanacca C, et al. MRI and neurological findings in macrocephaly–cutis marmorata telangiectatica congenita syndrome: report of ten cases and review of the literature. Genet Couns 2005; 16: 117–128.

50. Carrascosa JM, Ribera M, Bielsa I, et al. Cutis marmorata telangiectatica congenita or neonatal lupus? Pediatr Dermatol 1996; 13: 230–232.

51. Enjolras O, Riché MC, Merland JJ. Facial port-wine stains and Sturge–Weber syndrome. Pediatrics 1985; 76: 48–51.

52. Adamsbaum C, Pinton F, Rolland Y, et al. Accelerated myelination in early Sturge–Weber syndrome: MRI–SPECT

correlation. Pediatr Radiol 1996; 26: 759–762.

53. Pinton F, Chiron C, Enjolras O, et al. Early single photon emission computed tomography in Sturge–Weber syndrome. J Neurol Neurosurg Psychiatry 1997; 63: 616–621.

54. Chugani HT. The role of PET in childhood epilepsy. J Child Neurol 1994; 9: 82–88.

55. Ville D, Enjolras O, Chiron C, Dulac O. Prophylactic antiepileptic treatment in Sturge–Weber disease. Seizure 2002; 11: 145–150.

56. Enjolras O, Chapot R, Merland JJ. Vascular anomalies and the growth of limbs. J Pediatr Orthop B 2004; 13: 349–357.

57. Maari C, Frieden IJ. Klippel–Trenaunay syndrome: the importance of 'geographic stains' in identifying lymphatic disease and risk of complications. J Am Acad Dermatol 2004; 51: 391–398.

58. Greene AK, Kieran M, Burrows PE, et al. Wilms' tumor screening is unnecessary in Klippel–Trenaunay syndrome. Pediatrics 2004; 113: e326–e329.

59. Kundu RV, Frieden IJ. Presence of vascular anomalies with congenital hemihypertrophy and Wilms' tumor: an evidence-based evaluation. Pediatr Dermatol 2003; 20: 199–206.

60. Huiras EE, Barnes CJ, Eichenfield LF, et al. Pulmonary thromboembolism associated with Klippel–Trenaunay syndrome. Pediatrics 2005; 116: e596–e600.

61. Eerola I, Boon L M, Mulliken J B, et al. Capillary malformation arteriovenous malformation, a new clinical and genetic disorder caused by RASA1 mutations. Am J Hum Genet 2003; 73: 1240–1249.

62. Kassarjian A, Fishman SJ, Fox VL, Burrows PE. Imaging characteristics of blue rubber bleb nevus syndrome. Am J Roentgenol 2003; 181: 1041–1048.

63. Wiedemann HR, Burgio GR, Aldendorff P, et al. The Proteus syndrome. Eur J Pediatr 1983; 140: 5–12.

64. Hoeger PH, Martinez A, Maerker J, Harper JI. Vascular anomalies in Proteus syndrome. Clin Exp Dermatol 2004; 29: 222–230.

65. Nguyen D, Turner JT, Olsen C, Biesecker LG, Darling TN. Cutaneous manifestations of Proteus syndrome; Arch Dermatology 2004; 140: 947–953.

66. Turner JT, Cohen MM, Biesecker LG. Reassessment of the Proteus Syndrome literature: Application of diagnostic criteria to published cases. Am J Med Genet 2004: 130A: 111–122.

66a. Hall BD, de Lorimer A, Foster LH. A new syndrome of hemangiomatous branchial clefts, lip pseudoclefts, and unusual facial appearance. Am J Med Genet 1983; 14: 135–138.

67. Zergollen L, Hitrec V. Four siblings with Roberts syndrome. Clin Genet 1982; 21: 1–6.

68. Verdyck P, Holder-Espinasse M, Hul WV, Wuyts W. Clinical and molecular analysis of nine families with Adams–Oliver syndrome. Eur J Hum Genet 2003; 11: 457–463.

69. Martínez-Frías ML, Arroyo-Carrera I, Jiménez Munoz DN, et al. Síndrome de Adams–Oliver en nuestro medio: aspectos epidemiológicos. An Esp Pediatr 1996; 45: 57–61.

70. Dyall-Smith D, Ramsden A, Laurie S. Adams–Oliver syndrome: aplasia cutis congenita, terminal transverse limb defects, and cutis marmorata telangiectatica congenita. Australas J Dermatol 1994; 35: 19–22.

71. Romani J, Puig L, Aznar G, et al. Adams–Oliver syndrome with unusual central nervous system alterations. Pediatr Dermatol 1998; 15: 48–50.

72. Boon LM, Enjolras O, Mulliken JB. Congenital hemangioma: evidence of accelerated involution. J Pediatr 1996; 128: 329–335.

73. North PE, Waner M, James CA, et al. Congenital nonprogressive lemangioma: a distinct clinicopathologic entity unlike infertile hemangioma. Arch Dermatol. 2001; 137: 1607–1620.

74. Berenguer B, Mulliken JB, Enjolras O, et al. Rapidly involuting congenital hemangioma: clinical and histopathologic features. Pediatr Dev Pathol. 2003; 6: 495–510.

75. Mulliken JB, Enjolras O. Congenital hemangiomas and infantile hemangioma: missing links. J Am Acad Dermatol. 2004; 50: 875–882.

76. Enjolras O, Picard A, Soupre V. Hémangiomes congénitaux et autres tumeurs infantiles rares. Ann Chir Plast 2006; 51: 339–346.

77. Jacobs AH, Walton R. The incidence of birthmarks in neonate. Pediatrics 1976; 58: 218–222.

78. Pratt AG. Birthmarks in infants. Arch Dermatol Syphilol 1953; 67: 302–305.

79. Mulliken JB. Diagnosis and natural history of hemangiomas. In: Mulliken JB, Young AE, eds. Vascular birthmarks: hemangiomas and malformations. Philadelphia: WB Saunders, 1988; 41–62.

80. Hidano A, Nakajima S. Earliest features of the strawberry mark in the newborn. Br J Dermatol 1972; 87: 138–144.

81. Finn MC, Glowacki J, Mulliken JB. Congenital vascular lesions: clinical application of a new classification. J Pediatr Surg 1983; 18: 894–900.

82. Haggstrom AN, Drolet BA, Baselga E, et al. Prospective study of infantile hemangiomas: clinical characteristics predicting complications and treatment. Pediatrics 2006; 118: 882–887.

83. Enjolras O, Gelbert F. Superficial hemangiomas: associations and management. Pediatr Dermatol 1997; 14: 173–179.

84. Amir J, Metzker A, Krikler R, et al. Strawberry hemangioma in preterm infants. Pediatr Dermatol 1986; 3: 331–332.

85. Burton BK, Schulz CJ, Angle B, et al. An increased incidence of haemangiomas in infants born following chorionic villus sampling (CVS). Prenat Diagn 1995; 15: 209–214.

86. Frieden IJ, Haggstrom AN, Drolet BA, et al. Infantile hemangiomas: current knowledge, future directions, Proceedings of a Research workshop on infantile hemangiomas. April 7–9 2005, Bethesda Ma. Pediatr Dermatol 2005; 22: 383–406.

87. Blei F, Walter J, Orlow SJ, et al. Familial segregation of hemangiomas and vascular malformations as an autosomal dominant trait. Arch Dermatol 1998; 134: 718–722.

88. Payne MM, Moyer F, Marcks KM, et al. The precursor to the hemangioma. Plast Reconstr Surg 1966; 38: 64–67.

89. Liang MG, Frieden IJ. Perineal and lip ulcerations as the presenting manifestation of hemangioma of infancy. Pediatrics 1997; 99: 256–259.

90. Lister WA. The natural history of strawberry nevi. Lancet 1938; 1429–1434.

91. Waner M, North PE, Scherer KA, et al. The nonrandom distribution of facial hemangiomas. Arch Dermatol. 2003; 139: 869–875.

92. Chiller KG, Passaro D, Frieden IJ. Hemangiomas of infancy: clinical characteristics, morphologic subtypes and their relationship to race, ethnicity and sex. Arch Dermatol 2002; 138: 1567–1576.

93. Achauer BM, Chang C, Vander VM. Management of hemangioma of infancy: review of 245 patients. Plast Reconstr Surg 1997; 99: 1301–1308.

94. Haggstrom AN, Lammer EJ, Schneider RA, et al. Patterns of infantile hemangiomas: new clues to hemangioma pathogenesis and embryonic facial development. Pediatrics 2006; 117: 698–703.

95. Golitz LE, Rudikoff J, O'Meara OP. Diffuse neonatal hemangiomatosis. Pediatr Dermatol 1986; 3: 145–152.

96. Rahbar R, Nicollas R, Roger G, et al. The biology and management of subglottic hemangioma: past, present future. Laryngoscope 2004; 114: 1880–1891.

97. Boon LM, Burrows PE, Paltiel HJ, et al. Hepatic vascular anomalies in infancy: a twenty-seven-year experience. J Pediatr 1996; 129: 346–354.

98. Metry DW, Hawrot A, Altman C, et al. Association of solitary, segmental hemangiomas of the skin with visceral hemangiomatosis. Arch Dermatol 2004; 140: 591–596.

99. Stern JK, Wolf JE, Jarratt M. Benign neonatal hemangiomatosis. J Am Acad Dermatol 1981; 4: 442–445.

100. Holden KR, Alexander F. Diffuse neonatal hemangiomatosis. Pediatrics 1970; 46: 411–421.

101. Sheu B, Shyu M, Ling Y, et al. Prenatal diagnosis and corticosteroid treatment of diffuse neonatal hemangiomatosis. J Ultrasound Med 1994; 13: 495–499.

102. Fishman SJ, Burrows PE, Mulliken JB. Gastrointestinal manifestations of vascular anomalies in childhood: varied etiologies require multiple therapeutic modalities. J Pediatr Surg 1998; 33: 1163–1167.

103. Berman B, Lim HWP. Concurrent cutaneous and hepatic hemangiomata in infancy: report of a case and review of the literature. J Dermatol Surg Oncol 1978; 4: 869–873.

104. Kassarjian A, Zurakowski D, Dubois J, et al. Infantile hepatic hemangiomas: clinical and imaging findings and their correlation with therapy. Am J Roentgenol 2004; 182: 785–795.

105. Christison-Lagay ER, Burrows PE, Alomari A, et al. Hepatic hemangiomas: subtype classification and development of a clinical practice algorithm and registry. J Pediatr Surg 2007; 42: 62–67.

106. Orlow SJ, Isakoff MS, Blei F. Increased risk of symptomatic hemangiomas of the airway in association with cutaneous hemangiomas in a 'beard' distribution. J Pediatr 1997; 131: 643–646.

107. Drolet BA, Esterly NB, Frieden IJ. Hemangiomas in children. N Engl J Med 1999; 341: 173–181.

108. Burns AJ, Kaplan LC, Mulliken JB. Is there an association between hemangioma and syndromes with dysmorphic features? Pediatrics 1991; 88: 1257–1267.

109. Gorlin RJ, Kantaputra P, Aughton DJ, et al. Marked female predilection in some syndromes associated with facial hemangiomas. Am J Med Genet 1994; 52: 130–135.

110. Frieden IJ, Reese V, Cohen D. PHACE syndrome: the association of posterior fossa brain malformations, hemangiomas, arterial anomalies, coarctation of the aorta and cardiac defects, and eye abormalities. Arch Dermatol 1996; 132: 307–311.

111. Pascual-Castroviejo I, Viano J, Moreno F, et al. Hemangiomas of the head, neck, and chest with associated vascular and brain anomalies: a complex neurocutaneous syndrome. Am J NeuroRadiol 1996; 17: 461–471.

112. Burrows PE, Robertson, RL, Mulliken JB, et al. Cerebral vasculopathy and neurologic sequelae in infants with cervicofacial hemangioma: report of eight patients. Radiology 1998; 207: 601–607.

113. Reese V, Frieden IJ, Paller AS, et al. Association of facial hemangiomas with Dandy–Walker and other posterior fossa malformations. J Pediatr 1993; 122: 379–384.

114. Metry DW, Dowd CF, Barkovich AJ, Frieden IJ. The many faces of PHACE syndrome. J Pediatr 2001; 139: 470.

115. Metry DW, Haggstrom AN, Drolet BA, et al. A prospective study of PHACE association in infantile hemangiomas: demographic features, clinical findings and complications. Am J Med Genet 2006; 140: 975–986.

116. Geller JD, Topper SF, Hashimoto K, et al. Diffuse neonatal hemangiomatosis: a new constellation of findings. J Am Acad Dermatol 1991; 24: 816–818.

117. Vaillant L, Lorette G, Chantepie A, et al. Multiple cutaneous hemangiomas and coarctation of the aorta with right aotic arch. Pediatrics 1988, 81: 707–710.

118. Hersh JH, Waterfill D, Rutledge J, et al. Sternal malformation/ vascular dysplasia association. Am J Med Genet 1985; 21: 177–186.

119. Blei F, Orlow SJ, Geronemus RG. Supraumbilical mid-abdominal raphe, sternal atresia, and hemangioma in an infant. Pediatr Dermatol 1993; 10: 71–76.

120. Goldberg NS, Hebert AA, Esterly NB. Sacral hemangiomas and multiple congenital abnormalities. Arch Dermatol 1986; 122: 684–687.

121. Albright AL, Gartner C, Wiener ES, et al. Lumbar cutaneous hemangiomas as indicators of tethered spinal cords. Pediatrics 1989; 83: 977–980.

122. Huang SA, Tu HM, Harney JW, et al. Severe hypothyroidism caused by type 3 iodothyronine deiodinase in infantile hemangiomas. N Engl J Med 2000; 343: 185–189.

123. Konrad D, Ellis G, Perlman K. Spontaneous regression of severe acquired hypothyroidism associated with multiple liver hemangiomas. Pediatrics 2003; 112: 1424–1426.

124. Ho J, Kendrick V, Dewey D, Pacaud D. New insights into the pathophysiology of severe hypothyroidism in an infant with multiple hepatic hemangiomas. J Pediatr Endocrinol Metab 2005; 18: 511–514.

125. Bauland CG, van Steensel MA, Steijlen PM, et al. The pathogenesis of hemangiomas: a review. Plast Reconstr Surg 2006; 117: 29e–35e.

126. Boye E, Ying Y, Paranya G, et al. Clonality and altered behavior of endothelial cells from hemangioams. J Clin Invest 2001; 107: 745–752.

127. Walter JW, North PE, Waner M, et al. Somatic mutation of vascular endothelial growth factor receptors in juvenile hemangioma. Genes, Chromosomes Cancer 2002: 33: 295–303.

128. Yu Y, Brown LF, Mulliken JB, Bischoff J. Increased Tie2 expression, enhanced response to angiopoietin-1, and dysregulated angiopoietin-2 expression in hemangioma-derived endothelial cells. Am J Pathol 2001; 159: 2271–2280.

129. Walter JW, North PE, Waner M, et.al. Somatic mutation of vascular endothelial growth factor receptors in juvenile hemangioma. Genes, Chromosomes Cancer 2002: 33: 295–303.

130. Berg JN, Walter JW, Thisanagayam U, et al. Evidence for loss of heterozygosity of 5q in sporadic hemangiomas: are somatic mutations involved in hemangioma formation. J Clin Pathol 2001; 54: 249–252.

131. Bischoff J. Monoclonal expansion of endothelial cells in hemangioma: an intrinsic defect with extrinsic consequences? Trends Cardiovasc Med 2002; 12: 220–224.

132. Berard M, Ortega N, Carrier JL, et al. Vascular endothelial growth factor confers a growth advantage in vitro and in vivo to stromal cells cultured from neonatal hemangiomas. Am J Pathol 1997; 150: 1315–1326.

133. North PE, Waner M, Mizeracki A, Mihm MC. GLUT1: a newly discovered immunohistochemical marker for juvenile hemangiomas. Hum Pathol 2000; 31: 11–22.

134. North PE, Waner M, Mizeracki A, et al. A unique microvascular phenotype shared by juvenile hemangiomas and human placenta. Arch Dermatol 2001; 137: 559–570.

135. Barnes CM, Huang S, Kaipainen A, et al. Evidence by molecular profiling for a placental origin of infantile hemangiomas. Proc Natl Acad Sci USA 2005; 102: 19097–19102.

136. Enjolras O. L'hémangiome infantile, progrès biologiques et cliniques, stagnation des traitements. Lecture Journées Dermatologiques Paris December 6–10 2005. Ann Dermatol Venereol 2005; 132: 9SA25–27.

137. Chang J, Most D, Bresnick S, et al. Proliferative hemangiomas: analysis of cytokine gene expression and angiogenesis. Plas Reconstr Surg 1999; 103: 1–9.

138. Zhang L, Lin X, Wang W, et al. Circulating level of vascular endothelial growth factor in differentiating hemangioma from vascular malformation patients. Plast Reconstr Surg 2005; 116: 200–204.

139. Isik FF, Rand RP, Gruss JS, et al. Monocyte chemoattractant protein-1 mRNA expression in hemangiomas and vascular malformations. J Surg Res 1996; 61: 71–76.

140. Salcedo R, Ponce ML, Young HA, et al. Human endothelial cells express CCR2 and respond to MCP-1: direct role of MCP-1 in angiogenesis and tumor progression. Blood 2000; 96: 34–40.

141. Kraling BM, Razon MJ, et al. E-selectin is present in proliferating endothelial cells in human hemangiomas. Am J Pathol 1996; 148: 1181–1191.

142. Verkarre V, Patey-Mariaud de Serre N, Vazeux R, et al. ICAM-3 and E-selectin endothelial cell expression differentiate two phases of angiogenesis

in infantile hemangiomas. J Cutan Pathol 1999; 26: 17–24.

143. Ritter MR, Reinisch J, Friedlander SF, Friedlander M. Myeloid cells in infantile hemangioma. Am J Pathol 2006; 168: 621–628.

144. Tan ST, Velickovic M, Ruger BM, Davis BF. Cellular and extracellular markers of hemangioma. Plast Reconstr Surg 2000; 106: 529–538.

145. Marler JJ, Fishman SJ, Kilroy SM, et al. Increased levels of urinary matrix metalloproteinases parallels the extent and activity of vascular anomalies. Pediatrics 2005; 116: 38–45.

146. Dadras SS, North PE, Bertoncini J, et al. Infantile hemangiomas are arrested in an early developmental vascular differentiation state. Mod Pathol 2004; 17: 1068–1079.

147. Bielenberg DR, Bucana CD, Sanchez R, et al. Progressive growth of infantile cutaneous hemangiomas is directly correlated with hyperplasia and angiogenesis of adjacent epidermis and inversely correlated with expression of the endogenous angiogenesis inhibitor, IFN-beta. Int J Oncol 1999; 14: 401–408.

148. Ritter MR, Dorrell MI, Edmonds J, et al. Insulin-like growth factor 2 and potential regulators of hemangioma growth and involution identified by large-scale expression analysis. Proc Natl Acad Sci USA 2002; 99: 7455–7460.

149. Mancini AJ, Smoller BR. Proliferation and apoptosis within juvenile capillary hemangiomas. Am J Dermatopathol 1996; 18: 505–514.

150. Razon MJ, Kraling BM, Mulliken JB, Bischoff J. Increased apoptosis coincides with onset of involution in infantile hemangiomas. Microcirculation 1998; 5: 189–195.

151. Hasan Q, Ruger BM, Tan ST, et al. Clusterin/apoJ expression during the development of hemangiomas. Hum Pathol 2000; 31: 691–697.

152. Enjolras O, Mulliken JB. The current management of vascular birthmarks. Pediatr Dermatol 1993; 10: 311–333.

153. Burrows PE, Laor T, Paltiel H, Robertson RL. Diagnostic imaging in the evaluation of vascular birthmarks. Dermatol Clin 1998; 16: 455–488.

154. Folkman J, Mulliken JB, Ezekowitz RAB. Angiogenesis and hemangiomas. In: Oldham KT, Colombani PM, Foglia RP, eds. Surgery of infants and children: scientific principles and practice. Philadelphia: Lippincott-Raven, 1997; 569–580.

155. Glowacki J, Mulliken JB. Mast cells in hemangiomas and vascular malformations. Pediatrics 1982; 70: 48–51.

156. Folkman J. Clinical applications of research on angiogenesis. N Engl J Med 1995; 333: 1757–1763.

157. Robb R. Refractive errors associated with hemangiomas of the eyelids and orbit in infancy. Am J Ophthamol 1977; 83: 52–58.

158. Ceisler EJ, Santos L, Blei F. Periocular hemangiomas: what every physician should know. Pediatr Dermatol 2004; 21: 1–9.

159. Haik BG, Jakobiec F, Ellsworth RM, et al. Capillary hemangiomas of the lid and orbit: an analysis of the clinical features and therapeutic results in 101 cases. Ophthalmology 1979; 86: 760–789.

160. Hughes JA, Hill V, Patel K, et al. Cutaneous hemangioma: prevalence and sonographic characteristics of associated hepatic hemangioma. Clin Radiol 2004; 59: 273–280.

161. Enjolras O, Riche MC, Merland JJ, et al. Management of alarming hemangiomas in infancy: a review of 25 cases. Pediatrics 1990; 85: 491–498.

162. Frieden IJ, Eichenfield LF, Esterly NB, et al. Guidelines of care for hemangiomas of infancy. J Am Acad Dermatol 1997; 37: 631–637.

163. Frieden IJ. Which hemangiomas to treat – and how? Arch Dermatol 1997; 133: 1593–1595.

164. Tanner JL, Dechert MP, Frieden IJ. Growing up with a facial hemangioma: parent and child coping and adaptation. Pediatrics 1998; 101: 446–451.

165. Kim HJ, Colombo M, Frieden IJ. Ulcerated hemangiomas: clinical characteristics and response to therapy. J Am Acad Dermatol 2001; 44: 962–972.

166. Metz BJ, Rubenstein MC, Levy ML, et al. Response of ulcerated perineal hemangiomas of infancy to becaplermin gel, a recombinant human platelet-derived growth factor. Arch Dermatol 2004; 140: 867–870.

167. Bennett ML, Fleischer AB Jr, Chamlin SL, Frieden IJ. Oral corticosteroid use is effective for cutaneous hemangiomas: an evidence-based evaluation. Arch Dermatol 2001; 137: 1208–1213.

168. Boon, LM, MacDonald DM, Mulliken JB. Complications of systemic corticosteroid therapy for problematic hemangioma. Plast Reconstr Surg 1999; 104: 1616–1623.

169. George ME, Sharma V, Jacobson J, et al. Adverse effects of systemic glucocorticosteroid therapy in infants with hemangiomas. Arch Dermatol 2004; 140: 963–969.

170. Aviles R, Boyce TG, Thompson DM. Pneumocystis carinii pneumonia in a 3-month-old infant receiving high-dose corticosteroid therapy for airway hemangiomas. Mayo Clin Proc 2004; 79: 243–245.

171. Halliday HL. The effect of postnatal steroids on growth and development. J Perinat Med 2001; 29: 281–285.

172. Sloan GM, Reinisch JF, Nichter LS, et al. Intralesional corticosteroid therapy for infantile hemangiomas. Plast Reconstr Surg 1989; 83: 459–466.

173. Nelson LB, Melick JE, Harley R. Intralesional corticosteroid injections for infantile hemangiomas of the eyelid. Pediatrics 1984; 74: 241–245.

174. Schorr N, Seiff SR. Central retinal artery occlusion associated with periocular corticosteroid injection for juvenile hemangioma. Ophthalmol Surg 1986; 17: 229–231.

175. Egbert JE, Schwartz GS, Walsh AW. Diagnosis and treatment of an ophthalmic artery occlusion during an intralesional injection of corticosteroid into an eyelid capillary hemangioma. Am J Ophthalmol 1996; 121: 638–642.

176. Goyal R, Watts P, Lane CM, et al. Adrenal suppression and failure to thrive after steroid injections for periocular hemangioma. Ophthalmology 2004; 111: 389–395.

177. Elsas FJ, Lewis AR. Topical treatment of periocular capillary hemangioma. J Pediatr Opthalmol Strabismus 1994; 31: 153–156.

178. Cruz OA, Zarnegar SR, Myers SE. Treatment of periocular capillary hemangioma with topical clobetasol propionate. Ophthalmology 1995; 102: 2012–2015.

179. Garzon MC, Lucky AW, Hawrot A, et.al. Ultrapotent topical corticosteroid treatment of hemangiomas of infancy. J Am Acad Dermatol 2005; 52: 281–286.

180. Ezekowitz R, Mulliken JB, Folkman J. Interferon alfa-2a treatment for life threatening hemangiomas of infancy. N Engl J Med 1992; 326: 1456–1463.

181. Chang E, Boyd A, Nelson CC, et al. Successful treatment of infantile hemangiomas with interferon-alfa-2b. J Pediatr Hematol Oncol 1997; 19: 237–244.

182. Tamayo L, Ortiz D, Orozco-Covarrubias L, et al. Therapeutic efficacy of interferon alfa-2b in infants with life-threatening giant hemangiomas. Arch Dermatol 1997; 133: 1567–1571.

183. Dubois J, Hershon DJ, Carman L, et al. Toxicity profile of interferon alfa-2b in children: A prospective evaluation. J Pediatr 1999; 135: 782–785.

184. Barlow C, Priebe C, Mulliken JB, et al. Spastic diplegia as a complication of interferon alfa-2a treatment of hemangiomas of infancy. J Pediatr 1998; 132: 527–530.

185. Michaud AP, Bauman NM, Burke DK, et al. Spastic diplegia and other motor disturbances in infants receiving interferon alpha. Laryngoscope 2004; 114: 1231–1236.

186. Grimal I, Duveau E, Enjolras O, et al. Efficacité et danger de l'interféron-α dans le traitement des hémangiomes graves du nourrisson. Arch Pediatr 2000; 7: 163–167.

187. Martinez MI, Sanchez-Carpintero I, North PE, et al. Infantile hemangioma: clinical resolution with 5% imiquimod cream. Arch Dermatol 2002; 138: 881–884.

188. Sidbury R, Neuschler N, Neuschler E, et al. Topically applied imiquimod inhibits vascular tumor growth in vivo. J Invest Dermatol 2003; 121: 1205–1209.

189. Welsh O, Olazaran Z, Gomez M, et al. Treatment of infantile hemangiomas with short-term application of imiquimod 5% cream. J Am Acad Dermatol 2004; 51: 639–642.

190. Hazen PG, Carney JF, Engstrom CW, et al. Proliferating hemangioma of infancy: successful treatment with topical 5% imiquimod cream. Pediatr Dermatol 2005; 22: 254–256.

191. Haisley-Royster C, Enjolras O, Frieden IJ, et al. Kasabach–Merritt phenomenon: a retrospective study of treatment with vincristine. J Pediatr Hematol Oncol 2002; 24: 459–462. Erratum in: J Pediatr Hematol Oncol 2002; 24: 794.

192. Adams DM. The nonsurgical management of vascular lesions. Facial Plast Clin North Am 2001; 9: 601–608.

193. Payarols P, Masferrer P, Bellvert G. Treatment of life-threatening hemangiomas with vincristine. N Engl J Med 1995; 333: 69.

194. Hu B, Lachman R, Phillips J, et al. KasabachéMerritt syndrome-associated kaposiform hemangioendothelioma successfully treated with cyclophosphamide, vincristine, and actinomycin D. J Pediatr Hematol Oncol 1998; 20: 567–569.

195. Moore J, Lee M, Garzon M, et al. Effective therapy of a vascular tumor of infancy with vincristine. J Pediatr Surg 2001; 36: 1273–1276.

196. Fawcett SL, Grant I, Hall PN, et al. Vincristine as a treatment for a large haemangioma threatening vital functions. Br J Plast Surg 2004; 57: 168–171.

197. Enjolras O, Varotti E, Brévière GM, et al. Traitement par vincristine des hémangiomes graves du nourrisson. Arch Pediatr 2004; 11: 99–107.

198. Garden JM, Bakus AD, Paller AS. Treatment of cutaneous hemangiomas by the flashlamp-pumped pulsed dye laser: prospective analysis. J Pediatr 1992; 120: 555–560.

199. Hohenleutner S, Badur-Ganter E, Landthaler M, Hohenleutner U. Long-term results in the treatment of childhood hemangioma with the flashlamp-pumped pulsed dye laser: an evaluation of 617 cases. Lasers Surg Med 2001; 28: 273–277.

200. Ashinoff R, Geronemus RG. Failure of the flashlamp-pumped pulsed dye laser to prevent progression to deep hemangioma. Pediatr Dermatol 1993; 10: 77–80.

201. Batta K, Goodyear HM, Moss C, et al. Randomised controlled study of early pulsed-dye laser treatment of uncomplicated childhood haemangiomas: results of a 1-year analysis. Lancet 2002; 360: 521–527.

202. Witman PM, Wagner AM, Scherer K, et al. Complications following pulsed dye laser treatment of superficial hemangiomas. Lasers Surg Med 2006; 38: 116–123.

203. Morelli JG, Tan OT, Weston WL. Treatment of ulcerated hemangiomas with the pulsed tunable dye laser. Am J Dis Child 1991; 145: 1062–1064.

204. David LR, Malek MM, Argenta LC. Efficacy of pulse dye laser therapy for the treatment of ulcerated hemangiomas: a review of 78 patients. Br J Plast Surg 2003; 56: 317–327.

205. Berlien HP, Müller G, Waldschmidt J. Lasers in pediatric surgery. Prog Pediatr Surg 1990; 2: 5–22.

206. Cremer HJ, Djawari D. Fruththerapie der kutanen hemangiome mit der kontaktkryochirugie. Chir Praxis 1995; 49: 295–312.

207. Wilson-Jones E, Orkin M. Tufted angioma (angioblastoma): a benign progressive angioma not to be confused with Kaposi's sarcoma or low grade angiosarcoma. J Am Acad Dermatol 1989; 20: 214–225.

208. Catteau B, Enjolras O, Delaporte E, et al. Angiome en touffes sclérosant. A propos de 4 observations. Ann Dermatol Venereol 1998; 125: 682–687.

209. Lam WY, Mac-Moune Lai F, Look CN, et al. Tufted angioma with complete regression. J Cutan Pathol 1994; 21: 461–466.

210. Ishikawa K, Hatano Y, Ichikawa H., et al. The spontaneous regression of tufted angioma. A case of regression after two recurrences and a review of 27 cases reported in the literature. Dermatology 2005; 210: 346–348.

211. Léauté-Labreze C, Bioulac-Sage P, Labbé L, et al. Tufted angioma with platelet trapping syndrome: response to aspirin. Arch Dermatol 1997; 133: 1077–1079.

212. Zukerberg LR, Nickoloff BJ, Weiss SW. Kaposiform hemangioendothelioma of infancy and childhood: an aggressive neoplasm associated with Kasabach–Merritt syndrome and lymphangiomatosis. Am J Surg Pathol 1993; 17: 321–328.

213. Lyons LL, North PE, Mac-Moune Lai F, et al. Kaposiform hemangioendothelioma. A study of 33 cases emphasizing its pathologic, immunophenotypic, and biologic uniqueness from juvenile hemangioma. Am J Surg Pathol 2004; 28: 559–568.

214. Chu CY, Hsiao CH, Chiu HC. Transformation between kaposiform hemangioendothelioma and tufted angioma. Dermatology 2003; 206: 334–337.

215. Gruman A, Liang MG, Mulliken JB, et al. Kaposiform hemangioendothelioma without Kasabach–Merritt phenomenon. J Am Acad Dermatol 2005; 52: 616–622.

216. Kasabach HH, Merritt KK. Capillary hemangioma with extensive purpura, report of a case. Am J Dis Child 1940; 59: 1063–1070.

217. Enjolras O, Wassef M, Mazoyer E, et al. Infants with Kasabach–Merritt syndrome do not have 'true' hemangioma. J Pediatr 1997; 130: 631–640.

218. Tsang WYW, Chan JKC. Kaposi-like hemangioendothelioma: a distinctive vascular neoplasm of the retroperineum. Am J Surg Pathol 1991; 15: 982–989.

219. Niedt GW, Greco MA, Wieczorek R, et al. Hemangioma with Kaposi's sarcoma-like features: report of two cases. Pediatr Pathol 1989; 9: 567–575.

220. Vin-Christian K, McCalmont TH, Frieden IJ. Kaposiform hemangioendothelioma, an aggressive locally invasive vascular tumor that can mimic hemangioma of infancy. Arch Dermatol 1997; 133: 1573–1578.

221. Sarkar M, Mulliken JB, Kozakewich HPW, et al. Thrombocytopenic coagulopathy (Kasabach–Merritt phenomenon) is associated with kaposiform hemangioendothelioma and not with common infantile hemangioma. Plast Reconstr Surg 1997; 100: 1377–1386.

222. Raman S, Ramanujam T, Lim CT. Prenatal diagnosis of an extensive hemangioma of the fetal leg: a case report. J Obstet Gynecol Res 1996; 22: 375–378.

223. Enjolras O, Mulliken JB, Wassef M, et al. Residual lesions after Kasabach–Merritt phenomenon in 41 patients. J Am Acad Dermatol 2000; 42: 225–235.

224. Enjolras, M. Wassef, C. Dosquet, et al. Syndrome de Kasabach–Merritt sur angiome en touffes congénital. Ann Dermatol Venereol 1998; 125: 257–260.

225. North PE, Kahn T, Cordisco MR, et al. Multifocal lymphangioendotheliomatosis with thrombocytopenia: a newly recognized clinicopathologic entity. Arch Dermatol 2004; 140: 599–606.

226. Prasad V, Fishman S, Mulliken JB, et al. Cutaneovisceral angiomatosis with thrombocytopenia. Pediatr Dev Pathol 2005; 8: 407–419.

227. Enzinger FM, Weiss SW. Infantile myofibromatosis. In: Soft tissue tumors. St Louis: Mosby, 1995; 77–83.

228. Fletcher CDM. The evolving classification of soft tissue tumours: an update based on the new WHO classification. Histopathology 2006; 48: 3–12.

229. Perkins P, Weiss SW. Spindle cell hemangioendothelioma: an analysis of 78 cases with reassessment of its pathogenesis and biologic behavior. Am J Surg Pathol 1996; 20: 1196–1204.

230. Nakatsui TC, Schloss E, Krol A, Lin AN. Eccrine angiomatous hamartoma: report of a case and literature review. J Am Acad Dermatol 1999; 41: 109–111.

231. SanMartin O, Botella R, Alegre V, et al. Congenital eccrine angiomatous

hamartoma. Am J Dermatopathol 1992; 14: 161–164.

232. Nakatsui TC, Schloss E, Krol A, Lin AN. Eccrine angiomatous hamartoma: report of a case and literature review. J Am Acad Dermatol 1999; 41: 109–111.

233. Frieden IJ, Esterly NB. Pyogenic granulomas of infancy masquerading as strawberry hemangiomas. Pediatrics 1992; 90: 989–999.

234. Ho V, Krol A, Bhargava R, Osiovich H. Diffuse neonatal haemangiomatosis. J Paediatr Child Health 200; 36: 286–289.

235. Rothe MJ, Rowse D, Grant-Kels JM. Benign neonatal hemangiomatosis with aggressive growth of cutaneous lesions. Pediatr Dermatol 1991; 8: 140–146.

236. Patrice SJ, Wiss K, Mulliken JB. Pyogenic granuloma (lobular capillary hemangioma): a clinicopathologic study of 178 cases. Pediatr Dermatol 1991; 8: 267–276.

237. Pagliai KA, Cohen BA. Pyogenic granuloma in children. Pediatr Dermatol 2004; 21: 10–13.

Hypopigmentation Disorders

Yuin-Chew Chan, Yong-Kwang Tay

A diverse group of diseases present with hypopigmentation in neonates. A practical clinical approach would be to categorize them according to the distribution of the hypopigmentation: generalized, mosaic, or localized (Box 21-1). Some may be present at birth, but not noticed until later in infancy because neonates often have a lighter skin at birth than in later life.

Any defect occurring in melanocyte development, melanin synthesis and transport, or distribution of melanosomes to keratinocytes can result in a hypopigmentary disorder. Melanocytes originate from the neural crest and are located in the epidermis, hair bulb, eye (choroid, ciliary body, iris), inner ear (cochlea) and central nervous system (leptomeninges). Melanin is synthesized in melanosomes, which are organelles that share characteristics with lysosomes.

This chapter discusses a variety of clinical conditions causing hypopigmentary disorders in neonates, many of which have a genetic basis.

GENERALIZED HYPOPIGMENTATION OF SKIN, HAIR, AND EYES

Oculocutaneous Albinism

Oculocutaneous albinism (OCA) refers to a group of autosomal recessive disorders involving abnormal melanin synthesis. Affected individuals have absent or reduced pigmentation in the skin, hair, and eyes from birth. The color varies from white to brown, depending on ethnicity and the specific type of OCA. Ocular manifestations include nystagmus, photophobia, and decreased visual acuity. These are caused by decreased melanin within the eye or misrouting of optic nerve fibers. The affected neonate is typically less pigmented than unaffected siblings.

Historically, OCA was divided into two clinical types based on the presence or absence of tyrosinase, the rate-limiting enzyme in the melanin biosynthetic pathway.[1] Advances in molecular genetics have given rise to a more accurate classification and better understanding of pathogenesis.[2,3] In OCA, epidermal and follicular melanocytes are present in normal quantity and distribution but do not synthesize melanin adequately (Table 21.1).

Oculocutaneous Albinism Type 1

Oculocutaneous albinism type 1 (OCA1) is the second most common OCA worldwide.

Cutaneous Findings

In OCA1A there is marked generalized hypopigmentation at birth, with white hair and skin (Figs 21-1 and 21-2). As the child matures, the skin remains white. Nevi are nonpigmented and sun tanning does not occur. The hair may acquire a slightly yellowish tint as a result of denaturing of hair keratins.

In OCA1B the variable decrease in tyrosinase activity results in several clinical phenotypes: yellow, minimal pigment, platinum, and temperature sensitive. Individuals with OCA1B form pheomelanin, which requires less tyrosinase activity, and this results in some pigment production during the first and second decades of life.[4] Affected individuals have a similar appearance to those with OCA1A at birth, but with time develop some pigment. Hair color can change from white to light blond, and even progress to light brown in adolescence. With sun exposure, some individuals with OCA1B may be able to tan, although it is more common to burn without tanning. Pigmented nevi and freckles may develop.[5]

An interesting subtype of OCA1B is the temperature-sensitive phenotype in which the tyrosinase activity is seen mainly on the extremities. In these patients, the enzyme has no activity at 37°C, but some activity at 35°C. These individuals have white or lightly pigmented hairs on the scalp and trunk (axillae, pubic area) and darkly pigmented hair peripherally (legs, arms). The pattern is similar to that observed in Siamese cats.[4]

Extracutaneous Findings

In OCA1A the irises are pale blue at birth and throughout life. In bright light the entire iris can appear pink or red, which is caused by its translucency.[5] Severe photophobia results from a lack of retinal pigment. Other ocular abnormalities include decreased visual acuity, nystagmus, and strabismus.

In OCA1B the irises can progressively darken to light tan or brown.

In both subtypes, vision may remain stable or deteriorate with age.

Etiology/Pathogenesis

OCA1 is caused by loss-of-function mutations in the tyrosinase gene (*TYR*), which is mapped to chromosome 11q14-q21. The OCA1A subtype is characterized by mutations that result in complete loss of tyrosinase activity, whereas OCA1B is caused by mutations that result in markedly reduced tyrosinase activity (5–10% of the normal level).

Oculocutaneous Albinism Type 2

Oculocutaneous albinism type 2 (OCA2) is the most common OCA. It is most prevalent in people of African descent.[6]

Box 21-1 Hypopigmentary disorders in neonates

Generalized hypopigmentation involving skin, hair and eyes
Oculocutaneous albinism

Hermansky-Pudlak syndrome

Chediak-Higashi syndrome

Cross syndrome

Metabolic disorders
Phenylketonuria
Histidinemia
Homocystinuria

Generalized hypopigmentation involving skin and hair
Griscelli syndrome

Elejalde syndrome

Menkes disease and occipital horn syndrome

Mosaic hypopigmentation
Nevoid hypopigmentation (Hypomelanosis of Ito)

Nevus depigmentosus

Localized hypopigmentation
Piebaldism

Waardenburg syndrome

Tuberous sclerosis complex

Nevus anemicus

Postinflammatory hypopigmentation

Congenital halo nevi

Miscellaneous Hypopigmentation
Alezzandrini syndrome

Ziprkowski-Margolis syndrome

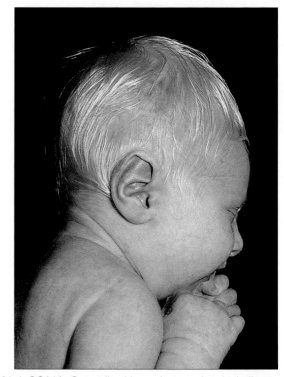

FIG. 21-1 OCA1A. Generalized hypopigmentation, including snow-white hair at birth.

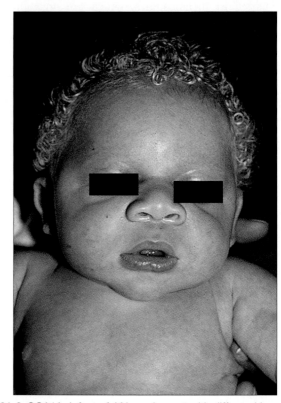

FIG. 21-2 OCA1A. Infant of African descent with diffuse skin and hair hypopigmentation.

Cutaneous Findings

There is a spectrum of clinical phenotypes, depending on the ethnic background and the dilution of hair and skin pigment, which may be minimal to moderate. Comparison with a first-degree relative may be necessary to distinguish the degree of lightening.[4] Most individuals are born with creamy white skin, and light yellow or blond hair. Depending on the individual's ethnic background, hair may also be reddish blond or brown. Pigmented birthmarks may be present. With maturity, the amount of pigment in the skin and hair tends to increase. In sun-exposed areas pigmented nevi and freckles can develop.

Extracutaneous Findings

The dilution of iris pigment may be mild to moderate. With age, the amount of pigment in the eyes tends to increase. Ocular manifestations are generally not as severe as those seen in OCA1A.[2] Visual acuity and nystagmus tend to improve with age.

OCA2 can be found in 1% of individuals with Prader–Willi and Angelman syndromes, which are associated with mental retardation and abnormal behaviour.[6]

Etiology/Pathogenesis

OCA2 results from loss-of-function mutations of the *P* gene, which is mapped to chromosome 15q11.2–q12.[7] The *P* gene encodes a melanosomal membrane protein. The specific function of the *P* protein is currently not known, but is believed to be involved in tyrosinase processing and transport.[8] The

melanocytes of affected individuals are able to synthesize some melanin, but the majority is yellow pheomelanin rather than black-brown eumelanin.

Prader–Willi syndrome involves deletions of the 15q region, including the *P* gene, on the paternally inherited copy of chromosome 15, whereas Angelman syndrome involves loss of the

TABLE 21-1 Classification of disorders with cutaneous and ocular albinism

	OCA 1A Tyrosinase negative	OCA 1B Tyrosinase positive	OCA 2 Tyrosinase positive	OCA 3 Rufous	OCA 4	HPS	CHS
Skin Color	White	White at birth, develop some pigmentation in first and second decades	Creamy white to brown at birth. Slight darkening with age	Light brown to red-bronze	Creamy white to brown at birth. Slight darkening with age	White to brown	Creamy white to slate grey
Pigmented nevi and freckles	Absent	Present	Present	Absent	Present	Many in exposed areas	Present
Hair color	White throughout life; may become light yellow	White to light yellow at birth; turns yellow or blonde in first few years	Light yellow, blond to brown at birth;m darkens with age	Light brown to red-brown. May darken with age	Silvery white to light yellow at birth. May darken in childhood	White, blonde to brown	Blonde to light brown; metallic silver grey sheen
Gene (mapping) Function	TYR gene (11q14-q21) Encodes tyrosinase	TYR gene (11q14-q21) Encodes tyrosinase	P gene (15q11.2-q12) May be involved in tyrosinase processing and transport	TYRP1 (9q23) Encodes dihydroxyindol carboxylic acid oxidase, a melanogenic enzyme	MATP (5p13.3) Encodes melasomal protein that likely functions as a transporter	HPS1: HPS1 (10q23.1) HPS2: AP3E1 (5q14.1) HPS3: HPS3 (3q24) HPS4: HPS4 (22c11.2-q12.2) HPS5: HPS5 (11p15-p13) HPS6: HPS6 (10c24.32) HPS7: DTNBP1 (6p22.3) 7 different gene mutations. Most encode proteins involved in biogenesis of lysosome-related proteins	LYST (1q42.1-q42.2) Encodes a large cytoplasmic protein which may function as an adapter protein that mediate intracellular membrane fusion reactions
Mouse model	Albino	Albino	Pink-eye dilution	Brown	Underwhite	HPS1: Pale-ear HPS2: Pear HPS3: Cocoa HPS4: Light-ear HPS5: Ruby eye 2 HPS6: Ruby eye HPS7: Sandy	Beige
Hair bulb melanosomes	Stages I, II	Stages I, II, III	Stages I, II, III	Stages I, II, III, IV	Stages I, II, III	Stages I, II, III	Macromelanosomes and normal to stage IV

maternally inherited allele. Deletion of one copy of the *P* gene associated with a mutation in the second copy results in OCA2 in these patients.[6]

Oculocutaneous Albinism Type 3

OCA3, previously called rufous OCA, is most commonly seen in people of African and Puerto Rican descent.[9,10]

Cutaneous Findings

At birth, individuals with this tyrosinase-positive OCA have light brown to red-brown skin and hair. With age, the hair becomes more pigmented. Mild sun tanning is possible.

Extracutaneous Findings

At birth, the irises are light brown and become more pigmented with age. Ocular manifestations are present, but less severe. Red reflex on transillumination of the iris and nystagmus are important clues to the diagnosis in dark-skinned people.

Etiology/Pathogenesis

OCA3 is due to loss-of-function mutations of tyrosinase-related protein-1 gene (*TYRP1*), which is mapped to chromosome 9q23.[11] The *TYRP1* gene encodes dihydroxyindol carboxylic acid oxidase, a melanogenic enzyme essential for eumelanin synthesis.[12]

Oculocutaneous Albinism Type 4

OCA4 is an OCA that was described only recently.[13] It is uncommon in German patients.[14] However, membrane-associated transporter protein (*MATP*) gene mutations were found in 24% of 75 unrelated Japanese patients with OCA, suggesting that OCA4 may be one of the most common types of OCA in Japan.[15]

Cutaneous Findings

The phenotype resembles that of OCA2 and the range of skin pigmentation is broad, from creamy white to brown. The hair is silvery white to light yellow at birth, and may darken in childhood.

Extracutaneous Findings

Ocular manifestations include nystagmus, decreased iris pigment with iris translucency, reduced retinal pigment, foveal hypoplasia associated with reduction in visual acuity, and strabismus.

Etiology/Pathogenesis

OCA4 results from mutations in the *MATP* gene, which is mapped to chromosome 5p13.3. The *MATP* gene encodes a melanosomal membrane protein that is likely to function as a transporter.[13] The similar functions of the *P* and *MATP* genes may explain the phenotypic resemblance of OCA2 and OCA4.

Differential Diagnosis

The diagnosis of OCA is usually made clinically and can be confirmed by DNA mutation analysis. Historically, the hair bulb incubator test for tyrosinase activity was used to differentiate between tyrosinase-positive and tyrosinase-negative OCA. In tyrosinase-negative albinism, there is the lack of pigment formation in hair bulbs when incubated with tyrosine, whereas in tyrosinase-positive albinism, pigment is produced. Prenatal diagnosis of OCA1 and OCA2 using DNA mutation analysis is available.

OCA can be differentiated from other disorders with cutaneous and ocular albinism by the absence of neurological defects, immunodeficiency, and bleeding diathesis.

Treatment and Care

No specific treatment is available for OCA. The importance of photoprotection, including sun avoidance, broad-spectrum sunscreen, protective eyewear and clothing, should be stressed to reduce the risk of photodamage and cutaneous malig-nancies. Early ophthalmologic evaluation and management is important. As cutaneous squamous cell carcinomas and basal cell carcinomas have been known to develop in all types of OCA, yearly examination by a dermatologist is recommended.

Hermansky–Pudlak syndrome

Hermansky-Pudlak syndrome (HPS) comprises seven genetically different autosomal recessive disorders characterized by tyrosinase-positive OCA, a bleeding diathesis, and a lysosomal ceroid storage disease affecting the viscera.[16–18] The majority of individuals affected are of Puerto Rican or Dutch descent. HPS type 1 is the most common.

Cutaneous Findings

The degree of pigmentary dilution in the skin and hair is highly variable. The color of the skin and hair ranges from white to brown.

Extracutaneous Findings

The degree of pigmentary dilution in the eyes is highly variable. Other ocular findings include nystagmus, reduced retinal pigment, and foveal hypoplasia with significant reduction in visual acuity. The nystagmus is most obvious during periods of fatigue or emotional change. The bleeding diathesis is caused by platelet storage pool deficiency and results in epistaxis, gingival bleeding, or bleeding after surgical procedures. Platelet numbers, prothrombin time, and partial thromboplastin time are normal but bleeding time is prolonged. The absence of dense bodies on electron microscopy of platelets is pathognomonic of HPS.[19] Lysosomal ceroid accumulation can result in interstitial pulmonary fibrosis, granulomatous colitis, cardiomyopathy, and renal failure. These life-threatening complications usually develop in adulthood.

Some patients with HPS type 2 have persistent neutropenia and suffer from recurrent bacterial infections.[20,21]

Etiology/Pathogenesis

Most of the HPS-related genes encode proteins involved in the biogenesis of lysosome-related organelles. Ceroid is produced by degradation of lipids and glycoproteins within lysosomes (Table 29-1).Ceroid accumulation in HPS suggests a defect in the elimination mechanisms of lysosomes.[22]

Differential Diagnosis

The diagnosis of HPS is made on clinical findings of oculocutaneous albinism, bleeding diathesis, and demonstration of absent dense bodies on electron microscopy of platelets. Molecular genetic testing of some HPS types, e.g. HPS1, HPS3, is available on a clinical basis. Differential diagnosis includes the Griscelli, Elejalde and Cross syndromes.

Treatment and Care

Photoprotection is important, as patients have a predisposition to develop basal cell carcinoma and squamous cell carcinoma. An examination by a dermatologist should be performed annually. Patients should avoid aspirin and trauma to minimize the chance of a bleeding episode. Platelet transfusions may be considered prior to surgical procedures. Cigarette smoking should be avoided, as this reduces pulmonary function and may hasten progression of pulmonary fibrosis.

Chediak–Higashi Syndrome

Chediak–Higashi syndrome (CHS) is an autosomal recessive disorder characterized by OCA, immunodeficiency, progressive neurological deterioration, and abnormal inclusions present in a wide variety of cells. This disorder has been identified in 10 species, including humans, the beige mouse, Hereford cattle, Aleutian mink, and killer whales.[23]

Cutaneous Findings

Compared to unaffected family members, the skin and the hair of affected individuals are both lighter in color. Cutaneous pigmentation is often slightly to moderately decreased. The hair is blond to light brown, often with a silvery tint (Fig. 21-3).

Recurrent skin and systemic pyogenic infections occur in early childhood. Cutaneous involvement usually manifests as a pyoderma, and there are a few reports of deeper involvement resembling pyoderma gangrenosum.[24]

Extracutaneous Findings

Loss of ocular pigmentation results in a translucent iris and pale retina, leading to photophobia and an increased red reflex. Visual acuity is normal, but strabismus and nystagmus are common.

Infections typically involve the skin, lungs, and upper respiratory tract. These intractable infections are often fatal before the age of 10 years. Common culprits include *Staphy-lococcus aureus*, *Streptococcus pyogenes*, and *Streptococcus pneumoniae*.

Progressive neurologic deterioration with clumsiness, abnormal gait, paresthesias, and dysesthesias is often apparent later in childhood. Other neurologic abnormalities include peripheral and cranial neuropathies, spinocerebellar degeneration, ataxia, seizures, decreased deep tendon reflexes, cranial nerve palsies, and motor weakness.[25–30]

Most patients with CHS eventually develop a lymphoproliferative syndrome ('accelerated phase') characterized by fever, hepatosplenomegaly, lymphadenopathy, pancytopenia, bleeding, and generalized lymphohistiocytic infiltrates.[26] Viral infections, particularly with the Epstein–Barr virus, have been implicated in causing the accelerated phase.[31,32]

Etiology/Pathogenesis

CHS results from mutations in the lysosomal trafficking regulator gene (*LYST*) gene. The *LYST* gene (1q42.1-q42.2) encodes a large cytoplasmic protein which appears to function as an adapter protein that mediates intracellular membrane fusion reactions.[33]

Natural killer (NK) cell function is drastically decreased. Diminished chemotaxis of granulocytes, monocytes, and lymphocytes has also been reported, as well as decreased antibody-dependent cytotoxicity and reduced suppressor T-cell function.[34–36] The resulting susceptibility to infections is caused by the combination of these factors.[37]

The diagnostic hallmark of CHS is the finding of giant lysosomal granules within leukocytes, melanocytes, platelets, and other cells due to uncontrolled fusion of lysosomes. In bone marrow myeloid cells, the giant granules appear prominent. In melanocytes, giant melanosomes result from uncontrolled fusion of melanosomes, and this failure to disperse melanin to adjacent keratinocytes accounts for the decrease in pigmentation.[38] On a cellular level, abnormal intracellular transport to and from the lysosomes has been detected.[39] Giant granules within the phagocytic cells cannot discharge their lysosomal and perioxidative enzymes into phagocytic vacuoles.[24,40] Prenatal diagnosis has been successfully performed using light microscopy by examining fetal hair shafts for characteristic clumping of melanosomes.[41]

Treatment and Care

Bone marrow transplantation (BMT) is the only definitive treatment for this disorder.[42] The NK cell defects and immunodeficiencies can be reversed, but the neurological deterioration and pigmentary dilution are not altered.[43,44]

Without BMT, patients who develop an accelerated phase usually die in childhood, usually from pyogenic infections or hemorrhage.[26] Patients who do not develop an accelerated phase tend to have fewer or no infections, but usually develop progressively debilitating neurologic manifestations.[45,46] Supportive treatments in early infancy include antibiotics for infections, and intravenous γ-globulin. Ascorbic acid has been shown to partially correct the granulocytic function in some patients.[34,35]

Cross Syndrome

Cross syndrome, or oculocerebral syndrome with hypopigmentation, is an oculocutaneous albinism associated with ocular anomalies, postnatal growth retardation, and neurological defects.[47–49] The inheritance is probably autosomal recessive.

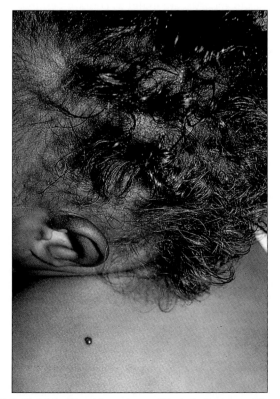

FIG. 21-3 Chediak–Higashi syndrome. The hair displays a silvery sheen.

Cutaneous Findings

The affected neonate has cutaneous generalized hypopigmentation and silvery hair.

Extracutaneous Findings

Ocular defects include microphthalmos, a small opaque cornea, and nystagmus. Neurological defects include mental retardation, ataxia, and spasticity.

Treatment and Care

Treatment is supportive.

Phenylketonuria

Phenylketonuria (PKU) is an autosomal recessive disorder that results from the impaired conversion of phenylalanine to tyrosine, which is caused by the absence of hepatic phenylalanine hydroxylase (PAH) activity. The absence of this enzyme leads to a build-up of the amino acid phenylalanine and its byproducts in the bloodstream and spinal fluid. The incidence in the United States is estimated at 1 in 10000 among caucasians.[50] It is most commonly observed in individuals of Scandinavian and northern European descent, with males and females equally affected. PKU without treatment results in mental retardation and oculocutaneous pigment dilution. Most affected individuals have blond hair, blue eyes, fair skin, photosensitivity, a musty body odor, and neurologic disturbances.[51]

Cutaneous Findings

At birth, the neonate appears normal but may have a musty odor secondary to urinary and sweat phenylacetic acid or phenylacetaldehyde. Caucasian children with PKU almost invariably have blond hair, blue eyes, fair skin, and photosensitivity. African-American and Asian children tend to be lighter in color than their parents and unaffected siblings. The ability to tan is normal. Endogenous eczema often develops in these patients.

Extracutaneous Findings

In affected babies, serum phenylalanine levels begin to rise on the third or fourth day of life. Newborn screening with the Guthrie inhibition assay test was implemented in the United States beginning in 1963, testing all newborns for PKU. Prenatal diagnosis is also possible by performing amniocentesis or chorionic villus sampling, with identification of the gene.[51] Untreated PKU results in neurologic defects, including mental retardation, seizures, psychosis, hyperreflexia, and growth retardation.

Etiology and Pathogenesis

Phenylalanine hydroxylase deficiency is caused by mutations in the *PAH* gene, with more than 400 different mutations identified so far.[52,53] Hypotheses to account for the decrease in skin and hair pigmentation include a competitive inhibition of the binding of tyrosine to tyrosinase by excess phenylalanine or a decreased amount of tyrosine.[54]

Treatment and Care

With a low-phenylalanine diet, the skin color, photosensitivity, odor, and eczema are reversible. Implementing a diet low in phenylalanine early in infancy can also dramatically reduce the mental retardation.[51] Although children with treated PKU typically have a lower IQ than the general population, affected individuals can be expected to have a low-normal to normal intelligence if blood phenylalanine is maintained at a reasonable level in early childhood.[55] Supplementation with tyrosine or tryptophan in the diet may be necessary. For women with PAH deficiency who are considering pregnancy, dietary restriction must be started before conception and continued throughout pregnancy.[56]

GENERALIZED HYPOPIGMENTATION INVOLVING SKIN AND HAIR

Griscelli Syndrome

Griscelli first described this syndrome in 1978.[57] It is a rare autosomal recessive syndrome that results in pigmentary dilution of the skin and hair, the presence of large clumps of pigment in hair shafts, and an accumulation of melanosomes in melanocytes. There are three types:

- Type 1 (GS1): association of hypopigmentation and neurological abnormalities, due to mutations of the *MYO5A* gene (15q21)[58,59]
- Type 2 (GS2): association of hypopigmentation and immunological abnormalities, due to *RAB27A* gene (4p13) mutation[60]
- Type 3 (GS3): only hypopigmentation, due to melanophilin (*MLPH*) gene (2q37) mutation.[61]

Cutaneous Findings[62–65]

In early childhood, individuals with all three types of GS have silvery gray hair, eyebrows, and eyelashes (findings that may also be present in the neonatal period), and skin hypopigmentation.[62–65]

Histologically, the hair shafts reveal uneven clumps of melanin, mainly in the medulla. Skin biopsy specimens reveal hyperpigmented oval melanocytes and poorly pigmented adjacent keratinocytes. On electron microscopic examination, epidermal melanocytes are found to contain perinuclear stage IV melanosomes. Adjacent keratinocytes contain only sparse melanosomes.[66]

Prenatal diagnosis of Griscelli syndrome has been accomplished by examination of hair from fetal scalp biopsies performed at 21 weeks' gestation, with confirmatory postabortion examination of the fetus revealing silvery hair and identical microscopic findings.[41]

Extracutaneous Findings[67]

Neurological defects in GS1 include intracranial hypertension, cerebellar signs, encephalopathy, hemiparesis, peripheral facial palsy, spasticity, hypotonia, seizures, psychomotor retardation, and progressive neurologic deterioration.[64–68]

Immunological abnormalities in GS2 result in severe pyogenic infections, due to defective release of cytotoxic lysosomal contents from hematopoietic cells, and a hemophagocytic syndrome.[66,69] There is combined T- and B-cell immunodeficiency. Frequent pyogenic infections, acute febrile episodes, neutropenia, and thrombocytopenia usually begin between 4 months of age and 4 years.[57,64,65,67,70–72] The hemophagocytic syndrome is characterized by acute onset of uncontrolled lymphocyte and macrophage activation, resulting in infiltration and hemophagocytosis in multiple organs and death.

Etiology/Pathogenesis

The *MYO5A*, *RAB27A* and *MLPH* genes encode respectively myosin 5a, rab27a and melanophilin, which form a complex that allows the transport of melanosomes on actin fibers and the docking of melanosomes on the dendritic tips.[61,73,74]

Differential Diagnosis

Differentiation from Chediak–Higashi syndrome can be made by pathognomonic light and electron microscopic features. Griscelli syndrome lacks the large cytoplasmic inclusions and granulocyte abnormalities that are characteristic of Chediak–Higashi syndrome. Both diseases, however, are associated with an accelerated phase and carry a poor prognosis without bone marrow transplantation.

Treatment and Care

Bone marrow transplant is most successful when performed early in the course of disease.[66,75]

Elojaldo Syndromo[76–78]

Elejalde syndrome, also called neuroectodermal melanolysosomal disease, is an autosomal recessive disorder characterized by silvery hair, hypopigmented skin, severe central nervous system dysfunction, and abnormal intracytoplasmic inclusions in fibroblasts, histiocytes, and lymphocytes.[76–78]

Cutaneous Findings

Neonates have silvery hair and generalized hypopigmentation of the skin, which may develop a bronze color after sun exposure.[79]

In homozygotes, abnormal melanolysosomes are found in melanocytes and keratinocytes, cultured fibroblasts, and histiocytes of bone marrow.

Extracutaneous Findings

Extracutaneous features include hypotonic facies, plagiocephaly, micrognathia, crowded teeth, a narrow high palate, pectus excavatum, and cryptorchidism. Neurological abnormalities range from severe hypotonia and the almost complete absence of movements, to seizures and spasticity. The age of onset of neurologic signs ranges from 1 month to 11 years.[78]

Differential Diagnosis[80–82]

Several authors have suggested that Elejalde syndrome in some patients and Griscelli syndrome type 1 are the same entity.[80–83]

Menkes' Disease and Occipital Horn Syndrome

Classic Menkes' disease is a multisystem disorder that manifests with hypopigmentation, hair abnormalities, failure to thrive, connective tissue changes, seizures, neurological degeneration, and death by the age of 3 years.[84] Most infants born with Menkes' disease appear normal for the first few months of life before showing a rapid decline in growth and neurologic development.

Cutaneous Findings

The cutaneous manifestations include alterations in hair, pigmentation, and elasticity of the skin.[85] The scalp hair may appear normal at birth, but by about 3 months of age it becomes sparse, light colored, lusterless, with a 'steel wool' quality. The hair is fragile and fractures easily, resulting in generalized alopecia (Fig. 21-4). Pili torti is the most common

hair shaft abnormality (Fig. 21-5), demonstrating a flattened appearance under light microscopy with multiple twists of 180° around the long axis of the shaft.[86] The twisted hairs result from excessive free sulfhydryl groups and a decrease in copper-dependent disulfide bonds. Cutaneous hypopigmenta-

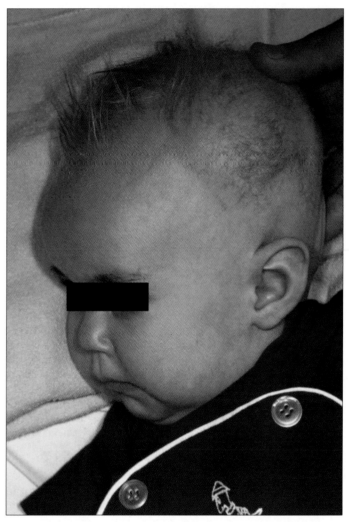

FIG. 21-4 Sparse, short, hypopigmented hair in Menkes' disease. (Reproduced with permission from Schachner L, Hansen R. Pediatric Dermatology, 3rd edn. Edinburgh: Mosby, 2003.)

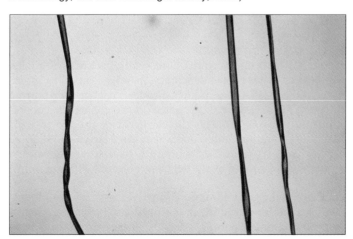

FIG. 21-5 Light microscopy showing pili torti. (Reproduced with permission from Schachner L, Hansen R. Pediatric Dermatology, 3rd edn. Edinburgh: Mosby, 2003.)

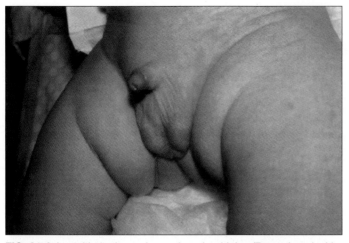

FIG. 21-6 Lax skin in the groins and on the thighs. (Reproduced with permission from Peterson J, Drolet BA, Esterly NB. Pediatr Dermatol 1998; 15: 137–139.)

TABLE 21-2 Effects of defective copper-dependent enzymes in Menkes Disease

Clinical Manifestations	Defective Enzyme (function)

Connective tissue abnormalities:
  Laxity of skin and joints
  Vascular abnormalities
  Bony abnormalities
  Bladder diverticulae
	Lysyl oxidase (cross-linkage of collagen and elastin)

Hypopigmentation	Tyrosinase (production of melanin)
Coarse, sparse brittle hair	Cross-linkase (cross-linkage of keratin)
Degeneration of myelin: seizures and spasticity	Superoxidase dismutase (detoxification of free radicals)
Deficient energy production: myopathy, ataxia, seizures	Cytochome C oxidase (electron transport)
Hypothalamic imbalances: hypothermia, dehydration, hypotension, somnolence	Dopamine ß hydroxylase (production of catecholamines)

tion is common, may be generalized or localized to the skin folds, and is caused by decreased tyrosinase, a copper-containing enzyme. The skin is lax, and this doughy laxity is most prominent over the posterior neck, eyebrows, and leg folds (Fig. 21-6).[85] Generalized puffiness of the cheeks and feet has been noted.

Extracutaneous Findings

Progressive neurodegeneration begins at about 2 months of age as a result of gliosis and demyelination of the cerebrum and cerebellum.[84] Patients present with seizures, hypothermia, developmental retardation, spontaneous subdural hematomas, muscle hypertonia, and feeding difficulties.[87] Urogenital problems include undescended testes, hydronephrosis, hydroureter, recurrent urinary tract infections, diverticula of the ureters and bladder, and rupture of the bladder. Skeletal abnormalities are manifested as wormian bones of the skull and spurring of long bone metaphyses. Connective tissue changes are evidenced by loose joints and tortuous blood vessels, such as the carotid and cerebellar arteries, which may cause intracranial hemorrhages. This increased tortuosity is secondary to fragmentation of the internal elastic lamina of the arteries. Low copper and ceruloplasmin levels in the serum and high copper levels in cultured fibroblasts are useful in the diagnosis.[88] Menkes' disease can be considered a disorder of copper maldistribution.

Etiology/Pathogenesis

Menkes' disease and occipital horn syndrome are rare, allelic, X-linked recessive copper deficiency disorders caused by mutations in the *ATP7A* gene, which encodes a copper-transporting P-type ATPase involved in transport of copper to copper-requiring proteins.[89,90] The clinical features are due to malfunction of one or more copper-requiring enzymes, such as lysyl oxidase, tyrosinase, cytochrome C oxidase, and dopamine β-hydroxylase, caused by the deficiency of the ATP7A protein[85] (Table 21-2).

Occipital horn syndrome, formerly classified as Ehlers–Danlos syndrome type IX, or X-linked cutis laxa, is now recognized as a milder form of Menkes' disease and is caused by mutations in the same gene. Occipital horn syndrome is characterized primarily by connective tissue abnormalities, including skin laxity, hyperextensible joints, urinary tract diverticuli,

hernias, and bony changes such as osteoporosis, arthrosis, and exostoses, such as the presence of a spike of ossification within the occipital insertion of the paraspinal muscles (occipital horns) which gives the syndrome its name.[91] Intelligence is normal or borderline, and patients can survive into adulthood. The milder phenotype results from the presence of low levels of functional ATP7A, unlike Menkes' disease, in which no normal ATP7A activity exists.[92,93]

Treatment and Care

Daily subcutaneous administration of copper-histidine has been shown to be helpful in preventing the severe neurodegenerative problems in some patients with Menkes' disease when the treatment is initiated early in life before the onset of significant neurological symptoms.[94,95] This treatment, however, does not prevent the development of connective tissue problems and should still be regarded as experimental.[95–97]

MOSAIC HYPOPIGMENTATION

Mosaicism refers to the presence of two or more genetically distinct cell lines within an individual. These cell lines may be due to X-inactivation, as is normal in all human females, or to postzygotic somatic mutation. When mosaicism affects the skin, the affected skin may show patchy hypopigmentation or hyperpigmentation in a linear or segmental distribution (Figs 21-7 and 21-8). (Pigmentary mosaicism associated with hyperpigmented disorders is discussed in Chapter 22, and other mosaic conditions in Chapter 26.) Segmental hypopigmented lesions may be seen as an isolated cutaneous skin condition or as part of a genetic syndrome. The presence of mosaicism can sometimes be documented by the karyotyping of lymphocytes from peripheral blood, or by fibroblast cultures from both involved and uninvolved skin, but in many cases chromosomal studies are normal, presumably because the defective gene is unable to be detected with currently available techniques.

In 1901 Blaschko characterized the distribution of segmental and linear skin abnormalities by examining patients with linear lesions and formulating a patterned composite diagram. He described these patterns as V-shaped or fountain-like over the spine, S-shaped or whorled on the anterior and lateral

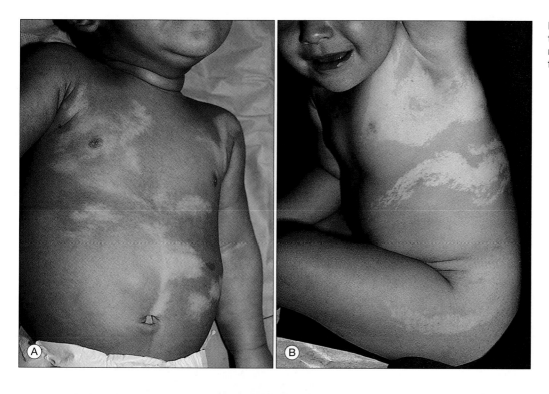

FIG. 21-7 Nevoid hypopigmentation. Whorls and streaks of macular hypopigmentation following lines of Blaschko.

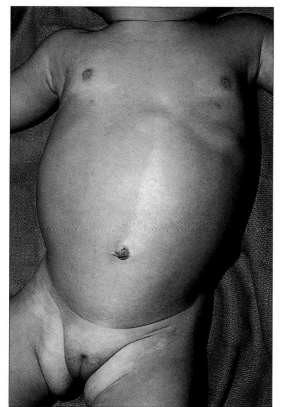

FIG. 21-8 Nevoid hypopigmentation without systemic anomalies. This child was otherwise well.

Nevoid Hypopigmentation, with or without Systemic Anomalies

In 1952 a Japanese dermatologist named Ito described a 21-year-old woman with hypopigmented cutaneous whorls and streaks.[100] As the distribution of the hypopigmentation was analogous to that of the hyperpigmented streaks observed in incontinentia pigmenti, he called the disorder incontinentia pigmenti achromians. To avoid confusion of these two unrelated entities, the preferred terminology later became 'hypomelanosis of Ito' (HI).[101]

HI is a descriptive term, rather than a diagnosis.[102] It is used for a phenotype with unilateral or bilateral hypopigmented streaks and whorls that follow the lines of Blaschko and which are present at birth or become apparent within the first 2 years of life (see Figs 21-7 and 21 8).[103] There may be associated systemic findings.

We advocate using the term 'nevoid hypopigmentation, with or without systemic anomalies' as it better reflects the heterogeneous nature of this group of disorders.

Cutaneous Findings

The hypopigmented whorls and streaks are distributed along the lines of Blaschko. They tend to be stable, although there are reported cases in which the pigmentary changes become more or less pronounced over time.[104] In some cases, both hypopigmented and hyperpigmented streaks are evident. Wood's lamp examination may help to determine the extent of the lesions in fair-skinned patients.

Extracutaneous Findings

Extracutaneous findings are variable, and include central nervous, musculoskeletal, and/or ocular abnormalities.[105] Defects of teeth, hair, nails, and sweat glands, as well as aplasia cutis, fibromas, and generalized or focal hypertrichosis, have been reported.[104,106,107] Additional abnormalities reported include limb-length discrepancies, facial hemiatrophy, scolio-

aspects of the trunk, and linear over the extremities (see Chapter 3) These lines should not be confused with dermatomes, which are the segments of skin that correspond to sensory innervation.[98] Hypopigmentation that follows the lines of Blaschko and segmental patterns is thought to reflect cellular migration during embryogenesis affecting pigmentation.[99]

sis, sternal abnormalities, dysmorphic facies, and genitourinary and cardiac anomalies. Nearly all of the defects are detectable by a thorough physical examination and regular follow-up. Infants should be observed for evidence of CNS involvement, reflected by developmental delay or seizures.[104] Most children with CNS involvement manifest with neurological abnormalities before 2 years of age.

Etiology/Pathogenesis

Chromosomal mosaicism has been found in about a third of patients. Multiple chromosomal abnormalities have been associated with HI, and most cases are sporadic and have negligible risk of recurrence.[101,106,108] On histologic examination, the hypopigmented areas have either normal or reduced numbers of melanocytes, and those melanocytes that are present demonstrate a reduction in the number of melanosomes.[109]

Differential Diagnosis

This includes nevus depigmentosus (also known as nevus achromicus) and Goltz syndrome. Patients with Goltz syndrome have both hyper- and hypopigmentation, as well as depressed areas of depigmentation following Blaschko's lines.

Treatment and Care

Cosmetic cover-up products such as Dermablend (Flori Roberts, Chicago, IL) or Covermark (Covermark Cosmetics, Rasbouck Heights, NJ) can be used to conceal the hypopigmented areas but are usually not needed. The use of sunscreens can prevent or lessen the accentuation of pigmentary differences.[104]

Nevus Depigmentosus
Cutaneous Findings

Nevus depigmentosus (nevus achromicus) is a well-circumscribed area of hypopigmentation that may occur as a small isolated (circular or rectangular) patch, or develop in a unilateral segmental distribution or follow the lines of Blaschko.[110] Hair within a nevus depigmentosus may also be hypopigmented, and the margins may be irregular or serrated. The isolated form is the most common (Fig. 21-9) and the lesions do not usually cross the midline.[111] The term depigmentosus is a misnomer because the lesions are actually hypopigmented, not completely depigmented, and become more prominent under Wood's lamp. They are usually present at birth or become evident shortly thereafter, and remain stable in size and shape. Increase in size is in proportion to the growth of the child. Some lesions may appear after 1 year of age.[111,112] Males and females are affected equally and there is no distinct pattern of inheritance.[110] The hypothesis is that during embryogenesis a clone of cells with a reduced melanogenic potential arises via a postzygotic somatic mutation.[98] The back and buttocks are the most commonly affected sites, followed by the chest and abdomen.[111]

Extracutaneous Findings

Systemic manifestations are rare in patients with nevus depigmentosus. Neurologic abnormalities such as seizures and mental retardation have been reported,[113] as well as ipsilateral hypertrophy of the extremities.[114] In a survey of 50 patients with nevus depigmentosus, none had any extracutaneous features on examination.[115] In two studies involving 29 patients with nevus depigmentosus, extracutaneous abnormalities were present in about 10% of the children.[112,116] Occasionally, lentigines can develop within the achromic nevi, and this could be explained by the reversion of a mutation in one of the genes involved in pigmentation.[117,118]

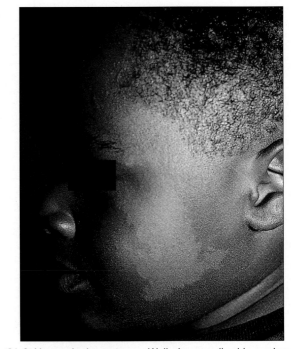

FIG. 21-9 Nevus depigmentosus. Well-circumscribed hypopigmented patch on the cheek that was present at birth.

Etiology/Pathogenesis

With dopa-staining, normal melanocytes are seen in nevus depigmentosus and electron microscopic studies suggest a reduced synthesis of melanosomes and also a defect in their transfer to the keratinocytes, which could account for the hypopigmentation.[119] Transfer of melanosomes from melanocytes to keratinocytes is essential for normal pigmentation.

Differential Diagnosis

Other entities with which nevus depigmentosus is sometimes confused include nevus anemicus, segmental vitiligo, hypopigmented lesions of tuberous sclerosis, and hypomelanosis of Ito.

The distinction between nevus depigmentosus and hypomelanosis of Ito may be artificial, as many patients with segmental hypopigmented macules also have linear pigmentary anomalies, similar to those seen in hypomelanosis of Ito, and underlying mosaicism is the common factor.[104] Patients currently diagnosed with either of these conditions might simply be categorized as having nevoid hypopigmentation with or without extracutaneous anomalies. Cytogenetic analysis, which entails analysis of peripheral blood lymphocytes and skin fibroblasts, should be considered in all patients with segmental or linear pigmentary abnormalities and extracutaneous abnormalities to look for chromosomal mosaicism.[104]

Treatment and Care

One patient with a nevus depigmentosus had partial repigmentation following autologous melanocyte grafting,[120] but otherwise there is no effective treatment. Cosmetic camouflage may be helpful.

LOCALIZED HYPOPIGMENTED DISORDERS

Piebaldism

Piebaldism is an autosomal dominant condition caused by defective cell proliferation and migration of melanocytes during embryogenesis.

Cutaneous Findings

Piebaldism is characterized by congenital depigmented white patches of skin and hair on the forehead, central chest and abdomen, upper arms and lower legs, with normally pigmented skin on the hands and feet (Fig. 21-10). A white forelock which consists of a tuft of white hair over the midfrontal scalp is present in 80–90% of patients and is associated with depigmentation of the underlying scalp.[121] Additional findings include poliosis of the eyebrows and eyelashes. The presence of islands of normally pigmented and hyperpigmented macules within the depigmented patches is typical and aids in the cli-nical diagnosis.[122] The lesions are generally stable in size and increase in proportion to the growth of the child, although in some cases spontaneous contraction or expansion with the appearance of new hyperpigmented macules has been reported.[123,124]

Light and electron microscopy studies show a complete absence of melanin and melanocytes in the epidermis and hair bulbs in the areas of leukoderma and poliosis.[119] The hyper-melanotic macules contain a normal number of melanocytes, but an abundance of abnormal melanosomes that are granular and spherical in shape.

Extracutaneous Findings[125–128]

Piebaldism is not typically associated with abnormalities of other organs, although associated mental retardation has been reported.[125] This may represent contiguous gene deletion syndromes, with inclusion of the *KIT* gene responsible for piebaldism as well as nearby genes whose absence result in neurologic deficits. There have been four reports of piebaldism associated with neurofibromatosis type 1.[126–128] Whether the simultaneous occurrence of these two dominantly inherited diseases is more than chance remains to be established.

Etiology/Pathogenesis

Piebaldism results from mutations of the *KIT* gene on chromosome 4q11-q12.[129] This codes for the tyrosine kinase transmembrane cellular receptor for mast/stem cell growth factor, a critical factor for melanoblast migration, proliferation, differentiation, and survival. The *KIT* proto-oncogenes consist of an extracellular ligand-binding domain, a transmembrane domain, and a cytoplasmic tyrosine kinase domain.[130] The severity of the clinical phenotype in piebaldism correlates with the site of the mutation within the *KIT* gene.[131,132] The most severe mutations tend to be dominant negative missense mutations involving the intracellular tyrosine kinase domain. Mutations causing an intermediate severity phenotype have largely been located at the transmembrane region, and the mildest phenotypes are those that occur in the amino terminal extracellular ligand-binding domain. Recently it has been shown that *KIT* activation induces the expression of a zinc-finger neural crest transcription factor SLUG, and that SLUG is necessary for the normal development of melanocytes, hematopoietic stem cells, and germ cells.[133] It has been shown that deletions in the SLUG (*SNA12*) gene on chromosome 8q11 are responsible for some cases of piebaldism that lacked mutations in *KIT*.[134]

Differential Diagnosis

Disorders with similar clinical presentations are vitiligo and Waardenburg syndrome. Vitiligo is acquired later in life, tends to progress, and has a different distribution. Waardenburg syndrome is the major entity in the differential diagnosis of piebaldism, and the patient should be examined for evidence of facial dysmorphism, heterochromia of the irides, and congenital sensorineural hearing loss.

Treatment and Care

Photoprotection of the depigmented patches is important, beginning early in life to protect the amelanotic areas from burning with sun exposure and to avoid skin cancers later on. Cosmetic camouflage or the use of a pigmenting tanning product such as dihydroxyacetone to camouflage the depigmented lesions are useful, although temporary.[135] PUVA therapy is generally disappointing,[136] but a combination of dermabrasion and split-thickness skin grafting followed by minigrafting[137] or the use of autologous cultured epidermal grafts[138] may be worthwhile in selected patients.

Waardenburg Syndrome

Waardenburg syndrome is a rare autosomal dominant disorder characterized by depigmented patches of the skin and hair, heterochromia iridis, congenital nerve deafness, and craniofacial anomalies. It is caused by the absence of melanocytes in the skin, hair, eyes, and stria vascularis of the cochlea, and is classified as a disorder of neural crest development.[139]

The estimated incidence of Waardenburg syndrome is 1 in 42000 in the Netherlands[140] and 1 in 20000 in Kenya.[141] It accounts for between 2% and 5% of cases of congenital deafness.[142] Both sexes and all races are equally affected.[143] Four types of Waardenburg syndrome have been described on clinical and genetic grounds (Box 21-2).

Cutaneous and Extracutaneous Findings

Affected persons have a depigmented patch, often V-shaped, on the central forehead in association with a white forelock.[140] Premature graying of the hair may occur. Depigmented patches with irregular borders containing hyperpigmented macules, resembling piebaldism, as well as hyperpigmented macules as normally pigmented skin, have been described.[143] Histology reveals a reduced number or complete absence of melanocytes

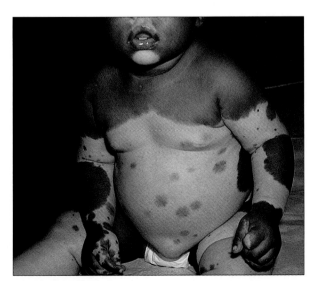

FIG. 21-10 Piebaldism.

Box 21-2 Types of Waardenburg Syndrome

Type 1:
1. Autosomal dominant
2. Dystopia canthorum
3. White forelock (poliosis)
4. Piebald skin lesions
5. Synophrys (thickening of medial eyebrows)
6. Broad nasal root
7. Hypoplasia of nasal alae
8. Heterochromia irides
9. Congenital sensorineural hearing loss
10. PAX 3 gene mutations (chromosome 2q35)

Type II:
1. Autosomal dominant
2. Similar features to type I, but lacks dystopia canthorum
3. MITF mutations (chromosome 3p12)

Type III (Klein-Waardenburg):
1. Autosomal dominant
2. Similar features to type I
3. Musculoskeletal abnormalities
4. PAX 3 gene mutations (chromosome 2q35)

Type IV (Shah-Waardenburg):
1. Autosomal recessive
2. Craniofacial abnormalities
3. No dystopia canthorum
4. Extensive depigmentation
5. Hirschsprung disease
6. Endothelin-3 gene mutations or one of its receptors, endothelin beta receptor (chromosome 13q22)

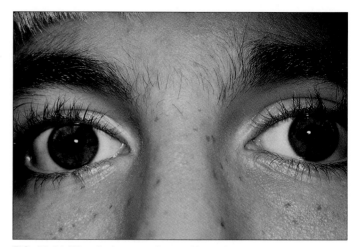

FIG. 21-11 Waardenburg syndrome. (Reproduced with permission from Bolognia, Jorizzo, Rapini. Dermatology 2003; 1: 960.)

Type IV Waardenburg syndrome (Shah–Waardenburg syndrome) is the association of Waardenburg syndrome with Hirschsprung disease (congenital aganglionic megacolon).[152]

Etiology/Pathogenesis

Waardenburg syndrome types 1 and 3 are allelic variants and due to mutations in the *PAX3* gene on chromosome 2q.[153] *PAX3* is one of a family of paired box genes that control neural crest differentiation by regulating the transcription of a number of other genes involved in embryological development. The neural crest gives rise not only to melanocytes but also to the bony and cartilaginous structures of the central face, accounting for the dysmorphic features associated with Waardenburg syndrome. Most mutations in *PAX3* result in Waardenburg syndrome type 1. Simple loss of function of one allele will result in the type 1 phenotype due to haploinsufficiency for the *PAX3* gene product (heterozygotes). A small fraction of *PAX3* mutations result in the more severe type 3 phenotype, and some of these patients are heterozygous for the *PAX3* mutation, suggesting a gene dosage effect.[154]

Waardenburg syndrome type 2 is caused by mutations in the gene encoding the microphthalmia association transcription factor (MITF), mapped to chromosome 3p.[155] The MITF gene product is a dimeric transcription factor of the basic–helix–loop–helix–leucine zipper class that is expressed in skin, hair follicles, retina and otic vesicles, and is involved in melanocyte differentiation. Type 2 Waardenburg syndrome is a heterogeneous group and some patients are heterozygous for mutations in the *MITF* gene, resulting in haploinsufficiency of the MITF protein due to loss of function mutations in one of the alleles of the *MITF* gene.[156] *MITF* is downstream of *PAX3*, and this hierarchy of effect explains the lesser facial abnormalities in Waardenburg syndrome type 2 compared to type 1.

Waardenburg syndrome type 4 is a rare autosomal recessive condition caused by mutations in the genes for endothelin-3 (*EDN3*), or one of its receptors, endothelin β receptor (*EDNRB*) or the *SOX10* gene.[157,158] All of these genes are functionally interrelated and contribute to the formation of the nervous system. *EDNRB* mutations are dosage sensitive: heterozygosity predisposes to isolated Hirschsprung disease, whereas homozygosity results in more complex neurocristopathies associating Hirschsprung disease and Waardenburg syndrome.[159]

within the depigmented areas.[144] Synophrys, or fusion of the medial eyebrows, is typical in Waardenburg syndrome. Heterochromia irides, or differently colored irises may be present, as well as sectorial areas of diminished pigment in a single iris[145] (Fig. 21-11). Type 1 Waardenburg syndrome is typified by the presence of dystopia canthorum, or an increase in the inner canthal distance, without change in the interpupillary distance. If the inner canthal distance divided by the interpupillary distance exceeds 0.6, dystopia canthorum is present.[145] In type 2 Waardenburg syndrome, dystopia canthorum is absent.[146] Additional facial features include a broad nasal root, hypoplastic alar cartilage, a thin upper lip and a protuberant lower lip.[140]

Congenital sensorineural hearing loss is a hallmark of all forms of Waardenburg syndrome and may be unilateral or bilateral.[140,146] Histopathologic examination of the inner ears has shown absent organs of Corti, atrophy of the spinal ganglion, and reduction of nerve fibers.[147] Hearing loss and heterochromia irides are more common in type 2 than in type 1 Waardenburg syndrome.[148] Rarely cleft lip and palate[149] and neural tube defects such as spina bifida[150] have been reported in association with Waardenburg syndrome.

Waardenburg syndrome type III (Klein–Waardenburg syndrome) is similar to type 1, but is also accompanied by musculoskeletal anomalies of upper limbs and pectoral areas.[151]

Differential Diagnosis

Piebaldism should be considered in patients with dominantly inherited patchy depigmentation. The pigmentary disturbances are very similar in both Waardenburg syndrome and piebaldism, but auditory and facial developmental anomalies are absent in piebaldism.[143] Fisch syndrome should be considered in cases of premature graying of the hair and congenital deafness.[160] The association of deafness and vitiligo with an autosomal recessive mode of inheritance is known as Rozycki syndrome.[161]

Treatment and Care

Physical findings suggestive of Waardenburg syndrome in neonates warrant a hearing evaluation, as detection of the associated deafness allows for early intervention with hearing aids and specialized education. Treatment options for the leukoderma are the same as those for piebaldism.

Tuberous Sclerosis Complex

Tuberous sclerosis complex (TSC) (see also Chapter 24) is an autosomal dominant condition with variable penetrance, characterized by cutaneous and neurologic abnormalities such as mental retardation and seizures as well as visceral hamartomas. Spontaneous mutations account for 66–86% of cases.[162,163] Estimates of prevalence range from 1:6000 to 1:10000.[164,165]

Criteria for diagnosis can be found in Box 21-3.[166]

Box 21-3 Diagnostic Criteria for Tuberous Sclerosis Complex

Major Features:

1. Facial angiofibromas or forehead plaque
2. Nontraumatic ungual or periungual fibroma
3. Hypomelanotic macules (three or more)
4. Shagreen patch (connective tissue nevus)
5. Multiple retinal nodular hamartomas
6. Cortical tuber
7. Subependymal nodule
8. Subependymal giant cell astrocytoma
9. Cardiac rhabdomyoma, single or multiple
10. Lymphangiomyomatosis
11. Renal angiomyolipoma

Minor Features:

1. Multiple randomly distributed pits in dental enamel
2. Hamartomatous rectal polyps
3. Bone cysts
4. Cerebral white matter radial migration lines
5. Gingival fibromas
6. Non-renal hamartoma
7. Retinal achromic patch
8. 'Confetti' skin lesions
9. Multiple renal cysts
   Definite TSC: either 2 major features or 1 major feature plus 2 minor features
   Probable TSC: one major plus 1 minor feature
   Possible TSC: either 1 major feature or 2 or more minor features
   (Roach ES, Gomez MR, Northrup H. J Child Neurol 1998; 13: 624–628)

Cutaneous Findings

Hypomelanotic macules or patches are the earliest sign of tuberous sclerosis complex and are present in up to 90% of patients.[163] The lesions are usually present from birth, but occasionally develop later in infancy or childhood. They have a partial rather than complete loss of pigmentation, and perifollicular pigmentation may be observed in some of them.[110] Multiple hypopigmented macules are of concern for TSC, although three or fewer may be a variant of normal and occur in otherwise healthy individuals.[167] Examination under Wood's lamp may be necessary to detect subtle lesions in fair-skinned individuals.[168] The hypopigmented macules can be polygonal (thumbprint), lanceovate (ash-leaf spot) or guttate (confetti-like)[169] (Figs 21-12 and 21-13). Confetti-like lesions appear as

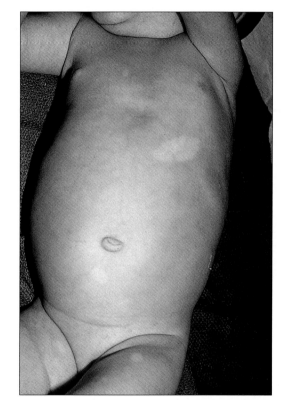

FIG. 21-12 Tuberous sclerosis. Hypopigmented macules and patches in an infant with cardiac rhabdomyoma.

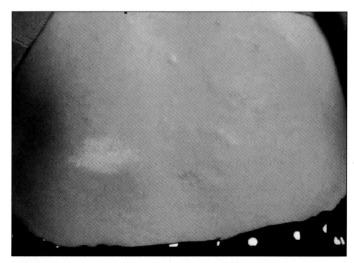

FIG. 21-13 Tuberous sclerosis. Hypopigmented macule with shagreen patch.

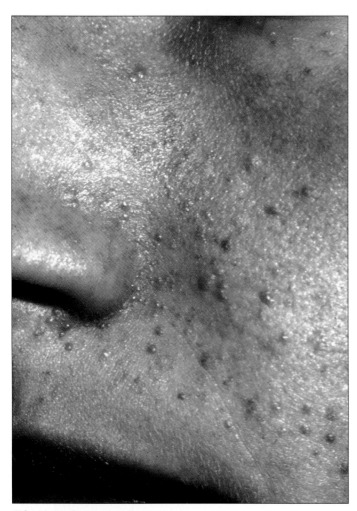

FIG. 21-14 Facial angiofibromas.

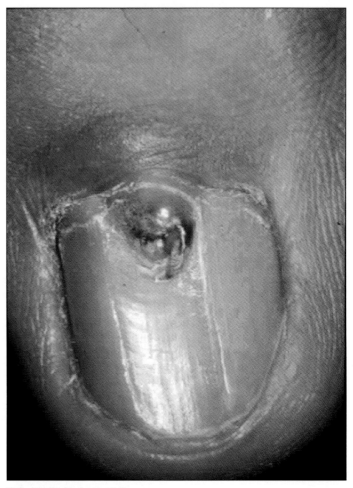

FIG. 21-15 Periungual fibromas.

multiple small areas of stippled hypopigmentation, typically on the extremities. Poliosis of scalp hair, eyebrows, or eyelashes may be seen in patients with TSC,[170] as well as circumscribed hypopigmentation of the iris or fundus.[171] Electron microscopy of the hypopigmented macules reveals smaller organelles and a reduction in the size and number of the melanosomes, which exist mainly in the unmelanized stages.[119]

Facial angiofibromas (adenoma sebaceum) are made up of vascular and connective tissue elements and are present in three-quarters of patients.[172] They are first noticed between the ages of 2 and 5 as a few small red papules on the malar area, and gradually become larger and more numerous, sometimes extending down the nasolabial folds and onto the chin (Fig. 21-14). A fibrous plaque may be seen on the forehead or scalp, is typically present from birth or early infancy, and has a similar histologic appear to an angiofibroma.[166] The shagreen patches, which are connective tissue nevi, are found in 20–30% of TSC patients, typically on the back or flank.[163] They appear as slightly raised areas with dimpling at areas of follicular openings, giving the appearance of 'orange peel' or 'gooseflesh'. Ungual and periungual fibromas are nodular or fleshy lesions that arise adjacent to or from underneath the nails (Fig. 21-15). Ungual fibromas usually occur in adolescents or adults, and are seen in 15–20% of TSC patients.[163] Although they are highly suggestive of TSC, these lesions may occasionally develop spontaneously[173] or after trauma. Examination of the mouth can reveal gingival fibromas and small dental enamel pits. Dental pits are more common in older patients with TSC than in unaffected individuals, and particularly affect the permanent teeth.[174]

Extracutaneous Findings

These include retinal hamartomas, seen in up to 87% of patients, and appear as classic mulberry lesions adjacent to the optic disc.[175] Most retinal lesions are clinically insignificant, although occasional patients may have visual impairment due to a large macular lesion, hamartoma enlargement, retinal detachment, or vitreous hemorrhage.

Up to two-thirds of TSC patients develop cardiac rhabdomyomas, detected by echocardiography.[163] The lesions tend to be multiple, and there is evidence that the majority regress with age.[176] Complications include congestive heart failure, cardiac arrhythmia, or cerebral thromboembolism.[177]

Renal involvement includes angiomyolipomas, which are benign tumors composed of varying amounts of vascular tissue, fat or smooth muscle, and occur in about two-thirds of TSC patients.[178] The prevalence of renal tumors increases with age, and larger lesions are more likely to become symptomatic than smaller tumors. Single or multiple renal cysts tend to appear earlier than the angiomyolipomas, and the combination of the two is characteristic of tuberous sclerosis complex.[163] Both angiomyolipomas and renal cysts are often asymptomatic and require no treatment. Hemorrhage is the most common complication of angiomyolipomas, causing hematuria and pain. Renal failure results from obstructive uropathy, or when cysts or tumors replace much of the normal renal parenchyma.

Pulmonary changes are rare, seldom cause symptoms, are five times more common in females, and tend to become clinically manifest in the second decade.[179] Recurrent spontaneous pneumothorax, dyspnea, cough, hemoptysis, and pulmonary failure are typical manifestations of pulmonary TSC.

Neurologic manifestations of TSC include mental retardation, seizures, and behavioral problems such as autism,[180] hyperkinesis, aggressiveness, and psychosis.[181] Neurologic lesions result from impaired cellular interaction, resulting in disrupted neuronal migration along radial glial fibers and abnormal proliferation of glial elements.[163] Neuropathologic lesions include subependymal nodules, cortical hamartomas, focal cortical hypoplasia, and heterotopic gray matter. The number of cortical tubers as observed by magnetic resonance imaging (MRI) has been shown to correlate with the severity of the cerebral dysfunction, with increased numbers of cortical tubers seen in patients with more severe cerebral disease.[182]

Etiology/Pathogenesis

Inactivating mutations in either of two tumor-suppressor genes – *TSC1* and *TSC2* – are the cause of this syndrome, with *TSC2* mutations accounting for 80–90% of all mutations.[183] *TSC1* contains 21 coding exons on chromosome 9q34 and encodes hamartin of 1164 amino acids; *TSC2* contains 41 exons on 16p13, which encodes tuberin of 1807 amino acids.[184,185] Recently, hamartin and tuberin were found to function as a complex that suppresses a major pathway for the stimulation of cell growth. The hamartin/tuberin complex inactivates GTPase Rheb, which is an activator of the growth-promoting protein kinases rapamycin (mTOR) and P70 s6 kinase (S6K).[186] Moreover, proto-oncogenes and tumor suppressors, such as *Ras* and *PTEN*, were found to regulate growth via the hamartin/tuberin complex.[187] Patients with *TSC1* mutations generally have milder disease than patients with *TSC2* mutations.[188]

Differential Diagnosis

Lesions that should be distinguished from the hypopigmented macules of TSC include nevus depigmentosus, nevus anemicus, postinflammatory hypopigmentation, pityriasis alba, tinea versicolor, and vitiligo.[167] Nevus depigmentosus is most easily confused with the hypopigmented macules of TSC.[110] A nevus depigmentosus can only be differentiated from a single ashleaf spot by the absence of other signs or symptoms of TSC.

Treatment and Care

Management is multidisciplinary. Special education may be required if mental retardation is present. Facial angiofibromas may be treated with the pulsed dye vascular laser. The more nodular lesions are best treated with the carbon dioxide laser, but slowly recur.[189] Examination of the parents and other family members of seemingly sporadic patients with TSC is indicated to exclude the possibility of a mild phenotype of which parents are not aware. Gonadal mosaicism is possible in around 2% of families where parents show no signs of TSC after full clinical evaluation.[190]

Nevus Anemicus

Cutaneous Findings

Nevus anemicus is a congenital vascular anomaly characterized by single or multiple hypopigmented patches with irregular margins, sometimes surrounded by satellite macules (Fig.

FIG. 21-16 Nevus anemicus.

21-16). It appears at birth or in early childhood, and is more common in women.[191,192] Although it occurs most commonly on the trunk, nevus anemicus has also been reported on the extremities and the head and neck.[192,193] It persists unchanged throughout life.

Extracutaneous Findings

Nevus anemicus may be seen in close association with port wine stains.[192] These twin anomalies may be a result of somatic recombination of allelic mutations for vasoconstriction and vasodilatation.[194] Phakomatosis pigmentovascularis, where vascular and pigmented nevi occur in association with nevus anemicus, has been used to support this concept.[195] Lesions of nevus anemicus occur with increased frequency in patients with neurofibromatosis.[191]

Etiology/Pathogenesis

Examination by light and electron microscopy reveals no abnormality, and the nevus is best characterized as a pharmacological abnormality, rather than an anatomical one.[193] The pallor is due to an increased local vascular reactivity to catecholamines. Donor dominance was demonstrated by grafting lesional skin from nevus anemicus to normal skin, which retained its pale appearance, emphasizing that nevus anemicus is due to increased sensitivity of the blood vessels to catecholamines rather than to increased sympathetic stimulation.[196]

Differential Diagnosis

Under diascopic pressure with a glass microscope slide, the lesion becomes indistinguishable from the blanched surrounding skin.[197] Wood's lamp examination does not accentuate the lesion, and rubbing or temperature change causes erythema in the surrounding area but not within the lesion itself. These maneuvers help to distinguish nevus anemicus from vitiligo, nevus depigmentosus, tuberous sclerosis macules, tinea versicolor, and leprosy.[198]

Treatment is cosmetic, and if desired the discoloration can be concealed with camouflage make-up.

Postinflammatory Hypopigmentation

Cutaneous Findings

Postinflammatory hypopigmentation refers to the partial loss of melanin in previously inflamed areas of skin. The hypochromic macules and patches usually appear in a mottled pattern in the distribution of the inflammatory process, and are more obvious in dark skin (Fig. 21-17).

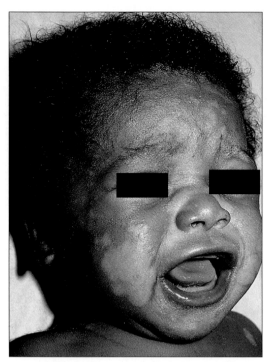

FIG. 21-17 Postinflammatory hypopigmentation secondary to seborrheic dermatitis. Once the inflammation is gone, the hypopigmentation improves.

Etiology/Pathogenesis

Postinflammatory hypopigmentation can appear in the newborn period after inflammatory conditions such as atopic dermatitis, seborrheic dermatitis, diaper dermatitis, pityriasis alba, psoriasis, pityriasis lichenoides, and infectious conditions.

Differential Diagnosis

Pityriasis alba is characterized by ill-defined, hypopigmented, minimally scaly macules and patches, commonly seen on the face without erythema or pruritus. It is common, being present in 25–40% of dark-skinned children,[199,200] and occasionally seen in the neonatal period. Histology reveals that the alterations found in the horny layer showed a dermatitic pattern, and the resulting hypopigmentation may be due to postinflammatory mechanisms.[201] Wood's lamp will enhance the hypopigmented areas in light skin and helps to distinguish depigmentation from hypopigmentation.

Treatment and Care

Treatment of the underlying cause of inflammation will improve the discoloration. In pityriasis alba repigmentation is achieved with avoidance of excessive sunlight and topical steroids applied daily for several weeks.

Congenital Halo Nevi
Cutaneous Findings

A halo nevus is a benign melanocytic nevus (usually a compound nevus) surrounded by a ring of depigmentation. Depig-

mented zones around nevi have also been reported with congenital nevi,[202,203] Spitz nevi, blue nevi, neurofibroma, and primary or metastatic malignant melanoma.[204]

Halo nevi are often multiple, usually occur on the trunk, and appear most commonly in young people. Vitiligo is often associated and develops at distant sites.[203] The condition is usually not inherited, although familial cases have been described.[205] The nevus tends to flatten and may eventually involute over a period of months, leaving an area of depigmentation that persists for several years, but which eventually may repigment.

Etiology/Pathogenesis

The nevus cells appear to be destroyed by cytotoxic CD8+ T lymphocytes recognizing class 1 HLA antigens on their surfaces.[206] This theory of an immunologic mechanism is supported by the fact that a lymphocytic infiltrate is seen around the nevus cells and the nevus cells show cytotoxic changes.[207] Unlike acquired halo nevi, congenital halo nevi may have an absence of inflammation on histology and may not involute.[202,203]

MISCELLANEOUS HYPOPIGMENTATION

Alezzandrini Syndrome

The syndrome is characterized by unilateral facial vitiligo, ipsilateral tapetoretinal degeneration, poliosis, and perceptual deafness.[208,209] Associated insulin-dependent diabetes mellitus and unilateral retinal detachment have been reported.[210]

Symptoms of visual loss begin gradually in one eye between the ages of 12 and 30 years. Vitiligo and poliosis of the scalp ipsilateral to the retinal lesions tend to occur 3–13 years after the visual decline.[210] A possible variant of this syndrome is the Vogt–Koyanagi–Harada Syndrome. Alezzandrini syndrome has only been reported in a small number of cases and has not been reported in neonates.

Ziprkowski–Margolis Syndrome
Cutaneous and Extracutaneous Findings

Ziprkowski–Margolis syndrome (albinism–deafness syndrome) is characterized by diffuse hypomelanosis of the skin and hair, except for the buttocks and genital region.[211,212] With time, multiple symmetrical macules of hyperpigmentation appear on the trunk and extremities, giving the skin a leopard-like appearance. Other features are heterochromic irides, congenital nerve deafness, and mutism. The syndrome was first reported in a Sephardi Jewish family of Moroccan origin.

Etiology/Pathogenesis

The mode of inheritance is X-linked recessive and the *ADFN* gene has been mapped to Xq26.3-27.1.[213] The mutation affects the migration of neural crest-derived precursors of the melanocytes. Female carriers of the diseases can demonstrate sensorineural hearing impairment.[214]

REFERENCES

1. King RA, Olds DP. Hairbulb tyrosinase activity in oculocutaneous albinism: Suggestions for pathway control and block location. Am J Hum Genet 1985; 20: 49–55.

2. King RA. Albinism. In: Nordlund JJ, Boissy RE, Hearing VJ, et al., eds. The pigmentary system. New York: Oxford University Press, 1998; 553–575.

3. Tomita Y, Suzuki T. Genetics of pigmentary disorders. Am J Med Genet 2004; 131C: 75–81.

4. Bolognia JL. Disorders of hypopigmentation: Update on

pathogenesis. Yale University/Glaxo Dermatology Lectureship Series in Dermatology, Glaxo: 1997.

5. King RA, Summers CG. Albinism. Dermatol Clin 1988; 6: 217–227.

6. Orlow SJ. Albinism: An update. Semin Cutan Med Surg 1997; 16: 24–29.

7. Ramsay M, Colman MA, Stevens G, et al. The tyrosine-positive oculocutaneous albinism locus maps to chromosome 15q11.2-q12. Am J Hum Genet 1992; 51: 879–884.

8. Toyofuku K, Valencia JC, Kushimoto T, et al. The etiology of oculocutaneous albinism (OCA) type II: the pink protein modulates the processing and transport of tyrosinase. Pigment Cell Res 2002; 15: 217–224.

9. King RA, Creel D, Cervenka J, et al. Albinism in Nigeria with delineation of new recessive oculocutaneous type. Clin Genet 1980; 17: 259–270.

10. King RA, Lewis RA, Townsend D, et al. Brown oculocutaneous albinism: clinical ophthalmological, and biochemical characterization. Ophthalmology 1986; 92: 1496–1505.

11. Boissy RE, Zhao H, Oetting WS, et al. Mutation in and lack of expression of tyrosinase-related protein-1 (TRP-1) in melanocytes from an individual with brown oculocutaneous albinism: a new subtype of albinism classified as 'OCA3.' Am J Hum Genet 1996; 58: 1145–1156.

12. Kobayashi T, Urabe K, Winder A, et al. Tyrosinase related protein 1 (TRP1) functions as a DHICA oxidase in melanin biosynthesis. EMBO J 1994; 13: 5818–5825.

13. Newton JM, Cohen-Barak O, Hagiwara N, et al. Mutations in the human orthologue of the mouse underwhite gene (uw) underlie a new form of oculocutaneous albinism, OCA4. Am J Hum Genet 2001; 69: 981–988.

14. Rundshagen U, Zuhlke C, Opitz S, et al. Mutations in the MATP gene in five German patients affected by oculocutaneous albinism type 4. Hum Mutat 2004; 23: 106–110.

15. Inagaki K, Suzuki T, Shimizu H, et al. Oculocutaneous albinism type 4 is one of the most common types of albinism in Japan. Am J Hum Genet 2004; 74: 466–471.

16. Hermansky F, Pudlak P. Albinism associated with hemorrhagic diathesis and unusual pigmented reticular cells in the bone marrow: report of two cases with histochemical studies. Blood 1959; 14: 162–169.

17. Gahl WA, Brantly M, Kaiser-Kupfer MI, et al. Genetic defects and clinical characteristics of patients with a form of oculocutaneous albinism (Hermansky–Pudlak syndrome). N Engl J Med 1998; 338: 1258–1264.

18. Passeron T, Mantoux F, Ortonne JP. Genetic disorders of pigmentation. Clin Dermatol 2005; 23: 56–67.

19. Witkop CJ, Krumwiede M, Sedano H, et al. Reliability of absent platelet dense bodies as a diagnostic criterion for Hermansky–Pudlak syndrome. Am J Hematol 1987; 26: 305–311.

20. Shotelersuk V, Dell'Angelica EC, Hartnell L, et al. A new variant of Hermansky–Pudlak syndrome due to mutations in a gene responsible for vesicle formation. Am J Med 2000; 108: 423–427.

21. Huizing M, Gahl WA. Disorders of vesicles of lysosomal lineage: the Hermansky–Pudlak syndromes. Curr Mol Med 2002; 2: 451–467.

22. Boissy RE, Nordlund JJ. Molecular basis of congenital hypopigmentary disorders in humans: a review. Pigment Res 1997; 10: 12–24.

23. Kahraman MM, Prieur DJ. Chediak–Higashi syndrome in the cat: prenatal diagnosis by evaluation of amniotic fluid cells. Am J Med Genet 1990; 36: 321–327.

24. Paller AS. Genetic disorders of the immune system. In: Schachner LA, Hansen RC, eds. Pediatric dermatology, 3rd edn. Philadelphia: Elsevier, 2003; 302–303.

25. Misra VP, King RM, Harding AE, et al. Peripheral neuropathy in the Chediak–Higashi syndrome. Acta Neuropathol 1991; 81: 354–358.

26. Blume RS, Wolff SM. The Chediak–Higashi syndrome: Studies in four patients and review of the literature. Medicine 1972; 51: 247–280.

27. Sheramata W, Kott SH, Cyr DP. The Chédiak–Higashi–Steinbrinck Syndrome. Arch Neurol 1971; 25: 289–294.

28. Weary PE, Bender AS. Chédiak–Higashi syndrome with severe cutaneous involvement: Occurrence in two brothers 14 and 15 years of age. Arch Intern Med 1967; 119: 381–386.

29. Barak Y, Nir E. Chédiak–Higashi syndrome. Am J Pediatr Hematol Oncol 1987; 9: 42–55.

30. Pettit RE, Berdal KG. Chédiak–Higashi syndrome. Neurologic appearance. Arch Neurol 1984; 41: 1001–1002.

31. Rubin CM, Burke BA, McKenna RW, et al. The accelerated phase of Chédiak–Higashi syndrome. An expression of the virus-associated hemophagocytic syndrome? Cancer 1985; 56: 524–530.

32. Kinugawa N. Epstein–Barr virus infection in Chédiak–Higashi syndrome mimicking acute lymphocytic leukemia. Am J Pediatr Hematol Oncol 1990; 12: 182–186.

33. Tchernev VT, Mansfield TA, Giot L, et al. The Chediak–Higashi protein interacts with SNARE complex and signal transduction proteins. Mol Med 2002; 8: 56–64.

34. Boxer LA, Watanabe AM, Rister M, et al. Correction of leukocyte function in Chédiak–Higashi syndrome by ascorbate. N Engl J Med 1976; 295: 1041–1045.

35. Weening RS, Schoorel EP, Roos D, et al. Effect of ascorbate on abnormal neutrophil, platelet, and lymphocyte function in a patient with the Chédiak–Higashi syndrome. Blood 1981; 57: 856–865.

36. Roder JC, Haliotis T, Klein M, et al. A new immunodeficiency disorder in humans involving NK cells. Nature 1980; 284: 553–555.

37. Nair MN, Gray RH, Boxer LA, et al. Deficiency of inducible suppressor cell activity in the Chédiak–Higashi syndrome. Am J Hematol 1987; 26: 56–66.

38. Amichai B, Zeharia A, Mimouni M, et al. Picture of the month. Arch Pediatr Adolesc Med 1997; 151: 425–426.

39. Brandt EJ, Elliot RW, Swank RT. Defective lysosomal enzyme secretion in kidneys of Chédiak–Higashi (beige) mice. J Cell Biol 1975; 67: 774–788.

40. Baetz K, Isaaz S, Griffiths GM. Loss of cytotoxic T lymphocyte function in Chédiak–Higashi syndrome arises from a secretory defect that prevents lytic granule exocytosis. J Immunol 1995; 154: 6122–6131.

41. Durandy A, Breton-Gorius J, Guy-Grand D, et al. Prenatal diagnosis of syndromes associating albinism and immune deficiencies (Chédiak–Higashi syndrome and variant). Prenat Diagn 1993; 13: 13–20.

42. Haddad E, Le Deist F, Blanche S, et al. Treatment of Chédiak–Higashi syndrome by allogenic bone marrow transplantation: Report of ten cases. Blood 1995; 85: 3328–3333.

43. Griscelli C, Virelizier JL. Bone marrow transplantation in a patient with Chédiak–Higashi syndrome. Birth Defects 1983; 19: 333–334.

44. Tardieu M, Lacroix C, Neven B, et al. Progressive neurologic dysfunctions 20 years after allogeneic bone marrow transplantation for Chediak–Higashi syndrome. Blood 2005; 106: 40–42.

45. Uyama E, Hirano T, Ito K, et al. Adult Chédiak–Higashi syndrome presenting as parkinsonism and dementia. Acta Neurol Scand 1994; 89: 175–183.

46. Misra VP, King RHM, Harding AE, et al. Peripheral neuropathy in the Chediak–Higashi syndrome. Acta Neuropathol 1991; 81: 354–358.

47. Courtens W, Broeckx W, Ledoux M, et al. Oculocerebral hypopigmentation syndrome (Cross syndrome) in a gypsy child. Acta Paediatr Scand 1989; 78: 806–810.

48. Cross HE, McKusick VA, Breen W. A new oculocerebral syndrome with hypopigmentation. J Pediatr 1967; 70: 398–406.

49. Fryns JP, Dereymaeker AM, Heremans G, et al. Oculocerebral syndrome with hypopigmentation (Cross syndrome): Report of two siblings born to consanguineous parents. Clin Genet 1988; 34: 81–84.

50. Lidsky AS, Robson KH, Thirumalachary C, et al. The PKU locus in man is on chromosome 12. Am J Hum Genet 1984; 36: 527–533.

51. Mineroff AD. Phenylketonuria. In: Nordlund JJ, Boissy RE, Hearing VJ, et al., eds. The pigmentary system. New York: Oxford University Press, 1998; 590–591.

52. Scriver CR, Hurtubise M, Konecki D, et al. PAHdb 2003: what a locus-specific knowledgebase can do. Hum Mutat 2003; 21: 333–344.

53. Scriver CR, Kaufman S. The hyperphenylalaninemias. In: Scriver CR, Beaudet AL, Sly SW, et al., eds. The metabolic and molecular bases of inherited disease, 8th edn. New York: McGraw-Hill, 2001.

54. Rosenberg LE. Inherited disorders of amino acid metabolism and storage. In: Isselbacher K, Braunwald E, Wilson J, et al., eds. Harrison's principles of internal medicine, 13th edn. New York: McGraw-Hill, 1994; 2117–2125.

55. Beasley MG, Costello PM, Smith I. Outcome of treatment in young adults with phenylketonuria detected by routine neonatal screening between 1964 and 1971. QJ Med 1994; 87: 155–160.

56. Platt LD, Koch R, Azen C, et al. Maternal phenylketonuria collaborative study, obstetric aspects and outcome: the first six years. Am Obstet Gynecol 1992; 166: 1150–1160.

57. Griscelli C, Durandy A, Guy-Grand D, et al. A syndrome associating partial albinism and immunodeficiency. Am J Med 1978; 65: 691–702.

58. Pastural E, Barrat FJ, Dufourcq-Lagelouse R, et al. Griscelli disease maps to chromosome 15q21 and is associated with mutations in the myosin-Va gene. Nature Genet 1997; 16: 289–292.

59. Menasche G, Fischer A, de Saint Basile G. Griscelli syndrome types 1 and 2. Am J Hum Genet 2002; 71: 1237–1238.

60. Menasche G, Pastural E, Feldmann J, et al. Mutations in RAB27A cause Griscelli syndrome associated with haemophagocytic syndrome. Nature Genet 2000; 25: 173–176.

61. Menasche G, Ho CH, Sanal O, et al. Griscelli syndrome restricted to hypopigmentation results from a melanophilin defect (GS3) or a MYO5A F-exon deletion (GS1). J Clin Invest 2003; 112: 450–456.

62. Orlow SJ. Genetic disorders of pigmentation. In: Schachner LA, Hansen RC, eds. Pediatric dermatology, 3rd edn. Philadelphia: Elsevier, 2003; 294–295.

63. Mancini AJ, Chan LS, Paller AS. Partial albinism with immunodeficiency: Griscelli syndrome: Report of a case and review of the literature. J Am Acad Dermatol 1998; 38: 295–300.

64. Haraldsson A, Weemaes CR, Bakkeren JM, et al. Griscelli disease with cerebral involvement. Eur J Pediatr 1991; 150: 419–422.

65. Gogus S, Topcu M, Kucukali T, et al. Griscelli syndrome: Report of three cases. Pediatr Pathol Lab Med 1995; 15: 309–319.

66. Klein C, Philippe N, Le Deist F, et al. Partial albinism with immunodeficiency (Griscelli syndrome). J Pediatr 1994; 125: 886–895.

67. Hurvitz H, Gillis R, Klaus S, et al. A kindred with Griscelli disease: spectrum of neurological involvement. Eur J Pediatr 1993; 152: 402–405.

68. Brismar J, Harfi HA. Partial albinism with immunodeficiency: A rare syndrome with prominent posterior fossa white matter changes. Am J Neuroradiol 1992; 13: 387–393.

69. Bizario JCS, Feldmann J, Castro FA, et al. Griscelli syndrome: characterization of a new mutation and rescue of T-cytotoxic activity by retroviral transfer of RAB27A gene. J Clin Immun 2004; 24: 397–410.

70. Siccardi AG, Bianchi E, Calligari A, et al. A new familial defect in neutrophil bactericidal activity. Helv Paediatr Acta 1978; 33: 401–412.

71. Brambilla E, Dechelette E, Stoebner P. Partial albinism and immunodeficiency: Ultrastructural study of haemophagocytosis and bone marrow erythroblasts in one case. Pathol Res Pract 1980; 167: 151–165.

72. Schneider LC, Berman RS, Shea CR, et al. Bone marrow transplantation (BMT) for the syndrome of pigmentary dilution and lymphohistiocytosis (Griscelli's syndrome). J Clin Immunol 1990; 10: 146–153.

73. Rogers SL, Karcher RL, Roland JT, et al. Regulation of melanosome movement in the cell cycle by reversible association with myosin V. J Cell Biol 1999; 146: 1265–1276.

74. Bahadoran P, Aberdam E, Mantoux F, et al. Rab27a: A key to melanosome transport in human melanocytes. J Cell Biol 2001; 152: 843–850.

75. Fischer A, Griscelli C, Friedrich W, et al. Bone marrow transplantation for immunodeficiencies and osteoporosis: European survey, 1968–1985. Lancet 1986; 2: 1080–1083.

76. Elejalde BR, Holguin J, Valencia A, et al. Mutations affecting pigmentation in man: I. Neuroectodermal melanolysosomal disease. Am J Med Genet 1979; 3: 65–80.

77. Elejalde BR, De Elejalde MM. Neuroectodermal melanolysosomal disease. In: Gomez MR, ed. Neurocutaneous diseases: A practical approach. Boston, MA: Butterworths, 1987; 254–260.

78. Duran-McKinster C, Rodriguez-Jurado R, Ridaura C, et al. Elejalde syndrome: A melanolysosomal neurocutaneous syndrome: Clinical and morphological findings in 7 patients. Arch Dermatol 1999; 135: 182–186.

79. Ivanovich J, Mallory S, Storer T, et al. 12-year-old male with Elejalde syndrome (neuroectodermal melanolysosomal disease). Am J Med Genet 2001; 98: 313–316.

80. Sanal O, Yel L, Kucukali T, et al. An allelic variant of Griscelli disease: presentation with severe hypotonia, mental–motor retardation, and hypopigmentation consistent with Elejalde syndrome (neuroectodermal melanolysosomal disorder). J Neurol 2000; 247: 570–572.

81. Menasche G, Fischer A, de Saint Basile G. Griscelli syndrome types 1 and 2. Am J Hum Genet 2002; 71: 1237–1238.

82. Anikster Y, Huizing M, Anderson PD, et al. Evidence that Griscelli syndrome with neurological involvement is caused by mutations in RAB27A, not MYO5A. Am J Hum Genet 2002; 71: 407–414.

83. Bahadoran P, Ortonne JP, Ballotti R, et al. Comment on Elejalde syndrome and relationship with Griscelli syndrome. Am J Med Genet 2003; 116A: 408–409.

84. Menkes JHM, Alter M, Steigleder GK, et al. A sex-linked recessive disorder with retardation of growth, peculiar hair and focal cerebral and cerebellar degeneration. Pediatrics 1962; 29: 764–779.

85. Peterson J, Drolet BA, Esterly NB. Menkes' kinky-hair syndrome. Pediatr Dermatol 1998; 15: 137–139.

86. Stratigos AJ, Baden HP. Unraveling the molecular mechanisms of hair and nail genodermatoses. Arch Dermatol 2001; 137: 1465–1471.

87. Hart DB. Menkes' kinky hair syndrome: an updated review. J Am Acad Dermatol 1983; 9: 145–152.

88. Kodama H, Murata Y, Kobayashi M. Clinical manifestations and treatment of Menkes disease and its variants. Pediatr Int 1999; 41: 423–429.

89. Levinson B, Gitschier J, Vulpe C, et al. Are X-linked cutis laxa and Menkes disease allelic? Nature Genet 1993; 3: 6.

90. Vulpe C, Levinson B, Whitney S, et al. Isolation of a candidate gene for Menkes disease and evidence that if encodes a copper-transporting ATPase. Nature Genet 1993; 3: 7–13.

91. Tsukahara M, Imaizumi K, Kawai S, et al. Occipital horn syndrome: report of a patient and review of the literature. Clin Genet 1994; 45: 32–35.

92. Moller LB, Tumer Z, Lund C, et al. Similar splice-site mutations of the ATP 7A gene lead to different phenotypes: Classical Menkes disease or occipital horn syndrome. Am J Hum Genet 2000; 66: 1211–1220.

93. Gu YH, Kodama H, Murata Y, et al. ATP 7A gene mutations in 16 patients with Menkes disease and a patient with occipital horn syndrome. Am J Med Genet 2001; 99: 217–222.

94. Sarkar B, Lingeratat-Walsh K, Clarke JTR. Copper-histidine therapy for Menkes disease. J Pediatr 1993; 123: 828–830.

95. Christodoulou J, Danks DM, Sarkar B, et al. Early treatment of Menkes disease with parenteral copper-histidine: Long-term follow-up of four treated patients. Am J Med Genet 1998; 76: 154–164.

96. Borm B, Moller LB, Hausser I, et al. Variable clinical expression of an identical mutation in the ATP 7A gene for Menkes disease/occipital horn syndrome in three affected males in a single family. J Pediatr 2004; 145: 119–121.

97. Sheela SR, Latha M, Liu P, et al. Copper-replacement treatment for symptomatic Menkes disease: ethical considerations. Clin Genet 2005; 68: 278–283.

98. Bolognia JL, Orlow SJ, Glick SA. Lines of Blaschko. J Am Acad Dermatol 1994; 31: 157–190.

99. Harre J, Millikan LE. Linear and whorled pigmentation. Int J Dermatol 1994; 33: 529–537.

100. Ito M. Incontinentia pigmenti achromians: A singular case of nevus depigmentosus systematicus bilateralis. Tohoku J Exp Med 1952; 55: 57–59.

101. Levine N. Pigmentary abnormalities. In: Schachner LA, Hansen RC, eds. Pediatric dermatology, 2nd edn. New York: Churchill Livingstone, 1995; 539–582.

102. Sybert VP. Hypomelanosis of Ito: A description, not a diagnosis. J Invest Dermatol 1994; 103: 141S–143S.

103. Ballmer-Weber BK, Inaebnit D, Brand CU, et al. Sporadic hypomelanosis of Ito with focal hypertrichosis in a 16-month-old girl. Dermatology 1996; 193: 63–64.

104. Loomis CA. Linear hypopigmentation and hyperpigmentation, including mosaicism. Semin Cutan Med Surg 1997; 16: 44–53.

105. Jelinek JE, Bart RS, Schiff, GM. Hypomelanosis of Ito ('incontinentia pigmenti achromians'): report of three cases and review of the literature. Arch Dermatol 1973; 107: 596–601.

106. Sybert VP, Pagon RA, Donlan M, et al. Pigmentary abnormalities and mosaicism for chromosomal aberration: association with clinical features similar to hypomelanosis of Ito. J Pediatr 1990; 116: 581–586.

107. Takematsu H, Sato S, Igarashi M, et al. Incontinentia pigmenti achromians (Ito). Arch Dermatol 1983; 119: 391–395.

108. Vormittag W, Ensinger C, Raff M. Cytogenetic and dermatoglyphic findings in a familial case of hypomelanosis of Ito (incontinentia pigmenti achromians). Clin Genet 1992; 41: 309–314.

109. Montagna P, Procaccianti G, Galli G, et al. Familial hypomelanosis of Ito. Eur Neurol 1991; 31: 345–347.

110. Pinto FJ, Bolognia JL. Disorders of hypopigmentation in children. Pediatr Clin North Am 1991; 38: 991–1017.

111. Lee HS, Chun YS, Hann SK. Nevus depigmentosus: Clinical features and histopathologic characteristics in 67 patients. J Am Acad Dermatol 1999; 40: 21–26.

112. Lernia VD. Segmental nevus depigmentosus: Analysis of 20 patients. Pediatr Dermatol 1999; 16: 349–353.

113. Sugarman GI, Reed WB. Two unusual neurocutaneous disorders with facial cutaneous signs. Arch Neurol 1969; 21: 242–247.

114. Dawn G, Dhar S, Handa S, et al. Nevus depigmentosus associated with hemihypertrophy of the limbs. Pediatr Dermatol 1995; 12: 286–287.

115. Dhar S, Kanwar AJ, Kaur S. Nevus depigmentosus in India: experience with 50 patients. Pediatr Dermatol 1993; 10: 299–300.

116. Nehal KS, PeBenito R, Orlow SJ. Analysis of 54 cases of hypopigmentation and hyperpigmentation along the lines of Blaschko. Arch Dermatol 1996; 132: 1167–1170.

117. Bolognia JL, Lazova R, Watsky K. The development of lentigines within segmental achromic nevi. J Am Acad Dermatol 1998; 39: 330–333.

118. Jagia R, Mendiratt V, Koranne RV, et al. Colocalized nevus depigmentosus and lentigines with underlying breast hypoplasia: a case of reverse mutation? Dermatol Online J 2004; 10: 12.

119. Jimbow K, Fitzpatrick TB, Szabo G, et al. Congenital circumscribed hypomelanosis: A characterization based on electron microscopic study of tuberous sclerosis, nevus depigmentosus and piebaldism. J Invest Dermatol 1975; 64: 50–62.

120. Gauthier Y, Surleve-Bazeille JE. Autologous grafting with noncultured melanocytes: A simplified method for treatment of depigmented lesions. J Am Acad Dermatol 1992; 26: 191–194.

121. Cooke JV. Familial white skin spotting (piebaldness) ('partial albinism') with white forelock. J Pediatr 1952; 41: 1–12.

122. Campbell B, Swift S. Partial albinism: nine cases in six generations. JAMA 1962; 181: 1103–1106.

123. Davis BK, Verdol LD. Expansion and contraction of hypomelanotic areas in human piebaldism. Hum Genet 1976; 34: 163–170.

124. Richards KA, Fukai K, Oiso N, et al. A novel KIT mutation results in piebaldism with progressive depigmentation. J Am Acad Dermatol 2001; 44: 288–292.

125. Sijmons RH, Kristoffersson U, Tuerlings JHAM, et al. Piebaldism in a mentally retarded girl with rare deletion of the long arm of chromosome 4. Pediatr Dermatol 1993; 10: 235–239.

126. Chang T, McGrae JD, Hashimoto K. Ultrastructural study of two patients with both piebaldism and neurofibromatosis 1. Pediatr Dermatol 1993; 10: 224–234.

127. Tay YK. Neurofibromatosis 1 and piebaldism: A case report. Dermatology 1998; 197: 401–402.

128. Angelo C, Cianchini G, Grosso MG, et al. Association of piebaldism and neurofibromatosis type 1 in a girl. Pediatr Dermatol 2001; 18: 490–493.

129. Giebel LB, Spritz RA. Mutation of the KIT (mast/stem cell growth factor receptor) protooncogene in human piebaldism. Proc Natl Acad Sci USA 1991; 88: 8696–8699.

130. Vandenbark GR, DeCastro CM, Taylor H, et al. Cloning and structural analysis of the human c-kit gene. Oncogene 1992; 7: 1259–1266.

131. Spritz RA, Holmes A, Ramesar R, et al. Mutations of the kit (mast/stem cell growth factor receptor) proto-oncogene account for a continuous range of phenotypes in human piebaldism. Am J Hum Genet 1992; 51: 1058–1065.

132. Ward KA, Moss C, Sanders DSA. Human piebaldism: relationship between phenotype and site of kit gene mutation. Br J Dermatol 1995; 132: 929–935.

133. Perez-Losada J, Sanchez-Martin M, Rodriguez-Garcia A, et al. The zinc-finger transcription factor SLUG contributes to the function of the SCF/c-Kit signaling pathway. Blood 2002; 100: 1274–1286.

134. Sanchez-Martin M, Perez-Losada J, Rodriguez-Garcia A, et al. Deletion of the SLUG (SNA12) gene results in human piebaldism. Am J Med Genet 2003; 122A: 125–132.

135. Suga Y, Ikejima A, Matsuba S, et al. Medical pearl: DHA application for camouflaging segmental vitiligo and piebald lesions. J Am Acad Dermatol 2002; 47: 436–438.

136. Spritz RA. Piebaldism, Waardenburg syndrome and related disorders of melanocyte development. Semin Cutan Med Surg 1997; 16: 15–23.

137. Njoo MD, Nieuweboer-Krobotova L, Westerhof W. Repigmentation of leucodermic defects in piebaldism by dermabrasion and thin split-thickness skin grafting in combination with minigrafting. Br J Dermatol 1998; 139: 829–833.

138. Guerra L, Primavera G, Raskovic D, et al. Permanent repigmentation of piebaldism by erbium: YAG laser and autologous cultured epidermis. Br J Dermatol 2004; 150: 715–721.

139. Read AP, Newton VE. Waardenburg syndrome. J Med Genet 1997; 34: 656–665.

140. Waardenburg PJ. A new syndrome combining developmental anomalies of the eyelids, eyebrows and nose root with pigmentary defects of the iris and head hair with congenital deafness. Am J Hum Genet 1951; 3: 195–253.

393

141. Hageman MJ. Waardenburg's syndrome in Kenyan Africans. Trop Geog Med 1978; 30: 45–55.

142. Nayak CS, Isaacson G. Worldwide distribution of Waardenburg syndrome. Ann Otol Rhinol Laryngol 2003; 112: 817–820.

143. Dourmishev AL, Dourmishev LA, Schwartz RA, et al. Waardenburg syndrome. Int J Dermatol 1999; 38: 656–663.

144. Ortonne JP. Piebaldism, Waardenburg's syndrome and related disorders. 'Neural crest depigmentation syndromes'? Dermatol Clin 1988; 6: 205–216.

145. Orlow SJ. Congenital and genetic disorders associated with hypopigmentation. Curr Probl Dermatol 1994; 6: 157–184.

146. Winship I, Beighton P. Phenotypic discriminants in the Waardenburg syndrome. Clin Genet 1992; 41: 181–188.

147. Friedman I, Fisch L. Deafness as part of an hereditary syndrome. J Laryngol Otol 1959; 73: 363–382.

148. Liu XZ, Newton VE, Read AP. Waardenburg syndrome type II: Phenotypic findings and diagnostic criteria. Am J Med Genet 1995; 55: 95–100.

149. Giacoia JP, Klein SW. Waardenburg's syndrome with bilateral cleft lip. Am J Dis Child 1969; 117: 344–348.

150. Kromberg JGR, Krause A. Waardenburg syndrome and spina bifida. Am J Med Genet 1993; 45: 536–537.

151. Klein D. Historical background and evidence for dominant inheritance of the Klein–Waardenburg syndrome. Am J Med Genet 1983; 14: 231–239.

152. Shah KN, Dalal SJ, Desai MP, et al. White forelock, pigmentary disorder of the irides, and long segment Hirschsprung disease: Possible variant of Waardenburg syndrome. J Pediatr 1981; 99: 432–435.

153. Hoth CF, Milunsky A, Lipsky N, et al. Mutations in the paired domain of the human PAX-3 gene cause Klein–Waardenburg syndrome (WS-III) as well as Waardenburg syndrome type 1 (WS1). Am J Hum Genet 1993; 52: 455–462.

154. Zlotogora J, Lerer I, Bar-David S, et al. Homozygosity for Waardenburg syndrome. Am J Hum Genet 1995; 56: 1173–1178.

155. Tassabehji M, Newton VE, Read AP. Waardenburg syndrome type 2 caused by mutations in the human microphthalmia (MITF) gene. Nature Genet 1994; 8: 251–255.

156. Nobukuni Y, Watanabe A, Takeda K, et al. Analyses of loss-of-function mutations of the MITF gene suggest that haploinsufficiency is a cause of Waardenburg syndrome type 2A. Am J Hum Genet 1996; 59: 76–83.

157. Edery P, Attie T, Amiel J, et al. Mutation of the endothelin-3 gene in the Waardenburg–Hirschsprung disease (Shah–Waardenburg syndrome). Nature Genet 1996; 12: 442–444.

158. Pingault V, Bondurand N, Kuhlbrodt K, et al. SOX 10 mutations in patients with Waardenburg–Hirschsprung disease. Nature Genet 1998; 18: 171–173.

159. Amiel J, Attie T, Jan D, et al. Heterozygous endothelin receptor B (EDNRB) mutations in isolated Hirschsprung disease. Hum Mol Genet 1996; 5: 355–357.

160. Fisch L. Deafness as part of an hereditary syndrome. J Laryngol Otol 1959; 73: 353–362.

161. Rozycki DL, Reuben RJ, Rapin I, et al. Autosomal recessive deafness associated with short stature, vitiligo, muscle wasting and achalasia. Arch Otolaryngol 1971; 93: 194–197.

162. Fleury P, de Groot WP, Delleman JW, et al. Tuberous sclerosis: The incidence of sporadic cases versus familial cases. Brain Dev 1980; 2: 107–117.

163. Roach ES, Delgado MR. Tuberous sclerosis. Dermatol Clin 1995; 13: 151–161.

164. Osborne JP, Fryer A, Webb D. Epidemiology of tuberous sclerosis. Ann NY Acad Sci 1991; 615: 125–127.

165. Wiederholt WC, Gomez MR, Kurland LT. Incidence and prevalence of tuberous sclerosis in Rochester, Minnesota, 1950 through 1982. Neurology 1985; 35: 600–603.

166. Roach ES, Gomez MR, Northrup H. Tuberous sclerosis complex consensus conference: Revised clinical diagnostic criteria. J Child Neurol 1998; 13: 624–628.

167. Vanderhooft SL, Francis JS, Pagon RA, et al. Prevalence of hypopigmented macules in a healthy population. J Pediatr 1996; 129: 355–361.

168. Fitzpatrick TB. History and significance of white markers: Earliest visible signs of tuberous sclerosis. Ann NY Acad Sci 1991; 615: 26–35.

169. Dohil MA, Baugh WP, Eichenfield LF. Vascular and pigmented birthmarks. Pediatr Clin North Am 2000; 47: 783–812.

170. McWilliam RC, Stephenson JB. Depigmented hair. The earliest sign of tuberous sclerosis. Arch Dis Child 1978; 53: 961–963.

171. Gutman I, Dunn D, Behrens M, et al. Hypopigmented iris spot. An early sign of tuberous sclerosis. Ophthalmology 1982; 89: 1115–1119.

172. Nickel WR, Reed WB. Tuberous sclerosis – special reference to the microscopic alterations in the cutaneous hamartomas. Arch Dermatol 1962; 85: 209–226.

173. Zeller J, Friedmann D, Clerici T, et al. The significance of a single periungual fibroma. Report of seven cases. Arch Dermatol 1995; 131: 1465–1466.

174. Sampson JR, Attwood D, al Mughery AS, et al. Pitted enamel hypoplasia in tuberous sclerosis. Clin Genet 1992; 42: 50–52.

175. Kiribuchi K, Uchida Y, Fukuyama Y, et al. High incidence of fundus hamartomas and clinical significance of a fundus score in tuberous sclerosis. Brain Dev 1986; 8: 509–517.

176. Smith HC, Watson GH, Patel RG, et al. Cardiac rhabdomyoma in tuberous sclerosis: their course and diagnostic value. Arch Dis Child 1989; 64: 196–200.

177. Konkol RJ, Walsh EP, Power T, et al. Cerebral embolism resulting from an intracardiac tumor in tuberous sclerosis. Pediatr Neurol 1986; 2: 108–110.

178. van Baal JG, Fleury P, Brummelkamp WH. Tuberous sclerosis and the relation with renal angiomyolipoma. A genetic study on the clinical aspects. Clin Genet 1989; 35: 167–173.

179. Dwyer JM, Hickie JB, Garvan J. Pulmonary tuberous sclerosis. Report of three patients and a review of the literature. QJ Med 1971; 40: 115–125.

180. Smalley SL, Tanguay PE, Smith M, et al. Autism and tuberous sclerosis. J Autism Dev Dis 1992; 22: 339–355.

181. Curatolo P, Cusmai R, Cortesi F, et al. Neuropsychiatric aspects of tuberous sclerosis. Ann NY Acad Sci 1991; 615: 8–16.

182. Goodman M, Lamm SH, Engel A, et al. Cortical tuber count: A biomarker indicating neurologic severity of tuberous sclerosis complex. J Child Neurol 1997; 12: 75–76.

183. Rendtorff ND, Bjerregaard B, Frodin M, et al. Analysis of 65 tuberous sclerosis complex (TSC) patients by TSC2 DGGE, TSCI/TSC2 MLPA, and TSC1 long-range PCR sequencing, and report of 28 novel mutations. Hum Mutat 2005; 25: 374–383.

184. Van Slegtenhorst M, de Hoogt R, Hermans C, et al. Identification of the tuberous sclerosis gene TSC1 on chromosome 9q34. Science 1997; 277: 805–808.

185. European Tuberous Sclerosis Consortium. Identification and characterization of the tuberous sclerosis gene on chromosome 16. Cell 1993; 75: 1305–1315.

186. Kwiatkowski DJ. Tuberous sclerosis: from tubers to mTOR. Ann Hum Genet 2003; 67: 87–96.

187. Potter CJ, Pedraza LG, Huang H, et al. The tuberous sclerosis complex (TSC) pathway and mechanism of size control. Biochem Soc Trans 2003; 31: 584–586.

188. Dabora SL, Jozwiak S, Franz DN, et al. Mutational analysis in a cohort of 224 tuberous sclerosis patients indicates increased severity of TSC2, compared with TSC1, disease in multiple organs. Am J Hum Genet 2001; 68: 64–80.

189. Papadavid E, Markey A, Bellaney G, et al. Carbon dioxide and pulsed dye laser treatment of angiofibromas in 29 patients with tuberous sclerosis. Br J Dermatol 2002; 147: 337–342.

190. Verhoef S, Bakker L, Tempelaars AMP, et al. High rate of mosaicism in tuberous sclerosis complex. Am J Hum Genet 1999; 64: 1632–1637.

191. Fleisher TL, Zeligman I. Nevus anemicus. Arch Dermatol 1969; 100: 750–755.

192. Katugampola GA, Lanigan SW. The clinical spectrum of naevus anaemicus and its association with port wine stains: report of 15 cases and a review of the literature. Br J Dermatol 1996; 134: 292–295.

193. Greaves MW, Birkett D, Johnson C. Nevus anemicus: a unique catecholamine-dependent nevus. Arch Dermatol 1970; 102: 172–176.

194. Happle R, Koopman R, Mier PD. Hypothesis: vascular twin naevi and somatic recombination in man. Lancet 1990; 335: 376–378.

195. Happle R. Allelic somatic mutations may explain vascular twin naevi. Hum Genet 1991; 86: 321–322.

196. Daniel RH, Hubler WR, Wolf JE, et al. Nevus anemicus. Donor-dominant defect. Arch Dermatol 1977; 113: 53–56.

197. Mountcastle EA, Diestelmeier MR, Lupton GP. Nevus anemicus. J Am Acad Dermatol 1986; 14: 628–632.

198. Ahkami RN, Schwartz RA. Nevus anemicus. Dermatology 1999; 198: 327–329.

199. Tay YK, Kong KH, Khoo L, et al. The prevalence and descriptive epidemiology of atopic dermatitis in Singapore school children. Br J Dermatol 2002; 146: 101–106.

200. Bassaly M, Milae A, Prasad AS. Studies on pityriasis alba. Arch Dermatol 1963; 88: 272–275.

201. Urano-Suehisa S, Tagami H. Functional and morphological analysis of the horny layer of pityriasis alba. Acta Dermatol Venereol 1985; 65: 164–167.

202. Berger RS, Voorhees JJ. Multiple congenital giant nevocellular nevi with halos: Clinical and electron microscopic study. Arch Dermatol 1971; 104: 515–521.

203. Brownstein MH, Kazam BB, Hashimoto K. Halo congenital nevus. Arch Dermatol 1977; 113: 1572–1575.

204. Kopf AW, Morrill SD, Silberberg I. Broad spectrum of leukoderma acquisitum centrifugum. Arch Dermatol 1965; 92: 14–35.

205. Herd RM, Hunter JAA. Familial halo naevi. Clin Exp Dermatol 1998; 23: 68–69.

206. Zeff RA, Freitag A, Grin CM, et al. The immune response in halo nevi. J Am Acad Dermatol 1997; 37: 620–624.

207. Gauthier Y, Surleve-Bazeille JE, Gauthier O, et al. Ultrastructure of halo nevi. J Cutan Pathol 1975; 2: 71–81.

208. Alezzandrini AA. Manifestations of tapeto-retinal degeneration, vitiligo, poliosis, grey hair and hypoacusia. Ophthalmologica 1964; 147: 409–419.

209. Cremona AC, Alezzandrini AA, Casala AM. Vitiligo, poliosis and unilateral macular degeneration. Arch Oftalmol Buenos Aires 1961; 36: 102–106.

210. Hoffman MD, Dudley C. Suspected Alezzandrini's syndrome in a diabetic patient with unilateral retinal detachment and ipsilateral vitiligo and poliosis. J Am Acad Dermatol 1992; 26: 496–497.

211. Ziprkowski L, Krakowski A, Adam A, et al. Partial albinism and deaf mutism due to a recessive sex-linked gene. Arch Dermatol 1962; 86: 530–539.

212. Margolis E. A new hereditary syndrome-sex linked deaf-mutism associated with total albinism. Acta Genet Stat Med 1962; 12: 12–19.

213. Shiloh Y, Litvak G, Ziv Y, et al. Genetic mapping of X-linked albinism-deafness syndrome (ADFN) to Xq26.3-q27.1. Am J Hum Genet 1990; 47: 20–27.

214. Fried K, Feinmesser M, Tsitsianov J. Hearing impairment in female carriers of the sex-linked syndrome of deafness with albinism. J Med Genet 1969; 6: 132–134.

22

Disorders of Hyperpigmentation and Melanocytes

Neil F. Gibbs, Hanspaul S. Makkar

Hyperpigmented lesions are common at birth and in the first few weeks of life. Lesions range from small macules to large hyperpigmented plaques. Some, such as mongolian spots, are frequently seen in newborns and are of little or no significance, whereas others may be signs of systemic diseases and genetic syndromes. In some cases hyperpigmented 'birthmarks' may not be evident at the time of birth but appear within weeks to months. At least part of the explanation for this may be the relatively light skin color of many infants at birth. Over time, melanocytes produce more pigment and differences between normal and hyperpigmented or hypopigmented anomalies become more evident. An approach based on lesional morphology and location may be useful (Table 22-1). Excellent review articles discuss congenital and genetic hyperpigmentation in more detail, and may be helpful supplements to this chapter.[1,2]

LOCALIZED HYPERPIGMENTATION – TAN-BROWN

Café au Lait Macules
Cutaneous Findings
Café au lait macules (CALM) are round to oval, tan to brown, flat, hairless lesions with distinct margins, ranging in size from a few millimeters to 15–20 cm in diameter, and can occur anywhere on the body (Figs 22-1 and 22-2). Most lesions in newborns are seen in the buttock area, whereas in older children they occur most commonly on the trunk.[2] Pigmentation is generally uniform. They are seen in 0.3–18% of neonates, with variation by ethnicity and race, and in 24–36% of older children.[3,4] Many or most are present at birth or develop in the first few months of life; they may increase in number and size with age.

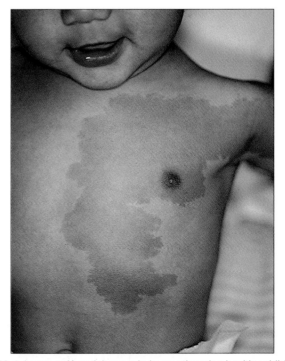

FIG. 22-1 Large café au lait macule in an otherwise healthy child. This pattern is sometimes referred to as 'segmental pigmentation disorder (see discussion on p. 399).

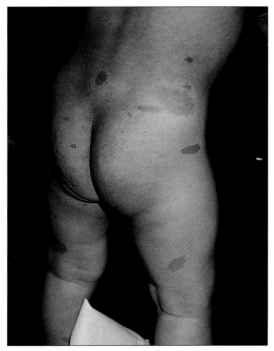

FIG. 22-2 Multiple café au lait macules on a child with NF1.

TABLE 22-1 Diagnosis using lesion morphology and location

Description of lesions	Location	Possible diagnoses
Blue-gray/blue-black patches	Torso Face Shoulder/neck Torso, in association with port wine stain	Mongolian spot Nevus of Ota Nevus of Ito Phakomatosis pigmentovascularis
Labial macules	Perioral More widespread facial Face/trunk Face	Peutz-Jeghers syndrome Carney syndrome LEOPARD syndrome Carney syndrome Centrofacial lentiginosis
Brown sharply defined patches or plaques		Congenital nevus Café au lait macule Congenital nevus
Small brown macules	Perioral/mucosal Widespread, non mucosal Central face/widespread Involves mucosa Axilliary/groin/neck only Central face only, not mucosa Clustered in a defined body area or segment. Background skin color normal Clustered in a defined body area or segment. Background skin color darker Single	Peutz-Jeghers syndrome LEOPARD syndrome Generalized lentiginosis Inherited patterned lentiginosis Carney syndrome Carney syndrome Neurofibromatosis Centrofacial lentiginosis Segmental lentiginosis Mosaicism Speckled lentiginous nevus Nevus spilus Congenital nevus
Linear hyperpigmentation in swirled or Blaschko pattern	Flat Raised	Linear and whorled nevoid hypermelanosis Epidermal nevus Incontinentia pigmenti Goltz syndrome Conradi-Hünermann syndrome Mosaicism Epidermal nevus Incontinentia pigmenti

Diagnosis is generally made on clinical grounds. On biopsy, CALM have increased epidermal melanin in both melanocytes and keratinocytes, without melanocytic proliferation, which readily distinguishes them from melanocytic nevi. Giant pigment granules may be present, but are not helpful in differentiating one cause of CALM (such as neurofibromatosis 1; NF1) from other causes.[5]

Differential Diagnosis

The differential diagnosis of CALM includes speckled lentiginous nevus (SLN, or nevus spilus), lentigo, congenital melanocytic nevus, Becker's nevus, and segmental pigmentation disorder. The distinction between SLN, congenital melanocytic nevi, and CALM usually becomes evident with time.

Extracutaneous Findings

The vast majority of patients with CALM have no associated extracutaneous abnormalities. A familial form of inherited CALM, without associated systemic abnormalities, has been mapped to chromosome 2p22-p21. Nonetheless, CALM can be markers for certain underlying disorders (Box 22-1), most commonly neurofibromatosis type 1.[6] Many additional genetically based disorders have been reported to have associated CALM on cutaneous examination. Watson's syndrome presents with multiple CALM, intertriginous freckling, short stature, pulmonary stenosis, and low intelligence, and is thought to be a subset or an allelic form of NF1. Large CALM may be seen in McCune–Albright syndrome. Other syndromes in which CALM appear to be strongly associated include neurofibromatosis type 2 (NF2) and ring chromosome syndrome.[2] Other conditions in which CALM may be seen, though with less strong associations, include tuberous sclerosis, Bloom syndrome, ataxia–telangiectasia syndrome, Silver–Russell syndrome, Jaffe–Campanacci syndrome, basal cell nevus syndrome, Gaucher disease, Turner syndrome, and Hunter syndrome.[7]

Treatment and Care

The significance of CALM is as a diagnostic aid to other disorders. Treatment is generally not necessary, but improvements have been reported with laser therapy and can be considered in disfiguring cases. Unfortunately, results are inconsistent. Although complete clearance can be seen, rapid recurrence may occur with sun exposure in some cases, and other CALM may actually darken and result in postinflammatory hyperpigmentation (usually temporary). Lasers, including Q-switched ruby, Q-switched alexandrite, and Q-switched Nd-YAG, can be used to treat CALM, but parents must be counseled regarding the unpredictability of responses and the need for multiple treatment sessions.[8]

Select Disorders Associated with Café-au-Lait Macules

Segmental Pigmentation Disorder

Segmental pigmentation disorder is one of the most common pigmentary birthmarks, although references to it are relatively sparse in the medical literature. It is really the hyperpigmented equivalent of a 'nevus depigmentosus' (see Chapter 21) Light-brown CALM occur in a segmental, block-like segmental pattern, most often on the trunk (Fig. 22-1, but other areas of the skin can also be affected. Lesions are typically solitary, but are occasionally multiple. They vary in size from several centimeters to much larger, and are usually larger than ordinary CALM. They usually have a homogeneous light to medium-brown color. Sharp delineation of lesions at the midline with a less distinctly defined lateral border is characteristic. Lesions tend to remain stable over time. The differential diagnosis includes zosteriform lentiginous nevus, linear and whorled nevoid hypermelanosis, and large CALM associated with either NF1 or McCune–Albright syndrome.[9] Segmental pigmentation disorder rarely has associated extracutaneous anomalies. As with CALM, laser therapy can be considered for lesions in prominent locations, such as the face, but results are inconsistent.

Neurofibromatosis

Neurofibromatosis refers to a group of distinct disorders involving neuroectodermal and mesenchymal derivatives, characterized by CALM and tumors of the nervous system. Neurofibromatosis 1 is by far the most common type, comprising 90% of all NF cases. Segmental neurofibromatosis 1 presents with a segmentally distributed CALM, with small CALM (so-called 'freckles' within it, and over time with development of neurofibromas. The neurofibromas themselves are rarely present in newborns or infants, however. The condition is thought to be caused by mosaicism. Neurofibromatosis type 2 is a genetically distinct autosomal dominant disorder, characterized by acoustic or central nervous system schwannomas. It may also present with CALM, although these lesions tend to be fewer and paler than in NF1.

Neonates with multiple CALM should be carefully evaluated for stigmata of NF1, including measuring and counting of lesions (Fig. 22-2). The presence of six or more CALM greater than 5 mm in diameter in infants and children is strong evidence of NF1, but at least one other criterion is needed for diagnosis. Axillary and/or inguinal 'freckling' (really small CALM) is usually absent at birth, but often present by age 2. Although small cutaneous neurofibromas are not typically present in the newborn period, plexiform neurofibromas can be, often appearing as a firm, brown-red plaque. A family history of NF or other syndromes should be sought, and parents examined when possible. Previously unrecognized findings in a parent may confirm the diagnosis. Macrocephaly is a not uncommon early sign in NF1. In one prospective study 75% of patients with six or more CALM who were followed for 2 years, and 89% of patients followed for 3 or more years, developed other signs of NF1.[7] Manifestations of NF1 may evolve over time, and neonates at risk or with presumptive evidence of disease should be monitored closely.[10] Awareness of the age-dependent nature of clinical signs and symptoms associated with NF1 is the key to providing appropriate anticipatory guidance.[11] A more extensive discussion of NF is found in Chapter 26.

McCune–Albright Syndrome

McCune–Albright syndrome refers to the triad of CALM, polyostotic fibrous dysplasia, and endocrine dysfunction. Clinical findings are quite variable, and not all patients will develop all three features. Neonatal presentation may be limited to cutaneous findings. CALM in McCune–Albright syndrome are usually larger than in NF1. Whereas previous descriptions have emphasized a jagged margin, said to resemble the 'coast of Maine,' the pattern is now recognized to correspond to a nevoid pattern, following the lines of Blaschko, albeit in broader lesions than those seen in other mosaic disorders, such as incontinentia pigmenti. Lesions may be unilateral or bilateral. They are often a somewhat darker brown than in other causes of CALM, though this is not consistent enough to be a diagnostic feature (Fig. 22-3). The skin lesions may be present at birth and can darken with time. Bony lesions are usually on the same side as unilateral CALM, consistent with the syndrome being a mosaic disorder.[12,13]

Extracutaneous findings may become manifest over time and include polyostotic fibrous dysplasia, where bone is replaced by fibrous tissue, resulting in asymmetry, bony growths, and pathological fractures. These are rarely seen at birth, more often developing in the first decade and frequently involving the face, hands, and legs. Multiple endocrine abnormalities have been reported, including precocious puberty, hyperthyroidism, Cushing syndrome, hypersomatotropism, hyperprolactinemia, and hyperparathyroidism.[14–16]

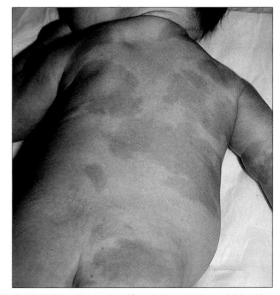

FIG. 22-3 Multiple patterned café au lait spots in a child with McCune–Albright syndrome.

McCune–Albright syndrome is more commonly recognized in females than in males. It is caused by a mutation of the *GNAS1* gene that encodes for the α subunit of the guanine nucleotide-binding protein, causing loss of GTPase activity and increased stimulation of the adenylate cyclase system, resulting in proliferation and autonomous hyperfunction of hormonally responsive cells.[12,15,19] This is an autosomal dominant mutation in which survival is only possible in individuals with a postzygotic somatic mutation with resulting mosaicism.[16,17]

As the clinical expression may be variable and segmental, diagnosis in newborns or young infants may be difficult. Radiological studies may not reveal bony abnormalities in the neonatal period. McCune–Albright syndrome must be differentiated from NF1. CALM of NF1 tend to be smaller and have a more scattered distribution.[12,13] Histologic study of the CALM does not help in differentiating McCune–Albright syndrome from other syndromes.[5,18]

Jaffe–Campanacci syndrome is evidenced by CALM with a 'coast of Maine' appearance, distributed unilaterally or diffusely, nonossifying fibromas (a condition distinct from polyostotic dysplasia), and multiple nevi.[1] The differential diagnosis also includes segmental pigmentation disorder.

The prognosis of McCune–Albright syndrome is generally good, but depends on the degree of bony and/or endocrine involvement. Close observation for endocrine abnormalities is appropriate. Referral for orthopedic and endocrine evaluation is recommended.[15] Many patients develop normal reproductive function. Development of malignancy is rare, and lifespan is usually normal. Extensive osseous dysplasia in the early years portends a poor prognosis.[13]

Silver–Russell Syndrome

Patients with Silver–Russell syndrome have a low birthweight, skeletal asymmetry, and a triangular facies. Some have been noted to have CALM and increased numbers of melanocytic nevi.[20]

Congenital Lingual Melanotic Macule

The congenital lingual melanotic macule is a rarely reported but distinct clinical entity, and should be considered in the differential diagnosis of pigmented lesions of the tongue.

Cutaneous Findings

Congenital lingual melanotic macules present at birth as solitary or multiple well-circumscribed brown to black macules on the dorsal surface of the tongue (Fig. 22-4). Growth tends to be commensurate with the growth of the neonate, and family history is negative for systemic disorders associated with mucosal hyperpigmentation. Characteristic histologic features include prominent basal hyperpigmentation with overlying hyperkeratosis. Melanocytes are normal in number, and do not display evidence of nesting or atypia.[21] Although it is typically benign in nature, a case of malignant transformation of histologically documented benign oral melanosis into oral melanoma has been reported.[22]

Treatment and Care

Because the number of reported cases is small, the approach to management cannot be generalized. Congenital lingual melanotic macules appear to be benign, but some authors advocate biopsy given their unclear potential for malignant transformation.

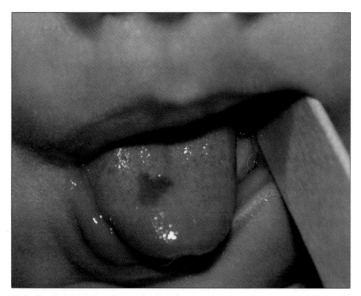

FIG. 22-4 Lingual melanotic macule.

DISORDERS OF DERMAL MELANOCYTOSIS

The following disorders, each characterized by a distinct blue-gray hyperpigmentation, share the common feature of the presence of melanocytes in the mid to lower dermis without proliferation of melanocytes in the upper dermis or at the dermoepidermal junction.

Mongolian Spots
Cutaneous Findings

Mongolian spots are well-defined, benign, brown, blue-gray or blue-black patches that are usually located over the sacrum or lower back (see Chapter 7). They are present at birth or early infancy in over 80% of African-American and Asian babies, with a lesser incidence in lighter-skinned races.[3,23] Mongolian spots can range in size from a few millimeters to more than 10 cm, and can be single or multiple.[23] The sacrococcygeal area is most commonly affected, but lesions may occur on the buttock, dorsal trunk, and extremities (Fig. 22-5).[23,24] Lesion color stabilizes in infancy, with the majority fading before adulthood.

Associations

Extensive mongolian spots can be seen in association with capillary vascular malformations (port wine stains) in so-called phakomatosis pigmentovascularis, and also in the metabolic disorders, GM1 gangliosidosis and mucopolysaccharidosis type II (Hurler syndrome; see discussion below).[1,25] Mongolian spots may also occasionally be seen directly contiguous to a structural malformation such as a cleft lip.

Histology reveals collections of greatly elongated, slender, spindle-shaped melanocytes scattered between the collagen bundles of the reticular dermis. The melanocytes generally lie parallel to the skin's surface, and melanophages are not observed.[5,18] Although other dermal melanocytic conditions may have similar microscopic appearance, clinical morphology and distribution will usually establish the diagnosis.

Pathogenesis

Dermal melanocytosis is thought to result from arrest in embryonal melanocyte migration from neural crest to epider-

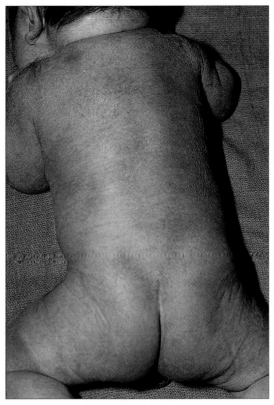

FIG. 22-5 Dermal melanocytosis/mongolian spot. Extensive involvement includes the trunk and lower extremity.

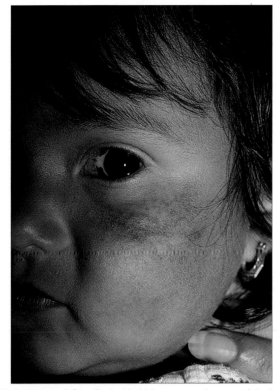

FIG. 22-6 Nevus of Ota. Periorbital blue-gray color associated with dermal melanocytosis.

mis. Why the lesions almost always occur in the same areas is not well understood.[3] The blue color, characteristic of dermal melanin, occurs as a result of the Tyndall phenomenon.

Differential Diagnosis

The diagnosis of mongolian spots is based on clinical morphology and location. Other disorders of dermal melanocytosis include nevus of Ito, nevus of Ota, and congenital blue nevus. Lesions of persistent dermal melanocytosis are usually more blue and more sharply demarcated than mongolian spots, and distribution and clinical context are helpful in differentiating them from nevus of Ito and Ota. The differential diagnosis occasionally includes CALM of congenital melanocytic nevi, but the blue-gray color usually helps in differentiation from these disorders. Biopsy can be helpful in verifying the dermal location of the melanocytes if the diagnosis is in doubt.

Treatment and Care

Most mongolian spots will fade over time, although the mechanism for this fading is not understood. Persistent lesions seldom require treatment. Laser treatment has been reported to achieve lightening, with varying degrees of success.[26]

As with CALM, dermal melanocytosis may sometimes serve as a marker of an underlying disorder. Extensive dermal melanocytosis has been reported in association with underlying disorders of lysosomal storage, most commonly GM1, gangliosidosis type1, and Hurler syndrome.[27] In contrast to the typical mongolian spot, dermal melanocytosis in patients with underlying metabolic disease tends to be extensive, with indistinct borders, posterior and anterior distribution, and persistence. Similarly, atypical mongolian spots have been associated with cleft lip. The etiology for this association is unclear but is

postulated to result from an error in nerve growth factor signaling.[27,28] Unusual, extensive or persistent mongolian spots may therefore warrant investigation for the presence of an associated disorder of lysosomal storage.

Nevus of Ota (Nevus Fuscoceruleus Ophthalmomaxillaris, Oculodermal Melanocytosis)

Periorbital dermal melanocytosis in the distribution of the first and second divisions of the trigeminal nerve is known as nevus of Ota. This is more common in Asians and the darker pigmented races and has a female preponderance.[29] Lesions are present at birth in 50% of affected individuals, with a second peak of onset around puberty.[29]

Cutaneous Findings

Nevus of Ota is characterized by unilateral blue-gray confluent macules and patchy hyperpigmentation in the distribution of the ophthalmic and maxillary branches of the trigeminal nerve. Unilateral lesions are typical, although bilateral lesions are described in approximately 5–10% of patients. Pigmentation of the ipsilateral sclera is common (Fig. 22-6). Less commonly, the oral or nasal mucosa, retina, leptomeninges, or iris may be involved.

Extracutaneous Findings

Malignant blue nevi and cutaneous malignant melanoma can rarely occur with nevus of Ota. CNS melanocytosis has been reported in association with nevus of Ota.[30] If ocular pigmentation is present, glaucoma may occur secondary to melanocytes in the ciliary body of the anterior chamber of the eye, impeding the normal flow of fluid.[24] In addition to reported associations with cutaneous melanoma, both uveal and choroidal melanomas are seen with nevus of Ota, making regular ophthalmologic evaluation mandatory.[31]

Finally, progressive ipsilateral sensorineural deafness has been reported in three patients with nevus of Ota.[32]

Differential Diagnosis

Differential diagnosis in the neonate includes facial CALM, speckled lentiginous nevus, congenital blue nevus, and ochronosis.

Pathogenesis

The etiology of nevus of Ota is presumed to be similar to that of mongolian spots, involving errors in melanocyte migration from the neural crest to the epidermis.[3,29,33]

The diagnosis is usually made clinically, based on appearance and location. Biopsy shows elongated dendritic melanocytes scattered among collagen bundles in the dermis. They are usually more numerous and superficial than in mongolian spots. At times, melanocytes surround the sheaths of adnexal structures.[5]

Treatment and Care

Unlike mongolian spots, nevus of Ota does not lighten or resolve with time, and may increase in size and color intensity.[29] An ophthalmologic evaluation is recommended if the periorbital skin is involved, and regular ophthalmologic examinations should be performed if ocular pigment is present.[1] If desired, treatment with pigmented lesion lasers (e.g. alexandrite or Q-switched ruby) may be considered to help lighten or cause resolution of the lesion, but recurrence after successful laser therapy has been reported.[34,35]

Nevus of Ito (Nevus Fuscoceruleus Acromiodeltoideus)

Cutaneous Findings

Nevus of Ito is a patchy blue-gray discoloration of the skin on the shoulder, supraclavicular, neck, upper arm, scapular, and deltoid areas of the body (Fig. 22-7).[29] The condition has the same features as nevus of Ota, but its location approximates the distribution of the posterior supraclavicular and lateral brachial cutaneous nerves. It is generally benign, but malignant melanoma/blue nevus can rarely develop.

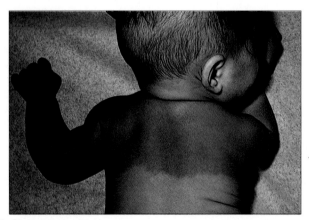

FIG. 22-7 Nevus of Ito.

Pathogenesis

The etiology is believed to be similar to that of mongolian spots and nevus of Ota (see previous discussion). Extracutaneous findings are not seen with nevus of Ito.

The diagnosis is usually made clinically, based on appearance and location. Elongated dendritic melanocytes scattered among collagen bundles in the dermis are noted on biopsy. They are usually more numerous and superficial than in mongolian spots. At times, melanocytes surround the sheaths of adnexal structures.[5,29,36]

Treatment and Care

Unlike mongolian spots, nevus of Ito does not lighten or resolve with time, and may increase in size and intensity of color.[29] Treatment with one of the pigment lasers has shown the potential for good results.[34,35]

Congenital Blue Nevus

A blue nevus is a hamartoma of dermal melanocytes. Congenital blue nevi are uncommon to rare. They may present in a similar fashion to large congenital melanocytic nevi, albeit with a blue-black color.

Cutaneous Findings

Classically, two forms of blue nevi have been described: common and cellular. Common blue nevi, which are uncommon as congenital lesions, typically present as 2–10 mm blue-black smooth macules or papules, most frequently on the scalp or face (although they can occur anywhere), and are rarely associated with complications.[5,37] Typical cellular blue nevi are acquired, may range between 2 and 20 mm, may be single or multiple, and are most commonly present on the buttock and sacrococcygeal areas.[38,39] Cellular blue nevi may exhibit aggressive benign growth that may be confused with a malignant tumor, but may also undergo malignant change. Congenital blue nevi are usually of the cellular type; larger lesions of the head (usually > 8 cm) may involve underlying muscle bone and dura.[5,38,39] Malignant melanoma may arise within giant congenital cellular blue nevi of the scalp, although incidence figures for this are unavailable owing to the rarity of these lesions. Combined nevi, with features of melanocytic nevi and blue nevi, and blue nevi developing within lentiginous lesions (e.g. congenital unilateral speckled lentiginous blue nevi) or dermal melanocytosis, have been reported.[40]

The diagnosis is usually suggested by the blue-black clinical appearance, but a biopsy may be needed. In the common form, dendritic melanocytes are found singly or in small aggregations in the reticular dermis, and may be clustered around adnexal structures, vessels, and nerves.[37,45] They resemble the cells in mongolian spot and in nevus of Ito, but their density is much greater. Melanophages are frequently observed. The cellular type has similar dendritic and spindled melanocytes, mixed in with cellular islands composed of closely aggregated, large, spindle-shaped cells with ovoid nuclei and abundant pale cytoplasm, often containing little or no melanin.[38,39]

Extracutaneous Findings

Familial multiple blue nevi may occur as part of Carney complex (the association of myxomas, endocrine overactivity, and spotty pigmentation that includes epithelioid blue nevi), or without associated abnormalities.[41]

Pathogenesis

The etiology is unknown. Blue nevi may represent a defect in embryogenesis with arrested migration of melanocytes from the neural crest to the epidermis.[3] In support of this theory is the predominant distribution of blue nevi on the scalp, sacrum, and dorsal hands and feet – all sites of residual pools of dermal melanocytes.[42]

Treatment and Care

For both types of blue nevi conservative surgical excision will usually suffice. In the absence of unusual or atypical features, clinically stable and small common blue nevi do not necessarily need to be removed. The common type is rarely malignant, but is sometimes removed based on appearance and/or dark color. The term 'malignant blue nevus' refers to a rare group of melanomas which can occur in association with common or cellular blue nevi, or arising de novo and resembling cellular blue nevi. As blue nevi sometimes share overlapping histologic features of melanoma, patients should be closely followed.[38,39,43] Dermoscopy of common blue nevi reveals uniform and dense blue coloring.[44]

MOSAIC CONDITIONS AND PATTERNED DYSPIGMENTATION (WHORLED AND SEGMENTAL HYPERPIGMENTATION)

Mosaic Conditions

A variety of hyperpigmented conditions may present in a segmental pattern or following lines of Blaschko (Box 22-2; see also Table 3-2). Many of these conditions are discussed in Chapter 26. Streaky, whorled macular hyperpigmentation is considered to be a physical representation of genomic mosaicism, and may be seen as an isolated cutaneous skin condition or as part of a more significant genetic disease (Fig. 22-8). For example, the X-linked condition incontinentia pigmenti often displays hyperpigmented streaks following the lines of Blaschko. Incontinentia pigmenti is an X-linked dominant condition, with affected females being heterozygous for the mutation with inactivation of one of the X-chromosomes, as predicted in the Lyon hypothesis. It is theorized that the pigmented whorls represent a clonal population of cells that arises during early development and progresses laterally, along the craniocaudal axis from the midline neuroectoderm. The peculiar but reproducible patterns reflect embryologic migration patterns, with linear appearance on the limbs, S-shapes on the chest, and V-shapes on the back. In addition to chromosome mosaicism, postzygotic somatic mutations of other chromosomes can create populations of genetically differing cells. Segmental hyperpigmented (or hypopigmented) lesions in patients without specific syndromic diagnoses may be caused by functional cutaneous mosaicism, and careful physical examination and follow-up is reasonable to assess for systemic problems (Fig. 22-9). A number of other conditions listed in this chapter (e.g. McCune–Albright syndrome) are due to mosaicism, but have been described under the headings pertaining to their cutaneous manifestations. An excellent review of mosaicism in cutaneous pigmentation has recently been published.[46]

Box 22-2 Conditions with hyperpigmentation having a 'lines of Blaschko' pattern

Epidermal nevus

Focal dermal hypoplasia (Goltz syndrome)

Human chimera

Incontinentia pigmenti

Linear and whorled hypermelanosis

Segmental hypermelanosis (Chromosomal mosaicism)

X-linked cutaneous amyloidosis, female carriers

X-linked chondrodysplasia punctata (Conradi–Hünermann disease)

Adapted from Bolognia JL, Orlow SJ, Glick SA. Lines of Blaschko. J Am Acad Dermatol 1994; 31: 157–190.

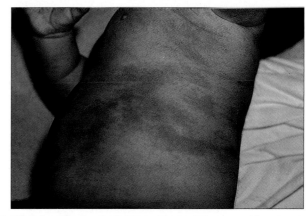

FIG. 22-8 Localized, whorled hyperpigmentation, considered a sign of cutaneous mosaicism. This child was clinically well.

Chimerism

Human chimerism is rare, but results from fusion of two or more genetically distinct zygotes. Chimerism may display pigmentation in a line of Blaschko distribution, checkerboard pattern, or asymmetric CALM.

Linear and Whorled Nevoid Hypermelanosis
Cutaneous Findings

Linear and whorled nevoid hypermelanosis is a term used to describe asymmetric epidermal hypermelanosis in streaky or swirl-like patterns (Fig. 22-10). These pigmented areas follow lines of Blaschko. Linear and whorled hypermelanosis appears at birth or within a few weeks of age without a preceding inflammatory event. Pigmentation may become more evident over the first few years of life and then stabilize, although fading with time has been observed in some individuals.[47–50] Some patients have hyperpigmentation admixed with hypopigmentation.[51]

Extracutaneous Findings

Linear and whorled nevoid hypermelanosis is usually a benign isolated condition. Patients with associated anomalies have been reported, although in most cases chromosomal analysis has not been performed to exclude mosaicism or chimerism, as has been described in extensive nevoid hypopigmentation (so-called hypomelanosis of Ito).[47] These anomalies include neurologic, cardiac, and musculoskeletal defects.

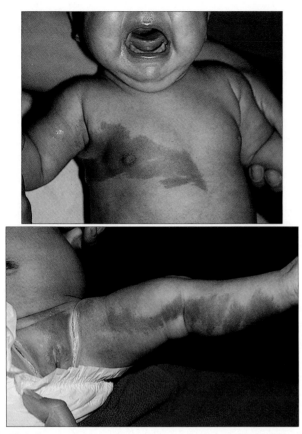

FIG. 22-9 Segmental hyperpigmentation affecting the right side of the face, chest and left leg.

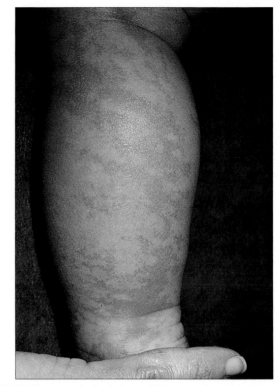

FIG. 22-10 Linear and whorled nevoid hypermelanosis.

Pathogenesis

Nevoid hypermelanosis is believed to be due to somatic mosaicism of neuroectodermal cells deriving from the neural crest, with the two skin colors representing two distinct populations of cells.[47,52]

Nevoid hypermelanosis is usually diagnosed clinically. Biopsy specimens demonstrate diffuse increased pigmentation of the epidermal basal layer and a slight increase in the number of melanocytes, without an increase in dermal melanophages or pigment incontinence.[5,47,48]

Differential Diagnosis

Nevoid hypermelanosis should be differentiated from other conditions with hyperpigmented lesions that follow Blaschko's lines, such as incontinentia pigmenti (third stage), linear epidermal nevus, nevoid hypermelanosis in human chimeras, Conradi–Hünermann syndrome, Goltz syndrome, and Naegeli–Franceschetti–Jadassohn syndrome.[49,50,52] These conditions may be excluded based on textural changes of the hyperpigmented areas and other clinical findings. Diffuse hypopigmentation, seen with extensive hypomelanosis of Ito, may be difficult to distinguish from nevoid hypermelanosis, as it may be hard to determine the patient's natural color and whether affected areas are pathologically lighter or darker.

Treatment and Care

No specific treatments have been described. Careful physical and developmental examinations are usually sufficient for detecting extracutaneous associations. If other anomalies exist, blood and skin fibroblast chromosomal analysis for mosaicism should be considered.[47,52]

Incontinentia Pigmenti (see also Chapter 26)

Incontinentia pigmenti is an X-linked dominant hereditary disorder characterized by streaky, linear, or splash-like cutaneous lesions following the lines of Blaschko that are usually present at birth or shortly thereafter (see Chapter 26). Also known as Bloch–Sulzberger syndrome, it is found almost exclusively in females as a result of prenatal lethality in males. Rare male cases may be due to XXY karyotype. Incontinentia pigmenti results from a mutation in nuclear factor-κB (NFκB) essential modulator (NEMO) and has been mapped to Xq28.

Cutaneous Findings

There are four classic stages in the skin. Patients may demonstrate only some of these, and overlap or 'skipping' of stages may occur. Neonates may be born with or develop the hyperpigmented lesions without signs of the preceding stages.[53,54] Stage 1 is an inflammatory vesicobullous stage with streaks of eosinophil-filled epidermal vesicles. It usually presents at birth or in the first few weeks of life, though later recurrences have been reported. A second stage with papules, pustules, verrucous, or lichenoid lesions usually appears within 2–6 weeks. These lesions may not correspond exactly to the same areas as stage 1, and usually resolve within weeks to months. A third stage of macular linear/whorled hyperpigmentation follows and gradually increases in intensity. There may be a fourth stage of hypopigmentation and atrophy that replaces the hyperpigmentation.

Extracutaneous Findings

Extracutaneous findings are common. Peripheral eosinophilia is often present during stage 1. Other organ system anomalies include defects of dentition (missing, pegged, and notched teeth), alopecia, ocular defects (retinal detachment, proliferative retinopathy, fibrovascular retrolental membrane, ciliary body atrophy, strabismus, cataracts, blindness, microphthalmia), central nervous system abnormalities (seizures, spastic paralysis, mental retardation), structural development problems (dwarfism, club foot, spina bifida, hemiatrophy, congenital hip dysplasia), nail dystrophy, hemarthrosis, various internal malignancies, and immunological problems.[53,54]

The differential diagnosis is stage dependent: in the neonatal period it includes epidermolysis bullosa, impetigo, and epidermolytic hyperkeratosis.

Clinical diagnosis can usually be made by the distinctive skin changes. The skin biopsy results will be different for each stage.[5] The first stage is characterized by epidermal vesicles and spongiosis with eosinophils.[55] Scattered dyskeratotic cells and whorls of squamous cells with central keratinization are found between vesicles. The second stage shows acanthosis, irregular papillomatosis, hyperkeratosis, and more dyskeratotic cells and squamous whorls, usually with pigment dilution, vacuolar alteration, and degeneration of the basal layer. Mild inflammatory infiltrate with melanin within melanophages in the upper dermis ('incontinent pigment') is seen in the second and third stages of the disease.

Phakomatosis Pigmentovascularis
(see also Chapter 20)
Cutaneous Findings

Phakomatosis pigmentovascularis is a term used to describe the simultaneous occurrence of congenital cutaneous pigmented lesions, including dermal melanocytosis, nevus spilus, and linear and whorled nevoid hyperpigmentation, in association with vascular malformations, particularly capillary vascular malformations (port wine stains).[25,56] Coexisting congenital triangular alopecia has been reported in cases of phakomatosis pigmentovascularis.[57]

A classification system with four types of phakomatosis pigmentovascularis has been proposed on the basis of the type of pigmented lesion, and each of these is subdivided on the basis of whether extracutaneous lesions are present (subtype 'b') or absent (subtype 'a') (Table 22-2).[1] The most common by far is type II, the concordance of dermal melanocytosis with port wine stains (Fig. 22-11). A simpler classification schema has recently been proposed, with only three distinctive categories, based on the type of associated vascular lesion.[58]

Extracutaneous Findings

Most of the coexistent extracutaneous abnormalities are those usually associated with each of the congenital birthmarks: Sturge–Weber syndrome with port wine stains in the trigeminal V1 distribution (and glaucoma, both with periorbital port wine stains and with nevus of Ota), and Klippel–Trenaunay syndrome with port wine stains on affected extremities. Addi-

TABLE 22-2 Classification schema of phakomatosis pigmentovascularis

Type	Vascular malformation	Pigmentary nevus
I	Port wine stain	Epidermal nevus
II	Port wine stain	Dermal melanocytosis (± nevus anemicus)
III	Port wine stain	Nevus spilus (± nevus anemicus)
IV	Port wine stain	Dermal melanocytosis and nevus spilus (± nevus anemicus)

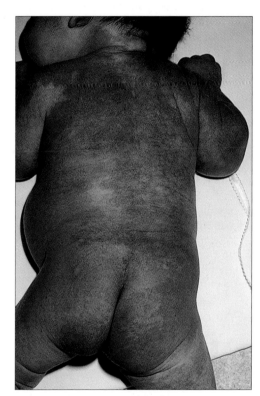

FIG. 22-11 Phakomatosis pigmentovascularis type II. Extensive dermal melanocytosis (mongolian spot) and port wine stain.

tional reported extracutaneous anomalies include hypoplastic larynx and subglottic stenosis, multiple granular cell tumors, iris mammillations, scoliosis, anemia, malignant polyposis, mental disturbances, psychomotor retardation, epilepsy, intracranial calcifications, and cerebral atrophy.

Pathogenesis

The pathogenesis of phakomatosis pigmentovascularis is not understood. Happle[58a] has proposed so-called 'twin-spotting' as an possible explanation, but this has not been proven (see discussion below).

Differential Diagnosis and Management

Proteus syndrome should be considered in the differential diagnosis of phakomatosis pigmentovascularis. Proteus syndrome may display coexisting epidermal and vascular nevi, though the presence of marked gigantism and asymmetry in proteus syndrome usually helps to distinguish the two. Laser treatments, such as pulsed dye laser for the port wine stain and one of the pigmented lesion lasers for the melanocytosis, may be helpful in reducing disfigurement.[1]

Phakomatosis Pigmentokeratotica

Phakomatosis pigmentokeratotica describes the simultaneous presence of epidermal nevus with pigmentary anomalies, including zosteriform lentiginous nevus, segmental lentigo, or nevus spilus. Its name emphasizes the analogy to phakomatosis pigmentovascularis.[59] The epidermal nevi may be organoid or sebaceous, and follow Blaschko's lines. Lentiginous elements may present in later life. Most reported cases have associated anomalies. These include neurologic abnormalities (seizures, retardation, hyperpathia, dysesthesia, hyperhidrosis), ophthalmologic abnormalities (including coloboma, lipodermoid of the conjunctiva, palpebral ptosis), and skeletal and limb defects (hemiatrophy, scoliosis, muscle weakness, gait disturbances). Basal cell epitheliomas may develop within sebaceous nevi, and ichthyosis-like hyperkeratosis has also been reported.[60] A report of malignant transformation in both nevus sebaceus and speckled lentiginous nevus underscores the need for serial examination in these patients.[61]

Pathogenesis

The pathogenesis of this condition is not known but as with phakomatosis pigmentovascuaris, Happle[58a] has hypothesized that the findings could be due to so-called twin-spotting. This genetic phenomenon occurs when paired patches of genetically distinct clones exist in a background of normal cells, and may result when organisms heterozygous for two different recessive mutations localized in close proximity on the same chromosome undergo somatic recombination, resulting in two homozygous daughter cells, which serve as stem cells for distinct clonal populations.[62] No experimental proof of twin-spotting has yet been demonstrated in humans.

Naegeli–Franceschetti–Jadassohn Syndrome

Naegeli–Franceschetti–Jadassohn syndrome is an autosomal dominantly inherited ectodermal dysplasia characterized by brown-gray reticulated hyperpigmentation beginning in early childhood, and a decreased ability to sweat. The pigmentation is more often on the abdomen, neck, and trunk, and less frequently on the flexures and face. Palmoplantar hyperkeratosis develops in late childhood.[63] Candidate gene loci map to chromosome 17q21.[64]

Striped Hyperpigmentation of the Torso
(see Chapter 7)

A case was described in an African-American neonate who had bands of horizontal pigmentation across the abdomen that appeared after birth (Fig. 22-12). At birth, the baby's skin had some slight thickening and scaling that decreased as the hyperpigmentation appeared. The dark stripes faded after a few months, and the skin became normal except for mild changes of ichthyosis vulgaris.[65] There were no known associations or signs of systemic disease. It was hypothesized that embryonal skin was unable to exfoliate normally, and that this was preceded by folding and fissuring of skin that promoted melanogenesis. Biopsy was not performed.

Congenital Curvilinear Palpable Hyperpigmentation

Congenital curvilinear palpable hyperpigmentation is a recently described unique pattern of hyperpigmentation confined to the

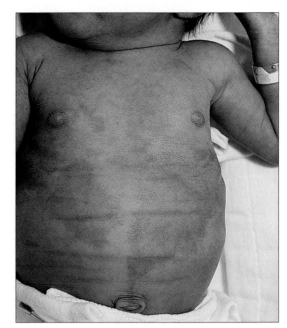

FIG. 22-12 Striped hyperpigmentation of the torso.

posterior aspect of the bilateral legs. It is characterized by a curvilinear loop configuration, palpability, neonatal onset, and bilateral posterior calf location. Lesions can mimic postinflammatory hyperpigmentation from trauma, or be secondary to child abuse from beating with a looped cord. Associated abnormal neurologic and developmental abnormalities have been reported.[66]

SPOTTY PIGMENTATION – DIFFUSE

Xeroderma Pigmentosum

Xeroderma pigmentosum (XP) is a severe, rare disease of autosomal recessive inheritance with clinical and cellular sensitivity to ultraviolet (UV) light, caused by decreased ability to repair DNA damage. Patients experience cutaneous and ocular photosensitivity and malignancies, with pigment abnormalities (Box 22-3).

Cutaneous Findings

The skin is normal at delivery, but changes can develop shortly thereafter depending on the amount of UV exposure. An early sign in some but not all affected infants is sunburn

---

Box 22-3 Summary of clinical features of xeroderma pigmentosum

- Autosomal recessive disease characterized by clinical and cellular sensitivity to ultraviolet light
- Normal skin at birth
- Sunburn with minimal sun exposure
- Skin findings with prolonged UV exposure include pigmented macules, achromic spots, telangiectasia and atrophy
- Most common skin malignancies include basal cell carcinomas, squamous cell carcinomas and melanoma
- Associated neurological problems in approximately 20% of patients

in spite of relatively minimal sun exposure. Patients with XP develop numerous pigmented macules (0.2–1 cm) on sun-exposed areas. The number of macules correlates with the degree of sun exposure and is seen even in individuals from more darkly pigmented races. Pigmented lesions may be brown, gray, or black, and may be so dense that they coalesce. Although they resemble freckles, they are actually solar lentigines and do not fade with time.[67] Each macule is a clone of cells derived from a single mutated melanocyte.[68] Achromic spots, which may represent mutated melanocytes that have lost their ability to synthesize melanin, may also develop. After continued exposure the skin enters a telangiectatic or atrophic stage. Skin malignancies may appear during the pigmented stage, but become more frequent in the atrophic stage. These include basal cell carcinomas, squamous cell carcinomas, and melanoma, as well as other rarer skin tumors.[68–70]

Extracutaneous Findings
Approximately 20% of patients have neurological problems, including low intelligence, cerebral and cerebellar dysfunction, peripheral neuropathy, basal ganglia involvement, hyporeflexia, spasticity, sensory defects, and progressive dementia.[68,69] An increase in internal malignancies has been reported.

Pathogenesis
Xeroderma pigmentosum is found in all races worldwide, and is (so far) divided into 10 complementation groups (A, B, C, D, E, F, G, H, I, and Variant) based on in-vitro cell fusion studies. Different races often have one dominant complementation group, and some groups consist of a single kindred. In groups A–I the cause is a genetic mutation (different in each group) that impairs removal of pyrimidine dimers in DNA damaged by UV because of a defect in endonuclease activity. Functional endonuclease recognizes and removes damaged DNA regions so that other enzymes can initiate DNA repair (unscheduled DNA synthesis). In the Variant form, initiation of repair occurs normally, but a later step in postreplication repair is defective.[68,69]

Differential Diagnosis
There are no findings of xeroderma pigmentosum at birth, as the skin is only damaged after exposure to UV light. A history of a young child developing erythema, lentigines, and increased pigmentation after UV exposure, particularly with conjunctivitis and photophobia, should prompt consideration of xeroderma pigmentosum. Other photosensitivity disorders, such as Cockayne syndrome (atrophy of the skin with telangiectasia) or trichothiodystrophy (brittle hair, ichthyosis, abnormal nails), should be easy to differentiate based on the clinical examination. Although erythropoietic protoporphyria has more burning pain and fewer skin findings, and erythropoietic porphyria (Günther) displays blistering, porphyrin screening is still recommended in suspected xeroderma pigmentosum cases. Hereditary polymorphous light eruption can cause similar symptoms, but without early malignancy. Peutz–Jeghers syndrome presents with the pigmented macules limited to the perioral skin and oral mucosa. Syndromes such as Rothmund–Thomson, Hartnup, or Bloom may display photosensitivity, but patients do not tend to have the hyperpigmented lesions of xeroderma pigmentosum.[71]

The histopathologic changes are nondiagnostic; lesional skin may show changes of severe photoaging, lentigines, or skin malignancy.[5] Specialized diagnostic tests may be performed from a specimen of nonlesional skin processed for cell culture. Some research laboratories may be able to confirm the diagnosis by demonstrating cellular UV sensitivity or unscheduled DNA repair, and may also be able to perform similar testing for prenatal diagnosis on cultured cells from amniocentesis if there is a family history of xeroderma pigmentosum.[72]

Treatment and Care
The severity of xeroderma pigmentosum varies, depending on the particular defect and the amount of UV exposure. The most severely affected usually die of cancer before 10 years of age. Management involves genetic counseling, meticulous light avoidance, protective clothing, sunscreen, sunglasses, window coatings, long hairstyles, and methylcellulose eye drops for moist corneas. Skin examinations need to be frequent and thorough to catch premalignant/malignant changes early so they can be treated with cryosurgery, topical antimitotic agents such as 5-fluorouracil, or surgery. In some patients, high-dose oral isotretinoin can prevent new cancer formation, but is associated with side effects, especially in children.[73] Treatment with topical liposome-encapsulated endonuclease has been reported to decrease the rate of formation of actinic keratoses and basal cell carcinomas.[74]

Cutaneous Mastocytosis (Urticaria Pigmentosa)

Cutaneous mastocytosis, or urticaria pigmentosa (UP; see Chapter 25), may develop in infancy or early childhood. Mastocytomas are usually yellow-orange in color, but occasionally present as a light brown to deeply pigmented infiltrative lesion mimicking a congenital melanocytic nevus. Urticaria pigmentosa is a multifocal form of mastocytosis characterized by up to hundreds of brown, reddish-brown or yellow macules, papules, and nodules composed of populations of cutaneous mast cells (see Figs 25-13 and 25-14). Lesions of UP are most commonly on the trunk and extremities, but may be anywhere on the body, although infrequently on the scalp, palms, soles, or mucous membranes. A characteristic finding is the development of erythema and an urticarial wheal with friction (Darier's sign). Vesicles or bullae may occur; recurrent blisters in the same anatomic location in the first few months of life should prompt consideration of mastocytosis. The age of onset varies. In one study, 15% of

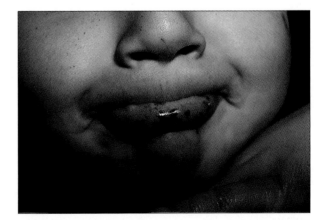

FIG. 22-13 Peutz–Jehger syndrome. Hyperpigmented labial macules.

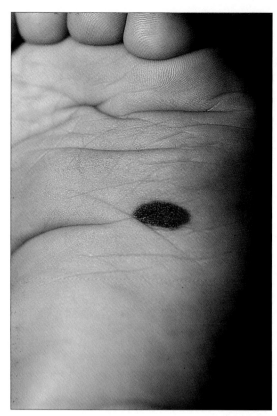

FIG. 22-14 Small congenital nevus.

patients had lesions at birth, and 64% of cases were apparent by age 6 months.[75]

The lesions tend to be larger on young children than adults, oval or round in shape, and usually between 1 and 10 mm in diameter.

The clinical appearance alone is often sufficient for diagnosis, especially if Darier's sign is present. Dermatographism of uninvolved skin occurs in 30–50% of all patients, owing to an increase in mast cells throughout the dermis of normal skin, but in itself is not diagnostic.[75,76] Histopathologic examination demonstrates an infiltrate of mast cells in the upper third of the dermis, generally located around capillaries. In the larger papules, the cells may be packed into tumor-like aggregates.

Postinflammatory Hyperpigmentation
Cutaneous Findings
Postinflammatory hyperpigmentation refers to brown macules and patches in the skin, seen after an inflammatory condition. Lesions consistent with postinflammatory hyperpigmentation have been seen at birth, and certainly may develop within the first few weeks of life. Common factors inducing postinflammatory hyperpigmentation in hospitalized neonates include the use of tape, adhesive monitor leads, and mechanical trauma, which may form distinct patterns. An indistinct pattern may form secondary to eczematous processes. Patients with darker skin types are more likely to develop postinflammatory hyperpigmentation than lighter skin types.

The dermoepidermal junction and basal layer are disrupted by epidermal injury (damaged epidermal keratinocytes and melanocytes). Melanin passes from its normal epidermal posi-

tion into the dermis and is engulfed by macrophages to form melanophages.[77] This dermal melanin is slow to break down, causing a delay in resolution of skin discoloration.

Differential Diagnosis
The diagnosis may be one of exclusion. A clinical history of brown macules or patches that occur subsequent to inflammation in a corresponding pattern is suggestive. If the preceding inflammatory event was not noted, however, the appearance of the pigmentation often gives few clues to the nature of the cause. A Wood's light examination accentuates epidermal melanin and can be useful in delimiting the extent of pigment alteration. Biopsy is rarely indicated, but when performed is characterized by melanophages in the superficial dermis along with a variably dense infiltrate of lymphohistiocytes around the superficial blood vessels and in dermal papillae. Necrotic keratinocytes and coarse collagen bundles are occasionally seen. There is increased pigment in the basal layer.[5,77]

The differential diagnosis of postinflammatory hyperpigmentation includes fixed drug eruption, which usually has more of a blue tint and appears after exposure to the causative drug. Postinflammatory hyperpigmentation may be seen as a sequela of transient neonatal pustular melanosis, either at birth or after resolution of pustular lesions (see Chapter 7). Interestingly, biopsy does not show dermal melanophages.[77] Striped hyperpigmentation of the torso may also be a postinflammatory phenomenon.[65]

Treatment and Care
Prevention includes the avoidance of frictional injury or inflammation. A low-potency topical steroid may help calm residual inflammation. Hyperpigmentation usually fades spontaneously with time, especially when the pigment is predominantly epidermal.

Universal Melanosis

There are several progressive conditions in which the patient demonstrates patches of hyperpigmentation at birth or during infancy. In addition to the skin, including the palms and soles, they involve the oral mucosa, conjunctiva, and sclera. Familial progressive hyperpigmentation displays hyperpigmentation in variably sized dots, whorls, streaks, and patches, not apparently following the lines of Blaschko,[78] whereas in universal acquired melanosis (carbon baby) the entire skin becomes deep black.[79] There are no known extracutaneous findings, and the etiologies are unknown.

Biopsy shows hyperpigmentation of the basal layer with pigment up to the stratum corneum. There are normal numbers of melanocytes, and some dermal melanophages.[78,79]

Differential Diagnosis
The clinical features, as well as the absence of significant melanin incontinence, should differentiate these conditions from incontinentia pigmenti, Naegeli–Franceschetti–Jadassohn syndrome, and linear and whorled nevoid hyperpigmentation.[78,79]

Poikiloderma (Box 22-4)

Poikiloderma is a cutaneous finding which characterizes a number of photosensitivity syndromes that can be present at birth, beginning as diffuse erythema and evolving into a red

The term poikiloderma describes a tetrad of cutaneous findings that include the following:

- Telangiectasia (permanent dilatation of capillaries, venules, and arterioles in the skin)
- Atrophy (cutaneous changes that result in thinning of epidermis, dermis, or both)
- Hyperpigmentation
- Hypopigmentation

reticulated dermatosis. It generally appears first on the cheeks, then spreads to the buttocks, extensor surfaces of hands, forearms, and legs.[80]

Poikiloderma can be seen in a number of syndromes, including poikiloderma congenitale (Rothmund–Thomson syndrome), Bloom syndrome, Kindler syndrome, and dyskeratosis congenita. It may be a later finding in conditions such as xeroderma pigmentosum, connective tissue disorders, Cockayne syndrome, and Fanconi anemia.[80]

Pathogenesis

The pathogenesis and etiology are unknown. It is a finding in a number of disorders with differing causes, and is exacerbated by light exposure.

Diagnosis

The diagnosis is made by the clinical appearance of the reticulated eruption. Biopsy results will differ depending on the severity. Abnormal findings include varying degrees of epidermal thinning, with hyperkeratosis, dilated vessels, hydropic degeneration of the basal layer, variable numbers of pigment-laden melanophages, and a band-like or perivascular lymphocytic infiltrate in the dermis.[5,80] Prognosis depends on the particular condition. Early recognition of the correct diagnosis, careful monitoring of the patient for associated abnormalities, and sun protection are all critical.[80]

METABOLIC CAUSES

Addison Disease and Adrenocortical-Unresponsiveness Syndrome

Addison disease is caused by deficiency of adrenocortical hormones. Changes in pigmentation, include diffuse tan, brown, or bronze darkening of all skin surfaces, especially exposed areas, and blue-black patches on mucous membranes. Associated signs and symptoms such as weakness, weight loss, and hypotension may be present. Hyponatremia, hyperkalemia, hypoglycemia, and eosinophilia accompany these changes. The prohormone pro-opiomelanocortin is secreted and cleaved, producing excessive ACTH and β-MSH (melanocyte-stimulating hormone). The increased level of β-MSH stimulates the production of melanin.[81,82]

Congenital insensitivity to functionally normal ACTH secretion has been termed ACTH-insensitivity syndrome, or adrenocortical-unresponsiveness syndrome.[83,84] Diffuse hyperpigmentation in the neonatal period may herald this condition before clinical hypoadrenalism. The histologic findings are nondiagnostic, and include increased amounts of melanin in the basal keratinocytes and often in the keratinocytes in the

upper spinous layer. The number of melanocytes is not increased.[5]

LENTIGINES

Spotty Pigmentation-Diffuse, With Lentigines
LEOPARD Syndrome (Multiple Lentigines Syndrome, Moynahan Syndrome) (Box 22-5)
LEOPARD is an acronym for a syndrome that includes lentigines, electrocardiographic conduction defects, ocular hypertelorism, pulmonary stenosis, abnormalities of genitalia, retardation of growth, and sensorineural deafness. It is a rare, autosomal dominant condition with variable expressivity involving multiple organ systems.[85] It results from a mutation in *PTPN 11*, a gene encoding the protein tyrosine phosphatase SHP2.[86] The mutation appears to have a dominant negative effect, interfering with growth factor/Erk-MAPK signaling.[87]

Cutaneous Findings

The lentigines may be present at birth, increasing in number until puberty, and are most numerous on the face, neck, upper trunk, upper arms, and diffusely elsewhere, but spare the mucous membranes.[85] CALM can also be seen in multiple lentigines syndrome.

On biopsy, the pigmented lesions are typical for lentigines, showing elongation of the rete ridges, an increase in concentration in melanocytes in the basal layer, an increase in the amount of melanin in both the melanocytes and the basal keratinocytes, and the presence of melanophages in the upper dermis.[5,85,89]

Extracutaneous Findings

A variety of extracutaneous abnormalities with variable expressivity have been associated.[85,88–90] Cardiac abnormalities include conduction defects and pulmonary or subaortic stenosis. Genital anomalies include gonadal hypoplasia, hypospadias, undescended testes, hypoplastic testes/ovaries, and delayed puberty. Short stature, pectus excavatum, kyphosis, ocular hypertelorism, mandibular prognathism, and other craniofacial defects constitute the skeletal abnormalities. Neurological findings include sensorineural deafness, mental retardation, seizures, abnormal nerve conduction, oculomotor defects, and an abnormal electroencephalogram (EEG).

Differential Diagnosis

Differential diagnosis includes both generalized and inherited patterned lentiginosis, Carney/NAME/LAMB syndrome (see the following discussion), and Peutz–Jeghers syndrome (see the following discussion). Xeroderma pigmentosa patients can

Lentigines
Electrocardiographic conduction defects
Ocular hypertelorism
Pulmonary stenosis
Abnormalities of genitalia
Retardation of growth
Sensorineural **D**eafness

have widespread lentigines, but these are related to UV exposure and are not present at birth.

Treatment and Care

In the neonatal period, evaluation of a suspected case should include complete physical examination for associated extracutaneous findings, electrocardiogram (ECG), hearing evaluation, and other studies as directed by symptomatology. Patients with suspected LEOPARD syndrome should have chest X-rays and ECGs periodically throughout childhood.[85] Associated abnormalities should be managed by the appropriate specialists, which may include cardiologists, audiologists, and urologists. Genetic counseling should be provided. There are reports of treatment of lentigines by cryotherapy and other surgical means.[91]

Carney/NAME/LAMB Syndrome

Several previously described syndromes have recently been consolidated under the classification of Carney syndrome, as it is now believed that they represent various manifestations of the same complex. These include the NAME syndrome (nevi, atrial myxoma, myxoid neurofibromata, ephelides) and the LAMB syndrome (lentigines, atrial myxoma, myxoid tumors, and blue nevi).[41]

Cutaneous Findings

Spotty pigmentation, mainly lentigines, is seen in the majority of patients (65%), but blue and junctional nevi may also occur.[41] The lentigines occur shortly after birth, have the highest concentration in the central face, and in contrast to LEOPARD syndrome, may involve the mucosa. They can also involve the neck, trunk, extremities, and genitalia. Associated nevi can either be congenital or appear later in infancy. Cutaneous myxomas, nontender dermal nodules, usually do not develop until the second decade of life, and typically are on the head and neck.[92,93] Psammomatous melanotic schwannomas may occur subcutaneously, but are usually in the nerve roots or GI tract and do not appear until the third decade of life.

Extracutaneous Findings

Extracutaneous associations include the presence of cardiac myxomas, endocrine disease (Cushing disease, acromegaly), testicular tumors and schwannomas.

Pathogenesis

This is an autosomal dominant-inherited multiple neoplasia disorder caused by a mutation in the *PRKAR1A* gene on chromosome 17q23.[94] Additional cases result from a mutation which maps to chromosome 2p.[73] *PRKAR1A* is a tumor-suppressor gene which encodes the regulatory subunit of protein kinase A (Box 22-6).

Biopsy reveals findings typical of lentigines (as described in Leopard syndrome).[5]

Differential Diagnosis

This condition needs to be differentiated from LEOPARD and Peutz–Jeghers syndromes. Neurofibromatosis is distinguished by freckling restricted to the axillary/groin/neck areas.[10] If a neonate has skin findings suggestive of Carney syndrome, ECG, echocardiography, and biopsy of a suspected blue nevus should be considered.[41]

Box 22-6 Carnex complex

Diagnosis of Carney complex requires two or more of the following:

- Spotty skin pigmentation (lentigines, nevi)
- Cutaneous myxomas
- Myxoid mammary fibroadenomas
- Primary pigmented nodular adrenocortical disease
- Testicular Sertoli cell tumors
- Pituitary adenomas with acromegaly or gigantism
- Cardiac myxomas
- Psammomatous melanotic schwannomas

Treatment and Care

Evaluation and treatment by cardiology, endocrinology, and urology is warranted. Genetic counseling should be offered.[95]

Localized, Spotty Pigmentation
Zosteriform Lentiginous Nevus

The term 'zosteriform lentiginous nevus' has been applied to a number of conditions with segmentally distributed hyperpigmentation, and it is best to think of this condition as a cutaneous finding which can be seen as a segmental manifestation of several pigmentary disorders, Clinical and semantic overlap exists with unilateral lentiginosis, segmental lentiginosis, lentiginous mosaicism, and speckled giant CALM. In the latter, partial, segmental forms of neurofibromatosis 1 may initially be diagnosed as zosteriform lentiginous nevus until later in life, when actual neurofibromas develop, allowing a diagnosis of segmental NF1 to be made.[96,97] Onset is generally at birth or in early childhood, although lesions may continue to evolve into adulthood. Lesions usually respect the midline. Histologic examination may be able to help differentiate cases which are truly lentigos from those with those with primarily increased basilar melanocytes. Some cases demonstrate both increase basilar melanin and small nests of melanocytes at the dermoepidermal junction, which has also been termed a 'jentigo' pattern. Axillary lesions may suggest the diagnosis of neurofibromatosis, though the unilateral or segmental cut-off and histology displaying increased number of melanocytes allow differentiation. Segmental lentiginosis is considered by many to be a distinct condition (see the following discussion).[98] Extracutaneous findings have been reported primarily in patients with segmental lentiginosis. Rare cases of melanoma arising within zosteriform lentiginous nevi have been reported.[99] Observation of lesions is reasonable because of the apparent rarity of malignancy, though excision might be considered if marked atypical nevus elements are present on biopsy. Therapy is usually not contemplated in newborns or early infancy; cryotherapy and various lasers may be of benefit in some patients.

Centrofacial Lentiginosis

These patients develop lentigines over the nose and cheeks in early childhood. The mucosa is spared, and there may be associated extracutaneous abnormalities. Neonatal presentation has not been reported.[100]

Segmental Lentiginosis (Partial Unilateral Lentiginosis, Lentiginous Mosaicism)

This rare pigmentary disorder consists of clustered lentigines in a segmental pattern. Lentigines may be present at birth or manifest in early childhood. Individual lesions are small, well-circumscribed, hyperpigmented macules grouped on a background of normal-appearing skin. This is in contrast to zosteriform lentiginous nevus, which has similar macules on a slightly hyperpigmented background.[96,97,101] Associated ipsilateral cerebrovascular hypertrophy and proliferation, and prominent neuropsychiatric findings with ipsilateral pes cavus have been reported.[102] There is speculation that affected individuals are mosaics of one of the more generalized lentigines syndromes.

Biopsy of lesions demonstrates findings typical of lentigo, including elongation of the rete ridges, an increase in the concentration of melanocytes in the basal layer, an increase in the amount of melanin in both the melanocytes and the basal keratinocytes, and the presence of melanophages in the upper dermis.[102] In a few cases the histological picture has appeared to represent a combination of lentigo and junctional nevus patterns.[96]

It may be difficult to distinguish segmental lentiginosis from zosteriform lentiginous nevus, agminated Spitz nevi, and segmental NF. Signs and symptoms that might indicate an alternative diagnosis should be looked for. Wood's light examination of the skin and skin biopsy may be indicated.[1] Cryotherapy and pigment lasers may be useful in removing the lentigines, if desired.[8] Prognosis depends on the specific systemic abnormalities.

Peutz–Jeghers Syndrome

Peutz–Jeghers syndrome is an autosomal dominantly inherited disorder with variable expressivity, characterized by mucocutaneous pigmentation and GI polyps. The lesions are dark-brown to black, 1–5 mm irregular macules that primarily involve the lips and buccal mucosa, but may also involve the palate, gingiva, face, fingers, elbows, palms, toes, and rarely even the periumbilical, perianal, or labial areas (Fig. 22-13).[103,104] There may be pigmented bands in the nail plates.[1] Hyperpigmented macules may be present at birth, but often develop later.

Later in life these patients develop hamartomatous polyps in the jejunum, ileum, colon, rectum, stomach, and duodenum, resulting in cramping pain, intussusception, and rectal bleeding. There can also be adenomatous polyps, and there is a slightly increased risk of gastrointestinal (GI) and other cancers, such as breast, cervix, uterus, lung, and testes in later life.[103,104]

A mutation has been identified in the gene for serine threonine kinase 11 (STK 11) on the short arm of chromosome 19. The disease manifestations are triggered by the loss of the functional copy of this gene in somatic cells. The mechanism by which this gene controls cellular differentiation is unknown.[105]

The histopathology of the pigmented lesions is typical for lentigines, that is, elongation of the rete ridges, increase in concentration of melanocytes in the basal layer, an increase in the amount of melanin in both the melanocytes and the basal keratinocytes, and the presence of melanophages in the upper dermis.[5] Abdominal pain, melena, or intussusception may be the presenting sign in older patients.[103,104] Facial lentigines

may also be seen during the neonatal period in LEOPARD syndrome, NAME/LAMB/Carney syndromes, and generalized lentiginosis. Labial melanosis may occur secondary to photo or sun damage, but would not involve the oral mucosa, nor be seen during the neonatal period.

Hematocrits and stool guaiacs should be performed at regular intervals in later childhood. Most of the GI polyps are not premalignant, but may cause symptoms requiring surgical intervention for relief. Referral to gastroenterology is prudent, as well as serial examination for malignancy of the GI tract and other associated organs. The cutaneous macules may fade after puberty, but the mucosal ones do not.[103,104] The macules may respond to treatment with liquid nitrogen or a pigment laser.

Bannayan–Riley–Ruvalcaba Syndrome

Bannayan–Riley–Ruvalcaba syndrome, a unifying term proposed to reflect overlap among three previously described conditions (Bannayan–Zonana, Riley–Smith, and Ruvalcaba–Myhre–Smith syndromes), is a condition with phenotypic variability having the common clinical features of macrocephaly with normal ventricular size, multiple subcutaneous and/or visceral lipomas, and vascular malformations, intestinal hamartomatous polyps, and lentigines of the penis and vulva.[106–108]

Pigmented macules, 2–6 mm in diameter, consistent with lentigines, occur on the glans and shaft of the penis. Lesions may be present at birth, or develop postnatally through adolescence.[107,109] Vulvar lesions have been reported in affected females. CALM, either single or multiple, may be observed. Other reported mucocutaneous findings include multiple subcutaneous lipomas, vascular malformations (termed hemangiomas in several reported cases), facial papules displaying features of trichilemmomas and verrucae, oral and perianal papillomas, acrochordons, acral keratoses, and acanthosis nigricans.

Macrocephaly (and macrosomia) is usually noted at birth or in early infancy. Central nervous system manifestations include hypotonia, developmental delay, mental retardation, seizures, arteriovenous malformations, meningiomas, and pseudopapilledema. Skeletal features include pectus excavatum, scoliosis and kyphoscoliosis, accelerated growth of digits, and a high arched palate. Hamartomatous polyps of the GI tract are seen in almost half of patients, but are not clinically significant in neonates. Lipid storage myopathy may present with increased limb size.[110] Ocular abnormalities include prominent Schwalbe lines and corneal nerves, strabismus, and amblyopia. Thyroiditis, adenomatous goiter, and thyroid carcinoma have been reported.

Autosomal dominant inheritance is observed, with sporadic occurrences and phenotypic variability. Germline mutations in PTEN, a tyrosine phosphatase and putative tumor suppressor gene, have been demonstrated in some families with Bannayan–Riley–Ruvalcaba syndrome, correlating with chromatin loss on chromosome 10q23. 33,111 Allelism with Cowden disease has been proposed. However, PTEN germline mutations were absent in several patients with sporadic Bannayan–Riley–Ruvalcaba syndrome.[112] Lipid-storage myopathy in a patient with Bannayan–Riley–Ruvalcaba syndrome has been attributed to long-chain L-3-Hydroxyacyl-coenzyme A dehydrogenase (L-CHAD) deficiency.[110]

Biopsy of the hyperpigmented penile macules display lentiginous hyperplasia of the epidermis with increased pigment in the basal layer and slight increase in melanocyte numbers. Cowden disease (multiple hamartoma syndrome) has many features in common, and may be allelic or have common genetic expression with Bannayan–Riley–Ruvalcaba syndrome, but it does not have neonatal manifestations. Lentiginosis with intestinal polyposis is seen with Peutz–Jeghers and Cronkhite–Canada syndromes, though the distribution of lentigines is different. Proteus syndrome (skull exostoses, epidermal nevi, pigmentary changes along Blaschko's lines, and palmoplantar masses) should be easily distinguishable. Recognition of the disease and specialty referral for management of systemic associations is appropriate.

PIGMENTARY VARIATIONS

Dyschromatosis

The dyschromatoses are a group of disorders characterized by both macular hyperpigmentation and hypopigmentation without atrophy or telangiectasia as seen in poikiloderma. Cases are extremely rare, and have been reported most commonly from Japan.[113] Dyschromatosis universalis hereditaria presents with generalized well-demarcated brown macules with variously sized hypopigmented macules. Cases have been reported with sparing of the face, hands, and feet, and generalized leukomelanoderma and leukotrichia have been observed.[114] Rare cases of universal dyschromia have been reported with small stature, high-tone deafness, idiopathic torsion dystonia, X-linked ocular albinism, photosensitivity, and neurosensory hearing loss.[115–117] Tissue histopathology shows increased epidermal melanin in the hyperpigmented areas without increased melanocyte numbers. Achromic skin shows an absence of melanin despite intact melanocytes, suggesting a disorder of melanosome production and distribution.[118] Dyschromatosis symmetrica hereditaria (reticulate acropigmentation of Dohi) presents with dyschromia restricted to sun-exposed skin, with distribution usually on the dorsal aspects of the extremities and face.[119] Findings generally develop after infancy. There is uncertainty if this condition is functionally related to the universal type.

Pigmentary Demarcation Lines

Pigmentary demarcation lines have been described and categorized into five types. They are most commonly seen in black and Asian individuals.[120,121] Type A (anterobrachial demarcation) is a line extending from the presternal area to the antecubital fossa on the dorsoventral surface of the upper arms. It is seen in 16–26% of black people and 6% of Japanese adults. Type B is on the lower extremities in the posteromedial position, and is seen in 40% of black adults. Type C is paired hypopigmented lines in a vertical direction from the clavicular area to the inferior sternal border. Type D is a hyperpigmented line on the mid back, occurring rarely in Asians. Type E is periareolar hypopigmentation, seen in 69% of black children and often becoming less noticeable with age.

Melanocytic Nevi

Congenital melanocytic nevi (CMN) are proliferations of nested melanocytes in the skin, present at birth or appearing in the first few months of life. Various classification schemes exist, and although not based on biologic principles, congenital

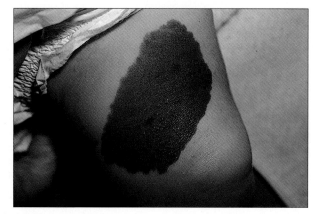

FIG. 22-15 Intermediate-sized congenital melanocytic nevus with irregular hyperpigmentation.

nevi are usually categorized based on the size of the largest lesional diameter.[122,123] Several definitions have been used to define large congenital nevi, the most common being a size of 20 cm or more in adolescents or adults. Small congenital nevi are lesions 1–1.5 cm or smaller (Fig. 22-14), and intermediate-sized lesions range from 1 to 1.5 cm up to 20 cm (Fig. 22-15). Assessment is generally based on adult size, and as lesions grow proportionately with the individual, those approximately 9 cm in diameter on the head or 6 cm on the body in a neonate may be considered large congenital melanocytic nevi (LCMN), or giant. Other names for LCMN include 'garment,' 'bathing trunk,' or 'giant hairy nevi.'

The nevi are tan, brown to dark brown macules, papules, or plaques at birth. Color is quite variable, some lesions having black or purple foci, whereas others are light tan, mimicking CALM. They may have a smooth, nodular, verrucous, or rough cobblestone-like texture. Lesions may or may not have hair, the presence or absence of which does not indicate malignant potential. The hairs may vary from light vellus to long, coarse, and darkly pigmented terminal hair. Scalp lesions may be cerebriform, similar to cutis verticis gyrata.

Small and Intermediate Congenital Nevi

Small nevi are seen in 1–2% of newborns, intermediate-sized lesions in 0.6%, and LCMN in no more than 0.02%.[124–126] The risk of developing melanoma in small and intermediate-sized CMN is quite controversial. Although prospective data are few, the risk of malignant melanoma arising within small and intermediate congenital melanocytic nevi is small. Although there are isolated reports of small congenital nevi progressing to melanoma, this is exceedingly rare before puberty. Early estimates ranged greatly, with several studies suggesting that there may not be a clinically significant increased risk for melanoma arising in banal-appearing, medium-sized CMN or small congenital nevi, whereas rare cases of prepubertal melanoma have been reported in intermediate-sized lesions.[127–130] More recent data have failed to detect an appreciable increased risk of melanoma in patients within small CMN, arguing against prophylactic excision of these lesions.[131] Even with this ongoing controversy there is widespread recognition that the risk in the neonatal period and early infancy is minimal, and the extent of lifetime risk, albeit somewhat uncertain, is low. Factors other than size that may confer an added risk of malignant transformation (e.g. family history, sun exposure) are unknown.

A number of congenital disorders include increased numbers of small congenital and acquired nevi as a clinical feature.[132] In many cases a critical reading of the literature raises the issue of whether the lesions described are truly melanocytic nevi or rather other melanocytic proliferations, such as lentigines, or freckles, and whether the nevi are truly an associated finding or merely a chance occurrence.

Differential Diagnosis

The differential diagnosis includes smooth muscle hamartoma, mastocytomas, nevus spilus, and in early life CALM. The histologic appearance may be the same as that of acquired nevi, or may show features diagnostic of congenital nevi.[130,133] Lesions may be junctional, compound, or intradermal, superficial, or deep. Features considered useful in differentiating congenital lesions from acquired nevi include the presence of melanocytes around and within hair follicles, sweat ducts, eccrine glands, vessel walls, and the perineurium of nerves, extension between collagen bundles in rows, or extension into deep reticular dermis or subcutis.[134] However, these features may be seen in acquired lesions, and it is unknown whether the features defining 'nevi with histologic pattern of the congenital type' are of any significance as risk markers for melanoma.[45]

Treatment and Care

Management of small and intermediate congenital nevi is controversial, as there are few studies on the natural history.[135,136] No consensus exists as to the management of small congenital nevi. In light of the very low prepubertal risk of melanoma, a conservative approach consisting of serial observation with photographic documentation may be appropriate. However, management may be individualized, with factors in decision making about surgical excision including the appearance of the lesion (color, presence of papules or nodules), its location, ease of excision (easily performed under local anesthesia versus staged excisions under general anesthesia), and the expected cosmetic result. Laser treatment (e.g. Q-switched or normal-mode ruby or other lasers) may be able to temporarily lighten small congenital nevi, but does not usually completely remove the melanocytes, and its use for this indication is controversial.[137]

Large Congenital Melanocytic Nevi

LCMN are most common on the posterior trunk, but may also be seen on the anterior and lateral trunk, head and neck, or extremities (Fig. 22-16).[138,139] Multiple small satellite CMN are seen in the majority of patients with LCMN and often continue to develop over time.[139,140] Dermatomal distribution of congenital nevi has been reported rarely.[147] LCMN may have multiple pink to purple areas that may mimic melanoma, or be mistaken for open neural tube defects or hemangiomas.[71] Erosions may be present at birth or in early infancy, and may represent benign superficial epidermal breakdown or melanoma (Fig. 22-17).[141,142] Intradermal nevi may develop within giant nevi as slow-growing, firm, asymptomatic nodules.

Extracutaneous Findings

Large congenital nevi of the scalp and dorsal axis are known to have an associated risk of central nervous system

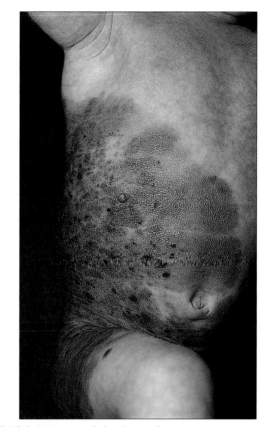

FIG. 22-16 Large congenital melanocytic nevus.

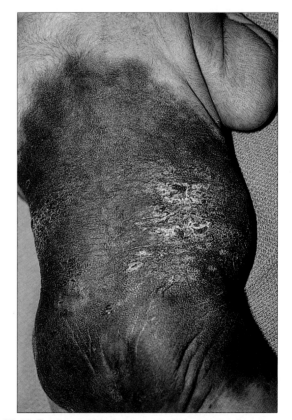

FIG. 22-17 Erosions within large congenital melanocytic nevus. Biopsy displayed features of a normal nevus of the congenital type.

melanocytosis (so-called neurocutaneous melanosis (NCM); see the following section). More recent data suggest that the major risk for symptomatic neurocutaneous melanosis disease is conferred by having multiple congenital nevi, either associated or unassociated with the presence of a giant nevus. A reduction in subcutaneous fat is quite common beneath giant congenital melanocytic nevi.[143] Limb hypoplasia has also been reported. Large CMN in the lumbosacral area may be associated with spinal dysraphism, including myelomeningocele.[144,145] Malignant tumors reported to arise within LCMN other than melanoma include rhabdomyosarcoma, liposarcoma, neuroblastoma, primitive neuroectodermal tumors, and mixed malignant neoplasms.[143,146,147]

Other malformations reportedly associated with LCMN include vascular malformations, supernumerary nipples, ear deformities, preauricular appendages, cryptorchidism, and club feet.[1] Large CMN (>10 cm) are reported in 2% of patients with NF1, a frequency greater than that in the general population. Care should be taken to distinguish pachydermatous overgrowth within LCMN from plexiform neurofibromas, as they are distinct entities.[141]

Cutaneous melanoma may arise from LCMN from both epidermal and nonepidermal sites.[148] The lifetime risk of melanoma associated with LCMN is difficult to determine precisely. Methodological problems in study design and hampering study comparisons include differing size definitions, histologic overdiagnosis of melanoma in the newborn period, varying ages of entry of patients into studies, and failure to consider the impact of surgical excision or partial excision. Most investigators, however, estimate the lifetime risk of melanoma in a patient with LCMN to be approximately 6–8%.[138,139,143,148–150] More recent published data suggest that this risk may be as low as 3%.[151] Onset of melanoma in utero has been reported. Approximately half of melanomas associated with LCMN may occur by 3–5 years of age, and the greatest risk for malignant transformation appears to be in the prepubertal years.[139] LCMN on the extremities appear to have a markedly lower risk of melanoma than those in an axial location. No cases of melanoma have been reported to have arisen from satellite nevi. Melanomas associated with LCMN appear to have a poorer prognosis than de novo melanomas, with earlier development of metastatic disease.[151]

Pathogenesis

Congenital nevi are proliferations of melanocytes and may be considered as hamartomas or benign neoplasms of melanocytic cells. Lesions that are clinically and histologically consistent with congenital nevi may appear weeks or months after birth, and it is believed that they were present in the skin but inapparent. Some have used the term tardive congenital nevi for these lesions. The mechanisms of malignant transformation of CMN are uncertain. Congenital nevi may have higher numbers of estrogen- and progesterone-binding cells than acquired melanocytic nevi, similar to malignant melanoma and dysplastic nevi.[153] Chromosomal abnormalities have been documented in some lesions; whereas LCMN are genetically polyclonal, melanomas arising within LCMN are monoclonal neoplasms.[152,154] The DNA content of melanocyte nuclei has shown more aneuploidy relative to acquired nevi.

Most CMN will grow proportionately with the anatomic site, though certain studies have found that some smaller lesions do not appear to grow with time, and that some will have disproportionately rapid expansion.[156–158] CMN may

evolve with change in texture and color. Some LCMN may decrease in pigment after birth, whereas others may darken with age, either focally or generally.[139,159] Papules and nodules may develop with time, most commonly in the first 2 years of life. Histologically, these lesions may be benign intradermal nevi, atypical melanocytic nevi with dysplasia, or unusual dysplastic or hamartoma-like lesions, including neurocristic dysplastic, neural crest hamartomas, spindle cell tumors, and neurofibromas.[139] Melanomas may present with similar nodules, although rapid growth, ulceration, and regional lymph node enlargement are more suggestive of melanoma.

The differential diagnosis is as listed previously for small and intermediate-sized congenital nevi. Melanoma arising within LCMN must be considered when there are lesional changes in color or the development of papules, nodules, or erosions, though all of these may simply indicate normal maturation of the lesion. Early lesions may appear identical to CALM, although speckled pigmentation or a papular component may differentiate CMN.

Pathology

The diagnosis of CMN (if in question) can readily be made with a skin biopsy, which demonstrates a benign proliferation of melanocytes in a nested pattern, which may extend from the superficial epidermis through the subcutaneous fat. Congenital nevi may have melanocytes that are fully intraepidermal in location (junctional melanocytic nevi), but more commonly melanocytes will be present in the reticular dermis and below. Dermal congenital nevi without an epidermal component may also be seen.[160] Common features in larger lesions include melanocytes around or within epithelial structures of adnexa (including hair follicles and eccrine ducts), nonepithelial adnexa (hair erectile muscle, smooth muscle, and nerve fascicles) and around venules.[159–162] Larger CMN display melanocytes situated in the lower two-thirds of the reticular dermis and in subcutaneous fat, and may extend into fascia, skeletal muscles, and occasionally lymph nodes. However, histologic features of small congenital nevi, although overlapping, may lack some of these patterns of melanocyte distribution.[133]

Differentiation from other pigmented lesions may be aided by use of staining techniques with antibodies to S100 protein and myelin basic protein: melanocytes are S100 positive, whereas myelin basic protein is negative.[153] Proliferative nodules and intensely pigmented areas arising in LCMN in the newborn period may resemble malignant melanoma both clinically and histologically, and require expert dermatopathology review to help differentiate from one another.[163]

Treatment and Care

The management of large CMN should be individualized, with consideration of the risk of melanoma, the risks and functional impact of surgery, disfigurement from the lesion or surgical intervention, and ease of observation of lesional changes. Although the data are insufficient to recommend prophylactic excision of all congenital nevi, many specialists recommend partial or complete excision of large CMN.[136,148] Surgical excision is often complex, requiring multiple operations, tissue expansion or grafting, and artificial skin replacement, and may not be technically feasible. Other surgical options that treat LCMN more superficially include curettage, which may be more effective in the first few weeks of life, dermabrasion, laser surgery (including carbon dioxide, ruby, and Q-switched lasers), cryosurgery, and electrocautery.[162,165–167]

Spontaneous resolution of giant congenital melanotic nevi may occur as a result of a vigorous host response to aberrant clone of melanocytes, which may suggest a possible future therapeutic option for those whose congenital nevi are not amenable to surgery.[168]

Neurocutaneous Melanosis

Neurocutaneous melanosis (NCM), also known as neurocutaneous melanocytosis or leptomeningeal melanosis, is a rare condition characterized by benign or malignant melanocytic infiltration of the leptomeninges associated with large or multiple (more than three) congenital melanocytic nevi.[169] CMN on the posterior midline trunk, most commonly in the lumbosacral area, or on the head and neck, are seen in virtually all patients with NCM. The appearance and histopathologic features of individual cutaneous lesions do not predict risk for NCM, but location and the number of CMN are strongly predictive of risk. In symptomatic cases macrocephaly may be seen as a result of hydrocephalus with or without increased intracranial pressure, which may be due to obstructed CSF flow, excess absorption due to subarachnoid infiltration by pigmented cells, or associated Dandy–Walker syndrome.[170] Leptomeningeal melanoma develops in 40–62% of symptomatic patients, often within the first few years of life, though delayed presentations after puberty are reported (Box 22-7).

With the availability of MRI scanning, more and more asymptomatic cases are recognized in as many as 25% of infants with LCMN involving the scalp, neck, and posterior midline trunk.[171] Although the course of these children is unknown, it may be that the findings correlate to the biology of cutaneous congenital nevi; lesions may be present that are melanocytic hamartomas, with some small risk of symptomatic or malignant change. Interestingly, children with neurologic alterations without evidence of NCM on CT or MRI scans have also been reported.[172] The diagnosis of NCM may be made using MRI with or without gadolinium contrast. Hyperintense regions on T_1-weighted images (T_1-shortening) most commonly involve the cerebellar hemispheres, pons, and anterior temporal horns, particularly the amygdala. A normal MRI does not fully rule out neurocutaneous melanosis, and cytologic examination of cerebrospinal fluid may be necessary. The differential diagnosis includes melanoma, including prenatal metastases.[170]

Although the pathogenesis of LCMN and NCM is not well understood, animal models suggest that aberrant expression of the hepatocyte growth factor/scatter factor (HGF/SF) may be involved.[173] The prognosis of symptomatic NCM is poor, with death occurring within 3 years in more than half of patients, and in 70% within 10 years. Not all patients die from melanoma, as structural damage from benign lesions may be severe enough to cause death. Neurosurgical consultation is appropriate, though procedures may be palliative. Spontaneous resolution of nodules presumed to be NCM has been reported, and the natural history of asymptomatic leptomeningeal melanosis is not fully known.

Congenital Malignant Melanoma

Fewer than 30 cases of congenital melanoma have been reported in the English language literature since 1925.[174] Congenital and neonatal melanoma may arise in utero secondary to transplacental transmission from metastatic maternal melanoma; in association with a giant congenital melanocytic nevus or with leptomeningeal melanocytosis; and de novo. Darkly pigmented, rapidly growing nodules, with or without ulceration, may be the initial signs of malignant melanoma arising in each of the above settings. Prenatal metastatic disease has been reported. Care should be taken to have pathologic specimens examined by an experienced dermatopathologist, as misdiagnosis of benign proliferative nodules within CMN as melanoma is not uncommon. Congenital melanoma is discussed in more detail in Chapter 25.

Speckled Lentiginous Nevus (Nevus Spilus)

Speckled lentiginous nevus (SLN), or nevus spilus, is an acquired or congenital lesion seen in 1.7 of 1000 newborns, although the prevalence in white schoolchildren and adults has ranged from 1.3% to 2.3%.[4,26] SLN are now considered to be part of the spectrum of congenital melanocytic nevi, as histology from biopsy specimens from these lesions demonstrates congenital features.[175]

Cutaneous Findings

SLN is a circumscribed patch of hyperpigmentation with smaller, darker pigmented macules or papules within the patch. Solitary, nonhairy, flat, light to medium-brown patches of pigmentation are generally present at birth or early infancy, resembling CALM. These are dotted by smaller dark-brown to black freckle-like areas of pigmentation that may not appear until later in childhood. Acquired lesions are not uncommon (Fig. 22-18). Size is quite varied, from 1 cm to more than 20 cm. More extensive lesions, including segmental, unilateral or generalized lesions, have been reported, and may involve a considerable proportion of the skin. Whereas the trunk and extremities are most commonly affected, SLN lesions that involve the upper and lower eyelids, termed divided nevi, have been reported and are presumed to develop prior to eyelid separation at 12–14 weeks' gestational age.[176] Speckled areas, generally 2–4 mm in size, may continue to develop in childhood.

Histologically, the tan to brown patches correspond to increased epidermal hyperpigmentation, often with macromelanosomes, or epidermal melanocytes with or without nest formation. Speckled darker areas correspond to junctional or dermal melanocytes. Blue nevi or spindle and epithelioid nevi have been described as variants of speckles.

Extracutaneous Findings

Nevus spilus may be seen in association with vascular malformations in phakomatosis pigmentovascularis types III and IV.

Box 22-7 Neurocutaneous melanosis

- Benign or malignant melanocytic infiltration of the leptomeninges
- Associated with multiple or large congenital melanocytic nevi
- May be symptomatic or asymptomatic
- Diagnosis may be made by MRI, with characteristic findings including hyperintense regions on T_1-weighted images in the cerebellar hemispheres, pons, and/or amygdala
- Associated risk of leptomeningeal melanoma

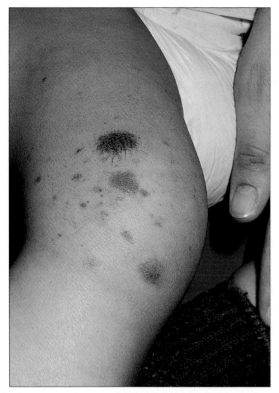

FIG. 22-18 Nevus spilus with faint brown hyperpigmented background and darker brown nevi within the affected area.

The speckled lentiginous nevus syndrome, a distinct phenotype characterized by large SLN, neurologic abnormalities (dysesthesia, muscular weakness, and hyperhidrosis), has recently been described. SLN syndrome most likely results from a mosaic phenotype as a consequence of loss of heterozygosity.[177,178]

Differential Diagnosis

Differential diagnosis includes CALM, light-colored congenital melanocytic nevi, Becker nevi, and the segmental (mosaic) form of NF1, although speckling is uncommonly seen in congenital melanocytic nevi or Becker nevi.

Treatment and Care

The risk of cutaneous melanoma associated with SLN is believed to be low. There are, however, several reported cases that describe malignant transformation, some of which have been fatal, although none in the neonatal period. In light of this, serial clinical observation, with photographic recording, especially of larger SLN, seems warranted. Additionally, atypical or changing areas within the SLN can be selectively excised, while balancing the untoward cosmetic effects of removing large areas of SLN. Although successful treatment has been reported with several laser modalities, including the Q-switched alexandrite (755 nm) and the Q-switched ruby (694 nm), the response appears to be at best partial and requires multiple treatment sessions.[179,180]

Spitz Nevi (Spindle and Epithelioid Cell Nevi)

Spitz nevi, also known as spindle and epithelioid nevi, or in the past as 'benign juvenile melanoma,' are a variant of mela-nocytic nevi which typically have a spindle and epithelioid cell histologic appearance. Spitz first described these lesions in 1948.[181]

Cutaneous Findings

Spitz nevi are commonly found in the first or second decade of life, and appear as hairless, red or brownish-red, smooth or verrucous, dome-shaped papules, 2–15 mm in size. Congenital Spitz nevi may be present at birth or develop within the first few months. Typically they present as an area of hyperpigmentation, usually described as a CALM, with subsequent development of multiple agminated Spitz nevi.[182–184] Multiple Spitz nevi are rare, and can occur as either disseminated lesions or grouped papules. This latter distribution is termed 'agminated Spitz nevi.' Furthermore, they have been reported in the following clinical contexts: disseminated; grouped on a background of normal skin; grouped on a background of hypopigmented skin; and grouped on a background of hyperpigmented skin.[185] Other presentations include isolated Spitz nevi present at birth, or developing within a compound nevus or congenital speckled lentiginous nevus.[186,187] There are no associated extracutaneous findings.

Histologic examination reveals collections of melanocytes with irregular cytoplasmic and nuclear shapes, in a spindle and epithelioid pattern. Surface telangiectasia may be prominent in lesions with a reddish color resembling vascular tumors.

Differential Diagnosis (Box 22-8)

The differential diagnosis of spindle and epithelioid nevi includes intradermal melanocytic nevi, pyogenic granulomas, juvenile xanthogranulomas, mastocytomas, and malignant melanoma.

Treatment and Care

Spitz nevi are benign melanocytic neoplasms, but share many clinical and histologic features with melanoma. Although there is apparently no malignant potential, regional lymph node involvement has been reported.[183]

Management is controversial, and there appears to be no consensus regarding the approach to these lesions.[188] Treatment should be individualized. Routine excision is advocated by some, because of concerns regarding the misdiagnosis of melanomas as Spitz nevi and uncertainty about the natural history of the tumors. Without excision, lesions may remain stable for years, evolve into compound nevi, flatten over time, or involute spontaneously. Similarly, some authors advocate complete excision of the involved areas of agminated nevi, whereas others report spontaneous involution.

Serial clinical observation, with photographic recording and dermoscopy, is an alternative approach to management in some patients. Dermoscopy, also known as epiluminescence microscopy, is a noninvasive, in vivo diagnostic tool which may enable the physician to visualize features of a pigmented lesion not otherwise discernible to the naked eye. The dermoscopic pattern common to Spitz nevi is the 'starburst' pattern, so-called because it resembles an exploding star.[189] Morphologic patterns may evolve within a single lesion over time, probably corresponding to the natural evolution in clinical morphology of Spitz nevi.[190]

Spitz nevi with atypical pathologic features should be evaluated by experienced dermatopathologists to rule out malignant melanoma. If atypia is confirmed, conservative re-excision is recommended.

REFERENCES

1. Salmon J, Frieden IJ. Congenital and genetic disorders of hyperpigmentation. Curr Probl Dermatol 1995; 7: 143–198.
2. Landau M, Krafchik B. The diagnostic value of café au lait macules. J Am Acad Dermatol 1999; 40: 877–890.
3. Jacobs A. Birthmarks. Pediatr Ann 1976; 5: 743–758.
4. McLean DI, Gallagher RP. 'Sunburn' freckles, café au lait macules, and other pigmented lesions of schoolchildren: The Vancouver Mole Study. J Am Acad Dermatol 1995; 32: 565–570.
5. Elder D. Lever's histopathology of the skin. Philadelphia: Lippincott-Raven, 1997; 970, 980.
6. Crowe FW, Schull WJ. Diagnostic importance of cafe-au-lait spots in neurofibromatosis. Arch Intern Med 1993; 91: 758–766.
7. Korf BR. Diagnostic outcome in children with multiple cafe au lait spots. Pediatrics 1992; 90: 924–927.
8. Shimbashi T, Kamide R, Hashimoto T. Long-term follow-up in treatment of solar lentigo and café au lait macules with Q-switched ruby laser. Aesthetic Plast Surg 1997; 21: 445–448.
9. Metzker A, Morag C, Weitz R. Segmental pigmentation disorder. Acta Dermatol Venereol 1983; 63: 167–169.
10. Riccardi VM. Neurofibromatosis: Clinical heterogeneity. Curr Probl Cancer 1982; 7: 1–34.
11. Committee on Genetics. Health Supervision for Children with Neurofibromatosis. Pediatrics 1995; 96: 368–372.
12. Levine MA. The McCune–Albright syndrome. The whys and wherefores of abnormal signal transduction. N Engl J Med 1991; 325: 1738–1740.
13. Roth JG, Esterly NB. McCune–Albright syndrome with multiple bilateral cafe au lait spots. Pediatr Dermatol 1991; 8: 35–39.
14. Yoshimoto M, Nakayama M, Baba T, et al. A case of neonatal McCune–Albright syndrome with Cushing syndrome and hyperthyroidism. Acta Paediatr Scand 1991; 80: 984–987.
15. Shenker A, Weinstein LS, Moran A, et al. Severe endocrine and nonendocrine manifestations of the McCune–Albright syndrome associated with activating mutations of stimulatory G protein GS. J Pediatr 1993; 123: 509–518.
16. Aarskog D, Tveteraas E. McCune–Albright's syndrome following adrenalectomy for Cushing's syndrome in infancy. J Pediatr 1968; 73: 89–96.
17. Happle R. The McCune–Albright syndrome: A lethal gene surviving by mosaicism. Clin Genet 1986; 29: 321–324.
18. Rieger E, Kofler R, Borkenstein M, et al. Melanotic macules following Blaschko's lines in McCune–Albright syndrome. Br J Dermatol 1994; 130: 215–220.
19. Olsen BR. 'A rare disorder, yes; an unimportant one, never.' J Clin Invest 1998; 101: 1545–1546.
20. Duncan PA, Hall JG, Shapiro LR, et al. Three-generation dominant transmission of the Silver–Russell syndrome. Am J Med Genet 1990; 35: 245–250.
21. Dohil MA, Billman G, Pransky S et al. The congenital lingual melanotic macule. Arch Dermatol. 2003; 139: 767–770.
22. Taylor CO, Lewis JS. Histologically documented transformation of benign oral melanosis into malignant melanoma: a case report. J Oral Maxillofac Surg. 1990; 48: 732–734.
23. Cordova A. The Mongolian spot: A study of ethnic differences and a literature review. Clin Pediatr 1981; 20: 714–719.
24. Jacobs A. The incidence of birthmarks in the neonate. Pediatrics 1976; 58: 218–222.
25. Ruiz-Maldonado R, Tamayo L, Laterza AM, et al. Phakomatosis pigmentovascularis: A new syndrome? Report of four cases. Pediatr Dermatol 1987; 4: 189–196.
26. Hisano A, Kasai K, Fukuzumi Y. An analysis of 114 patients with dermal melanocytosis on the trunk and extremities. Scand J Plast Reconstr Hand Surg 1999; 33: 231–236.
27. Hanson M, Lupski JR, Hicks J, et al. Association of dermal melanocytosis with lysosomal storage disease: clinical features and hypotheses regarding pathogenesis. Arch Dermatol 2003; 139: 916–920.
28. Tang TT, Esterly NB, Lubinsky MS, et al. GM1-gangliosidosis type 1 involving the cutaneous vascular endothelial cells in a black infant with multiple ectopic Mongolian spots. Acta Dermatol Venereol 1993; 73: 412–415.
29. Kopf AW, Bart RS. Malignant blue (Ota's?) nevus. J Dermatol Surg Oncol 1982; 8: 442–445.
30. Rahimi-Movaghar V, Karimi M. Meningeal melanocytoma of the brain and oculodermal melanocytosis (Nevus of Ota): Case report and literature review. Surg Neurol 2003; 59: 200–210.
31. Sharan S, Grigg JR, Billson FA. Bilateral naevus of Ota with choroidal melanoma and diffuse retinal pigmentation in a dark skinned person. Br J Ophthalmol. 2005; 89: 1529.
32. Alvarez-Cuesta CC, Raya-Aguado C, Vasquez-Lopez F, et al. Nevus of Ota associated with ipsilateral deafness. J Am Acad Dermatol. 2002; 47: S257–259.
33. Zigman AF, Lavine JE, Jones MC, et al. Localization of the Bannayan–Riley–Ruvalcaba syndrome gene to chromosome 10q23. Gastroenterology 1997; 113: 1433–1437.
34. Shimbashi T, Hyakusoku H, Okinaga M. Treatment of nevus of Ota by Q-switched ruby laser. Aesthetic Plast Surg 1997; 21: 118–121.
35. Raulin C, Schonermark MP, Greve B, Werner S. Q-switched ruby laser treatment of tattoos and benign pigmented skin lesions: A critical review. Ann Plast Surg 1998; 41: 555–565.
36. Okawa Y, Yokota R, Yamauchi A. On the extracellular sheath of dermal melanocytes in nevus fusco-ceruleus acromiodeltoideus (Ito) and Mongolian spot. An ultrastructural study. J Invest Dermatol 1979; 73: 224–230.
37. Radentz WH, Vogel P. Congenital common blue nevus. Arch Dermatol 1990; 126: 124–125.
38. Kawasaki T, Tsuboi R, Ueki R, et al. Congenital giant common blue nevus. J Am Acad Dermatol 1993; 28: 653–654.
39. Marano SR, Brooks RA, Spetzler RF, et al. Giant congenital cellular blue nevus of the scalp of a newborn with an underlying skull defect and invasion of the dura mater. Neurosurgery 1986; 18: 85–89.
40. Hofmann U, Wagner N, Grimm T, et al. [Linear and whorled nevoid hypermelanosis. Case report and review of the literature]. Hautarzt 1998; 49: 408–412.
41. Carney JA, Gordon H, Carpenter PC, et al. The complex of myxomas, spotty pigmentation, and endocrine

overactivity. Medicine (Baltimore) 1985; 64: 270–283.

42. de Giorgi V, Massi D, Brunasso G, et al. Eruptive multiple blue nevi of the penis: a clinical dermoscopic pathologic case study. J Cutan Pathol. 2004; 31: 185–188.

43. Maize JC Jr, McCalmont TH, Carlson JA, et al. Genomic analysis of blue nevi and related dermal melanocytic proliferations. Am J Surg Pathol. 2005; 29: 1214–20.

44. Dermoscopy of melanocytic neoplasms: blue nevi. Arch Dermatol 2004; 140: 1028.

45. Elder D, Elenitsas R. Benign pigmented lesions and malignant melanoma. In Elder D, et al...., eds. Lever's histopathology of the skin. Philadelphia: Raven Publishers, 1997: pp 626–630.

46. Lombillo VA, Sybert VP. Mosaicism in cutaneous pigmentation. Curr Opin Pediatr. 2005 Aug; 17: 494–500.

47. Van Gysel D, Oranje AP, Stroink H, et al. Phakomatosis pigmentovascularis. Pediatr Dermatol 1996; 13: 33–35.

48. Happle R, Hoffmann R, Restano L, et al. Phakomatosis pigmentokeratotica: A melanocytic-epidermal twin nevus syndrome. Am J Med Genet 1996; 65: 363–365.

49. Tadini G, Restano L, Gonzales-Perez R, et al. Phacomatosis pigmentokeratotica: Report of new cases and further delineation of the syndrome. Arch Dermatol 1998; 134: 333–337.

50. Koopman R. Concept of twin spotting. Am J Med Genet 1999; 85: 355–358.

51. Nehal KS, PeBenito R, Orlow SJ. Analysis of 54 cases of hypopigmentation and hyperpigmentation along the lines of Blaschko. Arch Dermatol. 1996 Oct; 132: 1167–1170.

52. Kalter DC, Griffiths WA, Atherton DJ. Linear and whorled nevoid hypermelanosis. J Am Acad Dermatol 1988; 19: 1037–1044.

53. Alvarez J, Peteiro C, Toribio J. Linear and whorled nevoid hypermelanosis. Pediatr Dermatol 1993; 10: 156–158.

54. Quecedo E, Febrer I, Aliaga A. Linear and whorled nevoid hypermelanosis. A spectrum of pigmentary disorders. Pediatr Dermatol 1997; 14: 247–248.

55. Akiyama M, Aranami A, Sasaki Y, et al. Familial linear and whorled nevoid hypermelanosis. J Am Acad Dermatol 1994; 30: 831–833.

56. Kubota Y, Shimura Y, Shimada S, et al. Linear and whorled nevoid hypermelanosis in a child with chromosomal mosaicism. Int J Dermatol 1992; 31: 345–347.

57. Kim HJ, Park KB, Yang JM, et al. Congenital triangular alopecia in phakomatosis pigmentovascularis: report of 3 cases. Acta Dermatol Venereol. 2000; 80: 215–216.

58. Happle R. Phacomatosis pigmentovascularis revisited and reclassified. Arch Dermatol 2005; 141: 385–388.

58a. Danarti R, Happle R. Paradominant inheritance of twin spotting: phacomatosis pigmentovascularis as a further possible example. Eur J Dermatol 2003; 13: 612.

59. Roberts JL, Morrow B, Vega-Rich C, et al. Incontinentia pigmenti in a newborn male infant with DNA confirmation. Am J Med Genet 1998; 75: 159–163.

60. Wagner A. Distinguishing vesicular and pustular disorders in the neonate. Curr Opin Pediatr 1997; 9: 396–405.

61. Martinez-Menchon T, Mahiques Santos L, Vilata Corell JJ, et al. Phakomatosis pigmentokeratotica: a 20-year follow-up with malignant degeneration of both nevus components. Pediatr Dermatol. 2005; 22: 44–447.

62. Thyresson NH, Goldberg NC, Tye MJ, et al. Localization of eosinophil granule major basic protein in incontinentia pigmenti. Pediatr Dermatol 1991; 8: 102–106.

63. Itin PH, Lautenschlager S, Meyer R, et al. Natural history of the Naegeli–Franceschetti–Jadassohn syndrome and further delineation of its clinical manifestations. J Am Acad Dermatol 1993; 28: 942–950.

64. Sprecher E, Itin P, Whittock NV, et al. Refined mapping of Naegeli–Franceschetti–Jadassohn syndrome to a 6 cM interval on chromosome 17q11.2-q21 and investigation of candidate genes. J Invest Dermatol. 2002; 119: 692–698.

65. Gibbs RC. Unusual striped hyperpigmentation of the torso. A sequel of abnormalities of epitrichial exfoliation. Arch Dermatol 1967; 95: 385–386.

66. Zhu YI, Fitzpatick JE, Weston WL. Congenital curvilinear palpable hyperpigmentation. J Am Acad Dermatol. 2005; 53: S162–164.

67. Kraemer KH. Xeroderma pigmentosum knockout mice: an immunologic tale. J Invest Dermatol 1996; 107: 291–292.

68. Robbins JH. Xeroderma pigmentosum. Defective DNA repair causes skin cancer and neurodegeneration. JAMA 1988; 260: 384–388.

69. Kraemer KH, Lee MM, Scotto J. Xeroderma pigmentosum. Cutaneous, ocular, and neurologic abnormalities in 830 published cases. Arch Dermatol 1987; 123: 241–250.

70. Masinjila H, Arnbjornsson E. Two children with xeroderma pigmentosum developing two different types of malignancies simultaneously. Pediatr Surg Int 1998; 13: 299–300.

71. Sybert V. Genetic skin disorders. New York: Oxford University Press, 1997.

72. Ramsay CA, Coltart TM, Blunt S, et al. Prenatal diagnosis of xeroderma pigmentosum. Report of the first successful case. Lancet 1974; 2: 1109–1112.

73. Kraemer KH, DiGiovanna JJ, Moshell AN, et al. Prevention of skin cancer in xeroderma pigmentosum with the use of oral isotretinoin. N Engl J Med 1988; 318: 1633–1637.

74. Yarosh D, Klein J, O'Connor A., et al. Effect of topically applied T4 endonuclease V in liposomes on skin cancer in xeroderma pigmentosum: a randomised study. Xeroderma Pigmentosum Study Group. Lancet 2001; 357: 926–929.

75. Soter NA. The skin in mastocytosis. J Invest Dermatol 1991; 96: 32S–39S.

76. Lazarus GS, Guzzo C, Lavker RM, et al. Urticaria pigmentosum: Nature's experiment in mast cell biology. J Dermatol Sci 1991; 2: 395–401.

77. Epstein JH. Postinflammatory hyperpigmentation. Clin Dermatol 1989; 7: 55–65.

78. Chernosky M, Anderson DE, Chang JP, et al. Familial progressive hyperpigmentation. Arch Dermatol 1971; 103: 581–598.

79. Ruiz-Maldonado R, Tamayo L, Fernandez-Diez J. Universal acquired melanosis. The carbon baby. Arch Dermatol 1978; 114: 775–778.

80. Collins P, Barnes L, McCabe M. Poikiloderma congenitale: Case report and review of the literature. Pediatr Dermatol 1991; 8: 58–60.

81. Williams G, Dluhy RG. Diseases of the adrenal cortex. In: Fauci AS, Braunwald E, Kasper D, et al., eds. Harrison's principles of internal medicine. New York: McGraw-Hill, 1998; 2051–2054.

82. Mulligan TM, Sowers JR. Hyperpigmentation, vitiligo, and Addison's disease. Cutis 1985; 36: 317–318, 322.

83. Migeon C, Kenny EM, Kowarski A, et al. The syndrome of congenital adrenocortical unresponsiveness to ACTH. Report of six cases. Pediatr Res 1968; 2: 501–513.

84. Moshang T Jr, Rosenfield RL, Bongiovanni AM, et al. Familial glucocorticoid insufficiency. J Pediatr 1973; 82: 821–826.

85. Gorlin RJ, Anderson RC, Moller JH. The Leopard (multiple lentigines) syndrome revisited. Birth Defects Orig Artic Ser 1971; 7: 110–115.

86. Legius E, Schrander-Stumpel C, Schollen E, et al. PTPN11 mutations in LEOPARD syndrome. J Med Genet 2002; 39: 571–574.

87. Kontaridis MI, Swanson KD, David FS, et al. PTPN11 (SHP2) mutations in leopard syndrome have dominant negative, not activating, effects. J Biol Chem 2005; 281: 6785–6792.

88. Lassonde M, Trudeau JG, Girard C. Generalized lentigines associated with multiple congenital defects (leopard syndrome). Can Med Assoc J 1970; 103: 293–294.

89. Nordlund JJ, Lerner AB, Braverman IM, et al. The multiple lentigines syndrome. Arch Dermatol 1973; 107: 259–261.

90. Arnsmeier SL, Paller AS. Pigmentary anomalies in the multiple lentigines

syndrome: Is it distinct from LEOPARD syndrome? Pediatr Dermatol 1996; 13: 100–104.

91. Rosenblum GA. Cryotherapy of lentiginous mosaicism. Cutis 1985; 35: 543–544.

92. Atherton DJ, Pitcher DW, Wells RS, et al. A syndrome of various cutaneous pigmented lesions, myxoid neurofibromata and atrial myxoma: The NAME syndrome. Br J Dermatol 1980; 103: 421–429.

93. Rhodes A, Silverman RA, Harrist TJ, et al. The 'LAMB' syndrome. J Am Acad Dermatol 1984; 10: 72–82.

94. Kirshcner LS, Carney JA, Pack SD, et al. Mutations of the gene encoding the protein kinase A type I-alpha regulatory subunit in patients with the Carney complex. Nature Genet 2000; 26: 89–92.

95. Stratakis C, Carney JA, Lin J, et al. Carney complex, a familial multiple neoplasia and lentiginosis syndrome. J Clin Invest 1996; 97: 699–705.

96. Marchesi L, Naldi L, Di Landro A, et al. Segmental lentiginosis with 'jentigo' histologic pattern. Am J Dermatopathol 1992; 14: 323–327.

97. Altman DA, Banse L. Zosteriform speckled lentiginous nevus. J Am Acad Dermatol 1992; 27: 106–108.

98. Trattner A, Metzker A. Unilateral dermatomal pigmentary dermatosis: A variant dyschromatosis? J Am Acad Dermatol 1993; 29: 1060.

99. Bolognia JL. Fatal melanoma arising in a zosteriform speckled lentiginous nevus. Arch Dermatol 1991; 127: 1240–1241.

100. Dociu I, Galaction-Nitelea O, Sirjita N, et al. Centrofacial lentiginosis. A survey of 40 cases. Br J Dermatol 1976; 94: 39–43.

101. Stewart DM, Altman J, Mehregan AH. Speckled lentiginous nevus. Arch Dermatol 1978; 114: 895–896.

102. Trattner A, Metzker A. Partial unilateral lentiginosis. J Am Acad Dermatol 1993; 29: 693–695.

103. Tovar JA, Eizaguirre I, Albert A, et al. Peutz–Jeghers syndrome in children: Report of two cases and review of the literature. J Pediatr Surg 1983; 18: 1–6.

104. Fernandez SM, Martinez Soto MI, Fernandez Lorenzo JR, et al. Peutz–Jehgers syndrome in a neonate. J Pediatr 1995; 126: 965–967.

105. Jenne DE, Reimann H, Nezu J, et al. Peutz–Jeghers syndrome is caused by mutations in a novel serine threonine kinase. Nature Genet 1998; 18: 38–43.

106. Cohen JM. Bannayan–Riley–Ruvalcaba syndrome: Renaming three formerly recognized syndromes as one etiologic entity. Am J Med Genet 1990; 35: 291.

107. Fargnoli M, Orlow SJ, Semel-Concepcion J, et al. Clinicopathologic findings in the Bannayan–Riley–Ruvalcaba syndrome. Arch Dermatol 1996; 132: 1214–1218.

108. Gorlin R, Cohen MM Jr, Condon LM, et al. Bannayan–Riley–Ruvalcaba syndrome. Am J Med Genet 1992; 44: 301–314.

109. Gretzula JC, Hevia O, Schachner LS, et al. Myhre–Smith–Ruvalcaba syndrome. Pediatr Dermatol 1988; 5: 28–32.

110. Fryburg JS, Pelegano JP, Bennett MJ, et al. Long-chain 3-hydoxylacyl-coenzymeA dehydrogenase (L-CHAD) deficiency in a patient with Bannayan–Riley–Ruvalcaba syndrome. Am J Med Genet 1994; 52: 97–102.

111. Arch E, Goodman BK, Van Wesep RA, et al. Deletion of PTEN in a patient with Bannayan–Riley–Ruvalcaba syndrome suggests allelism with Cowden disease. Am J Med Genet 1997; 275: 1943–1947.

112. Carethers J, Furnari FB, Zigman AF, et al. Absence of PTEN/ MMAC1 germ-line mutations in sporadic Bannayan–Riley–Ruvalcaba syndrome. Cancer Res 1998; 58: 2724–2726.

113. Urabe K, Hori Y. Dyschromatosis. Semin Cutan Med Surg 1997; 16: 81–85.

114. Schoenlaub P, Leroy JP, Dupre D, et al. [Universal dyschromatosis: a familial case]. Ann Dermatol Venereol 1998; 125: 700–704.

115. Yang JH, Wong CK. Dyschromatosis universalis with X-linked ocular albinism. Clin Exp Dermatol 1991; 16: 436–440.

116. Shono S, Toda K. Universal dyschromatosis associated with photosensitivity and neurosensory hearing defect. Arch Dermatol 1990; 126: 1659–1660.

117. Rycroft RJ, Calnan CD, Wells RS. Universal dyschromatosis, small stature and high-tone deafness. Clin Exp Dermatol 1977; 2: 45–48.

118. Kim NS, Im S, Kim SC. Dyschromatosis universalis hereditaria: An electron microscopic examination. J Dermatol 1997; 24: 161–164.

119. Oyama M, Shimizu H, Ohata Y, et al. Dyschromatosis symmetrica hereditaria (reticulate acropigmentation of Dohi): Report of a Japanese family with the condition and a literature review of 185 cases. Br J Dermatol 1999; 140: 491–496.

120. Grimes PE, Stockton T. Pigmentary disorders in blacks. Dermatol Clin 1988; 6: 271–281.

121. Selmanowitz VJ, Krivo JM. Pigmentary demarcation lines. Comparison of Negroes with Japanese. Br J Dermatol 1975; 93: 371–377.

122. Gari LM, Rivers JK, Kopf AW. Melanomas arising in large congenital nevocytic nevi: A prospective study. Pediatr Dermatol 1988; 5: 151–158.

123. Kopf AW, Bart RS, Hennessey P. Congenital nevocytic nevi and malignant melanomas. J Am Acad Dermatol 1979; 1: 123–130.

124. Castilla EE, da Graca Dutra M, Orioli-Parreiras IM. Epidemiology of congenital pigmented naevi: I. Incidence rates and relative frequencies. Br J Dermatol 1981; 104: 307–315.

125. Kroon S, Clemmensen OJ, Hastrup N. Incidence of congenital melanocytic nevi in newborn babies in Denmark. J Am Acad Dermatol 1987; 17: 422–426.

126. Walton RG, Jacobs AH, Cox AJ. Pigmented lesions in newborn infants. Br J Dermatol 1976; 95: 389–396.

127. Sahin S, Levin L, Kopf AW, et al. Risk of melanoma in medium-sized congenital melanocytic nevi: A follow-up study. J Am Acad Dermatol 1998; 39: 428–433.

128. Swerdlow AJ EJ, Qiao Z. The risk of melanoma in patients with congenital nevi: A cohort study. J Am Acad Dermatol 1995; 32: 595–599.

129. DaRaeve L, Danau W, DeBacker A, et al. Prepubertal melanoma in a medium-sized congenital naevus. Eur J Pediatr 1993; 152: 734–736.

130. Rhodes AR, Sober AJ, Day CL, et al. The malignant potential of small congenital nevocellular nevi. An estimate of association based on a histologic study of 234 primary cutaneous melanomas. J Am Acad Dermatol 1982; 6: 230–241.

131. Berg P, Lindelof B. Congenital melanocytic naevi and cutaneous melanoma. Melanoma Res 2003; 13: 441–445.

132. Marghoob AA, Orlow SJ, Kopf AW. Syndromes associated with melanocytic nevi. J Am Acad Dermatol 1993; 29: 373–390.

133. Everett MA. Histopathology of congenital pigmented nevi. Am J Dermatopathol 1989; 11: 11–12.

134. Caputo R, Ackerman AB, Sison-Torre EQ. Congenital melanocytic nevi in pediatric dermatology and dermatopathology. Philadelphia: Lea & Febiger, 1990; 331.

135. Williams ML, Pennella R. Melanoma, melanocytic nevi, and other melanoma risk factors in children. J Pediatr 1994; 124: 833–845.

136. Sweren R. Management of congenital nevocytic nevi: A survery of current practices. J Am Acad Dermatol 1984; 11: 629–633.

137. Chamlin SL, Williams ML. Moles and melanoma. Curr Opin Pediatr 1998; 10: 398–404.

138. Gari LM, Rivers JK, Kopf AW. Melanomas arising in large congenital nevocytic nevi: A prospective study. Pediatr Dermatol 1988; 5: 151–158.

139. Egan CL, Oliveria SA, Elenitsas R, et al. Cutaneous melanoma risk and phenotypic changes in large congenital nevi: a follow-up study of 46 patients. J Am Acad Dermatol 1998; 39: 923–932.

140. Castilla EE, da Graca Dutra M, Orioli-Parreiras IM. Epidemiology of congenital pigmented naevi: II. Risk factors. Br J Dermatol 1981; 104: 421–427.

141. Giam YC, Williams ML, Leboit PE, et al. Neonatal erosions and ulcerations in giant congenital melanocytic nevi. Pediatr Dermatol 1999; 16: 354–358.

142. Ruiz-Maldonado R, Tamayo L, Laterza AM, et al. Giant pigmented nevi: Clinical, histopathologic, and therapeutic considerations. J Pediatr 1992; 120: 906–911.

143. Arons MS, Hurwitz S. Congenital nevocellular nevus: A review of the treatment controversy and a report of 46 cases. Plast Reconstr Surg 1983; 72: 355–365.

144. James HE. Intrinsically derived deformational defects secondary to spinal dysraphism. Semin Perinatol 1983; 7: 253–256.

145. Hendrickson MR, Ross JC. Neoplasms arising in congenital giant nevi: Morphologic study of seven cases and a review of the literature. Am J Surg Pathol 1981; 5: 109–135.

146. Zuniga S, Las Heras J, Benveniste S. Rhabdomyosarcoma arising in a congenital giant nevus associated with neurocutaneous melanosis in a neonate. J Pediatr Surg 1987; 22: 1036–1038.

147. Reed W, Becker SW Sr, Becker SW Jr, et al. Giant pigmented nevi, melanoma, and leptomeningeal melanocytosis. Arch Dermatol 1965; 91: 100–119.

148. Rhodes A, Wood WC, Sober AJ, et al. Nonepidermal origin of malignant melanoma associated with a giant congenital nevocellular nevus. Plast Reconstr Surg 1981; 67: 782–790.

149. Marghoob AA, Schoenbach SP, Kopf AW, et al. Large congenital melanocytic nevi and the risk for the development of malignant melanoma. A prospective study. Arch Dermatol 1996; 132: 170–175.

150. DeDavid M, Orlow SJ, Provost N, et al. A study of large congenital melanocytic nevi and associated malignant melanomas: Review of cases in the New York University Registry and the world literature. J Am Acad Dermatol 1997; 36: 409–416.

151. Bett BJ. Large or multiple congenital melanocytic nevi: occurrence of cutaneous melanoma in 1008 persons. J Am Acad Dermatol 2005 May; 52: 793–797.

152. Quaba AA, Wallace AF. The incidence of malignant melanoma (0 to 15 years of age) arising in 'large' congenital nevocellular nevi. Plast Reconstr Surg 1986; 78: 174–181.

153. Ellis DL, Wheeland RG, Solomon H. Estrogen and progesterone receptors in congenital melanocytic nevi. J Am Acad Dermatol 1985; 12: 235–244.

154. Harada M, Suzuki M, Ikeda T, et al. Clonality in nevocellular nevus and melanoma: an expression-based clonality analysis at the X-linked genes by polymerase chain reaction. J Invest Dermatol 1997; 109: 656–660.

155. Stenzinger W, Suter L, Schumann J. DNA aneuploidy in congenital melanocytic nevi: suggestive evidence for premalignant changes. J Invest Dermatol 1984; 82: 569–572.

156. Nickoloff BJ, Walton R, Pregerson-Rodan K, et al. Immunohistologic patterns of congenital nevocellular nevi. Arch Dermatol 1986; 122: 1263–1268.

157. Rhodes A. Congenital nevomelanoctyic nevi: Histologic patterns in the first year of life and evolution during childhood. Arch Dermatol 1986; 122: 1257–1262.

158. Rhodes A, Albert LS, Weinstock MA. Congenital nevomelanocytic nevi: proportionate area expansion during infancy and early childhood. J Am Acad Dermatol 1996; 34: 51–62.

159. Ruiz-Maldonado R, Tamayo L, Laterza AM, et al. Giant pigmented nevi: clinical, histopathologic, and therapeutic considerations. J Pediatr 1992; 120: 906–911.

160. Zitelli JA, Grant MG, Abell E, et al. Histologic patterns of congenital nevocytic nevi and implications for treatment. J Am Acad Dermatol 1984; 11: 402–409.

161. Nickoloff B, Walton R, Pregerson-Rodan K, et al. Immunohistologic patterns of congenital nevocellular nevi. Arch Dermatol 1986; 26: 173–183.

162. Mark GJ, Mihm MC, Liteplo MG, et al. Congenital melanocytic nevi of the small and garment type. Clinical, histologic, and ultrastructural studies. Hum Pathol 1973; 4: 395–418.

163. Leech SN, Bell H, Leonard N, et al. Neonatal giant congenital nevi with proliferative nodules: a clinicopathologic study and literature review of neonatal melanoma. Arch Dermatol 2004; 140: 83–88.

164. Rhodes A, Silverman RA, Harrist TJ, et al. A histologic comparison of congenital and acquired nevomelanocytic nevi. Arch Dermatol 1985; 121: 1266–1273.

165. Casanova D, Bardot J, Aubert JP, et al. Management of nevus spilus. Pediatr Dermatol 1996; 13: 233–238.

166. Grevelink JM, van Leeuwen RL, Anderson RR, et al. Clinical and histological responses of congenital melanocytic nevi after single treatment with Q-switched lasers. Arch Dermatol 1997; 133: 349–353.

167. Rompel R, Moser M, Petres J. Dermabrasion of congenital nevocellular nevi: experience in 215 patients. Dermatology 1997; 194: 261–267.

168. Hogan DJ, Murphy F, Bremner RM. Spontaneous resolution of a giant congenital melanocytic nevus. Pediatr Dermatol 1988; 5: 170–172.

169. Kadonaga JN, Frieden IJ. Neurocutaneous melanosis: Definition and review of the literature. J Am Acad Dermatol 1991; 24: 747–755.

170. Schneiderman H, Wu AY, Campbell WA, et al. Congenital melanoma with multiple prenatal metastases. Cancer 1987; 60: 1371–1377.

171. Frieden IJ, Williams ML, Barkovich AJ. Giant congenital melanocytic nevi: Brain magnetic resonance findings in neurologically asymptomatic children. J Am Acad Dermatol 1994; 31: 423–429.

172. Ruiz-Maldonado R, del Rosario Barona-Mazuera M, Hidalgo-Galvan LR, et al. Giant congenital melanocytic nevi, neurocutaneous melanosis and neurological alterations. Dermatology 1997; 195: 125–128.

173. Kos L, Aronzon A, Takayama H, et al. Hepatocyte growth factor/scatter factor-MET signaling in neural crest-derived melanocyte development. Pigment Cell Res 1999; 12: 13–21.

174. Asai J, Takenaka H, Ikada S, et al. Congenital malignant melanoma: a case report. Br J Dermatol 2004; 151: 693–697.

175. Schaffer JV, Orlow SJ, Lazova R, et al. Speckled lentiginous nevus: within the spectrum of congenital melanocytic nevi. Arch Dermatol 2001; 137: 172–178.

176. Sato S, Kato H, Hidano A. Divided nevus spilus and divided form of spotted grouped pigmented nevus. J Cutan Pathol 1979; 6: 507–512.

177. Happle R. Speckled lentiginous nevus syndrome: delineation of a new distinct neurocutaneous phenotype. Eur J Dermatol 2002; 12: 133–135.

178. Vente C, Neumann C, Bertsch H. Speckled lentiginous nevus syndrome: report of a further case. Dermatology 2004; 209: 228–229.

179. Moreno-Arias GA, Bulla F, Vilata-Corell JJ, et al. Treatment of widespread segmental nevus spilus by Q-switched alexandrite laser (755 nm, 100 nsec). Dermatol Surg 2001; 27: 841–843.

180. Grevelink JM, White VR, Bonoan R, et al. Treatment of nevus spilus with the Q-switched ruby laser. Dermatol Surg 1997; 23: 365–369.

181. Spitz S. Melanomas of childhood 1948 [classic article]. CA Cancer J Clin 1991; 41: 40–51.

182. Hamm H, Happle R, Brocker EB. Multiple agminate Spitz naevi: Review of the literature and report of a case with distinctive immunohistological features. Br J Dermatol 1987; 117: 511–522.

183. Renfro L, Grant-Kels JM, Brown SA. Multiple agminate Spitz nevi. Pediatr Dermatol 1989; 6: 114–117.

184. Prose NS, Heilman E, Felman YM, et al. Multiple benign juvenile melanoma. J Am Acad Dermatol 1983; 9: 236–242.

185. Boer A, Wolter M, Kniesel L, et al. Multiple agminated Spitz nevi arising on a cafe au lait macule: review of the literature with contribution of another case. Pediatr Dermatol 2001; 18: 494–497.

186. Betti R, Inselvini E, Palvarini M, et al. Agminated intradermal Spitz nevi arising on an unusual speckled lentiginous nevus with localized lentiginosis: a continuum? Am J Dermatopathol 1997; 19: 524–527.

187. Aloi F, Tomasini C, Pippione M. Agminated Spitz nevi occurring within a congenital speckled lentiginous nevus. Am J Dermatopathol 1995; 17: 594–598.

188. Gelbard SN, Tripp JM, Marghoob AA, et al. Management of Spitz nevi: a survey of dermatologists in the United States. J Am Acad Dermatol 2002; 47: 224–230.

189. Marchell R, Marghoob AA, Braun RP, et al. Dermoscopy of pigmented Spitz and Reed nevi: the starburst pattern. Arch Dermatol 2005; 141: 1060.

190. Pizzichetta MA, Argenziano G, Grandi G, et al. Morphologic changes of a pigmented Spitz nevus assessed by dermoscopy. J Am Acad Dermatol 2002; 47: 137–139.

23

Lumps, Bumps, and Hamartomas

Julie S. Prendiville

LUMPS AND BUMPS

A wide variety of conditions affecting the skin and subcutaneous tissues present as papulonodular lesions, or 'lumps and bumps.' Benign and malignant neoplasms, hamartomas, and inflammatory and infectious disorders, as well as a number of infiltrative diseases, can be included in this category. Some of these conditions are discussed in detail in other chapters. This section deals with a group of nonmalignant disorders that present as discrete, circumscribed skin lesions in the newborn and young infant.

Fibromatoses

The fibromatoses represent a diverse collection of mesenchymal tumors characterized by fibroblastic–myofibroblastic proliferation.[1] They are locally invasive neoplasms that do not metastasize but which may recur following surgical excision. They vary in clinical behavior, from benign lesions that regress spontaneously to aggressive life-threatening tumors. They can be solitary or multifocal, and may exhibit skin, soft tissue, bone, or visceral involvement. Most of these tumors are sporadic, but some occur in a familial setting.

The fibromatoses are classified as juvenile or adult (Box 23-1).[1] The juvenile fibromatoses are a unique group of fibroblastic–myofibroblastic proliferations that present at birth or in the first years of life (Table 23-1), accounting for approximately 12% of pediatric soft tissue tumors.[1] Adult-type fibromatoses are occasionally observed in infancy and childhood.[1] The fibromatoses have also been subdivided according to the site of fibrous tissue overgrowth into superficial or fascial, and deep or musculoaponeurotic (desmoid type).[2]

Infantile Myofibromatosis

The term infantile myofibromatosis was introduced by Chung and Enzinger[3] in 1981 to designate a disorder previously described under numerous synonyms, including congenital multiple fibromatosis, diffuse congenital fibromatosis, multiple congenital mesenchymal tumors, and multiple vascular leiomyomas of the newborn. There are three clinical patterns of presentation: solitary infantile myofibroma; multicentric infantile myofibromatosis, with multiple lesions in the skin, soft tissues, and bone; and generalized infantile myofibromatosis, in which there is also visceral involvement.[1]

Cutaneous Findings

Over 80% of myofibromas present in the first 2 years of life, and 60% are apparent at birth or shortly thereafter.[3,4] Lesions may be superficial or deep, involving the skin, subcutaneous tissues, and muscle. They appear clinically as discrete, rubbery firm to hard nodules measuring from 0.5 to 7 cm in diameter (Fig. 23-1A). Cutaneous myofibromas may be skin colored or have a prominent vascular appearance, resembling hemangioma (Fig. 23-1B). Sites of predilection for solitary lesions are the head, neck, trunk, and upper extremities. In the multicentric and generalized forms there are multiple and widespread myofibromas, numbering from a few to over 100 (Fig. 23-2).[5] Skin and soft tissue lesions are asymptomatic and usually cause little morbidity. Rarely, a myofibroma presents with surface ulceration or an atrophic morphology (Fig. 23-3).[4,6] Joint contractures have been observed with extensive limb lesions.[7]

Extracutaneous Findings

In the multicentric form of the disease, myofibromas in the skin and soft tissues are associated with multiple lytic bone lesions. These may be extensive and can involve any bone.[5] Progression in size and number has been observed during infancy.[5] The bone tumors eventually stabilize, and spontaneous healing occurs with complete regression during the first few years of life. The development of sclerotic borders around lytic areas may be an early sign of regression.[5] In most cases there are no clinical signs or symptoms of bone disease. Pathologic fractures occur rarely and usually heal without residual deformity.[5] Vertebral body collapse has been described, with residual loss of vertebral height in early childhood.[5] There are reports of fatal spinal cord compression resulting from extension into the spinal canal.[8]

The much rarer generalized form of infantile myofibromatosis is characterized by involvement of visceral organs in addition to skin, soft tissue, and bone tumors. The gastrointestinal tract, heart, and lungs are most frequently affected. Involvement of the central nervous system is rare. Myofibromatosis in visceral organs is locally invasive and may severely compromise organ function. Cardiopulmonary, gastrointestinal, and hepatobiliary complications can be fatal, particularly in the newborn period or early infancy.[9]

Multiple skin and soft tissue tumors may occasionally occur in the absence of bone or visceral involvement.[1] Conversely, bone involvement has been observed in association with a single soft tissue lesion,[9] and uncommonly in the absence of skin lesions.[5]

Etiology and Pathogenesis

The pathogenesis is unknown. Most cases are sporadic. There are reports of familial occurrence with autosomal dominant inheritance.[10]

Box 23-1 Fibromatoses of the skin and soft tissues

Juvenile fibromatoses
Infantile myofibromatosis

Infantile desmoid-type fibromatosis

Fibromatosis colli

Infantile digital fibromatosis

Fibrous hamartoma of infancy

Gingival fibromatosis

Juvenile hyaline fibromatosis

Infantile systemic fibromatosis

Adult-type fibromatoses
Superficial

Dupuytren-type fibromatosis
   Palmar
   Plantar

Knuckle pads

Deep
Desmoid fibromatosis
   Intra-abdominal
   Abdominal
   Extra-abdominal

Diagnosis

Myofibromatosis may be suspected by the presence of firm, cutaneous and subcutaneous nodules. A biopsy is required to confirm the diagnosis. All three forms of infantile myofibromatosis show interlacing fascicles of spindle-shaped fibroblasts.[1] Central vascular areas resembling hemangiopericytoma are variably present. Focal necrosis, calcification, hyalinization, macrophages containing hemosiderin, and chronic inflammation may be seen.[1] A giant cell variant containing multiple multinucleated giant cells has also been described. There is positive immunoreactivity for vimentin and actin, consistent with the presumed myofibroblastic derivation of the tumor; desmin staining is variable. Electron microscopy shows cells with features of both fibroblasts and smooth muscle cells.

Infants with cutaneous myofibromas should be evaluated for bone and visceral involvement, particularly when there are multiple lesions. Recommended initial investigations include a skeletal survey, chest X-ray, echocardiogram, and abdominal imaging studies.[9]

Differential Diagnosis

Infantile myofibromatosis can be distinguished from other pediatric soft tissue tumors by histopathologic examination of biopsy material. These include other forms of fibromatosis, as well as congenital fibrosarcoma, leiomyoma and leiomyosarcoma, neurofibroma, metastatic neuroblastoma, hemangioma, hemangiopericytoma, chondromatosis, stiff skin syndrome, and nodular fasciitis.[1]

Treatment and Prognosis

The prognosis for infantile myofibromatosis is good in the absence of visceral involvement. Lesions in the skin and soft

---

TABLE 23-1 Juvenile Fibromatoses

	Location	Inheritance	Associated features	Course	Treatment
Infantile myofibromatosis	Solitary, multicentric or generalized	Sporadic, autosomal dominant, "?" autosomal recessive	Lytic bone lesions, visceral involvement	Spontaneous regression of bone and skin lesions; visceral lesions may be fatal	Await spontaneous regression, local excision if necessary; "?" chemotherapy or radiation for visceral lesions
Infantile desmoid-type fibromatosis	Any site	Usually sporadic, autosomal dominant	Other congenital anomalies	Locally invasive; does not metastasize; recurs after excision	Local excision with wide margins; "?" chemotherapy for non-resectable lesions
Fibromatosis colli	Neck	Rarely familial	None	Spontaneous regression	Physiotherapy
Infantile digital fibromatosis	Fingers and toes	Sporadic	None	Spontaneous regression reported; may recur	Await spontaneous regression; local excision if necessary
Fibrous hamartoma of infancy	Axillae, shoulders, chest wall	Sporadic	None	Does not regress	Local excision
Gingival fibromatosis	Gums	Autosomal dominant, recessive	Generalized hypertrichosis	May interfere with ability to eat, speak	Surgical debulking
Juvenile hyaline fibromatosis	Nodules on face and elsewhere	Autosomal recessive	Gingival hypertrophy, joint contractures	Chronic physical and cosmetic disability, overlaps with ISH	Supportive care, surgical excision of nodules if necessary
Infantile systemic hyalinosis (ISH)	Generalized thickening of skin	Autosomal recessive	Painful joint contractures, protein-losing enteropathy	Usually fatal within first few years of life	Supportive care

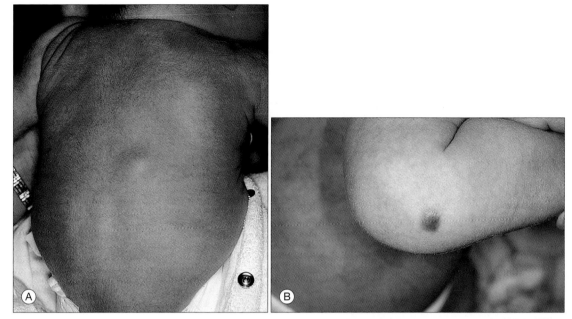

FIG. 23-1 (**A**) Flesh-colored nodule in infantile myofibromatosis. (**B**) Cutaneous myofibroma with a vascular appearance.

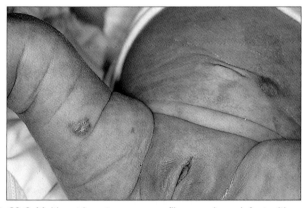

FIG. 23-2 Multicentric cutaneous myofibromas in an infant with extensive bone lesions. This case was familial, with autosomal dominant transmission.

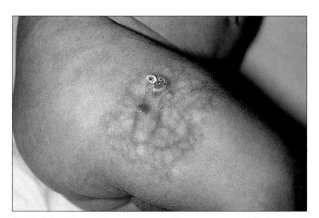

FIG. 23-3 Infantile myofibroma presenting as a congenital area of atrophy and telangiectasia with central red nodules, one of which was ulcerated.

tissues show spontaneous involution during the first few years of life, sometimes leaving residual areas of skin atrophy or hyperpigmentation. Bone lesions also regress spontaneously, usually without significant disability or residual radiologic change.[5] They do not interfere with enchondral bone growth.[5] The prognosis is grave for newborns with visceral disease, in whom a mortality rate of 76% has been documented.[9]

Surgical excision may be necessary to obtain tissue for diagnosis. Otherwise, excision should be limited to lesions that result in functional impairment or severe cosmetic disability.[7,9] The role of chemotherapy or radiation for symptomatic, recurrent, or nonresectable disease is not established. Successful treatment of life-threatening generalized infantile myofibromatosis using low-dose chemotherapy has been reported.[11]

Infantile Desmoid-Type or Aggressive Fibromatosis

Although desmoid fibromatosis has traditionally been considered a deep fibromatosis of adulthood, with abdominal, intra-abdominal, and extra-abdominal variants, a specific juvenile subset has become increasingly recognized.[1] Description of this entity under a variety of synonyms, including among others aggressive fibromatosis of infancy, musculoaponeurotic fibromatosis, desmoma, and fibrosarcoma grade 1 desmoid type, has led to confusion in the literature.[12] Up to 30% of juvenile desmoid tumors present in the first year of life, and congenital cases have been reported.[1,13]

Clinical Findings

Infantile desmoid-like or aggressive fibromatosis involves deep tissues and is generally extra-abdominal.[1] The usual clinical presentation is a slowly growing, nontender subcutaneous mass that has been present for weeks or months (Fig. 23-4). Sites of predilection in children are the head and neck, extremities, shoulder girdle, trunk, and hip regions. The abdomen, retroperitoneum, spermatic cord, and breast may also be involved. Rarely, there are multiple lesions. The tumor tends

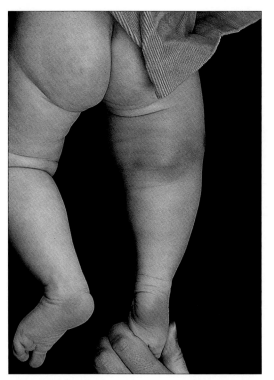

FIG. 23-4 Desmoid fibromatosis: firm mass on the thigh of an infant, diagnosed as 'aggressive fibromatosis of infancy.'

to be very locally aggressive, with infiltration of adjacent skeletal muscles, tendons, or periosteum, and erosion of bone.

Approximately 12% of pediatric patients with desmoid fibromatosis have other congenital abnormalities.[1] Adult-type intra-abdominal desmoid tumors are associated with Gardner syndrome and with familial adenomatous polyposis (FAP).[1,14] There are a few reports of desmoid tumors associated with Gardner syndrome in childhood, one of whom presented with a thoracic wall lesion in infancy.[15–17]

Etiology and Pathogenesis

The finding of minor radiologic bone abnormalities in 80% of patients with desmoids and 48% of their relatives suggests an autosomal dominant mode of inheritance.[1] Antecedent trauma, including surgery or irradiation, is reported in 12–63% of patients with all forms of desmoid tumor.[1] It is postulated that desmoid tumors are associated with a familial defect in the regulation of connective tissue and may be precipitated by multiple factors.[1,14,18] Desmoid fibromatosis in adults has been associated with mutations in the adenomatosis polyposis coli (APC) or β-catenin genes, but the significance of these findings in pediatric aggressive fibromatosis has not been established.[19]

Diagnosis

The tumor is composed of bundles of slender, uniform spindle cells surrounded by variable amounts of collagen. Cleft or slit-like blood vessels are variable in number and more abundant at the periphery. The fibrous proliferation may be indistinguishable from scar tissue, except that it infiltrates skeletal muscle and tendons.[1] Cellularity is variable. Some childhood lesions have an increased number of mitoses and greater cellularity.[1] Immunohistochemical and ultrastructural studies show that the lesion is composed of fibroblasts and myofibroblasts.

Differential Diagnosis

Myofibromatosis and other juvenile fibromatoses should be considered in the differential diagnosis. Keloid scars are more superficial than desmoid tumors. Cellular variants can be difficult to differentiate histologically from fibrosarcoma.

Treatment and Prognosis

The treatment of choice is local excision with wide margins if possible.[13–16,19] The recurrence rate varies from 30% to 80%.[1] Higher recurrence rates are associated with a young age at diagnosis, intralesional or marginal excision, mesenteric location, and associated Gardner syndrome. Microscopic features of high vascularity, myxoid foci, and abundant immature myofibroblasts are associated with a higher recurrence rate.[1] Treatment with combination chemotherapy and radiotherapy, or with tamoxifen and nonsteroidal anti-inflammatory agents, has been advocated for nonresectable lesions.[16,20] Mortality from locally aggressive desmoids is less than 10%.[1]

Fibromatosis Colli

Fibromatosis colli, or congenital muscular torticollis, is a congenital fibromatosis of the sternocleidomastoid muscle. It occurs in up to 0.4% of live newborns.[1] Males are affected more than females. It does not involve the skin.

Clinical Findings

A hard, nontender, lobulated subcutaneous mass is palpable in the lower third of the sternocleidomastoid muscle. The trapezoid muscle is sometimes involved. Following an initial rapid period of growth, the tumor stabilizes in size. Torticollis and facial asymmetry are variable and may be transient. There is a right-sided predominance, and 2–3% of cases are bilateral.[1]

Etiology and Pathogenesis

The pathogenesis is unknown. Birth trauma has been implicated, as 86% of cases have a history of complicated delivery; whether this is a cause or an effect of the tumor is not clear. Familial cases are rare.[1]

Diagnosis

Histologically, bands of fibroblasts with abundant collagen are intermingled with residual angulated skeletal muscle fibers. The diagnosis may be established by fine needle aspiration, which shows benign spindle cells and degenerating skeletal muscle fibers. Magnetic resonance imaging may also be useful.[21]

Differential Diagnosis

A combination of the typical location of the lesion in the neck and the characteristic histology is diagnostic. The clinical differential diagnosis includes lymphangioma, hemangioma, and malignant neoplasms. The histopathologic features may resemble those of a desmoid tumor.[1]

Treatment and Prognosis

The majority of lesions regress within the first year of life. Most resolve completely, but minor residual asymmetry or tightening of the sternocleidomastoid muscle is seen in 25% of cases.[1] Only 9% have persistence of the tumor and torticol-

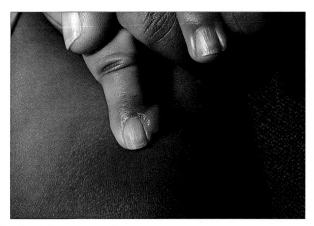

FIG. 23-5 Infantile digital fibroma presenting as a smooth, pink nodule.

lis. Physiotherapy is the treatment of choice. Surgery is rarely necessary unless the diagnosis is in doubt or the mass fails to resolve.

Infantile Digital Fibromatosis

Infantile digital fibromatosis is a recurring myofibroblastic proliferation of the fingers and toes. Synonyms for this tumor include digital fibrous tumor of Reye, digital fibrous swelling, recurring digital fibrous tumor of childhood, and inclusion body fibromatosis.[1]

Cutaneous Findings

Almost all lesions are diagnosed in infancy, and one-third are present at birth. Both sexes are affected equally. The typical lesion is an asymptomatic firm, smooth, pink nodule located on the lateral or dorsal aspect of the digit, measuring less than 3 cm in diameter (Fig. 23-5). Lesions are more common on the fingers than on the toes. The thumbs and great toes are spared. There is often deformity of the affected digit. There may be single or multiple nodules. Rarely, more than one digit is involved or extradigital lesions are seen.[22]

Extracutaneous Findings

Periosteal attachment is not unusual, but underlying bone erosion is rare.

Etiology and Pathogenesis

The pathogenesis is not known. Defective organization of actin filaments in myofibroblasts has been hypothesized.[1]

Diagnosis

Whorls and interdigitating sheets of uniform fibroblasts in a densely collagenous stroma are seen in the dermis or subcutis.[1] A unique feature is the presence of distinctive, eosinophilic, perinuclear cytoplasmic inclusions surrounded by a clear halo that stain red with a trichrome stain. Electron microscopy shows abundant cytoplasmic filaments that form whorled bodies; these are the ultrastructural correlate of the cytoplasmic inclusions. Immunostaining is positive for desmin, actin, vimentin, and keratin.

Differential Diagnosis

The digital location and the characteristic histology distinguish this lesion from other fibromatoses and pediatric soft tissue tumors.

Treatment and Prognosis

The local recurrence rate is 60–90% following surgical excision. Many tumors regress spontaneously within a few years.[22] Conservative management without surgery is appropriate unless there is functional impairment. The indications for surgical excision are controversial.[1,22] Mohs micrographic surgery to debulk the tumor has been performed.[23] Successful treatment with intralesional fluorouracil injections is reported in a 7-year-old child.[24]

Fibrous Hamartoma of Infancy

Fibrous hamartoma of infancy is a benign fibrous tumor that develops during the first 2 years of life.[25] Up to 20% are present at birth.[1] Occasional cases have been described in children between 2 and 10 years. Males are affected more frequently than females.

Cutaneous Findings

Fibrous hamartoma presents as a subcutaneous lesion located around the axillae, shoulders, and upper chest wall.[26] It may involve other sites, such as the inguinal region, extremities, and head and neck. It is usually a solitary nodule, measuring 2–5 cm in diameter, that feels lumpy to palpation. Occasionally, these lesions are multifocal. There are no symptoms.

Extracutaneous Findings

There are no systemic associations.

Etiology and Pathogenesis

Fibrous hamartoma of infancy is believed to represent a hamartomatous process rather than a true neoplasm. It is not familial.

Diagnosis

The hamartoma is located in the subcutaneous and musculoaponeurotic tissues.[25,26] Histopathologic examination reveals three characteristic elements: a fibrous component consisting of well defined fascicles of fibroblasts or disorderly fibroblasts in a collagenous stroma; mature adipose tissue; and myxoid mesenchymal tissue in a basophilic matrix. Electron microscopy reveals the presence of both fibroblasts and myofibroblasts, primitive mesenchymal cells, small blood vessels, and mature adipocytes.[1]

Differential Diagnosis

The clinical differential diagnosis of fibrous hamartoma of infancy includes cystic hygroma, hemangioma, and other soft tissue tumors. Identification of the three histologic components of this lesion distinguishes it from other fibroblastic proliferations.[26] A similar hamartoma with an admixture of fat and an absence of fibromyxoid tissue is described as lipofibromatosis.[27]

Treatment and Prognosis

There is no tendency to spontaneous regression. The treatment of choice is surgical excision. The recurrence rate is low, even with incomplete excision.[26]

Gingival Fibromatosis

This is a rare familial disorder that manifests at the time of eruption of the deciduous or permanent teeth.[1]

Cutaneous Findings

There is slowly progressive gingival enlargement that may cover the crowns of the teeth and result in difficulty in eating or speaking. It is associated with generalized hypertrichosis.

Extracutaneous Findings

Rarely there is associated mental retardation and epilepsy.

Etiology and Pathogenesis

Inheritance is most commonly autosomal dominant and the disorder has been mapped to loci on chromosomes 2 and 5.[28,29] Autosomal recessive and sporadic cases are also reported.[30]

Diagnosis

Mucosal biopsy shows coarse, interlacing collagen bundles with sparse fibroblasts and myofibroblasts. There may be calcification, ossification, abundant amorphous extracellular material, and cellular fibroblastic proliferation.[1]

Differential Diagnosis

The differential diagnosis includes phenytoin usage, chronic gingivitis, cherubism, juvenile hyaline fibromatosis, and other rare syndromes.[31] Gingival fibromatosis may be associated with skeletal anomalies and hepatosplenomegaly in the Zimmerman–Laband syndrome.[2,31]

Treatment and Prognosis

Treatment options include repeated surgical debulking of the gums or dental extraction.

Adult-Type Fibromatoses

The superficial fibromatoses of adulthood are the most common type of fibromatosis in the general population but are rare in infants and children. Fibromatosis may involve the palm (Dupuytren contracture), the plantar surface of the foot (Ledderhose disease), or the penis (Peyronie disease). Dupuytren-type fibromatosis of the palms and soles may be seen in childhood, and is occasionally congenital (Fig. 23-6).[1] Surgical excision is only necessary for diagnosis or for release of contractures. Knuckle pads are seen in older children and adolescents but not in infants.

Leiomyoma

Leiomyoma is a benign tumor of smooth muscle. Cutaneous leiomyoma may arise from the arrector pili muscle in hair follicles, the dartos muscle of the scrotum and labia majora, the erectile muscle of the nipple, and the muscular wall of veins (angioleiomyoma). Leiomyomas are uncommon in children and are extremely rare in the newborn period.[21,22]

Cutaneous Findings

Cutaneous leiomyomas appear as discrete papules or nodules with a pink or brown discoloration of the overlying skin. They are usually solitary but may be multiple. Rarely, a leiomyoma may present as a pedunculated mass at birth or as a papular plaque in early infancy.[33,34] Leiomyomas are often painful, particularly on exposure to cold.

Extracutaneous Findings

Most cutaneous leiomyomas are not associated with visceral disease. The multiple leiomyomas of the esophagus and tracheobronchial tree in Alport syndrome may be associated with female genital leiomyomas in older children and adults.[32] Leiomyomas that occur in immunocompromised children only rarely involve the skin or soft tissues.[35]

Etiology and Pathogenesis

Multiple cutaneous leiomyomas may be inherited as an autosomal dominant trait, but the etiology of other forms is unknown.

Diagnosis

The diagnosis is made by skin biopsy, which demonstrates whorls and bundles of well-differentiated spindle cells with cigar-shaped nuclei in the dermis. There is a variable collagenous component. The smooth muscle stains red with the Masson trichrome stain. Immunochemistry is positive for muscle-specific actin and desmin reactivity.

Differential Diagnosis

Leiomyoma must be distinguished from the fibroblastic and myofibroblastic proliferations of infancy and childhood, as well as from other spindle cell tumors such as neurofibroma and leiomyosarcoma. Immunohistochemistry may be helpful, as myofibroblastic tumors express smooth muscle actin more than muscle-specific actin or desmin.[32] The circumscribed spindle cell appearance of leiomyoma differs from the smooth muscle bundles of congenital smooth muscle hamartoma.

Treatment and Prognosis

Excision is curative for solitary lesions.

Neurofibromas and Other Neural Tumors

Cutaneous neurofibromas in infants and young children are most frequently associated with neurofibromatosis type 1 (NF1) (see Chapter 26). These benign tumors consist of Schwann cells, nerve fibers, and fibroblasts, and may be cutaneous, subcutaneous, or plexiform. Cutaneous and subcutaneous neurofibromas are rarely seen at birth but may sometimes appear within the first year of life. Plexiform neurofibromas are often present at birth and are considered pathognomonic of neurofibromatosis. There may be a large area of hyperpigmentation overlying the plexiform neurofibroma that predates the characteristic 'bag of worms' consistency of the tumor (Fig. 23-7). These lesions enlarge with time and can cause considerable cosmetic disfigurement, particularly on the face and around the eye. A plexiform neurofibroma in the neck may

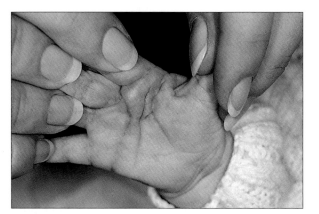

FIG. 23-6 Congenital fibromatosis of the palm.

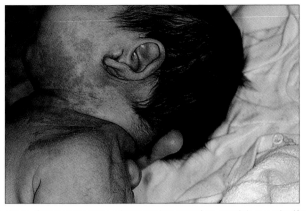

FIG. 23-7 Congenital area of hyperpigmentation overlying a plexiform neurofibroma in NF1.

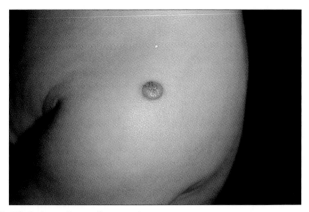

FIG. 23-8 Juvenile xanthogranuloma.

compromise airway function, and large lesions over the back are often associated with underlying spinal involvement.

Pacinian neurofibromas, or nerve-sheath myxomas, are uncommon tumors with components that resemble Vater–Pacini corpuscles.[36] Multiple hairy pacinian neurofibromas have been reported in children without NF1 and may be congenital.[36] Underlying skeletal anomalies may be associated with pacinian neurofibromas in a sacrococcygeal location.

In neurilemmomatosis, a syndrome reported in Japanese children, multiple cutaneous neurilemmomas derived from Schwann cells are present at birth or develop during childhood.[37] These lesions are a marker for development of central nervous system tumors in later childhood and adult life. Cutaneous neuromas or schwannomas associated with neurofibromatosis type 2 (NF2) may rarely present in early life.[38] The gene locus for neurilemmomatosis has been reported to lie within the NF2 gene region, suggesting that these two disorders may be the same disease.[39]

Non-Langerhans' Cell Histiocytoses

The non-Langerhans' cell histiocytoses encompass a diverse group of disorders in which there is proliferation of mononuclear phagocytes other than Langerhans' cells. Two variants, juvenile xanthogranuloma and benign cephalic histiocytosis, occur primarily in infants and young children. Other benign histiocytoses, such as papular xanthoma, xanthoma disseminatum, and generalized eruptive xanthoma, may rarely present in childhood, but are extremely unusual in infancy.[40,41]

Juvenile Xanthogranuloma

Juvenile xanthogranuloma is a benign, self-healing, non-Langerhans' cell histiocytosis characterized by solitary or multiple yellow-red papules and nodules in the skin and occasionally in other organs.[42] Although adults may be affected, it is predominantly a disorder of infancy and early childhood. There is an increased frequency of juvenile xanthogranuloma in children with NF1, juvenile myeloid leukemia, and urticaria pigmentosa.[43,44]

Cutaneous Findings

The typical juvenile xanthogranuloma is an asymptomatic, firm, well-demarcated papule or nodule that measures from 1 mm to 2 cm in diameter. Early lesions are pink or red in color, later changing to a distinctive yellow or orange-brown

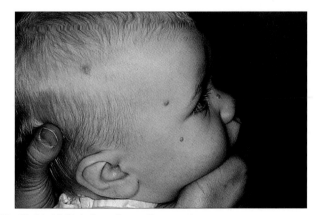

FIG. 23-9A Multiple juvenile xanthogranulomas.

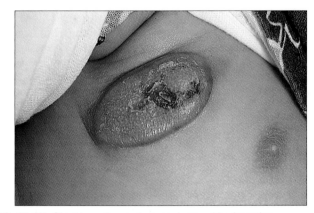

FIG. 23-9B Giant juvenile xanthogranuloma with ulceration.

(Fig. 23-8). There may be overlying telangiectasia with a purpuric appearance, and occasionally surface ulceration and bleeding with associated pruritus and discomfort. Solitary lesions with a hyperkeratotic surface, pedunculated or plaque-like morphology are also reported.[42] As many as 17% of juvenile xanthogranulomas are present at birth, and 70% develop within the first year of life.[42] The majority are solitary lesions. Multiple lesions may be few or number in the hundreds (Fig. 23-9A). They can be located at virtually any body site, but are most common on the head, neck, and upper trunk.

Juvenile xanthogranulomas may be classified as micronodular, measuring 2–5 mm, or macronodular, measuring 0.5–2 cm in diameter. An unusual variant is the giant juvenile xanthogranuloma, which measures from 2 to 10 cm in diameter (Fig. 23-9B).[45] These lesions are congenital or appear in early infancy and may have a greater propensity to ulcerate. Rarely, numerous micronodular lesions may present as a generalized lichenoid eruption.[46]

Extracutaneous Findings

Extracutaneous juvenile xanthogranuloma is rare, and less than 50% of these patients have associated cutaneous lesions.[47] The most frequent extracutaneous sites are the eye and orbit, central nervous system, liver/spleen, lung, oropharynx, and muscle. In contrast to cutaneous lesions, a systemic juvenile xanthogranuloma may produce symptoms related to a mass effect or infiltration of the involved organ. The incidence of ocular disease in patients with cutaneous lesions is 0.3–0.4%.[48] Eye lesions manifest as an asymptomatic mass on the iris, unilateral glaucoma, spontaneous hyphema, or color change of the iris. Risk factors for eye involvement include multiple lesions, age less than 2 years, and recently diagnosed disease.[48]

Juvenile xanthogranulomas are seen with increased frequency in patients with NF1. A triple association between juvenile chronic myeloid leukemia, juvenile xanthogranulomas, and NF1 has also been described (Fig. 23-10A & B).[43] Urticaria pigmentosa and juvenile xanthogranuloma have also been associated.[44]

Etiology

The etiology of juvenile xanthogranuloma is unknown. The precursor cell of the histiocytic proliferation is believed to be the interstitial/dermal dendrocyte.[49]

Diagnosis

The typical histologic appearance consists of a dense dermal infiltrate of foamy histiocytes with Touton giant cells. There is an admixture of other cell types, including lymphocytes, eosinophils, neutrophils, and foreign body giant cells, as well as infrequent mitoses. In early lesions there may be few or absent foam cells or Touton giant cells, with a variable number of spindle cells and numerous mitotic figures.[50] Immunohistochemistry shows negative staining for S100 and CD1a, and positive staining for factor X111a, CD68, CD163, fascin and CD14.[49] There are no Birbeck granules visible on ultrastructural examination.

Differential Diagnosis

Distinguishing a small juvenile xanthogranuloma from clinically similar lesions such as xanthoma, mastocytoma, Spitz nevus, and a number of other benign skin tumors may require a skin biopsy. Giant lesions may be mistaken for a hemangioma or malignant tumor. Early lesions that lack the characteristic lipid-laden histiocytes and Touton giant cells may resemble Langerhans' cell histiocytosis on histologic examination.[49,50] The absence of Birbeck granules and negative staining for S100 is characteristic of juvenile xanthogranuloma.

Treatment and Prognosis

Most cutaneous lesions resolve spontaneously over months or years and do not require treatment. Ulcerating, symptomatic, or large unsightly lesions may require surgical excision. Most lesions resolve completely, but some leave a residual area of hyperpigmentation or skin atrophy resembling anetoderma. Ocular and systemic lesions can be more problematic. Treatment options include observation, corticosteroids, surgical excision, radiation therapy, and chemotherapy.[42]

Benign Cephalic Histiocytosis

Benign cephalic histiocytosis is a non-Langerhans' cell histiocytosis characterized clinically by multiple brownish-yellow macules and papules on the face and adjacent areas. Some authors believe that benign cephalic histiocytosis is an early variant of micronodular juvenile xanthogranuloma.[51,52]

Cutaneous Findings

Lesions first appear between the ages of 2 months and 2 years.[42] The face is the site of predilection, but the scalp, neck, and ears can also be involved. Lesions may be scattered over the shoulders and upper arms.[53] Typical lesions are slightly raised, asymptomatic papules measuring 2–3 mm in diameter that vary from erythematous to light-brown or yellowish in color (Fig. 23-11). The mucous membranes are not involved.

Extracutaneous Findings

There are usually none, but there has been one report of associated diabetes insipidus.[54]

Diagnosis

Histologically, a monomorphous histiocytic infiltrate is located in the upper and mid-dermis. There may also be a few lymphocytes and eosinophils. Foamy macrophages and Touton giant cells are typically absent. Staining for S100 protein is negative. Electron microscopy reveals coated vesicles and comma- or worm-shaped bodies. Birbeck granules are absent.

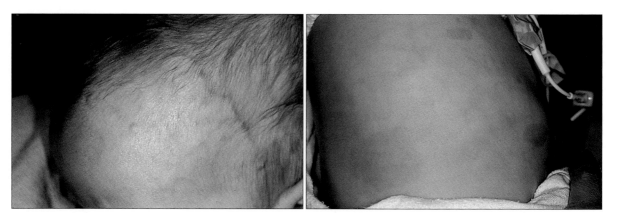

FIG. 23-10 (A) Multiple juvenile xanthogranulomas and (B) café au lait macules in a child with juvenile chronic myeloid leukemia.

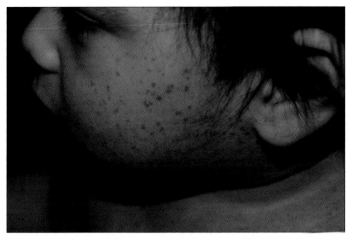

FIG. 23-11 Infant with benign cephalic histiocytosis.

Differential Diagnosis
The differential diagnosis includes juvenile xanthogranuloma, Langerhans' cell histiocytosis, and cutaneous mastocytosis. The lesions of mastocytosis have a similar color but urticate when rubbed (Darier's sign) and have a distinctive histology. Benign cephalic histiocytosis can be distinguished from Langerhans' cell histiocytosis by immunohistochemical stains and the absence of Birbeck granules on electron microscopy.

Treatment and Prognosis
There is no effective treatment. The skin lesions regress spontaneously over months to years. There may be residual hyperpigmentation and anetoderma-like atrophy.

CALCIFYING DISORDERS OF THE SKIN
Calcium deposition in the skin, or calcinosis cutis, is found in a diverse group of disorders. It is termed dystrophic calcification when calcium is deposited in abnormal or injured tissue in patients with no abnormality of calcium or phosphate metabolism. Metastatic calcification develops in normal tissues as a result of abnormal calcium and phosphorus metabolism. Idiopathic calcification occurs in the absence of any discernible tissue injury or metabolic abnormality. Iatrogenic calcification may develop as a complication of calcium infusions or the application of calcium-containing paste to abraded skin. Cutaneous ossification, in which normal bone is formed in the dermis and subcutaneous soft tissues, is termed osteoma cutis.

Dystrophic Calcification
Dystrophic calcification arises at sites of skin trauma or in association with inflammatory lesions, connective tissue disorders, skin tumors, and cysts. Calcinosis cutis on the heels is a not uncommon sequela of drawing blood by heel sticks during the neonatal period.[55,56] It presents some months later as one or more white papules or nodules, and usually resolves spontaneously by 18–30 months of age. Calcification may also occur in association with subcutaneous fat necrosis of the newborn.[57,58] Calcium deposition has been observed histologically both in the septa and within the fat lobules.[57,59] Widespread subcutaneous calcification may develop in cases of subcutaneous fat necrosis complicating hypothermic cardiac surgery.[58–60] Although hypercalcemia is a known complication

of subcutaneous fat necrosis, the majority of reported cases of soft-tissue calcification have occurred in normocalcemic patients. Conversely, most infants with subcutaneous fat necrosis and hypercalcemia do not show evidence of calcium deposition in biopsies taken from affected sites.[58]

Dystrophic calcification has been reported in the skin lesions of a newborn infant with intrauterine-acquired herpes simplex infection.[61] The calcification was present at birth and appeared to have developed in utero. A lethal disorder characterized by extensive congenital skin necrosis and follicular calcification has been described in three newborn females.[62] Dystrophic calcification may also occur as a complication of intralesional corticosteroid injection of infantile periocular hemangiomas.[63]

Metastatic Calcification
Metastatic calcification occurs when calcium salts are precipitated in normal tissues as a result of high serum calcium or phosphate levels. The calcium deposits usually consist of hydroxyapatite crystals. This is associated primarily with chronic renal insufficiency, in which ulceration of the skin may be caused by calcification of blood vessels, leading to ischemic skin necrosis, or by painful disseminated calcification of the dermis and subcutaneous tissues (calciphylaxis).[64] Chronic renal failure is also associated with benign nodular calcification. Calcium deposits in the skin may develop as a result of hypervitaminosis D, milk-alkali syndrome, and other causes of hypercalcemia and hyperphosphatemia.

Metastatic calcinosis in the skin is rarely seen in infancy and childhood.[65] In contrast, the cutaneous bone formation, or osteoma cutis, associated with Albright hereditary osteodystrophy frequently appears first in infancy or childhood and may present in the neonatal period. This metabolic disorder is discussed in the next section.

Idiopathic Calcification
Idiopathic calcification can be congenital or acquired. Congenital calcified nodules occur most frequently on the ear, but may be seen elsewhere on the face and limbs. These lesions are variously described as congenital calcified nodule of the ear, subepidermal calcified nodule, or solitary congenital nodular calcification of Winer.[66–68] Other types of idiopathic calcinosis cutis, such as idiopathic calcification of the scrotum or vulva, and the milia-like lesions associated with Down syndrome, present later in childhood or adolescence and are not seen in the newborn. There are rare reports of juxta-articular tumoral calcinosis in infancy.[69–72]

Calcified Ear Nodule
A solitary calcified nodule on the pinna or earlobe is the most common presentation of idiopathic calcinosis in the newborn (Fig. 23-12). These nodules may occur elsewhere on the face or limbs, and occasionally there is more than one. Auricular lesions developing after birth have also been described. There is a male preponderance.

Cutaneous Findings
The nodule is firm and measures 3–10 mm in diameter. The surface may be warty in appearance, or smooth and dome-shaped. The color is chalky white or yellow. Surface ulceration and discharge of calcified material may occur spontaneously

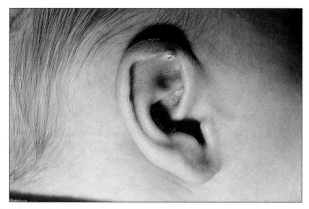

FIG. 23-12 Calcified ear nodule, also known as nodular calcification of Winer.

or as a result of trauma. There are usually no associated symptoms.

Extracutaneous Findings
Serum calcium and phosphate levels are normal. There are no systemic abnormalities.

Etiology and Pathogenesis
The pathogenesis of these lesions is not clear. Most authors believe that they represent dystrophic calcification following dermal damage from some unknown source. Proposed hypotheses include derivation from milia, syringomas, other sweat gland hamartomas, nevi, trauma, and ischemic injury.[67,68]

Diagnosis
The diagnosis is often made on the clinical appearance. Histologically, amorphous and/or globular masses of calcified material are seen in the papillary dermis and may extend to the reticular dermis. Foreign body giant cells may be observed in association with the calcified masses. The overlying epidermis shows a warty architecture with variable amounts of pseudoepitheliomatous hyperplasia. Ulceration and transepidermal elimination of calcium may occur.

Differential Diagnosis
Clinically, calcified nodules may be misdiagnosed as viral warts, molluscum contagiosum, pilomatrixomas, syringomas, and congenital inclusion cysts.

Treatment and Prognosis
If treatment is necessary, the nodule can be removed by curettage or excision. Calcified nodules sometimes recur following curettage or shave excision. Intralesional injection of triamcinolone at the time of shave excision has been suggested for recurrent lesions.[66]

Tumoral Calcinosis
Tumoral calcinosis is characterized by painless, calcified soft tissue nodules located close to large joints in otherwise healthy children and adults.[69–72] It may affect several family members and occurs most frequently in patients of African descent. There have been reports of tumoral calcinosis presenting in infancy, and two in the neonatal period.[71,73]

Cutaneous Findings
Tumoral calcinosis presents as progressively growing, lobulated masses in a juxta-articular location. The hip joints,

shoulders, and elbows are most frequently affected in older children and adults. A predilection for the anterior aspect of the knee has been noted in three infants.[71] Involvement of the buttock, axilla, and supraclavicular region has also been observed in infancy.[70,72] Lesions may be multifocal and occasionally bilateral. Rarely, ulceration of the overlying skin with discharge of a chalky-white substance may occur.[70] Large lesions may interfere with joint or muscle function.

Extracutaneous Findings
About one-third of patients with tumoral calcinosis have idiopathic hyperphosphatemia. Transient and marginally elevated serum phosphate levels were found in an affected infant.[61] Serum calcium levels are normal.

Etiology and Pathogenesis
Familial autosomal recessive tumoral calcinosis with hyperphosphatemia has been linked to mutations in the *GALNT3* gene on chromosome 2q24 and to the fibroblast growth factor-23 (*FGF-23*) gene.[74] Mechanical trauma is thought to play a role in some cases, based on the observation that lesions occur in areas of chronic mechanical trauma, particularly in Africans who carry heavy loads and sleep on hard floors.

Diagnosis
Radiographs show discrete, sometimes lobulated, calcified areas. There is no joint involvement, and the underlying bones appear normal. Excisional biopsy specimens usually show a well-encapsulated calcified mass, but there may be invasion of the surrounding musculature. Histologic examination reveals calcification, central necrosis, a chronic inflammatory cell infiltrate including multinucleate giant cells, and fibrosis.[69,72]

Treatment
Excision is the treatment of choice, but there may be recurrence after excision. Spontaneous resolution was observed in one infant after incisional biopsy of a supraclavicular mass.[72]

Iatrogenic Calcification

Iatrogenic calcinosis cutis (see Chapter 8) may result from intravenous infusion of calcium gluconate, with or without extravasation of the solution into the tissues. In addition to cutaneous calcification there may be an intense inflammatory response and occasionally soft tissue necrosis.[75]

Iatrogenic calcification has also been described following electrode placement for electroencephalography, electromyography, and brainstem auditory evoked potentials when calcium-containing electrode paste was applied to abraded skin.[76] Treatment is generally symptomatic, and resolution occurs spontaneously over several months.

Osteoma Cutis

Osteoma cutis is caused by heterotopic differentiation of osteoblasts in the dermis. It is classified as primary and secondary. In primary osteoma cutis there is no pre-existing skin pathology. In secondary osteoma cutis bone formation develops within scars, inflammatory lesions, skin tumors, hamartomas, or cysts.

Primary osteoma cutis may present in infancy as a manifestation of Albright hereditary osteodystrophy (AHO)[77] or progressive osseous heteroplasia (POH), both of which have been linked to mutations in the *GNAS1* gene.[78] Congenital plate-like osteoma cutis (POC)[79] and familial ectopic ossification or hereditary osteoma cutis may be variants of AHO and POH.[80]

Albright Hereditary Osteodystrophy

Albright hereditary osteodystrophy (AHO) is a genetic disorder that manifests clinically as pseudohypoparathyroidism (PHP) or pseudopseudohypoparathyroidism (PPHP). Both variants of the disorder have a similar phenotype. PHP is characterized by a lack of end-organ responsiveness to parathormone and variable degrees of hypocalcemia and hyperphosphatemia. In PPHP, serum calcium and phosphate levels are normal. PHP and PPHP may occur in the same kindred, and PPHP may progress to PHP in a single individual.[77]

Cutaneous Findings

Osteoma cutis is present in up to 42% of patients with PHP and PPHP. Lesions are usually first noted in infancy or childhood. They may be located anywhere on the body and have a predilection for sites of friction or mild trauma. The characteristic lesions are blue-tinged, stone-hard papules, nodules, or plaques that range in size from pinpoint to 5 cm in diameter. Early lesions may present as blue or erythematous macules (Fig. 23-13). Rarely, more extensive cutaneous ossification may occur (Fig. 23-14). Ulceration occurs occasionally.

Extracutaneous Findings

The characteristic phenotype of AHO includes short stature, round face, obesity, and brachydactyly, in particular a short-

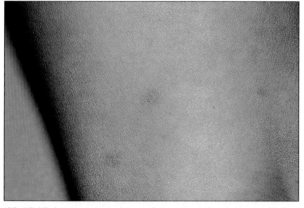

FIG. 23-13 Violaceous macules and papules of osteoma cutis in an infant with osteoma cutis with Albright hereditary osteodystrophy.

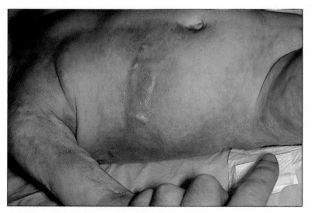

FIG. 23-14 Progressive osseous heteroplasia in an infant with familial Albright hereditary osteodystrophy at 1 year of age.

ened fourth metacarpal. Other manifestations include dental defects, short broad nails, cataracts, calcification of the basal ganglia, and mental retardation. These findings are easier to discern in late childhood and adulthood and are not usually manifest in infancy. Hypocalcemia may cause seizures and tetany. Some patients with PHP have evidence of other endocrine abnormalities such as hypogonadism or hypothyroidism.

Etiology and Pathogenesis

The metabolic changes in PHP result from a failure of receptors in renal and skeletal target tissues to respond to PTH. This resistance to the action of PTH is variable in PHP and absent in PPHP. End-organ resistance to PTH in the PHP variant of AHO (PHP type 1a) is associated with reduced expression or function of a guanine nucleotide stimulatory protein (Gs α) that is required for activation of adenylate cyclase by the hormone-bound receptor.[81] This protein is encoded by the *GNAS1* gene located on chromosome 20q13. Inheritance is by autosomal dominant transmission. AHO with hormone resistance (PHP type 1a) occurs only with maternal transmission of the genetic defect, whereas paternal imprinting results in PPHP or POH.[82] An AHO-like phenotype without end-organ resistance has been linked to mutations in 2q37.[83]

Diagnosis

Skin biopsy shows bone formation in the dermis and subcutis. Osteoblasts, osteocytes, and osteoclasts are present within the spicules of bone. When ossification is severe and progressive, a proliferation of spindle cells, resembling fibroblasts, may be prominent.

In PHP there is hypocalcemia, hyperphosphatemia, and an elevated serum PTH. In PPHP there is no discernible abnormality of calcium and phosphate metabolism. Urinary excretion of cAMP in response to intravenous infusion of PTH is impaired in most cases of PHP, but is normal in PPHP.

Radiologic abnormalities include ossification of the skin and subcutaneous tissues; shortening of the metacarpal, metatarsal, and phalangeal bones, notably the distal phalanx of the thumb and the fourth metacarpal; and cone epiphyses. Occasionally, there may be radiographic evidence of hyperparathyroidism or osteomalacia.

Differential Diagnosis

Hypocalcemia, hyperphosphatemia, and elevated levels of circulating PTH in the absence of renal disease, steatorrhea, and generalized osteomalacia are characteristic of PHP. A diagnosis of PPHP may be difficult to establish in infancy, particularly when there is no family history of AHO. The differential diagnosis includes POH, congenital plate-like osteoma cutis, and familial osteoma cutis in families without evidence of AHO.[80]

Treatment and Prognosis

Treatment of PHP is directed towards controlling hypocalcemia by careful administration and monitoring of calcium and vitamin D. Normocalcemic patients must be monitored closely and evaluated regularly for the development of cataracts or hypocalcemia. Mental retardation may be causally related to poorly controlled or undetected hypocalcemia. Patients should also be screened for hypothyroidism. There is no effective treatment for osteoma cutis. Surgical excision may be considered for individual lesions that cause pain or cosmetic disfigurement.

Progressive Osseous Heteroplasia

Progressive osseous heteroplasia (POH) is characterized by progressive heterotopic ossification of the skin and deeper soft tissues, including muscle.[78,84–86] It presents at birth or in early infancy with focal areas of dermal ossification that enlarge and coalesce to form larger nodules and plaques. Extension to the subcutaneous tissues and muscle often results in ankylosis of affected joints and growth retardation of involved limbs. There have been case reports of ossification limited to one half of the body or to a single limb.[85] Histologic examination reveals mainly intramembranous ossification similar to that seen in AHO, although foci of enchondral bone formation with cartilage are sometimes present. There is a female preponderance. POH may be sporadic or inherited as an autosomal dominant trait with phenotypic variability.[84] Familial cases have been linked to *GNAS1* mutations inherited exclusively from the father.[82,87]

POH is not associated with endocrine dysfunction or the skeletal and developmental abnormalities of Albright hereditary osteodystrophy. The heterotopic ossification in AHO is usually more superficial and limited to the dermis and subcutis. However, the clinical phenotype of POH is observed in families with AHO (see Fig. 23-14).[88] The relationship of AHO to POH and other forms of osteoma cutis awaits further understanding of mutations in the *GNAS1* gene and their effects on osteogenic differentiation in the skin and soft tissues.[89]

Congenital Plate-like Osteoma Cutis

Congenital plate-like osteoma cutis (POC) is a rare entity that occurs in infants with no abnormality of calcium or phosphate metabolism. Lesions present at birth or in the first year of life as a large, asymptomatic, skin-colored plaque, varying in size from 1 to 15 cm.[79] There are no predisposing events such as trauma or infection to explain the heterotopic ossification. The scalp is the site of predilection, but lesions may also be found on the limbs or trunk. There are no associated abnormalities. Radiographs reveal calcified sheets or nodules in the subcutaneous soft tissues. Histology shows mature spongy bone in the dermis and subcutis. There may be gradual progression of the lesion with time and clinical overlap with POH. It is proposed that the term congenital plate-like osteoma cutis should be reserved for nonprogressive, superficial lesions to distinguish this disorder from POH in which ossification extends deeper into muscle and is relentlessly progressive.[64] The finding of a *GNAS1* mutation in a child with severe progressive POC suggests it may be a variant of POH.[90] Treatment is by excision, if necessary and feasible. Recurrence after excision has been reported.

Pilomatrixoma

Pilomatrixoma, previously known as calcifying epithelioma of Malherbe, is a benign adnexal tumor derived from hair matrix cells. It commonly appears in children in the first decade of life and may be seen in infancy.[91,92] Familial occurrence is documented.[93] There is a slight female preponderance.[92]

Cutaneous Findings

The pilomatrixoma presents clinically as a slowly enlarging, hard nodule that is fixed to the skin but freely mobile over the underlying tissues. The overlying skin may be white, skin

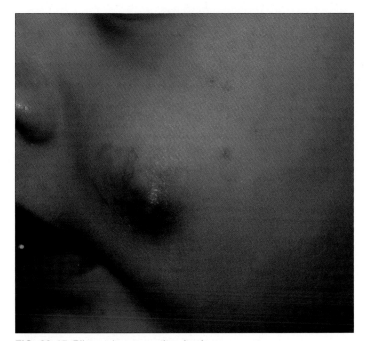

FIG. 23-15 Pilomatrixoma on the cheek.

colored, or have a blue-red discoloration. The size varies from 0.1 to 6 cm in diameter, with an average of about 1 cm.[92] Ulceration of the overlying skin occurs rarely and rapid enlargement due to bleeding within the lesion has been described.[94] Pilomatrixomas are seen most commonly on the head and neck (Fig. 23-15), but also appear on the trunk and extremities. They are usually solitary, but multiple and recurrent pilomatrixomas are well recognized and may be seen in otherwise healthy children. Multiple lesions can be associated with myotonic dystrophy, Gardner syndrome and the Rubinstein–Taybi syndrome.[91,95–98]

Extracutaneous Findings

Most patients with pilomatrixoma have no extracutaneous findings. Myotonic dystrophy and Gardner syndrome should be considered in children with multiple pilomatrixomas.[91,95–98]

Etiology and Pathogenesis

The tumor derives from cells in the hair matrix. Mutations in the β-catenin gene, a gene associated with colon cancer, have been demonstrated in pilomatrixomas.[99]

Diagnosis

The histology of pilomatrixoma is very characteristic, with two distinct types of cell, basophilic and shadow cells, located in the dermis or subcutis and surrounded by a fibrous capsule. The basophilic cells are seen at the periphery of the tumor and have rounded, darkly staining nuclei and scanty cytoplasm. The shadow cells are eosinophilic with a well-defined border and a central unstained area where the nucleus has been lost. Areas of keratinization may be seen, with foreign body giant cells and melanin pigmentation. Dystrophic calcification is a common finding and ossification occasionally occurs.

Differential Diagnosis

The clinical differential diagnosis includes other skin tumors, dermoid cyst, or a calcified nodule. Dermoid cysts are attached to underlying tissues rather than to the skin. A calcified nodule is hard to palpation and has a white surface discoloration; it can be difficult to distinguish clinically from a calcified pilomatrixoma. Ultrasound examination of pilomatrixomas shows a mass with an echogenic center and a hyperechoic rim at the junction of the dermis and subcutaneous fat.[100]

Treatment and Prognosis

Surgical excision with narrow margins or through a small skin incision is the treatment of choice. In asymptomatic lesions without progressive growth or recurrent inflammation, this may be deferred until the child is older and able to cooperate with excision under local anesthesia. Very superficial lesions may be amenable to incision and curettage. Spontaneous resolution is occasionally observed.

HAMARTOMAS

A hamartoma is a developmental abnormality of the skin in which there is an excess of one or more mature or nearly mature tissue structures normally found at that site.[101] The term nevus is often used synonymously, although not all 'nevi' are hamartomas (e.g. nevus anemicus, nevus depigmentosus). Whether a lesion is designated a hamartoma or a nevus depends largely on tradition.[102] An organoid nevus or organoid hamartoma refers to a malformation that consists of more than one type of tissue structure, and where identification of a single tissue of origin is not possible.[102]

Most hamartomas are isolated, sporadic malformations. They can be single or multiple, localized or extensive, and may be distributed in a linear or whorled pattern corresponding to the lines of Blaschko. Some arise from a postzygotic mutation in the embryo that leads to somatic mosaicism.[103] Others are manifestations of well-defined genetic disorders such as tuberous sclerosis. Epidermal hamartomas may be associated with underlying abnormalities in the central nervous system, skeleton, or other organs. Rarely, a postzygotic mutation that involves the germline results in transmission of generalized skin disease to subsequent offspring.[103,104]

Epidermal Nevus

The term epidermal nevus is used to encompass a group of hamartomas of ectodermal origin in which there is clinical and histologic overlap (Box 23-2). These include the nevus sebaceus, linear verrucous or keratinocytic epidermal nevus, inflammatory linear verrucous epidermal nevus (ILVEN), and nevus comedonicus. Other hamartomas that may be considered epidermal nevi are syringocystadenoma papilliferum, linear porokeratosis, Becker nevus, and the porokeratotic eccrine and ostial dermal duct nevus (porokeratotic eccrine nevus). Epidermal nevi also occur as a component of the Proteus syndrome and CHILD (congenital hemidysplasia with ichthyosiform nevus and limb defects) syndrome.[105] When applied without qualification, the term epidermal nevus usually refers to a linear verrucous or keratinocytic epidermal nevus. Epidermal nevi affect about 1:1000 people.[103]

Nevus Sebaceus

The nevus sebaceus (of Jadassohn) is an organoid hamartoma of appendageal structures that is usually evident at birth.[103] It occurs where pilosebaceous and apocrine structures are prominent and is considered to be a variant of epidermal nevus on the head and neck.[102,106] A nevus sebaceus is seen in 0.3% of newborns.[106]

Cutaneous Findings

The typical nevus sebaceus is a pink-yellow or yellow-orange plaque with a pebbly or velvety surface that is located on the scalp or face (Fig. 23-16). It varies in size from one to several centimeters and can be round, oval, or linear in shape. Lesions on the scalp present as a congenital area of circumscribed alopecia. There may be evolution from a slightly raised plaque at birth to a flat, almost macular lesion in infancy and childhood. A verrucous or cobblestone appearance develops in adolescence when the sebaceous and apocrine glands enlarge and proliferate.[101] Some lesions present with an atypical cerebriform (Fig. 23-17) or papillomatous morphology (Fig. 23-18). There can be some overlap between the morphology of a sebaceus nevus and an epidermal verrucous nevus on the head and neck. Both types of epidermal nevus may coexist at different sites when extensive lesions are present.

Box 23-2 Epidermal nevi

Organoid nevi
Nevus sebaceus
Syringocystadenoma papilliferum*[171]
Nevus comedonicus
Porokeratotic eccrine and ostial dermal duct nevus (porokeratotic eccrine nevus)

Keratinocytic (nonorganoid) nevi
Nonepidermolytic verrucous nevus
Epidermolytic verrucous nevus
Inflammatory linear verrucous epidermal nevus (ILVEN)
Linear porokeratosis

Often occurs in association with a nevus sebaceus.

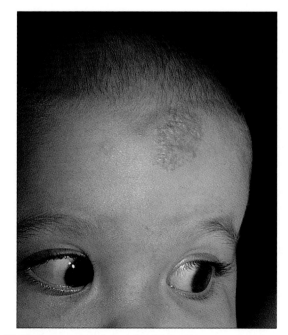

FIG. 23-16 Nevus sebaceus on the forehead.

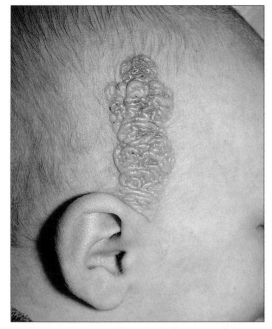

FIG. 23-17 Nevus sebaceus with a cerebriform morphology on the scalp.

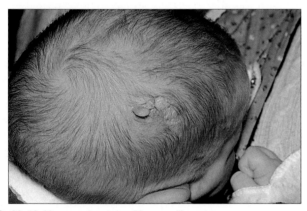

FIG. 23-18 Nevus sebaceus with a papillomatous appearance.

Extracutaneous Findings

Nevus sebaceus is usually an isolated lesion with no extracutaneous findings. Rarely, it is associated with other developmental abnormalities in a variable malformation syndrome known as the Schimmelpenning–Feuerstein–Mims syndrome,' 'nevus sebaceus syndrome' or 'epidermal nevus syndrome.[102,105,108] The nevus sebaceus can be of any size or shape but is often extensive or linear, with a distribution following the lines of Blaschko. Extracutaneous manifestations include mental retardation, seizures, coloboma of the eyelid, lipodermoids of the conjunctiva, choristomas, and other ophthalmologic and central nervous system abnormalities.[102,105,108–110] Skeletal, cardiac and genitourinary abnormalities, and vitamin D-resistant rickets are also reported.[102,105,111,112]

Etiology and Pathogenesis

The pathogenesis of this hamartoma is not known but is possibly linked to a postzygotic somatic gene mutation. Loss of heterozygosity in the *PTCH* gene has been documented.[113] There is no racial or gender predilection. There have been rare reports of familial lesions.[114,115] The nevus sebaceus (or epidermal nevus) syndrome occurs sporadically, and an autosomal lethal mutation that survives by mosaicism has been postulated.[116]

Diagnosis

The diagnosis is usually made on clinical grounds except in atypical cases. In infancy and childhood the characteristic histologic changes of nevus sebaceus are less developed than in adolescence and adulthood. Mature lesions show numerous sebaceous and apocrine glands in the dermis, with overlying epidermal hyperplasia. In infants the histologic findings are more subtle, with rudimentary hair follicles and immature glandular structures. It can sometimes be difficult to distinguish a linear nevus sebaceus from a verrucous epidermal nevus either histologically or clinically during childhood.

Differential Diagnosis

The differential diagnosis of a circumscribed area of alopecia on the scalp at birth includes aplasia cutis congenita and neural tube closure defects such as meningocele, encephalocele, and rests of heterotopic meningeal or brain tissue in the skin (see Chapter 9). Aplasia cutis congenita can be distinguished by the presence of atrophy and scarring, and in some cases ulceration of the skin at birth. Neural tube defects are located in or close to the midline at the vertex, nasal bridge, or lower occipital scalp. Both aplasia cutis congenita and neural tube closure defects may show a collarette of dark terminal hair in the newborn.[117]

Treatment and Prognosis

The nevus sebaceus has a propensity to develop neoplastic growths, most of which are benign appendageal tumors such as syringocystadenoma papilliferum, trichilemmoma, trichoblastoma, and apocrine cystadenoma. Malignant tumors include basal cell epithelioma, squamous cell carcinoma, and apocrine or sebaceous carcinoma.[118] These tumors are localized to the skin lesion and rarely metastasize, although they may be locally invasive.[119] They rarely occur in childhood. The lifetime risk of developing a superimposed malignant tumor is uncertain, and very high figures may be due to ascertainment bias.[118,119] More recent studies have found a lower incidence of malignant tumors than previously reported and suggest that benign follicular neoplasms such as trichoblastoma may have been misinterpreted as basal cell carcinoma in the past.[120–122] Changes that should lead one to suspect a neoplastic growth include surface ulceration or the development of a nodule within the lesion.

The need for prophylactic excision of a nevus sebaceus is controversial.[120–122] Decisions regarding surgery should be individualized. Excision may be performed in infancy or postponed until later childhood or adolescence. Continued observation may be preferable to surgery for extensive lesions that are difficult to excise with a good cosmetic result, particularly on the face.

Keratinocytic or Verrucous Epidermal Nevus

The verrucous epidermal nevus is a nonorganoid hamartoma of keratinocytes that may present at birth, within the first few years of life, or sometimes later.[105] There are a number of histologic variants including nonepidermolytic, epidermolytic and inflammatory linear epidermal nevus subtypes.[105]

Cutaneous Findings

The verrucous or keratinocytic epidermal nevus presents at birth or during early childhood and may continue to extend for a variable period.[105] Rarely, new lesions become apparent in adolescence or adult life. Lesions vary in extent from a small cluster or linear arrangement of pigmented, warty papules to widespread linear and swirled areas of pigmentation following the lines of Blaschko (Fig. 23-19). A linear epidermal nevus may involve an entire limb, half of the body in a unilateral distribution, or both sides of the trunk, limbs, and face in a symmetric pattern, with demarcation at the midline. Extensive bilateral lesions have been referred to historically as 'systematized epidermal nevus' or 'ichthyosis hystrix,' and unilateral lesions as 'nevus unius lateris.'

Keratinocytic nevi may have a macerated appearance at birth because of prolonged contact with amniotic fluid (Fig. 23-20). During childhood, the degree of verrucosity varies from subtle, almost flat pigmentation to a grossly elevated, warty appearance.[105] There is a tendency to become more verrucous with age, particularly during puberty. Epidermal nevi involving the head and neck often exhibit the morphology of a nevus sebaceus. Scalp lesions may also be associated with woolly hair nevus, and occasional epidermal nevi have overlying hypertri-

chosis.[123,124] A linear lesion that impinges on the nail matrix may cause dystrophy of the involved nail.

The linear inflammatory verrucous epidermal nevus (ILVEN) is a verrucous, erythematous lesion that can occur at any site, but is most often seen on the limbs or perineum in girls (Fig. 23-21). It is extremely pruritic and may simulate linear psoriasis or linear lichen planus. It is rarely present at birth, but may appear in the first months of life.

Extracutaneous Findings

The majority of epidermal nevi are isolated lesions with no evidence of extracutaneous disease. Multiple associated anomalies are seen in the 'epidermal nevus syndrome.'[102,105] Manifestations of this variable syndrome include developmental abnormalities of the central nervous system, skeleton, eye, and heart, as well as tumors of the genitourinary tract, precocious puberty, hyponatremia, and vitamin D-resistant rickets.[124–129]

In the Proteus syndrome, epidermal nevi occur in association with limb overgrowth, lipomatous lesions, cerebriform malformations of the feet, and cutaneous vascular

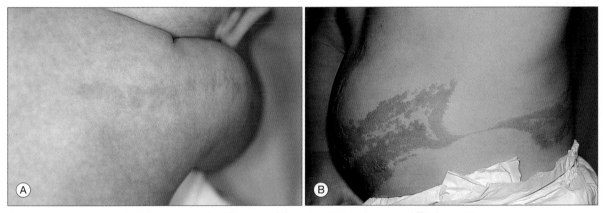

FIG. 23-19 Linear epidermal nevus following the lines of Blaschko (**A**), a shoulder and arm, and (**B**) the trunk.

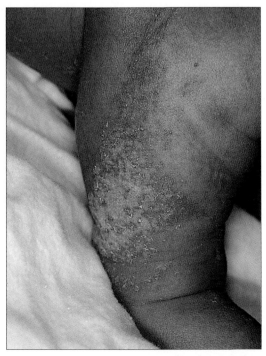

FIG. 23-20 Epidermal nevus on the leg shortly after delivery.

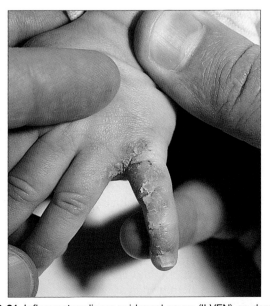

FIG. 23-21 Inflammatory linear epidermal nevus (ILVEN) on dorsal hand and finger.

anomalies.[105,116] The CHILD syndrome is characterized by verrucous lesions corresponding to the lines of Blaschko in conjunction with limb reduction defects.[105,116]

Diagnosis

The most common histologic pattern is that of a benign papilloma, with acanthosis, elongation of rete ridges, hyperkeratosis, and papillomatosis. This histologic appearance may be shared by viral warts, seborrheic keratosis, or acanthosis nigricans. Histology of lesions from the scalp may reveal features of a nevus sebaceus, especially after puberty. A subset of epidermal nevi shows the histologic features of epidermolytic hyperkeratosis, characterized by perinuclear vacuolization of keratinocytes and increased numbers of enlarged keratohyalin granules with overlying hyperkeratosis. In a less common variant there is acantholytic hyperkeratosis similar to that seen in Darier's disease.[130] Histologic findings in ILVEN include psoriasiform epidermal hyperplasia and an inflammatory infiltrate in the upper dermis.[105] The epidermal nevus of CHILD syndrome resembles ILVEN but may also have collections of foam cells in the upper dermis consistent with a verruciform xanthoma.[105]

Etiology and Pathogenesis

The distribution of lesions following the lines of Blaschko suggests somatic mosaicism. Chromosomal mosaicism has been demonstrated in a number of patients with linear verrucous epidermal nevi.[131,132] The concept of mosaicism is supported by observation of lesions with the histology of epidermolytic hyperkeratosis in the parents of children with bullous ichthyosiform erythroderma.[103,104] The same keratin 10 gene mutation was identified in lesional skin from parents with epidermal nevi, and in their offspring with generalized skin disease.[103] This phenomenon has not been observed with other epidermal nevi, suggesting that the genetic defects in these cases may be lethal if inherited.[116]Epidermal nevi are now thought to represent a phenotypic expression of several genetic defects due to postzygotic mutations, rather than a single disease. Whether the basic pathogenetic defect of nonepidermolytic lesions lies in the dermal fibroblast or in the keratinocyte is not known.

Differential Diagnosis

The differential diagnosis of a localized cluster of lesions includes viral warts, which do not commonly have a linear arrangement and regress spontaneously with time. Linear lesions at birth may be confused with the verrucous stage of incontinentia pigmenti. Linear keratinocytic nevi that develop during infancy and childhood differ in morphology, if not in distribution, from lichen striatus, a self-limiting disorder with an inflammatory, papular appearance and lichenoid histology. The differential diagnosis of ILVEN includes lichen simplex chronicus, linear psoriasis, and linear lichen planus, none of which is seen in the newborn period.

The CHILD syndrome and Proteus syndrome have distinctive clinical features. Happle[116] considers these two entities to be well-defined epidermal nevus syndromes. In phakomatosis pigmentokeratotica (PPK), the coexistence of an epidermal nevus of the nonepidermolytic type and a melanocytic speckled lentiginous nevus is frequently associated with neurologic and musculoskeletal anomalies (see Chapter 22).

Treatment and Prognosis

Unlike nevus sebaceus, the linear verrucous epidermal nevus is rarely associated with the development of superimposed benign or malignant tumors in adult life. Patients with epidermal nevi should be evaluated clinically and followed for developmental anomalies and other manifestations of the epidermal nevus syndrome.[105] When histologic examination shows epidermolytic hyperkeratosis, the patient should receive counseling about the possible risk of genetic transmission. The risk of transmission is not known.

Treatment may be requested for cosmetically disfiguring lesions but is generally undertaken in later childhood or adolescence. Excision of small lesions or localized areas of larger lesions may be feasible. Treatment of extensive lesions is difficult. Various destructive modalities, including CO_2 laser ablation, dermabrasion, or liquid nitrogen cryotherapy, have been attempted, but there may be recurrence.[105] The same is true for pharmacologic treatments such as topical or oral retinoids and 5-fluorouracil.[133]

Nevus Comedonicus

A nevus comedonicus is a developmental abnormality of the pilosebaceous unit that appears as a grouped or linear arrangement of small or large comedones. Lesions present at birth or during infancy in the majority of cases. Nevus comedonicus is considered a rare type of epidermal nevus.

Cutaneous Findings

Groups of enlarged follicular openings containing pigmented, comedone-like keratin plugs may be localized or extensive (Fig 23-22A, B). Most nevi are unilateral and located on the face or upper trunk. They frequently have a linear arrangement. Extensive lesions are distributed along the lines of Blaschko and are limited at the midline.[143,135] There may be associated white papules representing milia, closed comedones, or deeper follicular cystic structures. Later in childhood or adolescence these lesions may develop painful, inflammatory cystic nodules and acneiform scarring (Fig. 23-22C).[136] The coexistence of a nevus comedonicus and a verrucous epidermal nevus has been reported.[137] Comedone-like structures may also be seen within verrucous epidermal nevi.[105]

Extracutaneous Findings

In most cases there are no extracutaneous manifestations. Rarely, a nevus comedonicus is associated with central nervous system, skeletal, and ocular abnormalities.[136] In these cases, unilateral cataract and skeletal abnormalities are found on the same side of the body as the nevus.[136] The nevus comedonicus syndrome is considered a variant or subtype of the epidermal nevus syndrome.[105,116,136]

Etiology and Pathogenesis

Nevus comedonicus is a sporadic disorder and is not inherited. The pathogenesis is believed to involve somatic mosaicism.[116,135] A mutation in the fibroblast growth factor receptor 2 (FGFR2) gene detected in a nevus comedonicus suggests that this may represent a mosaic form of Apert syndrome.[138]

Diagnosis

The diagnosis is made on the clinical appearance of the lesion. Histopathologic examination reveals hyperkeratosis and acanthosis of the epidermis with widely dilated, keratin-filled,

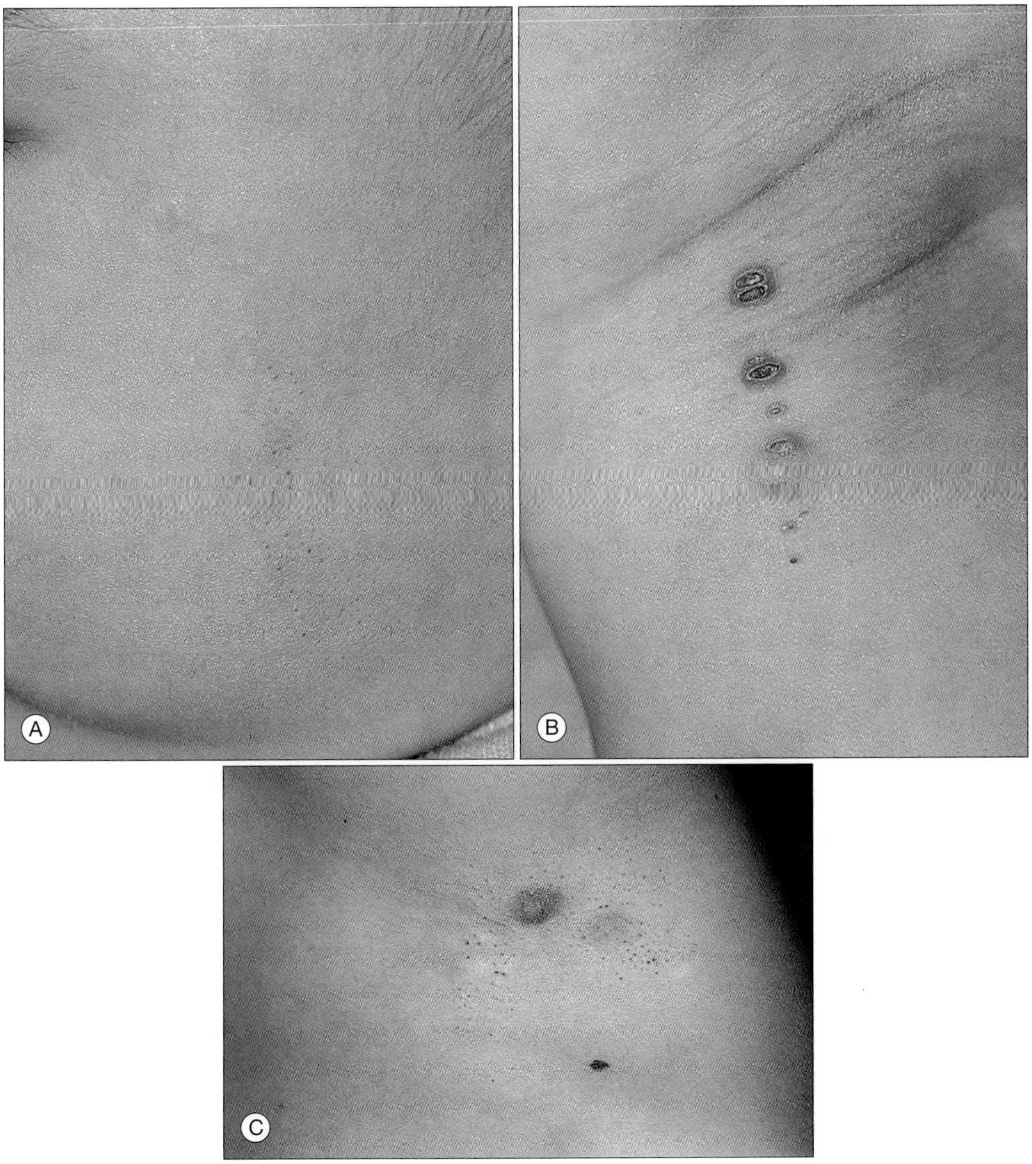

FIG. 23-22 Nevus comedonicus. (A) Open and closed comedones in a linear arrangement on the face of an infant. (B) Large pigmented follicular keratin plugs and a deep follicular cyst. (C) Comedones, inflammatory and noninflammatory cysts in an adolescent.

cystic structures. Epidermolytic hyperkeratosis may be observed in the keratinocytes of the follicular epithelial wall.[134,136]

Differential Diagnosis

The localized appearance of the lesion is very characteristic and unlikely to be mistaken for comedonal acne unless bilateral.[135] Porokeratotic eccrine ostial and dermal duct nevus presents with comedo-like lesions on the palms and soles and has distinctive histologic features. Inflammatory cysts may closely resemble cystic acne.

Treatment and Prognosis

Recurrent inflammation and scarring can cause cosmetic disfigurement. Treatment is difficult. Excision of smaller lesions is curative,[139] but inflammatory acneiform cysts may recur if excision is incomplete. Pharmacologic agents such as oral or topical retinoids are of minimal benefit. Topical and systemic antibiotics have been used to treat inflammatory lesions, with variable success.[135]

Porokeratotic Eccrine and Ostial Dermal Duct Nevus (Porokeratotic Eccrine Nevus)

The porokeratotic eccrine and ostial dermal duct nevus is a congenital hamartoma of the eccrine ducts. Although usually present at birth, lesions may first appear in later childhood or adult life.

Cutaneous and Extracutaneous Findings

This hamartoma is characterized clinically by grouped comedo-like keratotic papules or pits on a palm or sole.[140] Occasionally lesions may be more widespread with a linear distribution.[141,142] Keratotic papules and plaques located in sites other than the palms and soles resemble linear verrucous epidermal nevi.[141-144] There are no symptoms, but there may be associated anhidrosis. There are no recognized systemic manifestations.

Etiology and Pathogenesis

The pathogenesis is believed to represent a circumscribed disorder of keratinization localized to the acrosyringium.[141]

Diagnosis

Histologically, there are epidermal invaginations with parakeratotic plugs emerging from dilated eccrine ostia and surrounded by parakeratotic columns of cornoid lamellae.[143] The eccrine origin of the lesion is confirmed by positive staining for carcinoembryonic antigen (CEA).[141]

Differential Diagnosis

The clinical differential diagnosis includes linear porokeratosis, nevus comedonicus, and linear verrucous nevus. Histologically, punctate porokeratosis and linear porokeratosis of Mibelli can be distinguished by the lack of epidermal invaginations.

Treatment and Prognosis

Treatment with the UltraPulse CO_2 laser has been reported to be beneficial, although recurrence was noted.[141]

Congenital Smooth Muscle Hamartoma

Congenital smooth muscle hamartoma is a benign cutaneous developmental anomaly characterized by an excess of arrector pili muscle within the reticular dermis.[145] It is usually evident at birth or shortly thereafter. The estimated prevalence is 1 in 2600 live births, with a slight male preponderance.[146] Rarely, extensive involvement may be associated with the phenotype of the 'Michelin tire baby'.[147–149]

Cutaneous Findings

The typical congenital smooth muscle hamartoma presents as a lightly pigmented plaque or patch with overlying hypertrichosis (Fig. 23-23). The trunk, in particular the lumbosacral area, is the site of predilection, but lesions may also occur on the proximal limbs. Perifollicular papules are sometimes evident.[150] The overlying hair is vellus in type. Hypertrichosis is not invariable, and the hamartoma may present as a plaque of perifollicular papules with little or no increase in hair growth.[151] Transient elevation or a rippling movement of the lesion due to contraction of the muscle bundles can sometimes be elicited by rubbing or stroking the surface. Rarely, a congenital smooth muscle hamartoma has a linear configuration or presents with multiple lesions.[152,153]

Extracutaneous Findings

There are no systemic findings with localized lesions. There may be associated mental retardation, seizures, and other developmental abnormalities in children with extensive smooth muscle hamartoma as a manifestation of the 'Michelin tire baby' syndrome.[149] Unilateral hypoplasia of the breast and other cutaneous, muscular, or skeletal defects may be associated with smooth muscle hamartoma in the Becker nevus syndrome.[154]

Etiology and Pathogenesis

Congenital smooth muscle hamartoma is believed to represent aberrant development of pilar smooth muscle during fetal life. It has been suggested that the hamartoma involves other structures, such as neural tissue and hair.[150] The hypertrichosis appears to result from increased hair length and diameter rather than an increase in hair density.[151]

Diagnosis

Light microscopic examination of a skin biopsy specimen will establish the diagnosis if the clinical appearance is atypical. Numerous well-defined and variably oriented bundles of smooth muscle are seen within the reticular dermis. They may or may not be associated with follicular structures. Increased epidermal pigmentation may be observed.

Differential Diagnosis

The differential diagnosis of congenital smooth muscle hamartoma includes Becker nevus, nevus pilosus, leiomyoma, connective tissue nevus, solitary mastocytoma, plexiform neurofibroma, and congenital hairy melanocytic nevus. Smooth muscle may be observed in the dermis in Becker nevus, and a continuum between the two conditions has been proposed.[150] Unlike Becker nevus, the congenital smooth muscle hamartoma is always present at birth, does not show prominent epidermal changes, and may demonstrate abnormally whorled myofilaments on electron microscopy.[151]

A nevus pilosus, or hairy patch, shows no alteration in skin texture or pigmentation, and the hair is usually terminal in type. A congenital pigmented hairy nevus is more deeply pigmented, and the overlying hypertrichosis is composed of terminal hair. Leiomyoma is a circumscribed spindle-cell tumor. Connective tissue nevi and mastocytoma may be distinguished by skin biopsy.[151]

Prognosis

This hamartoma has no malignant potential and the prognosis is excellent. There is a tendency for the pigmentation and hair growth to become less noticeable with age.[146] Treatment is unnecessary unless there are cosmetic concerns in later life.

Congenital Becker Nevus and Becker Nevus Syndrome

Becker nevus is an organoid hamartoma characterized by a circumscribed area of hyperpigmentation and hypertrichosis. It is commonly located over the shoulder, chest, or scapula, and has a predilection for males. Although it is usually acquired in adolescence, a number of congenital cases of Becker nevus have been described.[154–157] Histopathologic examination reveals acanthosis and hyperpigmentation of the basal layer of the epidermis, as well as a variable dermal component consisting of smooth muscle bundles that resemble congenital smooth muscle hamartoma.

The Becker nevus syndrome refers to an association with unilateral hypoplasia of the female breast and ipsilateral skeletal defects such as hypoplasia of the shoulder girdle or

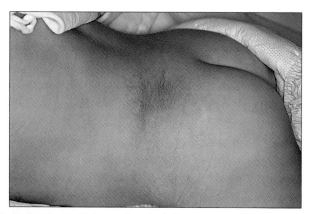

FIG. 23-23 Congenital smooth muscle hamartoma with overlying hypertrichosis.

arm. Other reported anomalies include supernumerary nipples, scoliosis, spina bifida occulta, congenital adrenal hyperplasia, and accessory scrotum.[154,156,158] The syndrome is twice as common in females, possibly because ipsilateral hypoplasia of the breast is easily recognized and reported.[154] A postzygotic mutation that gives rise to mosaicism may explain the location of the nevus and associated anomalies in a similar body region.[154] Although both the isolated nevus and the Becker nevus syndrome are generally sporadic, there have been a few reports of familial aggregation.[154,155] This phenomenon may be explained by paradominant inheritance. [105,159]

Michelin Tire Baby

The 'Michelin tire baby' is characterized by numerous transverse skin folds on all four limbs. These circumferential ringed creases may be associated with an underlying diffuse nevus lipomatosus or a smooth muscle hamartoma.[148] There have been two reports of autosomal dominant transmission.[149] There may be an association with other congenital defects, such as mental retardation, microcephaly, hemiplegia, hemihypertrophy, and chromosomal defects, suggesting a contiguous gene syndrome.[149,160] When the syndrome is associated with an underlying smooth muscle hamartoma there is often diffuse hyperpigmentation and hypertrichosis. In one such patient there were also moderate joint hyperextensibility and perifollicular papules.[148] No treatment is available. The skin folds usually diminish slowly as the child grows.[160]

Nevus Lipomatosus

Nevus lipomatosus cutaneous superficialis is a hamartoma composed of mature fat. Clinically, these lesions present at birth or later in childhood as an asymptomatic, soft or rubbery plaque with a polypoid or cerebriform appearance.[161,162] A linear arrangement of flesh-colored to yellow lesions in a zosteriform pattern is the most common presentation (Fig. 23-24). They are frequently observed in the lumbosacral or perineal areas, but can be located elsewhere. Histologic specimens show mature unencapsulated adipose tissue infiltrating between collagen bundles in the superficial and deep dermis. Similar features may be observed in the lipomatous lesions of encephalocraniocutaneous lipomatosis, focal dermal hypoplasia, or benign fat herniations on the feet of infants. Although asymptomatic, they may require excision for cosmetic reasons.

Connective Tissue Nevus

A connective tissue nevus is characterized by excessive deposition of one or both of the collagen or elastin components of dermal connective tissue. These hamartomas may occur sporadically, or as a familial disorder with autosomal dominant transmission.[163] Connective tissue nevi are also seen as a manifestation of genetic syndromes, notably the 'shagreen patch' or collagenoma in tuberous sclerosis, and the multiple elastic tissue nevi of Buschke–Ollendorff syndrome.[164] A connective tissue nevus may be present at birth, but most become evident during childhood or adolescence.

Cutaneous Findings

Connective tissue nevi present clinically as asymptomatic, firm, skin colored to yellowish nodules or plaques located on the trunk or limbs (Fig. 23-25). The surface of the lesion may be smooth or have a 'cobblestone,' 'leather-grain,' or 'peau d'orange' appearance. They may be solitary or multiple. A linear or 'zosteriform' morphology is sometimes observed.

Extracutaneous Findings

Osteopoikilosis is seen in association with elastic tissue nevi in the Buschke–Ollendorff syndrome.[164] The skin lesions in this condition may rarely be present at birth, but the distinctive bone changes are not reported in infancy. The collagenoma or 'shagreen patch' of tuberous sclerosis develops in later childhood, although other stigmata of the disease may be present at birth or in early infancy. Cardiomyopathy may occur in association with the multiple lesions of familial cutaneous collagenoma and with collagenomas and hypogonadism.[163] Multiple collagenomas in Down syndrome have been reported in adolescence.[165] A cerebriform collagenoma on the sole of the foot may be an isolated phenomenon or a component of Proteus syndrome.[166]

Etiology and Pathogenesis

The pathogenesis is unknown. In familial cutaneous collagenoma, the skin lesions are inherited as an autosomal dominant trait. Tuberous sclerosis and Buschke–Ollendorff syndrome are also inherited by autosomal dominant transmission. Somatic mosaicism may be postulated for sporadic lesions, particularly those with a linear distribution.

Diagnosis

Histologic examination of connective tissue nevi shows an excess of collagen or elastic tissue in the dermis. This may not

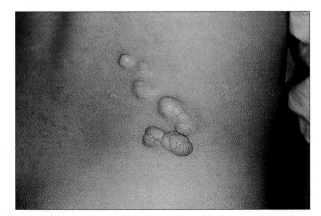

FIG. 23-24 Nevus lipomatosus with soft polypoid nodules on the lower back.

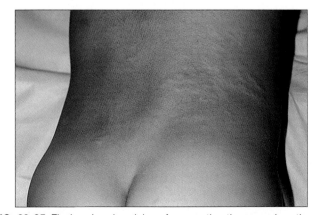

FIG. 23-25 Flesh-colored nodules of connective tissue nevi on the back.

be apparent unless a specimen of normal adjacent skin is obtained for comparison. Thus biopsies of connective tissue nevi are often reported as 'normal skin.' Special elastic stains are necessary to demonstrate the increased numbers of elastic fibers in elastic tissue nevi.

Differential Diagnosis

The differential diagnosis includes other cutaneous hamartomas, such as neurofibromas, leiomyomas, smooth muscle hamartomas, nevus lipomatosus, and epidermal nevus. These entities may be distinguished by histopathologic examination of a skin biopsy. A congenital mucinous nevus may be a variant of connective tissue nevus in which deposition of mucin (proteoglycan) in the dermis is the predominant histopathologic finding.[167]

Treatment and Prognosis

Connective tissue nevi are permanent lesions. They grow in proportion to the child's growth. There is no malignant potential and most do not require treatment. Surgical excision may occasionally be indicated for cosmetic reasons.

Acquired Raised Bands of Infancy

Acquired raised bands of infancy, also known as 'raised limb bands' were first reported by Meggitt and Harper in 2002.[168] Since then, several other cases have been reported in a relatively short period, suggesting that the condition may not be rare. Onset is typically within the first few weeks to months of life. The lesions are flesh-colored linear bands, which are

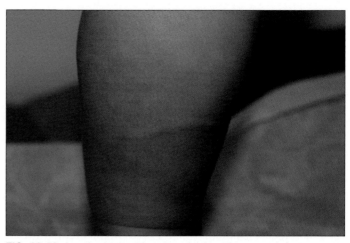

FIG. 23-26 Acquired raised band on the leg of a young infant.

typically horizontally oriented, slightly firm, and elevated above the skin surface. Linear atrophic skin lesions may also be present.[169] Most have been located on the extremities (Fig. 23-26), but the torso can also be involved. A relationship to amniotic bands has been proposed but is debatable. At least one familial case has been reported. Although some cases have occurred in premature infants with a perinatal history of placental abruption, they are also described in healthy term infants.[170] Limited information about the natural history suggests that the number of bands stabilizes in infancy, and these asymptomatic lesions persist.

REFERENCES

1. Coffin CM. Fibromyoblastic–myofibroblastic tumors. In: Coffin CM, Dehner LP, O'Shea PA, eds. Pediatric soft tissue tumors: A clinical, pathological, and therapeutic approach. Philadelphia: Williams & Wilkins, 1997; 133–178.
2. Enzinger FM, Weiss SW. Fibromatoses. In: Soft tissue tumors, 4th edn. St Louis: Mosby, 2001; 347–376.
3. Chung EB, Enzinger FM. Infantile myofibromatosis. Cancer 1981; 48: 1807–1818.
4. Stanford D, Rogers M. Dermatological presentations of infantile myofibromatosis: a review of 27 cases. Aust J Dermatol 2000; 41: 156–161.
5. Brill PW, Yandow DR, Langer LO, et al. Congenital generalized fibromatosis. Case report and literature review. Pediatr Radiol 1982; 12: 269–278.
6. Parker RK, Mallory SB, Baker GF. Infantile myofibromatosis. Pediatr Dermatol 1991; 8: 129–132.
7. Goldberg NS, Bauer BS, Kraus H, et al. Infantile myofibromatosis: A review of clinicopathology with perspectives on new treatment choices. Pediatr Dermatol 1988; 5: 37–46.
8. Wada H, Akiyama H, Seki H, et al. Spinal canal involvement in infantile myofibromatosis: Case report and review of the literature. J Pediatr Hematol Oncol 1998; 20: 353–356.

9. Wiswell TE, Sakas EL, Stephenson SR, et al. Infantile myofibromatosis. Pediatrics 1985; 76: 981–984.
10. Zand DJ, Huff D, Everman D, et al. Autosomal dominant inheritance of infantile myofibromatosis. Am J Med Genet 2004; 126: 261–266.
11. Gandhi MM, Nathan PC, Weitzman S, Levitt GA. Successful treatment of life-threatening generalized infantile myofibromatosis using low-dose chemotherapy. Pediatr Hematol Oncol 2003; 25: 750–754.
12. Keltz M, DiCostanzo D, Desai P, et al. Infantile (Desmoid-type) fibromatosis. Pediatr Dermatol 1995; 12: 149–151.
13. Martinez-Lage JF, Acosta J, Sola J, et al. Congenital desmoid tumor of the scalp: A histologically benign lesion with aggressive clinical behavior. Child's Nerv Sys 1996; 12: 409–412.
14. Pereyo NG, Heimer WL. Extraabdominal desmoid tumor. J Am Acad Dermatol 1996; 34: 352–356.
15. Faulkner LB, Hajdu SI, Kher U, et al. Pediatric desmoid tumor: Retrospective analysis of 63 cases. J Clin Oncol 1995; 13: 2813–2818.
16. Lachner H, Urban C, Benesch M, et al. Multimodal treatment of children with unresectable or recurrent desmoid tumors; An 11-year longitudinal observational study. J Pediatr Hematol Oncol 2004; 26: 518–522.

17. Fotiadis C, Tsekouras DK, Antonakis P, et al. Gardner's syndrome: A case report and review of the literature. World J Gastroenterol 2005; 11: 5408–5411.
18. Dormans JP, Spiegel D, Meyer J, et al. Fibromatoses in childhood: The desmoid/fibromatosis complex. Med Pediatr Oncol 2001; 37: 126–131.
19. Buitendijk A, van de Ven C, Dumans TG, et al. Pediatric aggressive fibromatosis: A retrospective analysis of 13 patients and review of literature. Cancer 2005; 104: 1090–1099.
20. Skapek SX, Hawk BJ, Hoffer FA, et al. Combination chemotherapy using vinblastine and methotrexate for the treatment of progressive desmoid tumor in children. J Clin Oncol 1998; 16: 3021–3027.
21. Eich GF, Hoeffel JC, Tschappeler H, et al. Fibrous tumors in children: imaging features of a heterogeneous group of disorders. Pediatr Radiol 1998; 28: 500–509.
22. Ishii N, Matsui K, Ichiyama S, et al. A case of infantile digital fibromatosis showing spontaneous regression. Br J Dermatol 1989; 121: 129–133.
23. Albertini JG, Welsch MJ, Conger LA, et al. Infantile digital fibroma treated with Mohs micrographic surgery. Dermatol Surg 2002; 10: 959–961.

24. Oh CK, Son HS, Kwon YW, et al. Intralesional fluorouracil injection in infantile digital fibromatosis. Arch Dermatol 2005; 141: 549–550.

25. Paller AS, Gonzalez-Crussi, Sherman JO. Fibrous hamartoma of infancy. Arch Dermatol 1989; 125: 88–91.

26. Dickey GE, Sotelo-Avila C. Fibrous hamartoma of infancy: current review. Pediatr Dev Pathol 1999; 2: 236–243.

27. Fetsch JF, Miettinen M, Laskin WB, et al. A clinicopathological study of 45 pediatric soft tissue tumors with an admixture of adipose tissue and fibroblastic elements, and a proposal for classification as lipofibromatosis. Am J Surg Pathol 2000; 24: 1491–1500.

28. Hart TC, Zhang Y, Gorry MC, et al. A mutation in the SOS1 gene causes hereditary gingival fibromatosis type 1. Am J Hum Genet 2002; 70: 943–954.

29. Ye X, Shi L, Cheng Y, et al. A novel locus for autosomal dominant hereditary gingival fibromatosis, GINGF3, maps to chromosome 2p22.3-p23.3. Clin Genet 2005; 68: 239–244.

30. Tagaki M, Yamamoto H, Mega H, et al. Heterogeneity in the gingival fibromatoses. Cancer 1991; 68: 2202–2212.

31. Davalos IP, Garcia-Cruz D, Garcia-Cruz MO. Zimmermann–Laband syndrome: further clinical delineation. Genet Couns 2005; 16: 283–290.

32. O'Shea PA. Myogenic tumors of soft tissue. In: Coffin CM, Dehner LP, O'Shea PA, eds. Pediatric soft tissue tumors: a clinical, pathological, and therapeutic approach. Philadelphia: Williams & Wilkins, 1997; 214–253.

33. Lupton GP, Naik DG, Rodman OG. An unusual congenital leiomyoma. Pediatr Dermatol 1986; 3: 158–160.

34. Henderson CA, Ruban A, Porter DL. Multiple leiomyomata presenting in a child. Pediatr Dermatol 1997; 14: 287–289.

35. Yang SS, Williams RJ, Bear BJ, et al. Leiomyoma of the hand in a child who has the human immunodeficiency virus: A case report. J Bone Joint Surg Am 1996; 78-A: 1904–1906.

36. McCormack K, Kaplan D, Murray JC, et al. Multiple hairy pacinian neurofibromas (nerve-sheath myxomas). J Am Acad Dermatol 1988; 18: 416–419.

37. Murato Y, Kumano K, Ugai K, et al. Neurilemmomatosis. Br J Dermatol 1991; 125: 466–468.

38. Mautner VF, Lindenau M, Baser ME, et al. Skin abnormalities in neurofibromatosis 2. Arch Dermatol 1997; 133: 1539–1543.

39. Iyengar V, Golomb CA, Schachner L. Neurilemmomatosis, NF2 and juvenile xanthogranuloma. J Am Acad Dermatol 1998; 39: 831–834.

40. Caputo R, Ermacora E, Gelmetti C, et al. Generalized eruptive histiocytoma in children. J Am Acad Dermatol 1987; 17: 449–454.

41. Jang KA, Lee HJ, Choi JH, et al. Generalized eruptive histiocytoma of childhood. Br J Dermatol 1999; 140: 174–176.

42. Hernandez-Martin A, Baselga E, Drolet BA, et al. Juvenile xanthogranuloma. J Am Acad Dermatol 1997; 36: 355–367.

43. Zvulunov A, Barak Y, Metzker A. Juvenile xanthogranuloma, neurofibromatosis, and juvenile chronic myelogenous leukemia. Arch Dermatol 1995; 131: 904–908.

44. Mann RE, Friedman KJ, Milgraum SS. Urticaria pigmentosa and juvenile xanthogranuloma: Case report and brief review of the literature. Pediatr Dermatol 1996; 13: 122–126.

45. Resnick SD, Woosly J, Azizkhan RG. Giant juvenile xanthogranuloma: Exophytic and endophytic variants. Pediatr Dermatol 1990; 7: 185–188.

46. Kolde G, Bonsmann G. Generalized lichenoid juvenile xanthogranuloma. Br J Dermatol 1992; 126: 66–70.

47. Freyer DR, Kennedy R, Bostrom BC, et al. Juvenile xanthogranuloma: Forms of systemic disease and their clinical implications. J Pediatr 1996; 129: 227–237.

48. Chang MW, Frieden IJ, Good W. The risk of intraocular juvenile xanthogranuloma: Survey of current practices and assessment of risk. J Am Acad Dermatol 1996; 34: 445–449.

49. Weitzman S, Jaffe R. Uncommon histiocytic disorders: the non-Langerhans cell histiocytoses. Pediatr Blood Cancer 2005; 45: 256–264.

50. Newman CC, Raimer SS, Sanchez RL. Nonlipidized juvenile xanthogranuloma: A histologic and immunohistochemical study. Pediatr Dermatol 1997; 14: 98–102.

51. Zelger BWH, Cerio R. Xanthogranuloma is the archetype of non-Langerhans cell histiocytosis. Br J Dermatol 2001; 145: 369–370.

52. Sidwell RU, Francis N, Slater DN, et al. Is disseminated juvenile xanthogranulomatosis benign cephalic histiocytosis? Pediatr Dermatol 2005; 22: 40–43.

53. Gianotti F, Caputo R. Histiocytic syndromes: a review. J Am Acad Dermatol 1985; 13: 383–404.

54. Weston WL, Travers SH, Mierau GW, et al. Benign cephalic histiocytosis with diabetes insipidus. Pediatr Dermatol 2000; 17: 296–298.

55. Sell EJ, Hansen RC, Struck-Pierce S. Calcified nodules of the heel: A complication of neonatal intensive care. J Pediatr 1985; 96: 473–475.

56. Leung A. Calcification following heel sticks. J Pediatr 1985; 106: 168.

57. Fretzin DF, Arias AM. Sclerema neonatorum and subcutaneous fat necrosis of the newborn. Pediatr Dermatol 1987; 4: 112–122.

58. Glover MT, Catterall MD, Atherton DJ. Subcutaneous fat necrosis in two infants after hypothermic cardiac surgery. Pediatr Dermatol 1991; 8: 210–212.

59. Chuang SD, Chiu HC, Chang CC. Subcutaneous fat necrosis of the newborn complicating hypothermic cardiac surgery. Br J Dermatol 1995; 132: 805–810.

60. Duhn R, Schoen E, Sui M. Subcutaneous fat necrosis with extensive calcification after hypothermia in two newborn infants. Pediatrics 1968; 41: 661–664.

61. Beers BB, Flowers FP, Sherertz EF, et al. Dystrophic calcinosis cutis secondary to intrauterine herpes simplex. Pediatr Dermatol 1986; 3: 208–211.

62. Ruiz-Maldonado R, Duran-McKinster C, Carrasco-Daza D, et al. Intrauterine epidermal necrosis: report of three cases. J Am Acad Dermatol 1998; 38: 712–715.

63. Carruthers J, Jevon G, Prendiville J. Localized dystrophic periocular calcification: A complication of intralesional corticosteroid therapy for infantile periocular hemangiomas. Pediatr Dermatol 1998; 15: 23–26.

64. Walsh JS, Fairley JA. Calcifying disorders of the skin. J Am Acad Dermatol 1995; 33: 693–706.

65. Zouboulis CC, Blume-Peytavi U, Lennert T, et al. Fulminant metastatic calcinosis with cutaneous necrosis in a child with end-stage renal disease and tertiary hyperparathyroidism. Br J Dermatol 1996; 135: 617–622.

66. Plott T, Wiss K, Raimer SS, et al. Recurrent subepidermal calcified nodule of the nose. Pediatr Dermatol 1988; 5: 107–111.

67. Evans MJ, Blessing K, Gray ES. Subepidermal calcified nodule in children: A clinicopathologic study of 21 cases. Pediatr Dermatol 1995; 12: 307–310.

68. Lai CH, Farah R, Mallory SB. Congenital calcinosis cutis of the ear. J Am Acad Dermatol 2003; 49: 122–124.

69. Bostrum B. Tumoral calcinosis in an infant. Am J Dis Child 1981; 135: 246–247.

70. Heydemann JS, McCarthy RE. Tumoral calcinosis in a child. J Pediatr Orthop 1988; 8: 474–477.

71. Greenberg SB. Tumoral calcinosis in an infant. Pediatr Radiol 1990; 20: 206–207.

72. Niall DM, Fogarty EE, Dowling FE, et al. Spontaneous regression of tumoral calcinosis in an infant: A case report. J Pediatr Surg 1998; 33: 1429–1431.

73. Polykandriotis EP, Beutel FK, Horch RE, Grunert J. A case of familial tumoral calcinosis in a neonate and review of the literature. Arch Orthop Traum Surg 2004; 124: 563–567.

74. Benet-Pages A, Orlik P, Strom TM, Lorenz-Depiereux B. An FGF23 missense mutation causes familial tumoral calcinosis with hyperphosphatemia. Hum Mol Genet 2005; 14: 385–390.

75. Sahn EE, Smith DJ. Annular dystrophic calcinosis cutis in an infant. J Am Acad Dermatol 1992; 6: 1015–1017.
76. Puig L, Rocamora V, Romani J, et al. Calcinosis cutis following calcium chloride electrode paste application for auditory-brainstem evoked potentials recording. Pediatr Dermatol 1998; 15: 27–30.
77. Prendiville JS, Lucky AW, Mallory SB, et al. Osteoma cutis as a presenting sign of pseudohypoparathyroidism. Pediatr Dermatol 1992; 9: 11–18.
78. Miller ES, Esterly NB, Fairley JA. Progressive osseous heteroplasia. Arch Dermatol 1996; 132: 787–791.
79. Sanmartin O, Alegre V, Martinez-Aparicio A, et al. Congenital platelike osteoma cutis: Case report and review of the literature. Pediatr Dermatol 1993; 10: 182–186.
80. Gardner RJM, Yun K, Craw SM. Familial ectopic ossification. J Med Genet 1988; 25: 113–117.
81. Patten JL, Johns JR, Valle D, et al. Mutation in the gene encoding the stimulatory G protein of adenylate cyclase in Albright's hereditary osteodystrophy. N Engl J Med 1990; 322: 1412–1419.
82. Shore EM, Ahn J, de Beur J, et al. Paternally inherited inactivating mutations of the GNAS1 gene in progressive osseous heteroplasia. N Engl J Med 2002; 246: 99–106.
83. Power MM, James RS, Barber JC, et al. RDCI, the vasoactive intestinal peptide receptor: A candidate gene for the features of Albright hereditary osteodystrophy associated with deletion of 2q37. J Med Genet 1997; 34: 287–290.
84. Kaplan KS, Craver R, MacEwan GD, et al. Progressive osseous heteroplasia: A distinct developmental disorder of heterotopic ossification. J Bone Joint Surg 1994; 76A: 425–436.
85. Schmidt AH, Vincent KA, Aiona MD. Hemimelic progressive osseous heteroplasia. J Bone Joint Surg 1994; 76A: 907–912.
86. Athanasou NA, Benson MK, Brenton DP, et al. Progressive osseous heteroplasia: A case report. Bone 1994; 15: 471–475.
87. Juppner H. The genetic basis of progressive osseous heteroplasia. N Engl J Med 2002; 346: 128–130.
88. Kaplan FS. Skin and bones. Arch Dermatol 1996; 132: 815–818.
89. Lietman SA, Ding C, Cooke DW, Levine MA. Reduction in Gsalpha induces osteogenic differentiation in human mesenchymal stem cells. Clin Orthop Relat Res 2005; 434; 231–238.
90. Yeh GL, Mathur S, Wivel A, et al. GNAS1 mutation and Cbfa1 misexpression in a child with severe congenital platelike osteoma cutis. J Bone Miner Res 2000; 15: 2063–2067.
91. Moehlenbeck FW. Pilomatricoma (calcifying epithelioma): a statistical study. Arch Dermatol 1973; 108: 532–534.
92. Pirouzmanesh ABS, Reinisch JF, Gonzalez-Gomez I, et al. Pilomatrixoma: a review of 346 cases. Plast Reconstruct Surg 2003; 112: 1784–1789.
93. Demircan M, Balik E. Pilomatricoma in children: a prospective study. Pediatr Dermatol 1997; 14: 430–432.
94. Julian CG, Bowers PW. A clinical review of 209 pilomatricomas. J Am Acad Dermatol 1998; 39: 191–195.
95. Geh JL, Moss Al. Multiple pilomatrixomata and myotonic dystrophy: a familial association. Br J Dermatol 1999; 52: 143–145.
96. Kopeloff I, Orlow SJ, Sanchez MR. Multiple pilomatricomas: report of two cases and review of the association with myotonic dystrophy. Cutis 1992; 50: 290–292.
97. Pujol RM, Casanova JM, Egido R, et al. Multiple familial pilomatricomas: a cutaneous marker for Gardner syndrome? Pediatr Dermatol 1995; 12: 331–335.
98. Cambiaghi S, Ermacora E, Brusasco A, et al. Multiple pilomatricomas in Rubenstein–Taybi syndrome: a case report. Pediatr Dermatol 1994; 11: 21–25.
99. Chan EF, Gat U, McNiff JM, et al. A common skin tumour is caused by activating mutations in beta-catenin. Nature Genet 1999; 21: 410–413.
100. Hughes J, Lam A, Rogers M. Use of ultrasonography in the diagnosis of childhood pilomatrixoma. Pediatr Dermatol 1999; 16: 341–344.
101. Poomeechaiwong S, Golitz LE. Hamartomas. Adv Dermatol 1990; 5: 257–288.
102. Solomon LM, Esterly NB. Epidermal and other congenital organoid nevi. Curr Probl Pediatr 1975; 6: 1–55.
103. Paller AS, Syder AJ, Chan Y-M, et al. Genetic and clinical mosaicism in a type of epidermal nevus. N Engl J Med 1994; 331: 1408–1415.
104. Nazarro V, Ermacora E, Santucci B, et al. Epidermolytic hyperkeratosis: Generalized form in children from parents with systematized linear form. Br J Dermatol 1990; 122: 417–422.
105. Happle R, Rogers M. Epidermal nevi. Adv Dermatol 2002; 18: 175–201.
106. Alper J, Holmes LB, Mihm MC. Birthmarks with serious medical significance: nevocellular nevi, sebaceous nevi, and multiple cafe au lait spots. J Pediatr 1979; 95: 696–700.
107. Vidaurri-de la Cruz H, Tamayo-Sanchez L, Duran-McKinster C, et al. Epidermal nevus syndromes: clinical findings in 35 patients. Pediatr Dermatol 2004; 4: 432–439.
108. Baker RS, Ross PA, Baumann RJ. Neurologic complications of the epidermal nevus syndrome. Arch Neurol 1987; 44: 227–232.
109. Davies D. Rogers M. Review of neurological manifestations in 196 patients with sebaceous naevi. Australas J Dermatol 2002; 43: 20–23.
110. Palazzi P, Artese O, Paolini A, et al. Linear sebaceous nevus syndrome: Report of a patient with unusual associated abnormalities. Pediatr Dermatol 1996; 13: 22–24.
111. Goldblum JR, Headington JT. Hypophosphatemic vitamin D-resistant rickets and multiple spindle and epithelioid nevi associated with linear nevus sebaceus syndrome. J Am Acad Dermatol 1993; 29: 109–111.
112. Oranje AP, Przyrembel H, Meradji M, et al. Solomon's epidermal nevus syndrome (Type: linear sebaceus nevus) and hypophosphatemic vitamin D-resistant rickets. Arch Dermatol 1994; 130: 1167–1171.
113. Xin H, Matt D, Qin JZ, et al. The sebaceous nevus: a nevus with deletions of the PTCH gene. Cancer Res 1999; 59: 1834–1836.
114. Benedetto L, Sood U, Blumenthal N, et al. Familial nevus sebaceus. J Am Acad Dermatol 1990; 23: 130–132.
115. Sahl WJ. Familial nevus sebaceus of Jadassohn: occurrence in three generations. J Am Acad Dermatol 1990; 22: 853–854.
116. Happle R. How many epidermal nevus syndromes exist? A clinicogenetic classification. J Am Acad Dermatol 1991; 25: 550–556.
117. Drolet BA, Prendiville J, Golden J, et al. Membranous aplasia cutis with hair collars: Congenital absence of the skin or neuroectodermal defect. Arch Dermatol 1997; 133: 1551–1554.
118. Wilson-Jones E, Heyl T. Naevus sebaceus: A report of 140 cases with special report of the development of secondary malignant tumours. Br J Dermatol 1970; 82: 99–117.
119. Domingo J, Helwig EB. Malignant neoplasms associated with nevus sebaceus of Jadassohn. J Am Acad Dermatol 1979; 1: 545–556.
120. Cribier B, Scrivener Y, Grosshans E. Tumors arising in nevus sebaceous: a study of 596 cases. J Am Acad Dermatol 2000; 42: 263–268.
121. Jaqueti G, Requena L, Sanchez Yus E. Trichoblastoma is the most common neoplasm developed in nevus sebaceous of Jadassohn: a clinicopathologic study of a series of 155 cases. Am J Dermatopathol 2000; 22: 108–118.
122. Santibanez-Gallerani, A, Marshall D, Duarte A-M, et al. Should nevus sebaceous of Jadassohn in children be excised? A study of 757 cases, and literature review. J Craniofac Surg 2003; 14: 658–660.
123. Tay Y-K, Weston WL, Ganong CA, et al. Epidermal nevus syndrome: association with central precocious puberty and woolly hair nevus. J Am Acad Dermatol 1996; 35: 839–842.
124. Allison MA, Dunn CL, Pedersen RC. Epidermal nevus syndrome: A neurologic variant with hemimeganencephaly, facial hemihypertrophy and gyral

malformation. Pediatr Dermatol 1998; 15: 59–61.

125. Grebe TA, Rinsen ME, Richter SF, et al. Further delineation of the epidermal nevus syndrome: Two cases with new findings and literature review. Am J Med Genet 1993; 47: 24–30.

126. Ivker R, Resnick SD, Skidmore RA. Hypophosphatemic vitamin D-resistant rickets, precocious puberty, and the epidermal nevus syndrome. Arch Dermatol 1997; 133: 1557–1561.

127. Moss C, Parkin JM, Comaish JS. Precocious puberty in a boy with a widespread linear epidermal nevus. Br J Dermatol 1991; 125: 178–182.

128. Rongioletti F, Rebora A. Epidermal nevus with transitional cell carcinomas in the urinary tract. J Am Acad Dermatol 1991; 25: 856–858.

129. Yu, TW, Tsau YK, Young C, et al. Epidermal nevus with hypermelanosis and chronic hyponatremia. Pediatr Neurol 2000; 22: 151–154.

130. Munro CS, Cox NH. An acantholytic dyskeratotic epidermal naevus with other features of Darier's disease on the same side of the body. Br J Dermatol 1992; 127: 168–171.

131. Stosiek N, Ulmer R, von den Driesch P, et al. Chromosomal mosaicism in two patients with epidermal verrucous nevus: demonstration of chromosomal breakpoint. J Am Acad Dermatol 1994; 30: 622–625.

132. Iglesias Zamora ME, Vazquez-Doval FJ. Epidermal naevi associated with trichilemmal cysts and chromosomal mosaicism. Br J Dermatol 1997; 137: 821–824.

133. Nelson BR, Kolansky G, Gillard M, et al. Management of linear verrucous epidermal nevus with topical 5-fluorouracil and tretinoin. J Am Acad Dermatol 1994; 30: 287.

134. Cestari T, Rubim M, Valentini BC. Nevus comedonicus: case report and brief review of the literature. Pediatr Dermatol 1991; 8: 300–305.

135. Vassiloudes PE, Morelli JP, Weston WL. Inflammatory nevus comedonicus in children. J Am Acad Dermatol 1998; 38: 834–836.

136. Patrizi A, Neri I, Fiorentini C, et al. Nevus comedonicus syndrome: a new pediatric case. Pediatr Dermatol 1998; 15: 304–306.

137. Kim SC, Kang WH. Nevus comedonicus associated with epidermal nevus. J Am Acad Dermatol 1989; 21: 1085–1088.

138. Munro CS, Wilkie AO. Epidermal mosaicism producing localized acne: somatic mutation in FGFR2. Lancet 1998; 352: 704–705.

139. Marcus J, Esterly NB, Bauer BS. Tissue expansion in a patient with extensive nevus comedonicus. Ann Plast Surg 1992; 29: 362–366.

140. Abell E, Read SI. Porokeratotic eccrine ostial and dermal duct naevus. Br J Dermatol 1980; 103: 435–441.

141. Leung CS, Tang WYM, Lam WY, et al. Porokeratotic eccrine ostial and dermal duct naevus. Br J Dermatol 1998; 138: 684–688.

142. Dogra S, Jain R, Mohanty SK, Handa S. Porokeratotic eccrine ostial and dermal duct nevus: unilateral systematized involvement. Pediatr Dermatol 2002; 19: 568–569.

143. Fernandez-Redondo V, Toribi J. Porokeratotic eccrine ostial and dermal duct nevus. J Cutan Pathol 1988; 15: 393–395.

144. Aloi F, Pippione M. Porokeratotic eccrine ostial and dermal duct nevus. Arch Dermatol 1986; 122: 892–895.

145. Prendiville JS, Esterly NB. Congenital smooth muscle hamartoma. J Pediatr 1987; 110: 742–744.

146. Zvulunov A, Rotem A, Merlob P, et al. Congenital smooth muscle hamartoma: Prevalence, clinical findings, and follow-up in 15 patients. AJDC 1990; 144: 782–784.

147. Sato M, Ishiwawa O, Miyachi Y, et al. Michelin tyre syndrome: A congenital disorder of elastic fibre formation. Br J Dermatol 1997; 136: 583–586.

148. Oku T, Iwasaki K, Fujita H. Folded skin with an underlying cutaneous smooth muscle hamartoma. Br J Dermatol 1993; 129: 606–608.

149. Schnur RE, Herzberg AJ, Spinner N, et al. Variability in the Michelin tire syndrome: A child with multiple anomalies, smooth muscle hamartoma, and familial paracentric inversion of chromosome 7q.102. J Am Acad Dermatol 1993; 28: 364–370.

150. Johnson MD, Jacobs AH. Congenital smooth muscle hamartoma. Arch Dermatol 1989; 125: 820–822.

151. Gagne EJ, Su WPD. Congenital smooth muscle hamartoma of the skin. Pediatr Dermatol 1993; 10: 142–145.

152. Grau-Massanes M, Raimer S, Colome-Grimmer M, et al. Congenital smooth muscle hamartoma presenting as a linear atrophic plaque: Case report and review of the literature. Pediatr Dermatol 1996; 13: 222–225.

153. Guillot B, Huet P, Joujoux JM, et al. Multiple congenital smooth muscle hamartomas. Ann Dermatol Venereol 1998; 125: 118–120.

154. Happle R, Koopman RJJ. Becker nevus syndrome. Am J Med Genet 1997; 68: 357–361.

155. Book SE, Glass AT, Laude TA. Congenital Becker's nevus with a familial association. Pediatr Dermatol 1997; 14: 373–375.

156. Lambert JR, Willems P, Abs R, et al. Becker's nevus associated with chromosomal mosaicism and congenital adrenal hyperplasia. J Am Acad Dermatol 1994; 30: 655–657.

157. Ferreira MJ, Bajanca R, Fiadeiro T. Congenital melanosis and hypertrichosis in a bilateral distribution. Pediatr Dermatol 1998; 15: 290–292.

158. Urbani CE, Betti R. Supernumerary nipple in association with Becker nevus vs. Becker nevus syndrome: A semantic problem only. Am J Med Genet 1998; 77: 76–77.

159. Happle R. Patterns on the skin. New aspects of their embryologic and genetic causes. Hautarzt 2004; 55: 960–968.

160. Saldana K, Mendiratta V, Kakar N, et al. Spontaneously improving Michelin Tire Baby Syndrome. Pediatr Dermatol 2003; 20: 150–152.

161. Wilson-Jones E, Marks R, Pongsehirun D. Naevus superficialis lipomatosus. Br J Dermatol 1975; 93: 121–133.

162. Lane JE, Clark E, Marzec T. Nevus lipomatosus cutaneous superficialis. Pediatr Dermatol 2003; 20: 313–314.

163. Uitto J, Santa Cruz DJ, Eisen AZ. Connective tissue nevi of the skin: Clinical, genetic and histopathologic classification of hamartomas of the collagen, elastin, and proteoglycan type. J Am Acad Dermatol 1980; 3: 441–461.

164. Verbov J, Graham R. Buschke–Ollendorff syndrome-disseminated dermatofibrosis with osteopoikilosis. Clin Exp Dermatol 1986; 11: 17–26.

165. Smith JB, Hogan DJ, Glass LF, et al. Multiple collagenomas in a patient with Down syndrome. J Am Acad Dermatol 1995; 33: 835–837.

166. Botella-Estrada R, Alegre V, Sanmartin O, et al. Isolated plantar cerebriform collagenoma. Arch Dermatol 1991; 127: 1589–1590.

167. Chang S-E, Kang S-K, Kim E-S, Lee M-W, et al. A case of congenital mucinous nevus: a connective tissue nevus of the proteoglycan type. Pediatr Dermatol 2003; 20: 229–231.

168. Meggitt SJ, Harper J, Lacour M, Taylor AE. Raised limb bands developing in infancy. Br J Dermatol 2002; 147: 359–363.

169. Dyer JA, Chamlin S. Acquired raised bands of infancy: association with amniotic bands. Pediatr Dermatol. 2005; 22: 346–349.

170. Lateo SA, Taylor AEM, Meggitt SJ. Raised limb bands developing in infancy. Br J Dermatol 2006; 154: 791–792.

171. Patterson JW, Straka BF, Wick MR. Linear syringocystadenoma papilliferum of the thigh. J Am Acad Dermatol 2001; 45: 139–141.

24

Disorders of the Subcutaneous Tissue

Bernard A. Cohen

The subcutaneous fat cushions the overlying skin, insulates and provides energy storage, and protects underlying soft tissue and bony structures. Although not fully functional at birth, a well-developed fatty layer is present in the neonate, even when premature.[1] Disorders of the fat can interfere with normal function and may have systemic implications.

The nomenclature and classification of subcutaneous fat disorders of the newborn are inconsistent and confusing. However, a number of entities have been recognized because of their distinctive clinical patterns, histopathology, biochemical markers, inheritance, and course. The clinician must distinguish disorders that are innocent and self-limiting from those that are associated with significant morbidity or underlying systemic disease.

SUBCUTANEOUS FAT NECROSIS OF THE NEWBORN

Subcutaneous fat necrosis of the newborn (SCFN) is an uncommon disorder that occurs primarily in full-term and postmature infants during the first few weeks of life. Although lesions can develop in infants with a normal delivery and neonatal course, SCFN has been associated with perinatal complications, including asphyxia, hypothermia, seizures, pre-eclampsia, meconium aspiration, and intrapartum medication.[2,3] Extensive subcutaneous fat necrosis has also been reported following induced hypothermia used in cardiac surgery.[4]

Although the first reports of SCFN appeared during the early 19th century, many investigators continued to use the terms scleroderma or scleredema to describe SCFN, as well as a number of diverse disorders of the subcutaneous tissue associated with the development of distinct nodules or widespread induration. Over a century later, the term subcutaneous fat necrosis was first applied to this clinically benign condition with histologic characteristics of fat necrosis.[3]

Cutaneous Findings

Affected infants typically present with one or several indurated, variably circumscribed, violaceous or red plaques or subcutaneous nodules from 1 to several centimeters in diameter on the buttocks, thighs, trunk, face, and/or arms (Figs 24-1 and 24-2). In some cases the nodules may be subtle, not associated with overlying color change, and only appreciated by careful palpation of the underlying fat. Rarely, large plaques may cover extensive areas of the trunk or extremities. However, lesions are usually freely movable over subjacent muscles and fascia. Although SCFN may be tender, affected infants are afebrile and usually asymptomatic.

Most SCFN regresses spontaneously without scarring over several weeks to months. Rarely nodules persist for over 6 months.[5] Occasionally fluctuance and abscess-like changes occur, resulting in spontaneous drainage and scar formation. Variable amounts of calcification develop, which can be appreciated radiographically.[6]

Etiology/Pathogenesis

Some investigators have proposed that SCFN results from hypoxic injury to fat caused by local trauma, particularly in the child with perinatal complications.[7,8] This is supported by the observation that fat necrosis occurs commonly over bony prominences. Others have suggested that the susceptibility to SCFN results from an increased proportion of the saturated fats palmitic and stearic acid, relative to the monounsaturated fat oleic acid in neonatal subcutaneous tissue.[5,7,9] Saturated fatty acids have a higher melting point than unsaturated fats, which may predispose newborn fat to crystallization at higher ambient temperatures than fat in older children and adults. Consequently, even in the setting of mild hypothermia, crystallization of fat may occur, with subsequent fat necrosis. Finally, an underlying defect in neonatal fat composition or metabolism, possibly related to immaturity, in the setting of perinatal stress may lead to fat necrosis.

Diagnosis

When subcutaneous nodules develop in an otherwise healthy newborn, the diagnosis of SCFN can be confirmed by the characteristic histopathologic findings of patchy areas of necrosis and crystallization of fat. The involved fat lobules contain pathognomonic needle-shaped clefts surrounded by a mixed inflammatory infiltrate composed of lymphocytes, histiocytes, fibroblasts, and foreign body giant cells.[3]

Although laboratory tests are usually normal, hypercalcemia is occasionally noted from 1 to 4 months after the appearance of skin lesions.[5,7-9] Rarely hypercalcemia is severe, and has been implicated in the deaths of three infants. Nephrocalcinosis, vomiting, failure to thrive, poor weight gain, irritability, and seizures can complicate hypercalcemia. Although the exact cause of hypercalcemia is unknown, several explanations, including elevated parathyroid hormone levels,

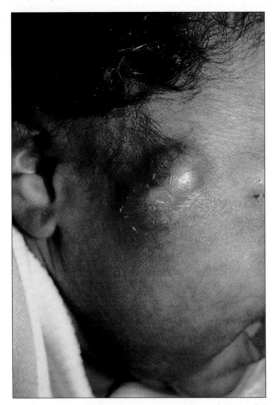

FIG. 24-1 Fat necrosis of the temple secondary to forceps injury.

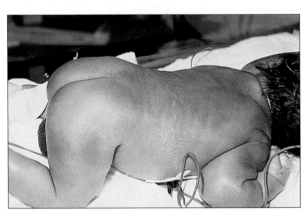

FIG. 24-2 Extensive fat necrosis involving the back, upper arm, and thigh. This infant also had transient thrombocytopenia.

prostaglandin E_2 release, calcium release from necrotic fat, and elevated levels of vitamin D, have been proposed. Calcitriol produced by macrophages in the inflammatory infiltrate of SCFN with increased calcium absorption in the gastrointestinal tract is the favored explanation.[2,3,7–9]

Soft tissue calcification may occur in the absence of hypercalcemia and can be detected radiographically. Tests of parathyroid function, vitamin D metabolites, and urinary prostaglandins may be useful in the evaluation of infants with hypercalcemia. Hypocalcemia with pseudohypoparathyroidism requiring therapy,[10] as well as hypertriglyceridemia and thrombocytopenia,[11] have also been reported in several children.

Differential Diagnosis

The subcutaneous nodules that follow the abrupt withdrawal of systemic steroids can be difficult to distinguish from those of SCFN. However, they usually occur on the cheeks, arms, and trunk 1–2 weeks after discontinuation of steroids. SCFN can be distinguished from sclerema neonatorum, lipograulomatosis, infectious panniculitis, and nodular panniculitis by the general wellbeing of the infant with SCFN and characteristic clinical and histopathologic features. Infants with sclerema neonatorum present with diffuse skin stiffness and severe multisystem disease. Deep soft tissue infections in neonates are usually associated with fever and other signs of sepsis. When hypercalcemia and/or soft tissue calcification is present, primary hyperparathyroidism, osteoma cutis, and calcification associated with Albright osteodystrophy should be excluded.

Management

In most infants with SCFN treatment is limited to parental reassurance and supportive measures.[2,7–9] Hypercalcemia, if present, may have clinical signs such as poor growth or irritability, or may be entirely asymptomatic. Monitoring of serum calcium levels for several months should be considered, especially with large areas of cutaneous involvement, or if symptoms are present. Treatment of hypercalcemia may require intravenous saline, calcium-wasting diuretics, and rarely intravenous corticosteroids. Etidronate therapy has also been reported to be successful in controlling severe hypercalcemia in SCFN.[9] Ulcerated lesions, which rarely occur in otherwise healthy infants, usually respond to topical antibiotics and bio-occlusive dressings.

SCLEREMA NEONATORUM

Sclerema neonatorum is a rare clinical finding rather than a distinct disorder that affects debilitated term and premature infants during the first 1–2 weeks of life.[3] It occasionally occurs in older infants up to 4 months of age with severe underlying disease.

Cutaneous Findings

Diffuse hardening of the skin usually appears suddenly on the third or fourth day of life, starting over the lower extremities, especially the calves, spreading to the thighs, buttocks, and cheeks, and eventually the trunk.[3,12–14] Sclerema eventually involves most of the skin, particularly in premature infants, with the exception of the palms, soles, and genitals. The skin feels cold, smooth, hard, and bound down. The joints are immobile, and the face appears mask-like.

Extracutaneous Findings

Affected infants are usually poorly nourished, dehydrated, hypotensive, hypothermic, and septic. Necrotizing enterocolitis, pneumonia, intracranial hemorrhage, hypoglycemia, and electrolyte disturbances are also often associated with sclerema.[3,12–16]

In most cases, sclerema is limited to the subcutaneous fat. However, in two infants autopsy revealed identical changes in the visceral fat.[17]

Etiology/Pathogenesis

The development of sclerema is probably a result of dysfunction of the neonatal enzymatic system involved in the conversion of saturated palmitic and stearic acids to unsaturated oleic acid. Immaturity of the neonatal lipoenzymes is further compromised by hypothermia, infection, shock, dehydration, and surgical and environmental stresses. The relative abundance of saturated fatty acids and depletion of unsaturated fatty acid allows for fat solidification to occur more readily, with the subsequent development of sclerema.[3]

Diagnosis

On gross pathologic examination, the subcutaneous tissue of affected infants is markedly thickened, firm, and lard-like, with fibrous bands seen to extend from the fat into the lower dermis. Microscopically, early lesions demonstrate distinctive lipid crystals within fat cells, forming rosettes of fine, needle-like clefts.[3] Although there is usually no inflammatory reaction to fat necrosis, occasionally some giant cells are present. Older lesions often show thickened septa, and rarely calcification.

Other laboratory findings in neonates with sclerema are nonspecific and usually reflect the underlying systemic medical problems. Thrombocytopenia, neutropenia, active bleeding, and worsening acidosis carry a poor prognosis.[3,15,16]

Differential Diagnosis

In healthy infants who develop widespread slowly progressive scleroderma-like plaques on the trunk and proximal extremities, the diagnosis of stiff skin syndrome should be considered (see next section). However, this is a primary disorder of fascia and, unlike sclerema, is not associated with systemic symptoms. The lack of inflammation and extensive involvement of the subcutis help to distinguish sclerema from SCFN and cold panniculitis, in which the lesions are localized and associated with exuberant granulomatous inflammation. Diffuse edema resulting from hemolytic anemia, renal, and/or cardiac dysfunction manifests as pitting edema, unlike sclerema. Congenital lymphedema or Milroy's disease is non-pitting and often widespread. However, in lymphedema the infant is otherwise healthy, and a skin biopsy reveals normal fat and dilated lymphatics. Erysipelas or lymphangitis is red, tender, and more localized than sclerema. Diffuse sclerodermatous changes associated with systemic sclerosis, which is extremely rare in the newborn, can also mimic sclerema. However, histology demonstrates characteristic hypertrophy and sclerosis of collagen, which eventually replaces the fat in scleroderma.

Treatment

Attention to the maintenance of a neutral thermal environment, electrolyte and water balance, adequate hydration and ventilation, and aggressive treatment of shock and infection in the modern nursery intensive care unit undoubtedly account for the extremely low incidence of sclerema today. Although most infants with sclerema succumb to sepsis and shock, reversal of the underlying systemic disease can result in recovery.

The role of systemic steroids in the management of infants with sclerema is controversial. Several investigators have reported a favorable outcome when exchange transfusion was combined with conventional therapy.[16]

STIFF SKIN SYNDROME

In 1971 Esterly and McKusick[18] described a disorder in infants and young children characterized by diffuse skin induration and thickening, with limitation of joint mobility, flexion contractures, and hypertrichosis. This condition, which has been called 'congenital fascial dystrophy' or the 'stiff skin syndrome' was further defined by Jablonska[19] as a generalized, noninflammatory disease of fascia without evidence of visceral or muscle involvement, immunologic abnormalities, or vascular hyperreactivity. Although most cases have been sporadic, disease affecting a mother and two siblings[18] and another family with a father, son and family members in four generations, support a hereditary transmission.[20]

Cutaneous Findings

Stiff skin syndrome presents in infancy or early childhood with scleroderma-like plaques initially affecting the trunk and proximal extremities, particularly the buttocks and thighs. Early on the condition may seem subtle and somewhat localized. Progression of the rock-hard indurated bound-down skin over large areas of the body, including the extremities, results in contractures, scoliosis, a narrow thorax, and a characteristic tiptoe gait. A variable increase in hair may be noted over areas of cutaneous involvement.[18–23]

Extracutaneous Findings

Orthopedic abnormalities result from the cutaneous and fascial plaques that produce contractures, especially over large joints. Although restrictive pulmonary changes and growth retardation have occasionally been reported, immunologic, visceral, bony, muscular, and vascular involvement is characteristically absent.[19,21–23]

Etiology/Pathogenesis

Although the cause is unclear, investigators have proposed a primary fibroblastic defect resulting in increased mucopolysaccharide deposition in the dermis, a primary fascial dystrophy resulting from increased collagen, and an inflammatory process.[19,21–23] Some patients with stiff skin syndrome have been noted to have increased myofibroblastic activity in fascia, with overproduction of type VI collagen. Similar findings have been observed in extra-abdominal desmoid tumors, juvenile hyaline fibromatosis, scleroderma, and the tight skin mouse model which is transmitted in an autosomal dominant pattern and is located on chromosome 2.[24] Further characterization of the TSK gene defect will hopefully lead to a better understanding of stiff skin syndrome, which also demonstrates an autosomal dominant inheritance pattern.

Diagnosis

In infants and young children with progressive bound-down plaques beginning on the trunk, limited joint mobility, and no evidence of systemic disease, stiff skin syndrome should be considered. Varying histologic changes from patient to patient and in the same patient over time may reflect different triggers which result in similar clinical findings.[21–24] In some cases thickening of the collagen in the fascia was noted, whereas in others the fascia was normal and increased mucopolysaccharide deposition was found in the dermis. Noninflammatory sclerosis in the deep reticular dermis extending into the subcutaneous fat has also been noted.

Differential Diagnosis

Firm woody induration of the skin with joint contractures may occur in geleophysic dysplasia, progeria, neonatal mucolipidosis II, and Farber's lipomatosis. These disorders can be distinguished from stiff skin syndrome by their characteristic clinical, histologic, biochemical, and genetic findings. The clinical features of scleroderma overlap with some cases of stiff skin syndrome, but thickening of the fascia does not occur in scleroderma. Eosinophilic fasciitis, which presents with acral scleroderma-like changes, can also be distinguished by characteristic clinical features, course, and histology. Sclerema neonatorum and subcutaneous fat necrosis of the newborn demonstrate a distinctive panniculitis and clinical course, and infantile systemic hyalinosis can be distinguished by the presence of hyaline deposits in the skin, multiorgan failure, and death in early childhood. In milder cases, the condition may mimic a connective tissue nevus, smooth muscle hamartoma, or myofibroma.

Treatment

Although the disorder is usually slowly progressive, in some patients lesions have been noted to stabilize or improve. Treatment is generally limited to supportive and rehabilitative care.

PANNICULITIS CAUSED BY PHYSICAL AGENTS

Although physical agents may contribute to the development of SCFN and sclerema neonatorum, a number of environmental factors can cause direct injury to the fat. Cold, heat, mechanical trauma, and chemical injury can lead to the formation of nodules in the fat. The overlying epidermis is usually unaffected in cold and mechanical trauma, whereas bullae, erosions, and ulcerations from epidermal and dermal necrosis characterize heat and chemical insults.

Cold Panniculitis

The development of panniculitis following exposure to subfreezing temperatures was first noted over 50 years ago by Haxthausen, who described four young children and an adolescent with facial plaques.[25,26] In his paper he referred to several earlier reports of hardening of the fat associated with cold exposure and the application of ice directly to the skin.[27,28] Similar cases have been reported following the use of ice to induce hypothermia before cardiac surgery,[27] and the application of ice bags to the face for management of supraventricular tachycardia.[28,29] Popsicle panniculitis is a term coined by Epstein in 1970[30] to refer to a specific subset of cold panniculitis triggered by infants sucking on flavored ice. Although lesions may develop in older children and adults, most cases occur in infants under 1 year.

Cutaneous Findings

Symmetric, tender, indurated nodules and plaques 1–3 cm in diameter typically appear on the cheeks of infants 1–2 days after cold exposure.[25,26,29–31] The overlying skin appears red to violaceous (Fig. 24-3), and the infant is otherwise well. In a study by Rotman[26] the application of an ice cube to the volar aspect of the forearm of an 8-month-old girl resulted in mild transient erythema for 15 minutes. A red plaque developed 12–18 hours later and resolved after 13 days. Lesions usually soften, flatten, and heal over 2–3 weeks, leaving postinflammatory pigmentary changes, particularly in darkly pigmented individuals.

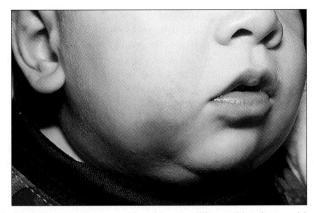

FIG. 24-3 Erythematous nodule of panniculitis resulting from cold exposure (popsicle).

Etiology/Pathogenesis

As in subcutaneous fat necrosis of the newborn and sclerema neonatorum, exposure to low ambient temperatures is thought to result in crystallization of the subcutaneous tissue in infants, which is relatively high in saturated fats compared to that of older children and adults. Applying ice to the skin for 50 seconds results in nodules in all newborns, but only in 40% of 6-month-olds, and only occasionally in 9-month-olds.[30] In 1966 Duncan[32] described a child in whom nodules followed the application of ice for several minutes at 6 months of age, and 8 minutes at 18 months of age. When the child was 22 months old, ice applied for 15 minutes did not trigger panniculitis. The resistance to cold injury correlates with the relative increase in unsaturated fats in the subcutaneous tissue of older infants and children.

Diagnosis

The development of subcutaneous nodules in any neonate or young infant exposed to ice or subfreezing temperatures in the preceding 1–3 days should suggest the diagnosis of cold panniculitis. Histologic changes evolve over several days.[32] The earliest changes 24 hours after cold injury include an infiltrate of macrophages and lymphocytes at the dermoepidermal junction extending into the dermis and fat. At 48 hours the inflammation is more intense and fat necrosis is present. Lipid from ruptured fat cells forms large cystic structures surrounded by histiocytes, neutrophils, and lymphocytes. These changes become more pronounced over the next few days, and subside completely in 2 weeks.

Other laboratory studies, including blood counts, cold agglutinins, cryoglobulins, and general chemistry studies, are usually normal.

Differential Diagnosis

The history of cold exposure in an otherwise healthy infant will help to distinguish cold panniculitis from other causes of subcutaneous nodules. Clinical lesions of SCFN can overlap with those of cold panniculitis. Although a skin biopsy is not usually necessary to distinguish these two disorders, the distribution of nodules and histological changes is usually distinctive. Cellulitis should also be considered in any child with tender red facial nodules. However, the lack of progression of lesions or fever in a healthy-appearing infant is against the diagnosis of infection.

Post-steroid panniculitis can be clinically indistinguishable from cold panniculitis.[33] Subcutaneous nodules or plaques appear on the cheeks of infants within 2 weeks of rapidly discontinuing high-dose systemic steroids after a prolonged course. A biopsy reveals granulomatous inflammation in the fat lobules and needle-shaped clefts within histiocytes identical to those of SCFN. However, in a child with the typical history a biopsy is unnecessary, and nodules resolve over a period of months without treatment.

Treatment and Course
Although skin lesions are self-limiting and no treatment is recommended, early recognition of cold panniculitis is important to prevent unnecessary parental anxiety or laboratory studies. Nodules heal in 1–3 weeks without scarring.

MECHANICAL TRAUMA

Cutaneous Findings
Firm, subcutaneous nodules may follow blunt trauma to the skin, especially in areas prone to trauma where the fat is in close proximity to the underlying bone.[34] This occurs most commonly on the cheeks in children between 6 and 12 years old. However, nodules can also develop in infants and over other bony prominences after accidental or deliberate injury.

Diganosis
Traumatic fat injury should be considered in any child with subcutaneous nodules over injury-prone areas. Skin biopsies will demonstrate fat necrosis with granulomatous inflammation. However, a biopsy is usually not necessary.

Treatment and Course
Nodules slowly resolve over 6–12 months without treatment. In some patients localized lipoatrophy can lead to a depression with normal overlying epidermis and dermis.

INJECTION-SITE GRANULOMA

Cutaneous Findings
Firm, tender, subcutaneous nodules commonly appear 1–2 days after vaccinations in the buttocks or thighs in infants, and in the deltoid area in older children and adults.[35] Although lesions occasionally result from direct trauma to the subcutaneous tissue when the needle is accidentally placed in the fat, some patients develop aluminum granulomas when an aluminum-adsorbed vaccine is used.

Diagnosis
The diagnosis is apparent when one or several nodules develop in a vaccination injection site. Skin biopsies demonstrate characteristic findings, including lymphoid follicles with germinal centers and a dense surrounding infiltrate of lymphocytes, histiocytes, plasma cells, and eosinophils. Staining for aluminum is also positive, confirming the diagnosis.[35]

Differential Diagnosis
Other foreign material injected into the skin can produce panniculitis, with nodule formation and fat necrosis. This can occur with certain medications and intravenous fluid extravasation.[36] Munchausen syndrome by proxy should be considered when recurrent panniculitis with associated cellulitis and/or ulceration occurs in an otherwise healthy infant without a clear diagnosis.

Treatment and Course
Injection-site granulomas usually resolve without scarring within 2 weeks. Occasionally liponecrosis leads to ulceration and/or lipoatrophy, with persistent dimpling of the skin.

INFECTIOUS PANNICULITIS

Although this entity usually occurs in immunocompromised adults, there are rare reports of affected children in the pediatric and infectious disease literature.[37,38] In infants, infectious panniculitis can occur as an extension of primary cutaneous infection or direct hematogenous dissemination to fat.

Cutaneous Findings
Septic emboli produce tender, red, subcutaneous nodules that are usually confined to one area, such as a portion of an extremity, but widespread dissemination can occur (Fig. 24-4).

In primary cutaneous infection, superficial tissue destruction by the invading organism and ischemia from invasion of local blood vessels and lymphatics leads to necrosis and ulceration of the skin and deeper soft tissue structures.

Extracutaneous Findings
Infected children are febrile, irritable, and appear ill. There may be other signs of systemic infection or sepsis. Although infectious panniculitis is more common in immunocompromised individuals,[39] it has rarely been reported in immunocompetent children.[37]

Etiology/Pathogenesis
Infectious panniculitis has been associated with Gram-positive (*Staphylococcus aureus*, *S. epidermidis*, *Streptococcus* sp.) and Gram-negative (*Pseudomonas* sp., *Klebsiella* sp., *Fusobacterium*, *Fusarium*) bacteria, fungi (*Candida* sp., *Nocardia* sp.), and atypical mycobacteria.

Diagnosis
Skin biopsies from subcutaneous nodules reveal a mixed septal–lobular panniculitis with infiltration by neutrophils.[37–39]

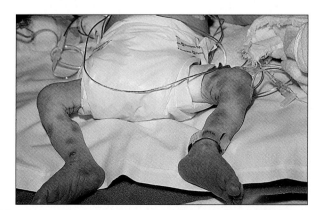

FIG. 24-4 Multiple nodules of panniculitis in an infant with *Escherichia coli* sepsis.

Special stains demonstrate organisms scattered throughout fat lobules. Blood cultures and cultures of other body fluids may also be positive.

Differential Diagnosis

Other conditions to be considered in the setting of possible panniculitis associated with fever include erythema nodosum, Henoch–Schönlein purpura (HSP), and cellulitis. The most difficult of these to exclude is erythema nodosum, an immunologically mediated phenomenon commonly associated with streptococcal and other infections. In erythema nodosum, the panniculitis occurs primarily in the fat septa, and the infecting organisms are not found in the skin nodules. HSP is not usually associated with fever, and skin biopsy shows leukocytoclastic vasculitis.

Treatment and Course

Treatment should be directed against the specific organism. Skin biopsy for pathology and cultures, blood cultures, and other appropriate cultures will hopefully identify a specific organism and direct antibiotic and/or antifungal therapy.

TUMORS OF FAT

Tumors of fat include a number of neoplasms and hamartomatous malformations. A specific diagnosis is important to distinguish between those disorders with isolated cutaneous findings and those with systemic implications.

Lipoma

Cutaneous Findings

Although lipomas represent the most common tumor of the mesenchyme in adults, they are rare in infants. Lipomas are soft, rounded or lobulated, mobile, slightly compressible, subcutaneous tumors with smooth margins (Fig. 24-5). Lumbo-sacral lipomas are usually congenital and occur in conjunction with intraspinal lipomas and anomalies of the spine (Fig. 24-6).[40-43] They are often softer and less discrete than lipomas found in other sites.

Extracutaneous Findings

In 1967 Lassman and James[40] described 26 cases of lumbosacral lipomas associated with laminar defects on X-ray and spinal anomalies at surgery. The recognition of lipomas as markers of underlying spinal dysraphism has been re-emphasized by a number of investigators.[40-43] Conversely, most cases of intraspinal lipoma are associated with congenital lumbosacral cutaneous markers, including lipoma, myelocele closure scar, hairy patch, vascular lesions, and dimpling[42] (see also Chapter 9).

Diagnosis

The presence of a soft, spongy congenital mass in the lumbosacral area is characteristic, and requires a radioimaging evaluation to exclude anomalies of the underlying cord and bony spine. Ultrasound is a reliable noninvasive screening tool for infants during the first 6 months of life. In older children, or when the findings are equivocal on ultrasound, MRI may be required.[44,45] Histologic findings are typical of lipomas in other sites and show mature adipocytes within a thin connective tissue capsule.

Treatment, Course, and Management

Although the need for surgical management of intraspinal lipomas associated with lumbosacral lipomas is controversial, it should be recognized that the development of neurologic impairment can be delayed for years.[40-43] Unfortunately, many patients present in later childhood and adolescence with neurologic defects in the lower extremities, including weakness and foot deformities. Consequently, immediate neurosurgical evaluation and long-term neurologic follow-up are required.

Nevus Lipomatosus Cutaneous Superficialis

Nevus lipomatosus cutaneous superficialis (NLCS) is a malformation of the subcutaneous tissue consisting of multiple or solitary papules, usually occurring on the lower trunk, buttocks, or upper thighs.[46-49] Based on the paucity of reports, NLCS is either rare or underdiagnosed. In 1921 Hoffmann and Zurhelle[49] described the original case of a 25-year-old man

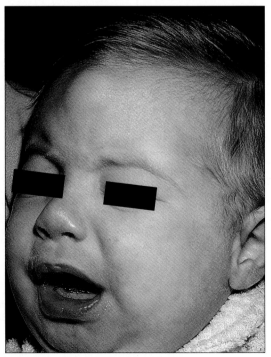

FIG. 24-5 Lipoma of the forehead in a young infant.

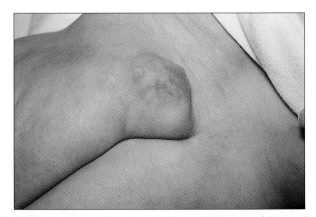

FIG. 24-6 Lumbosacral lipoma associated with lipoma of the cord. Note the deviation of the gluteal cleft.

with multiple papules on the left buttock. In 1975 Jones and Marks[49a] summarized the findings of an additional 40 cases subsequently reported in the literature, and 20 of their own patients. A number of other reports have expanded our understanding of the clinical expression and pathogenesis of NLCS.

Cutaneous Findings

Most patients report that lesions were present at birth or appeared in the first two decades of life.[46–49] NLCS typically presents as multiple, soft, skin-colored to yellowish lobules that may coalesce into plaques with a cerebriform surface. Unilateral involvement of the buttock is most common, but plaques may extend to the adjacent skin of the upper thigh or lower back. Lesions may be confined to the upper thigh, lower back, hip, or abdomen. Usually lesions do not cross the midline, but bilateral involvement of opposing surfaces of the buttocks has been reported. Once formed, papules usually remain stable. However, new lobules may develop slowly for decades.

Solitary nevi have been described at various sites, including the scalp, ear, and neck, but these lesions probably represent fibromas or polypoid fibrolipomas rather than true NLCS.

Extracutaneous Findings

NLCS is not usually associated with extracutaneous findings.[46–49] Cases reported with bony, dental, and other anomalies probably represent focal dermal hypoplasia (Goltz syndrome), which can be confused clinically and histologically with NLCS. However, there are several reports of NLCS associated with pigment anomalies, including café au lait spots and hypopigmented macules.

Etiology/Pathogenesis

Although the origin of NLCS is unclear, electron microscopic studies support the hypothesis of several investigators that the hamartomatous lesion arises from pluripotential vascular elements in the dermis.[47] The presence of varying amounts of other connective tissue components also suggests a relationship with connective tissue nevi.

Diagnosis

Although the clinical appearance of NLCS varies, the presence of typical nodules and plaques in the pelvic girdle region should suggest the diagnosis. Histopathology shows some hyperkeratosis and acanthosis of the epidermis and a marked increase in mature fat cells throughout the dermis.[47,49] Adipocytes are most prominent in the reticular dermis, where they are arranged in clusters and interspersed by broad, interwoven, collagen bundles. However, they may extend into the papillary dermis, and the distinction between the dermis and subcutaneous fat may be poorly defined. Although the remainder of the dermis often appears normal, other connective tissue anomalies, including thickening of collagen and elastic fibers, and increased numbers of fibroblasts and blood vessels with a perivascular mononuclear infiltrate, may also develop.

Differential Diagnosis

The varying clinical findings explain the wide range of clinical diagnoses suspected before skin biopsy. These include pigmented nevi, supernumerary nipples, lipomas, neurofibromas, connective tissue nevi, sebaceous nevi, epidermal nevi, and warts.

Encephalocraniocutaneous lipomatosis and congenital diffuse lipomatosis ('Michelin tire baby') may represent distinctive variants of NLCS (see the following discussion).

Treatment, Course, and Management

Although new lobules may develop in adolescence and adult life, NLCS is usually static and not associated with pain, pruritus, or other symptoms. Consequently, treatment is not necessary, but surgical excision, particularly for small lesions, gives a good cosmetic result. Moreover, excision should be considered in lesions that demonstrate progressive growth.[50]

Encephalocraniocutaneous Lipomatosis

In encephalocraniocutaneous lipomatosis (ECL), unilateral cerebral malformations are associated with ipsilateral scalp, face, and eye lesions.[51] Since the first description of this congenital neurocutaneous disorder in 1970 by Haberland and Perou,[52] 12 cases with similar clinical and histologic findings have been reported.[53–55]

Cutaneous Findings

Soft, spongy, hairless, pink to yellowish tumors characteristically involve the scalp, often in a linear configuration, but may extend to the legs and paravertebral area.[51–55] Although lesions are usually unilateral, bilateral involvement has been reported. Papular and polypoid nodules, often contiguous to the scalp lesions, are constant features on the face of affected infants. Atrophic hairless patches may also be present on the scalp and face.[51]

Extracutaneous Findings

Characteristic papules and nodules on the bulbar conjunctivae show histologic features of desmoid tumors.[51] Anomalies of the hyaloid vessel system, lens, and cornea are also common.[56]

Cerebral defects are usually ipsilateral to the main cutaneous scalp lesions and include ventricular dilatation and cerebral atrophy.[51,57] Other anomalies, including arachnoidal cyst, pontocerebellar lipoma, porencephaly, agenesis of the corpus callosum, and paramedullary lipomas, have also been described.

Etiology/Pathogenesis

There is no evidence of genetic transmission or chromosomal aberration, and all cases have been sporadic. Happle[58] proposed that ECL might be caused by a lethal autosomal mutation that survives in the mosaic state.

Diagnosis

Biopsies of the cutaneous nodules show normal epidermis overlying a dermis with irregularly shaped collagen fibers that extend into the subcutis and form large fibrous septa associated with increased amounts of fat.[51–55] These histologic features typical of fibrolipoma seen in children with characteristic cutaneous, ocular, and cerebral features should suggest the diagnosis of ECL.

Differential Diagnosis

The clinical features of ECL may overlap with those of focal dermal hypoplasia (Goltz syndrome), oculoauricular vertebral dysplasia (Goldenhar syndrome), Schimmelpenning syndrome, oculocerebrocutaneous (Dellman) syndrome, Proteus syndrome, and the epidermal nevus syndrome. However, careful analysis of clinical and histologic features will help to distinguish these neurocutaneous genodermatoses.

Treatment and Course

The care of affected children is determined by neurologic symptoms, which range from normal to global neurodevelopmental retardation, unilateral spasticity, and mental retardation.[51] Seizures are variable and may develop later in childhood. Moreover, the severity of neurologic symptoms does not seem to correlate with the extent of cutaneous involvement. Ocular and cutaneous lesions appear to be static and amenable to surgical repair. Children without clinical evidence of neurologic involvement should be screened for occult spinal anomalies.[57]

Congenital Diffuse Lipomatosis

Congenital diffuse lipomatosis (Michelin tire baby) was initially referred to by Ross in 1969, who described a child with ringed creases of the skin reminiscent of the mascot of the French tire manufacturer Michelin.[59] Since then a number of cases of this rare hamartomatous disorder have been reported, demonstrating the variability of clinical and histologic findings.[59–64]

Cutaneous Findings

Symmetric ringed creases of the extremities may be associated with hirsutism of the arms, legs, shoulders, and buttocks (Fig. 24-7).[59–63] The palmar and plantar skin may also demonstrate excessive folding. Although scalp hair is usually normal, long curled eyelashes and thick eyebrows are typical.

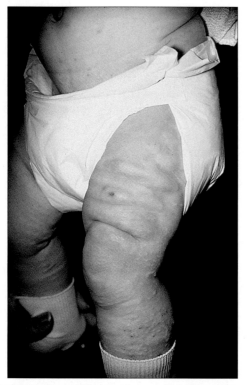

FIG. 24-7 Multiple ringed creases of congenital diffuse lipomatosis. (From Novice FM, Collison DW, Burgdorf WHC, Esterly NB. Handbook of genetic skin disorders. Philadelphia: WB Saunders, 1994.)

Extracutaneous Findings

Although affected children may be otherwise normal, a number of anomalies have been reported.[59–63] Facial dysmorphisms have included epicanthal folds, hypertelorism, an antimongoloid slant to the eyes, a flat nasal bridge, and low-set ears. Variable oral anomalies, including cleft lip and palate, a high-arched palate, dental hypoplasia, and micrognathia, are common. Orthopedic defects such as rocker-bottom feet, metatarsus abductus, coxa valga, genu valgus, overlapping of toes, and pectus excavatum may require surgical intervention. Psychomotor delay and the development of seizures are also variable.

Etiology/Pathogenesis

Although no specific chromosomal abnormality has been identified in congenital diffuse lipomatosis, autosomal dominant inheritance has been noted in two families in which the cutaneous findings occurred as isolated defects.[62] In two other patients with multiple associated anomalies, unrelated cytogenetic defects were found.[60] Further studies may help to detect a Michelin tire baby gene, although this syndrome may represent disparate disorders with similar phenotypic expression.

Diagnosis

Skin biopsies from the extremities of affected children have shown changes in the dermis consistent with nevus lipomatosus cutaneous superficialis or smooth muscle hamartoma.[60,61] A recent report in which histopathology showed fragmented elastic fibers and decreased deposition of elastin on electron microscopy suggests that some cases may result from a primary defect in elastic fibers.[61]

Differential Diagnosis

Although congenital diffuse lipomatosis may be confused histologically with localized smooth muscle hamartoma, Becker nevus, and nevus lipomatosis cutaneous superficialis, the diffuse, symmetric, and dramatic cutaneous findings are distinctive.

Treatment, Course, and Management

Management of affected individuals depends on the presence of associated anomalies. Clinicians should look carefully for oral and orthopedic anomalies, which may require early surgical intervention. Neurodevelopmental parameters will also require long-term follow-up.

Congenital Pedal Papules

Congenital papules or nodules of the plantar surface of the feet have been described under a variety of names, including congenital pedal papules, congenital piezogenic-like papules, plantar fibromatosis of the heel, 'podalic papules of the newborn,' and precalcaneal fibrolipomatous hamartoma.[65–67]

Cutaneous Findings

Pedal nodules are asymptomatic, symmetric, flesh-colored nodules of the medial plantar surface of the feet, generally 0.5–1.5 cm in size (Fig. 24-8). They are ill defined and may go unnoticed by parents. Lesions undergo minimal change over time, though proportionate growth may be seen.

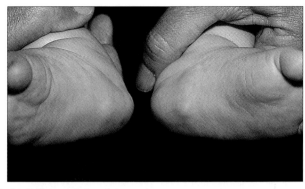

FIG. 24-8 Congenital pedal papules.

Etiology/Pathogenesis

The pathogenesis is uncertain. Possible etiologies include a hamartomatous condition or a developmental defect in the plantar aponeurosis. The nodules may occur in a familial pattern.[68] Histopathology displays increased mature adipocytes in the mid and deep dermis within fibrous sheaths.

Diagnosis and Differential Diagnosis

The diagnosis is a clinical one. Differential diagnosis includes piezogenic papules seen on the lateral surface of the feet in older children, fibrous hamartoma of infancy, and aponeurotic fibroma.

Treatment and Course

Although the natural history is not fully known, lesions seem to persist over time. Treatment is unnecessary.

Lipoblastoma and Lipoblastomatosis

Lipoblastoma is a term first used by Jaffe[69] in 1926 to describe recurrent fatty tumors of the groin in infants and young children. Van Meurs[70] subsequently wrote of his experience with an infant with a lipomatous tumor in the right axilla that required four surgeries over a 2-year period before she was free of recurrence. Histologic changes from biopsies over the 2-year period in Van Meurs case demonstrated maturation from a tumor comprised primarily of lipoblasts to a mature lipoma. In 1973 Chung and Enzinger[71] reported a large series of lipomatous tumors in infancy and proposed that the term lipoblastoma be used to describe the well-encapsulated variant and that lipoblastomatosis be reserved for unencapsulated infiltrating lesions.

Cutaneous Findings

Clinically, the tumors are soft, subcutaneous or deep, soft tissue masses ranging in size from 1 to 12 cm in diameter.[72–74] Although cases have been diagnosed in children as old as 10 years, most appear before 3 years of age, and congenital tumors are common. The most common location is the extremities (Fig. 24-9), followed by the trunk and face. However, unusual sites, including the parotid gland, mediastinum, and tonsils, have been reported.

Etiology and Pathogenesis

Although the cause of lipoblastoma is unknown, recent reports demonstrate an association with rearrangements of chromo-

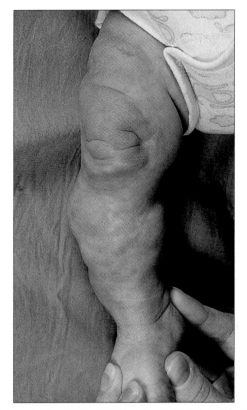

FIG. 24-9 Lipoblastomatosis involving the entire leg and foot, present from birth.

some band 8q 11–13 which targets the gene *PLAG1*.[75] Electron microscopic findings suggest a close resemblance to human fetal adipose tissue.[76] Some investigators propose that lipoblastoma results from the continued proliferation of fetal lipoblasts in the postnatal period. This is supported by observations of histologic maturation of adipose cells in recurrent tumors.

Diagnosis

Histologically lipoblastoma is encapsulated or well circumscribed, whereas in lipoblastomatosis the tumor infiltrates surrounding normal structures.[71–73] The diagnostic feature is the presence of lobules of mature and immature fat cells, primitive mesenchymal cells, and lipoblasts with varying degrees of differentiation. The lobules are separated by fibrous septa containing small blood vessels, hyaline collagen, and fibroblasts. There is no evidence of atypia, and mitotic figures are rare.

Differential Diagnosis

Lipoblastomatosis should be differentiated from liposarcoma, an exceedingly rare tumor in children under 10 years of age.[73] Although histologic distinction is occasionally difficult, the lack of cytologic atypia and mitotic figures and the presence of a uniform growth pattern and extensive lobulation favor lipoblastoma.

Treatment and Course

Encapsulated tumors represent the majority of lesions and generally respond well to simple excision. However, in some series lipoblastomatosis accounts for nearly a third of cases.

Metastases do not occur, but recurrences are common. Although extensive infiltration into local muscle and fascial structures precludes complete excision, in most cases maturation of recurrent tumor results in a favorable outcome.

LIPODYSTROPHIES

The lipodystrophies are a rare group of disorders characterized by complete or partial loss of fat. The congenital variants are inherited in an autosomal recessive pattern and express variable abnormalities in carbohydrate and lipid metabolism and insulin resistance.

Leprechaunism

Donohue and Uchida[77,78] were the first to describe this rare syndrome when they reported their observations on two sisters of consanguineous parents with intrauterine growth retardation, gnome-like facies, and severe endocrine dysfunction evidenced by emaciation, enlargement of the breasts and clitoris, and histologic changes in the ovaries, pancreas, and breasts.[79] Leprechaunism was the term applied to the elfin facial features and poor growth characteristic of this disorder.

The incidence of this autosomal recessive disorder has been estimated at 1 in 4 million live births, and the prevalence of the carrier state as at least 1 in 1000 individuals.[80]

Cutaneous Findings

In a review of 31 patients with leprechaunism reported since the original description by Donohue in 1948, Elsas[81] summarized the clinical findings, including severe growth retardation; an elfin face with large, protuberant, low-set ears; depressed nasal bridge with a broad nasal tip and flared nares; thick lips; distended abdomen; relatively large hands, feet, nipples, and genitalia; and abnormal skin with hyperpigmentation, café au lait spots, hypertrichosis, acanthosis nigricans, pachyderma, and decreased subcutaneous fat (Fig. 24-10).[81–83] The virtual absence of fat gives a cachectic appearance, with wrinkled skin hanging loosely over the skeletal frame.

Etiology and Pathogenesis

Initially leprechaunism was identified as a primary endocrinologic disorder because of the associated cystic changes of the gonads and hyperplasia of the islet cells of the pancreas. In the 1970s and 1980s laboratory advances led to the identification of severe insulin resistance resulting from a genetic defect of the insulin receptor system in infants with leprechaunism.[81,82] Using molecular genetic techniques, the first defect in the insulin receptor gene was discovered in a child with leprechaunism in 1988.[84] Subsequently, multiple mutations have been described, indicating that there is great genetic heterogeneity in this disorder. Overactivation of insulin-like growth factor-1 (IGF-1) by high levels of insulin and lack of functional insulin receptors in a number of organ systems lead to growth failure, lipodystrophy, and other cutaneous findings.

Diagnosis

The diagnosis can be made by DNA analysis of fibroblasts grown in culture from skin biopsies from affected infants. Specific mutations in the insulin receptor gene can be identified. Prenatal diagnosis is possible by similar evaluation of chorionic villus biopsy specimens.

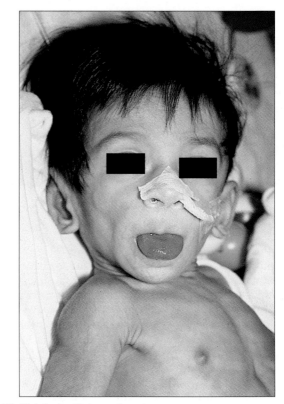

FIG. 24-10 Infant with leprechaunism.

Differential Diagnosis

Leprechaunism shares many features with congenital total lipoatrophy, including insulin resistance, absence of subcutaneous fat, acanthosis nigricans, and hyperpigmentation. However, the elfin facies, wrinkled skin, and other cutaneous markers are distinctive.

Treatment and Course

Postnatal growth is invariably poor, and affected children are severely motor and mentally retarded. Infants rarely survive beyond the first few months of life unless they have some residual insulin receptor function.

Congenital Generalized Lipodystrophy (Seip–Berardinelli Syndrome)

Congenital generalized lipodystrophy (CGL) was first described by Berardinelli in 1954, and in greater detail by Seip in 1959.[85,86] In 1996 Seip published a follow-up study of the original patients and summarized the findings from over 90 cases reported in the literature.[87]

Cutaneous Findings

A complete absence of subcutaneous fat and marked muscular hypertrophy are evident at birth and persist through adolescence. The skin tends to become coarse, particularly in boys, and patients often develop warty fibromas on the upper half of the body.[79,85,87] Acanthosis nigricans develops to a variable degree in early childhood but disappears in adolescence. Excessive, curly scalp hair and hypertrichosis are also common.

Extracutaneous Features

An anabolic state develops, with increased height velocity, advanced bone and dental age, muscular hypertrophy, masculine body build, acromegaloid stigmata, organomegaly, and enlarged genitals.[85–87] Growth velocity is already advanced at birth and continues throughout childhood. The absence of facial fat pads and enlarged muscles gives adolescent girls a female 'body-builder' look.

Patients tend to be hypermetabolic with a voracious appetite, increased energy consumption, and associated hyperhidrosis and decreased heat tolerance. Cardiac muscle hypertrophy is also present at birth and may result in progressive hypertrophic cardiomyopathy with decrease in cardiac function. Most patients with CGL demonstrate mild to moderate developmental delay and mental retardation.

Etiology and Pathogenesis

Although the cause is unknown, clinical and biochemical findings point to a mutation in a gene controlling the transport and storage of glucose and fatty acids in subcutaneous tissue.[87] Recent studies suggest that the primary cause may be a defect in the insulin receptor or postreceptor mechanisms.

Diagnosis

This is a well-characterized disorder inherited in an autosomal recessive fashion, with clinical and metabolic features that allow for diagnosis at birth. However, CGD syndrome is genetically heterogeneous, allowing for some variation in phenotypic expression.

Metabolic features include insulin resistance, hyperinsulinemia, hypertriglyceridemia, and nonketotic diabetes. Skin biopsies demonstrate a marked decrease in adipocyte size and number.[87] Unlike the subcutaneous fat, glycogen and triglycerides are abundant in the liver, where variable amounts of connective tissue with liver cirrhosis have been noted. Hypertriglyceridemia varies from patient to patient, but tends to increase at puberty and with increased dietary fat consumption. In childhood, glucose and insulin levels tend to be normal except with large glucose challenges. However, at or shortly after puberty glucose metabolism deteriorates, with the development of clinical diabetes with hyperinsulinemia, elevated serum glucose, and glycosuria.

Differential Diagnosis

CGL can be distinguished from other lipodystrophies by the characteristic clinical and metabolic findings.

Treatment and Course

Treatment is complex and should emphasize dietary measures to control energy consumption, hyperglycemia, and hypertriglyceridemia.[87] Appetite suppressants have been used with some success. Therapy is further complicated by moderate to severe mental retardation in most individuals with CGL. Despite therapy, many patients die in childhood of liver cirrhosis or associated complications and/or cardiomyopathy.

Carbohydrate-Deficient Glycoprotein Syndrome

Although carbohydrate-deficient glycoprotein syndrome (CDGS) represents a heterogeneous group of disorders, all share clinical features that result from a defect in the synthesis of N-linked oligosaccharides.[88–90] This entity was first recognized by Jaeken in 1980,[91] who reported monozygotic twins with psychomotor retardation, increased CSF protein, delayed nerve conduction velocity, thyroxine-binding deficiency, and increased serum arylsulfatase A activity. Carbohydrate analysis of a number of subsequent patients resulted in identification of the common defect in N-linked glycoproteins.

Cutaneous Findings

Dysmorphic features typical of CDGS appear in infancy, including inverted nipples and an abnormal distribution of fat over the suprapubic region and labia majora.[88–90] Peculiar fat pads, which tend to disappear in later childhood, are noted on the superior lateral portion of the buttocks. Lipoatrophy can be marked on the rest of the buttocks, and lipoatrophic streaks often extend down the legs. Variable facial dysmorphisms include a high nasal bridge, prominent jaw, and large pinnae.

Extracutaneous Findings

Neurologic features of CDGS include hypotonia, hyporeflexia, and alternating esotropia.[87] Infants often suck poorly and present with feeding difficulties. Even when nutritional intake is good, lipoatrophy gives many children an emaciated appearance. Although most infants are full term and appropriate weight for gestational age, developmental delay and failure to thrive usually occur by 3 months of age.

Significant coagulopathy may result in stroke-like episodes, and hepatomegaly with hepatic dysfunction is common. Renal cysts, pericardial effusions, pericardial tamponade, and hypertrophic obstructive cardiomyopathy have been reported.

Although the central nervous system involvement tends to be static, musculoskeletal complications, including muscular atrophy, contractures, and spinal deformities, progress in later childhood and adulthood. In girls, defective peptide hormone glycosylation results in hypogonadotrophic hypogonadism with failure to undergo pubertal sexual development. Males are virilized at puberty, but may exhibit decreased testicular volume. Other endocrinologic findings result from hyperglycemia-induced growth hormone release, hyperprolactinemia, and insulin resistance.

Etiology and Pathogenesis

A recessive mode of inheritance is supported by several cases. Recent genetic studies have demonstrated linkage to a locus on chromosome 16 p.[87,92] Although a common clinical phenotype is recognized, at least four different defects in N-linked oligosaccharide synthesis have been identified, and more types are expected to emerge. In subtypes 1 and 2, specific enzymatic deficiencies have been identified.

Diagnosis

Typical clinical features seen in association with the presence of abnormally glycosylated serum proteins, typically transferrin detected by cathodal migration on serum isoelectric focusing, may allow for diagnosis in the neonatal period. Other serum glycoproteins also show abnormal bands on isoelectric focusing.

Prenatal diagnosis of CDGS type 1A by lysosomal enzyme analysis of amniotic fluid and genetic linkage analysis of cultured amniocytes was recently reported.[92]

Differential Diagnosis

Although other lipodystrophies should be considered, the clinical features are usually distinctive. When dysmorphic features are subtle, biochemical studies are required to distinguish CDGS from related disorders.

Treatment and Course

Supportive treatment is necessary to avoid complications from the central nervous system, as well as ophthalmologic and hematologic manifestations of CDGS. Mannose has been used to deal with some of the acute crises of infancy, including intractable seizures, severe coagulopathy, and pericardial effusions, but does not change the dismal prognosis.

Farber Lipogranulomatosis

Farber disease is a rare autosomal recessive disorder of lipid metabolism that usually presents with a fatal course in early infancy.[90,93,94] Although skin, joint, and laryngeal symptoms associated with neurodegeneration are characteristic, some patients may present with later onset of primarily neurologic findings.

Clinical Findings

Tender, red, subcutaneous nodules and swelling appear during the first few weeks of life over joints and areas of trauma, particularly the wrists and ankles. Granulomatous infiltration of the larynx results in a weak, hoarse cry.[93,94] Infants are usually irritable, and psychomotor retardation is severe. Reticuloendothelial involvement may produce generalized lymphadenopathy and marked hepatosplenomegaly.

Etiology and Pathogenesis

In Farber disease, ceramide, a normal intermediate in the metabolism of gangliosides and structurally important sphingolipids and glycolipids, accumulates as a result of a deficiency of lysosomal acid ceramidase.[93] Variable storage of ceramide occurs in visceral organs and brain white matter.

Diagnosis

The biochemical defect can be demonstrated in kidney, liver, cultured fibroblasts, and leukocytes.[93,94] Prenatal diagnosis is also possible by amniocentesis and chorionic villus sampling.

Differential Diagnosis

In the young infant the diagnosis can usually be made clinically when the classic findings are present. However, when various aspects are missing, Farber disease can be confused with juvenile rheumatoid arthritis, multicentric reticulohistiocytosis, and juvenile hyaline fibromatosis.[94] Ceramide levels are normal in all of these conditions.

Treatment and Course

The clinical course is usually characterized by recurrent fever and pulmonary infiltrates, with death occurring by 2 years of age. Rarely patients present with later onset of neurologic disease followed by extraneuronal granulomas in skin and viscera. Some patients with little or no involvement of the central nervous system develop normally and survive longer.

REFERENCES

1. Holbrook KA. Structure and function of the developing human skin. In: Goldsmith LE, ed. Physiology, biochemistry and molecular biology of the skin, 2nd edn. Vol 1. New York: Oxford University Press, 1991; 63.
2. Scales JW, Krowchuk DP, Schwartz RP, et al. An infant with firm fixed plaques. Arch Dermatol 1998; 134: 425–426.
3. Fretzin DF, Arias AM. Sclerema neonatorum and subcutaneous fat necrosis of the newborn. Pediatr Dermatol 1987; 4: 112–122.
4. Rosbotham JL, Johnson A, Haque KN, et al. Painful subcutaneous fat necrosis of the newborn associated with intrapartum use of a calcium channel blocker. Clin Exp Dermatol 1998; 23: 19–21.
5. Silverman AK, Michels EH, Rasmussen JE. Subcutaneous fat necrosis in an infant occurring after hypothermic cardiac surgery. J Am Acad Dermatol 1986; 15: 331–336.
6. Duhn R, Schoen E, Sui M. Subcutaneous fat necrosis with extensive calcification after hypothermia in two newborn infants. Pediatrics 1968; 41: 661–664.
7. Hicks MJ, Levy ML, Alexander J, et al. Subcutaneous fat necrosis of the newborn and hypercalcemia: A case report and review of the literature. Pediatr Dermatol 1993; 10: 271–276.
8. Fernandez-Lopez E, Garcia-Dorado J, de Unamuno P, et al. Subcutaneous fat necrosis of the newborn and idiopathic hypercalcemia. Dermatology 1990; 180: 250–254.
9. Rice AM, Rivkees SA. Etidronate therapy for hypercalcemia in subcutaneous fat necrosis of the newborn. J Pediatr 1999; 134: 349–351.
10. Karochristou K, Siahanidou T, Kakouvon-Tsivitanidou T, et al. Subcutaneous fat necrosis of the newborn associated with hypocalcemia in a neonate. J Perinatol 2006; 26: 64–66.
11. Tran JT, Sheth AP. Complications of subcutaneous fat necrosis of the newborn: a case report and review of the literature. Pediatr Dermatol 2003; 20: 257–261.
12. Kellum RE, Ray TL, Brown GR. Sclerema neonatorum. Arch Dermatol 1968; 97: 372–376.
13. Horsfield MB, Yardley H. Sclerema neonatorum. J Invest Dermatol 1965; 44: 326–332.
14. Warwick WJ, Ruttenberg HD, Quie PG. Sclerema neonatorum, a sign, not a disease. JAMA 1963; 184: 680.
15. Gupta AK, Shashi S Mohon M, et al. Epidemiology of *Pseudomonas aeruginosa* infection in a nursery intensive care unit. J Trop Pediatr 1993; 39: 32–36.
16. Gupta P, Murali MV, Furidi MM, et al. Clinical profile of *Klebsiella* septicemia in neonates. Indian J Pediatr 1993; 60: 568–572.
17. Zeck P, Madden EM. Sclerema neonatorum of both internal and external adipose tissue. Arch Pathol 1946; 41: 166.
18. Esterly NB, McKusick VA. Stiff skin syndrome. Pediatrics 1971; 47: 360–369.
19. Jablonska S, Groniowski J, Krieg T, et al. Congenital fascial dystrophy – a noninflammatory disease of fascia: the stiff skin syndrome. Pediatr Dermatol 1984; 2: 87–97.
20. Singer H, Valle D, Rogers J, Thomas GH. The stiff skin syndrome: new genetic and biochemical investigations. [Abstract] Birth Defects Org Art Ser XIII (3B) 1977: 254–255.
21. Kikuchi I, Inoue S, Hamada K, Ando H. Stiff skin syndrome. Pediatr Dermatol 1985; 3: 48–53.
22. Fidzianska A, Jablonska S. Congenital fascial dystrophy: abnormal composition of the fascia. J Am Acad Dermatol 2000; 43: 797–802.
23. Gilaberte Y, Sainz-de-Santamaria MC, Farcia-Latasa FJ, et al. Stiff skin syndrome: a case report and review of the literature. Dermatology 1995; 190: 148–151.
24. Jablonska S, Schubety J, Kikuchi I. Congenital fascial dystrophy: stiff skin

syndrome – a human counterpart of the tight-skin mouse. J Am Acad Dermatol 1989; 21: 943–950.

25. Haxthausen H. Adiponecrosis e frigore. Br J Dermatol 1941; 53: 83.

26. Rotman H. Cold panniculitis in children. Arch Dermatol 1966; 94: 720–721.

27. Collins HA, Stahlman M, Scott HW Jr. The occurrence of subcutaneous fat necrosis in an infant following induced hypothermia used as an adjuvant in cardiac surgery. Ann Surg 1953; 138: 880–885.

28. Mimouni F, Merlob P, Metzker A, et al. Supraventricular tachycardia: The icebag technique may be harmful in newborn infants. J Pediatr 1983; 103: 337.

29. Ter Poorten JC, Hebert AA, Ilkiw R. Cold panniculitis in a neonate. J Am Acad Dermatol 1995; 33: 383–385.

30. Epstein EH Jr, Oren ME. Popsicle panniculitis. N Engl J Med 1970; 282: 966–967.

31. Lowe IB Jr. Cold panniculitis in children. Am J Dis Child 11968; 115: 709–713.

32. Duncan WC, Freeman RG, Heaton CL. Cold panniculitis. Arch Dermatol 1966; 94: 722–724.

33. Silverman RA, Newman AJ, LeVine MJ, et al. Poststeroid panniculitis: A case report. Pediatr Dermatol 1988; 5: 92–93.

34. Buswell WA. Traumatic fat necrosis of the face in children. Br J Plast Surg 1979; 32: 127–128.

35. Fawcett HA, Smith NP. Injection-site granuloma due to aluminum. Arch Dermatol 1984; 120: 1318–1322.

36. Forstrom L, Winkelmann RK. Factitial panniculitis. Arch Dermatol 1974; 110: 747–750.

37. Pao W, Duncan KO, Bolognia JL, et al. Numerous eruptive lesions of panniculitis associated with group A *Streptococcus* bacteremia in an immunocompetent child. Clin Infect Dis 1998; 27: 430–433.

38. Patterson J, Brown PO, Broecker LR. Infection-induced panniculitis. J Cutan Pathol 1989; 161: 183–193.

39. Patterson JW, Brown PC, Broecker AH. Infection-induced panniculitis. J Cutan Pathol 1989; 16: 183–193.

40. Lassman LP, James CC. Lumbosacral lipomas: critical survey of 26 cases submitted to laminectomy. J Neurol Neurosurg Psychiatry 1967; 30: 174–181.

41. Harrist TJ, Gary DL, Kleinman GM, et al. Unusual sacrococcygeal embryologic malformation with cutaneous manifestation. Arch Dermatol 1982; 118: 643–648.

42. Goldberg NS, Hebert AA, Esterly NB. Sacral lipomas: The need for neurologic and radiologic evaluation. Arch Dermatol 1987; 123: 711–712.

43. Lhowe D, Ehrlich MC, Chapman PH, et al. Congenital intraspinal lipomas: Clinical presentation and response to therapy. J Pediatr Orthop 1987; 7: 531–537.

44. Azzoni R, Gerevini S, Cabitza P. Spinal cord sonography in newborns: anatomy and diseases. J Pediatr Orthop B 2005; 14: 185–188.

45. Hughes JA, DeBruyn R, Patel K, Thompson D. Spinal ultrasound in spinal dysraphism. Clin Radiol 2003; 58: 227–233.

46. Park HJ, Park CJ, Yi TY, et al. Nevus lipomatosus cutaneous superficialis. Int J Dermatol 1997; 36: 435–437.

47. Raymond JL, Stoebner P, Amblard P. Nevus lipomatosus cutaneous superficialis, an electron microscopic study of 4 cases. J Cutan Pathol 1980; 7: 295–301.

48. Orteau CH, Hughes JR. Nevus lipomatosus cutaneous superficialis: Overlap with connective tissue naevi [Letter]. Acta Dermatol Venereol 1996; 76: 243–245.

49. Jones EW, Marks R, Pongsehirun D. Nevus superficialis lipomatosus, a clinicopathological report of 20 cases. Br J Dermatol 1975; 93: 121–133.

49a. Jones EW, Marks R, Pongsehirun D. Naevus superficialis lipomatosus. A clinicopathological report of twenty cases. Br J Dermatol 1975; 93: 121–133.

50. Knuttel R, Silver EA. A cerebriform mass on the right buttock. Dermatol Surg 2003; 29: 780–781.

51. Grimalt R, Ermacora E, Mistura L, et al. Encephalocraniocutaneous lipomatosis: Case report and review of the literature. Pediatr Dermatol 1993; 10: 164–168.

52. Haberland C, Perou M. Encephalocraniocutaneous lipomatosis. A new example of ectodermal dysgenesis. Arch Neurol 1970; 22: 144–155.

53. Fishman MA, Chang CS, Miller JE. Encephalocraniocutaneous lipomatosis. Pediatrics 1978; 61: 580–582.

54. Miyao M, Saito T, Yamamoto Y, Kamoshita S. Encephalocraniocutaneous lipomatosis: A recently described neurocutaneous syndrome. Childs Brain 1984; 11: 280–284.

55. Fishman MA. Encephalocraniocutaneous lipomatosis. J Child Neurol 1987; 2: 186–193.

56. Rubegni P, Risulo M, Sbano P, et al. Encephalocraniocutaneous lipomatosis (Haberland syndrome) with bilateral cutaneous and visual involvement. Clin Exp Dermatol 2003; 28: 387–390.

57. Lasierra R, Valencia I, Carapeto FJ, et al. Encephalocraniocutaneous lipomatosis: neurologic manifestatations. J Child Neurol 2003; 18: 725–729.

58. Happle R. How many epidermal nevus syndromes exist? J Am Acad Dermatol 1991; 25: 550–556.

59. Ross CM. Generalized folded skin with an underlying lipomatous nevus. Arch Dermatol 1969; 100: 320–323.

60. Schnur RE, Herzberg AJ, Spinner N, et al. Variability in the Michelin tire syndrome, a child with multiple anomalies, smooth muscle hamartoma and familial paracentric inversion of chromosome 7q. J Am Acad Dermatol 1993; 28: 364–370.

61. Sato M, Ishikawa O, Miyachi Y, et al. Michelin tyre syndrome: A congenital disorder of elastic fibre formation? Br J Dermatol 1997; 136: 583–586.

62. Kunze J, Riehm H. A new genetic disorder: Autosomal dominant multiple benign ring-shaped skin creases. Eur J Pediatr 1982; 138: 301–313.

63. Gardner EW, Miller HM, Lowney ED. Folded skin associated with underlying nevus lipomatous. Arch Dermatol 1979; 115: 978–979.

64. Kharfi M, Zaraa I, Chaouechi S, et al. Michelin Tire syndrome: a report of 2 siblings. Pediatr Dermatol 2005; 22: 245–249.

65. Eichenfield LF, Cunningham BC, Friedlander SF. Congenital piezogenic-like papules. Ann Dermatol 1998; 125: 182.

66. Larralde De Luna M, Ruiz Leon J, Cabrera HN. [Pedal papules in newborn infants]. [Spanish] Med Cutan Ibero Lat Am 1987; 15: 135–139.

67. Larregue M, Varbres P, Echard P, et al. Precalcaneal congenital fibrolipomatous hamartoma. Vth Int Congress Pediatric Dermatology, September, 1996.

68. Fangman WL, Prose NS. Precalcaneal congenital fibrolipomatosus hamartomas: report of occurrence in half brothers. Pediatr Dermatol 2004; 21: 655–656.

69. Jaffe RH. Recurrent lipomatous tumors of the groin: Liposarcoma and lipoma pseudomyxomatodes. Arch Pathol 1926; 1: 381–387.

70. Van Meurs DP. The transformation of an embryonic lipoma to common lipoma. Br J Surg 1947; 34: 282–284.

71. Chung EF, Enzinger FM. Benign lipoblastomatosis: an analysis of 35 cases. Cancer 1973; 32: 482–492.

72. Mahour GH, Bryan BJ, Isaacs H. Lipoblastoma and lipoblastomatosis – a report of six cases. Surgery 1988; 104: 577–579.

73. Mentzel T, Calonje E, Fletcher CD. Lipoblastoma and lipoblastomatosis: A clinicopathological study of 14 cases. Histopathology 1993; 23: 527–533.

74. Jung SM, Chang DY, Lao CL, et al. Lipoblastoma/lipoblastomatosis: a clinicopathologic study of 16 cases in Taiwan. Pediatr Surg Int 2005; 21: 809–812.

75. Brandal P, Bjerkehagen B, Heim J. Rearrangement of chromosome region 8q 11–13 in lipomatous tumours: correlation with lipomatous morphology. J Pathol 2006; 208: 388–394.

76. Gaffney EF, Vellios F, Hiliary K, et al. Lipoblastoma ultrastructure of two cases and relationship to human fetal white adipose tissue. Pediatr Pathol 1986; 5: 207–216.

77. Donohue WL, Uchida IA. Leprechaunism: A euphemism for a rare familial disorder. J Pediatr 1954; 45: 505–519.

78. Donohue WL. Dysendocrinism. J Pediatr 1948; 32: 739–748.

79. Musso C, Cochran E, Moran SA, et al. Clinical course of genetic diseases of

insulin receptor (type A and Rabson–Mendenhall syndromes): a 30-year prospective. Medicine (Baltimore) 2004; 83: 209–222.

80. Taylor SI. Lilly lecture: Molecular mechanism of insulin resistance. Diabetes 1992; 41: 1473–1490.

81. Elsas LJ, Endo F, Strumlauf E, et al. Leprechaunism: An inherited defect in high-affinity insulin receptor. Am J Human Genet 1985; 37: 73–88.

82. Kosztolanyi F. Leprechaunism/Donohue syndrome/insulin receptor gene mutations: A syndrome delineation story from clinicopathological description to molecular understanding. Eur J Pediatr 1997; 156: 253–255.

83. Ozbey H, Ozbey N, Tunnessen W. Picture of the month: Leprechaunism. Arch Pediatr Adolesc Med 1998; 1998; 152: 1031–1032.

84. Kadowaki T, Bevins CL, Cama A. Two mutant alleles of the insulin receptor gene in a patient with extreme insulin resistance. Science 1998; 240: 787–790.

85. Berardinelli W. An undiagnosed endocrinometabolic syndrome: Report of 2 cases. J Clin Endocrinol 1954; 14: 193–204.

86. Seip M. Lipodystrophy and gigantism with associated endocrine manifestations: A new diencephalic syndrome? Acta Pediatr Scand 1959; 48: 555–574.

87. Seip M, Trugstad O. Generalized lipodystrophy, congenital and acquired (lipoatrophy). Acta Pediatr 1996; Suppl 413: 2–28.

88. Jaeken J, Stibler H, Hagberg B. The carbohydrate-deficient glycoprotein syndrome. Acta Paediatr Scand 1991; 375: 5S–71S.

89. Krasnewich D, Gahl WA. Carbohydrate-deficient glycoprotein syndrome. Adv Pediatr 1997; 44: 109–139.

90. Collins AE, Ferriero DM. The expanding spectrum of congenital disorders of glycosylation. J Pediatr 2005; 147: 728–730.

91. Jaeken J, Vanderschueren-Lodewyckx M, Casaer P. Familial psychomotor retardation with markedly fluctuative serum prolactin, FSH and GH levels, partial TBG deficiency, increased CSF protein: a new syndrome? Pediatr Res 1980; 14: 129.

92. Charlwood J, Clayton P, Keir G, et al. Prenatal diagnosis of the carbohydrate-deficient glycoprotein syndrome type 1A (CDG1A) by a combination of enzymology and genetic linkage analysis after amniocentesis or chorionic villus sampling. Prenat Diagn 1998; 18: 693–699.

93. Rutledge P. Gangliosidoses and related lipid storage diseases. In: Rimoin DL, Connor JM, Pyeritz RE, eds. Emery and Rimoin's principles and practice of medical genetics, 3rd edn. New York: Churchill Livingstone, 1996; 2113–2114.

94. Antonarakis SE, Valle D, Hugo M, et al. Phenotypic variability in siblings with Farber disease. J Pediatr 1984; 104: 406–409.

25

Neoplastic and Infiltrative Diseases

Neil S. Prose, Richard J. Antaya

Skin disorders characterized by infiltrative lesions can be present at birth or develop during the first few months of life. Some represent frank neoplasms, both benign and malignant, whereas others are the result of metabolic errors. In most instances, diagnosis is facilitated by skin biopsy, in which certain cell types can be identified by special stains and immunologic markers. Others require special enzyme assays for definitive diagnosis.

NEOPLASTIC DISORDERS

Leukemia

Congenital leukemia is a rare hematologic disorder. Of the two distinct types, acute nonlymphocytic leukemia is far more common than the lymphocytic variety. To differentiate congenital leukemia from the several infectious and proliferative disorders that can easily mimic this condition, the following diagnostic criteria are employed:

1. The presence of immature white cells in the blood
2. Infiltration of these cells into extrahematopoietic tissues
3. The absence of diseases that can cause leukemoid reactions (such as erythroblastosis fetalis and a variety of congenital infections)
4. The absence of chromosomal disorders that are associated with 'unstable' hematopoiesis (such as trisomy 21).[1,2]

Cutaneous Findings
The cutaneous manifestations of congenital leukemia consist of petechiae, ecchymoses, and skin nodules. The firm nodules are usually 1–2.5 cm in diameter and blue to purple in color (Fig. 25-1A, B). They are often widely spread over the skin surface, although congenital leukemia may present as a single cutaneous lesion. Diffuse calcinosis cutis in an infant with congenital acute monocytic leukemia has been reported.[3] Congenital monoblastic leukemia may be manifested by 'blueberry muffin' lesions,[4] and Darier's sign has been observed.[5] The clinical signs and symptoms include hepatosplenomegaly, pallor, lethargy, and respiratory distress. Lymphadenopathy occurs in some infants.

Diagnosis
Biopsy of a cutaneous lesion reveals a dense pleomorphic mononuclear cell infiltrate in the dermis and subcutaneous fat. Atypical mitotic figures may be present. The diagnosis of congenital leukemia can usually be confirmed by a complete blood count, bone marrow aspirate, and radiographs of the skull and long bones.

In every case, cytogenetic studies must be performed to exclude the possibility of transient myeloproliferative disorder, which is usually associated with trisomy 21.[6] This disorder is also associated with a diffuse vesiculopustular eruption[7,8] (see Chapter 10).

Treatment and Course
Congenital leukemia, when untreated, is almost always a lethal neoplastic disorder. Treatment alternatives include chemotherapy and bone marrow transplant. Because of the severe side effects of these therapies in the neonate, and the occasional occurrence of complete spontaneous remission, some authors advocate the initial postponement of treatment, and the initiation of chemotherapy only when the malignancy interferes with vital parameters.[9,10]

Langerhans' cell histiocytosis

Langerhans' cell histiocytosis (LCH), a rare proliferative disorder, may be present at birth or may develop during the first few months of life. The estimated incidence of neonatal LCH is 9/1 000 000 in infants less than 1 year of age, with disease presentation during the first month of life in about 6%.[11,11a] The spectrum of clinical presentations, and the clinical course, is extremely varied and ranges from the simple presence of one or several nodules, widespread crusted papules and vesicles, to severe, progressive multisystem disease.

Cutaneous Findings
The most frequent cutaneous presentation consists of multiple widespread vesiculopustules with umbilication and a hemorrhagic crust.[12–16] Lesions tend to favor the scalp, trunk, diaper area, and skin folds (Fig. 25-2A). They may begin as subtle brown or pink papules, and evolve into crusted or purpuric lesions (Fig. 25-2B). Papular lesions may coalesce into areas of superficial ulceration with oozing, especially in intertriginous areas. Characteristic lesions also include fissures behind the ears, and crusting and oozing of the external ear canals. The scalp is a frequent site of involvement, and the coalescence of crusted and scaling lesions may lead to partial alopecia. Presentation as a 'blueberry muffin baby,' with cutaneous hematopoiesis, has been reported.[17] Nodules and

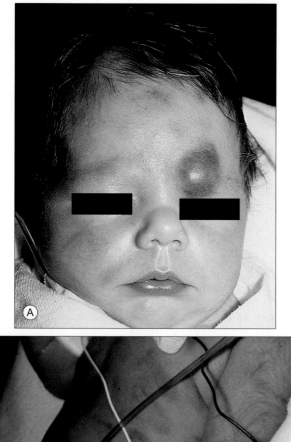

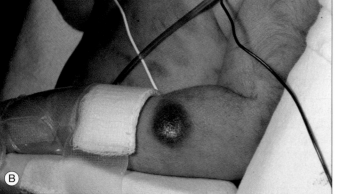

FIG. 25-1 (A) The large nodule above the eye of this neonate represented a manifestation of congenital leukemia resulting from acute lymphocytic leukemia. **(B)** Congenital acute myelogenous leukemia with purpuric nodules and areas of macular purpura.

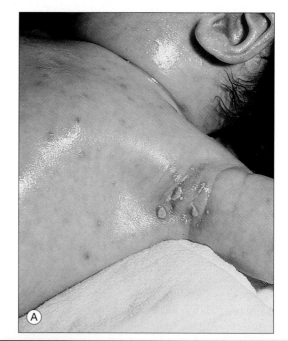

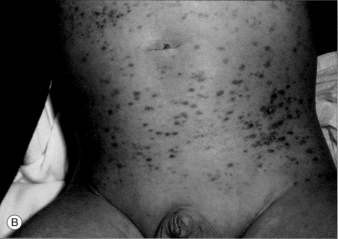

FIG. 25-2 (A) Multiple pustules and erosions are evident in this young infant with Langerhans' cell histiocytosis and multisystem involvement. **(B)** Extensive LCH with purpuric and crusted papules.

petechiae, which may involve the palms and soles, are also observed.

Oral lesions are relatively common, and may develop before skin lesions. They may appear as superficial ulcerations or erosions, but these are often associated with underlying alveolar bone disease. Other oral manifestations include gingival bleeding, facial swelling, and pain. Premature exfoliation and eruption of teeth, and destruction of alveolar bone are characteristic. Involvement of the vulva and vagina may also occur. Nail involvement consists of subungual pustules, paronychia, onycholysis, and longitudinal grooving. Permanent nail dystrophy may result.[18]

Congenital 'Self-Healing' Langerhans' Cell Histiocytosis

In 1973, Hashimoto and Pritzker[19] described a disorder characterized by congenital papulonodular and papulovesicular skin lesions which they termed 'self-healing reticulohistiocy-

tosis.' It was subsequently determined that these cells were composed of S100-positive histiocytes and eosinophils, and this form is now recognized as a variant of LCH. Most affected infants have lesions at the time of birth without evidence of other organ system involvement (Figs 25-3 and 25-4).[19] Skin lesions typically resolve spontaneously, without sequelae.[20–22] However, skin relapse, bone disease, late-onset diabetes insipidus, and even progression to severe LCH has now been reported in children who present with these clinical findings.[25] Therefore Hashimoto–Pritzker disease should be considered a mild form of LCH, which is most cases is self-healing, but patients who present with only papular or nodular skin lesions in the newborn period should also be closely monitored for the later development of extracutaneous disease.

Extracutaneous Findings

The majority of infants with all forms of congenital or neonatal Langerhans' cell histiocytosis will show evidence of multisystem disease.[23–25]

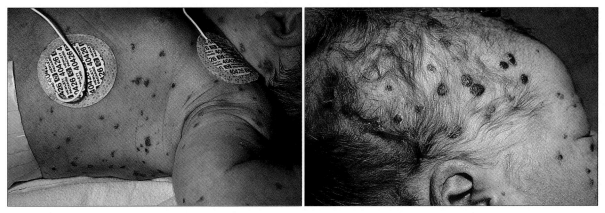

FIG. 25-3 Multiple crusted papules are typical of the 'self-healing' variant of congenital Langerhans' cell histiocytosis.

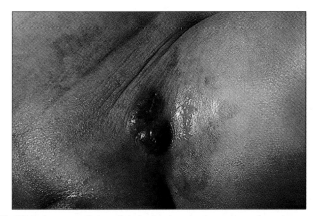

FIG. 25-4 A congenital nodule in the inguinal area was found on biopsy to be congenital Langerhans' cell histiocytosis. It resolved without further sequelae.

Bone lesions are the most frequent noncutaneous manifestation of LCH. Findings may include asymptomatic lytic lesions, deformation, fracture, or medullary compression. The skull is a common site, and disease in that location manifests on X-ray as punched-out lesions in the cranial vault. Mastoid involvement may lead to mastoid necrosis, and destruction of the ossicles may result in deafness.

Intercranial disease may cause exophthalmos and diabetes insipidus. Lymph node involvement is seen in a significant percentage of patients, and tends to occur in the cervical chain.

Pulmonary disease may be associated with cough and tachypnea. Other findings include bulla formation and diffuse interstitial fibrosis.

Invasion of the liver may cause mild cholestasis, but eventually evolve to sclerosing cholangitis. Severe fibrosis of the liver results in ascites, jaundice, and liver failure. Involvement of the spleen may worsen the severity of thrombocytopenia.

Gastrointestinal disease is reported to occur in a small percentage of patients.[26] Characteristic findings are vomiting, diarrhea, protein-losing enteropathy, and failure to thrive secondary to malabsorption.

The most common endocrine manifestation is diabetes insipidus. This occurs most often in children with extensive disease and involvement of the skull. Langerhans' cells may also infiltrate the thyroid and pancreas.

Diagnosis

Biopsy of a cutaneous lesion reveals a diffuse infiltration of histiocytes with abundant eosinophilic cytoplasm and eccentric, indented nuclei. In some cases the nuclei may appear pleomorphic or atypical. Cells are S100 and CD-1a positive, and electron microscopy reveals the presence of Langerhans' granules in a significant percentage of histiocytes.

Preliminary laboratory evaluation of the patient with biopsy-proven skin lesions must include a complete blood count (CBC), serum electrolytes, urine specific gravity, and assessment of liver function. Examination of the bone marrow may show the presence of increased histiocytes. Skeletal survey, chest radiographs, and magnetic resonance imaging (MRI) may be used to determine the extent of bone, pulmonary, liver, spleen, and CNS involvement.

Differential Diagnosis

The pustular and intertriginous lesions of LCH in neonates and infants may be confused with candidiasis, seborrheic dermatitis, psoriasis and scabies. Congenital LCH must also be differentiated from other neoplastic disorders, such as leukemia and lymphoma; from congenital infections, especially herpes simplex; and from those viral disorders associated with blueberry muffin lesions.

Treatment and Course

The majority of children with infantile LCH develop multisystem disease. The prognosis seems to be better in infants born with LCH, but multisystem disease is still possible, and such infants must be followed to assure that they do not develop extracutaneous disease later on. Survival in the past few decades has improved from 57% to 74%.[11,11a] Single system disease has a significantly higher rate of survival (94%), but patients with initial liver involvement have a much poorer prognosis, with a 25% 5-year survival.[11a] In children with LCH limited to the skin, a 'wait and see' approach should be accompanied by careful monitoring for disease progression. Children in this category may benefit from therapy with mild to moderate-strength topical corticosteroids. Children with multisystem disease are treated with chemotherapy or with bone marrow, stem cell, or cord blood transplant.

Familial Hemophagocytic Lymphohistiocytosis

Familial hemophagocytic lymphohistiocytosis (FHL) is an autosomal recessive disorder that most often presents during the first year of life.[27] Some children have been noted to have an evanescent macular and papular skin eruption, sometimes associated with episodes of fever (Fig. 25-5). Most patients have pronounced hepatosplenomegaly, and many develop symptoms related to CNS involvement. Diagnosis is made by the detection of a nonmalignant mixed lymphohistiocytic proliferation in the reticuloendothelial system, with evidence of hemophagocytosis. Without treatment, FLH is usually rapidly fatal. Chemotherapy and bone marrow transplant are the preferred therapies.

Infantile Fibrosarcoma

Congenital/infantile fibrosarcoma is a rare tumor that occurs most frequently on the extremities. Lesions are seen less commonly on the head, neck, and trunk, and may also occur in the retroperitoneum.[28] The tumor may be present at birth, or may develop during early infancy. Infantile fibrosarcoma is associated with a high incidence of the *TEL/TRKC* fusion gene.[29]

Cutaneous Findings

Fibrosarcoma most often presents as a soft tissue mass, sometimes with rapid growth. The overlying skin may be tense,

shiny, and erythematous, and ulceration may occur (Fig. 25-6).[30]

Diagnosis

MRI is useful in defining the extent of the lesion, but the diagnosis is based on histology. Histologic examination reveals a highly cellular fibroblastic proliferation, with sizeable vascular clefts and occasional myxoid degeneration and hemorrhagic necrosis.[31]

Differential Diagnosis

Clinically, infantile fibrosarcomas are easily confused with either hemangiomas or vascular/lymphatic malformations.[32,33] Transient consumptive coagulopathy mimicking Kasabach–Merritt phenomenon has been reported, causing confusion with other vascular tumors[33a] (see Chapter 20). The differential diagnosis also includes rhabdomyosarcoma and infantile myofibromatosis.

Treatment and Course

Most authors suggest that the risk of metastasis, especially in cutaneous lesions, is considerably lower in infants (approximately 8%) than in older patients.[34] Treatment consists of wide local excision. Chemotherapy has been used in some patients to reduce the lesion mass preoperatively, and for lesions that are not resectable.[35] Close follow-up, to monitor for the presence of local recurrence and metastatic disease, is mandatory.

Dermatofibrosarcoma Protuberans

Dermatofibrosarcoma protuberans (DFSP) is a fibrohistiocytic tumor with low metastatic potential and a high incidence of local recurrence. Congenital DFSP is rare, but several cases have been reported.[36,37] Another neoplastic disorder, giant cell fibroblastoma, can also present in early infancy (Fig. 25-7). Some authors consider this to be a variant of DFSP; others consider it to be a separate entity, but believe that hybrids of giant cell fibroblastoma and DFS may sometimes occur.

Cutaneous Findings

Characteristically, DFSP begins as an atrophic plaque surrounded by an area of bluish discoloration. Over time, as the cellular proliferation extends into the deep dermis and subcutaneous tissues, nodules develop on the plaque surface (Fig. 25-8). Similar to the lesions seen in older patients, congenital

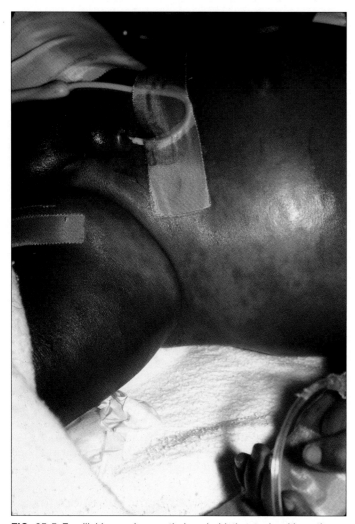

FIG. 25-5 Familial hemophagocytic lymphohistiocytosis with erythematous macules and abdominal distension.

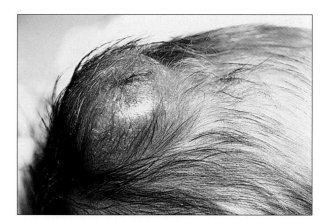

FIG. 25-6 Infantile fibrosarcoma of the scalp in a 15-day-old boy.

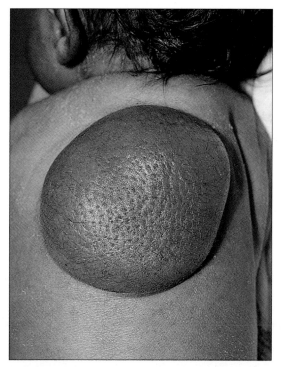

FIG. 25-7 Giant cell fibroblastoma, considered a variant of dermatofibrosarcoma protuberans.

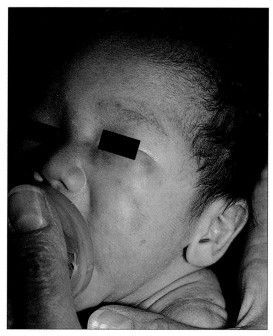

FIG. 25-9 Congenital neuroblastoma: blue nodules on the face. (Courtesy of Dr. Bari Cunningham.)

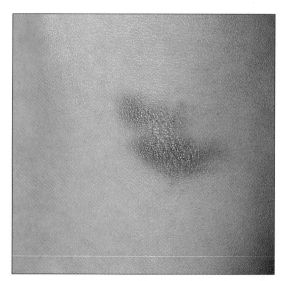

FIG. 25-8 Nodular, plaque-type dermatofibrosarcoma protuberans.

DFSP occurs most commonly on the trunk and proximal extremities.[38]

Diagnosis

Histologically, DFSP is characterized by the presence of spindle cells in a well-defined and uniform storiform pattern. Focal myxoid change and scarring may occur. Tumor cells express vimentin, but are negative for S100 protein, epithelial membrane antigen, and smooth muscle actin.[39]

Differential Diagnosis

Clinically, the differential diagnosis of congenital DFSP includes fibrous hamartoma of infancy, infantile myofibroma-tosis, lipoblastoma (see Chapter 24), and vascular tumors and malformations. Neuro-fibroma and fibrous histiocytoma may mimic DFSP histologically.

Treatment

Because of the high risk of recurrence, adequate surgical margins must be obtained. Mohs micrographic surgery is an alternative approach in some patients.[40]

Neuroblastoma

Cutaneous Findings

Neuroblastoma is among the most common solid tumors of early childhood, and may present at birth or in early infancy. In stage IV-s neuroblastoma cutaneous metastases present as bluish, firm papules and nodules on the trunk and extremities (Fig. 25-9). Several authors have reported that these lesions may blanch after palpation, and that the blanching persists for 30–60 minutes.[41,42] This phenomenon has been related to the localized release of catecholamines. Periorbital ecchymoses, secondary to orbital metastases, may also occur.

Extracutaneous Findings

Metastatic disease, characterized by fever, hepatomegaly, and failure to thrive, is often present at the time of diagnosis. The primary lesion is usually located in the upper abdomen, arising within the adrenal gland, and may be detected as an enlarging mass.

Diagnosis

Diagnosis of the cutaneous lesions is based on histologic examination. The dermal or subcutaneous infiltrate consists of small cells with scanty cytoplasm and heterochromatic nuclei. Pseudorosettes and mature ganglion cells are present in differentiated lesions. Immunoperoxidase staining may establish the presence of neuron-specific proteins.

Although most cases of neuroblastoma are sporadic, autosomal dominant inheritance may occur. Concordance in monozygotic twins has also been reported.[43] The location and extent of the primary lesion is most often established by computed tomography (CT) or MRI. Increased urinary catecholamines are present in the majority of patients.

Differential Diagnosis

Clinically and histologically, the lesions of neuroblastoma must be differentiated from leukemia and lymphoma. In addition, the blueberry muffin appearance of some lesions may mimic congenital rubella or cytomegalovirus infection.

Treatment and Course

The prognosis of neuroblastoma depends on the age of the patient and the extent of the disease (stages I to IV-s). The survival rate at 2 years in children who are diagnosed under the age of 1 year exceeds 80%. In some patients, especially with stage IV-s, spontaneous differentiation to neural ganglion cells and regression without treatment have been reported. The choice of treatment depends on staging and patient age, and consists of various combinations of surgery, radiation therapy, and chemotherapy.[44]

Rhabdomyosarcoma

Rhabdomyosarcoma presents most commonly as a tumor of the head and neck. Other locations include the genitourinary tract, extremities, and trunk (Fig. 25-10A, B). Two percent of cases are present at birth. An association between rhabdomyosarcoma and both neurofibromatosis type 1 and major congenital abnormalities has been observed.[45] Rhabdomyosarcoma arising in children with giant congenital melanocytic nevi has also been reported.[45a]

A cutaneous origin of rhabdomyosarcoma is rare. Most commonly, extension of the tumor into the dermis results in the evolution of a nodule or plaque.[46] Facial lesions are most common, and these must be differentiated clinically from dermoid cysts, hemangiomas, and inflammatory disorders. Histologically, there is a dermal infiltrate of small blue cells with occasional differentiation toward rhabdomyoblasts. The presence of desmin staining with immunoperoxidase may help to differentiate these lesions from neuroblastoma and lymphoma.

Treatment is based on the extent of local, regional, and distant disease, and consists of combinations of surgery, radiation, and chemotherapy. Combined modality therapy results in a long-term survival of greater than 50%.[47]

Congenital Melanoma

Congenital malignant melanoma may develop in several different clinical situations:[48,49]

1. Congenital malignant melanoma arising de novo. Malignant melanoma may present at birth as a nodular, darkly pigmented, and rapidly growing skin lesion, sometimes with ulceration.[50,51] In these neonates there is no clinical or histologic evidence of an underlying congenital melanocytic nevus, and there is no maternal history of melanoma (Fig. 25-11).
2. Congenital malignant melanoma arising in a giant congenital melanocytic nevus. In these patients, ulcerated and nonulcerated nodules may be present in the congenital

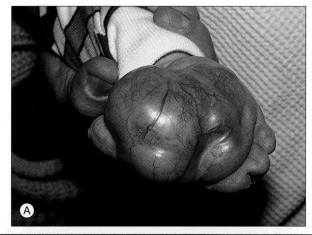

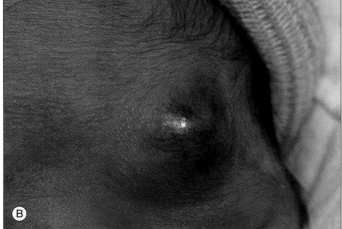

FIG. 25-10 (A) Rhabdomyosarcoma. A firm, vascular-appearing tumor of the hand. (B) Alveolar rhabdomyosarcoma on the forehead of a 6-day-old infant with multifocal disease at birth.

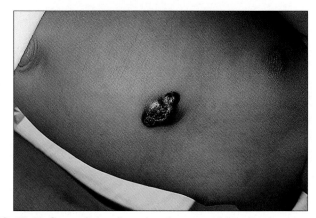

FIG. 25-11 Congenital malignant melanoma, arising de novo on normal skin.

melanocytic nevus and on adjoining skin. The presence of prenatal metastatic disease has been noted to occur in some children.[52,53]
3. Congenital malignant melanoma arising from leptomeningeal melanocytosis. Children with leptomeningeal melanocytosis may have a high lifetime incidence of metastatic malignant melanoma. Rarely, these metastatic cutaneous lesions may be present at birth.

4. Congenital malignant melanoma secondary to maternal melanoma. Transplacental transmission from a mother with metastatic disease may occur.[54] Typically, the skin lesions are multiple pigmented macules, papules, and nodules, and there may be multiorgan involvement.

The diagnosis of malignant melanoma is made by excisional biopsy of the suspicious lesion, and the cellular and architectural features are similar to those seen in melanoma in older patients. However, a wide variety of benign and malignant tumors, with small round cell, spindled, neural, and epithelioid components, have been observed within congenital melanocytic nevi.[51] In addition, histologic changes within a benign, congenital melanocytic nevus may include displaced large melanocytes within the epidermis, and heterogeneous patterns of melanocytic hyperplasia.[52] In some cases, findings of this type have led to an incorrect diagnosis of malignant melanoma. Biopsies of congenital melanocytic nevi, especially in the neonate, must therefore be interpreted with caution.[55–57]

The evaluation of children with all forms of melanoma must include a complete evaluation for local and distant lymph node involvement. Metastases are most frequently seen in the CNS, bones, lungs, and liver.

Treatment is based on lesion thickness and the stage of the disease. Therapeutic options include lymph-node dissection of enlarged draining regional nodes and chemotherapy for metastatic disease.[53] Lesions arising de novo have an unpredictable prognosis, and long-term survival has been reported in children who developed both local recurrences and metastatic lesions. Melanomas arising in congenital melanocytic nevi appear to have a significantly worse prognosis. Congenital malignant melanoma secondary to maternal melanoma is usually fatal, but spontaneous regression has been reported to occur.[54]

Congenital Teratoma

Congenital teratomas most frequently present as masses in the cervical, nasopharynx, or sacrococcygeal region.[58] These benign tumors, which are derived from elements of all three germinal layers, result in significant morbidity and mortality because of their location, size, and tendency to cause airway obstruction. The differential diagnosis includes dermoids and lymphatic or vascular malformations. Treatment consists of complete surgical excision.

INFILTRATIVE DISORDERS

Mastocytosis

Mastocytosis refers to a spectrum of conditions characterized by the infiltration of benign mast cells in the skin or other organs. Fifty-five percent of cases develop during the first 2 years, and an additional 10% develop before puberty.[59] Cases developing after puberty are classified as adult onset. Both sexes are affected equally. Mastocytoma, urticaria pigmentosa (UP), and diffuse cutaneous mastocytosis (DCM) are most likely to affect neonates and infants (see the following discussion). Mastocytoma is the most common clinical manifestation of mastocytosis. UP is less common, and DCM, the most severe form, is rare. Most cases are sporadic; however, there have been several reports of UP affecting multiple family members, and some believe diffuse cutaneous mastocytosis

can be inherited in an autosomal dominant fashion.[59–61] Telangiectasia macularis eruptiva perstans (TMEP) has also been reported rarely in the neonatal period, but usually begins during adulthood.

Cutaneous Findings

Most patients with mastocytosis exhibit Darier's sign, which is the development of an urticarial wheal and flare after firm stroking of lesional skin. This cutaneous finding represents the response to physical disruption of the granular contents of mast cells, particularly histamine. Rarely, flushing and hypotension have resulted from stroking of a large lesion, or from surgery. Dermatographism, the formation of linear urticarial plaques following scratching of uninvolved skin, is also seen. However, this nonspecific finding also occurs in up to 5% of the normal population. A variety of physical stimulants and drugs can evoke mast cell degranulation, resulting in urtication, bulla formation, or systemic manifestations (flushing, hypotension, or shock) (Box 25-1).

Many patients have no symptoms, but when present, the major presenting symptom is pruritus. It may be periodic or unremitting. Excoriations may be observed. In children less than 2 years of age vesicles and bullae occur, and are observed in all forms of cutaneous mastocytosis except telangiectasia macularis eruptiva perstans. The tendency to blister diminishes over 1–3 years. In one series, generalized flushing was observed in 65% of patients with all forms of the disease.[62]

Mastocytoma

Mastocytoma most often appears in the first 3 months of life. It presents as one or several isolated, skin-colored to light brown, 1–5 cm, oval to round macules or slightly elevated nodules or plaques (Fig. 25-12). Some lesions have a pink or

---

Box 25-1 Histamine-releasing triggers to avoid in mastocytosis

Drugs
Narcotics (opiates): codeine, meperidine, morphine, dextromethorphan etc.

Aspirin (acetylsalicylic acid) and related analgesics

Alcohol

Polymyxin B

D-tubocurarine*

Iodine-containing radiologic contrast dyes

Cholinergic medications (scopolamine etc.)

Thiamine

Physical stimuli
Pressure or friction

Temperature changes (especially bathing)

Sunlight

Other
Venoms (IgE-mediated hymenoptera venom)

Polymers (dextran)

Biological peptides (substance P, somatostatin)

General anesthesia is not contraindicated but should be approached cautiously; lorazepam has been shown to be safe for routine sedation in infants.

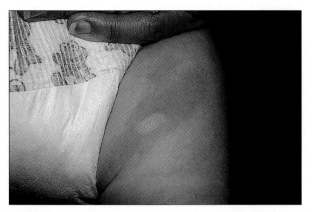

FIG. 25-12 Mastocytoma on the leg of a young infant with a centrally urticated plaque with surrounding flare, demonstrating a positive Darier's sign.

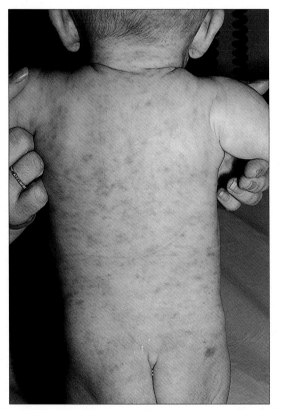

FIG. 25-13 Multiple lesions of urticaria pigmentosa in a 1-month-old infant.

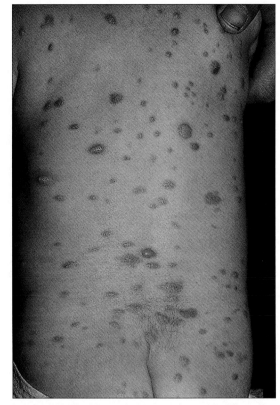

FIG. 25-14 Focal blister formation in an infant with diffuse cutaneous mastocytosis.

ent. Any cutaneous surface may be affected, including mucous membranes, but most are on the trunk. Additional lesions of UP may develop for several months after the initial diagnosis is made.

Diffuse Cutaneous Mastocytosis

Diffuse cutaneous mastocytosis (DCM) is characterized by widespread infiltration of mast cells throughout the skin (Figs 10-12 and 25-14). It presents in the first 3 years of life, and is characterized by generalized thickening and palpable edema of the skin with or without the presence of typical UP lesions. The skin may be normal in color or display a reddish-yellow hue. The first sign of DCM most often is hemorrhagic bullae and erosions, sometimes following minor trauma. Severe dermatographism with resultant bullae and flushing may also occur.

Telangiectasia Macularis Eruptiva Perstans (TMEP)

Infantile TMEP presents with congenital or acquired asymptomatic, 1–4 cm, sharply defined, round or oval, telangiectatic, red-brown patches that resemble small capillary malformations. The patches blanch with pressure, but Darier's sign is reportedly negative. The few documented cases have remained stable over time, and multiple family members can be affected.[63]

Extracutaneous Findings

Hepatosplenomegaly, lymphadenopathy, or skeletal lesions caused by mast cell hyperplasia occur infrequently in infants

yellow hue. Any cutaneous surface may be affected, and the trunk, upper extremities, and neck are favored locations. Most new lesions appear within 2 months of the initial lesion, but individual lesions may enlarge for several months.

Urticaria Pigmentosa

Urticaria pigmentosa generally develops between 3 and 9 months of life. The lesions appear as multiple, fixed, reddish-brown, hyperpigmented macules, papules, and nodules (Fig. 25-13) that have a tendency to coalesce into plaques and often exhibit increased skin markings. Early lesions of UP may mimic recurrent urticaria until pigmentation becomes appar-

with DCM or UP.[64] Associated systemic findings in infants with these forms of the disease include diarrhea, vomiting, abdominal pain, bone pain, headache, hypotension, and rarely shock. Prolonged bleeding in the skin and GI tract may occur, and is more frequent in infants with DCM. In these children, heparin from mast cells acts as a local anticoagulant. Elevated levels of circulating histamine, which stimulates gastric acid secretion, may result in gastric ulceration and gastrointestinal hemorrhage.[65] Children with DCM have the highest incidence of visceral mast cell disease and associated systemic manifestations. UP in infants is rarely (<3%) associated with visceral involvement, and visceral involvement does not appear to occur in children with cutaneous mastocytomas. The incidence of allergic disease is not increased in children with mastocytosis, but the severity of allergic reactions may be increased. Evaluation for systemic mastocytosis via a bone marrow biopsy should only be considered for children who develop disease after 2 years of age, or infants who present with either hepatosplenomegaly, unexplained lymphadenopathy, abnormal complete blood count or a baseline serum total tryptase levels of >20 ng/ml (normal is ~5 ng/ml).

Etiology/Pathogenesis

The cause of mastocytosis is unknown. A mutation in the c-kit proto-oncogene has been identified in some patients. C-kit codes for KIT, the membrane receptor for stem cell factor, and is expressed on mast cells, melanocytes, and hematopoietic stem cells. This mutation may contribute to the characteristic proliferation of mast cells, the hyperpigmentation of the skin seen in cutaneous mastocytosis, or the myeloproliferative diseases observed in some patients with mastocytosis.[66]

Diagnosis

The clinical presentation and characteristic cutaneous lesions usually allow for easy diagnosis. Skin biopsy should be performed when the diagnosis is unclear or when bullae are the main feature. Histopathologic sections may demonstrate variable degrees of mast cell infiltration in the dermis, around blood vessels, and within skin appendages. Bullae, when present, are subepidermal.

Determination of plasma histamine or tryptase levels may be useful in infants at high risk of GI bleeding, as in DCM.[65] Clinical evidence of extracutaneous mastocytosis should guide any additional diagnostic studies (ultrasound, bone and liver/spleen scans, GI endoscopy, skeletal survey, and bone marrow evaluation).[67] The usefulness of studies performed empirically is limited, and they do not appear to provide any prognostic information.[59]

Differential Diagnosis

Mastocytomas should be differentiated from xanthomas, juvenile xanthogranulomas, and congenital nevi. Infestation with Sarcoptes scabei presenting with pruritic, red-brown nodules that exhibit a Darier's sign may be mistaken for mastocytosis. Differentiating characteristics include more severe pruritus, lack of other lesions with other morphologies (e.g. paucity of macules and plaques commonly observed with UP), and distribution favoring covered and intertriginous areas in scabetic nodules.[68] Where bullae are prominent or lesions are atypical, biopsy is indicated to differentiate mastocytosis from the immunobullous diseases, epidermolysis bullosa, or other infiltrative disorders.

Treatment and Care

The course of most cases of pediatric mastocytosis is benign and the prognosis generally favorable. Solitary mastocytomas have not been reported to progress to systemic involvement.[67] More than 50% of childhood cases of urticaria pigmentosa resolve by adolescence, and the remainder experience a marked reduction in cutaneous symptoms.[62,69] Fifteen to 30% of patients whose disease persists into adulthood develop systemic involvement, which is similar to the rate observed in adult-onset disease.[62] Children presenting with congenital bullous UP or DCM have a higher risk for sudden death, usually from circulatory collapse.[70]

Treatment is aimed at reducing pruritus and, in some children, minimizing blister formation. The regular use of H_1 antihistamines such as hydroxyzine is effective in treating pruritus, bullae, flushing, and abdominal pain. The addition of H_2 blockers and oral disodium cromoglycate may be effective for patients with gastrointestinal signs or symptoms.[71-73]

Solitary mastocytomas may be treated with a short course of a superpotent topical steroid, and very problematic lesions may be excised. Rare instances of circulatory collapse as a result of systemic histamine release should be treated with careful fluid management and intravenous epinephrine.[73] A self-injectable epinephrine device may be prescribed for children with a history of such episodes.[59] PUVA therapy is effective for severe UP and DCM.[74] Parents should be provided with a list of substances that stimulate mast cell activity and which should therefore be avoided (see Box 25-1).

Infantile Systemic Hyalinosis and Juvenile Hyaline Fibromatosis

Infantile systemic hyalinosis (ISH) and juvenile hyaline fibromatosis (JHF) are rare, progressive, autosomal recessive diseases. They are allelic and represent part of a spectrum, rather than two distinct entities. Clinical manifestations which are noted at birth or in early infancy include papular and nodular skin lesions (Fig. 25-15A), joint contractures (Fig. 25-15B), skeletal and soft tissue lesions, gingival hyperplasia (Fig. 25-15C), and growth retardation.

Cutaneous Findings

Several distinct characteristic skin lesions are observed in JHF. Small, skin-colored, pearly papules are found predominantly on the ears, neck, and paranasal folds, where they may coalesce to form thin plaques (Fig. 25-15A). Translucent-appearing larger papules and nodules are found around the nose, behind the ears, and on the tips of digits. These may have a gelatinous consistency. Papillomatous perianal lesions, resembling condylomata, have been observed in some patients.[75]

Extracutaneous Findings

The most consistent and earliest extracutaneous manifestation of JHF are joint flexion contractures, especially of the knees and elbows. Many patients become severely disabled by these progressively severe contractures. Gingival hypertrophy is seen in nearly all patients, and the majority have osteolytic bone lesions and osteoporosis.[76] JHF generally does not involve the viscera; however, there is considerable clinical and histologic overlap with the more severe disease infantile systemic hyalinosis (ISH). In ISH there are hyaline deposits in multiple organs, recurrent infections, and death within the first 2 years of life.[75]

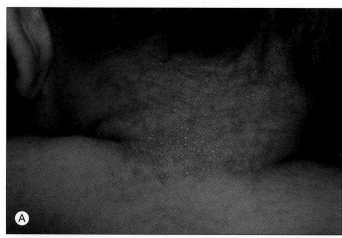

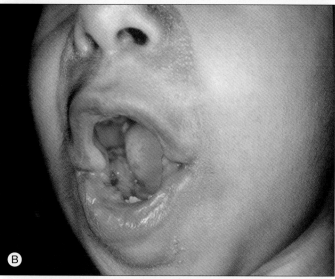

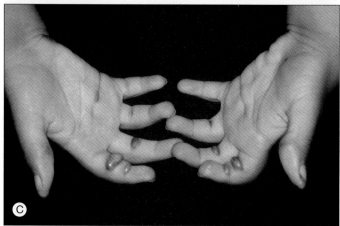

FIG. 25-15 (**A**) Young child with juvenile hyaline fibromatosis with characteristic small papules on the nape. (**B**) A 7-year-old patient with juvenile hyaline fibromatosis. Gingival hypertrophy, fibromas of the vermillion and cutaneous lips, decreased oral aperture, and papules on the chin coalescing paranasally into small plaques are evident. (**C**) Same patient with fibromas of the fingers and hands with flexion contractures.

Etiology and Pathogenesis

JHF and ISD are caused by mutations in the gene encoding capillary morphogenesis protein-2 (*CMG-2*), an integrin-like cell surface receptor for laminins and type IV collagen.[77,78] The hyaline deposition may be composed of type IV collagen or

represent leakage of plasma components through the basement membrane, but this remains unresolved.

On routine histology, the dermal papules show thinning of the epidermis and a dermis occupied by abundant, amorphous, PAS-positive, diastase-resistant material containing wavy filamentous elements. Cells with oval or spindle-shaped nuclei are embedded in this stroma, imparting a chondroid appearance. These fibroblastic cells often display PAS-positive cytoplasmic vacuoles. Ultrastructurally, the fibroblastic stromal cells display a hyperplastic and dilated rough endoplasmic reticulum with collections of smooth-surfaced cisternae filled with tangled microfilaments.[75] Osteoporosis and osteolytic bone lesions are observed on radiographic examination of most patients. Routine laboratory evaluations are normal.

Differential Diagnosis

The differential diagnosis should first include Winchester syndrome, a rare autosomal recessive condition that has many overlapping features with JHF, including joint contractures, dwarfism, hypertrophic lips and gingivae, severe osteoporosis, thickened leathery skin, and corneal opacities.[79] Lipoid proteinosis may be distinguished from JHF by a distinctly different histology, a characteristic hoarse cry, and a more benign clinical course.

Treatment and Course

The course is progressive. Excluding those most severely affected with hyaline material in the viscera, most patients survive into adulthood with severe physical deformities due to joint contractures, delayed motor development, and skin nodules that recur after surgical excision. Treatment, which is unsatisfactory, includes excision of skin lesions, repeated gingivectomy, and systemic corticosteroids for joint symptoms. At least one patient has been treated with interferon-α, with some reduction and softening of the smaller fibromas only (personal communication, Ruiz-Maldonado and Duran).

Farber Disease

Farber disease, or Farber lipogranulomatosis, is a rare, progressive, autosomal recessive mucolipidosis. The disorder primarily involves the musculoskeletal, respiratory, integumentary, and nervous systems of affected infants, and onset occurs in the first year of life.[80]

Cutaneous Findings

The characteristic cutaneous features include multiple subcutaneous nodules, flesh-colored papules, and periarticular tumors or nodules. Coarse facial features and xanthoma-like papules on the face and hands have also been reported. The resultant granulomatous inflammation is a common but unexplained finding which may be due to decreased apoptosis of inflammatory cells secondary to increased intracellular ceremide.[81]

Extracutaneous Findings

Painful, deforming joint swelling with restriction of movement, particularly of the distal interphalangeal and metacarpal joints, is characteristic. Infants frequently exhibit marked failure to thrive, recurrent infections, a hoarse cry attributed to laryngomalacia, dyspnea, noisy breathing, and hyperirritability. Impairment of cognitive development, seizures, hepatosplenomegaly, macroglossia, recurrent fevers, and hyporeflexia are variably present.

Etiology and Pathogenesis

Farber lipogranulomatosis is caused by a deficiency of the lysosomal acid ceramidase, with resultant progressive accumulation of ceramide-containing nodules in tissues. The characteristic clinical presentation and the detection of low levels of acid ceramidase are diagnostic of Farber disease. Light microscopic examination of skin and other affected tissues is nonspecific, demonstrating foam cells and a granulomatous infiltrate. This inflammation is hypothesized to be due to altered receptor-mediated apoptosis by intracellular ceramide accumulation.[82] Several characteristic structures are observed ultramicroscopically, probably resulting from the accumulation of ceramide in cells. Curvilinear tubular bodies – comma-shaped, tubular structures consisting of two single membranes separated by a clear space – are observed in dermal fibroblasts among other affected cells. Banana bodies, variably membrane-bound structures that have a spindle and usually curved shape, are found predominantly in Schwann cells of peripheral nerves.[81]

Diagnosis

Radiologic examination reveals diffuse osteopenia, underdevelopment of terminal phalanges, and reduced long bone diameters.[82] The diagnosis should be confirmed by detection of deficient lysosomal acid ceramidase activity in leukocytes, fibroblasts, or other tissues.

Differential Diagnosis

The differential diagnosis includes metabolic storage diseases, particularly other mucolipidoses. Some cases have been misdiagnosed as juvenile rheumatoid arthritis because of the severe joint involvement seen early in the course.

Treatment and Course

Most patients die of progressive neurologic deterioration early in the first decade of life. Hematopoietic stem cell transplantation was successfully performed in two infants without CNS involvement (type 2/3 disease), but allogeneic bone marrow transplant failed to halt the progression of Farber disease with CNS involvement (type 1).[82] Various other treatments, including corticosteroids and radiotherapy, have been attempted and are ineffective. The potassium–titanyl–phosphate (KTP) laser has been used for treatment of severe oral lesions.[83]

Because transmission is autosomal recessive, genetic counseling is mandatory. Prenatal diagnosis, performed by assaying acid ceramidase levels in skin cells cultured from amniotic fluid, is now possible.[84]

I-Cell Disease

I-cell disease, or mucolipidosis II, is a severe autosomal recessive storage disorder of lysosomal enzyme localization. The skeletal and central nervous systems are most severely affected, but characteristic skin changes also occur. I-cell disease exhibits signs and symptoms of both the mucopolysaccharidoses, particularly Hurler syndrome, and the sphingolipidoses. The term I-cell, or inclusion cell, refers to the presence of cytoplasmic inclusions associated with lysosomes. Onset occurs at birth, and disease progression results in death during the first decade.

Cutaneous Findings

The most notable cutaneous findings are the facial features: small orbits and prominent eyes, thickening of the eyelids with a prominent venous pattern, and fullness of the lower face with rounded cheeks. Many small telangiectases impart a ruddy appearance to the cheeks. Patients often exhibit a fish-mouth appearance in profile as a result of prominent maxillary bones. The neck is short, and the skin has a thickened and rigid texture, particularly on the neck and ears. Gingival hypertrophy, not present in Hurler syndrome, is progressive and severe.

Extracutaneous Findings

Neonates commonly exhibit intrauterine growth retardation, with birth weights often below 2500 g. Linear growth is below normal and ceases at 1 year of age. Orthopedic problems manifesting as dysostosis multiplex are common presenting features. Inguinal hernias, especially in boys, may be noted at birth, and patients of both sexes have frequent upper respiratory tract infections and hepatosplenomegaly. All patients experience severe psychomotor retardation, and the majority neither walk unaided nor develop more than primitive language skills. There is progressive stiffness of all joints, first apparent in the shoulders, with decreased mobility by 2 years of age.[85]

The long bones of affected infants younger than 6 months display periosteal cloaking, possibly due to repeated new bone formation. Also observed are cone-shaped phalanges and abnormalities of the skull and pelvis.[86]

Etiology and Pathogenesis

I-cell disease is caused by an underlying defect in N-acetyl-glucosamine-1-phosphotransferase, an enzyme involved in the synthesis of a mannose-6-phosphate marker of hydrolases normally found in lysosomes. Because newly synthesized lysosomal enzymes are not marked correctly, the mannose-6-phosphate receptor-dependent transport fails, and the enzymes are secreted out of cells instead of being targeted to lysosomes. This results in failed lysosomal degradation of macromolecules, simulating a catabolic enzyme defect.[87] Fibroblast lysosomal enzymes are deficient in patients with I-cell disease, whereas the serum levels of the same enzymes are markedly elevated.[88] The finding that some tissues have normal levels of lysosomal enzymes suggests that there may be an alternative method for targeting lysosomal hydrolases in these tissues.[89] The defective phosphotransferase gene has been mapped to chromosome 4q.

Diagnosis

The diagnosis of I-cell disease is suggested by detection of an increase in the activity of several hydrolases in plasma. It is confirmed by dermal fibroblast cultures, which show the characteristic cytoplasmic inclusions (I-cells) in the cultured cells. These cytoplasmic inclusions stain positively for PAS and Sudan black, but almost negatively for Alcian blue, suggesting that the inclusion bodies represent an abnormal accumulation of glycolipid.[86] Reduced activity of lysosomal hydrolases in the fibroblasts provides additional confirmation of the diagnosis.

Differential Diagnosis

I-cell disease shares most of the clinical features of Hurler syndrome, including coarse facial features, severe psychomotor retardation, and skeletal dysplasia. However, patients with

I-cell disease do not exhibit mucopolysaccharides in their urine. Gingival hypertrophy and vacuolated peripheral blood lymphocytes, characteristic of I-cell disease, are not present in Hurler disease.

Treatment and Course

Death in early childhood is usually secondary to pulmonary infection or congestive heart failure. Bone marrow transplantation appears to slow neurologic and cardiac progression, but does not alter the skeletal disease.[90] Because of the recessive inheritance pattern, genetic counseling should be offered. Successful prenatal diagnosis has been accomplished by demonstrating elevated enzyme levels in amniotic fluid in conjunction with enzyme assays from cultured amniotic fluid cells and by electron microscopy showing marked vacuolation in chorionic villus cells.[91,92]

Mucopolysaccharidoses

The mucopolysaccharidoses (MPSs) are a heterogeneous group of rare lysosomal storage disorders that display several variable clinical features, including coarse facies, skeletal abnormalities, mental retardation, corneal clouding, and hepatosplenomegaly. The degree of progression varies among the diseases, as does the constellation of clinical and laboratory findings. Each disease results from the deficiency of one specific lysosomal enzyme, but all are characterized by accumulation of mucopolysaccharides (glycosaminoglycans) in lysosomes and excessive amounts of mucopolysaccharides in the urine.[93] Sanfilippo syndrome is the most common, and has an incidence of about 1 : 25 000. This is contrasted with Sly syndrome, of which only 40 cases have been reported worldwide.[94]

Cutaneous Findings

The most characteristic cutaneous feature, manifest in all types of MPS, is coarse, thickened skin. This cutaneous alteration combines with underlying craniofacial abnormalities to impart coarse facial features. Patients have a thick nose with a depressed nasal bridge, thick tongue and lips, short neck,

and macrocephaly. The severity of the facial abnormalities is variable, and the most striking features are observed in Hurler and Hunter syndromes. Coarse facies may not be present in young infants.[95] Patients also display variable degrees of coarse hair and generalized hirsutism.

Apart from Sanfilippo syndrome, which presents with synophrys, Hunter syndrome is the only MPS that regularly presents with specific cutaneous findings. Children with Hunter syndrome may develop firm, discrete or coalescing ivory-colored papules on the arms or symmetrically distributed between the angles of the scapulae and the posterior axillary lines. Recently, this same finding was described in a patient with Hurler–Scheie syndrome.[96] Another finding occasionally reported in Hunter syndrome is usually widespread dermal melanocytosis (see Chapter 22).

Extracutaneous Findings

Infants may appear normal at birth, but usually develop characteristic findings in the first few years of life. Each disease has its own array of clinical findings; however, the most important extracutaneous features are mental retardation, deafness, hyperactivity/behavior problems, stiff joints, skeletal dysplasia, kyphoscoliosis, corneal clouding, valvular and coronary heart disease, hepatosplenomegaly, noisy breathing, and lower respiratory tract infections. Table 25-1 lists the cardinal characteristics and pertinent negative findings for each disorder.

The skeletal abnormalities in the MPSs are referred to as dysostosis multiplex and comprise the following elements: large, thickened skull with premature closure of lambdoid and sagittal sutures; shallow orbits; enlarged J-shaped sellae; and anterior hypoplasia of the lumbar vertebrae. In addition, the long bones display enlarged diaphyses, irregular metaphyses, and poor development of the epiphyseal centers.

Etiology and Pathogenesis

Each type of MPS is caused by a deficiency of a specific lysosomal enzyme responsible for the degradation of mucopolysaccharides. This deficiency results in excessive accumulation of

---

TABLE 25-1 Classification and features of the mucopolysaccharidoses*

Eponym	MPS number	Main clinical features (and pertinent negatives)	Urinary mucopolysaccharide
Hurler	I-H	IH, UH, HSM, SS, JS, URI, MR, HL, HD, DM, CC, Hc	DS, HS
Hurler–Scheie	I-H/S	HL, JS, CC, HD, Mg, no MR	DS, HS
Scheie	I-S	JS, HD, CC, no MR, no SS	DS, HS
Hunter (severe)	II-A	SP, IH, UH, HSM, SS, JS, URI, MR, HL, DM, RD, Hc, no CC	DS, HS
Hunter (mild)	II-B	SP, HL, JS, HD, mild CC, no MR	DS, HS
Sanfilippo	III A-D	MR (onset 3–4 yrs), mild HSM, mild DM, synophrys	HS†
Morquio (classic)	IV-A	SD, SS, CC, no MR	KS
Maroteaux–Lamy	VI	IH, UH, SS, JS, URI, HD, HSM, HLHc, DM, CC, no MR	DS
Sly	VII	IH, UH, HSM, SS, JS, URI, MR, HL, HD, Hc, DM, CC‡	DS, HS

*Some subtypes omitted.

†May be missed due to small amount.

‡Large variability of phenotypes observed.

CC, corneal clouding; DM, dysostosis multiplex; DS, dermatan sulfate; Hc, hydrocephalus; HD, heart disease; HL, hearing loss; HS, heparan sulfate; HSM, hepatosplenomegaly; IH, inguinal hernia; JS, joint stiffness; KS, keratan sulfate; Mg, micrognathism; MR, mental retardation; RD, retinal degeneration; SD, spondyloepiphyseal dysplasia; SP, skin papules; SS, short stature; UH, umbilical hernia; URI, upper respiratory tract infections.

the mucopolysaccharides dermatan sulfate, heparan sulfate, and keratan sulfate throughout the body. The deficient enzyme has been elucidated for each disease, and the genetic loci for several have been mapped.[97] All have an autosomal recessive inheritance, except for Hunter syndrome, which is X-linked recessive. Excluding an increased incidence of Hunter syndrome in the Jewish population in Israel and Morquio syndrome in French-Canadians, MPSs appear to affect all ethnic groups equally.

Diagnosis

The testing of urine for glycosaminoglycans is the basis for screening patients suspected of having MPS. If screening tests are positive for glycosaminoglycans, a quantitative analysis should be performed to confirm the presence of MPS. The type and quantity of urinary glycosaminoglycans, combined with the child's clinical presentation, are used to determine the most appropriate enzyme assay to establish definitively the specific type of MPS.[93]

The enzymatic diagnosis should be determined in all patients in whom MPS is suspected. Lysosomal enzyme analysis may be carried out using serum, leukocytes, or cultured cells. In all the MPSs, histopathologic examination of skin with Alcian blue, colloidal iron, or Giemsa stain reveals metachromatic granules in fibroblasts, and occasionally in keratinocytes and in the secretory and ductal cells of eccrine glands. In addition, the cutaneous papules, mostly seen in Hunter syndrome, exhibit extracellular dermal deposits of metachromatic material.[97]

Differential Diagnosis

The mucolipidoses are the most important group of diseases to be differentiated from the MPSs. I-cell disease (mucolipidosis II) shares most of the clinical features of Hurler syndrome, but patients with I-cell disease do not exhibit urine mucopolysaccharides or acceleration of skeletal growth around 1 year of age.

Treatment, Course, and Management

The natural course of the more severe forms is progressive, and death resulting from respiratory or cardiac complications often occurs during the second decade. Some types, such as Scheie syndrome, have a normal life expectancy. Bone marrow transplantation lessens the severity and slows the progression of most cases.[94,98] Treatment of patients with MPS I using enzyme replacement therapy with recombinant human α-L-iduronidase reduces lysosomal storage in the liver and levels of urinary glycosaminoglycan excretion, and improves respiratory function and exercise tolerance.[99,100] Because this enzyme does not cross the blood–brain barrier, most likely it will not influence the central nervous manifestations.[101]

Otherwise, management revolves around supportive care. Physical therapy and nighttime splinting may prevent contractures. Special education and frequent audiologic evaluation should be instituted. Many patients benefit from hearing aids. Echocardiograms are recommended to evaluate for valvular abnormalities. Surgical interventions, including corneal transplants for cloudy corneas, cardiac valve replacement, ventriculoperitoneal shunts for communicating hydrocephalus, tracheostomies for obstructive sleep apnea, and occasionally herniorrhaphies, may be helpful. Patients may possess atlantoaxial joint instability, and injury to the head or spine may result in paralysis. Because of this potentially devastating complication, all patients at risk should undergo careful evaluation, and spinal fusion is recommended for those who are severely affected.

Prenatal diagnosis is performed by enzyme assays of cultured amniotic cells, or of cells obtained in chorionic villus sampling.[102] Prenatal genetic mutational analysis is used less frequently.

Lipoid Proteinosis

Lipoid proteinosis (hyalinosis cutis et mucosae, or Urbach–Weithe syndrome) is a rare, nonfatal, autosomal recessive disorder characterized by deposition of amorphous hyaline material around dermal blood vessels. Cutaneous lesions progress from infancy throughout childhood and become characteristic for this disease by adulthood. Even though any system can be involved, the upper aerodigestive tract, skin, and central nervous system are most commonly affected.

Cutaneous Findings

The cutaneous lesions are rarely present at birth but tend to occur in the first few years of life. Initially they have varied morphologies, such as erosions, small blisters, crusts and thin papules, which may have features suggestive of impetigo, acne, or varicella. These lesions subsequently develop hypertrophic, and less often atrophic, scarring. Over time the face and trauma-prone sites develop yellowish infiltrated papules and nodules, reminiscent of cutaneous changes observed with porphyria. Scalp lesions may result in scarring alopecia.

Over years the majority of patients will display the characteristic small beaded papules along the eyelid margins (moniliform blepharosis) and lips; however, this is not typically observed in young children. In addition to these findings, less distinctive firm papules may develop on the neck, armpits, hands, elbows, and knees. Similar lesions may involve the oral mucosa, with resultant loss of teeth and various degrees of ankyloglossia.

Extracutaneous Findings

Hoarseness and a weak cry secondary to thickened vocal cords may be present at birth and are usually the first signs of the disease. Even though virtually every organ has been reported to be involved, lipoid proteinosis runs a chronic benign course. Apart from the laryngeal and mucosal involvement, the central nervous system is most commonly affected, resulting in seizures or behavioral changes. Frequently, intracranial calcifications, most often in the temporal lobes, are noted on radiographs from affected individuals.

Etiology and Pathogenesis

Pathogenic mutations have been found in the extracellular matrix protein 1 gene (ECM1).[103] Studies have shown that ECM1 is also a target antigen for autoantibodies in patients with the acquired disease lichen sclerosus. The precise function of ECM1 is still unknown, but this glycoprotein appears to have a role in the regulation of blood vessel physiology and anatomy in the skin.

Diagnosis and Differential Diagnosis

Routine histology of affected skin demonstrates deposition of amorphous eosinophilic, PAS-positive, hyaline-like material forming concentric rings around microvasculature of the dermis. The mucosa, especially the larynx, and internal organs may likewise be affected. Ultrastructurally, there is disruption and reduplication of the basement membrane around blood vessels and at the dermoepidermal junction. Lipoid proteinosis must first be differentiated from erythropoietic protoporphyria. Lesions in sun-protected and mucosal sites when porphyrin levels are normal assist in this distinction. Other diseases to consider in the differential include papular mucinosis, amyloidosis, cutaneous xanthomas, and leprosy. The rare finding of persistent hoarseness in infancy should be differentiated from congenital hypothyroidism, congenital dysphonia, junctional epidermolysis bullosa, and Farber lipogranulomatosis (see previous section).

Treatment, Course, and Management

There is no generally accepted treatment. Mucosal stripping of the vocal cords can temporarily relieve hoarseness, and dermabrasion has been performed on skin lesions. Dimethyl sulfoxide, D-pencillamine and etretinate have reportedly been attempted, with varying responses.[104] The overall course is generally benign, with progression throughout childhood and stabilization in early adulthood therefore supportive care is a rational approach.

REFERENCES

1. Francis JS, Sybert VP, Benjamin, DR. Congenital monocytic leukemia: Report of a case with cutaneous involvement, and review of the literature. Pediatr Dermatol 1989; 6: 306–311.
2. Resnik KS, Brod BB. Leukemia cutis in congenital leukemia. Arch Dermatol 1993; 129: 1301–1306.
3. Lestringant GG, Masouye I, El-Hayek M, et al. Diffuse calcinosis cutis in a patient with congenital leukemia and leukemia cutis. Dermatology 2000; 200: 147–150.
4. Gottesfeld E, Silverman A, Coccia PF, et al. Transient blueberry muffin appearance of a newborn with congenital monoblastic leukemia. J Am Acad Dermatol 1989; 21: 347–351.
5. Yen A, Sanchez R, Oblender M, et al. Leukemia cutis: Darier's sign in a neonate with acute lymphoblastic leukemia. J Am Acad Dermatol 1996; 34: 375–378.
6. Bhatt S, Schreck R, Graham JM, et al. Transient leukemia with trisomy 21: Description of a case and review of the literature. Am J Genet 1995; 58: 310–314.
7. Solky BA, Yang CF, Xu X, et al. Transient myeloproliferative disorder causing a vesiculopustular eruption in a phenotypically normal neonate. Pediatr Dermatol 2004; 21: 551.
8. Viros A, Garcia-Patos V, Aparicio G, et al. Sterile neonatal pustulosis associated with transient myeloproliferative disorder in twins. Arch Dermatol 2005; 141: 1053–1054.
9. van den Berg H, Hopman AH, Kraakman KC, et al. Spontaneous remission in congenital leukemia is not related to (mosaic) trisomy 21: case presentation and literature review. Pediatr Hematol Oncol 2004; 21: 135–144.
10. Dinulos JG, Hawkins DS, Clark BS, et al. Spontaneous remission of congenital leukemia. J Pediatr 1997; 131: 300–303.
11. Minkov M, Prosch H, Steiner M, et al. Langerhans cell histiocytosis in neonates. Pediatr Blood Cancer 2005; 45: 802–807.

11A. Alston RD, Tatevossian RG, McNally RJ, et al. Incidence and survival of childhood Langerhans' cell histiocytosis in Northwest England from 1954 to 1998. Pediatr Blood Cancer 2006; [Epub ahead of print].
12. Stiakaki E, Giannakopoulou C, Kouvidi E, et al. Congenital systemic Langerhans' cell histiocytosis (Report of two cases). Haematologia 1997; 28: 215–222.
13. Esterly NB, Maurer HS, Gonzalez-Crussi F. Histiocytosis X: A seven-year experience at a children's hospital. J Am Acad Dermatol 1985; 13: 481–496.
14. Enjolras O, Leibowitch M, Bocanini F, et al. Congenital cutaneous Langerhans' cell histiocytosis; a seven cases report. Ann Dermatol Venereol 1992; 119: 111–117.
15. The French Langerhans' Cell Histiocytosis Study Group. A multicentre retrospective survey of Langerhans' cell histiocytosis: 348 cases observed between 1983 and 1993. Arch Dis Child 1996; 75: 17–24.
16. Munn S, Chu AC. Langerhans' cell histiocytosis of the skin. Hematol Oncol Clin North Am 1998; 12: 269–286.
17. Shaffer MP, Walling HW, Stone MS. Langerhans' cell histiocytosis presenting as blueberry muffin baby. J Am Acad Dermatol 2005; 53: S143–146.
18. De Berker D, Lever LR, Windebank K. Nail features in Langerhans' cell histiocytosis. Br J Dermatol 1994; 130: 523–527.
19. Hashimoto K, Pritzker MS. Electron microscopic study of reticulohistiocytoma; an unusual case of congenital, self-healing reticulohistiocytosis. Arch Dermatol 1973; 107: 263–270.
20. Herman LE, Rothman KF, Harawi S, et al. Congenital self-healing reticulohistiocytosis. Arch Dermatol 1990; 126: 210–212.
21. Hashimoto K, Takahashi S, Lee RG, et al. Congenital self-healing reticulohistiocytosis. J Am Acad Dermatol 1984; 11: 447–454.

22. Kapila PK, Grant-Kels JM, Allred C, et al. Congenital, spontaneously regressing histiocytosis: Case report and review of the literature. Pediatr Dermatol 1985; 2: 312–317.
23. Longaker MA, Frieden IJ, LeBoit PE, et al. Congenital 'self-healing' Langerhans' cell histiocytosis: the need for long term follow-up. J Am Acad Dermatol 1994; 31: 910–916.
24. Arico M, Egeler RM. Clinical aspects of Langerhans' cell histiocytosis. Hematol Oncol Clin North Am 1998; 12: 247–258.
25. Schmitz L, Favara BE. Nosology and pathology of Langerhans' cell histiocytosis. Hematol Oncol Clin North Am 1998; 12: 221–247.
26. Geissmann F, Thomas C, Emile JF, et al. Digestive tract involvement in Langerhans' cell histocytosis. The French Langerhans' Cell Histiocytosis Study Group. J Pediatr 1996; 129: 836–845.
27. Henter, J-I, Arico M, Elinder G, et al. Familial hemophagocytic lymphohistiocytosis. Hematol Oncol Clin North Am 1998; 12: 417–433.
28. Soule EH, Pritchard DJ. Fibrosarcoma in infants and children. Cancer 1977; 40: 1711–1721.
29. Loh ML, Ahn P, Perez-Atayde AR, et al. Treatment of infantile fibrosarcoma with chemotherapy and surgery: results from the Dana-Farber Cancer Institute and Children's Hospital, Boston. J Pediatr Hematol Oncol 2002; 24: 722–726.
30. Balsaver AM, Butler JJ, Martin RG. Congenital fibrosarcoma. Cancer 1967; 20: 1607–1616.
31. Chung EB, Enzinger FM. Infantile fibrosarcoma. Cancer 1976; 38: 729–739.
32. Hayward PG, Orgill DP, Mulliken JB, et al. Congenital fibrosarcoma masquerading as lymphatic malformation: Report of two cases. J Pediatr Surg 1995; 30: 84–88.
33. Boon LM, Fishman SJ, Lund DP, et al. Congenital fibrosarcoma masquerading as congenital hemangioma: Report of two cases. J Pediatr Surg 1995; 30: 1378–1381.

33A. Muzaffar AR, Friedrich JB, Lu KK, Hanel DP. Infantile fibrosarcoma of the hand associated with coagulopathy. Plast Reconstr Surg 2006; 117: 81e–86e.

34. Neifeld JP, Berg JW, Godwin D, et al. A retrospective epidemiologic study of pediatric fibrosarcomas. J Pediatr Surg 1978; 13: 735–739.

35. Ferguson WS. Advances in the adjuvant treatment of infantile fibrosarcoma. Exp Rev Anticancer Ther 2003; 3: 185–191.

36. Kahn TA, Liranzo MO, Vidimos AT, et al. Pathological case of the month. Arch Pediatr Adolesc Med 1996; 150: 549–550.

37. Annessi G, Cimitan A, Girolomoni G, et al. Congenital dermatofibrosarcoma protuberans. Pediatr Dermatol 1993; 10: 40–42.

38. Terrier-Lacombe MJ, Guillou L, Maire G, et al. Dermatofibrosarcoma protuberans, giant cell fibroblastoma, and hybrid lesions in children: clinicopathologic comparative analysis of 28 cases with molecular data – a study from the French Federation of Cancer Centers Sarcoma Group. Am J Surg Pathol 2003; 27: 27–39.

39. McKee PH, Fletcher CD. Dermatofibrosarcoma protuberans presenting in infancy and childhood. J Cutan Pathol 1991; 18: 241–246.

40. Hobbs ER, Wheeland RG, Bailin PL, et al. Treatment of dermatofibrosarcoma protuberans with Mohs micrographic surgery. Ann Surg 1988; 207: 102–107.

41. Hawthorne HC, Nelson JS, Witzleben CL, et al. Blanching subcutaneous nodules in neonatal neuroblastoma. J Pediatr 1970; 77: 297–300.

42. Lucky AW, McGuire J, Komp DM. Infantile neuroblastoma presenting with cutaneous blanching nodules. J Am Acad Dermatol 1982; 6: 389–391.

43. Boyd TK, Schofield DE. Monozygotic twins concordant for congenital neuroblastoma: Case report and review of the literature. Pediatr Pathol Lab Med 1995; 15: 931–940.

44. Brodeur GM, Prithcard J, Berthold F. Revisions of the international criteria of neuroblastoma diagnosis. J Clin Oncol 1993; 11: 1466–1477.

45. Yang P, Grufferman S, Khoury MJ, et al. Association of childhood rhabdomyosarcoma with neurofibromatosis type I and birth defects. Gen Epidemiol 1995; 12: 467–474.

45A. Ilyas EN, Goldsmith K, Lintner R, Manders SM. Rhabdomyosarcoma arising in a giant congenital melanocytic nevus. Cutis 2004; 73: 39–43.

46. Wiss K, Solomon A, Raimer S, et al. Rhabdomyosarcoma presenting as a cutaneous nodule. Arch Dermatol 1988; 124: 1687.

47. Maurer HM, Gehan EA, Hayes DM, et al. The Intergroup Rhabdomyosarcoma Study II. Cancer 1993; 71: 1904–1922.

48. Ceballos PI, Ruiz-Maldonado R, Mihm MC. Melanoma in children. N Engl J Med 1995; 332: 656–662.

49. Trozak DJ, Rowland WD, Hu F. Metastatic malignant melanoma in prepubertal children. Pediatr Clin 1973; 191–204.

50. Prose NS, Laude TA, Heilman ER, et al. Congenital malignant melanoma. Pediatrics 1987; 79: 967–970.

51. Ruiz-Maldonado R, Orozco-Covarrubias L. Malignant melanoma in children. Arch Dermatol 1997; 133: 363–371.

52. Naraysingh V, Busby GO. Congenital malignant melanoma. J Pediatr Surg 1986; 21: 81–82.

53. Schneiderman H, Wu AY, Campbell WA. Congenital melanoma with multiple prenatal metastases. Cancer 1987; 60: 1371–1377.

54. Cavell B. Transplacental metastasis of malignant melanoma. Acta Pediatr 1963; 146: 37–40.

55. Hendrickson MR, Ross JC. Neoplasms arsing in giant congenital nevi. Morphologic study of seven cases and a review of the literature. Am J Surg Pathol 1981; 5: 109–135.

56. Silvers DN, Helwig EB. Melanocytic nevi in neonates. J Am Acad Dermatol 1981; 4: 166–175.

57. Ceballos PI, Ruiz-Maldonado R, Mihm MC. Melanoma in children. N Engl J Med 1995; 332: 656–662.

58. April MM, Ward RF, Garelick JM. Diagnosis, management, and follow-up of congenital head and neck teratomas. Laryngoscope 1998; 108: 1398–1401.

59. Kettelhut BV, Metcalfe OD. Pediatric mastocytosis. J Invest Dermatol 1991; 96: 15s–18s.

60. Stein DH. Mastocytosis: a review. Pediatr Dermatol 1986; 3: 365–375.

61. Boyano T, Carrascosa T, Val J, et al. Urticaria pigmentosa in monozygotic twins. Arch Dermatol 1990; 126: 1375–1376.

62. Caplan RM. The natural course of urticaria pigmentosa. Arch Dermatol 1963; 87: 146–157.

63. Neri I, Guareschi E, Guerrini V, Patrizi A. Familial telangiectasia macularis eruptiva perstans. Pediatr Dermatol 2005; 22: 488–489.

64. Lucaya J, Perez-Candela V, Celestina A, et al. Mastocytosis with skeletal and gastrointestinal involvement in infancy. Two case reports and a review of the literature. Radiology 1979; 131: 363–366.

65. Kettelhut BV, Metcalfe DD. Plasma histamine concentration in the evaluation of pediatric mastocytosis. J Pediatr 1987; 111: 419–421.

66. Shah PY, Sharma V, Worobec AS, et al. Congenital bullous mastocytosis with myeloproliferative disorder and c-kit mutation. J Am Acad Dermatol 1998; 39: 119–121.

67. Kettelhut BV, Metcalfe DD. Pediatric mastocytosis. Ann Allergy 1994; 73: 197–202.

68. Mauleón-Fernández C, Sáez-de-Ocariz M, Rodriguez-Jurado R, et al. Nodular scabies mimicking urticaria pigmentosa in an infant. Clin Exp Dermatol 2005; 30: 595–596.

69. Azana MJ, Torrelo A, Mediero IG, et al. Urticaria pigmentosa: A review of 67 pediatric cases. Pediatr Dermatol 1994; 11: 102–106.

70. Murphy M, Walsh D, Drumm B, Watson R. Bullous mastocytosis: a fatal outcome. Pediatr Dermatol 1999; 16: 452–455.

71. Kettelhut BV, Berkebile C, Bradley D, et al. A double-blind placebo controlled, crossover trial of ketotifen versus hydroxyzine in the treatment of pediatric mastocytosis. J Allergy Clin Immunol 1989; 83: 866–870.

72. Horan RF, Sheffer AL, Austen KF. Cromolyn sodium in the management of systemic mastocytosis. J Allergy Clin Immunol 1990; 85: 852–855.

73. Turk J, Oates JA, Roberts LJ. Intervention with epinephrine in hypotension associated with mastocytosis. J Allergy Clin Immunol 1983; 71: 189–192.

74. Smith ML, Orton PW, Chu H, et al. Photochemotherapy of dominant, diffuse, cutaneous mastocytosis. Pediatr Dermatol 1990; 7: 251–255.

75. Kan AE, Rogers M. Juvenile hyaline fibromatosis: an expanded clinicopathologic spectrum. Pediatr Dermatol 1989; 6: 68–75.

76. Fayad MN, Yacoub A, Salman S, et al. Juvenile hyaline fibromatosis: Two new patients and review of the literature. Am J Med Genet 1987; 26: 123–131.

77. Dowling O, Difeo A, Ramirez MC, et al. Mutations in capillary morphogenesis gene-2 result in the allelic disorders juvenile hyaline fibromatosis and infantile systemic hyalinosis. Am J Hum Genet 2003; 73: 957–966.

78. Hanks S, Adams S, Douglas J, et al. Mutations in the gene encoding capillary morphogenesis protein 2 cause juvenile hyaline fibromatosis and infantile systemic hyalinosis. Am J Hum Genet 2003; 73: 791–800.

79. Winchester P, Grossman H, Lim WN, et al. A new acid mucopolysaccharidosis with skeletal deformities simulating rheumatoid arthritis. Am J Roentgenol 1969; 106: 121–128.

80. Farber S. A lipid metabolic disorder – disseminated 'lipogranulomatosis' a syndrome with similarity to, and important difference from, Niemann–Pick and Hand–Schuller–Christian diseases. Am J Dis Child 1952; 84: 499–500.

81. Abenoza P, Sibley RK. Farber's disease: A fine structural study. Ultrastruct Pathol 1987; 11: 397–403.

82. Vormoor J, Ehlert K, Groll AH, et al. Successful hematopoietic stem cell transplantation in farber disease. J Pediatr 2004; 144: 132–134.

83. Haraoka G, Muraoka M, Yoshioka N, et al. First case of surgical treatment of Farber's disease. Ann Plast Surg 1997; 39: 405–410.

84. Fensome AH, Benson PF, Neville BR, et al. Prenatal diagnosis of Farber's disease. Lancet 1979; 2: 990–992.

85. Leroy JG, Martin JJ. Mucolipidosis II (I-cell disease): Present status of knowledge. Birth Defects Orig Artic Ser 1975; 11: 283–293.

86. Terashima Y, Tsuda K, Isomura S, et al. I-cell disease: Report of three cases. Am J Dis Child 1975; 129: 1083–1090.

87. McDowell G, Gahl WA. Inherited disorders of glycoprotein synthesis: Cell biological insights. Proc Soc Exp Biol Med 1997; 215: 145–157.

88. Leroy JG, Demars RI. Mutant enzymatic and cytological phenotypes in cultured human fibroblasts. Science 1967; 157: 804–806.

89. von Figura K, Haslik A, Pohlmann R, et al. Mutations affecting transport and stability of lysosomal enzymes. Enzyme 1987; 38: 144–153.

90. Grewal S, Shapiro E, Braunlin E, et al. Continued neurocognitive development and prevention of cardiopulmonary complications after successful BMT for I-cell disease: a long-term follow-up report. Bone Marrow Transplant 2003; 32: 957–960.

91. Aula P, Rapola J, Autio S, et al. Prenatal diagnosis and fetal pathology of I-cell disease (mucolipidosis type II). J Pediatr 1975; 87: 221–226.

92. Carey WF, Jaunzems A, Richardson M, et al. Prenatal diagnosis of mucolipidosis II – electron microscopy and biochemical evaluation. Prenat Diagn 1999; 19: 252–256.

93. Muenzer J. Mucopolysaccharidoses. Adv Pediatr 1986; 33: 269–302.

94. Matsuyama T, Sly WS, Kondo N, et al. Treatment of MPS VII (Sly syndrome) by allogeneic BMT in a female with homozygous A619V mutation. Bone Marrow Transplant 1998; 21: 629–634.

95. Hirschhorn K, Willner J. Disorders of metabolism. In: Spitz JL, ed. Genodermatoses: a full-color clinical guide to genetic skin disorders. Baltimore: Williams & Wilkins, 1996; 266–267.

96. Schiro JA, Mallory SB, Demmer L, et al. Grouped papules in Hurler–Scheie syndrome. J Am Acad Dermatol 1996; 35: 868–870.

97. Maize J, Metcalf J. Metabolic diseases of the skin. In: Elder D, Elenitsas R, Jaworsky C, et al., eds. Lever's histopathology of the skin, 8th edn. Philadelphia: Lippincott-Raven, 1997; 393.

98. Vellodi A, Young EP, Cooper A, et al. Bone marrow transplantation for mucopolysaccharidosis type I: Experience of two British centres. Arch Dis Child 1997; 76: 92–99.

99. Kakkis ED, Muenzer J, Tiller GE, et al. Enzyme-replacement therapy in mucopolysaccharidosis I. N Engl J Med 2001; 344: 182–188.

100. Wraith JE, Clarke LA, Beck M, et al. Enzyme replacement therapy for mucopolysaccharidosis I: a randomized, double-blinded, placebo-controlled, multinational study of recombinant human alpha-L-iduronidase (laronidase). J Pediatr 2004; 144: 581–588.

101. Wraith JE, Hopwood JJ, Fuller M, et al. Laronidase treatment of mucopolysaccharidosis I. BioDrugs 2005; 19: 1–7

102. Fensom AH, Benson PF. Recent advances in the prenatal diagnosis of the mucopolysaccharidoses. Prenat Diagn 1994; 14: 1–12.

103. Hamada T, McLean WH, Ramsay M, et al. Lipoid proteinosis maps to 1q21 and is caused by mutations in the extracellular matrix protein 1 gene (ECM1). Hum Mol Genet 2002; 11: 833–840.

104. Gruber F, Manestar D, Stasic A, Grgurevic Z. Treatment of lipoid proteinosis with etretinate. Acta Dermatol Venereol 1996; 76: 154–155.

26

Selected Hereditary Diseases

Dean S. Morrell, Craig N. Burkhart, Dawn Siegel

Our understanding of disease inheritance is rapidly evolving. This chapter discusses selected hereditary diseases with significant cutaneous manifestations, including neurocutaneous syndromes, disorders of laxity and redundant skin, mosaic disorders, photosensitivity disorders, ectodermal dysplasias, chromosomal disorders, and selected miscellaneous diseases. Many other inherited disorders are discussed in other chapters. Several textbooks and websites discuss genetic diseases in a comprehensive fashion. The reader is referred to OMIM (On-line Mendelian Inheritance in Man; http://www.ncbi.nlm.nih.gov/entrez/query.fcgi?db=OMIM) in addition to other excellent textbook resources.

NEUROCUTANEOUS SYNDROMES

Many disorders share neurologic and dermatologic findings. Disorders for which the major diagnostic features occur in the skin and in which the neurologic abnormalities figure significantly are referred to as neurocutaneous syndromes. A variety of conditions are included in this category. Many textbooks and reviews offer different listings of included disorders. The most universally accepted conditions under this heading are neurofibromatosis, tuberous sclerosis, and Sturge–Weber syndrome (see Chapter 20). We also include cerebello-trigeminal dermal dysplasia.

Neurofibromatosis Type 1

Neurofibromatosis 1 (NF1, MIM +162200) is a disorder characterized by multiple congenital and age-related abnormalities of tissue proliferation. Seven consensus criteria for the diagnosis of NF1 were established at the 1988 NIH conference as a guideline for clinical diagnosis (Box 26-1).[1] The cutaneous manifestations were chosen because of their high prevalence in adults, and noncutaneous features were selected to add specificity.

In 95% of affected individuals a diagnosis can be made by age 11 by clinical evaluation alone.[2] However, NF1 is a difficult condition to diagnose in the infant owing to the high incidence of sporadic mutations, variability of clinical expression, and age-related penetrance of individual clinical manifestations. Hence, anticipatory guidance counseling should be provided in all established and suspected cases of NF1.[3] Recognition of the possible age-related concerns may allow early diagnosis of medical complications that would otherwise be overlooked in standard health care.

Cutaneous Findings

Café au lait macules (CALM) are light to dark brown sharply defined macules on almost any skin surface (Fig. 26-1A).[2] Approximately 80% of individuals with neurofibromatosis will have over five such macules by the first year of life:[4] these are the major sign of NF1 evident in children under 5 years of age.[5,6] CALM may be present at birth, develop during early infancy, or take several years to develop. They continue to appear throughout childhood, especially after significant sun exposure. Infants with six or more café au lait macules larger than 5 mm in diameter which are not confined to a single segmental region should be evaluated and managed as though they have NF1, even without other signs of NF1, as the likelihood is high that they will develop other diagnostic signs (such as intertriginous 'freckling') with time. At puberty, if other features are lacking the approach and diagnosis can be reconsidered.

Crowe's sign is axillary and inguinal 'freckling' which may be present during infancy, but which often does not appear until late toddler/childhood years or later (Fig. 26-1B). These 'freckles' are really very small café au lait macules, rather than true ephilides. Although freckling on the neck and trunk is also common in NF1, it is not accepted as a diagnostic criterion.

Peripheral neurofibromas are infrequent in childhood NF1, occurring in only 14% of children less than 10 years of age.[7] However, it has been suggested that a subset of children with large deletions of the NF1 gene typically present with multiple neurofibromas in early childhood.[8]

Plexiform neurofibromas may present at birth or soon thereafter,[9] but occur in only 1% or less of patients and may be difficult to detect (Figs 26-1C and 23-7). There may be an orange-hued area or vascular stain, a coarse texture to the overlying skin, and increased overlying hair growth. Facial plexiform neurofibromas in particular often present only as mild asymmetric fullness of the face. Plexiform neurofibromas may grow rapidly and interdigitate with and surround normal structures. Radiologic imaging and neurosurgical consultation should be considered if lesions are extensive or close to major nerve bundles.

Extracutaneous Findings

Optic gliomas are astrocytomas arising anywhere along the optic pathway. These lesions tend to arise in infancy or early childhood. Half of the tumors are symptomatic, causing loss of visual acuity, decreased field of view, agitation and behavioral changes, or interference with the hypothalamopituitary axis.[4] Symptomatic optic gliomas are almost always

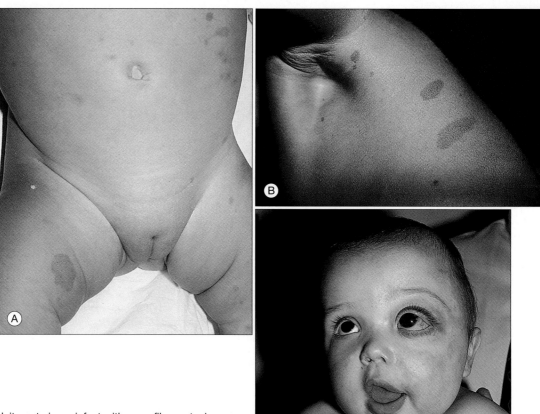

FIG. 26-1 (A) Multiple café-au-lait spots in an infant with neurofibromatosis. (B) Axillary freckling and multiple café-au-lait spots. (C) Plexiform neurofibroma of the left orgit causing proptosis. Note the slight skin thickening and faint hyperpigmentation. (Courtesy of Dr VP Sybert.)

Box 26-1 NIH consensus criteria for neurofibromatosis 1[1]

- ≥6 café-au-lait macules >5 mm in greatest diameter in prepubertal individuals or >15 mm in greatest diameter after puberty
- ≥2 neurofibromas of any type, or ≥1 plexiform neurofibromas
- Axillary/inguinal freckling (Crowe's sign)
- Tumor of the optic nerve pathway (optic glioma)
- ≥2 Lisch nodules (iris hamartomas)
- Distinctive osseous changes (e.g. sphenoid wing dysplasia or pseudoarthrosis)
- First-degree relative with NF1

diagnosed by 3 years of age. There is consensus that patients with NF1 require regular ophthalmologic examination, but the need for routine MRI scanning in asymptomatic children without signs of the presence of an optic glioma is controversial.[2]

Lisch nodules are pigmented iris hamartomas that rarely present in infants. They are best seen on slit lamp examination and do not result in functional disability. Only 20% of individuals under 5 years of age with NF1 have Lisch nodules. Congenital glaucoma occurs in less than 0.05% of individuals with NF1 and may present with an ipsilateral neurofibroma of the eyelid.

Macrocephaly is a relatively common finding, seen in 25% of cases, and can be an early clue to diagnosis. Relatively short stature has also been reported. These findings are seen with greater frequency than the more specifically diagnostic skeletal changes, pseudoarthrosis and sphenoid wing dysplasia. Congenital pseudoarthrosis represents failure of union after fracture and affects 5% or fewer of newborns or infants with NF1.[4] It is always unilateral and most commonly presents in the tibia as anterolateral bowing. Ultimately, pseudoarthrosis can progress to severe deformity. Sphenoid wing dysplasia is a unilateral defect of the orbit present in approximately 5% of individuals with NF1 and results in a change in orbit structure. Approximately half of those with sphenoid wing dysplasia develop an ipsilateral temporal–orbital plexiform neurofibroma, and half of individuals presenting with a temporal–orbital tumor have an underlying plexiform neurofibroma.[4]

Etiology/Pathogenesis

NF1 is due to an autosomal dominant mutation localized to chromosome 17 resulting in defects in neurofibromin, a tumor suppressor protein that stimulates hydrolysis of guanosine triphosphate (GTP) bound to *ras*.[10] Half of these mutations are inherited and the other half are sporadic.

Differential Diagnosis and Diagnosis

Café au lait macules may be found in many other conditions, including segmental pigmentary disorder and McCune–Albright syndrome (see Chapter 22). Autosomal dominant multiple café-au-lait macules are diagnosed in adults who have multiple CALM but no other features of NF1, but such a diagnosis cannot be made in infancy, with the possible exception of occurrence in a well-defined pedigree. Gene testing for NF1 is available from several commercial and research laboratories (see www.genetests.org for specific information). Decisions regarding whether laboratory-based NF testing is appropriate are best made in conjunction with a geneticist and genetic counselor.

Treatment and Care

Patients with neurofibromatosis require age-related anticipatory guidance counseling and regular follow-up with a pediatrician, ophthalmologist, orthopedist, neurologist, and dermatologist (Box 26-2). Ophthalmologists and neurologists should evaluate for optic nerve pathway tumors and glaucoma. Pseudoarthroses when present require prompt orthopedic evaluation, as the critical time for fracture and poor healing is infancy to early childhood.[4] Periodic evaluation for scoliosis is also needed. Regular physical examinations should include careful measurement of blood pressure because of a higher incidence of hypertension secondary to renovascular disease, vasoactive secreting tumors, and coarctation of the aorta.[4] Head circumference should be followed because of the risk of hydrocephalus and the occurrence of macrocephaly without hydrocephalus.[11]

Careful developmental assessment is a key part of management, as the risk of neurologic abnormalities and learning disabilities is increased.

Although dermal neurofibromas never transform to a malignant phenotype and should only be excised if they are symptomatic or disfiguring, plexiform neurofibromas require close evaluation. Skin should be palpated carefully as plexiform neurofibromas usually remain below the surface. MRI scans should be obtained to determine the extent of plexiform neurofibromas. Serial imaging may be necessary to assess potential growth. Pain and/or growth may herald malignant transformation, but this is exceedingly rare in infancy. Neurologic compromise may result from perineural extension, however, and neurology and/or neurosurgery may need to be consulted for plexiform lesions near neurovascular structures (such as the neck, axilla and spinal area.[4] Orbitotemporal neurofibromas may be better managed by numerous surgical procedures over time; plastic surgery should be involved early for management of these tumors.

Tuberous Sclerosis

Tuberous sclerosis (TSC, MIM #191100) is a multisystem disorder characterized by hamartomas, often in association with seizures and mental retardation. Owing to the variability

---

Box 26-2 Care plan: extracutaneous manifestations of neurofibromatosis 1

- Routine history and physical by a pediatrician
- Yearly blood pressure monitoring
- Baseline and periodic ophthalmologic examination
- Routine neurologic and developmental evaluation
- Regular head circumference monitoring
- Genetic counseling

---

in clinical features and causative mutations, some prefer the designation tuberous sclerosis complex for this disorder.

Cutaneous Findings

Hypomelanotic macules are usually present at birth or within the first few months of life. Classically, they present as an 'ash leaf macule,' an oval area with reduction in pigment (Fig. 26-2A). These areas can also be irregular in outline and shape, or very small and guttate (confetti-like) (Fig. 26-2B). In fair skinned infants Wood's lamp examination may be necessary to detect these lesions. They can also occur on the scalp, with lightening of the hair within the patch. They are found in almost 90% of TSC patients, but may disappear in adult life.

A single, hypopigmented macule without other features of TSC in an infant should not cause concern,[12] but multiple lesions should lead to further investigation. A single lesion or several lesions occurring along the lines of Blaschko suggests the diagnosis of nevoid hypopigmentation rather than TSC (see Chapter 21). Often the neurologic, cardiac, or renal features of TSC raise the question of TSC in a neonate, at which time a complete skin examination is performed, revealing hypopigmented macules. Every infant with infantile spasms, cardiac rhabdomyomas, or renal cysts should undergo a complete skin examination under both ambient and Wood's lamp illumination.

Angiofibromas typically appear after 4 years of age and are not pathognomonic for TSC. They also have been described in MEN1[13] and Birt–Hogg–Dube syndrome, and as an isolated autosomal dominant disorder.

Forehead plaques are connective tissue nevi which present as firm slightly raised lesions that are commonly erythematous and may initially resemble a hemangioma. They may be present at birth or appear shortly thereafter over the scalp, face, or neck.

Shagreen patches may also resemble hemangiomas when first developing, but usually present with firm, palpable thickened dermal plaques (Fig. 26-2C). Typically, these lesions occur in the lumbar region as a roughened area of erythematous skin with a rubbery consistency. They range in size from a few millimeters to 15 cm in diameter, and generally appear by adolescence. Periungual fibromas are uncommon in the first decade.

Extracutaneous Findings

Seizures occur in more than 60–80% of patients with TSC.[14,15] Conversely 4–50% of infants with infantile spasms have TSC.[15,16] TSC patients with early onset of seizures (less than 2 years of age) or infantile spasms have an elevated risk for mental retardation. Overall, 38–50% of affected patients with seizures develop mental retardation,[17,18] whereas this is rare in those without epilepsy.

Renal cysts, angiomyolipomas, and cardiac rhabdomyomas are findings in newborns and infants that suggest TSC. Cardiac rhabdomyomas are often discovered on routine antenatal ultrasound; 30–50% of infants with TSC have cardiac rhabdomyomas, and 80–90% of infants with these lesions have TSC.[19,20] They are rarely symptomatic and typically regress spontaneously.[21] An expert panel at the Tuberous Sclerosis Consensus Conference (1998) recommended a baseline electrocardiogram both at the time of diagnosis and prior to surgery, as cardiac rhabdomyomas can be associated with pre-excitation and arrhythmias on the electrocardiogram.[22]

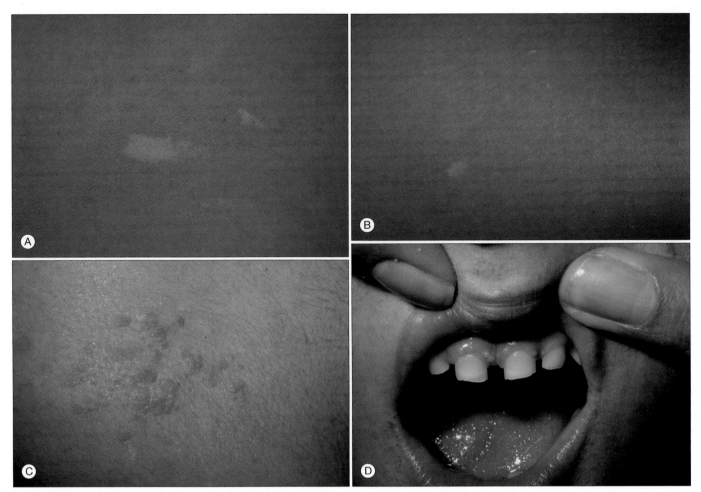

FIG. 26-2 (**A**) Ashleaf macules are often present at birth or noted early in infancy. (**B**) Confetti hypopigmentation typically becomes more common over time. (**C**) Shagreen patch: large shagreen patches may be congenital, whereas smaller ones typically develop over time. (**D**) Gingival fibromas are a less common feature, but occasionally develop in young children.

The most common renal manifestation of TSC is angiomyolipomas. They are identified in approximately 17% of children under 2 years of age and 92% aged 14–18 years.[23] By adulthood, they become bilateral and often too numerous to count. Fortunately, they rarely cause symptoms.[24,25] Renal cysts also increase in number and size with age, without causing symptoms.[26,27] However, some patients harbor a contiguous deletion of the *TSC2* and *PKD1* genes,[28] leading to end-stage renal disease in early adult life owing to autosomal dominant polycystic kidney disease. Hence, all patients newly diagnosed with TSC should have renal imaging to identify possible coexisting polycystic kidney disease.

Etiology/Pathogenesis

TSC may be caused by an autosomal dominant mutation in the *TSC1* gene (encoding hamartin) or the *TSC2* gene (encoding tuberin). The two proteins form a complex that is involved with the phosphoinositide-3-kinase (PI3K) signaling pathway, which regulates cell growth and proliferation.[29]

Differential Diagnosis

In general, characteristic skin lesions in a patient with seizures and/or mental retardation establish a diagnosis of TSC. Specific clinical diagnostic criteria for TSC were most recently revised at the Tuberous Sclerosis Complex Consensus Conference in 1998 (Box 26-3).[30] Features considered major criteria are believed to have a higher degree of specificity for tuberous sclerosis.[22]

Treatment and Care

Recommendations based on knowledge of the natural history of TSC have been made according to a United States Consensus Conference held in 1998 (Box 26-4).[22] The Scottish Clinical Genetics Service (http://www.genisys.hw.ac.uk/cgibin/WebObjects/genisys) and the UK Tuberous Sclerosis Association (http://www.tuberous-sclerosis.org/professionals/guidelines.shtml) have also created clinical guidelines. Neurology and/or neurosurgery should be consulted for management of seizures, brain tumors, and shunting of obstructive hydro-

Box 26-3 Clinical diagnostic criteria for tuberous sclerosis[30]

Major features
- Facial angiofibromas or forehead plaque
- Nontraumatic ungual fibroma
- ≥3 hypomelanotic macules
- Shagreen patch
- Multiple retinal nodular hamartomas
- Cortical tuber*
- Subependymal nodule
- Subependymal giant cell astrocytoma
- Cardiac rhabdomyoma
- Renal angiomyolipoma or pulmonary lymphangiomyomatosis**

Minor features
- Multiple randomly distributed pits in dental enamel
- Hamartomatous rectal polyps
- Bone cysts
- Cerebral white matter radial migration lines*
- Gingival fibromas
- Nonrenal hamartoma
- Retinal achromic patch
- 'Confetti' skin lesions
- Multiple renal cysts

Diagnostic requirements
- Definite diagnosis: two major features or one major and two minor features
- Probable diagnosis: one major and one minor feature
- Possible diagnosis: one major or two minor features

*Cerebral cortical dysplasia and cerebral white matter migration tracts count as one feature rather than two when they occur together.
**Other features of TSC must be present for a definite diagnosis when lymphangiomyomatosis and renal angiomyolipomas are both present.

Box 26-4 Care plan for tuberous sclerosis: testing recommendations in the neonate or infant at time of diagnosis
- Age-appropriate neurologic and developmental assessment
- Ophthalmic examination
- Neurologic consultation
- Cardiac evaluation
- Renal ultrasonography
- Cranial CT or magnetic resonance imaging

cephalus. Ophthalmology should examine patients to assist in confirming the diagnosis. Renal ultrasound is important to screen for patients who may have coexisting polycystic kidney disease. Some recommend echocardiography at diagnosis for confirmation (cardiac rhabdomyomas) and to screen for aortic aneurysms.[31] This is not standard practice, however, as the risk of developing cardiac dysfunction is small in asymptomatic patients, and no controlled trials have been carried out to confirm its value in these individuals.

Although treatment of facial angiofibromas was formerly delayed until adolescence, when the lesions have stabilized, early use of vascular lasers may limit their progression. Pulsed dye laser has been recommended for flat erythematous angiofibromas, and both KTP and carbon dioxide laser are used to treat more elevated lesions.[32] Fibrous forehead plaques are generally left untreated, but can also be treated with lasers or surgery.

Cerebello-Trigeminal Dermal Dysplasia

Cerebello-trigeminal dermal dysplasia (Gomez–Lopez–Hernandez syndrome, MIM 601853)[33] is a rare condition characterized by cerebellar, trigeminal nerve, and scalp abnormalities. Seven patients have been described to date. Alopecia appears on the scalp at birth, most often symmetrically in the parieto-occipital region. Later in life, patients may develop multiple facial scars secondary to self-injury related to trigeminal anesthesia.

Cerebellar alterations can be detected clinically and characteristic structural abnormalities are seen on both CT and MRI.[33,34] Patients have retardation of motor and mental development. Anesthesia occurs in the trigeminal distribution and cornea. The skull is asymmetric, with midfacial hypoplasia and low-set ears. Fifth finger clinodactyly, corneal opacities, and short stature have been reported in all patients to date.[33] Failure of migration and multiplication from a specific ectodermal region have been hypothesized to cause this syndrome.[35]

The differential diagnosis includes healed areas of aplasia cutis congenita; however, other signs of disease become evident in patients with cerebello-trigeminal dermal dysplasia as the individuals age. Consultation with a neurologist for evaluation and treatment of motor development delay, and neuropsychiatric evaluation and with an ophthalmologist for corneal abnormalities is recommended.

DISORDERS WITH SKIN LAXITY AND REDUNDANT SKIN

Soft, hyperelastic skin, lax skin, or redundant skin, with or without bruising, fragility, or abnormal healing, is seen in a variety of related and distinct inherited disorders. Most are clinically evident in infancy or early childhood, but a correct diagnosis may be delayed until later in childhood.

Cutis Laxa

Cutaneous Findings
Cutis laxa is a term that encompasses the clinical finding of loose, nonelastic skin that droops rather than stretches (Fig. 26-3). The skin is inelastic and does not spring back to place on release of tension. Three forms with different inheritance patterns have been described (Table 26-1). Loss of skin elasticity is progressive, and sagging may not be evident in the newborn, although in autosomal recessive disease flaccid skin is often evident at birth.[36] Autosomal dominant cutis laxa patients tend to develop skin laxity in later childhood.[37]

Extracutaneous Findings
All three forms may present in the newborn with skin changes, joint laxity, and abdominal and inguinal hernias. Pulmonary

emphysema may develop either during childhood or later in the course of disease.[36] In X-linked cutis laxa, bladder and gastrointestinal diverticuli can occur. Many newborns present with congenital dislocation of the hip. The characteristic long-bone and occipital exostoses (occipital horns) occur over time. Autosomal recessive disease is often more severe than the other forms, with flaccid skin evident at birth, early-onset emphysema, and vascular abnormalities such as aortic aneurysms or pulmonary artery/valve stenosis.[36] Death from com-

plications related to emphysema may occur early in infancy. The autosomal dominant form typically has fewer internal manifestations and a normal lifespan.[37]

Etiology/Pathogenesis

The disorder may be inherited or acquired. Only inherited forms are discussed in this chapter. Of the inherited forms, autosomal dominant, autosomal recessive, and X-linked forms have been described. The X-linked type is caused by mutations in the *ATP7A* gene leading to a deficiency in copper transport adenosine triphosphatase, MNK.[38] This results in malfunction of several copper-dependent enzymes, including lysyl oxidase, which is responsible for collagen cross-linking.[39]

Mutations in the elastin (*ELN*) gene have been found in some families with autosomal dominant cutis laxa.[40,41] Mutations in the fibulin 5 (*FBLN5*) gene have been found in individuals with autosomal dominant[42–44] and autosomal recessive cutis laxa.[45] Fibulin 5 is involved in the organization and stabilization of elastic fibers.[46]

Differential Diagnosis

Ehlers–Danlos syndrome (EDS) has similar skin laxity, but has the elastic recoil lacking in cutis laxa. Unlike in EDS, vascular fragility and problems with wound healing are lacking. Cutis laxa may also present as a component of other genetic disorders (Table 26-2). Acquired cutis laxa is often late onset and

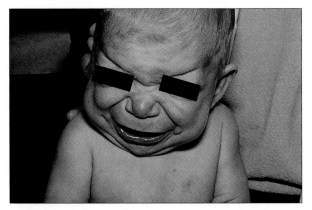

FIG. 26-3 Infant with cutis laxa. Droopy appearing face. (Courtesy of Dr VP Sybert.)

TABLE 26-1 Features of congenital cutis laxa[36]

Inheritance	Gene/protein	Cardiopulmonary abnormalities	Other abnormalities
Autosomal dominant	*ELN*/elastin, *FBLN5*/fibulin 5, others	None or emphysema	Ventral hernias, ligamentous laxity, gastrointestinal diverticuli
Autosomal recessive	*FBLN5*/fibulin 5, others	Severe emphysema, cor pulmonale, aortic aneurysm, pulmonary artery/valve stenosis	Ventral and diaphragmatic hernias, growth retardation, widened fontanelle, hip dislocation, gastrointestinal and genitourinary diverticuli
X-linked recessive (Ehlers–Danlos IX or occipital horn disease)	*ATP7A*/MNK	Tortuous carotid arteries	Occipital and long-bone exostoses, broad clavicles, shortening of long bones, osteopenia, joint laxity, chronic diarrhea, bladder diverticuli

TABLE 26-2 Genetic disorders with cutis laxa[48]

Disease	Inheritance	Other cutaneous findings	Extracutaneous findings
Costello syndrome	Autosomal dominant	Excessive wrinkling, deep creases at hands, feet, and neck Papillomata on nares, mouth, anus Acanthosis nigricans Coarse faces, thick lips, macroglossia	Hyperextensible digits Occasional abnormal glucose metabolism Failure to thrive Relative macrocephaly Short stature Mental retardation Hypertrophic cardiomyopathy
DeBarsy syndrome	Autosomal recessive	Progeroid facies Cutaneous atrophy	Short stature Frontal bossing Prominent nose and ears Hyperextensible small joints Choreoathetoid movements Mental retardation
Lenz–Majewski hyperostotic dwarfism	Unknown	Cutaneous atrophy Large ears	Generalized hyperostosis Proximal symphalangism Syndactyly Brachydactyly Mental retardation Hypertelorism Enamel hypoplasia

associated with drug exposure to penicillin, D-penicillamine,[47] or isoniazid. Alternatively, acquired disease may develop from crops of well-demarcated inflammatory plaques in association with fever, malaise, and peripheral neutrophilia or eosinophilia.[48] This form, which has sometimes been called 'Marshall syndrome' has been reported in infancy.[49] Areas of loose wrinkled skin are also evident in the so-called 'prune belly syndrome' where lax skin is seen in association with renal anomalies and hypoplastic abdominal musculature (Fig. 26-4).[50]

The diagnosis is confirmed by elastin staining (Verhoff–van Gieson, orcein) of a skin biopsy. X-linked disease has abnormally large collagen fibrils with normal elastic fibers, whereas autosomal disease has reduced elastin, an abnormal dense amorphous component, and variation in collagen fibril diameter with collagen 'flowers.' Low serum ceruloplasmin or copper levels may also help in the diagnosis of affected boys.[36]

Treatment and Care

All patients should have a complete physical examination for associated abnormalities, chest radiography to screen for emphysema and cardiomyopathy, and echocardiography for potential cardiac valve involvement (Box 26-5). Pulmonary function tests should be considered for early detection of emphysema. As solar elastosis aggravates cutaneous disease, sun protection should be emphasized.[51] Early parenteral copper-histidine replacement may prolong life and delay the onset of symptoms in patients with the X-linked form.[52]

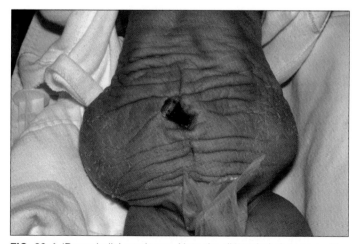

FIG. 26-4 'Prune-belly' syndrome. Note the distended abdomen with prominent skin laxity.

Box 26-5 Care plan: cutis laxa

- Complete physical examination
- Chest X-ray
- Consider pulmonary function tests
- Echocardiogram
- Surgical consult for diverticuli, rectal prolapse, and hernias
- Sunscreen protection
- Possible parenteral copper-histidine replacement (X-linked)

DeBarsy Syndrome

This rare condition is characterized by very lax, wrinkled skin and a progeroid facies with thin hair, thin skin, and lack of subcutaneous fat, present at birth without progression over time. A prominent vascular pattern is probably due to the thin dermis. Affected infants also have intrauterine growth retardation and poor postnatal growth. The hands are held in fists, whereas other joints are typically lax. Mental retardation is present; choreoathetosis develops over time. Eye findings include cataracts, strabismus, and myopia. The mode of inheritance is uncertain. Elastic fibers are decreased or frayed. Infants with other forms of cutis laxa do not have the progeroid appearance seen in this condition.[53]

Ehlers–Danlos Syndromes

The Ehlers–Danlos syndromes (EDS) are a group of inherited connective tissue disorders characterized by articular hypermobility, skin extensibility, and tissue fragility. A significant number of individuals with all types of EDS have cardiac abnormalities.[54] Originally classified as 11 separate disorders,[55] a new nomenclature has reduced these divisions to six (Table 26-3).[56]

Cutaneous Findings

Babies with the classic type of EDS have soft, velvety, extensible skin that feels like pudding and is very fragile with bruising and splitting secondary to minimal trauma. Wounds are slow to heal, quickly dehisce, and often resolve with cigarette paper-like atrophic scars. Patients with kyphoscoliosis-type and arthrochalasia-type EDS have less prominent skin fragility, bruisability, and dermal hyperextensibility than those with classic EDS.[54] Patients with the periodontal form have similar skin findings to those in classic EDS, but additionally have excessive wrinkling of the palms and soles. Over time, the skin becomes hyperpigmented and markedly atrophic. In dermatopraxis-type EDS patients skin is characterized by extreme fragility and is sagging, redundant, and not stretchable.

Rather than having the extensible and doughy skin seen in classic EDS, the skin in vascular-type EDS is thin and translucent with a visible vascular pattern (Fig. 26-5). It is not fragile and heals normally, but bruising is still common. Patients have a typical facial appearance, characterized by a thin nose, thin lips, and prominent eyes. Unless the disorder is already known to be in the family, none of these features is likely to be appreciated in the newborn or young infant.

Extracutaneous Findings

Forty percent of neonates with EDS are delivered prematurely.[57] All forms of EDS have joint hypermobility with joint dislocations; congenital dislocation of the hip occurs in the classic, vascular, and arthrochalasia types. Although the prevalence is unknown, cardiac and aortic abnormalities seem to be much more common than in the general population. This is most evident in patients with the vascular type of EDS, who are at high risk for rupture of medium-sized arteries, aorta, and bowel, either spontaneously or following minor trauma. Special precautions should be taken when performing surgery on these patients.[58]

TABLE 26-3 Clinical features, inheritance patterns, and biochemical defects of the Ehlers–Danlos syndromes[51]

Villefranche classification (1997)	Berlin classification (1988)	Cutaneous features	Extracutaneous features	Inheritance	Biochemical defects
Classic type	I (gravis), II (mitis)	Soft, hyperextensible skin; thin atrophic scars	Hypermobile joints; prematurity	AD	Type V collagen or tenascin-X
Hypermobility type	III	Soft skin	Large and small joint hypermobility	AD	Unknown
Vascular type (Sack–Barabas)	IV (arterial–ecchymotic)	Thin, translucent skin with visible veins; easy bruising; absence of skin and joint extensibility	Arterial, bowel, and uterine rupture	AD	Type III collagen
Kyphoscoliosis type	VI	Soft, hyperextensible skin	Muscle hypotonia; scoliosis; joint laxity	AR	PLOD1 gene (lysyl hydroxylase)
Arthrochalasia type	VIIA, VIIB arthrochalasia multiplex		Congenital hip dislocation, severe joint hypermobility	AD	Type I collagen
Dermatosporaxis type	VIIC	Severe skin fragility; sagging redundant skin		AR	Type I collagen N-peptidase
Other variants	VIII (periodontal)	Soft, hyperextensible skin; chronic purple-hued scarring over shins	Generalized periodontitis	AD	Unknown
	V (X-linked)	Soft, hyperextensible skin; easy bruising; thin atrophic scars		XLR	Unknown
	X		Joint laxity; clotting disorder	AR	Unknown

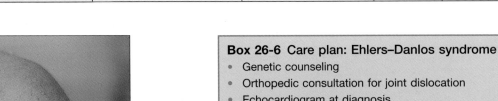

FIG. 26-5 Prominent visible venous pattern in EDS IV. (From Sybert VP. Genetic skin disorders. New York: Oxford University Press, 1997.)

Etiology/Pathogenesis

EDS is caused by mutations in various collagens, collagen-processing genes, and tenascin-X, which is a connective tissue protein. Autosomal dominant, autosomal recessive, and X-linked recessive inheritance has been described, depending on the subgroup (Table 26-3).

Differential Diagnosis

Cutis laxa also has hyperextensible skin, but it is loose and sagging, whereas the skin in EDS is elastic and recoils. Although patients with Marfan syndrome may also have mild to moderate joint hypermobility, the skin in newborns with Marfan syndrome does not show distinctive findings in this age group as it may in EDS.

Box 26-6 Care plan: Ehlers–Danlos syndrome
- Genetic counseling
- Orthopedic consultation for joint dislocation
- Echocardiogram at diagnosis
- Consider high-dose ascorbic acid
- Skin protection from trauma

Treatment and Care

Treatment of EDS is mostly supportive and preventative (Box 26-6). Large doses of ascorbic acid (a cofactor of lysyl hydroxylase), 2–4 g/day, have been used in patients with kyphoscoliosis-type EDS, with clinical response.[59] Specific therapies are not routinely used in other subtypes, although some physicians recommend high-dose ascorbic acid for all subtypes.[60]

A cardiovascular examination should be performed on all patients. Those with evidence of abnormalities or any patient with the vascular form of EDS should have an echocardiogram. Alternatively, some recommend echocardiography at diagnosis for all patients, to assess aortic size.[54]

Because of tissue friability, surgical procedures are difficult, with dehiscence and wound breakdown being common. Although scars will still spread over time, a combination of adhesive tape, skin closure surgical adhesive tape, absorbable running subcuticular suturing, increased density of sutures, or cyanoacrylate adhesives may facilitate healing. Pseudotumor formation may be prevented by applying pressure bandages to hematomas. Parents should be instructed on how to protect the infant from trauma.

MOSAIC DISORDERS

Our understanding of the genetics of mosaicism and its impact on skin development is increasing. In general, asymmetric and/or linear skin changes may be attributed to mosaicism, which can be result of distinct cell lines or X inactivation. Female carriers of X-linked disorders such as incontinentia pigmenti express pigment changes along the lines of Blaschko. Children mosaic for chromosomal aneuploidy may have hyperpigmentation or hypopigmentation along the lines of Blaschko, or in other patterns, such as a phylloid (leaf-like) or checkerboard appearance. These cutaneous patterns represent the endpoint of cell migration during embryogenesis.

Incontinentia Pigmenti

Cutaneous Findings

Incontinentia pigmenti (IP, MIM #308300)[61] is an X-linked dominant multisystem disorder with characteristic cutaneous manifestations. Classically, the skin changes occur in four stages: vesicular, verrucous, hyperpigmented, and atrophic. A patient may not develop all stages, and several stages may overlap.

In the newborn period, affected infants develop small, clustered blisters on an erythematous base, scattered along the lines of Blaschko (Fig. 26-6A). This stage usually resolves by 4–6 months of age, but milder, short-lived eruptions may continue during the first year of life or longer, sometimes associated with an acute febrile illness.[62] The second phase occurs as warty, hyperkeratotic, linear lesions (Fig. 26-6B, C), typically resolving by 6 months.[61] The presence and extent of the third, hyperpigmented, stage is highly variable (Fig. 26-6D) but is often unrelated to the distribution of the previous stages. Hyperpigmented streaks and whorls may coalesce to resemble 'Chinese writing figures.' By the age of 16, most pigmented lesions will have faded.[62] The last hypopigmented/atrophic stage becomes apparent with resolution of the lesions from the first three stages and demonstrates loss of hair and sweat glands. The face is usually spared in all stages. Alopecia and nail dystrophy are common.

The histopathology of IP is stage specific. Blisters show intercellular edema and intraepidermal vesicles filled with eosinophils, along with dyskeratotic keratinocytes. Patients may have peripheral eosinophilia or leukocytosis as well. Warty lesions show hyperkeratosis, papillomatosis, and mild dyskeratosis. In areas of hyperpigmentation, pigment-laden melanophages are evident in the dermis and focal dyskeratosis may also be present.

Extracutaneous Findings

Other organ systems are variably affected. The most characteristic ocular finding is retinal vascular proliferation,[63] which can result in bleeding, fibrosis, retinal detachment,[64] and in 10% of patients enough scarring to produce permanent visual impairment.[62] All neonates with IP need prompt and periodic evaluation by an experienced ophthalmologist. The magnitude of risk of central nervous system abnormalities is controversial but probably lower than previously believed, with current estimates varying from 10% to 30%.[61,65] Nevertheless, careful neurologic and developmental examinations should be carried out on all affected infants. Neonates do not display the dental anomalies seen later in life, which include missing or malformed teeth. Eosinophilia is found in more than 70% of patients. Multiple other malformations have been described in patients with IP, but it is questionable whether they are related or coincidental.

Etiology/Pathogenesis

IP results from mutations in the X chromosomal gene NEMO (NF-κB essential modulator),[66] which is involved in immune, inflammatory, and apoptotic pathways.[67] The mutation is believed to be lethal in affected 46,XY males, but male cases have been reported in the setting of XXY genotype, and other cases in males are presumably due to somatic mosaicism or half-chromatid mutations.

Differential Diagnosis

In the newborn, IP must be differentiated from other causes of blistering, including infectious (bacteria and herpes simplex virus), erythema toxicum, and epidermolysis bullosa (see Chapter 10). The warty phase of IP is unique, but may be confused with a linear epidermal nevus. Linear and whorled nevoid hypermelanosis may appear identical to stage 3 of IP. Although history helps to distinguish between the two conditions, a biopsy may be necessary, as stage 3 IP has occurred as late as 15 months of age without any antecedent skin changes.

Treatment and Care

The skin changes of IP do not require any treatment other than hygiene for blisters to prevent secondary infection. Baseline eye examination by an ophthalmologist and a full neurological assessment with anticipatory evaluation for the possibility of neurologic deficits are appropriate. Dental evaluation should be considered after teeth erupt.

Focal Dermal Hypoplasia of Goltz

Cutaneous Findings

Focal dermal hypoplasia (FDH, MIM %305600) is characterized by congenital linear or reticulated atrophic, hypo- or hyperpigmented lesions following the lines of Blaschko, often with prominent telangiectases (see Fig. 26-7A).[68,69] Fat herniations, hyperkeratosis, aplasia cutis, and scarring with pinpoint pore-like depressions may occur within these lesions (Fig. 26-7B).[70] The skin lesions are usually regarded as essential for the diagnosis, but cases without skin involvement have been reported.[71] Biopsy of affected areas reveals dermal hypoplasia with upward extension of subcutaneous fat almost to normal epidermis.

Other common findings include raspberry-like papillomas, which are commonly found on the perineum, vulva, anus, or lips. These vascular papillomas usually develop over time, but may be present at birth.[72] Nails are often dystrophic, and hair may be sparse and brittle.

Extracutaneous Findings

After skin disease, skeletal abnormalities constitute the second most constant manifestation of FDH and include limb reduction, asymmetric growth, small stature, and split-hand/split-foot malformations ('lobster-claw' deformity).[70] Vertical striations in metaphyses of long bones (osteopathia striata) may be seen in many patients and is a useful index for diagnosis.[73,74] Ocular abnormalities affect approximately 40% of patients and range from strabismus to microphthalmia.[70] Teeth are commonly malformed or absent. Less commonly

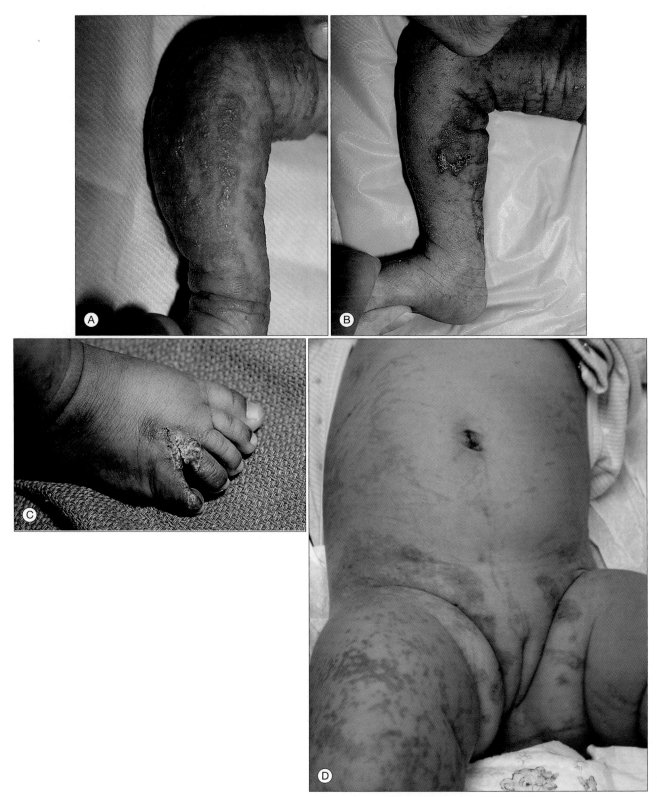

FIG. 26-6 Incontinentia pigmenti. (**A**) Erythematous, linear vesicles. (**B**) Vesicles, verrucous plaques, and early hyperpigmentation in a neonate. (**C**) Verrucous phase. (**D**) Widespread hyperpigmentation (phase 3) in a young infant; note that a few vesicles are also present.

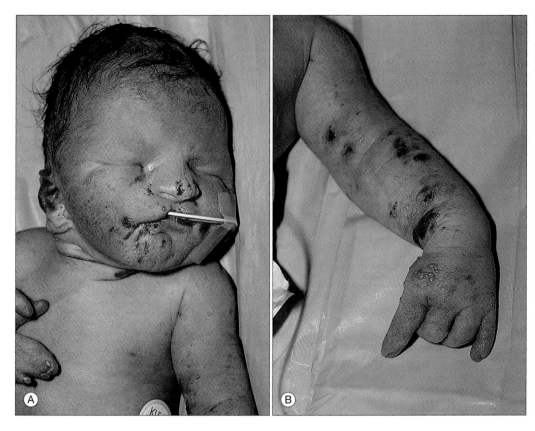

described findings include clavicular anomalies, abdominal wall defects, renal anomalies, and congenital heart defects.[70,75,76]

Etiology/Pathogenesis

FDH is X-linked dominant and presumed lethal in hemizygous males. Lyonization of the X chromosome may explain the cutaneous Blaschko linear distribution. Rare cases in males may arise from somatic mosaicism and half-chromatid mutations.[76,77]

Differential Diagnosis

The diagnosis of FDH is clinical, with histologic and radiographic corroboration (see above). Skin lesions of FDH do not blister and are static in comparison with IP. There is no epiphyseal stippling in FDH as in Conradi–Hunermann–Happle syndrome (X-linked dominant chondrodysplasia punctata), which also has linear ichthyosis and follicular atrophoderma as opposed to the telangiectases, hypo-/hyperpigmentation, and/or dermal atrophy of FDH. Distal extremities are not involved in MIDAS (microphthalmia, dermal aplasia, and sclerocornea) syndrome, and herniations of fatty tissue are not found. The initial skin changes of linear porokeratosis and porokeratotic eccrine and ostial dermal duct nevus may also resemble FDH, but evolution over time and histopathology can help to distinguish these conditions.

Treatment and Care

After a complete physical examination looking for possible systemic manifestations, the management of FDH is mainly symptomatic. Infants should be evaluated by dermatology, ophthalmology, and orthopedic surgery as needed because of the common occurrence of skeletal, cutaneous, and ophthal-

mologic disease. Other anomalies should be investigated in symptomatic individuals.

Proteus Syndrome

Proteus syndrome (MIM #176920) consists of segmental or mosaic overgrowth of body parts. Common complications include skeletal asymmetry, soft tissue overgrowth of the feet, linear epidermal nevi, vascular malformations, and tumor predisposition (see also Chapter 20).

Cutaneous Findings

Almost all individuals with Proteus syndrome have a dermatologic manifestation.[78] Over 40% of affected neonates will demonstrate at least some evidence of the disease at birth, such as epidermal nevi or vascular malformations.[79] The three main cutaneous findings are epidermal nevi, vascular malformations, and soft subcutaneous masses. Epidermal nevi are usually linear and verrucous,[80] but may only be hyper- or hypopigmented.[81–85] Malformations may be venous, capillary, and/or lymphatic. The connective tissue nevus, also known as cerebriform lesion, or moccasin lesion when on the sole of the foot, is caused by hyperplasia of cutaneous and subcutaneous tissues. The tissue is very firm and may also occur on the hands, perinasal area, or near the canthus. Prominent cutaneous venous structures may occur as a result of patchy dermal hypoplasia. Macrodactyly and lipomas may also be seen.[86]

Extracutaneous Findings

Overgrowth in Proteus syndrome is disproportionate, asymmetric, progressive, distorting, and persistent (Fig. 26-8). Overgrowth can occur in areas of the body that were completely normal at birth and involve bones, cartilage, muscle,

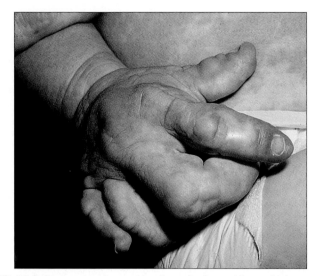

FIG. 26-8 Proteus syndrome. Hemihypertophy and lipomatosis. (Courtesy of Dr VP Sybert.)

> **Box 26-7 Diagnostic criteria for Proteus syndrome[136]**
> **General criteria**: Mosaic, *and* progressive, *and* sporadic
> **Category A:** Cerebriform connective tissue nevus
> **Category B:**
> 1. Epidermal nevus
> 2. Disproportionate overgrowth in two of: limbs, skull, external auditory canal, vertebrae, or viscera
> 3. Bilateral ovarian cystadenomas or monomorphic adenomas of the parotid gland in children
> **Category C:**
> 1. Dysregulated adipose tissue (lipoatrophy or lipomas)
> 2. Vascular malformations (capillary, venous, or lymphatic)
> 3. Facial phenotype (long face, dolichocephaly, downslanting palpebral fissures, low nasal bridge, wide or anteverted nares, open mouth at rest)
>
> *All three general criteria plus either one from A, two from B, or three from C required to make a diagnosis of Proteus syndrome.*

and connective tissues. Although much more dramatic postnatally, at least some overgrowth and asymmetry are present at birth in 17.5%.[79] Orifices may be affected, leading to respiratory obstruction, conductive hearing loss, or gastric outlet obstruction. Lungs may be involved with cystic degeneration, leading to an increased risk of pneumonia.[87] Patients are also predisposed to deep venous thrombosis and pulmonary embolism.[88] The central nervous system is most commonly affected by hemimegalencephaly (unilateral enlargement of the brain), but most patients are asymptomatic.[89] Ophthalmologic findings[90] are common and range from strabismus to epibulbar hamartomas. Ovarian cystadenomas and cystic lesions of the epididymis are also common.

Etiology/Pathogenesis
The cause of Proteus syndrome remains unknown. It is suggested that it represents a somatic mosaicism that is lethal in the nonmosaic state.[91] The role of *PTEN* mutations in Proteus syndrome is debated.[89]

Differential Diagnosis
Diagnostic criteria have been developed, which should be followed (Box 26-7). Most patients diagnosed with Proteus syndrome and referred to the National Institutes of Health do not meet published diagnostic criteria.[79,92–94] Several other disorders share asymmetric hypertrophy with Proteus syndrome. The most common disorder misdiagnosed as Proteus syndrome is hemihyperplasia with multiple lipomatosis, which is more common than Proteus syndrome and distinguished by the relative lack of severe progressive overgrowth and lack of pronounced cerebriform connective tissue nevi on the foot.[89,95] Other features of Proteus syndrome, such as vascular malformations, lipomas, and epidermal nevi, are seen in both conditions. Maffucci syndrome consists of multiple enchondromatosis (which may be confused with hyperostosis) and vascular malformations.[96] Klippel–Trenaunay syndrome consists of vascular malformations with overgrowth, typically in the same segment. Axillary freckling and neurofibromas help distinguish neurofibromatosis from Proteus syndrome.

Treatment and Care
Treatment of Proteus syndrome is often difficult. Orthopedic, ophthalmologic, neurologic, and pediatric care must be individualized. A multidisciplinary approach is needed to address all aspects of the disease adequately. Orthopedic surgery should be consulted before functional deficits become apparent.

Epidermal Nevus Syndrome (see also Chapter 23)

The sporadic association of epidermal nevi with developmental abnormalities in other organ systems constitutes epidermal nevus syndrome (ENS, MIM 163200).

Epidermal nevi vary according to their predominant component and include nevus sebaceus (sebaceous glands), nevus comedonicus (hair follicles) and verrucous nevus (keratinocytes). Multiple other mucocutaneous findings may occur simultaneously with the epidermal nevus. Central nervous, ocular, and musculoskeletal systems are predominantly affected. However, a wide range of abnormalities may occur within each of these systems, and occasionally other organ systems may be involved. ENS occurs sporadically. ENS should be considered in any patient with extensive epidermal nevi or epidermal nevi associated with systemic abnormalities. The possibility that an epidermal nevus is a component of another syndrome, such as Proteus, CHILD (congenital hemidysplasia with ichthyosiform nevus and limb defects), or phakomatosis pigmentovascularis, should be considered. Patients suspected of having ENS should have a thorough physical evaluation with special attention to the musculoskeletal, neurologic, ocular, and cardiovascular systems. Management should be multidisciplinary, depending on the findings of the physical examination.

MIDAS Syndrome

Microphthalmia, dermal aplasia, and sclerocornea (MIM #309801) are the hallmarks of MIDAS or MLS (microphthalmia and linear skin defects). Dermal aplasia typically presents as atrophic linear scars on the face, scalp, and neck

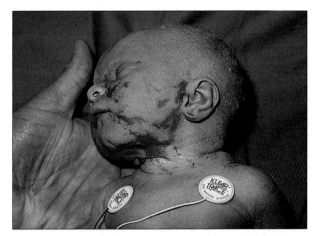

FIG. 26-9 Microphthalmia/linear skin defects. Atrophic linear scars on the face and neck.

(Fig. 26-9).[97] The skin shows irregular, linear, erythematous areas of atrophic skin similar in appearance to fresh lesions of aplasia cutis congenita. Eye defects are usually bilateral and include microphthalmia, corneal opacities, and orbital cysts. Congenital heart disease and neurologic abnormalities may be found.[98]

MIDAS syndrome is an X-linked dominant disorder caused in some cases by a deletion at the Xp 22.3 locus.[99]

In contrast to FDH, aplastic skin lesions are limited to the upper half of the body. Fat herniation and other manifestations of FDH, such as papillomas, clefting of the hands or feet, syndactyly, and coloboma, do not occur in MIDAS syndrome.

Patients should have complete physical and ophthalmic examinations, with treatment individualized to the patient.

PHOTOSENSITIVITY DISORDERS AND MISCELLANEOUS METABOLIC DISORDERS

Although some inherited skin disorders are exacerbated by sun exposure, few are noted to do so in the neonate or young infant. Congenital erythropoietic porphyria (Gunther disease) is discussed in Chapter 19, Hartnup disorder in Chapter 15, and xeroderma pigmentosum in Chapter 22. In this chapter, we will discuss Bloom syndrome and Rothmund–Thomson syndrome.

Bloom Syndrome
Cutaneous Findings
Bloom syndrome (congenital telangiectatic erythema, MIM #210900)[100] may present within the first 3 weeks of life as erythema and telangiectases develop on the cheeks in a butterfly distribution. Skin involvement spreads with exposure to sunlight to the nose, eyelids, forehead, ears, and lips. Progressive atrophy and actinic pigmentary changes ensue. Other cutaneous findings may include café-au-lait macules, areas of hypopigmentation, and/or acanthosis nigricans.

Extracutaneous Findings
Immunodeficiency is manifested primarily by severe recurrent pneumonia and gastrointestinal infections, which may lead to vomiting and diarrhea during infancy. Hypoglobulinemia, dys-

functional helper T cells, and abnormal delayed hypersensitivity may be found. Patients are born at full term with low birthweight and subsequent severe failure to thrive.[101] Other features include a long and narrow head with characteristic facies consisting of a narrow, prominent nose, hypoplastic malar areas, and a receding chin. After infancy patients may develop internal malignancies, diabetes, and reduced fertility.[102]

Etiology/Pathogenesis
Bloom syndrome is an autosomal recessive disorder most frequently found in Ashkenazi Jews. It is caused by mutations in BLM, a helicase of the RecQ family.[103]

Differential Diagnosis
Others disorders with photosensitivity typically have other distinguishing clinical features which help to distinguish them from Bloom syndrome. Neonatal lupus erythematosus has positive serologic markers for anti-SSA or SSB. More pronounced poikiloderma and differing associated malformations and facial features are found in Rothmund–Thomson syndrome. Xeroderma pigmentosum is characterized more by freckling and less by telangiectases on sun-exposed areas. Cockayne syndrome patients have a senile appearance, with cataracts, retinopathy, sensorineural deafness, and progressive neurologic deterioration. Metabolic disorders such as Hartnup disease and erythropoietic protoporphyria have other characteristic features.

Cytogenetic analysis can be used to confirm the diagnosis. Bloom syndrome patients have a high frequency of chromosomal breakage, sister chromatid exchanges, and quadriradial configurations.

Treatment and Care
Sun avoidance and the use of sunscreens may reduce photosensitive eruptions. Cosmetics may hide facial telangiectases. Appropriate antibiotic therapy may be needed for treatment of frequent bacterial gastrointestinal and respiratory infections. Periodically, patients should be evaluated by hematology/oncology for possible neoplastic disease. Endocrinologists should be consulted regarding management of short stature.

Rothmund–Thomson Syndrome
Cutaneous Findings
Rothmund–Thomson syndrome (RTS, MIM #268400) is a rare autosomal recessive genodermatosis characterized primarily by a sun-sensitive eruption, usually beginning between 3 and 6 months, but which may appear soon after birth or as late as 2 years. Beginning as erythema, edema, and blistering on the cheeks and face (acute phase), skin findings spread to the buttocks and flexural aspects of the extremities, sparing the chest, back, and abdomen. Over months to years, skin involvement develops into permanent reticulated pigmentation, telangiectases, and areas of punctuate dermal atrophy (poikiloderma). Patients may have sparse to absent hair, eyelashes, and/or eyebrows, and abnormal nails and dentition.[104] In later life, hyperkeratosis and frank photosensitivity develop in about one-third of patients. Nonmelanoma skin cancers have an estimated prevalence of 5%, which can occur at any age but generally earlier than in the general population.[105]

Extracutaneous Findings

Skeletal abnormalities are found in many patients and include dysplasias (abnormal trabeculation and/or irregular metaphyses, osteoporosis, absent or malformed bones, and delayed bone formation). Limb reduction defects, such as absent or malformed thumbs, radii, and ulnae, are reported in 4–11% of cases.[106]

Other physical findings have variable frequencies, reported as juvenile cataracts (45–47%), hypogonadism (29–94%), defective dentition (27–59%), and osteosarcoma (3–9%).[106]

Etiology/Pathogenesis

RTS is an autosomal recessive chromosomal instability syndrome. Of clinically diagnosed cases, 66% have mutations in the *RECQL4* gene, a member of the RecQ family of DNA helicases.[107] Although the function of *RECQL4* is not completely understood, it appears to be involved in DNA replication and chromosomal segregation.[108]

Differential Diagnosis

A definitive diagnosis of RTS is made clinically, based on the characteristic appearance and pattern of development of skin findings described above. If skin involvement is atypical, either in appearance, distribution, or pattern of onset and spread, a probable diagnosis of RTS can be made when two other features of RTS are present (e.g. a positive family history, osteosarcoma, skin cancer, skeletal abnormalities, cataract, sparse hair, or small stature). The poikiloderma that accompanies the telangiectases of RTS distinguish it from Fanconi, Bloom, and ataxia–telangiectasia syndromes. Nevertheless, one should consider diagnostic tests to exclude these syndromes during the work-up (i.e. increased sister chromatid exchange for Bloom syndrome, increased diepoxybutane (DEB)-induced chromosome breakage for Fanconi anemia, and increased α-fetoprotein for ataxia–telangiectasia).[109]

Treatment and Care

Neonates with RTS should be protected from the sun and have sunscreens with UVA and UVB protection applied daily. The eyes should be examined by an ophthalmologist at diagnosis, and annually thereafter. At the time of diagnosis, families should be counseled for the signs of osteosarcoma, including bone pain, swelling, or an enlarging lesion on a limb.[109] Because of concerns that areas of bone change may undergo malignant transformation, some suggest long-bone radiographs be obtained by age 3, with annual follow-up for dysplastic lesions.[110]

ECTODERMAL DYSPLASIAS

There are over 100 rare syndromes whose primary features involve alterations in two or more of the structures that derive from the embryonic ectoderm, which include developmental defects in hair, teeth, nails, sweat glands, and the lens of the eye. These are referred to as 'ectodermal dysplasias.' Although most are infrequent to rare in absolute terms, some of the more common are discussed in this chapter. The National Foundation for Ectodermal Dysplasia can be a great support for families and provides information to professionals caring for children with a wide variety of ED types (www.nfed.org).

Hypohidrotic Ectodermal Dysplasia

Hypohidrotric ectodermal dysplasia, (HED, Christ–Siemens–Touraine syndrome, MIM #305100)[111] is most often an X-linked recessive condition and is the most common form of ED encountered by clinicians.

Cutaneous Findings

Patients with hypohidrotic ectodermal dysplasia often present at birth with a collodion membrane or marked scaling of the skin, which may be misconstrued as a marker of congenital ichthyosis or of postmaturity.[112] After membrane shedding, the skin is soft, thin, and light-colored with fine periorbital wrinkling (Fig. 26-10). Patients have an increased frequency of atopic dermatitis, particularly periorbital dermatitis. Even in the neonatal period, the hair tends to be either absent or sparse, short, and blond. Nails are usually normal.

In cases without a positive family history, repeated bouts of unexplained fevers most often bring infants with HED to medical attention. As the infants produce little to no sweat, they cannot make the appropriate physiologic response to increased environmental temperature, resulting in core temperature elevation. Diminished or absent sweat pores may be appreciated both clinically and histologically.

Extracutaneous Findings

Most infants with HED have a typical facies that is easily recognizable to educated family members and/or physicians, characterized by a square forehead with frontal bossing, a flattened nasal bridge with prominent nostrils, wide cheekbones with flat malar ridges, a relatively thick everted lower lip, prominent chin, and small, pointed, low-lying ears. Lacrimal and mucous glands are hypoplastic, leading to reduced tearing or epiphora, chronic nasal discharge, and an increased frequency of otitis media and respiratory tract infections. As the teeth are not present in the neonatal period, the typical peg-shaped or missing teeth cannot be used to aid in diagnosis, but dental X-rays can demonstrate these findings, even in young infants.

Etiology/Pathogenesis

Most patients are male and carry the X-linked recessive form; however, mutations in several individual genes may lead to identical developmental abnormalities of the hair and glands.

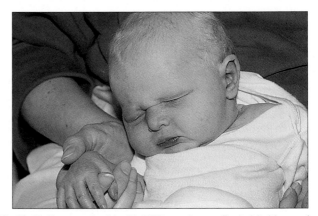

FIG. 26-10 Two-week-old with HED syndrome. Periorbital hyperpigmentation is evident. (From Sybert VP. Genetic skin disorders. New York: Oxford University Press, 1997.)

These include ectodysplasin-A1 (Eda-A1), Eda-A1 receptor (Edar), ectodysplasin-A2, Eda-A1 receptor (Xedar), and NF-κB essential modulator (NEMO).[113–116] Female carriers of ectodysplasin mutations show varied manifestations following the lines of Blaschko.

Differential Diagnosis

When an affected male is born to a family with other affected members, the diagnosis of HED is readily recognized. If there is no family history, repeated bouts of fever may be thought to have an infectious source and scaling at birth may be misdiagnosed as congenital ichthyosis. Clinical examination of mothers may detect the carrier state. Hypohidrosis may be found in another group of ectodermal dysplasias resulting from autosomal dominant mutations in p63 (Rapp–Hodgkin syndrome, AEC syndrome, EEC syndrome, limb–mammary syndrome, or ADULT syndrome), but that group has associated facial clefting and split-hand/foot malformations.[117,118]

Treatment and Care

Temperature must be carefully regulated with cool baths, air conditioning, light clothing, spray-mist bottles to dampen clothing during activities, and avoidance of warm environments (Box 26-8).[119] Some families find commercially available cooling suits to be helpful. Reduced glandular secretion may be treated with lubricating eye drops and nasal irrigation. Treatment of recurrent otitis media, respiratory infections, atopic dermatitis, and asthma should be individualized. Dental disease should be managed early.

Hidrotic Ectodermal Dysplasia

Cutaneous Findings

Also known as Clouston syndrome, hidrotic ectodermal dysplasia (MIM #129500) is an autosomal dominant form of hidrotic or 'sweating' ectodermal dysplasia characterized by nail dystrophy, hyperkeratosis of the palms and soles, and hair defects.[120,121] Affected newborns may have milky-white-appearing nails and dry skin, or may show no clinical signs. Chronic paronychial infections frequently develop. Hair may be normal during infancy and childhood, and the diagnosis may not be recognized until abnormal sparse, fine, and brittle hair is detected or progressive nail dystrophy develops.

Extracutaneous Findings

The terminal phalanges may be tufted. Individuals show normal sweating, facies, and dentition.

Etiology/Pathogenesis

Autosomal dominant mutations in connexin 30 (GJB6) cause the disorder.[122]

Box 26-8 Care plan: hypohidrotic ectodermal dysplasia

- Avoid overheating
- Consult dentistry
- Treat ophthalmic, ENT, pulmonary, and dermatologic disease as symptoms dictate
- Recommend families contact National Foundation for Ectodermal Dysplasias

Differential Diagnosis

Although it is a relatively common form of ectodermal dysplasia, it is not a diagnosis likely to be made in the newborn period in the absence of a positive family history. Nail dystrophy may be the only manifestation in one-third of patients. Swollen, tufted terminal phalanges may aid in diagnosis. One should differentiate hidrotic ectodermal dysplasia from pachyonychia congenita and other palmoplantar keratodermas (see Chapters 18 and 29).

Treatment and Care

Keratolytics and surgical debridement may be effective for keratoderma. Paronychial infections can be treated with antibiotics or anticandidal agents as appropriate.

Ectodermal Dysplasia due to p63 mutations

Several forms of ectodermal dysplasias with overlapping clinical features have been found to be due to mutations in p63, a transcription factor that is structurally related to p53, localized to gene locus 3q27. These include Rapp–Hodgkin syndrome, ectrodactyly, ectodermal dysplasia, and cleft lip/palate syndrome 3; ankyloblepharon–ectodermal defects–cleft lip/palate syndrome, acrodermato–ungual–lacrimal–tooth syndrome, limb–mammary syndrome, and nonsyndromic split-hand/foot malformation are caused by mutations in p63 as well.[123,124]

Ankyloblepharon–Ectodermal Dysplasia–Clefting (AEC) Syndrome

This syndrome (AEC, Hay–Wells syndrome, MIM #106260) is an uncommon form of ectodermal dysplasia with autosomal dominant inheritance.[125]

Cutaneous Findings

The upper and lower eyelids of the newborn have fine strands of skin between them (so-called ankyloblepharon) which are pieces of tissue that can be thick or thin, may tear spontaneously, or require surgical lysis (Fig. 26-11A). They are a cardinal feature of this condition, but are not mandatory for diagnosis. During the newborn period, the rest of the skin is erythematous and fissured with a collodion membrane appearance, resembling bullous congenital ichthyosiform erythroderma with peeling, erythema, and erosions (Fig. 26-11B) (see also Chapters 10 and 18). After the membrane has shed over the first few weeks, the underlying skin is dry and thin. Recurrent scalp infections, erosions, and granulation tissue may have their onset in early infancy and are present in two-thirds to three-quarters of older infants, children, and adults with this condition.[126] The hair is sparse and coarse. Sweating is usually not significantly affected. Nail dystrophy is variable. The nails can be thickened and malformed, thin or absent.

Extracutaneous Findings

Cleft palate, with or without cleft lip, is the third major sign of AEC syndrome, occurring in 80% of affected newborns. The reported hypodontia associated with the condition may reflect the degree of severity of the clefting, rather than a primary ectodermal defect.

A few males with AEC have had hypospadias. External ear malformations are described in some patients. Supernumerary

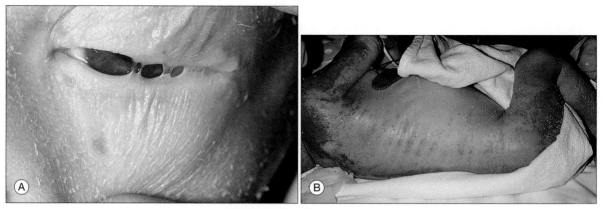

FIG. 26-11 (**A**) Fine strands of tissue between eyelids in AEC syndrome. (From Sybert VP. Genetic skin disorders. New York: Oxford University Press, 1997.) (**B**) Cracking erosions of skin of body in AEC. (From Vanderhooft SL, Stephan MJ, Sybert VP. Severe skin erosions and scalp infections in AEC syndrome. Pediatr Dermatol 1993; 10: 334–340.)

nipples and ectopic breast tissue occur in a minority of cases. There may be tear duct abnormalities and recurrent lid inflammation.

Etiology/Pathogenesis
AEC is caused by a mutation in p63 (see discussion above).

Differential Diagnosis
Other diagnoses to be considered when presented with an infant with cleft palate and a collodion membrane include EEC (ectodermal dysplasia, ectrodactyly, cleft lip/palate syndrome), distinguished by its limb involvement, and Rapp–Hodgkin syndrome. Chronic dermatitis of the scalp is possibly less frequent in Rapp–Hodgkin ectodermal dysplasia.[127] Not surprisingly, there is considerable overlap between Rapp–Hodgkin and AEC, as they are allelic. The presence of ankyloblepharon can distinguish the two, being a key characteristic of AEC, but now that the genetics of the conditions is appreciated a true distinction may not be truly necessary.

Treatment and Care
Treatment is limited to surgical management of eyelid involvement and oral facial clefting. The use of light emollients may speed the shedding of dry, cracking neonatal skin. Careful handling of the scalp and prompt attention to secondary bacterial infection may decrease long-term complications. Patients will require ongoing ocular hygiene.

Ectrodactyly–Ectodermal Dysplasia–Clefting Syndrome (EEC)

Cutaneous Findings
Cutaneous findings in EEC syndrome are mild. Fair skin and fine, sparse, light-colored hair are common features. Nails overlying abnormal and occasionally normal phalanges are dystrophic. Skin may be dry with occasional hypohidrosis.

Extracutaneous Findings
Ectrodactyly (abnormal development of the median rays of the hands and feet) serves to distinguish this disorder from other ectodermal dysplasias and occurs in 80–100% of affected individuals. Depending on the series, cleft palate with or without cleft lip occurs in 70–100% of patients.[128,129] Lacrimal duct hypoplasia or atresia is seen in over 90% of affected individuals, leading to excessive tearing, conjunctivitis, and blepharitis.[130-132] Genitourinary malformations affect over a third of patients. Chronic otitis media with secondary hearing loss occurs in 50%.[133]

Etiology/Pathogenesis
Three forms of EEC have been described, EEC1 (129900), EEC2 (602077), and EEC3 (604292). Most individuals harbor mutations in p63, a tumor-suppressor gene (see discussion above).[134]

Differential Diagnosis
The diagnosis of EEC is self-evident when all three features are present. In the absence of limb defects, other ectodermal dysplasias associated with oral facial clefting, including Hay–Wells, Rapp–Hodgkin, and limb–mammary syndromes, need to be considered. Other diseases with limb defects include odontotrichomelic syndrome, which presents with severe absence deformities of the limbs, and Adams–Oliver syndrome (aplasia cutis congenita with limb defects), which has neither clefting nor ectodermal defects other than localized absence of skin.

Treatment and Care
Treatment is mainly surgical. Consultations may include plastic surgery for cleft palate, orthopedics for limb repair, ENT for otitis media and hearing loss, ophthalmology for symptoms related to lacrimal duct hypoplasia, and urology for possible genitourinary malformations.

CHROMOSOMAL DISORDERS

Turner syndrome

Turner syndrome (Ullrich–Turner syndrome) occurs in approximately 1 in 3000 females and is caused by sex chromosome aneuploidy. Lymphedema, short stature, gonadal dysfunction, and cardiac malformations are the characteristic features (Box 26-9).

Cutaneous Findings
Lymphatic abnormalities are a common presenting manifestation of Turner syndrome (TS). Fetal edema, viewed on ultrasound, can lead to the prenatal diagnosis. Any infant presenting

Box 26-9 Clinical features: Turner syndrome

Dermatologic associations
Congenital lymphedema
Low posterior hairline
Webbed neck
Pigmented nevi
Cutis vertices gyrata
Hypoplastic, concave nails

Extracutaneous manifestations
Gonads:
  Infertility
  Streak gonads
Musculoskeletal:
  Short stature
  Shield chest
  Widely spaced nipples
  Micrognathia
Cardiac malformations:
  Bicuspid aortic valve
  Coarctation
Renal malformations
Autoimmune thyroiditis
Mental retardation

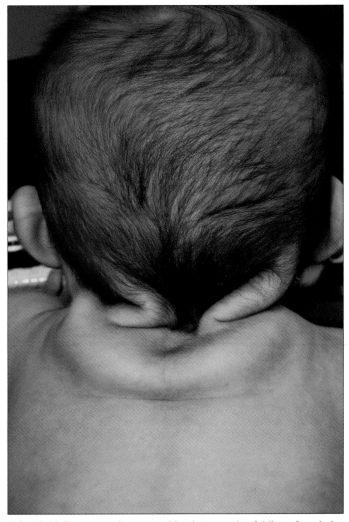

FIG. 26-12 Turner syndrome resulting in excessive folding of nuchal skin (From Charrow J. A 1-year-old girl with 'puffy feet.' Pediatr Ann 2006; 35: 546–548.)

with congenital lymphedema of the extremities or neck requires a karyotype analysis (Fig. 26-12). Lymphatic defects result in many clinical manifestations, including pterygium coli (webbing of the neck), redundant neck folds, and a low hairline over the nape.[135] Nails may become hypoplastic and concave, with an increased insertion angle secondary to lymphedema.[136] Cutis verticis gyrata or congenital areas of fixed skin folds are also presumed to be caused by in utero entrapment and fixation of edematous skin.[137] Acral edema usually resolves by age 2, but may persist or recur in childhood in a minority of patients. No sequelae of lymphedema, such as cellulitis or elephantiasis nostras verrucosa, have been reported.[135]

Benign melanocytic nevi are increased in number in TS, with one study showing the average number of nevi to be 115[138] versus 20–40 per person in the general population.[139] The nevi are not dysplastic clinically or histologically, and patients do not appear to have an increased risk of developing malignant melanoma.[140]

Other cutaneous stigmata including alopecia areata, café au lait macules, a tendency to keloid, psoriasis, and vitiligo are of questionable increased frequency.[135] A subset of patients who are mosaics for their chromosome alterations present with pigmentary alterations along the lines of Blaschko.

Extracutaneous Findings
The physical phenotype of patients with TS is highly variable, with many patients appearing physically normal except for short stature.[141] Nevertheless, several clinical features related to bone deformities may be found, including a square-shaped 'shield' chest with widely spaced nipples, cubitus valgus, chondrodysplasia of the distal radial epiphysis (Madelung's deformity), and brachymetacarpalia/tarsalia.[135] Additional features

include micrognathia, downward displacement of the outer corner of the eyes and epicanthic folds, low-set ears, and a high arched palate.

Etiology/Pathogenesis
Turner's syndrome is a sporadic disease of females characterized by the absence of all or part of the second X chromosome. TS is often diagnosed incidentally by amniocentesis or chorionic villous sampling performed for unrelated reasons.[142] However, many infants are diagnosed prenatally based on the ultrasonic finding of fetal edema or an abnormal triple screen. Other ultrasonic findings may include nuchal translucency, cystic hygroma, coarctation of the aorta, renal anomalies, growth retardation, and fetal hydrops.[143] Up to one-third of affected girls are diagnosed as newborns based on puffy hands and feet or redundant nuchal skin.[142] Another third have edema at birth, but it is commonly overlooked until adolescence or adulthood.

Differential Diagnosis
The main differential is Noonan syndrome or other chromosomal abnormalities leading to short stature.

Box 26-10 Clinical features: trisomy 21

Dermatologic associations
Cutis marmorata

Transient neonatal leukemoid reaction

Elastosis perforans serpiginosa

Multiple syringomas

Milia-like calcinosis

Alopecia areata

Folliculitis

Extracutaneous manifestations
Short stature

Hypotonia

Cardiac malformations:
 Ventral septal defect
 Atrioventricular communis

Duodenal atresia

Mental retardation

Alzheimer disease

Leukemia

Box 26-11 Clinical features: trisomy 18

Dermatologic associations
Skin redundancy

Cutis marmorata

Hirsutism of forehead and back

Nail hypoplasia

Low arch dermal ridge pattern on fingertips

Scalp defects (rare)

Extracutaneous manifestations
Cerebellar hypoplasia

Agenesis of corpus callosum

Malformed ears

Overriding fingers/clenched hand

Short sternum

Cardiac defects

Box 26-12 Clinical features: trisomy 13

Dermatologic associations
Scalp defects (parieto-occipital)

Loose skin on posterior neck

Transverse palmar crease on hand

Hyperconvex narrow fingernails

Forehead hemangioma

Extracutaneous manifestations
Cleft lip/palate

Holoprosencephaly

Polydactyly

Abnormal helices

Deafness

Cardiac ventricular septal defect

Cryptorchidism

Treatment and Care

Baseline evaluation of patients diagnosed with Turner syndrome should include physical examination, echocardiography, renal ultrasound, thyroid function tests, and a hearing screen. Patients should be also be monitored for ovarian failure, growth issues, and psychosocial issues.[142]

Trisomy 21

In 1959 Down syndrome (MIM 190685) was found by Lejeune et al.[144] to be caused by the presence of three copies of chromosome 21. In most instances Down syndrome is sporadic, the risk increasing with increased maternal age. The chromosome has been sequenced and is estimated to contain over 200 genes.[145] Despite considerable effort to determine which features, if any, of Down syndrome are due to dosage effects of specific genes, none have so far been identified.

Cutaneous Findings

There are many phenotypic changes associated with Down syndrome (Box 26-10). One feature relevant to evaluation in the newborn period is a pustular eruption which can occur in the setting of a transient neonatal leukemoid reaction, which occurs in as many as 10% of newborns with Down syndrome.[146] Most cases resolve spontaneously; however, children with Down syndrome are also at risk for the development of acute leukemia, both ALL and AML (see Chapter 10). Other cutaneous associations in Down syndrome include elastosis perforans serpiginosa, multiple syringomas, alopecia areata, milia-like idiopathic calcinosis cutis, and crusted scabies, but these rarely if ever occur in the neonatal period or early infancy.[147]

Trisomy 18

Trisomy 18 (Edwards syndrome) occurs in approximately 1 in 3600–8500 live births. It is fatal by 1 year of age in 90% of cases. Characteristic features (Box 26-11) include overriding fingers, nail hypoplasia, short hallux, and distinctive facial appearance. Neurologic features include cerebellar hypoplasia and agenesis of the corpus collosum.[148] Skin findings include redundancy, hirsutism of the forehead and back, and cutis marmorata. Scalp defects have also been reported. G-banded karyotype can be used to confirm the diagnosis. The differential diagnosis includes fetal akinesia sequence, which is characterized by polyhydramnios, characteristic facial features, joint contractures, and overriding fingers.

Trisomy 13

Trisomy 13 (Patau syndrome) was first reported in 1960 and is a cause of multiple congenital anomalies occurring in approximately 1 in 10000–20000 live births (Box 26-12). Orofacial clefts, holoprosencephaly, microphthalmia, and postaxial polydactyly are the cardinal features. Parieto-occipital aplasia cutis of the scalp is also a diagnostic feature. Minor findings include hemangioma on the forehead, anterior cowlick, loose skin, and abnormal ears.[148]

MISCELLANEOUS DISORDERS

Noonan Syndrome

Noonan syndrome (MIM #163950) shares with Turner syndrome the features of congenital lymphedema, broad or webbed neck, low posterior hairline, short stature, and cardiac malformations (Box 26-13).

Cutaneous Findings

The neonate with Noonan syndrome is unlikely to have skin manifestations other than nuchal webbing that lead to diagnosis. Keratosis pilaris atrophicans faciei (ulerythema oophryogenes), characterized by horny, whitish, hemispherical, or acuminate papules at the opening of pilosebaceous follicles, is generally noted in older children, but may manifest itself at a few months after birth in the external third of the eyebrows.[149]

Some children with Noonan syndrome have multiple café-au-lait macules and/or lentigines. Several patients with both neurofibromatosis type 1 and Noonan syndrome have been reported,[150] leading to the designation neurofibromatosis/Noonan syndrome. However, a recent case report showed the concurrence of both an NF1 mutation and a PTPN11 mutation, demonstrating that this may only reflect the chance association of the two phenotypes.[151]

Extracutaneous Findings

Patients have a characteristic facial appearance that is most striking in the newborn period,[152] consisting of a tall forehead, ptosis, downslanting palpebral fissures, low-set, posteriorly rotated ears, and a high palate. They also have a unique chest shape of superior pectus carinatum and inferior pectus excavatum. Coagulation defects occur in approximately one-third of patients with Noonan syndrome.[153] The classic cardiac lesion in Noonan syndrome is pulmonic stenosis, in contrast to bicuspid aortic valve and coarctation of the aorta in Turner syndrome. Karyotype analysis revealing the presence of two full sex chromosomes also distinguishes Noonan syndrome.

Box 26-13 Clinical features: Noonan syndrome

Dermatologic associations
Webbed neck
Cutis vertices gyrata
Ulerythema oophyogenes
Koilonychia
Thick, curly and wooly hair
Prominent fetal finger pads

Extracutaneous manifestations
Short stature
Craniofacial:
  Ptosis
  Downslanting palpebral fissures
  High palate
Cardiac pulmonic stenosis
Cryptorchidism

Etiology/Pathogenesis

Noonan syndrome is caused by mutations in the PTPN11 gene, which encodes the signal transduction molecule Src-homology tyrosine phosphatase 2 (SHP-2).[154] Although Noonan syndrome is inherited as an autosomal dominant condition, nearly half of cases arise sporadically. Of note, PTPN11 mutations are associated with juvenile myelomonocytic leukemia, and infants with Noonan syndrome may have an increased risk of developing a myeloproliferative disorder.[155] PTPN11 mutations are also the genetic basis of LEOPARD syndrome (multiple lentigines syndrome; see Chapter 22).[156]

Differential Diagnosis

Cardiofaciocutaneous syndrome (CFC) (see below) overlaps considerably with Noonan syndrome and there is much debate about whether or not it is a separate condition.[157] Mental retardation, skin abnormalities, and gastrointestinal problems tend to be more severe in the former. Facial features tend to be more coarse in CFC, with the additional finding of earlobe creases and absence of the characteristic blue or blue-green eyes of Noonan syndrome.[152] Costello syndrome has a similar phenotype characterized by short stature, coarse face, pulmonic stenosis, and short neck (see below).

Treatment and Care

Patients with Noonan syndrome should be monitored for growth deficiency and developmental delay. Echocardiography can be used to evaluate and monitor cardiac malformations. Coagulopathy work-up should be performed if the patient has a history of easy bruising or prolonged bleeding.

Cardiofaciocutaneous Syndrome

Cardiofaciocutaneous (CFC) syndrome (MIM 115150) is characterized by short stature, congenital heart defects, mental retardation, ectodermal abnormalities and a characteristic facial appearance (Box 26-14).

Cutaneous Findings

Numerous cutaneous findings have been reported in CFC. In 2004, Weiss et al.[158] reviewed the cutaneous manifestations in 58 patients with CFC syndrome. All had dermatologic findings. The most common manifestations in over half of the patients were sparse, curly hair and hyperkeratosis (Fig. 26-13). Additional findings were dry skin (23.4%), eczematous skin (17%), keratosis pilaris (10.6%), and seborrheic dermatitis (8.5%). Less frequent findings included loose skin, papillomas, acanthosis nigricans, pigmented nevi and café au lait macules. Of note, hemangiomas were reported in 21.4% of patients.[159]

Extracutaneous Findings

Grebe et al.[157] identified two patients with a severe phenotype of cardiofaciocutaneous syndrome to refine the diagnostic criteria. In addition to the cutaneous findings listed above, they used the following features: macrocephaly, characteristic facial appearance, growth retardation, cardiac defects, neurologic impairment, gastrointestinal dysfunction, ocular abnormalities, and a history of polyhydramnios. Kavamura et al.[160] took this a step further and developed a CFC Index based on the frequencies of 82 clinical traits to aid in the diagnosis.

> **Box 26-14 Clinical features: cardiofaciocutaneous syndrome**
>
> **Dermatologic associations**
> Sparse, curly hair
> Lack of eyebrows and eyelashes
> Hyperkeratotic, dry skin
> Eczematous skin
> Keratosis pilaris
> Seborrheic dermatitis
>
> **Extracutaneous manifestations**
> Craniofacial:
>   Macrocephaly
>   Prominent forehead
>   Bitemporal narrowing
>   High palate
>   Shallow orbital ridge
> Growth retardation
> Cardiac defects:
>   Atrial septal defect
>   Pulmonic stenosis
> Neurologic impairment
> Gastrointestinal dysfunction
> Ocular abnormalities
> History of polyhydramnios

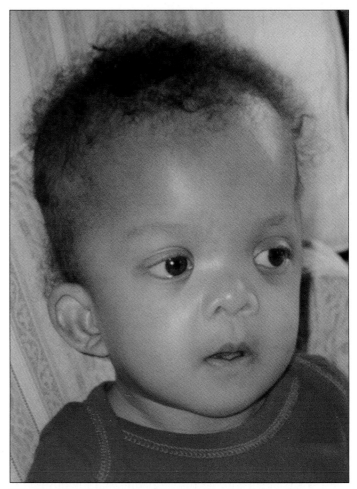

FIG. 26-13 Cardiofaciocutaneous syndrome in an infant with a confirmed *BRAF* mutation. The sparse curly hair and eyebrows and characteristic facial features are evident. (Courtesy of Brenda Conger, CFC International.)

Etiology/Pathogenesis

CFC syndrome is caused by mutations in either the *KRAS* or the *BRAF* genes.[161,162] These mutations were discovered in part because of the similarity of the phenotypic features of Noonan and Costello syndromes, both of which were known to have mutations involving the *RAS–RAF–ERK* pathway.

Differential Diagnosis

Given insights into genetics and pathogenesis, it is not surprising that the main differential diagnoses for CFC syndrome include Noonan and Costello syndromes.

Costello Syndrome

Costello syndrome (MIM #218040) is a rare multiple congenital abnormality syndrome associated with failure to thrive, developmental delay, and an increased risk of malignancy. Inheritance is autosomal dominant.

Cutaneous Findings

Several cutaneous stigmata have been described, including cutis laxa (especially the hands and feet), dark skin pigmentation, papillomas (perioral, nasal, and anal regions), acanthosis nigricans, palmar nevi, and deep palmar creases. Nails may be thin and brittle, with koilonychias, and hair may be curly, sparse, and especially thin over the anterior skull.

Extracutaneous Findings

Normal size at birth is often followed by postnatal growth failure. Macrocephaly, developmental delay, a distinctive facies, and various cardiac and cardiovascular defects are among the many features of the syndrome.

Etiology/Pathogenesis

The condition is caused by mutations in the *HRAS* gene, at 11p15.5.[163]

Riley–Day Syndrome

Riley–Day syndrome (familial dysautonomia, hereditary sensory and autonomic neuropathy III; MIM 223900) is an autosomal recessive condition seen almost exclusively in Ashkenazi Jews (Box 26-15). In older children, excessive drooling and sweating, often in response to inappropriate stimuli, occur, as do orthostatic hypotension and labile hypertension. Other complications tend to occur in later childhood and adult life. Survival is reduced, and almost one-fifth of those affected die in infancy or childhood.

Cutaneous Findings

The diagnostic significance of absence of tearing, a cardinal feature of Riley–Day syndrome, is usually not appreciated in young infants, as overflow tearing does not develop until 2–3 months of age in normal infants. Affected babies often have blotching and mottling of the skin. This usually appears after a month of age and within the first year or so, as do bouts of hyperpyrexia. Emotional excitement often precipitates the appearance of the red blotches. In familial dysautonomia the indifference or insensitivity to pain results in progressive self-mutilation, biting of the tongue, loss of teeth, burns, and ulcers. Mechanically induced ulceration of the tongue and granulation tissue growths (Riga–Fede disease) in teething infants have been reported. There is absence of fungiform papillae on the tongue and a decrease in the ability to taste.

Extracutaneous Findings
Although affected individuals are usually not diagnosed until several years of age, generalized signs appear within the newborn period in over 80% of patients.[164] These features include breech birth in one-quarter, intrauterine growth retardation, hypotonia, respiratory insufficiency, and poor feeding with swallowing difficulty and aspiration. Unexplained episodes of fever and failure to thrive, aspiration pneumonia, and repeated episodes of vomiting are typical. Deep tendon reflexes are invariably absent.

Etiology/Pathogenesis
The gene for Riley–Day syndrome has been mapped to 9q31. Mutations in the *IKBKAP* gene have been demonstrated.[165,166] There appears to be a decrease in survival of sensory, sympathetic, and some parasympathetic nerves.

Differential Diagnosis
Faced with an infant with unexplainable hyperpyrexia, sweating abnormalities, and failure to thrive, the primary differential diagnosis is hypohidrotic ectodermal dysplasia versus Riley–Day syndrome. Injection of histamine (1:10000) does not elicit a flare response in Riley–Day syndrome. The flare response can be used to discriminate between the two conditions, as can the presence of teeth on a panorex examination of the jaw. The astute physician, aware of the feature of random blotching and mottling of the skin, may be able to make the diagnosis of Riley–Day syndrome in an infant whose multiplicity of problems have failed to lead to the correct diagnosis.

Treatment and Care
The involvement of multiple subspecialists in addition to close follow-up with the primary care provider is important. Delivery of proper nutrition though feeding tubes, use of artificial tears, and avoidance of aspiration are necessary. Referral to neurology and orthopedics for specialized care is recommended.

Coffin–Siris syndrome

Cutaneous Findings
Several ectodermal manifestations have been reported in Coffin–Siris syndrome (MIM 135900). These include a hypoplastic or absent fifth fingernail and toenail, and hypertrichosis on the body with sparse scalp hair (Box 26-16). Eyebrows tend to be thick and eyelashes long (see Chapter 28).

Extracutaneous Findings
The facial features of Coffin–Siris are characterized by coarse facies with a flat nasal bridge, wide mouth, micrognathia, thick lips and abnormal ears. Developmental delay and mental retardation are common findings. Almost all patients have an absent or hypoplastic fifth phalanx on the hands and feet. Short stature and delayed bone age are also characteristic. Delayed dentition and cardiac defects have also been reported.[167]

Etiology/Pathogenesis
Coffin–Siris syndrome has sporadic occurrence and the etiology is unknown. Most cases have had normal karyotypes. The diagnosis is based on clinical findings.

Differential Diagnosis
The differential diagnosis includes fetal hydantoin syndrome, fetal alcohol syndrome, and Cornelia de Lange syndrome.[167]

Treatment and Care
Patients with Coffin–Siris syndrome have been reported to have frequent upper respiratory and ear infections.[167] Younger infants may have feeding problems. Work-up should include hand radiographs to assess for hypoplastic or absent phalanges on the fifth digit. Cardiac evaluation is recommended to rule out cardiac malformations. Karyotyping is useful to exclude other multiple malformation and mental retardation syndromes. Additional work-up should include renal ultrasound, ophthalmologic evaluation, and hearing screen.

MITOCHONDRIAL DISORDERS

Mitochondrial enzyme abnormalities are characterized by an unexplained association of symptoms with multiple involved organs that have no common embryologic origin or biologic function. An increasing number of involved organs and systems during the course of disease is characteristic. In recent years, the causative mutations for many mitochondrial disorders have been described. Mitochondrial disorders have a heterogeneous group of findings, such as poor growth, vomiting, developmental delay, renal tubular dysfunction, and seizures. Therefore, the diagnosis is often delayed for many months. Over the past several years, cutaneous findings have begun to be recognized in mitochondrial diseases.

Cutaneous Findings

The most common cutaneous findings in patients with mitochondrial disease include lipomas, alopecia, mottled pigmentation or poikiloderma, erythematous patches, hypertrichosis, and acrocyanosis.[168,169] The alopecia seems to be related to hair shaft abnormalities, fractures (trichoschisis), twists (pili torti), and trichorrhexis nodosa. The mottled or reticulated pigmentation is most commonly in sun-exposed areas, such as the neck, dorsal arms, and forehead. Hypertrichosis has frequently been noted in Leigh syndrome.

Extracutaneous Findings

Neurologic features may include seizures, developmental delay, myoclonus, and ataxia. Skeletal muscle is involved, resulting in myopathy and hypotonia. Sideroblastic anemia and pancytopenia can be hematologic complications. The endocrine manifestations include hypoparathyroidism, growth deficiency, and diabetes mellitus. Cardiomyopathy and conduction defects are the cardiac manifestations. In addition, sensorineural deafness and lactic acidosis may be present.[170]

Etiology/Pathogenesis

Mitochondria are ubiquitous and are the main organelle responsible for producing energy in cells. Several different mutations in the mitochondrial DNA (mtDNA) have been identified resulting in a variety of diseases, including Leigh syndrome (subacute necrotizing encephalopathy) and MELAS (mitochondrial encephalomyopathy, acidosis, and stroke-like episodes), and NARP (neurogenic muscle weakness, ataxia and retinitis pigmentosa). Mitochondrial DNA mutations can be either inherited or acquired. Acquired mutations may be related to ultraviolet-induced damage and may play a role in aging.[171]

Treatment and Care

Evaluation should include plasma lactate, pyruvate and ketone body levels, head CT or MRI, and muscle biopsy for histology and for genetic analysis of the mitochondrial DNA. Treatment is supportive.

REFERENCES

1. National Institute of Health Consensus Development Conference. Neurofibromatosis: Conference statement. Arch Neurol 1988; 45: 575–578.
2. Friedman JM, Gutmann DH, MacCollin M, et al. Neurofibromatosis: phenotype, natural history, and pathogenesis, 3rd edn. Baltimore: Johns Hopkins Press, 1999.
3. Carey JC. Health supervision and anticipatory guidance for children with genetic disorders (including specific recommendations for trisomy 21, trisomy 18, and neurofibromatosis). Pediatr Clin North Am 1992; 39: 25–53.
4. Viskochil D. Neurofibromatosis type 1. In: Cassidy SB, Allanson JE, eds. Management of genetic syndromes, 2nd edn. Hoboken, NJ: John Wiley, 2005; 369–384.
5. Obringer A, Meadows A, Zackai E. The diagnosis of neurofibromatosis-1 in the child under the age of 6 years. Am J Dis Child 1989; 14: 717–719.
6. Whitehouse D. Diagnostic value of the café-au-lait spot in children. Arch Dis Child 1966; 41: 316–319
7. North K. NF type 1 in childhood. In: International review of child neurology series. London: MacKeith Press, 1997.
8. Leppig K, Kaplan P, Viskochil D, et al. Familial neurofibromatosis 1 microdeletions: Cosegregation with distinct facial phenotype and early onset of neurofibromata. Am J Med Genet 1997; 73: 197–204.
9. Huson S, Harper P, Compston D, et al. Von Recklinghausen neurofibromatosis. A clinical and population study in southeast Wales. Brain 1998; 111: 1355–1381.
10. Martin G, Viskochil D, Bollag G, et al. The GAP-related domain of the NF1 gene product interacts with ras p21. Cell 1990; 63: 843–849.
11. Paller A. Neurofibromatosis I: Clinical pearls. In: Spitz JL ed. Genodermatoses: a clinical guide to genetic skin disorders. Philadelphia: Lippincott Williams & Wilkins, 2005: 83.
12. Vanderhooft S, Francis J, Pagon R, et al. Prevalence of hypopigmented macules in a healthy population. J Pediatr 1996; 129: 355–361.
13. Darling T, Skarulis M, Steinberg S, et al. Multiple facial angiofibromas and collagenomas in patients with multiple endocrine neoplasia type 1. Arch Dermatol 1997; 133: 853–857.
14. Webb D, Fryer A, Osborn J. Morbidity associated with tuberous sclerosis: a population study. Dev Med Child Neurol 1996; 38: 146–155.
15. Sidenvall R, Eeg-Olofsson O. Epidemiology of infantile spasms in Sweden. Epilepsia 1995; 36: 572–574.
16. Webb D, Osborne J. tuberous sclerosis. Arch Dis Child 1995; 72: 471–474.
17. Gomez M. Tuberous sclerosis, 2nd edn. New York: Raven Press, 1988.
18. Webb D, Fryer A, Osborne J. On the incidence of fits and mental retardation in tuberous sclerosis. J Med Genet 1991; 28: 395–397.
19. Webb D, Thomas R, Osborne J. Cardiac rhabdomyomas and their association with tuberous sclerosis. Arch Dis Child 1993; 68: 367–370.
20. Bosi G, Lintermans J, Pellgrino P, et al. The natural history of cardiac rhabdomyomas with and without tuberous sclerosis. Arch Pediatr 1996; 85: 928–931.
21. Smith HC, Watson GH, Patel RG, et al. Cardiac rhabdomyomata in tuberous sclerosis: Their coarse and diagnostic value. Arch Dis Child 1989; 64: 196–200.
22. Roach ES, DiMario FJ, Kandt RS, et al. Tuberous Sclerosis Consensus Conference: Recommendations for diagnostic evaluation. National Tuberous Sclerosis Association. J Child Neurol 1999; 14: 401–407.
23. Jozwiak S, Schwartz RA, Janniger CK, et al. Usefulness of diagnostic criteria of tuberous sclerosis complex in pediatric patients. J Child Neurol 2000; 15: 652–659.
24. Webb DW, Kabala J, Osborne JP. A population study of renal disease in patients with tuberous sclerosis. Br J Urol 1994; 74: 151–154.
25. Cook JA, Oliver K, Mueller RF, et al. A cross sectional study of renal involvement in tuberous sclerosis. J Med Genet 1996; 33: 480–484.
26. Ewalt DH, Sheffield E, Sparagana SP, et al. Renal lesion growth in children with tuberous sclerosis complex. J Urol 1998; 160: 141–145.
27. Casper KA, Donnelly LF, Chen B, et al. Tuberous sclerosis complex: Renal imaging findings. Radiology 2002; 225: 451–456.

28. Sampson JR, Mahashwar MM, Aspinwall R, et al. Renal cystic disease in tuberous sclerosis: Role of the polycystic kidney disease 1 gene. Am J Hum Genet 1997; 61: 843–851.

29. Kwiatkowski DJ. Tuberous sclerosis: From tubers to mTOR. Ann Hum Genet 2003; 67: 87–96.

30. Roach ES, Gomez MR, Northrup H. Tuberous sclerosis complex consensus conference: Revised clinical diagnostic criteria. J Child Neurol 1998; 13: 624–628.

31. Jost CJ, Gloviczki P, Edwards WD, et al. Aortic aneurysms in children and young adults with tuberous sclerosis: Report of two cases and review of the literature. J Vasc Surg 2001; 33: 639–642.

32. Papadavid E, Markey A, Bellaney G, et al. Carbon dioxide and pulsed dye laser treatment of angiofibromas in 29 patients with tuberous sclerosis. Br J Dermatol 2002; 147: 337–342.

33. Munoz MV, Santos AC, Graziadio C, et al. Cerebello-trigeminal-dermal dysplasia (Gomez–Lopez–Hernandez syndrome): Description of three new cases and review. Am J Med Genet 1997; 72: 34–39.

34. Orlow SJ. Cutaneous findings in craniofacial malformation syndromes. Arch Dermatol 1992; 128: 1379–1386.

35. Gomez MR. Cerebello-trigemino-dermal dysplasia. In: Gomez MR, ed. Neurocutaneous diseases. New York: Raven Press, 1987; 145–148.

36. Ringpfeil F. Selected disorders of connective tissue: pseudoxanthoma elasticum, cutis laxa, and lipoid proteinosis. Clin Dermatol 2005; 23: 41–46.

37. Damkier A, Brandup F, Starklint H. Cutis laxa: autosomal dominant inheritance in five generations. Clin Genet 1991; 39: 321–329.

38. Kaler SG, Gallo LK, Proud VK, et al. Occipital horn syndrome and a mild Menkes phenotype associated with splice site mutations at the MNK locus. Nature Genet 1994; 8: 195–202.

39. Peltonen L, Kuivaniemi H, Palotic A, et al. alterations in copper and collagen metabolism in the Menkes syndrome and a new subtype of the Ehlers–Danlos syndrome. Biochemistry 1983; 22: 6156–6163.

40. Tassabehji M, Metcalfe K, Hurst J, et al. An elastin gene mutation producing abnormal tropoelastin and abnormal elastic fibres in a patient with autosomal dominant cutis laxa. Hum Mol Genet 1998; 7: 1021–1028.

41. Zhang MC, He L, Giro M, et al. Cutis laxa arising from frameshift mutations in exon 30 of the elastin gene (ELN). J Biol Chem 1999; 274: 981–986.

42. Nakamura T, Lozano PR, Ikeda Y, et al. Fibulin-5/DANCE is essential for elastogenesis in vivo. Nature 2002; 415: 171–175.

43. Yanagisawa H, Davis EC, Starcher BC, et al. Fibulin-5 is an elastin-binding protein essential for elastic fibre development in vivo. Nature 2002; 415: 168–171.

44. Markova D, Zou Y, Ringpfeil F, et al. Genetic heterogeneity of cutis laxa: a heterozygous tandem duplication within the fibulin-5 (FBLN5) gene. Am J Hum Genet 2003; 72: 998–1004.

45. Loeys B, Van Maldergem L, Mortier G, et al. Homozygosity for a missense mutation in fibulin-5 (FBLN5) results in a severe form of cutis laxa. Hum Mol Genet 2002; 11: 2113–2118.

46. Johnson JP, Golabi M, Norton ME, et al. Costello syndrome: Phenotype, natural history, differential diagnosis, and possible cause. J Pediatr 1998; 133: 441–448.

47. Hill VA, Seymour CA, Mortimer PS. Pencillamine-induced elastosis perforans serpiginosa and cutis laxa in Wilson's disease. Br J Dermatol 2000; 142: 560–561.

48. Paller AS, Mancini AJ. Hereditary disorders of the dermis. In: Paller AS, Mancini AJ eds. Hurwitz clinical pediatric dermatology, 3rd ed. Philadelphia: Elsevier, 2006; 129–144.

49. Hwang ST, Williams ML, McCalmont TH, Frieden IJ. Sweet's syndrome leading to acquired cutis laxa (Marshall's syndrome) in an infant with alpha 1-antitrypsin deficiency. Arch Dermatol 1995; 131: 1175–1177.

50. Bogart MM, Arnold HE, Greer KE. Prune-belly syndrome in two children and review of the literature. Pediatr Dermatol. 2006; 23: 342–345.

51. Uitto J. Cutis laxa: clinical pearls. In: Spitz JL, ed. Genodermatoses: a clinical guide to genetic skin disorders. Philadelphia: Lippincott Williams & Wilkins, 2005; 142–143.

52. Kaler SG. Diagnosis and therapy of Menkes syndrome, a genetic form of copper deficiency. Am J Clin Nutr 1998; 67: 1029S–1034S.

53. Karnes PS, Shamban AT, Olsen DR, et al. De Barsy syndrome: report of a case, literature review, and elastin gene expression studies of the skin. Am J Med Genet 1992; 42: 29–34.

54. Wenstrup RJ, Hoechstetter LB. Ehlers–Danlos syndromes. In: Cassidy SB, Allanson JE, eds. Management of genetic syndromes. Hoboken, NJ: Wiley, 2005; 211–223.

55. Beighton P, De Paepe A, Danks D, et al. International nosology of heritable disorders of connective tissue, Berlin, 1986. Am J Med Genet 1988; 29: 581–594.

56. Beighton P, De Paepe A, Steinmann B, et al. Ehlers–Danlos syndromes: revised nosology, Villefranche, 1997. Am J Med Genet 1998; 77: 31–37.

57. Lind J, Wallenburg HC. Pregnancy and the Ehlers–Danlos syndrome: A retrospective study in a Dutch population. Acta Obstet Gynecol Scand 2002; 81: 293–300.

58. Freeman RK, Bird H. The surgical complications of Ehlers–Danlos syndrome. Am Surg 1996; 62: 869–873.

59. Elsas LJ 2nd, Miller RL, Pinnell SR. Inherited human collagen lysyl hydroxylase deficiency: Ascorbic acid response. J Pediatr 1978; 92378–384.

60. Uitto J. Ehlers–Danlos syndrome: clinical pearls. In: Spitz JL ed. Genodermatoses: a clinical guide to genetic skin disorders. Philadelphia: Lippincott Williams & Wilkins, 2005; 136.

61. Carney RJ. Incontinentia pigmenti: a world of statistical analysis. Arch Dermatol 1976; 112: 535–542.

62. Donnai D. Incontinentia pigmenti. In: Cassidy SB, Allanson JE, eds. Management of genetic syndromes. Hoboken, NJ: Wiley, 2005; 309–314.

63. Goldberg MF, Custis PH. Retinal and other manifestations of incontinentia pigmenti (Bloch–Sulzberger syndrome). Ophthalmology 1993; 100: 1645–1654.

64. Wald KJ, Mehta MC, Katsumi O, et al. Retinal detachments in incontinentia pigmenti. Arch Ophthalmol 1993; 111: 614–617.

65. Landy SJ, Donnai D. Incontinentia pigmenti (Bloch–Sulzberger syndrome). J Med Genet 1993; 30: 53–59.

66. Smahi A, Courtois G, Vabres P, et al. Genomic rearrangement in NEMO impairs NF-kappaB activation and is a cause of incontinentia pigment. Nature 2000; 405: 466–472.

67. International Incontinentia Pigmenti (IP) Consortium. Genomic rearrangement in NEMO impairs NF-kappaB activation and is a cause of incontinentia pigmenti. Nature 2000; 405: 466–472.

68. Skaria A, Feldmann R, Hauser C. The clinical spectrum of focal dermal hypoplasia. Hautarzt 1995; 46: 779–784.

69. Terezhalmy GT, Moore WS, Bsoul SA, et al. Focal dermal hypoplasia. Quintessence Int 2002; 33: 706–707.

70. Hall EH, Terezhalmy GT. Focal dermal hypoplasia syndrome. Case report and literature review. J Am Acad Dermatol 1983; 9: 443–451.

71. Ayme S, Fraser FC. Possible examples of the Goltz syndrome (focal dermal hypoplasia) without linear areas of skin hypoplasia. Birth Defects 1982; 18: 59–65.

72. Goltz RW. Focal dermal hypoplasia syndrome. An update. Arch Dermatol 1992; 128: 1108–1111.

73. Howell JB, Reynolds J. Osteopathia striata. A diagnostic osseous marker of focal dermal hypoplasia. Trans St John's Hosp Dermatol Soc 1974; 60: 178–182.

74. Happle R, Lenz W. Striation of bones in focal dermal hypoplasia: manifestation of functional mosaicism? Br J Dermatol 1977; 96: 133–138.

75. Samejima N, Ito S, Nakajima S, et al. Omphalocele and focal dermal

hypoplasia. Zeitschr Kinderchir 1981; 34: 284–289.

76. Han XY, Wu SS, Conway DH, et al. Truncus arteriosus and other lethal internal anomalies in Goltz syndrome. Am J Med Genet 2000; 90: 45–48.

77. Moss C. Mosaicism and linear lesions. In: Bolognia JL, Jorizzo JL, Rapini RP, eds. Dermatology. Edinburgh: Mosby, 2003; 869–885.

78. Cohen MM Jr, Neri G, Weksberg R. Proteus syndrome. In: Overgrowth syndromes. New York: Oxford University Press, 2002; 75–110.

79. Turner JT, Cohen MM Jr, Biesecker LG. A reassessment of the Proteus syndrome literature: Application of diagnostic criteria on published cases. Am J Med Genet 2004; 130A: 111–122.

80. Mucke J, Willgerodt H, Kunzel R, et al. Variability in the Proteus syndrome: report of an affected child with progressive lipomatosis. Eur J Pediatr 1985; 143: 320–323.

81. Costa T, Fitch N, Azouz EM. Proteus syndrome: report of two cases with pelvic lipomatosis. Pediatrics 1985; 76: 984–989.

82. Clark RD, Donnai D, Rogers J, et al. Proteus syndrome: an expanded phenotype. Am J Med Genet 1987; 27: 99–117.

83. Viljoen DL, Saxe N, Temple-Camp C. Cutaneous manifestations of the Proteus syndrome. Pediatr Dermatol 1988; 5: 14–21.

84. Samlaska CP, Levin S, James WD, et al. Proteus syndrome. Arch Dermatol 1989; 125: 1109–1114.

85. Viljoen DL, Nelson MM, de Jong G, et al. Proteus syndrome in Southern Africa: natural history and clinical manifestations in six individuals. Am J Med Genet 1987; 27: 87–97.

86. Happle R, Steijlen PM, Theile U, et al. Patchy dermal hypoplasia as a characteristic feature of Proteus syndrome. Arch Dermatol 1997; 133: 77–80.

87. Newman B, Urbach AH, Orenstein D, et al. Proteus syndrome: Emphasis on the pulmonary manifestations. Pediatr Radiol 1994; 24: 189–193.

88. Slavotinek AM, Vacha SJ, Peters KF, et al. Sudden death caused by pulmonary thromboembolism in Proteus syndrome. Clin Genet 2000; 58: 386–389.

89. Biesecker LG. Proteus syndrome. In: Cassidy SB, Allanson JE, eds. Management of genetic syndromes. Hoboken, NJ: Wiley, 2005; 449–456.

90. Burke J, Bowell R, O'Doherty N. Proteus syndrome: ocular complications. J Pediatr Ophthalmol Strabismus 1988; 25: 99–102.

91. Happle R. Lethal genes surviving by mosaicism: A possible explanation for sporadic birth defects involving the skin. J Am Acad Dermatol 1987; 16: 899–906.

92. Biesecker LG, Happle R, Mulliken JB, et al. Proteus syndrome: Diagnostic criteria, differential diagnosis, and patient evaluation. Am J Med Genet 1999; 84: 389–395.

93. Cohen MM Jr, Turner JT, Biesecker LG. Proteus syndrome: Misdiagnosis with PTEN mutations. Am J Med Genet 2003; 122A: 323–324.

94. Cohen MM Jr, Turner JT, Biesecker LG. Reply to Kirk et al. Reassessment of the Proteus syndrome literature: application of diagnostic criteria to published cases. Am J Med Genet 2004; 130A: 216–217.

95. Biesecker LG, Peters KF, Darling TN, et al. Clinical differentiation between Proteus syndrome and hemihyperplasia: Description of a distinct form of hemihyperplasia. Am J Med Genet 1998; 79: 311–318.

96. Cohen MM Jr, Neri G, Weksberg R. Maffucci syndrome. In: Overgrowth syndromes. New York: Oxford University Press, 2002; 125–129.

97. Al-Gazali L, Mueller R, Caine A, et al. Two 46,XX,t(X; Y) females with linear skin defects and congenital microphthalmia: a new syndrome at Xp22.3. J Med Genet 1990; 27: 59–63.

98. Happle R, Daniels O, Koopman RJ. MIDAS syndrome (microphthalmia, dermal aplasia, and sclerocornea): An X-linked phenotype distinct from Goltz syndrome. Am J Med Genet 1993; 47: 710–713.

99. Ballabio A, Andria G. Deletions and translocations involving the distal short arm of the human X chromosome: Review and hypotheses. Hum Mol Genet 1992; 1: 221–227.

100. Bloom D. The syndrome of congenital telangiectatic erythema and stunted growth. J Pediatr 1966; 68: 103–113.

101. Wolkenstein P, Latarjet J, Roujeau JC, et al. Randomised comparison of thalidomide versus placebo in toxic epidermal necrolysis. Lancet 1998; 352: 1586–1589.

102. Tsai RJ, Li LM, Chen JK. Reconstruction of damaged corneas by transplantation of autologous limbal epithelial cells. N Engl J Med 2000; 343: 86–93.

103. Tristani-Firouzi P, Petersen MJ, Saffle JR, et al. Treatment of toxic epidermal necrolysis with intravenous immunoglobulin in children. J Am Acad Dermatol 2002; 47: 548–552.

104. Kraus BS, Gottlieb MA, Meliton HR. The dentition in Rothmund's syndrome. J Am Dent Assoc 1970; 81: 895–915.

105. Marin-Bertolin S, Amorrortu-Belayos J, Aliaga BA. Squamous cell carcinoma of the tongue in a patient with Rothmund–Thomson syndrome. Br J Plast Surg 1998; 51: 646–648.

106. Pujol LA, Erickson RP, Heidenreich RA, et al. Variable presentation of Rothmund–Thomson syndrome. Am J Med Genet 2000; 95: 204–207.

107. Wang LL, Ganavarapu A, Kozinetz CA, et al. Association between osteosarcoma and deleterious mutations in the RECQL4 gene in Rothmund–Thomson syndrome. J Natl Cancer Inst 2003; 95: 669–674.

108. Larizza L, Magnani I, Roversi G. Rothmund–Thomson syndrome and RECQL4 defect: Splitting and lumping. Cancer Lett 2005; (in press.)

109. Wang LL, Levy ML, Lewis RA, et al. Clinical manifestations in a cohort of 41 Rothmund–Thomson syndrome patients. Am J Med Genet 2001; 102: 11–17.

110. Cumin I, Cohen J, Mechinaud F, et al. Rothmund–Thomson syndrome and osteosarcoma. Med Pediatr Oncol 1996; 26: 414–416.

111. Clarke A, Phillips D, Brown R, et al. Clinical aspects of X-linked hypohidrotic ectodermal dysplasia. Arch Dis Child 1987; 62: 989–996.

112. Executive and Scientific Advisory Boards of the National Foundation for Ectodermal Dysplasias. Scaling skin in the neonate: A clue to the early diagnosis of X-linked hypohidrotic ectodermal dysplasia (Christ–Siemens–Touraine syndrome). J Pediatr 1989; 114: 600.

113. Mikkola ML, Theselff I. Ectodysplasin signaling in development. Cytokine Growth Factor Rev 2003; 14: 211–224.

114. Kere J, Srivastava AK, Montonen O, et al. X-linked anhidrotic (hypohidrotic) ectodermal dysplasia is caused by mutation in a novel transmembrane protein. Nature Genet 1996; 13: 409–416.

115. Munoz F, Lestringant G, Sybert V, et al. Definitive evidence for an autosomal recessive form of hypohidrotic ectodermal dysplasia clinically indistinguishable from the more common X-linked disorder. Am J Hum Genet 1997; 61: 94–100.

116. Headon DJ, Emmal SA, Ferguson BM, et al. Gene defect in ectodermal dysplasia implicates a death domain adapter in development. Nature 2001; 414: 913–916.

117. van Bokhoven H, Hamel BC, Bamshad M, et al. p63 Gene mutations in EEC syndrome, limb–mammary syndrome, and isolated split hand–split foot malformation suggest a genotype–phenotype correlation. Am J Hum Genet 2001; 69: 481–492.

118. Brunner HG, Hamel BC, Van Bokhoven H. The p63 gene in EEC and other syndromes. J Med Genet 2002; 39: 377–381.

119. Dhanrajani PJ, Jiffry AO. Management of ectodermal dysplasia: A literature review. Dent Update 1998; 25: 73–75.

120. Clouston H. A hereditary ectodermal dysplasia. Can Med Assoc J 1929; 21: 18–31.

121. Smith SB, Ervin JW. What is your diagnosis? Hidrotic ectodermal dysplasia. Cutis 2003; 71: 190, 224–225.

122. Lamartine J, Munhoz Essenfelder G, Kibar Z, et al. Mutations in GJB6 cause hidrotic ectodermal dysplasia. Nature Genet 2000; 26: 142–144.

123. Itin PH, Fistarol SK. Ectodermal dysplasias. Am J Med Genet Part C (Semin Med Genet) 2004; 131: 45–51.

124. Brunner HG, Hamel BC, Bokhoven HvH. P63 gene mutations and human developmental syndromes. Am J Med Genet 2002; 112: 284–290.

125. Hay R, Wells R. The syndrome of ankyloblepharon, ectodermal defects and cleft lip and palate: An autosomal dominant condition. Br J Dermatol 1976; 94: 277–289.

126. Vanderhooft S, Stephan M, Sybert V. Severe skin erosions and scalp infections in AEC syndrome. Pediatr Dermatol 1993; 10: 334–340.

127. Fosko SW, Stenn KS, Bolognia JL. Ectodermal dysplasias associated with clefting: significance of scalp dermatitis. J Am Acad Dermatol 1992; 27: 249–256.

128. Buss PW, Hughes HE, Clarke A. Twenty-four cases of the EEC syndrome: Clinical presentation and management. J Med Genet 1995; 32: 716.

129. Roelfsema NM, Cobben JM. The EEC syndrome: A literature study. Clin Dysmorphol 1996; 5: 115.

130. Fosko SW, Stenn KS, Bolognia JL. Ectodermal dysplasias associated with clefting: significance of scalp dermatitis. J Am Acad Dermatol 1992; 27: 249–256.

131. Rodini ESO, Richieri-Costa A. EEC syndrome: report on 20 new patients, clinical and genetic considerations. Am J Med Genet 1990; 37: 42–53.

132. McNab AA, Potts MJ, Welham RAN. The EEC syndrome and its ocular manifestations. Br J Ophthalmol 1989; 73: 261–264.

133. Spitz JL. Disorders of hair and nails. In: Spitz JL ed. Genodermatoses: a clinical guide to genetic skin disorders. Philadelphia: Lippincott Williams & Wilkins, 2005; 273–301.

134. Celli J, Duijf P, Hamel BC, et al. Heterozygous germline mutations in the p53 homolog p63 are the cause of EEC syndrome. Cell 1999; 99: 143.

135. Lowenstein EJ, Kim KH, Glick SA. Turner's syndrome in dermatology. J Am Acad Dermatol 2004; 50: 767–776.

136. Kaplowitz PB, Chernausek SD, Horn JA. Fingernail angle in girls with Ullrich–Turner syndrome. Am J Med Genet 1993; 46: 570–573.

137. Larralde M, Gardner SS, Torrado MV, et al. Lymphedema as a postulated cause of cutis verticis gyrata in Turner syndrome. Pediatr Dermatol 1998; 15: 18–22.

138. Lemli L, Smith DW. The Xo syndrome. A study of the differentiated phenotype in 25 patients. J Pediatr 1963; 63: 577–588.

139. Bataille V, Snieder H, MacGregor AJ, et al. Genetics of risk factors for melanoma: an adult twin study of nevi and freckles. J Natl Cancer Inst 2000; 92: 457–463.

140. Gibbs P, Brady BM, Gonzalez R, Robinson WA. Nevi and melanoma: lessons from Turner's syndrome. Dermatology 2001; 202: 1–3.

141. Sybert VP. Turner syndrome. In: Cassidy S, Allanson J, eds. Management of genetic syndromes. Hoboken, NJ: Wiley, 2005; 589–606.

142. Sybert VP, McCauley E. Turner's syndrome. N Engl J Med 2004; 351: 1227–1238.

143. Ranke MB, Saenger P. Turner's syndrome. Lancet 2001; 358: 309–314.

144. Lejeune J, Turpin R, Gautier M. [Mongolism; a chromosomal disease (trisomy).]. Bull Acad Natl Med 1959; 143: 256–265.

145. Hattori M, Fujiyama A, Taylor TD, et al. The DNA sequence of human chromosome 21. Nature 2000; 405: 311–319.

146. Burch JM, Weston WL, Rogers M, Morelli JG. Cutaneous pustular leukemoid reactions in trisomy 21. Pediatr Dermatol 2003; 20: 232–237.

147. Scherbenske JM, Benson PM, Rotchford JP, James WD. Cutaneous and ocular manifestations of Down syndrome. J Am Acad Dermatol 1990; 22: 933–938.

148. Carey J. Trisomy 18 and trisomy 13 syndromes. In: Cassidy S, Allanson J, eds. Management of genetic syndromes, 2nd edn. Hoboken, NJ: Wiley, 2005; 555–568.

149. Sybert VP. Genetic skin disorders. New York: Oxford University Press, 1997.

150. Allanson JE, Hall JG, Van Allen MI. Noonan phenotype associated with neurofibromatosis. Am J Med Genet 1985; 21: 457–462.

151. Bertola DR, Pereira AC, Passetti F, et al. Neurofibromatosis–Noonan syndrome: molecular evidence of the concurrence of both disorders in a patient. Am J Med Genet A 2005; 136: 242–245.

152. Allanson JE. Noonan syndrome. In: Cassidy SB, Allanson JE, eds. Management of genetic syndromes. Hoboken, NJ: Wiley, 2005; 385–398.

153. Witt DR, Hoyme HE, Zonana J, et al. Lymphedema in Noonan syndrome: clues to pathogenesis and prenatal diagnosis and review of the literature. Am J Med Genet 1987; 27: 841–856.

154. Tartaglia M, Mehler EL, Goldberg R, et al. Mutations in PTPN11, encoding the protein tyrosine phosphatase SHP-2, cause Noonan syndrome. Nature Genet 2001; 29: 465–468.

155. Kratz CP, Niemeyer CM, Castleberry RP, et al. The mutational spectrum of PTPN11 in juvenile myelomonocytic leukemia and Noonan syndrome/myeloproliferative disease. Blood 2005; 106: 2183–2185.

156. Digilio MC, Conti E, Sarkozy A, et al. Grouping of multiple-lentigines/LEOPARD and Noonan syndromes on the PTPN11 gene. Am J Hum Genet 2002; 71: 389–394.

157. Grebe TA, Clericuzio C. Neurologic and gastrointestinal dysfunction in cardio-facio-cutaneous syndrome: identification of a severe phenotype. Am J Med Genet 2000; 95: 135–143.

158. Weiss G, Confino Y, Shemer A, Trau H. Cutaneous manifestations in the cardiofaciocutaneous syndrome, a variant of the classical Noonan syndrome. Report of a case and review of the literature. J Eur Acad Dermatol Venereol 2004; 18: 324–327.

159. Wieczorek D, Majewski F, Gillessen-Kaesbach G. Cardio-facio-cutaneous (CFC) syndrome – a distinct entity? Report of three patients demonstrating the diagnostic difficulties in delineation of CFC syndrome. Clin Genet 1997; 52: 37–46.

160. Kavamura MI, Peres CA, Alchorne MM, Brunoni D. CFC index for the diagnosis of cardiofaciocutaneous syndrome. Am J Med Genet 2002; 112: 12–16.

161. Ion A, Tartaglia M, Song X, et al. Absence of PTPN11 mutations in 28 cases of cardiofaciocutaneous (CFC) syndrome. Hum Genet 2002; 111: 421–427.

162. Niihori T, Aoki Y, Narumi Y, et al. Germline KRAS and BRAF mutations in cardio-facio-cutaneous syndrome. Nature Genet 2006; 38: 294–296.

163. Kerr B, Delrue MA, Sigaudy S et al. Genotype–phenotype correlation in Costello syndrome; HRAS mutation analysis in 43 cases. J Med Genet 2006; [Epub ahead of print].

164. Axelrod FB, Porges RF, Sein ME. Neonatal recognition of familial dysautonomia. J Pediatr 1987; 110: 946–948.

165. Anderson SL, Coli R, Daly IW, et al. Familial dysautonomia is caused by mutations of the IKAP gene. Am J Hum Genet 2001; 68: 753–758.

166. Slaugenhaupt SA, Blumenfeld A, Gill SP, et al. Tissue-specific expression of a splicing mutation in the IKBKAP gene causes familial dysautonomia. Am J Hum Genet 2001; 68: 598–605.

167. Fleck BJ, Pandya A, Vanner L, et al. Coffin–Siris syndrome: review and presentation of new cases from a questionnaire study. Am J Med Genet 2001; 99: 1–7.

168. Bodemer C, Rotig A, Rustin P, et al. Hair and skin disorders as signs of mitochondrial disease. Pediatrics 1999; 103: 428–433.

169. Flynn MK, Wee SA, Lane AT. Skin manifestations of mitochondrial DNA syndromes: case report and review. J Am Acad Dermatol 1998; 39: 819–823.

170. Birch-Machin MA. Mitochondria and skin disease. Clin Exp Dermatol 2000; 25: 141–146.

171. Pang CY, Lee HC, Yang JH, Wei YH. Human skin mitochondrial DNA deletions associated with light exposure. Arch Biochem Biophys 1994; 312: 534–538.

27

Neonatal Mucous Membrane Disorders

Denise W. Metry, Adelaide A. Hebert

Examination of the mucous membranes is an important, yet often overlooked, part of the neonatal evaluation. In this chapter we discuss abnormal cutaneous findings of the oral, genital, and ocular systems. Many of these abnormalities provide important clues to the diagnosis of underlying disease and/or developmental syndromes in the newborn infant.[1]

DISORDERS OF THE ORAL MUCOUS MEMBRANES (Table 27-1)

Bohn's Nodules

Bohn's nodules are multiple, small cystic structures found along the lingual gum margins and lateral palate (Fig. 27-1). These lesions are commonly found in up to 85% of newborn infants. Bohn's nodules most likely develop from epithelial remnants of salivary gland tissue or from remnants of the dental lamina. However, some authors refute this idea because mucinous glands are rarely found on the lateral edge of the gingival margins. Bohn's nodules are felt to be asymptomatic and occur more often in full-term infants than in premature newborns.[2-5]

Congenital Epulis

The congenital epulis is a rare, benign tumor of the newborn. Clinically, the lesion is a solitary soft nodule, measuring from 1 to several millimeters in diameter, and often pedunculated. The lesion represents a hamartoma of the alveolar ridge.[6] The epulis forms over the gingival margin, most frequently along the anterior maxillary ridge or the incisor/canine.[7,8] The rate of alveolar placement of these lesions on the maxilla rather than the mandible is 1:2.[6] Female infants are more often affected, with a female to male ratio of 3:2. Fetal ovarian estrogen levels were originally thought to account for this predominance, but this concept has been challenged.[9] Currently there is no known cause of these lesions and no teratogenic or genetic association has been reported.

Histologic examination shows tightly packed granular cells surrounded by a prominent fibrovascular network. The absence of pseudoepitheliomatous hyperplasia and neural elements differentiates the epulis from a granular cell myoblastoma.

Lesions may regress spontaneously over time. However, difficulties with feeding and respiration can occur with large or multiple lesions.[10] Simple excision is curative; recurrences have not been reported.

Congenital Ranula

The congenital ranula is a very rare type of mucocele that results from an obstructed, imperforate, or atretic sublingual or submandibular salivary gland duct. Lesions are found specifically on the anterior floor of the mouth, lateral to the lingual frenulum. The overlying mucosa may be normal in color or have a translucent blue hue. These retention cysts are asymptomatic.

Ranulae may resemble mucous retention cysts, dermoid cysts, or cystic hygromas. Differentiation of a ranula from a mucous retention cyst can be confirmed only by histopathologic examination. Although the mucous retention cyst is a true cyst lined by epithelium, the ranula is a pseudocyst.

Ranulae may rupture spontaneously during feeding and sucking; however, obstructed ducts should be treated early with marsupialization. In some cases, failure to operate may lead to sialadenitis. If surgery is warranted, the risk of recurrence postoperatively is minimal.[11,12]

Granular Cell Tumor

The granular cell tumor, first described in 1926, was originally thought to arise from skeletal muscle and was hence named a granular cell myoblastoma.[13] However, more recent immu-

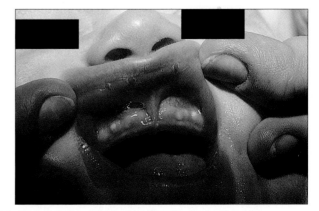

FIG. 27-1 Bohn's nodules along the upper alveolar ridge.

TABLE 27-1 Benign Papular Lesions of the Tongue/Oral Mucosa

Lesion	Morphology	Most common location
Bohn's nodules	Multiple, small cysts	Gingival margin, lateral palate
Congenital epulis	Pedunculated, soft nodule from 1 mm to several cm in diameter	Gingival margin
Congenital ranula	Translucent, firm papule or nodule	Anterior floor of mouth, lateral to lingual frenulum
Epstein's pearls	Multiple, tiny (< few mm) cysts	Median palatal raphe
Eruption cysts	Circumscribed, fluctuant swelling; may have bluish-red to black surface if hemorrhage has occurred	Alveolar ridge of mandible or maxilla
Granular cell tumor	Small (<3 cm in diameter), firm, flesh-colored nodule	Tongue
Hemangiomas	Red to blue, soft to semi-firm nodule	Lips, buccal mucosa, palate
Lymphangiomas	Translucent papules or nodule	Tongue
Neurofibromas	Soft, flesh-colored nodule	Tongue
Venous malformations	Bluish, compressible nodule; often intermittently painful	Oropharynx
White sponge nevus	White plaque with thick, folded surface	Buccal mucosa

nohistochemical testing suggests a neural origin.[14] Intraoral granular cell tumors most commonly occur on the tongue, but may also affect the lips and gingiva. The lesion is typically a solitary, small (<3 cm), firm, asymptomatic nodule, with a smooth, nonulcerated surface. These lesions may rarely cause obstruction of the oral cavity.[15] The differential diagnosis includes other benign neural neoplasms (neuromas, neurofibromas), and vascular tumors (hemangiomas, venous malformations).[16–19] Histologically, large, eosinophilic granular cells are arranged in clusters and fascicles. Pseudoepitheliomatous hyperplasia of the overlying epithelium may be present, mimicking squamous cell carcinoma.[20] Although the majority of granular cell tumors are entirely benign, these tumors can be locally invasive and metastases have been rarely reported. Surgical excision is recommended and curative. Recurrences are uncommon.[21]

Epstein's Pearls

Epstein's pearls are benign cystic lesions that occur along the median palatal raphe, most commonly at the junction of the hard and soft palates (Fig. 27-2). Lesions are multiple and small, ranging in size from less than a millimeter to several millimeters in diameter. The overall appearance is similar to that of Bohn's nodule, but the location and etiology make this a distinct entity. Epstein's pearls are common, occurring in 60–85% of newborn infants. Japanese newborns are most commonly affected (up to 92%), followed by Caucasians and African-Americans.[3,22,23]

Epstein's pearls are epidermal inclusion cysts formed during the fusion of the soft and hard palates, and contain desquamated keratin within their lumina. They are considered the counterpart of milia, which are commonly seen on the faces of neonates. No therapy is indicated, as most lesions rupture spontaneously within the first few weeks to months of life.[2,3,22]

Eruption Cysts

An eruption cyst (or eruption hematoma) is a circumscribed fluctuant swelling that develops over the site of an erupting

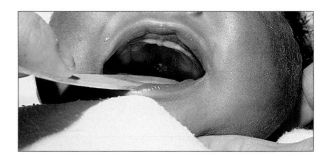

FIG. 27-2 Epstein's pearls of the hard palate.

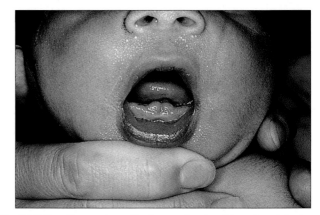

FIG. 27-3 Eruption cysts on the lower alveolar ridge of an infant.

tooth (Fig. 27-3). Lesions in the newborn may occur secondary to natal or neonatal teeth, but these cysts are more commonly associated with the eruption of deciduous or permanent teeth. Eruption cysts most commonly develop on the alveolar ridge of the maxilla or mandible. Size varies with the type of tooth overlaid, but most lesions are approximately 0.6 cm in diameter. The surface of the cyst may appear flesh-colored or have a bluish-red to blue-black color if the cyst cavity contains blood. Although removal of the tissue overlying the tooth may aid in its eruption, most eruption cysts resolve spontaneously within several weeks without treatment.[24]

Infantile hemangiomas

Hemangiomas of the oral mucosa in newborns most commonly develop within the first few days to weeks of life, generally over the lips, buccal mucosa, or palate (Fig. 27-4). Superficial lesions consist of bright red papules, nodules or plaques, whereas deeper lesions are generally flesh colored, and may have a bluish hue or overlying telangiectasias. Lesions with a combination of both superficial and deep features are also common.

Hemangiomas of the oral cavity are prone to trauma, which can lead to ulceration and/or bleeding, particularly during the newborn period. The lip can also be a high-risk location for scarring, particularly when lesions ulcerate or are superficial and cross the vermillion border. There is also a known association between hemangiomas in a cervicofacial, or 'beard' distribution (preauricular skin, chin, anterior neck, or lower lip) and airway hemangioma. At-risk infants should be followed closely during the newborn period for the development of stridor or other signs of airway compromise, in which case direct visualization of the airway can provide a definitive diagnosis.[25]

Treatment indications and options for hemangiomas are discussed in Chapter 20. Ulceration of a lip hemangioma can be particularly difficult to manage owing to the challenges of wound care in this location, and because associated pain can interfere with feeding. Such cases may require additional management with corticosteroids, laser, or excisional surgery.[26]

Lymphatic Malformations

Lymphatic malformations (LM) are benign, structural malformations of lymphatic vessels, and are much less common than hemangiomas. They are congenital, but sometimes do not manifest until later in childhood. No known sexual predilection or hereditary predisposition exists. Unlike hemangiomas, LM remain static or undergo slow expansion over time, and rarely undergo any significant degree of involution.[27–29]

The cervicofacial region is a common site for LM. Lesions may be localized, diffuse or multiple in distribution, and may be microcystic ('lymphangioma'), macrocystic ('cystic hygroma') or combined. Microcystic lesions of the skin present as translucent papules or nodules, which often turn red or purpuric due to intralesional bleeding. The most common location for

intraoral LM is the tongue, although the lips, buccal mucosa, palate, or alveolar ridges may also be affected. LM of the tongue (Fig. 27-5) most commonly affect the dorsal anterior two-thirds and may result in macroglossia and difficulties with feeding and speech.[28–30] Large macrocystic or combined LM of the posterior triangle of the neck, which often present as fluctuant, flesh-colored tumors, may also involve the floor or the mouth and submandibular space. Bacterial cellulitis occurring within cervicofacial LM is potentially dangerous because of the risks of airway compromise. In such instance, systemic antibiotics should be administered at the first sign of swelling, pain, redness, or systemic toxicity.

Histologically, LM consist of multiple lymphatic channels lined by single or multiple layers of endothelial cells. Treatment is rarely necessary in first year of life, and is generally reserved for lesions causing functional compromise or cosmetic deformity. MRI is the best means of determining lesion extent and microcystic or macrocystic morphology, which is generally necessary before decisions regarding treatment can be made. The mainstay of therapy for LM includes surgery and/or sclerotherapy, though cure is rarely achieved except for the smallest, most well-localized lesion. Attempts at surgical resection are often accompanied by a variety of intraoperative and postoperative complications, including recurrence. Sclerotherapy with agents such as absolute ethanol, sodium tetradecylsulfate, or OK-432 (a killed strain of group A *Streptococcus pyogenes*) is not effective for microcystic lesions, but can be used for treatment of macrocystic LM, alone or in conjunction with surgical techniques. Microcystic LM of the tongue can also be treated with laser photocoagulation, though this is also a temporary measure.[31,32]

Neurofibromas

A neurofibroma is a tumor of neural origin, which may occur as an isolated finding or in association with the syndrome of neurofibromatosis. Neurofibromatosis may be difficult to

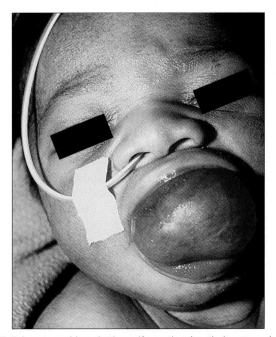

FIG. 27-5 Large, oral lymphatic malformation (cystic hygromas) may result in life-threatening respiratory distress.

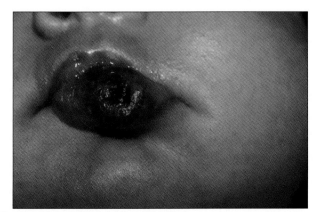

FIG. 27-4 Hemangioma of the lower lip.

diagnose in the newborn period, when many of the features of the syndrome are not yet evident.

Neurofibromas may be found on the skin or within the oral cavity, although intraoral lesions are exceedingly rare in the newborn. The most common intraoral location is the tongue, though tumors have also been observed over the buccal mucosa and palate. Oral lesions are typically asymptomatic, slow-growing, soft nodules, of the same color as the surrounding mucosa. Neurofibromas range in size from a few millimeters to a few centimeters in diameter. Histologically, the tumor is unencapsulated and composed of Schwann cells, perineural cells, and fibroblasts. Neurofibromas are benign and can be electively surgically excised with little risk of recurrence.[33,34]

Venous Malformations

Venous malformations (VM) are slow-flow structural anomalies of the venous vasculature, which are generally present at birth but may not manifest until later in childhood. Lesions most commonly involve the face and oropharynx, but may occur in any anatomic location. Though usually solitary, lesions may be multiple, especially when associated with the autosomal dominant, familial cutaneous–mucosal VM syndrome, or blue rubber bleb nevus syndrome, both characterized by small dome-shaped lesions. VMs are bluish, compressible nodules, which slowly refill upon release and are often intermittently painful. Lesions may result in skeletal alterations, such as facial asymmetry, dental malalignment, open mouth deformity, and bony hypertrophy.

The best means of establishing the diagnosis and determining the extent of tissue involvement is with MRI. In addition, the presence of phleboliths is highly characteristic of the diagnosis. Extensive lesions may be complicated by a localized, intravascular coagulopathy, characterized by a normal or moderately low platelet count and fibrinogen, increased D-dimers, and normal prothrombin and partial thromboplastin times.

VMs characteristically undergo slow expansion over time. Treatment is rarely necessary in first year of life, and is generally reserved for those lesions causing functional compromise or cosmetic deformity. Depending on the location and size of the lesion, surgical excision and/or sclerotherapy can be considered.[35]

White Sponge Nevus (of Cannon)

White sponge nevus is a rare, benign condition inherited as an autosomal dominant trait. Typical lesions are asymptomatic white plaques in which the oral mucosa appears thickened and folded, with a spongy texture (Figs 27-6 and 29-10). The most common location for a white sponge nevus is on the buccal mucosa, often in a bilateral distribution. Extraoral locations, such as labial, nasal, vaginal, esophageal, and anal mucosa, are uncommon, and such lesions usually do not occur in the absence of oral involvement.[36] The white sponge nevus is most often present at birth or discovered during early childhood.[37]

The clinical differential diagnosis of white sponge nevus includes candidiasis, leukoderma, leukoplakia, lichen planus, and local irritation. It is sometimes seen in association with pachyonychia congenita. However, the clinical and histologic findings are usually characteristic enough to differentiate this condition from other white mucosal lesions.[38] The histopa-

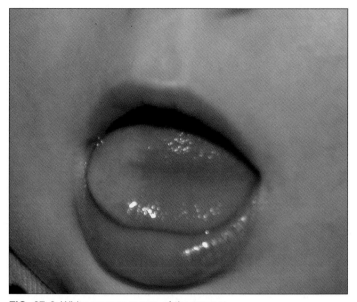

FIG. 27-6 White sponge nevus of the tongue.

thology of a white sponge nevus shows epithelial thickening with hyperkeratosis and acanthosis. The suprabasal cells exhibit intracellular edema with pyknotic nuclei and compact aggregates of keratin intermediate filaments within the upper spinous layer.[39]

Natal Teeth

Natal teeth are defined as teeth present at birth and must be differentiated from neonatal teeth, which erupt during the first month of life. The reported incidence of both natal and neonatal teeth varies widely, but is decidedly rare. Both may occur in either premature or term infants. However, natal teeth occur three times more often than neonatal teeth and are twice as common in females. Two-thirds of natal teeth occur in pairs. The most common location for natal teeth is at the sites of the central mandibular incisors (85%), followed by the maxillary incisors (11%) (Fig. 27-7).[40–42]

Although the exact etiology for natal teeth remains unknown, it appears that the primary tooth bud develops in a more superficial location than normal, and therefore erupts prematurely.[43] Many syndromes have been associated with natal teeth (Table 27-2), and newborns with this finding should be examined carefully. Other reported associations include congenital syphilis, endocrine disturbances, febrile systemic illness, hypovitaminosis, and pyelitis during pregnancy.[7]

Natal teeth usually represent deciduous rather than supernumerary teeth, which can be distinguished by radiography. Supernumerary teeth are extraneous teeth, which should be extracted as they may interfere with normal tooth eruption. The lower central incisors are normally the first teeth in the oral cavity to erupt. The condition of Riga-Fede describes a traumatic ulcerative lesion of the tongue or frenulum, produced when an infant rakes the tongue over the primary lower incisors, which may be mobile and/or have poorly formed crowns (Fig. 27-8). This condition may be related to pain insensitivity, and has been associated with familial dysautonomia.[7,44]

Treatment of natal teeth is dependent on morphology, the amount of root development, and mobility. If the tooth is only minimally loose, it will tend to stabilize over time and can be left in place. Problematic teeth should be extracted to prevent trauma or aspiration.[45,46]

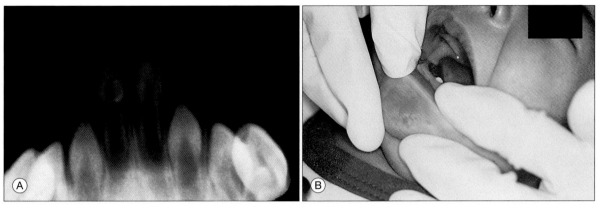

FIG. 27-7 (**A**) Radiograph of natal teeth. (**B**) Natal teeth on the lower alveolar ridge of an infant.

TABLE 27-2 Syndromes Associated With Natal Teeth

Syndrome	Associated anomalies	Inheritance/chromosomal abnormality/prevalence
Ellis-van Creveld (chondroectodermal dysplasia)	Bilateral postaxial polydactyly of hands, chondrodysplasia of long bones resulting in acromesolic dwarfism, ectodermal dysplasia affecting nails/teeth, congenital heart malformation	Autosomal-recessive Not known $7/1 \times 106$
Hallermann-Streiff	Dyscephaly, hypotrichosis, micro-ophthalmia, cataracts, beaked nose, micrognathia, proportionate short stature	Sporadic Not known 150 cases to date
Pachyonychia congenita (Jadassohn-Lewandowsky or Jackson-Lawler)	Dystrophic nails, palmoplantar keratosis, hyperhidrosis, follicular keratosis, oral leukokeratosis, cutaneous cysts	Autosomal-dominant Not known $0.07/1 \times 106$ 9:5 male to female
Pallister-Hall (hypothalamic hamartoblastoma)	Hypothalamic hamartoblastoma, craniofacial abnormalities, postaxial polydactyly, cardiac and renal defects	Sporadic Not known 13 cases to date 8:5 male to female
Weidemann-Rautenstrauch	Endocrine dysfunction, aged facies, frontal and biparietal bossing, small facial bones, sparse scalp hair, prominent scalp veins, small beaked nose, low-set ears	Autosomal-recessive Not known 1 case to date
Natal teeth, patent ductus arteriosus, intestinal pseudoobstruction	Dilatation/hypermobility of small bowel, short or microcolon without obstruction, incomplete rotation of midgut, patent ductus arteriosus	X-linked recessive Not known 2 cases to date, brothers

From Hebert AA, Berg JH. Mucous membrane disorders. In Schachner LA, Hansen RC, eds. Pediatric dermatology, 2nd edition. New York: Churchill Livingstone, 1995.

Sucking Calluses

Sucking calluses (or sucking pads) develop on the lips or buccal mucosa as solitary, oval thickenings (Fig. 27-9). When these lesions are congenital, they are indicative of vigorous sucking in utero. Presentation after birth is more common in breastfed black infants. Histology reveals a thickened epidermis secondary to intracellular edema and hyperkeratosis. Sucking calluses involute spontaneously within a few days or weeks after birth, or on cessation of breastfeeding.[5,22]

Congenital Fistulae of the Lower Lip

Congenital fistulae of the lower lip (or lip pits) are rare developmental anomalies. The estimated frequency of lower lip pits in Caucasians is uncommon, with approximately 1 in 100 000 persons affected; the frequency in the black population is rare.

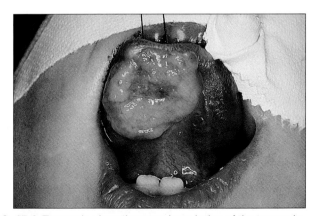

FIG. 27-8 Traumatic ulcerative granuloma lesion of the tongue in Riga-Fede syndrome.

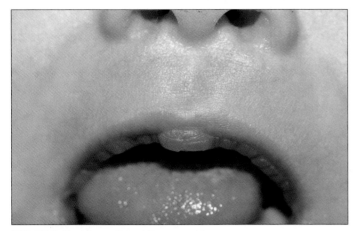

FIG. 27-9 Sucking callus of the upper lip.

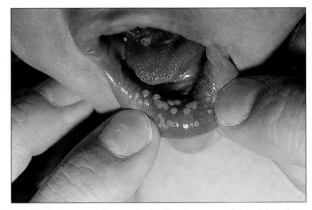

FIG. 27-10 Sebaceous hyperplasia (Fordyce spots) involving the lower gingiva.

Clinically, bilateral indentations are seen on the vermilion portion of the lower lip. The pits are usually 1 cm apart and equidistant from the midline. The defect results from incomplete closure of the furrows on the fetal mandibular process. The pits range in depth from a few millimeters to 25 mm; longer fistulae can transverse the orbicularis oris muscle. The proximal opening of the fistula at the lip may extrude saliva, either spontaneously or during mastication. Histologically, the fistula lumen is lined by stratified squamous epithelium, similar to lip mucosa. At the distal end of the fistula, scattered acini of mucinous glands with tubular ducts are present. True salivary glands are not seen.[23,47]

Congenital fistulae are inherited as an autosomal dominant trait with an estimated penetrance of 80–100%. The presence of a single fistula is considered an incomplete expression of the trait and not a separate entity. Less severe forms may occur and present as simple elevations of a portion of the vermillion border or as an isolated ptosis of the lower lip.[48] The evaluation of a patient with lower lip pits should include a search for other possible anomalies. Lip pits are strongly associated with the formation of cleft lip and/or palate. This association approaches 80% and is now referred to as the Van de Woude syndrome. Newborn infants with single lip pits are at equal risk with those having double pits for associated clefting. Congenital fistulae of the lip are only treated to correct visible deformity or to eradicate significant aberrant salivation.[23,47–51] The best time for surgical repair of the lower lip may be between 10 and 12 months of age. Surgical intervention at this time also helps with parental concerns to normalize the appearance of their child.[51]

Sebaceous Hyperplasia of the Lip (Fordyce Spots or Granules)

Fordyce spots are collections of normal sebaceous glands within the oral cavity. Lesions appear as white to yellow macules and papules visible through the transparent oral mucosa. The papules measure 1–3 mm and may be clustered (Fig. 27-10). Plaques form when large numbers of sebaceous glands coalesce. Sebaceous hyperplasia is most commonly seen on the upper lip, but may also be evident on the buccal mucosa, tongue, gingiva, or palate. No treatment is warranted, as these lesions are asymptomatic, resolve spontaneously, and are of no medical consequence.[23] Superpulsed CO_2 laser has been reported to be safe and effective in a small number of cases.[52]

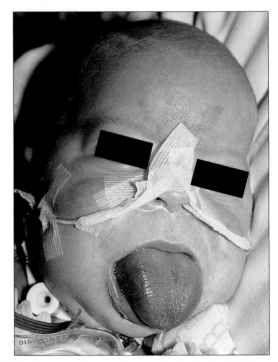

FIG. 27-11 Macroglossia in an infant with Beckwith–Weidemann syndrome.

Annulus Migrans (Geographic Tongue)

Annulus migrans (or geographic tongue) is a common condition that may present as early as 2 weeks of life. Another name for this condition is benign migratory glossitis. Characteristically, multiple erythematous patches surrounded by white, polycyclic borders are seen over the dorsum of the tongue. The lesions are often migratory and transient in nature. The etiology of annulus migrans is most likely reactive in nature; reported associated disorders have included psoriasis (especially pustular), Reiter's syndrome, atopic and seborrheic dermatitis, and spasmodic bronchitis of childhood. Histologically, geographic tongue is indistinguishable from pustular psoriasis or Reiter's syndrome. Therapy of this benign condition is generally unsuccessful and unwarranted.[23,53]

Macroglossia

Macroglossia is defined as a resting tongue that protrudes beyond the teeth or gum line (Figs 27-11 and 27-12). When

Box 27-1 Primary and secondary causes of macroglossia

Primary
Muscular hypertrophy

Secondary

Congenital
Lymphangioma
Hemangioma
Vascular malformations
Beckwith-Weidemann syndrome
Trisomy 4p syndrome
Triploidy syndrome
Trisomy 21 syndrome (Down syndrome)
Fetal face syndrome (Robinow syndrome)

Metabolic storage disease
Mucopolysaccharidoses II, III, IV
Generalized gangliosidosis S
Glycogen storage disease
Endocrine disorders
Congenital hypothyroidism

Tumors
Granular cell tumor
Neurofibroma

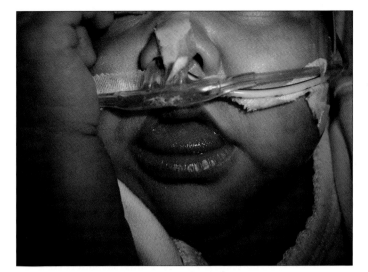

FIG. 27-12 Protruding tongue from macroglossia.

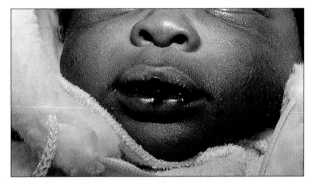

FIG. 27-13 Macular hyperpigmentation involving the lower lip.

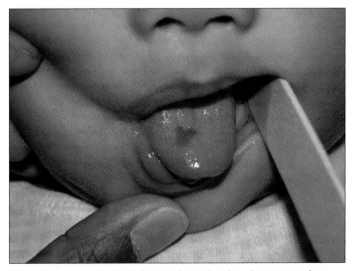

FIG. 27-14 Lingual melanotic macule on the dorsal tongue surface.

this is present in a newborn, a thorough evaluation should be performed to rule out genetic, metabolic, or other possibly contributing factors. True macroglossia may be 'primary,' whereby the tongue is enlarged due to hyperplasia or hypertrophy of normal lingual structures, or, more commonly, 'secondary' to an underlying process, as with a lymphangioma or in amyloidosis (Box 27-1).

True macroglossia must be distinguished from pseudomacroglossia. In pseudomacroglossia, the tongue is normal size but functionally enlarged as a result of a small or inferiorly displaced mandible. This situation occurs in the Pierre–Robin syndrome, and is also seen in some newborns ultimately diagnosed with cerebral palsy.

An enlarged tongue may affect feeding, speech, and respiration. In later infancy, macroglossia may also cause malocclusion as a result of increased pressure on the teeth.

Surgical trimming or reduction of the tongue is often effective in reducing tissue bulk. However, therapeutic intervention, when feasible, should be aimed at treating any underlying cause[23] (Fig. 27-12).

Macular Pigmentation

Macular pigmentation of the oral mucosa is a normal variant found in darker-skinned persons. Several patterns of pigmentation may occur. Most commonly, a pigmented band is present at the junction of the free and attached alveolar mucosa. Patchy pigmentation may also be evident over the buccal mucosa, on the lips, and on the floor of the mouth (Fig. 27-13). When the tongue is involved, which is rare, the pigment is localized to the filiform papillae. The increased pigmentation occurs as a result of an increase in melanocytic activity rather than an increase in the number of melanocytes. No therapy is necessary.[54]

Lingual Melanotic Macule

Congenital lingual melanotic macules have been observed as solitary or multiple, well-circumscribed, brown lesions on the dorsal surface of the tongue at birth that grow proportionately to the tongue (Fig. 27-14). Histological features are those of increased basal pigmentation with minimal melanocytic hyperplasia and mild pigment incontinence. It is distinct from macular pigmentation, and appears to be a benign process. The diagnosis of congenital lingual melanotic macule should be considered if the pigmented macules are present at birth and grow proportionately with the child.[55]

Acatalasemia

Acatalasemia is a genetically heterogeneous disease characterized by an inherited absence of the enzyme catalase. Affected infants are unable to degrade endogenous or exogenous hydrogen peroxide, which accumulates, resulting in oxidation deprivation. The soft tissues of the mouth and nasal mucosa are preferentially affected, leading to ulceration, necrosis, and in severe cases gangrene. The physical examination is otherwise normal. The diagnosis is confirmed by the absence of blood catalase. Therapy consists of meticulous oral hygiene, early removal of diseased teeth and tonsils, and the administration of systemic antibiotics as necessary to control bacterial proliferation.[23,56]

Orofacial–Digital Syndrome, Type I

Orofacial–digital (OFD) syndrome is a rare and complex condition. Seven types are currently recognized. Oral abnormalities are the most consistent and characteristic findings of type I OFD (also known as Papillon–Leage–Psaume syndrome). Features may include multiple hyperplastic frenulae between the buccal mucosa and alveolar ridge, cleft lip (45%) or palate (80%), a lobated or bifid tongue (30–40%) with small hamartomas (70%) (Fig. 27-15), dental caries, and/or anomalous anterior teeth. Distinguishing facial features are frontal bossing, hypoplasia of the malar bones and alar cartilages, a broad nasal root, and milia of the ears. Skeletal findings include asymmetric shortening of digits, clinodactyly and brachydactyly of the hands (45%), and unilateral polydactyly (25%) of the feet. Infants may also have a dry, rough scalp with significant alopecia.

This form of OFD is part of a heterogeneous group of PFD syndromes.[57] The *OFDI* gene is named Cxof5 (Xp22.2-22.3). The condition is seen in one in 50 000 live births.

Newborns with OFD type I may also have internal manifestations, the most common of which are multiple renal, hepatic, or pancreatic cysts. OFD I is considered a distinct subset of this syndrome because of the X-linked dominant inheritance pattern and this association with polycystic kidney disease.[57]

Significant CNS abnormalities, especially agenesis or absence of the corpus callosum, also occur. The overall prognosis is poor: one-third of affected patients die within the first year of life. Therapy must be individualized based on the presence of visceral anomalies. Surgical intervention may be necessary to ensure proper feeding and oral communication.[23,58,59]

Oral and Genital Ulcerations with Immunodeficiency

The presentation of oral and genital ulcers in a newborn may be a sign of underlying congenital immunodeficiency (Fig. 27-16). In particular, ulcers in these locations appear to be a distinctive marker and are often the presenting feature of severe combined immunodeficiency disease with T- and B-cell lymphopenia (T-B-SCID) in Athabascan-speaking American Indian infants.[60] In this population, ulcers are typically punched-out and deep, albeit without invasion to underlying

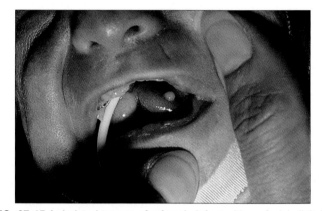

FIG. 27-15 Lobulated tongue of a female infant with orofacial–digital I syndrome.

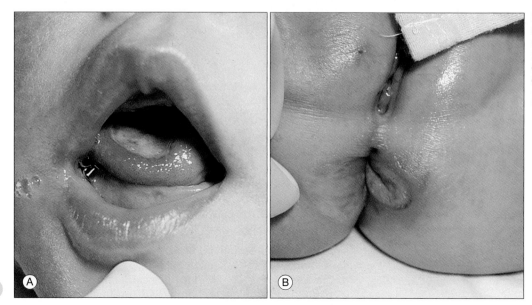

FIG. 27-16 (A) Oral ulceration associated with immunodeficiency. (B) Genital ulceration associated with immunodeficiency. (From Kwong PC, O'Marcaigh AS, Howard R, et al. Oral and genital ulceration: a unique presentation. Arch Dermatol 1999; 135: 927–931.)

structures, and do not result in functional sequelae or significant scarring. This is to be distinguished from the condition neonatal noma, which is a rare condition of preterm infants in developing countries. Neonatal noma causes aggressive orofacial tissue gangrene, accompanied by a high mortality rate, and is most commonly associated with *Pseudomonas aeruginosa* sepsis.[61,62] In contrast, the ulcers found in American Indian children with T-B-SCID are most likely a result of T-cell immunodeficiency combined with a genetic predisposition. In such children, treatment of the underlying condition with bone marrow transplantation results in resolution of the ulcers. Early recognition and diagnosis can lead to prompt intervention and prevention of complications.[60]

Ectopic Thyroid Tissue

Ectopic thyroid tissue is defined by the development of thyroid tissue outside the usual pretracheal position (inferior to the thyroid cartilage). This abnormality results from an arrest or irregularity in thyroid descent during embryologic development. Ectopic thyroid tissue, also referred to as a thyroglossal duct cyst, may be classified as lingual, sublingual, pretracheal, or substernal. Lingual is the most common type, representing over 90% of cases. A lingual thyroglossal duct cyst presents as a painless, nodular mass in the cervical midline or at the base of the tongue between the circumvallate papillae and the epiglottis. Lesions may be present at birth or develop in early infancy. However, most become evident during the first or second decades of life, at which time associated symptoms may occur.[63–66]

Thyroglossal duct cysts are a rare but serious cause of airway obstruction in newborns and infants: mortality rates of up to 43% have been reported. Although usually asymptomatic, lesions may be associated with cough, dysphagia, hemorrhage, or pain. If a cutaneous tract is present, mucous drainage can occur.

Ectopic thyroid tissue occurs in fewer than 1 in 100 000–300 000 persons. The incidence is much more common among patients with thyroid disease.[64–67] The extraglandular tissue secretes chemically normal thyroid hormone, but in quantities sometimes insufficient to meet metabolic needs. Hypothyroidism occurs in up to one-third of patients; thus serum TSH, T_4, and T_3 levels should be measured in all suspected cases.[65] If the quantity of thyroid hormone is insufficient, a compensatory increase of TSH from the anterior pituitary will lead to hypertrophy of the thyroid tissue. Thyroid hormone supplementation is indicated if clinical hypothyroidism develops, or to reduce the size of an enlarged thyroid tissue mass. Some authors suggest thyroid hormone supplementation on discovery of a thyroglossal duct cyst to prevent such complications.[65,68–71]

Surgical treatment may be necessary, particularly where hemorrhage occurs or medical measures fail. A preoperative thyroid scan can assist in localizing the ectopic thyroid tissue. If the duct cannot be adequately excised because of its size, marsupialization may be attempted.[66]

DISORDERS OF THE GENITAL MUCOUS MEMBRANES

Labial Adhesions

Labial adhesions are exceedingly rare during the newborn period. The rarity of this finding has been attributed to the presence of maternal estrogens at birth. Infants between the ages of 13 and 23 months are most commonly affected, with an incidence of 3.3%. Clinically, a thin membrane extends between the labia, which may partially or completely conceal the vaginal opening. Recommended treatments include A and D ointment for asymptomatic cases, and topical estrogen cream or ointment if urinary or vaginal drainage is impaired.[72,73]

Perianal Pyramidal Protrusion

Perianal pyramidal protrusion is an increasingly recognized entity characteristically located on the perineal median raphe, anterior to the anus. Clinically the lesion is pyramidal in shape, with a smooth, red, or rose-colored surface (Fig. 27-17). The average age at presentation is 14.1 months, and 94% occur in females. Histologic examination shows epidermal acanthosis, marked edema in the upper dermis, and a mild dermal inflammatory infiltrate.[74] The pathogenesis is unknown, but some cases have been related to constipation and lichen sclerosus et atrophicus.[75,76] This condition is not associated with child abuse. Differential diagnosis includes genital warts, granulomatous lesions of inflammatory bowel disease, rectal prolapse, hemorrhoids, acrochordons, and perineal midline malformation. Although most lesions show spontaneous reduction without any specific treatment, treating associated constipation may hasten resolution.[74,77,78]

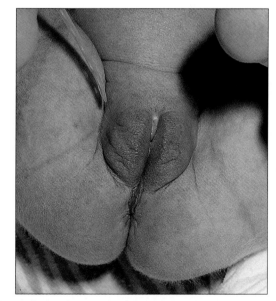

FIG. 27-17 Perianal pyramidal protrusion in a female infant.

Pyoderma Gangrenosum

Pyoderma gangrenosum (PG) is an ulcerative skin disorder most commonly seen on the lower legs of adults. In adults, it is often associated with an underlying systemic disease, especially ulcerative colitis, Crohn's disease, or leukemia. The condition is rare in children (4% of cases), and rarer still in infants less than 2 years of age. Diagnosis in infancy is challenging because of the atypical location of lesions (perianal or genital) and the lack of associated systemic illness. Differential diagnosis in infancy includes ecthyma gangrenosum caused by *Pseudomonas* infection, herpes simplex infection, and severe diaper dermatitis. Successful treatment has been reported with systemic, topical, and intralesional corticosteroids.[79]

Urethral Retention Cyst

The urethral retention cyst is an inclusion cyst that forms at the urethral opening in newborn boys. This lesion is simply a milium, which develops either as a result of friction or from remnants of epithelial tissue trapped along a line of skin fusion. No therapy is necessary, as the white, firm, smooth-surfaced papule will rupture spontaneously and be shed during the first weeks of life. These cysts are not likely to cause urinary retention or symptoms.[80]

DISORDERS OF THE OCULAR MUCOUS MEMBRANES

Behçet's Disease

Behçet's disease is a complex, multisystem disease characterized clinically by the presence of oral aphthae and at least two of the following: genital aphthae, synovitis, cutaneous pustular vasculitis, posterior uveitis, or meningoencephalitis.

Although uncommon, pediatric Behçet's disease does occur. Neonatal cases have been described in which affected mothers had oral and genital ulcerations during pregnancy.[81,82] A case of transient neonatal Behçet's disease with life-threatening complications has been reported.[83] In comparison with adults, oral and genital ulcers are less common in children with Behçet's disease. Uveitis, however, is more common. As in adults, ocular lesions in children pose a serious threat because they may lead to blindness.[84]

Colobomata

The term coloboma describes a defect such as a notch, gap, fissure, or hole caused by the loss of ocular tissue or an ocular structure. (Fig. 27-18) Colobomata may occur as an isolated anomaly, but are most frequently associated with chromosomal defects, especially trisomies 13 and 18, often in association with significant central nervous system abnormalities.[85]

Infants with the CHARGE syndrome (congenital heart disease, choanal atresia, growth and/or mental retardation, genital hypoplasia, ear anomalies and/or deafness) have a 79% incidence of colobomata.[86,88] Colobomata may occasionally be associated with an impaired vision. Retinal colobomas are also a regular feature of the CHIME syndrome (see Chapter 18).

Congenital Obstruction of the Nasolacrimal Duct

Congenital obstruction of the nasolacrimal duct is the most common abnormality of the lacrimal system in children. Up to 6% of newborn infants are affected. Symptoms typically begin shortly after birth and are variable. Many infants will have only a wet-looking eye or overflow tearing, but most will have recurrent infections manifested by reflux or mucopurulent material from the lacrimal sac. The majority of nasolacrimal duct obstructions clear spontaneously. Simple medical management with antibiotics and massage may hasten resolution. When spontaneous resolution does not occur, ophthalmologic probing and/or irrigation may be required.[89,90]

Glaucoma

Glaucoma is defined as abnormal elevation of intraocular pressure, which may cause damage to the eye and changes in visual function. In infants, the principal signs of glaucoma are tearing, conjunctival hyperemia, photophobia, blepharospasm, corneal clouding, and an enlargement of the cornea and globe, referred to as buphthalmos (Fig. 27-19). Glaucoma in infants is usually due to a developmental disorder in which residual mesodermal tissue impedes the drainage of aqueous humor from the anterior chamber. This primary or simple congenital glaucoma is probably a multifactorial, recessively inherited condition. Other major causes of glaucoma in children are trauma, intraocular hemorrhage, ocular inflammatory disease, and intraocular tumors.

Infantile glaucoma has been associated with a variety of other ocular conditions as well as a number of systemic dis-

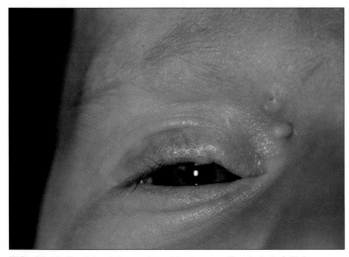

FIG. 27-18 Eyelid coloboma is evident, as well as a hair follicle hamartomas.

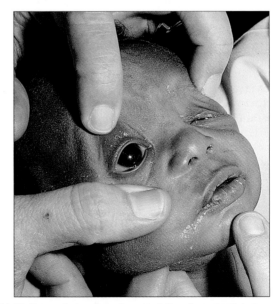

FIG. 27-19 Corneal clouding characteristic of congenital glaucoma.

orders. Those systemic disorders relevant to the dermatologist include the Sturge–Weber syndrome, neurofibromatosis, the congenital infection (TORCH) syndromes, and juvenile xanthogranulomas.

Ocular manifestations of the Sturge–Weber syndrome include a port wine stain (nevus flammeus) involving the eyelids; dilatation and tortuosity of the conjunctival, scleral, and retinal vessels; angiomatous lesions of the uveal tract; and glaucoma.[85] Childhood glaucoma occurs in 45% of children if both the ophthalmic and maxillary divisions of the trigeminal are involved.[91] In some children signs of glaucoma may develop later in infancy, and long-term monitoring of children at risk is advised.

Ocular manifestations associated with neurofibromatosis include plexiform neurofibromas of the eyelid (often presenting with ptosis), optic gliomas or meningiomas, pulsatile exophthalmos secondary to bony defects of the orbital wall, and Lisch nodules (yellowish-brown hamartomas of the iris). Glaucoma, most frequently unilateral, is uncommon. The mechanism of glaucoma development in neurofibromatosis is often unclear, but may be associated with developmental abnormalities of the orbital tissue, plexiform neurofibromas of the eyelid, or neurofibromas of the uvea.

Children with the congenital infection (TORCH) syndromes may develop glaucoma in infancy or later in life. This occurs as a result of intraocular inflammation, except in the case of congenital rubella, in which anomalies of the optic angle have been found.

The most frequent systemic complication found in infants with multiple juvenile xanthogranulomas other than neurofibromatosis type 1 is involvement of the iris and epibulbar area with this histiocytic tumor. Complications include glaucoma, hemorrhage, and blindness.[85,91,92]

Mucocele of the Lacrimal Sac

The mucocele of the lacrimal sac is a rare anomaly. It presents at birth or shortly thereafter as a bluish, cystic swelling located just below the medial canthus. The lesion is typically about 1 cm in diameter and may be confused with a hemangioma because of its color. Blockage of both the proximal and distal ends of the lacrimal drainage system leads to the accumulation of mucus within the lacrimal sac. The natural course is variable. In some cases the blockage may open spontaneously, but many lesions become infected and/or inflamed with erythema, edema, and surrounding cellulitis. Treatment includes gentle application of warm compresses and systemic antibiotics if infection is suspected. Mucoceles unresponsive to conservative treatment may require ophthalmologic probing.[89]

Seborrheic Blepharitis

Seborrheic blepharitis is an inflammatory condition of the eyelid margin. In infants, seborrheic blepharitis usually occurs in association with dermatitis of the scalp (termed cradle cap) or diaper area, and is most commonly seen between the second and 10th weeks of life. The lid margins are typically erythematous and scaly, with accumulation of debris at the base of the lashes. The severity of the blepharitis usually correlates with degree of dermatitis and rarely may cause a superficial, marginal keratitis.

Treatment consists of warm water compresses and gentle cleansing using a dilute amount of an isotonic (baby) shampoo. If necessary, a soft-bristled toothbrush can be used to mechanically remove the scale. A low-potency, nonfluorinated corticosteroid (hydrocortisone) or sulfacetamide ointment may then be gently massaged into the lid margin. These procedures should be repeated daily until the blepharitis has subsided.[93]

REFERENCES

1. del Rosario Rioboo Crespo M, del Pozo PP, Garcia RR. Epidemiology of the most common oral mucosal diseases in children. Med Oral Patol Otal Cir Bucal 2005; 10: 376–387.
2. Cambiaghi S Gelmetti C. Therapy for Bohn's nodules is unnecessary, since spontaneous involution or shedding is the rule. Int J Dermatol 2005; 44: 753–754.
3. Paller AS, Mancini A. Hurwitz clinical pediatric dermatology, 3rd edn. Philadelphia: Elsevier Saunders, 2006; 23.
4. Kula KS, Josell SD. Oral problems. In: McMillan JA, Feigin RD, DeAngelis CD, Douglas Jones M, eds. Oski's pediatrics: principles and practice, 4th edn. Philadelphia: Lippincott Williams & Wilkins, 2006; 781–800.
5. Hebert AA, Haneke E. Mucous membrane disorders. In: Schachner LA, Hansen RC, eds. Pediatric dermatology, 3rd edn. Philadelphia: Mosby, 2003; 447–489.
6. Olson JL, Marcus JR, Zuker RM. J Craniofac Surg 2005; 16: 161–164.
7. Dilley DC, Siegel MA, Budnick S. Diagnosing and treating common oral pathologies. Pediatr Clin North Am 1991; 38: 1227–1264.
8. Zuker RM, Buenechea R. Congenital epulis: Review of the literature and case report. J Oral Maxillofac Surg 1993; 51: 1040–1043.
9. Al-Qattan MM, Clarke HM. Congenital epulis: evidence against the intrauterine estrogen stimulus theory. Ann Plast Surg 1994; 33: 320–321.
10. Raissaki, MT, Segkos N, Prokopakis, EP, et al. Congenital granular cell tumor (epulis). J Comput Assist Tomogr 2005; 29: 520–523.
11. Steelman R, Weisse M, Ramadan H. Congenital ranula. Clin Pediatr 1998; 37: 205–206.
12. Yuca K, Bayram I, Cankaya H, et al. Pediatric intraoral ranulas: an analysis of nine cases. Yohoku J Exp Med 2005; 205: 151–155.
13. Buley ID, Gatter KC, Kelly PM, et al. Granular cell tumors revisited. An immunohistochemical and ultrastructural study. Histopathology 1988; 12: 263.
14. Junquera LM, deVincente JC, Vega JA, et al. Granular-cell tumours: an immunohistochemical study. Br J Oral Maxillofac Surg 1997; 35: 180–184.
15. Bilen TB, Alaybeyoglu N, Arsian A, et al. Obstructive congenital granular cell tumor. Int J Pediatr Otorhinolaryngol 2004; 68: 1567–1571.
16. Noonan JD, Horton CE, Old WL, Stokes TL. Granular cell myoblastoma of the head and neck. Am J Surg 1979; 138: 611–614.
17. Peterson LJ. Granular-cell tumor: review of the literature and report of a case. Oral Surg 1974; 37: 728–735.
18. Robinson HBG, Miller AS, eds. Colby, Kerr and Robinson's color atlas of pathology. St Louis: JB Lippincott, 1990; 149.
19. Brannon RB, Anand PM. Oral granular cell tumors: an analysis of 10 new pediatric and adolescent cases and a review of the literature. J Clin Pediatr Dent 2004; 29: 69–74.
20. Reed RJ, Argenyi Z. Tumors of neural tissue. In: Elder D, Elenitsas R, Jaworsky C, Johnson B, eds. Lever's histopathology of the skin, 8th edn. Philadelphia: Lippincott-Raven, 1997; 994.

21. Kershisnik M, et al. Granular cell tumors. Ann Otol Rhinol Laryngol 1994; 103: 416–419.

22. Weston WL, ed. Neonatal dermatology. In: Color textbook of pediatric dermatology. St Louis: Mosby, 1991; 224, 227.

23. Hebert AA, Berg JH. Mucous membrane disorders. In: Schachner LA, Hansen RC, eds. Pediatric dermatology, 2nd edn. New York: Churchill Livingstone, 1995; 469–537.

24. Peters R, Schock RK. Oral cysts in newborn infants. Oral Surg 1971; 7: 10–14.

25. Orlow SJ, Isakoff MS, Blei F. Increased risk of symptomatic hemangiomas of the airway in association with cutaneous hemangiomas in a 'beard' distribution. J Pediatr 1997; 131: 643–646.

26. Frieden IJ. Which hemangiomas to treat – and how? Arch Dermatol 1997; 133: 1593–1595.

27. Eisen D, Lynch D. Developmental disorders. In: The mouth: Diagnosis and treatment. St Louis: Mosby, 1998; 48.

28. Shafer WG, Hine MK, Levy BM, eds. Benign and malignant tumors of the oral cavity. In: A textbook of oral pathology, 4th edn. Philadelphia: WB Saunders, 1983; 159–160.

29. Stal S, Hamilton S, Spira M. Hemangiomas, lymphangiomas, and vascular malformations of the head and neck. Otolaryngol Clin North Am 1986; 19: 769–884.

30. Levin SL, Jorgeson RJ, Jarvey BA. Lymphangiomas of the alveolar ridges in neonates. Pediatrics 1976; 58: 881–884.

31. Edwards PD, Rahbar R, Ferraro NF, et al. Lymphatic malformation of the lingual base and oral floor. Plast Recostr Surg 2006; 115: 1906–1915.

32. Hebert AA, Lopez MC. Oral lesions in pediatric patients. In: Advances in dermatology. Vol 12. St Louis: Mosby, 1997: p 181.

33. Chrysomali E, Papanicolaou SI, Dekker NP, Regezi JA. Benign neural tumors of the oral cavity. Oral Surg Oral Med Oral Pathol Oral Radiol Endod 1997; 84: 381–390.

34. Geist JR, Gander DL, Stefanac SJ. Oral manifestation of neurofibromatosis type I and II. Oral Surg Oral Med Oral Pathol 1992; 73: 376–382.

35. Grevelink SV, Mulliken JB. Vascular anomalies. In: Freedberg IM et al., eds. Fitzpatrick's dermatology in general medicine, 5th edn. New York: McGraw-Hill, 1999; 1175–1194.

36. Fitzgerald JF, Troncone R, Iwanczak F, et al. Clinical quiz. J Pediatr Gastroenterol Nutr 2004; 38: 151–153.

37. Krajewska IA, Moore L, Brown LH. White sponge nevus presenting in the esophagus. Case report and literature review. Pathology 1992; 24: 112–115.

38. Eisen D, Lynch D. Genodermatoses. In: The mouth: diagnosis and treatment. St Louis; Mosby, 1998; 193–194.

39. Miller CS, Craig RM. White corrugated mucosa. J Am Dental Assoc 1988; 117: 345–347.

40. Bodenhoff J. Dentitio connatalis et neonatalis. Odont Tidskr 1959; 67: 645–695.

41. Kates GA, Needleman HL, Holmes LB. Natal and neonatal teeth: a clinical study. JADA 1984; 109: 441–443.

42. Zhu J, King D. Natal and neonatal teeth. J Dent Child 1995; 3: 123–128.

43. Nelson WE, ed. Disorders of the teeth associated with other conditions. In: Nelson's textbook of pediatrics. Philadelphia: WB Saunders, 1996; 1039.

44. Eichenfield LF, Honig PJ, Nelson L. Traumatic granuloma of the tongue (Riga-Fede disease): Association with familial dysautonomia. J Pediatr 1990; 116: 742–744.

45. Cohen RL. Clinical perspectives on premature tooth eruption and cyst formation in neonates. Pediatr Dermatol 1984; 1: 301–306.

46. Shafer WG, Hine MK, Levy BM, eds. Developmental disturbance of oral and paraoral structures. In: A textbook of oral pathology, 4th edn. Philadelphia: WB Saunders, 1983; 64.

47. Iregbulem LM. Congenital lower lip sinuses in Nigerian children. Br J Plast Surg 1997; 50: 649–650.

48. Ranta A, Rintala A. Correlations between microforms of the van der Woude syndrome and cleft palate. Cleft Palate J 1983; 20: 158–162.

49. Mohrenschlager M, Kohler LD, Vogt HJ, Ring J. Congenital lower lip pits – a very rare syndrome? Report of two cases and review of the literature. Cutis 1998; 61: 127–128.

50. Velez A, Gorslay M, Buchner A, et al. Congenital lower lip pits (Van der Woude Syndrome). J Am Acad Dermatol 1995; 3: 520–521.

51. Capon-Degardin N, Martinot-Duquennoy, V, Auvray G, Pellerin P. Eur J Pediatr Surg 2003; 13: 92–96.

52. Ocampo-Candiani J, Villareal_Rodriquez A, Quinones-Fernandez AG, et al. Treatment of Fordyce spots with CO_2 laser. Dermatol Surg 2003; 29: 869–871.

53. Cambiaghi, S, Colonna C, Caballi, R. Geographic tongue in two children with nonpustular psoriasis. Pediatr Dermatol 2005; 22: 83–85.

54. Amir E, et al. Physiologic pigmentation of the oral mucosa in Israeli children. Oral Surg Med Oral Pathol 1991; 71: 396–398.

55. Dohil MA, Billman G, Pransky S, Eichenfield, LF. The congenital lingual melanotic macule. Arch Dermatol 2003; 139: 767–770.

56. Ogata M. Acatalasemia. Hum Genet 1991; 86: 331–340.

57. Thauvin-Robinet C, Cossee M, Cormier-Daire V, et al. Clinical, molecular, and genotype–phenotype correlation studies from 25 cases of oral–facial–digital syndrome type 1: A French and Belgian collaborative study. J Med Genet 2006; 43: 54–61.

58. Larralde de Luna M, Raspa ML, Ibargoyen J. Oral–facial–digital type I syndrome of Papillon–Leage and Psaume. Pediatr Dermatol 1992; 9: 52–56.

59. Patrizi A, Orlandi C, Neri I, et al. What syndrome is this? Oral–facial–digital type I. Pediatr Dermatol 1999; 16: 329–331.

60. Kwong PC, O'Marcaigh AS, Howard R, et al. Oral and genital ulceration: a unique presentation of immunodeficiency in Athabascan-speaking American Indian children with severe combined immunodeficiency. Arch Dermatol 1999; 135: 927–31.

61. Ghosal SP, Gupta PC, Muhherjee AK. Noma neonatorum: Its aetiopathogenesis. Lancet 1978; 2: 289–290.

62. Juster-Reicher A, Mogilner BM, Levi G, et al. Neonatal noma. Am J Perinatol 1993; 10: 409–411.

63. Damiano A, Glickman AB, Rubin JS, Cohen AF. Ectopic thyroid tissue presenting as a midline neck mass. Int J Pediatr Otorhinolaryngol 1996; 34: 141–148.

64. Krishnamurthy GT, Bajd WH. Lingual thyroid associated with Zenker's and vallecular diverticula: report of a case and review of the literature. Arch Otolaryngol 1972; 96: 171–175.

65. Leung AK, Wong AL, Robson WL. Ectopic thyroid gland simulating a thyroglossal duct cyst: a case report. Can J Surg 1995; 38: 87–89.

66. Fanaroff AA, Martin RJ, eds. The respiratory system. In: Neonatal–perinatal medicine: diseases of the fetus and infant. Vol 2. St Louis: Mosby, 1997; 1068.

67. Temmel AF, Baumgartner WD, Steiner E, et al. Ectopic thyroid gland simulating a submandibular tumor. Am J Otolaryngol 1998; 19: 342–344.

68. Neinas, FW, Gorman CA, Devine KD, Woolner LB. Lingual thyroid: clinical characteristics of 15 cases. Ann Intern Med 1973; 79: 205–210.

69. Hulse JA, Grant DB, Clayton BE, et al. Population screening for congenital hypothyroidism. Br Med J 1980; 280: 675–678.

70. Jones JA. Lingual thyroid. Br J Oral Maxillofac Surg 1986; 24: 58–62.

71. Kansal P, Sakati N, Rifai A, Woodhouse N. Lingual thyroid: diagnosis and treatment. Arch Intern Med 1987; 147: 2046–2048.

72. Leung AK, Robson WL, Tay-Uyboco J. The incidence of labial fusion in children. J Paediatr Child Health 1993; 29: 235–236.

73. Starr NB. Labial adhesions in childhood. J Paediatr Child Health 1996; 10: 26–27.

74. Kayashima K, Kitoh M, Ono T. Infantile perianal pyramidal protrusion. Arch Dermatol 1996; 132: 1481–1484.

75. Merigou D, Labreze C, Lamireau T, et al. Infantile perianal pyramidal protrusion: A marker of constipation? Pediatr Dermatol 1998; 15: 143–144.

76. Cruces MJ, DeLaTorre C, Losada A, et al. Infantile pyramidal protrusion as a manifestation of lichen sclerosus et

atrophicus. Arch Dermatol 1998; 134: 1118–1120.

77. Fleet SL, Davis LS. Infantile perianal pyramidal protrusion: Report of a case and review of the literature. Pediatr Dermatol 2005; 22 : 151–152.

78. Miyamoto T, Inoue S, Hagari Y, et al. Clinical cameo: infantile perianal pyramidal protrusion with hard stool history. Br J Dermatol 2004; 151: 229.

79. Graham JA, Hansen KK, Rabinowitz LG, Esterly NB. Pyoderma gangrenosum in infants and children. Pediatr Dermatol 1994; 11: 10–17.

80. Yaffe D, Zissin R. Cowper's glands duct: radiographic findings. Urol Radiol 1991; 13: 123–125.

81. Fain O, Mathieu E, Lachassinne E, et al. Neonatal Behçet's disease. Am J Med 1995; 98: 310–311.

82. Jog S, Patole S, Koh G, et al. Unusual presentation of neonatal Behcet's disease. Am J Perinatol 2001; 18: 287–291.

83. Stark AC, Bhakta B, Chamberlain MA, et al. Life threatening transient neonatal Behçet's disease. J Rheumatol 1997; 36: 700–702.

84. Kaklamani V, Vaiopoulos G, Kaklamanis PG. Behçet's disease. Semin Arthritis Rheum 1998; 27: 197–217.

85. Martyn LJ, DiGeorge A. Pediatric ophthalmology. Pediatr Clin North Am 1987; 34; 1530–1536.

86. Tellier AL, Cormier-Daire V, Abadie V, et al. CHARGE syndrome: Report of 47 cases and review. Am J Med Genet 1998; 76: 402–409.

87. Searle LC, Graham JM Jr, Prashad C, et al. CHARGE syndrome from birth to adulthood: An individual reported on from 0 to 33 years. Am J Med Genet A 2005; 133: 344–349.

88. Edwards BM, Kileny PR, van Riper LA. CHARGE syndrome: A window of opportunity for audiologic intervention. Pediatrics 2002; 110: 119–126.

89. Calhoun JH. Problems of the lacrimal system in children. Pediatr Clin North Am 1987; 34: 1457–1465.

90. Forbes BJ, Khazaeni LM. Evaluation and management of an infant with tearing and eye discharge. Pediatr Case Rev 2003; 3: 40–43.

91. Stevenson RF, Thomson HG, Marin JD. Unrecognized ocular problems associated with port-wine stain of the face in children. Can Med Assoc J 1974; 111: 953–954.

92. Sena DF, Finzi S, Rodgers K, et al. Founder mutations of CYP1B1 gene in patients with congenital glaucoma from the United States and Brazil. J Med Genet 2004; 41: e6.

93. Hurwitz S. Eczematous eruptions in childhood. In: Clinical pediatric dermatology, 2nd edn. Philadelphia: WB Saunders, 1993; 62.

28

Hair Disorders

Maureen Rogers, Li-Chuen Wong

This chapter covers neonatal hair patterns, genetic hair shaft abnormalities, and the conditions in which hypo- or hypertrichosis are present in the neonatal period. There are many syndromes in which hypotrichosis or atrichia occur, and those in which it is a prominent feature are discussed. Localized alopecia can occur physiologically, with trauma, and as a nevoid disorder, either alone or associated with other nevi. Diffuse hypertrichosis can occur alone or as part of various syndromes. Localized hypertrichosis may occur with other nevi, but also may be a marker for serious neural tube closure defects (see also Chapter 9).

SCALP HAIR WHORLS

Ninety-five to 98% of normal Caucasian infants have a single hair whorl in the parietal area,[1,2] usually clockwise but inconsistent in position. The remainder have a double parietal whorl. Only 10% of African-American individuals with short curly hair have a parietal whorl.[2] A mild frontal upsweep or 'cowlick' is present in 7% of normal infants.[1] Hair patterns may be very abnormal in infants with structural abnormalities of the brain, demonstrating a striking frontal upsweep and absent or aberrant parietal whorls.[1] Multiple parietal whorls occur with increased frequency in developmentally delayed children, and their presence in the neonate may be an early sign of dysmorphic features.[3] Results of a recent study of hair whorl orientation and handedness suggests that a single gene controls these traits.[4]

THE HAIRLINE

The frontal hairline of neonates is lower than in older children, a feature most striking in racial groups in which there is profuse hair at birth. These terminal hairs on the brow are gradually replaced over the first 12 months of life by vellus hairs. Displacement of the hairline may be a dysmorphic feature. A low frontal hairline is a feature of several syndromes, including Costello, Cornelia de Lange (Brachmann–de Lange), Coffin–Siris, Fanconi, and fetal hydantoin syndromes. The syndromes in which a low posterior hairline occurs include Noonan, Turner, Kabuki, Cornelia de Lange, and fetal hydantoin syndromes.

HETEROCHROMIA OF SCALP HAIR

This may be noted at birth as a result of several clinical situations.[5] In piebaldism there is a white forelock, which will be obvious in a dark-haired neonate. A congenital melanocytic nevus may present as a tuft of dark hair, which is often also longer than the surrounding normal hair. In hereditary, usually autosomal dominant, heterochromia there may, for example, be a tuft of red hair in a dark-haired neonate or a dark tuft in a fair individual. There has recently been a report of a diffuse heterochromia of scalp hair, present from birth, with black and red hairs evenly distributed over the scalp.[5]

HAIR SHAFT ABNORMALITIES

A diverse group of conditions can result in hair shaft abnormalities. Some are associated with extracutaneous disease, whereas others affect only the hair itself. These conditions have been reviewed in detail by Whiting,[6] Price,[7] and Rogers.[8,9]

Monilethrix

Monilethrix is an autosomal dominant condition that produces a beaded appearance of the hair.[6–8] On microscopy, spindle-shaped 'nodes' separated by constricted internodes are seen (Fig. 28-1). The nodes have the diameter of normal hair and may be medullated, whereas the internodes are narrower and usually nonmedullated, and are the sites of fracture. Mutations in two hair specific keratins, hHb1 and hHb6, have been identified in these patients.[10] However, the exclusion of mutations in these genes in some families indicates further genetic heterogeneity. The hair is usually normal at birth but is replaced within weeks by affected hairs that are dry, dull, and brittle, breaking spontaneously and leaving a stubble-like appearance (Fig. 28-2). The hairs may break almost flush with the scalp or may attain lengths of 0.5–2.5 cm, or occasionally longer. Follicular keratosis is commonly associated and may involve the scalp, face, and limbs.

Pili Torti

This is characterized by groups of three or four regularly spaced twists of the hair shaft on its own axis (Fig. 28-3).[6–8] Microscopically, twists are seen, each 0.4–0.9 mm in width, occurring usually in groups of three or more at irregular intervals. Twists are almost always through 180°, although some are through 90° or 360°. The hair shaft is somewhat flattened. Pili torti may occur as an isolated phenomenon, with onset at birth or in the early months of life. The hair is usually fairer than expected and is spangled, dry, and brittle, breaking at different lengths (Fig. 28-4). It may stand out from the scalp and tends to be short, especially in areas subject to trauma.

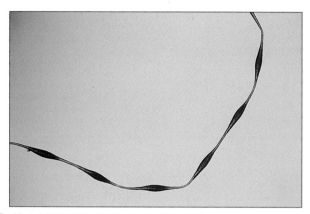

FIG. 28-1 Monilethrix. Microscopic appearance.

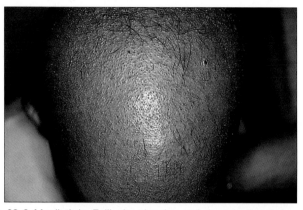

FIG. 28-2 Monilethrix. Follicular plugging and short, broken hairs.

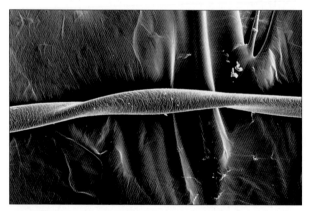

FIG. 28-3 Pili torti. Electron microscopic appearance.

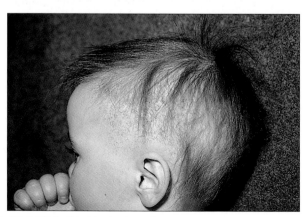

FIG. 28-4 Pili torti in Menkes' syndrome.

Pili torti can occur alone or as a manifestation of defined syndromes, some of which are identifiable in the neonatal period. Menkes syndrome is an X-linked recessive condition caused by mutations in a gene encoding for a protein believed to be a copper-transporting P-type ATP-ase,[11] and the multiple abnormalities are due to decreased bioavailability of copper, with resultant functional deficiencies of copper-dependent enzymes. In the early months of life, scalp and eyebrow hair becomes kinky, coarse, and sparse. Lax, pale skin, hypotonia, and early neurodegenerative changes may already be seen in the neonatal period. In Bazex syndrome, inherited as an X-linked dominant trait,[12] congenital hypotrichosis with pili torti is associated with follicular atrophoderma and multiple facial milia, both of which may also be present from birth. These patients have an increased susceptibility to the development of basal cell carcinomas. In Bjornstad syndrome pili torti is associated with sensorineural deafness and occasionally mental retardation.[13] In later childhood normal hair may replace the affected hairs, with a considerable improvement in appearance. Both autosomal dominant and recessive inheritance patterns have been reported. Recently the gene for the syndrome has been mapped to chromosome 2 in a family with an autosomal recessive mode of inheritance.[13] In Crandall syndrome, probably inherited as an X-linked recessive trait, congenital hypotrichosis with pili torti is associated with sensorineural deafness and hypopituitarism (Fig. 28-5).[14] Pili torti may occur also in Rapp–Hodgkin syndrome, although pili canaliculi is the more characteristic finding.

Trichorrhexis Nodosa

The term trichorrhexis nodosa (TN) refers to the light microscopic appearance of a fracture with splaying out and release of individual cortical cells from the main body of the hair shaft, producing an appearance suggestive of the ends of two brushes pushed together (Fig. 28-6).[6–8] When the break occurs, the brush-like end is clearly seen. Electron microscopy shows the disrupted cuticle and splaying of cortical cells. The defect renders the hair very fragile, and it breaks readily with trauma – or sometimes probably spontaneously. In congenital autosomal dominant TN, the hair is usually normal at birth but is replaced within a few months with abnormal, fragile hair. Trichorrhexis nodosa was found in eight of 25 children with mitochondrial disorders in the absence of skin manifestations, suggesting that hair examination may be a useful diagnostic

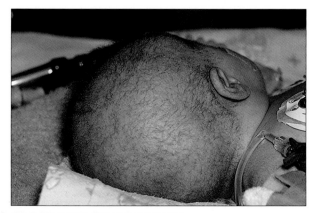

FIG. 28-5 Pili torti in Crandall syndrome.

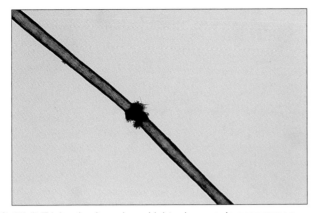

FIG. 28-6 Trichorrhexis nodosa. Light microscopic appearance.

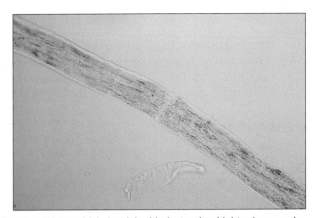

FIG. 28-8 Trichoschisis in trichothiodystrophy. Light microscopic appearance.

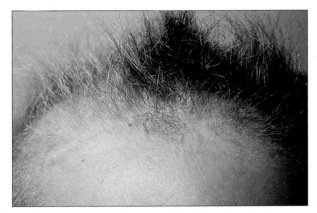

FIG. 28-7 Short, broken, dull hair in trichothiodystrophy.

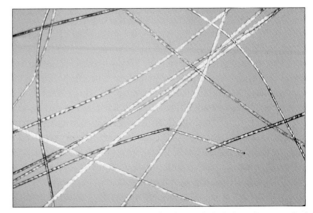

FIG. 28-9 'Tiger tail' appearance of light and dark bands on polarizing microscopy of hair in trichothiodystrophy.

tool when these disorders are suspected.[15] Secondary TN may occur in the condition of intractable diarrhea of infancy.[16]

Trichothiodystrophy

The term trichothiodystrophy refers to the sulfur-deficient brittle hair that is a marker for a neuroectodermal symptom complex occurring in a group of autosomal recessive genetic disorders.[17,18] There is considerable genetic heterogeneity in trichothiodystrophy.[19] Named syndromes that fit into this spectrum include Tay, Pollitt, Sabinas brittle hair, and Marinesco Sjögren syndromes. The words describing the various clinical features of the condition have led to other mnemonic names, including BIDS, IBIDS, and PIBIDS (see also Chapter 18).[17,18] The major clinical features seen in this group of conditions are brittle hair, ichthyosis, short stature, decreased fertility, intellectual impairment, photosensitivity with a DNA repair defect (due to mutations in the *XPD ECCR2 DNA* repair/transcription gene),[20–22] and osteosclerosis. Features that may be evident in the neonatal period are intrauterine growth retardation, severe infections, congenital cataracts, nail dystrophy, facial dysmorphism, a collodion baby phenotype, and the characteristic fragile, dull, short, disordered hair involving the scalp hair, eyebrows, and eyelashes (Fig. 28-7).[23,24] On light microscopy the hair has a wavy, irregular outline and a flattened shaft, in which twists like a folded ribbon occur. Two types of fracture are seen: an atypical trichorrhexis nodosa and trichoschisis, a clean, transverse fracture (Fig. 28-8). Using crossed polarizers, light and dark bands are seen when the hair is

aligned in one of the polarizer directions – the so-called tiger-tail appearance (Fig. 28-9). This may be absent at birth and is not fully developed until 3 months of age.[25] Scanning electron microscopy shows irregular ridging and fluting and a disordered, reduced, or absent cuticle scale pattern.

Woolly Hair

This is tight, curly hair that differs considerably from other areas of scalp hair and that of family members. It is usually abnormal from birth. Fragility of the hair is rarely significant in this condition. A wide variety of changes are described in shaft cross-sectional shape, follicle morphology, and cuticular appearance on scanning electron microscopy. The pathogenesis is unclear and may vary from case to case. There are three main groups, one autosomal recessive, and one autosomal dominant, and one localized and sporadic, the woolly hair nevus. The condition is important to define early because there are many associations. Diffuse woolly hair has been associated with ocular abnormalities, some present at birth:[26] keratosis pilaris atrophicans,[27] Noonan syndrome,[27] and giant axonal neuropathy.[28] Mutations in the desmosomal proteins plakoglobin and desmoplakin have been demonstrated in syndromes incorporating arrhythmogenic cardiomyopathy, palmoplantar keratoderma, and woolly hair.[29,30] In addition, desmoplakin mutations have been described in a syndrome with congenital fragile skin, palmoplantar keratoderma, hyperkeratotic plaques on the trunk and limbs, and woolly hair.[31]

Woolly hair nevus has been associated with ocular abnormalities[26] and epidermal nevi, usually away from the site of the woolly hair nevus and sometimes quite extensive.

Uncombable Hair

This is a condition defined by its clinical features.[7,9,32] Synonyms are spun-glass hair, pili canaliculi, and pili trianguli et canaliculi. In the classic clinical form the hair is a light silvery-blond, paler than expected. It is frizzy, stands away from the scalp, and cannot be combed flat. It is often 'spangled' or glistening. It is usually normal in length, quantity, and tensile strength. The onset may be with the first terminal growth or later. Eyebrows, lashes, and body hair are normal. There are reports suggesting both dominant and recessive inheritance patterns. Scanning electron microscopy best demonstrates the characteristic shallow grooving or flattening of the surface.[32] These areas are often discontinuous and change orientation many times along the length of the hair, occurring on different faces of the hair at different points. Cross-sectional microscopy shows triangular, reniform, and other unusual shapes. It is now clear that longitudinal grooving of hair shafts and/or irregular cross-section are not specific for the clinical entity of uncombable hair. Most children with uncombable hair are otherwise normal; the findings have been demonstrated in a variety of other syndromes with congenital onset, including progeria, Marie Unna hypotrichosis,[33] Rapp–Hodgkin syndrome,[34] orofacial digital syndrome type I,[35] ectrodactyly ectodermal dysplasia and clefting syndrome,[35] and hypohidrotic ectodermal dysplasia.[35] The classic clinical appearance of spun-glass or uncombable hair would seem to depend on the proportion of abnormal hairs.

Pili Annulati

This hair shaft abnormality, which may be present at birth, does not result in significant hair fragility. The hair looks pleasantly shiny, and on close observation alternating bright and dark bands are seen.[36] There are usually no associated abnormalities. The condition may be sporadic or inherited, usually as a dominant characteristic. The bright areas are due to light scattered from clusters of air-filled cavities within the cortex, and in a hair mount, viewed with transmitted light, the light areas appear as dark patches. Scanning electron microscopy shows longitudinal wrinkling and folding in bands corresponding to the abnormal areas, possibly due to the evaporation of air in the spaces when the hair is coated in the vacuum. Transmission electron microscopy demonstrates multiple holes within the cortex.

Trichorrhexis Invaginata

This is the characteristic hair shaft abnormality of Netherton syndrome, an autosomal recessive condition due to mutations in the *SPINK5* gene, which encodes for the serine protease inhibitor *LEKTI*[37] (see also Chapter 18). Although the severity varies considerably, the clinical and microscopic findings are present from birth. In the severely affected neonate, the hair may be extremely sparse or even absent altogether (Fig. 28-10).

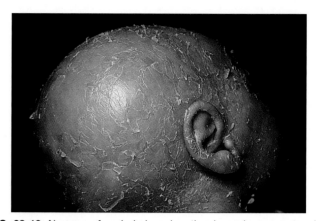

FIG. 28-10 Absence of scalp hair and erythroderma in a neonate with Netherton syndrome.

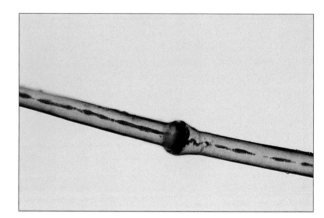

FIG. 28-11 Trichorrhexis invaginata in Netherton syndrome. Light microscopic appearance.

What hair is present is short and dull and breaks easily. The changes may affect eyebrows, eyelashes, and general body hair.[9]

Microscopically, a ball-and-socket configuration with various patterns is seen (Fig. 28-11). The classic 'bamboo hair' occurs when the soft abnormal hair shaft wraps around a firmer distal shaft, producing the appearance of a shallow invagination of the distal into the proximal shaft. There is a tulip-like form with a deeper invagination and longer sides of the 'cup.'[7] Circumferential strictures may be found, representing the earliest stage of the invagination. The term golf-tee hair has been given to the expanded proximal end of an invaginate node after a break has occurred. Thin vellus hairs may show multiple invaginations, the so-called 'canestick hairs.'[38] A helical pattern of twisting with obliquely running parallel invaginations has recently been described.[39]

DIFFUSE ALOPECIA OR HYPOTRICHOSIS (Box 28-1)

Hypotrichosis with Hair Shaft Abnormalities

As discussed in the previous section, many hair shaft abnormalities present in the neonatal period or in early infancy with significant hypotrichosis.

Box 28-1 Diffuse alopecia or hypotrichosis

- Hypotrichosis with major hair shaft abnormalities
- Congenital alopecia or hypotrichosis without other defects
- Atrichia congenita
- Congenital hypotrichosis
- Marie Unna hypotrichosis
- Atrichia with papular lesions
- Congenital hypotrichosis and milia
- Hypotrichosis in ectodermal dysplasias
  - Hidrotic ectodermal dysplasia
  - Hypohidrotic ectodermal dysplasia
  - Anhidrotic ectodermal dysplasia with immunodeficiency
  - Ankyloblepharon ectodermal dysplasia and clefting syndrome and Rapp–Hodgkin syndrome
  - Bazex–Dupre–Christol syndrome
  - Congenital atrichia with nail dystrophy, abnormal facies and retarded psychomotor development
  - Ectodermal dysplasia/skin fragility syndrome
- Hypotrichosis with ichthyoses
  - Ichthyoses presenting as the collodion baby phenotype
  - Congenital ichthyosis, follicular atrophoderma, hypotrichosis and hypohidrosis
  - Keratitis, ichthyosis and deafness syndrome
  - Ichthyosis follicularis, congenital atrichia and photophobia
- Hypotrichosis with hereditary mucoepithelial dysplasia
- Hypotrichosis with premature aging syndromes
- Hypotrichosis with immunodeficiency syndromes

Isolated Congenital Alopecia or Hypotrichosis without other Defects

There appear to be several distinct genotypes within this group, with recessive, dominant, and X-linked inheritance patterns being represented.[40–44]

Those with recessive inheritance are in general the most severe and congenital in onset. In some pedigrees, there is a total absence of hair (congenital atrichia, atrichia congenita, alopecia universalis congenita) and on biopsy no hair follicles are found. Mutations in the *hairless* gene on chromosome 8 have been demonstrated in some families.[40]

In some dominant pedigrees the hair is present but extremely sparse (congenital hypotrichosis, hypotrichosis simplex), with biopsy demonstrating a few scattered, miniaturized follicles occurring in decreased numbers; only the scalp is involved, the hair elsewhere being normal. In some of these pedigrees mutations have been found in corneodesmin, a keratinocyte adhesion molecule.[45]

Marie Unna Hypotrichosis

The hair in this autosomal dominant condition is usually sparse or absent at birth, but it is not until early childhood that the characteristic coarse, wiry hair appears, showing flattening and irregularly distributed twisting on microscopy.[46,47] In some cases the condition has been mapped to chromosome 8p21 in the vicinity of the *hairless* locus, but the *hairless* gene

has been excluded by direct sequencing.[46] In other cases linkage to chromosome 1 has been demonstrated, suggesting this is a genetically heterogeneous condition.[48]

Atrichia With Papular Lesions

This is a distinctive association of congenital atrichia and tiny, white papules.[49] Atrichia of the scalp may be present from birth or appear in early childhood. In most cases, fetal hair is shed in the first 3 months of life and never replaced; eyebrows and eyelashes may or may not be involved. The papular lesions, which occur diffusely but predominate on the face and scalp, are not present in the neonatal period. Histopathology shows the papules to represent keratin-filled follicular cysts in contact with the overlying epidermis. Recent work has demonstrated mutations in the *hairless* gene on chromosome 8, as seen also in alopecia universalis congenita.[44]

Congenital Hypotrichosis and Milia

In this condition, which bears some clinical similarity to atrichia with papular lesions, there is hypotrichosis with sparse, coarse hair, and multiple milia are present at birth on the face and sometimes also the limbs and trunk. Study of a large pedigree suggests X-linked dominant inheritance.[50]

Hypotrichosis With Juvenile Macular Dystrophy

Hair that is short and sparse from birth is a feature of this rare autosomal recessive disorder in which progressive macular degeneration can lead to blindness during the first to fourth decades. The hair may be morphologically normal or show a variety of nonspecific shaft abnormalities. The disease results from mutations in *CDH3* encoding P-cadherin.[51]

Hypotrichosis–Lymphedema–Telangiectasia Syndrome

Congenital hypotrichosis is a feature of this condition, accompanied later in life by lymphedema and telangiectasia. Mutations have been found in the transcription factor gene *SOX18*.[52]

Hypotrichosis Associated With Ectodermal Dysplasias

Hypotrichosis is an important feature in many ectodermal dysplasias,[53] but often becomes obvious only after the neonatal period. A selection of conditions in which there may be congenital or early-onset severe hypotrichosis or atrichia will be considered here.

Hidrotic Ectodermal Dysplasia (Clouston syndrome)

Hypotrichosis of a variable and sometimes very severe degree of scalp hair, eyebrows, eyelashes, and body hair is usually present at birth.[54] Any hair present is fine and fragile. Later significant features are leukoplakia, nail dystrophy, and palmoplantar keratoderma. The condition is caused by mutations in *GJB6*, coding connexin 30.[54] Recently a phenotype resembling Clouston syndrome but with the additional feature of deafness has been linked to mutations in *GJB2*, coding connexin 26. This phenotype was quite different from the keratitis–ichthyosis–deafness syndrome, which is also caused by *GJB2* mutations.[54]

Hypohidrotic Ectodermal Dysplasia

This condition may be inherited in an X-linked pattern due to mutations in a gene named *EDA* which encodes ectodysplasin, or in an autosomal pattern due to mutations in a gene named *downless*, encoding a protein which functions as an ectodysplasin receptor.[46]

Marked hypotrichosis of all hair-bearing areas may be evident in the neonatal period; hair that is present is fine and fair, and often shows pili canaliculi on microscopy. Other features that may be evident in the neonatal period include impaired heat regulation, diffuse scaling of skin, hypoplastic or absent nipples, and the typical facies with a depressed nasal bridge and prominent brow.[55] Rouse et al.[56] have reported that scalp biopsies from patients with hypohidrotic ectodermal dysplasia (HED) demonstrate an absence of eccrine structures in the majority of cases. Their absence is diagnostic of HED, and their presence suggests that the patient does not have this disorder. As the eccrine apparatus is fully formed by the third trimester this test should be reliable in the neonate.[56]

Anhidrotic Ectodermal Dysplasia With Immunodeficiency

This is an X-linked condition due to mutations in the *NEMO* gene.[57] The features are hypotrichosis or atrichia, hypohidrosis or anhidrosis, and later hypodontia or anodontia along with recurrent bacterial infections.

Ankyloblepharon, Ectodermal Dysplasia and Clefting Syndrome and Rapp–Hodgkin Syndrome

At birth in the ankyloblepharon, ectodermal dysplasia, and clefting syndrome (AEC, Hay–Wells) the scalp is usually red and scaly with extensive erosions and crusts, and there is a severe hypotrichosis[58] (Fig. 28-12). Other neonatal features include a generalized erythroderma with or without erosive lesions, ankyloblepharon filiforme, lacrimal duct atresia, cleft palate and lip, and hypoplastic nails. It seems very likely that Rapp–Hodgkin[59,60] and AEC syndromes are variable expressions of the same entity, with reported cases of Rapp–Hodgkin syndrome sharing all the features of AEC apart from the ankyloblepharon.[61] Mutations in the *p63* gene on chromosome 3 have been found in AEC syndrome.[53]

Bazex–Dupre–Christol Syndrome

The main features of this probably X-linked dominant condition are congenital hypotrichosis, milia with onset in the first 3 months of life, the later appearance of follicular atrophoderma as the milia are shed, and early development of basal cell carcinomas.[12] Microscopic hair shaft examination may show trichorrhexis nodosa and an irregular twisting.

Congenital Atrichia With Nail Dystrophy, Abnormal Facies, and Retarded Psychomotor Development

In this condition, after the shedding in the first weeks of life of an initial sparse cover of hair, there is almost total alopecia with only tiny vellus hairs being evident; scalp biopsy demonstrates atrophy of hair follicles and rudimentary hair shafts.[62] Nail dystrophy and an abnormal facies with a broad nasal bridge, hypertelorism, a broad nose, and a long philtrum are other congenital features.

Ectodermal Dysplasia/Skin Fragility Syndrome

Mutations in the desmosomal protein plakophilin have been demonstrated in an ectodermal dysplasia, with sparse hair, skin fragility, hypohidrosis, palmoplantar keratoderma, and hyperkeratotic plaques elsewhere.[46,53]

Hypotrichosis associated with Ichthyoses
(see also Chapter 18)

Ichthyoses Presenting as the Collodion Baby Phenotype

In this group of conditions, which includes autosomal recessive and autosomal dominant forms of lamellar ichthyosis, congenital ichthyosiform erythroderma, and lamellar ichthyosis of the newborn (self-healing collodion baby), the hair is often either absent or shed in the early weeks of life with the collodion scale (Fig. 28-13).

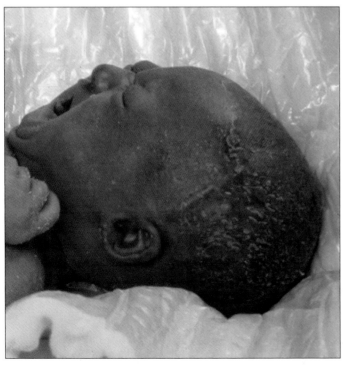

FIG. 28-12 Crusted scalp and alopecia in ankyloblepharon–ectodermal dysplasia–clefting (AEC) syndrome.

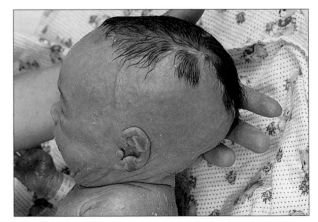

FIG. 28-13 Alopecia in neonate with lamellar ichthyosis.

Congenital Ichthyosis, Follicular Atrophoderma, Hypotrichosis and Hypohidrosis

This combination of traits has been described as a new autosomal recessive genodermatosis.[63,64] Hypotrichosis of scalp, eyebrows, and eyelashes is evident in the neonatal period, and the ichthyosis and follicular atrophoderma are both also congenital. Woolly hair was an additional feature in one case.[64]

Keratitis, Ichthyosis and Deafness Syndrome

Severe hypotrichosis of scalp, eyebrows, and eyelashes may be evident at birth (Fig. 28-14). Other congenital features include spiny follicular plugs, perioral furrowing, reticulate hyperkeratosis of the palms and soles, widespread thickened erythematous plaques, and hearing loss. The condition is usually caused by mutations in *GJB2*, encoding connexin 26.[45,54] A recent interesting case was reported with phenotypic features of KID syndrome but with congenital atrichia rather than hypotrichosis, in which the characteristic connexin 26 mutation was absent but a connexin 30 mutation, as seen in Clouston syndrome, was demonstrated.[65]

Ichthyosis Follicularis, Congenital Atrichia and Photophobia (IFAP)

From birth these individuals demonstrate keratotic follicular papules, atrichia, or severe hypotrichosis and photophobia.[66]

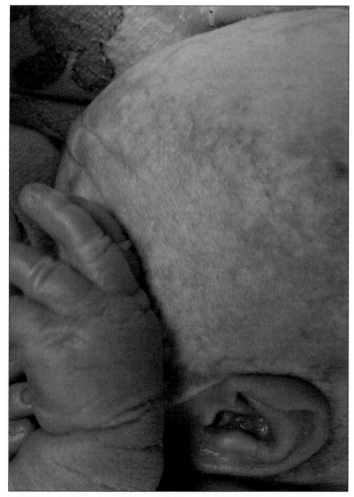

FIG. 28-14 Alopecia and thick scale in keratitis–ichthyosis–deafness (KID) syndrome. (Courtesy of Dr Virginia Sybert, Seattle, USA.)

A variety of other features can be present and there are pedigrees suggesting both X-linked recessive and autosomal dominant inheritance. Happle[67] suggests there may be more than one syndrome within this designation.

Hypotrichosis With Hereditary Mucoepithelial Dysplasia

Hereditary mucoepithelial dysplasia is a dominantly inherited disease characterized by congenital nonscarring hypotrichosis with coarse abnormal hair, gingival erythema, severe keratitis, follicular keratotic papules, and periorificial psoriasiform plaques.[68] It has been suggested that this and IFAP may be the same condition,[69] but there are sufficiently different features to make it likely they are separate entities. Searches for abnormal expression of gap junction and desmosomal proteins have so far been unrewarding.[68]

Hypotrichosis With Premature Aging Syndromes

Although the onset of obvious hypotrichosis is often delayed until several years of age in these conditions, in some cases of Hutchison–Gilford progeria, Cockayne syndrome, and Rothmund–Thomson syndrome, sparse hair is evident in early infancy. A severe neonatal progeroid syndrome has been described in which severe hypotrichois is evident at birth, along with redundant skin, absent subcutaneous fat, and prominent blood vessels.[70]

Hypotrichosis With Immunodeficiency Syndromes

In cartilage hair hypoplasia syndrome, sparsity of scalp, eyebrow, and eyelash hair is often evident in the neonatal period, together with short limbs and prenatal growth failure.[71] A human homologue of the *nude* mouse has recently been identified with mutations in the *winged helix nude* gene leading to complete absence of all hair and severe immunodeficiency.[46] Alopecia is also often a striking feature of a heterogeneous group of congenital immunodeficiency conditions presenting with erythroderma, failure to thrive, and diarrhea in early infancy, which includes Omenn syndrome and severe combined immunodeficiency-associated congenital graft-versus-host disease.[72–74]

LOCALIZED ALOPECIA (Box 28-2)

Trauma

Alopecia in the neonatal period may occur in areas of scalp damaged by instrumentation, such as forceps, scalp monitors, and vacuum extractor, and also around a caput succedaneum (see Chapter 8).

Neonatal Occipital Alopecia

A well-defined patch of alopecia commonly develops in the occipital area in the early months of life (Fig. 28-15). This has been attributed to pressure or friction due to sleeping in a supine position and/or rubbing against the bedding surface, but is explained more fully by an understanding of the patterns of

Box 28-2 Localized alopecia

- Trauma
- Neonatal occipital alopecia
- Triangular alopecia
- With other nevoid conditions
  - Aplastic nevus
  - Sebaceous nevus
  - Congenital melanocytic nevus
- Meningocele, encephalocele, heterotopic meningeal and brain tissue
- Membranous aplasia cutis
- Alopecia areata
- Localized alopecia as part of syndromes
  - Hallermann–Streiff syndrome
  - X-linked dominant conditions

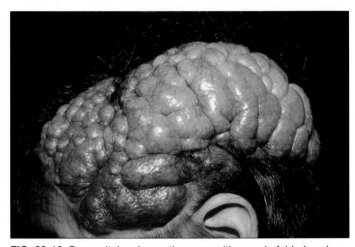

FIG. 28-16 Congenital melanocytic nevus with grossly folded scalp and alopecia. (Courtesy of Dr Marcelo Ruvertoni, Montevideo, Uruguay.)

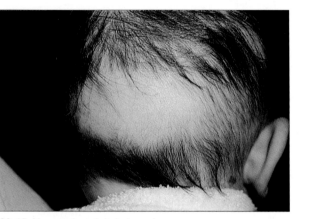

FIG. 28-15 Neonatal occipital alopecia.

hair cycle evolution in fetal and early neonatal life.[75] By 20 weeks of gestation there are well-developed hair follicles containing anagen hairs all over the scalp. Although the hair roots enter catagen and then telogen in a progressive manner from frontal to parietal areas at 26–28 weeks' gestation, the roots in the occipital area remain in anagen until around the time of birth, when they abruptly enter telogen. These hairs inevitably fall 8–12 weeks later. Thus neonatal occipital alopecia is really a form of localized telogen effluvium. Often there are considerable numbers of hairs in the parietal area still in telogen at birth, and a more extensive postnatal alopecia can occur, leaving hair only on the vertex. In pigmented races there is a delay in onset of these physiologic changes, most roots are still in anagen at birth, and the mean diameter of the hairs is greater than in fair-complexioned neonates. For these reasons the hair is often prolific at a time when the fair neonates are developing significant alopecia.

Triangular Alopecia

This noncicatricial circumscribed area of hypotrichosis is triangular or lance-shaped and is positioned in the frontotemporal area, with the base facing the temporal edge of the hairline but sometimes separated from it by a small fringe of normal hair.[76] It is unilateral in 80% of cases. It is a hypotrichosis

rather than a true alopecia because vellus hairs are present in the affected area. Occasionally a few terminal hairs are retained. Although the condition usually occurs sporadically it may very rarely affect several members of a family, and Happle[77] has suggested it may be a paradominant trait; he notes that it has occurred in association with phakomatosis pigmentovascularis, providing further evidence that it may result from loss of heterozygosity.[77] Histopathologic examination of transverse sections of a biopsy specimen demonstrates that the majority of follicles are vellus; a normal number of follicles are present, but their size is abnormal for the scalp.[76] The condition certainly may be congenital and may be noted in the neonatal period in infants with abundant scalp hair, in whom it is often erroneously ascribed to forceps trauma. Whether it is always congenital is disputed.[76]

Localized Alopecia Associated With Other Nevoid Conditions

Aplastic Nevus (Minus Nevus)

This is a nevoid condition in which there is a complete absence of skin appendages in an area of otherwise normal skin.[78]

Sebaceous Nevus

These nevi are characteristically hairless. Sometimes the nevus is so flat and subtle that it is only recognized as such later, and the presentation is as a patch of congenital alopecia.

Congenital Melanocytic Nevus (see also Chapter 22)

These lesions are usually associated with hypertrichosis, but large, folded lesions on the scalp causing an appearance of cutis verticis gyrata may have sparse covering hair (Figs 28-16 and 28-20).

Cranial Meningoceles, Encephaloceles and Heterotopic Meningeal or Brain Tissue (see also Chapter 9)

These present characteristically as tumors or cysts that are either hairless or have sparse overlying hair. There is often a surrounding collar of long hair. Membranous aplasia cutis, which is in the same spectrum, representing a forme fruste of neural tube defect, presents as a hairless plaque, sometimes also with a collar of longer hair (see the following discussion).

Alopecia Areata

This condition is very rarely encountered in early infancy, but has been reported in neonates. De Viragh et al.[79] reported a case in which a patch of alopecia, with histology typical of alopecia areata, was present at birth in a premature infant. Several other cases have subsequently been reported.[80]

Localized Alopecia Associated With Syndromes

Hallermann–Streiff Syndrome

The hair may be normal at birth, but in some cases the typical alopecia, located in the frontal and parietal areas over the cranial sutures, may be evident in early months together with atrophic facial skin and multiple craniofacial and ocular abnormalities.[81]

X-linked Dominant Conditions

Several rare syndromes caused by X-linked dominant genes that interfere with hair growth produce a mosaic pattern of alopecia in affected females as a result of functional X-chromosome mosaicism.[82] The hemizygous males with these conditions rarely survive. The conditions include incontinentia pigmenti, focal dermal hypoplasia (Goltz syndrome), X-linked dominant chondrodysplasia punctata, orofacial digital syndrome, and CHILD syndrome. The alopecia in these conditions has a patchy distribution, sometimes obviously linear or spiral as it follows the lines of Blaschko.[82]

DIFFUSE HYPERTRICHOSIS

The term hypertrichosis refers to increased hair, whereas hirsutism specifically refers to increased hair in hormonally responsive areas of skin (such as the axillae, pubic area, and beard area). Hirsutism in neonates and young infants is rare and is virtually always a result of congenital endocrine disorders. Hypertrichosis, on the other hand, can result from a wide variety of conditions.

Primary Hypertrichosis

There is much confusion about congenital hypertrichosis occurring alone or with only occasional associations, because of the wide variety of designations given and the poor clinical descriptions in the early literature. Baumeister et al.,[83] and more recently Garcia Cruz et al.,[84] have attempted to clarify the classification, but some confusion persists. However, several apparently individual entities can be separated out (Box 28-3).

Transient Diffuse Hypertrichosis

Lanugo is the fine unmedullated hair that is present in the fetus. The hairs are several centimeters long and usually nonpigmented.[85] Growth occurs on the entire body, including the face. This hair is normally shed at around 7–8 months' gestation. However, in some neonates, especially if premature, diffuse lanugo hair is still present and is most marked on the

---

Box 28-3 Diffuse hypertrichosis

- Primary hypertrichosis
- Transient diffuse hypertrichosis
- Hypertrichosis lanuginosa
- Prepubertal hypertrichosis
- X-linked hypertrichosis
- Ambras syndrome
- Hypertrichosis as part of other genetically determined disorders
  - Hypertrichosis with gingival fibromatosis
  - Hypertrichosis with osteochondrodysplasia
  - Hypertrichosis, pigmentary retinopathy and facial anomalies
  - Hypertrichosis with cone rod dystrophy
  - Hypertrichosis with congenital cataract and mental retardation
  - Coffin–Siris syndrome
  - Cornelia de Lange syndrome
  - Leprechaunism
  - Seip–Berardinelli syndrome (congenital generalized lipodystrophy)
  - Rubinstein–Taybi syndrome
  - Barber–Say syndrome
- Drug-induced hypertrichosis
  - Fetal alcohol syndrome
  - Maternal minoxidil
  - Diazoxide

---

shoulders, posterior trunk, cheeks and sometimes ears (Fig. 28-17). This is then shed in the early weeks of life.

Hypertrichosis Lanuginosa

This rare condition is characterized by prolonged retention of lanugo hair. The infant is born with a coat of profuse, long, silky, fine, hair on all the usual hair-bearing areas.[86–89] It may reach 10 cm in length and blends with the terminal hair of scalp and eyebrows (Fig. 28-18). There may be accentuation in certain areas, particularly over the spine and on the pinnae. Profuse growth in the ear may lead to infection and reduced hearing, and needs to be cleared. Matted hair in the diaper area is particularly troublesome, and shaving or laser hair removal in this and other areas may be indicated. A 40–80% reduction in hair has been noted in laser-treated areas using low fluences to minimize pain.[90,91] At puberty there may be no conversion to terminal hair in secondary sexual hair areas, with long, fine, lanugo hairs growing in the beard, pubic, and axillary areas. Although about one-third of cases are sporadic, autosomal dominant inheritance is well established.[84,86,87] However, a single family with possible autosomal recessive inheritance has also been reported.[88] Most patients are free of other abnormalities, but congenital glaucoma,[89] skeletal,[92] and dental[87,90] abnormalities, including neonatal teeth, have been observed.

Prepubertal Hypertrichosis

A series has been reported[93] of otherwise healthy children, with no clinical evidence of endocrinopathy, having general-

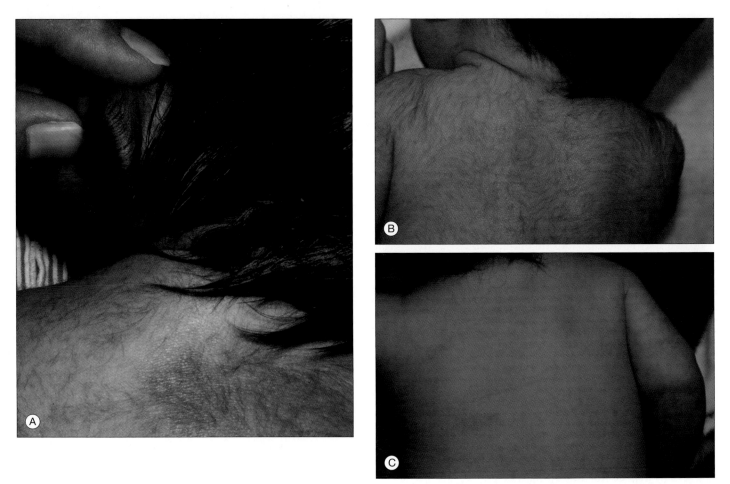

FIG. 28-17 (**A**) Transient neonatal hypertrichosis with marked involvement of the helix and adjacent skin. (**B**) Two-week-old with diffuse lanugo hair on the back. (**C**) At age 4 months this hair is no longer present.

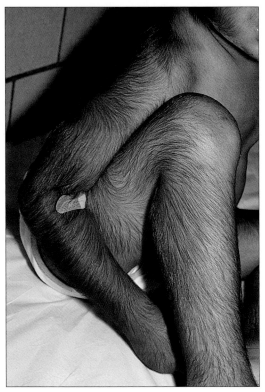

FIG. 28-18 Hypertrichosis lanuginosa.

ized hypertrichosis present from birth and increasing in severity in early childhood. There is terminal hair growth on the temples, spreading across the brow and merging with bushy eyebrows, and also profusely on the back and proximal limbs.[93] The pattern does not resemble hirsutism and hair growth on the back is in an inverted fir tree distribution, centering on the spine. It is not clear whether this represents an abnormality or whether it is an extreme form of the normal range of hair growth, resembling as it does the patterns of hair growth seen regularly in some racial groups.[93] However, a recent study has demonstrated that testosterone levels and the free androgen index are increased in patients compared to controls. This suggests that an endocrine imbalance may indeed be the basis for this condition.[94]

X-Linked Dominant Hypertrichosis

A pedigree has been reported with probable X-linked dominant inheritance where affected members have generalized terminal hair hypertrichosis present at birth.[95] The face, pubic area, back, and upper chest are most involved, but the palms, soles, and mucosae are spared. There is no gingival hyperplasia. After puberty there may be an improvement on the trunk and limbs. This condition has recently been mapped to a 22-cm interval between *DXS425* and *DXS1227* on chromosome Xq24-q27.1.[96]

Ambras Syndrome

Baumeister et al.[97] have delineated what they regard as a unique form of diffuse congenital hypertrichosis which has been previously reported under a variety of names, and have demonstrated a balanced structural chromosomal aberration in a patient with this condition. It has been designated Ambras syndrome in reference to the first documented case. The hair, which may demonstrate pigmentation and medullation, is said to be vellus rather than lanugo. The hypertrichosis is most marked on the face, nose, ears, and shoulders, and the forehead, eyelids, cheeks, and preauricular regions show hair of variable lengths.[84] The palms, soles, mucous membranes, dorsal terminal phalanges, labia minora, prepuce, and glans penis are always spared.[84] The hypertrichosis persists throughout life. A number of dysmorphic facial features (coarse face, wide intercanthal distance, broad palpebral fissures, broad interalar distance and anteverted nares) and dental abnormalities (andontia and delayed secondary dentition) may be present.[84,98] An autosomal dominant inheritance is proposed, with the causative gene mutation found on chromosome 8q22-q24.[84,98]

Hypertrichosis as Part of Other Genetically Determined Disorders

Many syndromes have hypertrichosis as a feature, and in some of these it is present in the neonatal period. A selection of these conditions is considered here.

Hypertrichosis With Gingival Fibromatosis

Hypertrichosis and gingival fibromatosis may occur as a dominantly inherited trait.[84,99] The hypertrichosis is usually of terminal hair, but may be relatively mild. It can be present at birth or develop during early infancy, but in up to half of the reported cases the hypertrichosis begins at puberty.[92] The gingival hyperplasia appears later in childhood. Other clinical features include a coarse facies with a wide, flat nose, thick lips, and large ears.[84]

Several patients have been reported with epilepsy and mental retardation in association with severe hypertrichosis and gingival fibromatosis.[100] Most cases are familial, and although some heterogeneity is postulated the inheritance is usually autosomal dominant. The gingival fibromatosis in this condition usually presents in the second decade but has been reported in infancy. The hypertrichosis is congenital, and the hair varies from fine to coarse and is pigmented. The face, arms, and lumbosacral area are most severely affected. It is possible that these conditions are within a single spectrum.

Further overlap is suggested with the Laband syndrome of gingival hyperplasia, dysplasia of the terminal phalanges, hepatosplenomegaly, and facial dysmorphism, with the recent report of marked congenital hypertrichosis as an additional feature in one patient.[101]

Hypertrichosis With Osteochondrodysplasia

This rare syndrome (Cantu syndrome) is the combination of diffuse congenital hypertrichosis, congenital macrosomia, cardiomegaly which may also be present at birth, and a variety of skeletal changes.[84,102-105] The hair changes from lanugo to postnatal hair, which continues to grow in length and diameter, extending all over the body but sparing the palms, soles, and mucosae.[84] It is most marked on the face, with involvement of the forehead and thick eyebrows, and there is a low posterior cervical hairline. Other features include mild mental retardation, macrocephaly, global cardiomegaly due to cardiomyopathy (sometimes complicated by pericarditis with effusion),[84] and a variety of skeletal changes, including a wide posterior fossa in the skull, a verticalized base of the cranium, narrow thorax, broad ribs, bilateral coxa valga, a short distal phalanx of the thumbs and first toes, and hypertrophy of the first metatarsals.[84,104,105] Most cases are autosomal dominant.[105]

Hypertrichosis With Congenital Eye Disorders
Hypertrichosis, Pigmentary Retinopathy, and Facial Anomalies

An apparently distinct form of congenital hypertrichosis has been reported in one male patient.[106] At birth, long, fine, dark hair covered the shoulders, back, buttocks, and limbs; the chest and abdomen were relatively spared. A biopsy from an arm showed a smooth muscle proliferation suggestive of smooth muscle hamartoma. Associated findings were pigmentary retinopathy and dysmorphic facial features. The finding of hypopigmented and hyperpigmented streaks following Blaschko's lines on the limbs suggested mosaicism, but this could not be confirmed on chromosomal studies of lymphocytes and skin fibroblasts.[106]

Hypertrichosis With Cone/Rod Dystrophy

In 1999, Jalili[107] reported two female cousins with Leber's amaurosis, with cone/rod dystrophy and congenital hypertrichosis.[84] They had severe retinal dystrophy with visual impairment from birth and profound photophobia in the absence of night blindness. Trichomegaly, bushy eyebrows with synophrys, and excessive facial and body hair, including hypertrophied circumareolar hair on the breast, were present. An autosomal recessive inheritance pattern was proposed.[107]

Hypertrichosis With Congenital Cataracts and Mental Retardation

A new autosomal recessive syndrome characterized by congenital lamellar cataracts, generalized hypertrichosis on the back, shoulders, and face, and mental retardation (CAHMR syndrome) was reported in 1992.[108] Associated findings were a low hairline, high narrow palate, macrodontia, and pectus excavatum.[108]

Coffin–Siris Syndrome

Hypertrichosis is a feature in many cases,[109,110] particularly of the face and back; there is a low frontal hairline, bushy laterally displaced eyebrows, and long eyelashes, but often sparse scalp hair. Also evident in the neonatal period are absence or hypoplasia of the nails and distal phalanges of the fifth fingers and toes, microcephaly, facial dysmorphism, and low birthweight. Short stature is common, as is delayed bone age. Spinal anomalies are also frequently seen, including sacral dimples, spina bifida occulta, scoliosis, and kyphosis. Mental retardation becomes evident later. The region 7q32-34 is a candidate region for the gene responsible for this syndrome.[111]

Cornelia de Lange Syndrome

There is a mild generalized hypertrichosis with low frontal and occipital hairlines, thick eyebrows, synophrys, and long, upturned lashes (Fig. 28-19). The hair on the lateral elbows

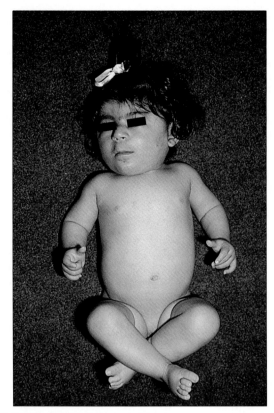

FIG. 28-19 Cornelia de Lange syndrome.

and sacral area may be very long and fine. Other features notable in the neonatal period include congenital livedo, low birthweight, feeding difficulties, increased susceptibility to infection, and an unusual low-pitched growling cry. There is a distinctive facies with hypertelorism, an antimongoloid slant of the palpebral fissures, long philtrum, and thin lips. Other features in occasional cases include micromelia and phocomelia, cryptorchidism, and hypospadias.

Leprechaunism

These infants have coarse, curly scalp hair, and 75% of cases have extensive body and facial hypertrichosis.[112] There is low birthweight, wrinkled loose skin with reduced or absent subcutaneous fat, acanthosis nigricans, periorificial rugosity of skin, thick lips, gingival hypertrophy, large low-set ears, and hypertrophic external genitalia.

Seip–Berardinelli Syndrome (Congenital Generalized Lipodystrophy)

Hypertrichosis of the face, neck, and limbs may be present at birth. There is thick, curly scalp hair with a low frontal hairline. Other features that may be evident in the neonatal period include deficiency of subcutaneous fat, acanthosis nigricans, organomegaly, and hypertrophy of genitalia.

Rubenstein–Taybi Syndrome

In Rubenstein–Taybi syndrome hypertrichosis of the trunk, limbs, and face occurs in two-thirds of cases.[113,114] The eyebrows are highly arched and the eyelashes unusually long. There are downward-sloping palpebral fissures and mental retardation. Other features evident in the neonatal period include capillary vascular malformations, pilomatrixomas, keloid formation, beaked nose, hypertelorism, cryptorchidism,

broad thumbs and great toes, and sometimes broad terminal phalanges of the other digits. This syndrome is sporadic in nature and has been linked to a microdeletion at 16p13.3 encoding the CREB-binding protein gene.[114]

Barber–Say Syndrome

In this rare syndrome, extensive generalized hypertrichosis, most marked over the forehead and back, is associated with redundant atrophic skin showing changes of premature aging, coarse face with bilateral ectropion, hypertelorism, absent eyebrows and lashes, bulbous nose with anteverted nares, macrostomia, abnormal ears, ectropion, hypoplastic nipples, and failure to thrive.[84,115] Other features, less frequently reported, include strabismus, nystagmus, mental retardation, small teeth, and high arched palate.[84]

Drug-Induced Neonatal Hypertrichosis

Fetal Alcohol Syndrome

Neonatal hypertrichosis is an occasional feature of this condition.[116,117] The infant is small and microcephalic with dysmorphic facial features, including short palpebral fissures, microphthalmia, midfacial hypoplasia, and a long philtrum.

Maternal Minoxidil

Maternal use of minoxidil during pregnancy has been associated with a striking hypertrichosis of the back and extremities in the neonate, accompanied by multiple dysmorphic facial features, uneven fat distribution, omphalocele, and cardiac anomalies.[109,118]

Diazoxide

Diazoxide is commenced in babies with hyperinsulinemia as soon as the diagnosis is established, usually in the first week of life; hypertrichosis of brow, limbs, and back becomes obvious in the first 4 weeks of treatment and is dose dependent.

LOCALIZED CONGENITAL HYPERTRICHOSIS

Localized hypertrichosis may occur in association with certain nevi or developmental abnormalities (Box 28-4).

Congenital Melanocytic Nevus

Congenital melanocytic nevi may be covered with dense, dark terminal hair at birth over part or all of their surface (Fig. 28-20). In areas other than the scalp, the degree of hairiness is usually proportional to the degree of elevation of the lesion. On the scalp, however, even very flat lesions often have a dense covering of hair that is longer, darker, and coarser than the surrounding scalp hair.

Congenital Smooth Muscle Hamartoma

These nevi present most commonly as congenital, slightly elevated, pebbly, firm skin-colored or slightly pigmented plaques, with local hypertrichosis.[119,120] Most occur on the trunk or the proximal extremities, but other areas, including the scalp,[121] may be affected. A pseudo-Darier sign of transient piloerection or elevation of the lesion after it is rubbed is a characteristic feature. Extensive hypertrichosis overlying diffuse, widespread, smooth muscle hamartomas has also been

* Congenital melanocytic nevus
* Congenital smooth muscle hamartoma
* Hypertrichosis over plexiform neurofibroma
* Tufted angioma
* Hypertrichosis with spinal fusion abnormalities
* Familial cervical hypertrichosis with kyphoscoliosis
* Associated with cranial meningoceles, encephaloceles, and heterotopic meningeal or brain tissue
* Nevoid hypertrichosis
* Hemihypertrophy with hypertrichosis
* Scrotal hair
* Anterior cervical hypertrichosis
* Hairy cutaneous malformations of palms and soles
* Hypertrichosis cubiti
* Ectopic cilia
* Distichiasis

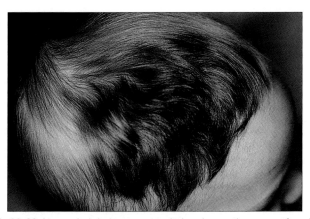

FIG. 28-20 Long, dark hair on congenital melanocytic nevus of scalp.

reported.[122,123] Histopathologic examination demonstrates a proliferation of variably oriented smooth muscle bundles, often associated with hair follicles. There may also be epidermal changes of acanthosis and papillomatosis, as seen in Becker nevus.

Becker nevus usually presents in late childhood or adolescence as a patch of thickened, pigmented, hypertrichotic skin. Congenital cases have been reported, although usually lacking hypertrichosis in the neonatal period.[124] These nevi are uncommon in females.[120] An unusual presentation with congenital bilaterally symmetric lesions, hypertrichotic at birth, has been reported.[125] Some believe that congenital smooth muscle hamartoma and Becker nevus are in a spectrum,[119] but others feel they are distinct entities.[126]

Plexiform Neurofibroma

The skin over these lesions is often notable for a patch of hyperpigmentation with an irregular border and hypertrichosis of varying degree.[127] A prominent paraspinal hair whorl may also occur at the site of a deep mediastinal plexiform neuro-

fibroma.[128] A similar paraspinal whorl has been described in a patient with a posterior mediastinal ganglioneuroma.[129] Erythema may also be a feature, leading to confusion with vascular tumors such as tufted angiomas and kaposiform haemangioendotheliomas, that may themselves have associated focal hypertrichosis.

Tufted Angioma

This is a rare benign vascular tumour found particularly on the neck and upper trunk regions, as well as the abdomen, groin, and lower limbs. Most commonly they present as dusky red to violaceous, indurated, subcutaneous plaques or nodules; 30% of lesions are tender.[130] Some have been associated with focal hyperhidrosis and/or hypertrichosis.[131]

Hypertrichosis With Spinal Fusion Abnormalities

Isolated hypertrichosis in the lumbosacral region may be a normal variant and is usually genetically or racially determined. It should be distinguished from hypertrichosis associated with an underlying spinal abnormality. This presents at birth as a tuft of long, silky hair (faun tail) with or without the presence of other cutaneous markers, such as a dimple, sinus tract, aplasia cutis, lipoma with deviation of the gluteal fold, capillary malformation, hemangioma, or a pigmented nevus.[132–134] These cutaneous lesions may be found in the presence of clinical spina bifida with myelomeningocele (Fig. 28-21), but are particularly helpful as markers for occult spinal dysraphism. Two or more congenital midline skin lesions constitute a particularly strong marker for spinal dysraphism.[134] Hypertrichosis associated with spinal fusion abnormalities may also occur less commonly over other areas of the spine.

Familial Cervical Hypertrichosis With Kyphoscoliosis

A family has been reported with congenital localized hypertrichosis of the cervical area overlying a kyphoscoliosis without other spinal or cutaneous abnormalities.[135] The inheritance pattern was autosomal dominant.

Hypertrichosis With Cranial Meningoceles, Encephaloceles, and Heterotopic Meningeal or Brain Tissue

These conditions are described in detail in Chapter 9. They are often marked by a peripheral collar of hair (Fig. 28-22), a tuft of hair nearby, or overlying hair.[133] In scalp lesions the hair is longer, thicker, and often darker than the surrounding normal hair. An associated vascular stain may also be present.[136] With lesions away from the scalp, the presence of hair may be an indication that one is dealing with a neural lesion (Figs 28-23 and 28-24). Prominent hair follicle orifices may also be a feature. It is now clear that the membranous form of aplasia cutis, which may also demonstrate a hair collar and which can occur on the face[133,137,138] as well as the scalp, is a form fruste of a neural tube closure defect and in the same spectrum as cranial meningoceles, encephaloceles, and heterotopic brain tissue.[133] A patient has been reported with a congenital patch of hypertrichosis over the lumbar area, well away from the spine, overlying what was demonstrated histologi-

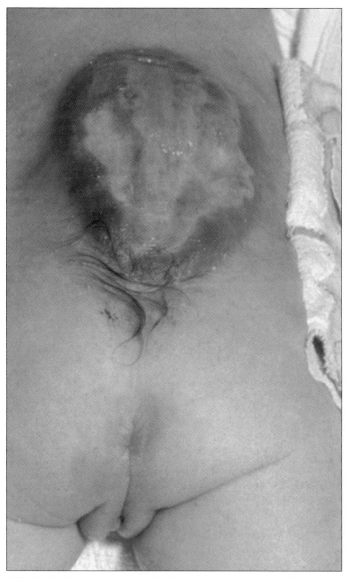

FIG. 28-21 Faun tail nevus (tuft of long fine hair) in association with spina bifida with myelomeningocele.

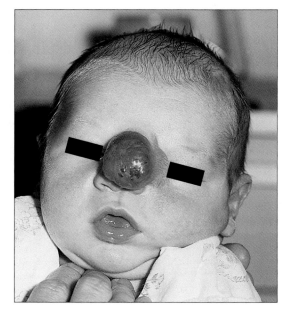

FIG. 28-23 Encephalocele with surrounding hypertrichosis.

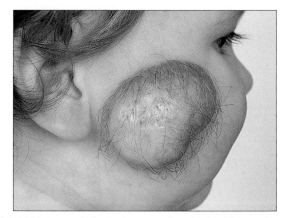

FIG. 28-24 Heterotopic brain tissue on the cheek with prominent hair follicle orifices and superimposed hypertrichosis.

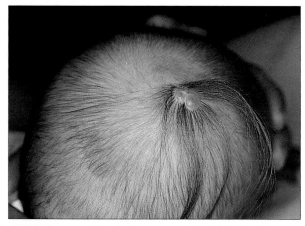

FIG. 28-22 Heterotopic brain tissue on scalp with hair collar.

cally to be meningeal tissue; in this case, displacement of meningeal cells along nerves during embryogenesis is postulated as the mechanism, rather than entrapment of meningeal membranes at the time of closure of the neural tube.[139]

Nevoid Hypertrichosis

Several patients have been reported with single or multiple localized patches of terminal hair growing from skin of normal color and texture (Fig. 28-25).[120,140,141] Presentation is usually at or soon after birth, although the development of additional patches after puberty has been described. The color of the hair is typically the same as that of the scalp, but rarely the hair may be paler or there may be premature graying. In one case, underlying lipoatrophy was found in some patches.[140] Additional abnormalities seen in another patient included areas of lipoatrophy and streaky depigmentation away from the areas of hypertrichosis, developmental delay and seizures, congenital lung cysts, congenital malrotation of the gut, and multiple

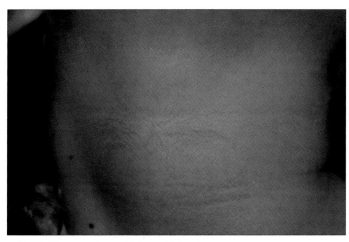

FIG. 28-25 Area of nevoid hypertrichosis.

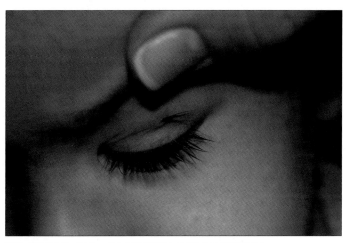

FIG. 28-26 Ectopic cilia. (Courtesy of Dr Amy Gilliam.)

skeletal, dental, and ocular abnormalities.[141] This constellation of findings did not fit into any recognized syndrome. The excess hair can be treated with laser.[142]

Hemihypertrophy With Hypertrichosis

Hemihypertrophy is a rare congenital disorder in which the whole of one side of the body or, less commonly, part of one side of the body is enlarged. Serious associated malformations include Wilms' tumor and tumors of the brain and adrenals. The skin is often normal, but cutaneous abnormalities reported include pigmentation, telangiectasia, abnormal nail growth, and hypertrichosis, which can be very striking.[143,144]

Scrotal Hair

Several infant boys have been reported who developed scrotal hair within the first 3 months of life in the absence of clinical or biochemical evidence of excess androgen production.[145–147] The condition is not progressive and most cases are sporadic. It is most likely caused by an increased hypersensitivity of scrotal hair follicles in affected infants to the normal 'physiological' high concentrations of testosterone seen in early infancy.[147] As concentrations decrease later in infancy the scrotal hair disappears or diminishes. Although this is a benign condition, it should be regarded only as a diagnosis of exclusion and all infants with signs of androgenization should be fully investigated.

Anterior Cervical Hypertrichosis

A congenital patch of hypertrichosis localized to the front of the neck at the sternal notch has been described and the inheritance pattern is most likely autosomal recessive.[92,148] Although usually an isolated finding, it may be associated with peripheral sensory and motor neuropathy,[149] and sometimes retinal abnormalities.[150]

Hairy Cutaneous Malformations of Palms and Soles

There have been reports of the familial occurrence of hair growth on circumscribed areas of the palms and soles.[151] In one family, the skin in the area showed exaggerated markings in a geometric pattern. The condition was present at birth and persisted throughout life. Histopathology demonstrated the presence of ectopic hair follicles and some increase in the amount of elastic fibers in the dermis.

Hypertrichosis Cubiti

In 'hairy elbows syndrome' lanugo hairs are present symmetrically at birth or develop during infancy on the extensor surfaces of the elbows, extending from midhumerus to midforearm.[92,152] This syndrome is not usually associated with other anomalies and most frequently only represents a cosmetic problem. There have, however, been isolated case reports of hypertrichosis cubiti associated with short stature.[152]

Ectopic Cilia

The eyelashes or cilia are modified hairs originating from follicles on the margins of the eyelids. The rarest of all cilial anomalies is ectopic placement. The locations of the ectopic cilia fall into two distinct groups: those originating anterior to the tarsal plate and those arising from the posterior surface of the tarsus. Ectopic cilia arising anterior to the tarsal plate are all seen within the lateral quarter of the lid, with multiple hairs (15–20) surrounding a pit, and the bulbs of the follicles being tightly adherent to the underlying tarsus (Fig. 28-26). Ectopic cilia originating from the posterior surface of the tarsal plate presents with a single lash seen beneath the conjunctiva; the position on the lid varies. The two forms of lesion have different etiologic origins.[153]

Distichiasis

This term refers to lashes arising from the meibomian gland orifices. This can occur as a result of eyelid inflammation, but there is an inherited congenital form in which there is a double row of lashes, the normal row and a row arising from meibomian gland orifices. This condition can be inherited alone or more commonly as part of lymphedoma–distichiasis syndrome. Mutations in the *FOXC2* gene have been identified in both groups, suggesting they are phenotypic varieties of the same disorder.[154]

REFERENCES

1. Smith DW, Gong BT. Scalp hair patterning as a clue to early fetal brain development. J Pediatr 1973; 83: 374–380.

2. Wunderlich RC, Heerema NA. Hair crown patterns of human newborns. Clin Pediatr 1975; 14: 1045–1049.

3. Tirosh E, Jaffe M, Dar H. The clinical significance of multiple hair whorls and their association with unusual dermatoglyphics and dysmorphic features in mentally retarded Israeli children. Eur J Pediatr 1987; 146: 568–570.

4. Klar AJS. Human handedness and scalp hair-whorl direction develop from a common mechanism. Genetics 2003; 165: 269–276.

5. Lee WS, Lee IW, Ahn SK. Diffuse heterochromia of scalp hair. J Am Acad Dermatol 1996; 35: 823–825.

6. Whiting D. Structural abnormalities of the hair shaft. J Am Acad Dermatol 1987; 16: 1–25.

7. Price VH. Structural abnormalities of the hair shaft. In: Orfanos C, Happle R, eds. Hair and hair diseases. Berlin: Springer Verlag, 1990; 363–422.

8. Rogers M. Hair shaft abnormalities: Part I. Aust J Dermatol 1995; 36: 179–186.

9. Rogers M. Hair shaft abnormalities: Part II. Aust J Dermatol 1996; 37: 1–11.

10. Djabali K, Panteleyev AA, Lalin T et al. Recurrent missense mutations in the hair keratin gene hHb6 in monilethrix. Clin Exp Dermatol 2003; 28: 206–210.

11. Chelly J, Tumer Z, Tonnesen T, et al. Isolation of a candidate gene for Menkes disease that encodes a potential heavy metal binding protein. Nature Genet 1993; 3: 14–19.

12. Goetyn M, Geerts M-L, Kint A, et al. The Bazex–Dupre–Christol syndrome. Arch Dermatol 1994; 130: 337–342.

13. Selvaag E. Pili torti and sensorineural hearing loss. A follow-up of Bjornstad's original patients and a review of the literature. Eur J Dermatol 2000; 10: 91–97.

14. Crandall B, Samec L, Sparkes RS, et al. A familial syndrome of deafness, alopecia and hypogonadism. J Pediatr 1973; 82: 461–465.

15. Silengo M, Valenzise M, Spada M, et al. Hair anomalies as a sign of mitochondrial disease. Eur J Pediatr 2003; 162: 459–461.

16. Landers MC, Schroeder TL. Intractable diarrhea of infancy with facial dysmorphism, trichorrhexis nodosa and cirrhosis. Pediatr Dermatol 2003; 20: 432–435.

17. Itin PH, Pittelkow MR. Trichothiodystrophy: review of sulfur-deficient brittle hair syndromes and association with the ectodermal dysplasias. J Am Acad Dermatol 1990; 22: 705–717.

18. Itin PH, Sarasin A, Pittelkow MR. Trichothiodystrophy: Update on the sulfur deficient brittle hair syndromes. J Am Acad Dermatol 2001; 44: 891–920.

19. Nakabayashi K, Amann D, Ren Y et al. Identification of C7orf11 (TTDN1) gene mutations and genetic heterogeneity of non-photosensitive trichothiodystrophy. Am J Med Genet 2005; 76: 510–516.

20. Taylor EM, Broughton BC, Botta E, et al. Xeroderma pigmentosum and trichothiodystrophy are associated with different mutations in the XPD(ERCC2) repair/transcription gene. Proc Natl Acad Sci USA 1997; 94: 8658–8663.

21. Weeda G, Eveno E, Donker I, et al. A mutation in the XPB/ERCC3 DNA repair transcription gene, associated with trichothiodystrophy. Am J Hum Genet 1997; 60: 320–329.

22. Nishiwaki Y, Kobayashi N, Imoto K et al. Trichothiodystrophy fibroblasts are deficient in the repair of ultraviolet-induced cyclobutane pyrimidine dimers and (6–4) photoproducts. J Invest Dermatol 2004; 122: 526–532.

23. Petrin JH, Meckler KA, Sybert VP. A new variant of trichothiodystrophy with recurrent infections, failure to thrive and death. Pediatr Dermatol 1998; 15: 31–34.

24. Tolmie JL, de Berker D, Dawber R, et al. Syndromes associated with trichothiodystrophy. Clin Dysmorphol 1994; 3: 1–14.

25. Brusasco A. The typical 'tiger-tail' pattern of the hair shaft in trichothiodystrophy may not be evident at birth. Arch Dermatol 1997; 133: 249.

26. Taylor A. Hereditary woolly hair with ocular involvement. Br J Dermatol 1990; 123: 523–526.

27. Neild VS, Pegum JS, Wells RS. The association of keratosis pilaris atrophicans and woolly hair, with or without Noonan's syndrome. Br J Dermatol 1984; 110: 357–362.

28. Ouvrier RA. Giant axonal neuropathy. Brain Dev 1989; 11: 207–214.

29. McCoy G, Protonotarios N, Crosby A, et al. Identification of a deletion in plakoglobin in arrhythmogenic right ventricular cardiomyopathy with palmoplantar keratoderma and woolly hair (Naxos disease). Lancet 2000; 42: 319–327.

30. Cheong JEL, Wessagowit V, McGrath JA. Molecular abnormalities of the desmosomal protein desmoplakin in human disease. Clin Exp Dermatol 2005; 30: 261–266.

31. Whittock NV, Wan H, Morley SM, et al. Compound heterozygosity for non-sense and mis-sense mutations in desmoplakin underlies skin fragility/woolly hair syndrome. J Invest Dermatol 2002; 118: 232–238.

32. Hicks J, Metry DW, Barrish J, Levy M. Uncombable hair (cheveux incoiffables, pili trianguli et canaliculi) syndrome: Brief review and role of scanning electron microscopy in diagnosis. Ultrastruct Pathol 2001; 25: 99–103.

33. Marren P, Wilson C, Dawber RPR, et al. Hereditary hypotrichosis (Marie-Unna type) and juvenile macular degeneration. Clin Exp Dermatol 1992; 17: 189–191.

34. Camacho F, Ferrando J, Pichardo AR, et al. Rapp–Hodgkin syndrome with pili canaliculi. Pediatr Dermatol 1993; 10: 54–57.

35. Micali GM, Cook B, Blekys I, et al. Structural hair abnormalities in ectodermal dysplasia. Pediatr Dermatol 1990; 7: 27–32.

36. Giehl KA, Ferguson DJP, Dawber RPR, et al. Update on detection, morphology and fragility in pili annulati in three kindreds. J Eur Acad Dermatol Venereol 2004; 18: 654–658.

37. Ong C, O'Toole EA, Ghali L, et al. LEKTI demonstrable by immunohistochemistry of the skin: a potential diagnostic test for Netherton syndrome. Br J Dermatol 2004; 151: 1253–1257.

38. Menne T, Weisman K. Canestick lesions of vellus hair in Netherton's syndrome. Arch Dermatol 1985; 121: 451.

39. Lurie R, Ben-Zion G. Helical hairs: A new hair anomaly in a patient with Netherton's syndrome. Cutis 1995; 55: 349–352.

40. Baden HP, Kubilus J. Analysis of hair from alopecia congenita. J Am Acad Dermatol 1980; 3: 623–626.

41. Ahmad M, Abbas H, Haque S. Alopecia universalis as a single abnormality in an inbred Pakistani kindred. Am J Med Genet 1993; 46: 369–371.

42. Pinheiro M, Freire-Maia N. Atrichias and hypotrichosis: a brief review with description of a recessive atrichia in two brothers. Hum Hered 1985; 35: 53–55.

43. Kenue RK, al-Dhafri KS. Isolated congenital atrichia in an Omani kindred. Dermatology 1994; 188: 72–75.

44. Sprecher E. Genetic hair and nail disorders. Clin Dermatol 2005; 23: 47–55.

45. Van Steensel MAM, van Geel M, Steiljen PM. Molecular genetics of hereditary hair and nail disease. Am J Med Genet 2004; 131C: 52–60.

46. Irvine AD, Christiano AM. Hair on a gene string: recent advances in understanding the molecular genetics of hair loss. Clin Exp Dermatol 2001; 26: 59–71.

47. Roberts JL, Whiting DA, Henry D. Marie Unna congenital hypotrichosis: Clinical description, histopathology, scanning electron microscopy of a

previously unreported large pedigree. J Invest Dermatol 1999; 4: 261–267.

48. Yang S, Gao M, Cui Y, et al. Identification of a novel locus for Marie Unna hereditary hypotrichosis to a 17.5 cM interval at 1p21.1–1q21.3. J Invest Dermatol 2005; 125: 711–714.

49. Zlotogorski A, Panteleyev AA, Aita VM, et al. Clinical and molecular diagnostic criteria of congenital atrichia with papular lesions. J Invest Dermatol 2001; 117: 1662–1665.

50. Rapelanoro R, Taieb A, Lacombe D. Congenital hypotrichosis and milia: Report of a large family suggesting X-linked dominant inheritance. Am J Med Genet 1994; 52: 487–490.

51. Indelman M, Leibu R, Jammal A, et al. Molecular basis of hypotrichosis with juvenile macular dystrophy in two siblings. Br J Dermatol 2005; 153: 635–638.

52. Irrthum A, Devriendt K, Chitayat D, et al. Mutations in the transcription factor gene SOX18 underlie recessive and dominant forms of hypotrichosis-lymphedema-telangiectasia. Am J Hum Genet 2002; 72: 1470–1478.

53. Itin PH, Fistarol SK. Ectodermal dysplasias. Am J Med Genet 2004; 131C: 45–51.

54. Van Steensel MAM. Gap junction diseases of the skin. Am J Med Genet 2004; 131C: 12–19.

55. Clarke A, Phillips DIM, Brown R, et al. Clinical aspects of X-linked hypohidrotic ectodermal dysplasia. Arch Dis Child 1987; 62: 989–996.

56. Rouse C, Siegfried E, Breer W, et al. Hair and sweat glands in families with hypohidrotic ectodermal dysplasia. Arch Dermatol 2000; 140: 850–855.

57. Ku CL, Dupuis-Girod S, Dittrich AM, et al. NEMO mutations in two unrelated boys with severe infections and conical teeth. Pediatrics 2005; 115: e615–619.

58. Vanderhooft SL, Stephan MJ, Sybert VP. Severe skin erosions and scalp infections in AEC syndrome. Pediatr Dermatol 1993; 10: 334–340.

59. Felding IB, Bjorklund LJ. Rapp–Hodgkin ectodermal dysplasia. Pediatr Dermatol 1990; 7: 126–131.

60. Camacho F, Ferrando J, Pichardo AR, et al. Rapp–Hodgkin syndrome with pili canaliculi. Pediatr Dermatol 1993; 10: 54–57.

61. Cambiaghi S, Tadini G, Barbareschi M, et al. Rapp–Hodgkin syndrome and AEC syndrome: Are they the same entity? Br J Dermatol 1994; 130: 97–101.

62. Vogt BR, Traupe H, Hamm H. Congenital atrichia with nail dystrophy, abnormal facies and retarded psychomotor development in two siblings: A new autosomal recessive syndrome? Pediatr Dermatol 1988; 5: 236–242.

63. Lestringant GG, Kuster W, Frossard PM, et al. Congenital ichthyosis, follicular atrophoderma, hypotrichosis and hypohidrosis: a new genodermatosis? Am J Med Genet 1998; 75: 186–189.

64. Tursen U, Kaya T, Ikizoglu G, et al. Genetic syndrome with ichthyosis: congenital ichthyosis, follicular atrophoderma, hypotrichosis and wooly hair; second report. Br J Dermatol 2002; 147: 614–606.

65. Jan AY, Amin S, Ratajcak P, et al. Genetic heterogeneity of KID syndrome: Identification of a Cx30 gene (GJB6) mutation in a patient with KID syndrome and congenital atrichia. J Invest Dermatol 2004; 122: 1108–1113.

66. Megarbane H, Zablit C, Waked N, et al. Ichthyosis follicularis, alopecia and photophobia (IFAP) syndrome: report of a new family with additional features and review. Am J Med Genet 2004; 124A: 323–327.

67. Happle R. What is IFAP syndrome? Am J Med Genet 2004; 124A: 328.

68. Boralevi F, Haftek M, Vabres P, et al. Hereditary mucoepithelial dysplasia: clinical ultrastructural and genetic study of eight patients and literature review. Br J Dermatol 2005; 153: 310–318.

69. Rothe MJ, Lucky AW. Are ichthyosis follicularis and hereditary mucoepithelial dystrophy related diseases? Pediatr Dermatol 1995; 12: 195.

70. Korniszewski L, Nowak R, Okniniska-Hoffmann E, et al. Wiedemann–Rautenstrauch (neonatal progeroid) syndrome: New case with normal telomere length in skin fibroblasts. Am J Med Genet 2001; 103: 144–148.

71. Makitie O, Sulisalo T, de la Chapelle A, et al. Cartilage–hair hypoplasia. J Med Genet 1995; 32: 39–43.

72. Pruszowski A, Bodemer C, Fraitag S, et al. Neonatal and infantile erythrodermas: a retrospective study of 51 patients. Arch Dermatol 2000; 136: 875–880.

73. Ricci, G, Patrizi A, Specchia F. Omenn syndrome. Pediatr Dermatol 1997; 14: 49–52.

74. Farrell A, Scerri L, Stevens A, et al. Acute graft-versus-host disease with unusual cutaneous intracellular vacuolation in an infant with severe combined immunodeficiency. Pediatr Dermatol 1995; 12: 311–313.

75. Cutrone M, Grimalt R. Transient neonatal hair loss: a common transient neonatal dermatosis. Eur J Pediatr 2005; 164: 630–632.

76. Trakimas C, Sperling LC, Skelton HG, et al. Clinical and histologic findings in temporal triangular alopecia. J Am Acad Dermatol 1994; 31: 205–209.

77. Happle R. Congenital triangular alopecia may be categorized as a paradominant trait. Eur J Dermatol 2003; 13: 346–347.

78. Schoenfeld RJ, Mehregan AH. Aplastic nevus – the 'minus nevus'. Cutis 1973; 12: 386–389.

79. de Viragh PA, Giannada B, Levy ML. Congenital alopecia areata. Dermatology 1997; 195: 96–98.

80. Lenane P, Pope E, Krafchik B. Congenital alopecia areata. J Am Acad Dermatol 2005; 52: S8–11.

81. Cohen JJ. Hallermann–Streiff syndrome: A review. Am J Med Genet 1991; 41: 488–489.

82. Happle R. Genetic defects involving the hair. In: Orfanos CE, Happle R, eds. Hair and hair diseases. Berlin: Springer-Verlag, 1989; 345.

83. Baumeister FAM, Schwartz HP, Stengel-Rutkowski S. Childhood hypertrichosis: Diagnosis and management. Arch Dis Child 1995; 72: 457–459.

84. Garcia-Cruz D, Figuera LE, Cantu JM. Inherited hypertrichoses. Clin Genet 2002; 61: 321–329.

85. Gworys B, Domagala Z. The typology of the human fetal lanugo on the thorax. Ann Anat 2003; 185: 383–386.

86. Felgenhauer WR. Hypertrichosis lanuginosa universalis. J Genet Hum 1969; 17: 1–44.

87. Freire-Maia N, Felizali J, de Figueiredo AC, et al. Hypertrichosis lanuginosa in a mother and son. Clin Genet 1976; 10: 303–306.

88. Janssen TAE, de Lange C. Hypertrichosis (trichostasis) lanuginosa. Ned Tijdschr Geneesk 1946; 90: 198.

89. Judge MR, Rice NSC, Christopher A, et al. Congenital hypertrichosis lanuginosa and congenital glaucoma. Br J Dermatol 1991; 124: 495–497.

90. Partridge JW. Congenital hypertrichosis lanuginosa: Neonatal shaving. Arch Dis Child 1987; 62: 623–625.

91. Littler CM. Laser hair removal in a patient with hypertrichosis lanuginosa congenita. Dermatol Surg 1997; 23: 705–707.

92. Vashi R, Mancini A, Paller A. Primary generalized and localized hypertrichosis in children. Arch Dermatol 2001; 137: 877–884.

93. Barth JH, Wilkinson JD, Dawber RPR. Prepubertal hypertrichosis: Normal or abnormal? Arch Dis Child 1988; 63: 666–668.

94. Gryngarten M, Bedecarras P, Ayuso S, et al. Clinical assessment and serum hormonal profile in prepubertal hypertrichosis. Horm Res 2000; 54: 20–25.

95. Macias-Flores MA, Garcia-Cruz D, Rivera H, et al. A new form of hypertrichosis inherited as an X-linked dominant trait. Hum Genet 1984; 66: 66–70.

96. Figuera LE, Pandolfo M, Dunne PW, et al. Mapping of the congenital generalized hypertrichosis locus to chromosome Xq24-q27.1. Nature Genet 1995; 10: 202–207.

97. Baumeister FAM, Egger J, Schildhaure MT, et al. Ambras syndrome: Delineation of a unique hypertrichosis universalis congenita and association

with a balanced pericentric inversion (8)(p11.2; q22). Clin Genet 1993; 44: 121–128.

98. Tadin-Strapps M, Warburton D, Baumeister FA, et al. Cloning of the breakpoints of a de novo inversion of chromosome 8, inv (8)(p11.2q23.1) in a patient with Ambras syndrome. Cytogenet Genome Res 2004; 107: 68–76.

99. Lee IJ, Im SB, Kim D-K. Hypertrichosis universalis congenita: A separate entity, or the same disease as gingival fibromatosis? Pediatr Dermatol 1993; 10: 263–266.

100. Kiss P. Gingival fibromatosis, mental retardation, epilepsy and hypertrichosis. Dev Med Child Neurol 1990; 32: 459–460.

101. Lacombe D, Bioulac-Sage P, Sibout M, et al. Congenital marked hypertrichosis and Laband syndrome in a child: Overlap between the gingival fibromatosis-hypertrichosis and Laband syndromes. Genet Couns 1994; 5: 251–256.

102. Cantu JM, Garcia-Cruz D, Sanchez-Corona J, et al. A distinct osteochondrodysplasia with hypertrichosis. Hum Genet 1982; 60: 36–41.

103. Nevin NC, Mulholland HC, Thomas P. Congenital hypertrichosis, cardiomegaly and mild osteochondrodysplasia. Am J Med Genet 1996; 66: 33–38.

104. Garcia-Cruz D, Sanchez-Corona J, Nazara Z, et al. Congenital hypertrichosis, osteochondrodysplasia and cardiomegaly: Further delineation of a new genetic syndrome. Am J Med Genet 1997; 69: 138–151.

105. Herman TE, McAlister WH. Cantu syndrome. Pediatr Radiol 2005; 35: 550–551.

106. Pivnick EK, Wilroy RS, Martens PR, et al. Hypertrichosis, pigmentary retinopathy and facial anomalies: A new syndrome? Am J Med Genet 1996; 62: 386–390.

107. Jalili IK. Cone-rod congenital amaurosis associated with congenital hypertrichosis: an autosomal recessive condition. J Med Genet 1999; 26: 504–510.

108. Temtamy SA, Sinbawy AHH. Cataract, hypertrichosis and mental retardation (CAHMR): a new autosomal recessive syndrome. Am J Med Genet 1992; 41: 432–433.

109. Gleck BJ, Pandya A, Vanner L, et al. Coffin–Siris syndrome: review and presentation of new cases from a questionnaire study. Am J Med Genet 2001; 99; 1–7.

110. Levy P, Baraitser M. Coffin–Siris syndrome. J Med Genet 1991; 28: 338–341.

111. McGhee EM, Klump CJ, Bitts SM, et al. Candidate region for Coffin–Siris syndrome at 7q32–34. Am J Med Genet 2000; 93: 241–243.

112. Roth SI, Schedewie HK, Herzberg VK, et al. Cutaneous manifestations of leprechaunism. Arch Dermatol 1981; 117: 531–535.

113. Selmanowitz VJ, Stiller MJ. Rubinstein–Taybi syndrome. Arch Dermatol 1981; 117: 504–506.

114. Hsiung SH. Rubinstein–Taybi syndrome (broad thumb-hallux syndrome). Dermatol Online J 2004; 10: 2.

115. Santana SM, Alvarez FP, Frias JL, et al. Hypertrichosis, atrophic skin, ectropion and macrostomia (Barber–Say) syndrome: Report of a new case. Am J Med Genet 1993; 47: 20–23.

116. Blum A, Loser H, Dehaene P, et al. Fetal alcohol syndrome (FAS) in dermatology: an overview and an evaluation. Eur J Dermatol 1999; 9: 341–345.

117. Kvigne VL. Leonardson GR. Neff-Smith M, et al. Characteristics of children who have full or incomplete fetal alcohol syndrome. J Pediatr 2004; 145: 635–640.

118. Kaler SG, Patrinos ME, Lambert GH, et al. Hypertrichosis and congenital anomalies associated with maternal use of Minoxidil. Pediatrics 1987; 79; 434–436.

119. Johnson MD, Jacobs AJ. Congenital smooth muscle hamartoma. Arch Dermatol 1989; 125: 820–822.

120. Vergani R, Betti R, Martino P, et al. Giant nevoid hypertrichosis in an Iranian girl. Pediatr Dermatol 2002; 19: 64–66.

121. Knable A, Treadwell P. Pigmented plaque with hypertrichosis on the scalp of an infant. Pediatr Dermatol 1996; 13: 431–433.

122. Glover MT, Malone M, Atherton DJ. Michelin-tire baby syndrome resulting from diffuse smooth muscle hamartoma. Pediatr Dermatol 1989; 6: 329–331.

123. Larregue M, Vabre P, Cavaroc Y, et al. Hamartome diffus des muscles arrecteurs et hypertrichose lanugineuse congénitale. Ann Dermatol Venereol (Paris) 1991; 118: 796–798.

124. Danarti R, Konig A, Salhi A, et al. Becker's nevus syndrome revisited. J Am Acad Dermatol 2004; 51: 965–969.

125. Ferreira MJ, Bajanca R, Fiadeiro T. Congenital melanosis and hypertrichosis in a bilateral distribution. Pediatr Dermatol 1998; 15: 290–292.

126. Gagne EJ, Su WPD. Congenital smooth muscle hamartoma of the skin. Pediatr Dermatol 1993; 10: 142–145.

127. Ettl A, Marinkovic M, Koornneef L. Localized hypertrichosis associated with periorbital neurofibroma; clinical findings and differential diagnosis. Ophthalmology 1996; 103: 942–948.

128. Pivnik EK, Lobe TE, Fitch SJ, et al. Hair whorl as an indicator of a mediastinal plexiform neurofibroma. Pediatr Dermatol 1997; 14: 196–198.

129. Flannery DB, Howell CG. Confirmation of the Riccardi sign. Proc Greenwood Genet Centre 1986; 6: 161.

130. Wong SN, Tay YK. Tufted angioma: a report of five cases. Pediatr Dermatol 2002; 19: 388–393.

131. Herron M, Coffin CM, Vanderhooft SL. Tufted angiomas: variability of the clinical morphology. Pediatr Dermatol 2002; 19: 394–401.

132. Guggisberg D, Hadj-Rabia S, Viney C, et al. Skin markers of occult spinal dysraphism in children. Arch Dermatol 2004; 140: 1109–1115.

133. Drolet B. Cutaneous signs of neural tube malformations. Semin Cutan Med Surg 2004; 23: 125–137.

134. Schropp C, Sorensen N, Collmann H, Krauss J. Cutaneous lesions in occult spinal dysraphism – correlation with intraspinal findings. Childs Nerv Syst 2005; (Epub ahead of print).

135. Reed OM, Mellette JR, Fitzpatrick JE. Familial cervical hypertrichosis with underlying kyphoscoliosis. J Am Acad Dermatol 1989; 20: 1069–1072.

136. Herron M, Coffin CM, Vanderhooft SL. Vascular stains and hair collar sign associated with congenital anomalies of the scalp. Pediatr Dermatol 2005; 22: 200–205.

137. Stone N, Burge S. Focal facial dermal dysplasia with a hair collar. Br J Dermatol 1998; 139: 1136–1137.

138. Wells JM, Weedon D. Focal facial dermal dysplasia or aplasia cutis congenita: a case with a hair collar. Australas J Dermatol 2001; 42: 129–131.

139. Penas PF, Jones-Caballero M, Garcia-Diez A. Cutaneous heterotopic meningeal nodules. Arch Dermatol 1995; 131: 731.

140. Cox NH, McClure JP, Hardie RA. Naevoid hypertrichosis – report of a patient with multiple lesions. Clin Exp Dermatol 1989; 14: 62–64.

141. Rogers M. Naevoid hypertrichosis. Clin Exp Dermatol 1981: 16: 74.

142. Cheung ST, Lanigan SW. Naevoid hypertrichosis treated with alexandrite laser. Clin Exp Dermatol 2004; 29: 435–436.

143. Hurwitz S, Klaus SN. Congenital hemihypertrophy with hypertrichosis. Arch Dermatol 1971; 103: 98–100.

144. Akarsu S, Coskun BK, Aydin AM, et al. Congenital hemihypertrophy with hemihypertrophy. J Dermatol 2005; 32: 478–481.

145. Diamond FB, Shulman DI, Root AW. Scrotal hair in infancy. J Pediatr 1989; 114: 999–1001.

146. Slyper AH, Esterly NB. Nonprogressive scrotal hair growth in two infants. Pediatr Dermatol 1993; 10: 34–35.

147. Bragonier R, Karabouta Z, Crowne L. Transient scrotal hair growth in infancy. Postgrad Med J 2005; 81: 412.

148. Braddock SR, Jones KL, Bird LM, et al. Anterior cervical hypertrichosis: A

dominantly inherited isolated defect. Am J Med Genet 1995; 55: 498–499.

149. Trattner A, Hodak E, Sagie-Lerman T, et al. Familial congenital anterior cervical hypertrichosis associated with peripheral sensory and motor neuropathy. A new syndrome? J Am Acad Dermatol 1991; 25: 767–770.

150. Garty BZ, Snir M, Kremer I, et al. Retinal changes in familial peripheral sensory and motor neuropathy associated with anterior cervical hypertrichosis. J Pediatr Ophthalmol Strabismus 1997; 34: 309–312.

151. Jackson CE, Callies QC, Krull EA, et al. Hairy cutaneous malformations of the palms and soles. Arch Dermatol 1975; 111: 1146–1149.

152. Visser R, Beemer FA, Veenhoven RH, et al. Hypertrichosis cubiti: Two new cases and a review of the literature. Genet Couns 2002; 13: 397–403.

153. MacQuillan A, Hamilton S, Grobbelaar, A. Angiosomes, clefts, and eyelashes. Plast Reconstr Surg 2004; 113: 1400–1403.

154. Brooks BP, Dagenais SL, Nelson CC, et al. Mutation of the FOXC2 gene in familial distichiasis. J Am Assoc Pediatr Ophthalmol Strabismus 2003; 7: 354–357.

29

Nail Disorders

Robert A. Silverman

Nails are specialized cutaneous appendages composed of hard keratins similar to those found in hair, and are unique to primates. In humans, nails function as a stabilizing unit to aid in tactile sensation, grasping, and scratching. Well-manicured or adorned nails in adolescents and adults may be perceived as an attribute of social acceptability and serve as a source of personal satisfaction. Although abnormalities of the nails are rare, they may affect an individual's self-esteem and their relationships with others. Abnormal nails in a neonate may be indicative of a more widespread inherited or sporadic syndrome, or they may be a localized congenital malformation. In either case, parents of a newborn may be concerned about their infant's nails, sometimes out of proportion to the magnitude of any other problems that may be present. Investigation and consultations to uncover any associated illness and to allay any untoward parental anxiety are warranted.

The nail unit is composed of a rectangular nail plate bordered by proximal and lateral nail folds[1] (Fig. 29-1). The cuticle attaches the proximal nail fold to the nail plate. This acellular membrane is tightly adherent and prevents invasive microorganisms reaching the underlying matrix. The lunula (half moon) represents the distal portion of the nail's proliferative matrix. The ventral side of the nail plate has longitudinal ridges that orient the direction of growth from the root over a complementary grooved nail bed. At birth, the dorsal surface of the nail displays unique, somewhat oblique ridges as well. These ridges become parallel and disappear slowly, and over time the surface becomes smooth. The distal free edge of the plate separates from the bed at the hyponychium. The shape of the nail plate is convex. It is normally thickest at its proximal portion and thins distally. The size of the nail plate is determined by the size and growth of the underlying distal phalanx. Because embryologic development occurs in a cephalocaudal direction, it is not surprising that at birth, especially in premature infants, toenails may be smaller than fingernails. In premature infants less than 32 weeks' gestation, nail plates may not extend beyond the distal groove of the hyponychium. In postmature infants, such as macrosomic infants or infants of diabetic mothers, the nail plate may extend well beyond the hyponychium. In adults, it is estimated that fingernails grow 0.1 mm/day and toenails grow 1 mm/month. Similar data in newborns and infants are not available. Box 29-1 lists pathologic factors that affect nail growth.

The anatomic structure of the nail unit is affected by many disease states.[1] Conditions may be primary or secondary, localized or generalized, congenital or acquired, inherited, associated with syndromes, known genetic defects or drug exposures, and infectious or systemic disease. Nail morphogenesis begins during the 9th week of gestation and is completed by the end of the second trimester (see Chapter 1).

BEAU'S LINES

Beau's lines are transverse grooves or moat-like depressions that extend across the nail plate from one lateral nail fold to the other.[2,3] This deformity is a manifestation of nail matrix arrest and is first observed adjacent to the proximal nail fold. Beau's lines slowly move toward the distal free edge of the nail plate as nail growth resumes. If the rate of nail growth is known, one can estimate the date of nail matrix arrest by measuring the distance between the proximal nail fold and the Beau's line. Causes of Beau's lines include high fevers caused by infection, severe cutaneous inflammatory diseases such as Stevens–Johnson syndrome or Kawasaki disease, a reaction to medications, and acrodermatitis enteropathica. Beau's lines may occur in infants, 4–10 weeks of age, as a result of the stress of delivery. They have also been reported at birth as a result of intrauterine stress in a premature infant[4] (Fig. 29-2). Although Beau's lines should develop on all fingernails and toenails, they are usually most prominent on the thumbs and great toe nails because of their slower rate of growth.

Onychomadesis refers to proximal separation of the nail plate from the nail bed. Latent onychomadesis occurs when the nail separates some time after a profound interruption in nail growth. Causes are similar to those that produce Beau's lines and may occur during the neonatal period as well.

ALTERATIONS IN NAIL SHAPE

There is a close interaction between the formation of epidermal appendages and mesoderm during embryologic development. Therefore it is not surprising that there are many alterations of nail shape that are linked with distant or underlying malformations of bone. It is not uncommon for newborns to have variations of the normal convex curvature of the nail. Koilonychia refers to nails that exhibit a concave or spoon shape.[5] This may be a normal variant in newborns, especially when it involves the great toe nails. As the child grows and the distal phalanges lengthen, koilonychia gradually improves. Recently a case of koilonychia, dome-shaped femoral epiphyses, and platyspondylia has been described.[6] It is widely accepted that koilonychia in infants and toddlers may be indicative of iron deficiency. According to some investigators, koilonychia may precede clinical or laboratory evidence of anemia.[7] However, no well-controlled studies of iron deficiency in large numbers of infants with and without koilonychia have been

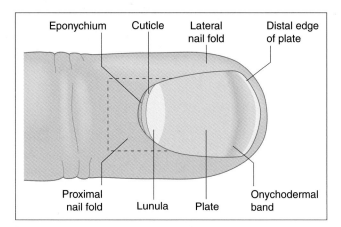

Eponychium   Cuticle   Lateral nail fold   Distal edge of plate

Proximal nail fold   Lunula   Plate   Onychodermal band

FIG. 29-1 Dorsal view of the nail unit. (From Gonzales-Servas A. Scher & Daniel Nails: therapy diagnosis, surgery, 2nd edn. New York: WB Saunders, 1997.)

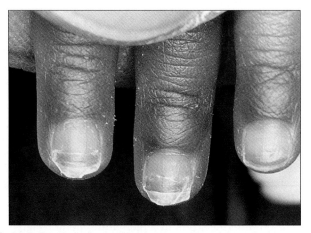

FIG. 29-2 Beau's lines are transverse grooves of the nail plate that represent a brief reduction of growth from the nail matrix.

Box 29-1 Pathologic factors that alter nail growth

Slower
Severe infections
Prolonged illness
Hypothyroidism
Malnutrition
Congestive heart failure
Ischemia
Nerve injury

Faster
Arteriovenous shunts
Erythroderma
Hyperthyroidism

reported, and improvement of nail shape with the administration of iron has not been documented. Familial koilonychia has rarely been reported.[8] It has been described with other ectodermal defects such as monilethrix, palmoplantar keratoderma, and steatocystoma multiplex, as well as Turner syndrome.[9]

Other deformities in nail shape include pincer nails, claw nails, and racquet nails. Pincer nails are characterized by a transverse overcurvature of the nail plates.[10] The condition is usually acquired, but some cases may result from an inherited developmental anomaly. If the convex transverse overcurvature is prominent, nails may appear similar to those in patients with pachyonychia congenita and occasionally may be quite painful. Congenital claw-like nails have also been reported.[11] The nail plates have a dorsal convexity and then curve downward to resemble onychogryphosis. This is usually noted on the second to fourth toes and may be associated with a cleft hand. Hypoplasia of the distal phalanx with absence of the ossification center is observed on radiographs of the affected digits.[12] Correction of the deformity is desirable because of the tendency toward recurrent bleeding and ulceration of the tip of the toe. Some authors distinguish claw nails from another isolated ungual anomaly, congenital curved nail of the fourth toe.[13] Nails in these cases are normal thickness and have a longitudinal overcurvature. This trait may be sporadic or inherited, and is also associated with underlying distal phalangeal deformities.[14] It may not come to medical attention until traumatic dystrophy later in childhood. Racquet nails occur when the width of the nail plate exceeds its length, also referred to as brachyonychia. It may be a sign of foreshortening of the terminal phalanx and may be associated with other congenital anomalies.[15]

Clubbing is a curved or beak-like deformity of the nail unit that accompanies hypertrophy and hyperplasia of the fibrovascular support stroma of the distal phalanx. It is an acquired sign of both systemic and hereditary diseases.[16] In neonates or infants, clubbing may be an early manifestation of cyanotic congenital heart disease, bronchopulmonary diseases, or HIV disease.[17,18]

ALTERATIONS IN NAIL SIZE

Anonychia refers to the absence of nails. The most widely known association is with nail–patella syndrome (see subsequent discussion). Isolated congenital anonychia has been reported in families with both autosomal recessive[19,20] and autosomal dominant inheritance (OMIM 206800: Online Mendelian Inheritance in Man (www.ncbi.nlm.nih.gov/Omim/)). Rudimentary nail units may be evident, but the underlying phalangeal structure is normal. Anonychia and hypoplasia of the nails may be observed with absence of the distal phalanges and foreshortening of the affected digits (Fig. 29-3). Anonychia has been reported with limb defects (OMIM 106990),[21] ectrodactyly,[22] flexural pigmentation (OMIM 106750),[23] isolated to the thumbnails (OMIM 188200),[24] and with sensorineural hearing loss (OMIM 124480, 220500).[25] These latter cases have been termed DOOR syndrome (deafness, onycho-osteodystrophy, and retardation). Elevated urinary amino acids have been detected in some patients with DOOR syndrome.[23] Anonychia of the fifth fingers and toenails is characteristic of Coffin–Siris syndrome (OMIM 135900).[26] Other features include growth and mental retardation, generalized hypertrichosis and scalp hypotrichosis, lax joints, and abnormal facies. Anonychia, nail hypoplasia, and other nail anomalies, such as double nails (Fig. 29-4), may occur as isolated findings.[27]

Infants with junctional and dystrophic forms of epidermolysis bullosa (EB) frequently have anonychia at birth (Fig. 29-5).[28] Subungual hemorrhages, onycholysis (separation of

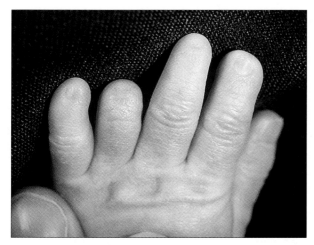

FIG. 29-3 Anonychia with absence of the distal phalanx and fore-shortening of the digit.

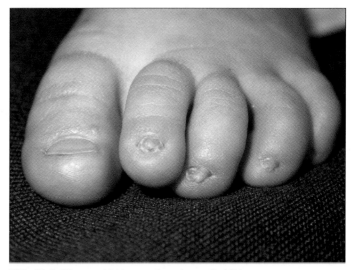

FIG. 29-6 Micronychia in an otherwise well child.

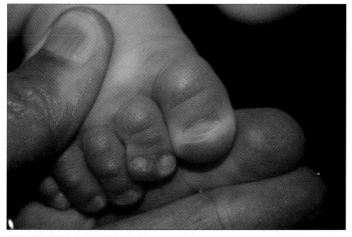

FIG. 29-4 Double nail anomaly.

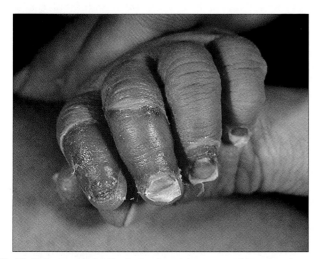

FIG. 29-5 Anonychia of the index finger in a case of junctional epidermolysis bullosa.

the nail plate from the nail bed) and onychomadesis precede nail loss. One or more fingernails are usually affected. The periungual tissues and nail beds are frequently swollen and inflamed. Granulation tissue develops quickly. Meticulous hygiene, application of topical antibiotics, and wound care with synthetic dressings may optimize regrowth if possible. It is the author's opinion that in utero sucking of the fingers results in most of the nail disease that is present at birth in EB.

MICRONYCHIA

Small nails may be localized to one or a few digits or involve all of the nail fields (Fig. 29-6). Conditions associated with micronychia are listed in Table 29-1.[29-33] Current theory suggests that at least some forms of micronychia, such as in fetal alcohol syndrome and exposure to anticonvulsants, are due to inhibition of retinoic acid synthesis during early embryologic development.[34,35] Selected specific causes of micronychia are discussed in subsequent sections.

NAIL–PATELLA SYNDROME

Nail–patella syndrome (OMIM 161200), also known as hereditary osteo-onychodysplasia (HOOD), is an autosomal dominant genodermatosis characterized by nail hypoplasia present at birth, chronic progressive nephropathy, and hypoplastic patellae that may result in debilitating osteoarthritis. This disorder has a high degree of penetrance and widely variable expressivity.[36] Nail disease is usually the only manifestation in neonates. However, there are rare reports of infants with proteinuria, signifying the early onset of renal pathology.[37]

Ungual manifestations are most prominent on the ulnar sides of the thumbs and index fingers, and to a lesser degree on other digits. They include micronychia, hemionychia, and occasionally anonychia. If present, a triangularly shaped lunula with a distal apex is nearly pathognomonic for the condition.[38] Nail plates may be thin and display koilonychia, which can lead to frequent chipping and splitting later in childhood.

Skeletal deformities are not visible until ossification centers develop. Parents may be screened for small, easily subluxed patellae, characteristic posterior iliac horns, hypoplasia of the proximal radius and ulna, scoliosis, and thickened scapulae. Generally, patients with nail–patella syndrome are not identified until early adulthood, when knee dislocation, pain, and gait disturbances bring them to medical attention.[39]

TABLE 29-1 Micronychias

Disorder	Clinical manifestations
Nail-patella syndrome	Small or absent patellas, iliac horns, triangular lunulas
Congenital onychodysplasia	
Ectodermal dysplasias	Variable sweating, hair and tooth abnormalities
Congenital malalignment of index fingers	None, Except underlying phalangeal malformation
Fetal Teratogens	
Alcohol	Microcephaly, short palpebral fissures, maxillary hypoplasia
Hydantoins (and other anticonvulsants)	Short stature, retardation, hypertelorism, depressed nasal bridge, cardiac anomalies, mucosal changes
Polychlorinated biphenyls	Natal teeth, pigment anomalies, mucosal changes
Warfarin	Nasal hypoplasia, stippled epiphyses
Coffin-Siris syndrome	Hypoplasia of the fifth digit, lax joints, blepharoptosis
Dyskeratosis Congenita	Hyperpigmentation and hypopigmentation, Γanconi-like anemia, blepharitis, leukoplakia, XLR* (OMIM30500)
Chromosome Abnormalities	
Trisomies	3q, 8, 13, 18
Turner syndrome	XO, webbed neck, nevi, lymphedema, coarctation of the aorta
Noonan syndrome	XY male with a Turner phenotype and pulmonic stenosis
Amniotic bands	Hypoplasia of the distal phalanx associated with aplasia cutis

*X-linked recessive inheritance.

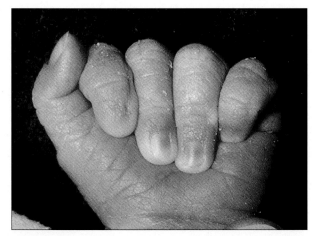

FIG. 29-7 Absence or hypoplasia of the nail unit of the index fingers is characteristic of congenital onychodysplasia of the index fingers.

Renal disease that presents as asymptomatic proteinuria is the most serious manifestation of nail–patella syndrome. It is usually not apparent until adulthood, but a newborn and a 2-year-old child with nephrosis have been reported.[40] Renal biopsies have uncovered glomerulonephritis secondary to glomerular basement membrane zone thickening from collagen fibril deposition. These findings have even been noted in a spontaneously aborted 18-week-old fetus.[41]

Other manifestations include heterochromic irides, colobomas, microcorneas, glaucoma,[42] popliteal pterygia, and mild mental deficiency. It has been suggested that these, as well as other findings such as colon cancer, in specific kindreds may be a result of contiguous gene defects, translocations, or other genetic aberrations.[43] Complications from cerebral and large vessel dilation have also been reported, and are also caused by collagenous basal lamina reduplication.[44]

Mutations in the LIM homeodomain protein gene *Lmx1b* have been demonstrated in the region of 9q34 and result in the nail–patella syndrome.[45] This gene is responsible for dorsoventral body pattern formation during fetal development. It is linked to the ABO blood group and had been believed to be an abnormality in *COL5A1*, which is necessary for the production of collagen type V, an important component in the glomerular and other basement membrane zones.[46]

CONGENITAL ONYCHODYSPLASIA OF THE INDEX FINGERS

Congenital onychodysplasia of the index fingers (COIF), also known as Iso and Kikuchi syndrome, was first described in 1969.[47,48] Original cases were congenital, limited mainly to the index fingers, and characterized by anonychia, micronychia, and/or polyonychia (Fig. 29-7). They were nonfamilial and nonhereditary, and without underlying bone or joint abnormalities. Since that time the clinical criteria have been changed or expanded to encompass a number of additional observations.[49]

Although the index fingers are most commonly affected, onychodystrophy has been reported on other fingers and toes.[50,51] Malalignment, 'rolled micronychia,' hemionychogryphosis, onychoheterotopia, and polyonychia with syndactyly have also been detailed. Unlike nail–patella syndrome, abnormalities in the nail unit are more prominent on the radial aspects of the digits. A Y-shaped bifurcation of the distal phalanx on lateral radiographs is frequent and is characteristic of the condition.[52] Familial cases have also been documented.[53]

The pathogenesis of congenital onychodysplasia is poorly understood. An abnormal vascular supply, anomalies from an abnormal grip, external deformation from pressure against the cranium, exposure to teratogens, and genetic influences have been implicated by a number of authors.[54] It is quite possible that the clinical findings may be explained by any of these theories if the inciting event occurs at a specific time during the embryologic development of the nail unit.

ONYCHOATROPHY

Onychoatrophy refers to a progressive reduction in size and thickness of the nail unit. The term is usually used to describe acquired dissolution of ungual structures and should not be used synonymously with micronychia, although some authors do so. Inflammatory disorders, which are observed in older children and adults and rarely documented in newborns, such as Stevens–Johnson syndrome or graft-versus-host disease, may result in onychoatrophy. Infants with congenital disorders that have a progressive phenotype, such as acrogeria or dyskeratosis congenita, can have onychoatrophy as well. Occlusion of the digital artery by emboli may result in phalangeal necrosis and destruction of nail structures. Other postnatal vascular insults, such as extensive aplasia cutis congenita or disseminated intravascular coagulation from homozygous protein C deficiency, could potentially have similar effects.

ECTOPIC NAILS

Onychoheterotopia, or ectopic nails, occurs when ungual tissue develops on areas other than the dorsal aspect of the distal phalanx.[54] Cases that have been reported tend to involve the palmar surface of the fifth fingers.[55–58] They have been both sporadic and reported in siblings, suggesting possible autosomal recessive inheritance. Other abnormalities of the hand may also be present, including underlying osseous malformations. A circumferential nail of the fifth finger has been documented in association with a deletion in the long arm of chromosome 6.[59] This tubular defect may occur on other digits as well.[60] The presence of a circumferential nail is frequently observed at the tip of the fused digits of the hand in acrocephalosyndactyly or Apert syndrome (OMIM 101200).[61] Synonychia and fusion of all of the toes are also observed in this sporadic condition, which is caused by mutations in the gene encoding fibroblast growth factor receptor-2 (*FGFR-2*) found on the chromosomal locus 10q26 (Fig. 29-8).[62]

HYPERTROPHY OF THE NAIL

Large nails with anatomically normal nail units may be observed in newborns with macrodactyly. Conditions that display macronychia include epidermal nevus syndrome, Proteus syndrome, Maffucci syndrome, Klippel–Trenaunay–Weber syndrome, and gigantism. Patients with the ectrodactyly–ectodermal dysplasia–cleft lip/palate (EEC) syndrome also may have a large nail on the fused digits. Several terms are used to describe different types of enlarged nails. Onychauxis refers to nails that exhibit thick nail plates but retain a normal overall size and shape. Onychogryphosis is present when the nail plate thickens and develops an inferior overcurvature. If nail growth is uneven, the plate deviates obliquely and takes on the appearance of a ram's horn. The nail plates are usually discolored and display oyster-like striations across the surface. Although onychogryphosis is usually observed on toenails in the elderly or on digits that have been permanently injured,

hereditary autosomal dominant and congenital forms involving both the fingernails and toenails have been reported.[55,56] Hemionychogryphosis has been seen in cases of congenital malalignment of the great toe nails and COIF. Pachyonychia refers to thickening and superior deviation of the nail plate owing to the accumulation of subungual hyperkeratosis. This may be observed in older patients with psoriasis or onychomycosis, but the term is classically used to describe the inherited condition pachyonychia congenita.

PACHYONYCHIA CONGENITA

Pachyonychia congenita is characterized by hard, thick nails that angle upwards at their distal free edge because of a massive accumulation of keratin in the ventral nail plate. The lateral borders curve under and give the plates a pincer-like appearance (Fig. 29-9). Unlike onychogryphosis, the nails of pachyonychia congenita have a smooth surface. Although pachyonychia congenita syndrome is transmitted as an autosomal dominant trait with a high degree of penetrance, full expressivity may not become evident until later childhood or adulthood. Infants with pachyonychia congenita initially display a yellowish-brown discoloration of the nails. Thickening from subungual hyperkeratosis occurs gradually over months to years.

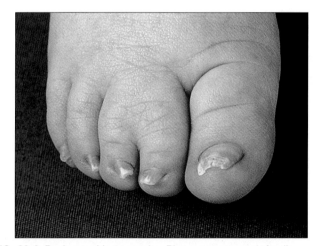

FIG. 29-9 Pachyonychia congenita. Pincer appearance of nails.

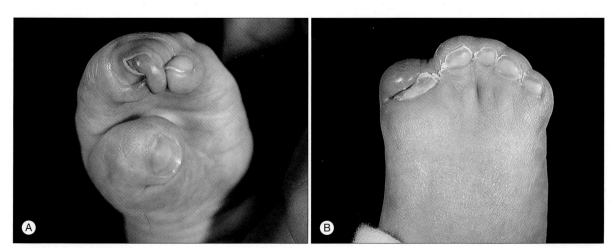

FIG. 29-8 (**A**) Fused second to fourth digits of the hand of a patient with Apert syndrome who had a single circumferential nail. (**B**) Synonychia and syndactyly of the toes in a patient with Apert syndrome.

It is now accepted that patients with pachyonychia congenita can be classified into one of two syndromes that have one of several genetic defects in hard keratin.[57] Mutations in keratin 16 (located on chromosome 17) or in keratin 6A (located on chromosome 12) have been found in type I, the Jadassohn–Lewandowski variant. As newborns, these patients may have foamy white mucosal plaques of oral leukokeratosis (Fig. 29-10). During childhood debilitating palmoplantar keratoderma, hyperhidrosis, and secondary bullae develop. Clusters of rough, dry, spiny papules become evident over the body, particularly on the elbows and knees, similar to psoriasis. Later, there may be eruption of epidermoid cysts. Type II patients with the Jackson–Lawler form of the disease have abnormalities in the keratin 17 gene (found on chromosome 17) or keratin 6B (found on chromosome 12). Natal teeth with milia, minimal oral leukokeratosis, cylindromas, steatocystomas, and milder keratoderma are present in these cases. A registry and support group for patients and their families with pachyonychia congenita is now available (http://www.pachyonychia.org/index.html).

INGROWN TOENAILS

There are three types of ingrown toenail in neonates. Congenital malalignment of the nails of the great toe presents with a trapezoid-shaped nail plate that deviates laterally with respect to the longitudinal axis of the distal phalanx (Fig. 29-11).[58]

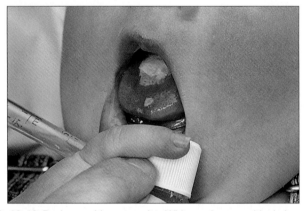

FIG. 29-10 Pachyonychia congenita. White oral mucosal leukokeratotic plaques.

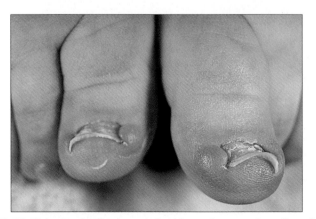

FIG. 29-11 Ingrown nails characterized by erythema and swelling of the medial nail folds in a case of congenital malalignment of the great toe nails.

Cases may be unilateral, bilateral, sporadic, or inherited as an autosomal dominant trait.[59] Recurrent damage to the nail matrix occurs when the child is old enough to crawl and walk. This damage is manifested by multiple transverse ridges, discoloration caused by infection and hemorrhage, paronychia, onycholysis, and nail loss.[60] Mild degrees of malalignment may improve over time.[61] However, when marked deviation of the nail plate results in the distal free edge embedding into the soft tissues of the hyponychium, surgical rotation of the misdirected matrix may be necessary to prevent chronic long-term disability.[62]

Congenital hypertrophy of the lateral nail folds of the hallux may present at birth or in the first month of life as red, firm, enlarged masses of tissue that may cover significant amounts of the nail plate.[63] If the induration persists, it may become painful or infected when the infant begins to crawl or walk. The condition usually remits spontaneously. A 2-week trial of a potent topical steroid solution (e.g. fluocinonide twice daily) would not be unreasonable if surgical reduction of the excess tissue is contemplated.

Embedding of the distal free margin of the nail plate into the soft tissue of the hyponychium is not uncommon. A prominent ridge of tissue may form a wall that results in embedding or superior deflection of the nail plate. Most neonates outgrow these findings by 6 months of age.[64] Some authors believe that factors such as sleeping prone, especially when the child begins to kick actively, and tight-fitting sleepers may predispose the older infant to paronychia.[65]

PARONYCHIA AND INFECTIOUS NAIL DYSTROPHY

Infections of the nail unit in neonates are extremely important to identify and treat promptly because of the possibility of irreversible damage to the nail matrix. Once the protective cuticle or hyponychium are compromised, then the matrix, an area of relative immune privilege, can be easily invaded.[66] Acute paronychia presents with red, swollen, tender nail folds. Purulent material accumulates in the periungual groove and can extend under the nail plate. Chronic paronychia manifests with painless swelling of the nail fold, loss of the cuticle, and the development of granulation tissue. Organisms responsible for paronychia include *Candida* spp.,[67] *Staphylococcus*, *Streptococcus*, *Veillonella* (in neonates),[68] anaerobes, saprophytes, and herpes simplex. Paronychia is most common on the fingers as a result of developmentally appropriate sucking or mouthing of the digits. Systemic diseases associated with paronychia include mucocutaneous candidiasis, DiGeorge syndrome, acrodermatitis enteropathica, Langerhans' cell histiocytosis,[69] and HIV infections.[70] Once diagnostic tests have been completed (e.g. cultures, Gram stain, potassium hydroxide preparation, and Tzanck preparation), treatment can be started. Burrow's solution soaks aid in gentle debridement of infected tissues. In mild cases, twice-daily use of topical solutions such as clindamycin or clotrimazole is indicated. Several days of concomitant applications of a topical steroid solution may reduce any pain and swelling. In more severe cases, purulent material may have to be surgically drained and granulation tissue may need to be cauterized.

Onychomycosis is extremely rare in neonates. Congenital candidiasis localized to the nails has been reported in premature and term newborns (Fig. 29-12).[71,72] Topical applications

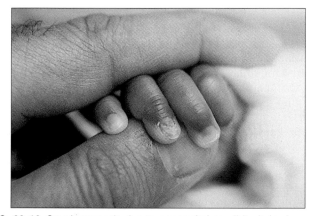

FIG. 29-12 Onychomycosis due to congenital candidiasis is characterized by punctate leukonychia, pits, brittleness, and chipping of the surface of the nail plate. (Courtesy Dr Lloyd Krammer, INOVA Fairfax Hospital for Children.)

of ciclopirox olamine nail lacquer were sufficient to clear the infection, unlike nail infections in most adults. The dermatophyte *Trichophyton rubrum* was isolated from the nails of a 4-month-old who may have acquired the organism as a neonate.[73]

ONYCHOLYSIS

Separation of the nail plate from the nail bed is known as onycholysis. This usually occurs at the distal free edge of the nail plate, but may be observed laterally as well. The separation creates a narrow space that can fill with keratin, exogenous debris, or fluids such as water or saliva. The air pocket of the cleft gives an onycholytic nail a grayish-white color. Onycholysis is a physical sign for which there are numerous causes (Box 29-2).

CHROMONYCHIA

Nail dyschromia may be due to discoloration of the nail plate or nail bed[74] (Table 29-2). The causes of nail discoloration may be exogenous, secondary to local infectious agents, systemic drugs or diseases, primary skin diseases, or ungual neoplasms (Fig. 29-13). The shape of the discolored area depends upon how and where in the nail unit the pigment is deposited, and the duration of the pigment deposition.

Leukonychia (white nails) is the most common type of nail dyschromia.[75] It should not be confused with onycholysis. Total or subtotal leukonychia may be inherited as an autosomal dominant trait.[76] Partial leukonychia on the distal portion of the nail apparatus may be a sign of congenital candidiasis limited to the nail plates.[77] Proximal partial leukonychia is also a sign of subungual onychomycosis from dermatophytes or other fungi.[78] Transversely striated leukonychia in a longitudinal band may be observed after a febrile illness, similar to Beau's lines. Multiple striations are associated with successive events that affect the matrix, including the administration of chemotherapeutic agents,[79] the classic Mees' lines of heavy metal intoxication, or Muehrcke's paired lines of hypoalbuminemia. Muehrcke's lines have also been described in the presence of zinc deficiency. Partial leukonychia in which the proximal portion of the nail is white has several eponyms.

Box 29-2 Causes of onycholysis

Systemic
Thyroid disease
Iron deficiency
Erythropoietic protoporphyria

Congenital/hereditary
Partial hereditary onycholysis
Ectodermal dysplasias
Periodic shedding of the nails
Leprechaunism

Primary skin diseases
Epidermolysis bullosa
Psoriasis

Medications*
Indomethacin
Retinoids
Antibiotics
Chemotherapy

Local causes
Thermal injury (pulse oximeters)
Trauma

Infections
Candida

*Directly or in combination with ultraviolet light (photo-onycholysis).
Modified from Baran R, Dawber RPR. Diseases of the nails and their management, 2nd edn. Oxford: Blackwell Scientific Publications, 1994; 59.

TABLE 29-2 Chromonychia (Nails with abnormal color)

Condition	Color	Other features
Hematomas	Purple	Observed on fingers, similar to sucking blisters (Fig. 29-9)
Endocarditis	Purple	Splinter shaped
Phototoxicity	Purple	Drugs, porphyrias
Hyperbilirubinemia	Yellow-brown	Scleral icterus
Yellow nail syndrome	Yellow	Lymphedema, respiratory disease, nephrotic syndrome
Pernicious anemia	Blue-gray	Macrocytosis
Onychomycosis	Gray-green	Aspergillus, Pseudomonas
Candidiasis	White	
PCB exposure	Brown-gray	
Addison's/Cushing's disease	Brown	

They include Lindsay's half-and-half nails of uremia, and Terry's nails secondary to cirrhosis or congestive heart failure. Leukonychia may also be a sign of malnutrition or iron deficiency anemia. Punctate leukonychia is manifested by small, irregular white spots. It is usually caused by repeated minor trauma to the nail matrix.

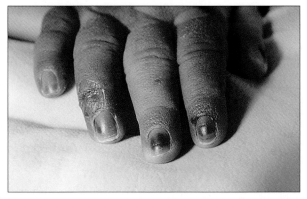

FIG. 29-13 A dusky violaceous hue of the nail beds resulting from ecchymoses and an eroded blister caused by vigorous intrauterine sucking.

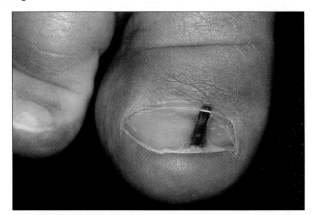

FIG. 29-14 A longitudinal pigmented band of the nail plate develops from a nevoculluar nevus in the nail matrix.

Single longitudinal pigmented bands of the nail in children are due to melanocytic lesions located in the nail matrix (Fig. 29-14).[80] Multiple longitudinal pigmented bands are common in dark-skinned persons but are unusual in children. Multiple brown bands may be observed in fetal hydantoin syndrome, Addison and Cushing disease, Peutz–Jegher syndrome, HIV, and after exposure to maternal chlorpromazine ingestion or other maternally ingested drugs.[81] A study of longitudinal pigmented bands in 100 individuals found that 22 had nail matrix nevi.[82] Twelve patients had lesions present at birth, and most were located on the fingernails. The bands were different shades, from light tan to black, and their width varied from 2 mm to the breadth of the entire nail plate. Periungual pigmentation (Hutchinson's sign) was present in many of these benign lesions. In a series of eight cases of longitudinal melanonychia in children, four were present at birth.[83] No cases of melanoma were documented in either series. There have even been isolated reports of spontaneous regression of ungual nevi.[84] To date, six cases of melanoma of the nail unit in young children have been reported.[85] Most cases of suspected ungual melanomas are probably benign Spitz nevi. Their pathology should be interpreted with caution, even by dermatopathologists. Most experts in nail diseases do not recommend biopsy of longitudinal pigmented bands unless a previously stable lesion undergoes progressive, rapid change. Biopsy specimens should be obtained from children who are predisposed to develop malignancies (e.g. xeroderma pigmentosum or dysplastic nevus syndrome). Improperly performed biopsies can lead to permanent nail dystrophy.

REFERENCES

1. Baran R, Dawber RPR. Diseases of the nails and their management, Oxford: Blackwell Scientific Publications, 1994.
2. Silverman R, Baran R. Nail and appendageal abnormalities. In: Schachner LA, Hansen RC, eds. Pediatric dermatology, 3rd edn.. Philadelphia: Elsevier Ltd., 2003; 12: 574.
3. Turano AF. Transverse nail ridging in early infancy. Pediatrics 1968; 41: 996–997.
4. Wolf D, Wolf R, Goldberg MD. Beau's lines, a case report. Cutis 1982; 29: 191–194.
5. Yinnon AM, Matalon M. Koilonychia of the toenails in children. Int J Dermatol 1988; 27: 685–687.
6. Nguyen V, Buka RL, Roberts B, et al. Koilonychia, dome-shaped epiphyses, and vertebral playtspondylia. J Pediatr 2005; 147: 112–114.
7. Hogan GR, Jones B. The relationship of koilonychia and iron deficiency in infants. J Pediatr 1970; 77: 1054–1057.
8. Crosby DL, Petersen MJ. Familial koilonychia. Cutis 1989; 44: 209–210.
9. Bumpers RD, Bishop ME. Familial koilonychia: a current case. Arch Dermatol 1980; 116: 845–846.
10. Chapman RS. Overcurvature of the nails: an inherited disorder. Br J Dermatol 1973; 89: 211–213.

11. Egawa T. Congenital claw-like fingers and toes. Plast Reconstr Surg 1977; 59: 569–574.
12. Takeshi M, Tadao K, Ogawa Y, et al. Claw nail deformity of the toe accompanied with cleft hand. J Plast Reconstr Surg 1998; 101: 427–430.
13. Iwasa M, Hirose T, Matsuo K. Congenital curved nail of the fourth toe. Plast Reconstr Surg 1991; 553–554.
14. Lin Y-C, Wu Y-H, Scher R. Congenital curved nail of the fourth toe: Three different clinical presentations. Pediatr Dermatol (in press).
15. Johnson CF. Broad thumbs and broad great toes with facial abnormalities and mental retardation. Pediatrics 1966; 68: 942.
16. Baran R, Dawber RPR. Diseases of the nails and their management, 2nd edn. Oxford: Blackwell Scientific Publications, 1994; 324–327.
17. Silverman RA. Nail and appendageal disorders. In: Schachner LA, Hansen RC, eds. Pediatric dermatology, 2nd edn. London: Churchill Livingstone, 1995; 629.
18. Katz BZ. Finger clubbing as sign of HIV infection in children [letter]. Lancet 1997; 349: 575.

19. Hopsu-Havu VK, Jansen CT. Anonychia congenita. Arch Dermatol 1973; 107: 752–753.
20. Teebi AS, Kaurah P. Total anonychia congenita and microcephaly with normal intelligence: a new autosomal-recessive syndrome? Am J Med Genet 1996; 66: 257–260.
21. Nevin NC, Thomas PS, Eady DJ, et al. Anonychia and absence/hypoplasia of distal phalanges (Cook's syndrome): report of a second family. J Med Genet 1995; 32: 638–641.
22. Rahbari H, Heath L, Chapel TA. Anonychia with ectrodactyly. Arch Dermatol 1975; 111: 1482–1483.
23. Verbov J. Anonychia with bizarre flexural pigmentation – an autosomal dominant dermatosis. Br J Dermatol 1975; 92: 469–474.
24. Strandskov HH. Inheritance of absence of thumbnails. J Hered 1939; 30: 53–54.
25. Robinson GC, Miller JR, Bensimon JR. Familial ectodermal dysplasia with sensorineural deafness and other anomalies. Pediatrics 1962; 30: 797–802.
26. Qazi QH, Heckman LS, Markouizos D, et al. The Coffin–Siris syndrome. J Med Genet 1990; 27: 333–336.
27. Seitz CS, Hamm H. Congenital brachydactyly and nail hypoplasia: clue

to bone-dependent nail formation. Br J Dermatol. 2005 Jun; 152: 1339–1342.

28. Bruckner-Tuderman L, Schnyder UW, Baran R. Nail changes in epidermolysis bullosa: clinical and pathogenic considerations. Br J Dermatol 1995; 132: 339–344.

29. Crain LS, Fitzmaurice NE, Mondry C. Nail dysplasia and fetal alcohol syndrome. Am J Dis Child 1983; 137: 1069.

30. D'Souza SW, Robertson IG, Donnai D. Fetal phenytoin exposure, hypoplastic nails, and jitteriness. Arch Dis Child 1990; 65: 320.

31. Hsu MM, Mak CP, Hus CC. Follow-up of skin manifestations in Yu-Cheng children. Br J Dermatol 1995; 132: 427–432.

32. Thakker JC, Kothari SS, Deshmu KL, et al. Hypoplasia of nails and phalanges: a teratogenic manifestation of phenobarbitone. Indian Pediatr J 1991; 28: 73.

33. Jàger-Roman E, Deichl A, Jakob S, et al. Fetal growth, major malformations, and minor anomalies in infants born to women receiving valproic acid. J Pediatr 1986; 108: 997.

34. Duester GA. Hypothetical mechanism for fetal alcohol syndrome involving ethanol inhibition of retinoic acid synthesis at the alcohol dehydrogenase step. Alcohol Clin Exp Res 1991; 15: 568–572.

35. Fex G, Larsson K, Andersson A, et al. Low serum concentration of all-trans and 13-cis retinoic acids in patients treated with phenytoin, carbamazepine, and valproate: possible relation to teratogenicity. Arch Toxicol 1995; 69: 572–574.

36. Lucas GL, Opitz JM. The nail–patella syndrome: clinical and genetic aspects of 5 kindreds with 38 affected family members. J Pediatr 1966; 68: 273–288.

37. Simila S, Vesa L, Wasz-Hockert O. Hereditary onycho-osteodysplasia (the nail–patella syndrome) with nephrosis-like renal disease in a newborn boy. Pediatrics 1970; 46: 61–65.

38. Daniel CR III, Osment LS, Noojin RO. Triangular lunulae: a clue to nail–patella syndrome. Arch Dermatol 1980; 116: 448–449.

39. Carbonara P, Kane AC, Alpert M. Hereditary osteo-onychodysplasia (HOOD). Am J Med Sci 1964; 248: 139–151.

40. Browning MC, Weidner N, Lorentz WB Jr. Renal histopathology of the nail–patella syndrome in a two-year-old boy. Clin Nephrol 1988; 29: 210–213.

41. Drut RM, Chandra S, Latorraca R, et al. Nail–patella syndrome in a spontaneously aborted 18-week fetus: ultrastructural and immunofluorescent study of the kidneys. Am J Med Genet 1992; 43: 693–696.

42. Lichter PR, Richards JE, Downs CA, et al. Cosegregation of open-angle glaucoma and the nail–patella syndrome. Am J Ophthalmol 1997; 124: 506–515.

43. Gilula LA, Kantor OS. Familial colon carcinoma in nail-patella syndrome. Am J Roentgenol 1975; 123: 783–790.

44. Burkhart CG, Bhumbra R, Iannone AM. Nail–patella syndrome: a distinctive clinical and electron microscopic presentation. J Am Acad Dermatol 1980; 3: 251–256.

45. Dreyer SD, Zhou G, Baldini A, et al. Mutations in LMX1B cause abnormal skeletal patterning and renal dysplasia in nail patella syndrome. Nature Genet 1998; 19: 47–50.

46. Greenspan DC, Byers MG, Eddy RL, et al. Human collagen gene COL5A1 maps to the q34.2 q34.3 region of chromosome 9, near the locus for nail–patella syndrome. Genomics 1992; 12: 836–837.

47. Iso R. Congenital nail defects of the index finger and reconstructive surgery. Orthop Surg (Tokyo) 1969; 20: 1383–1384.

48. Baran R, Stroud JD. Congenital onychodysplasia of the index fingers. Iso and Kikuchi syndrome. Arch Dermatol 1984; 120: 243–244.

49. Prais D, Horev G, Merlob P. Prevalence and new phenotypic and radiologic findings in congenital onychodysplasia of the index finger. Pediatr Dermatol 1999; 16: 201–204.

50. Youn SH, Kwon OS, Park KC, et al. Congenital onychodysplasia of the index fingers – Iso–Kikuchi syndrome. A case involving the second toenail. Clin Exp Dermatol 1996; 21: 457–458.

51. Kikuchi I. Congenital onychodysplasia of the index fingers: a case involving the thumbnails. Semin Dermatol 1991; 10: 7–11.

52. Miura T, Nakamura R. Congenital onychodysplasia of the index fingers. J Hand Surg 1990; 15A: 793–797.

53. Millman AJ, Strier RP. Congenital onychodysplasia of the index fingers. Report of a family. J Am Acad Dermatol 1982; 7: 57–65.

54. Kikuchi I. Congenital onychodysplasia of the index fingers: a case involving the thumbnails. Semin Dermatol 1991; 10: 7–11.

55. Schmidt H. Total onychogryphosis traced during six generations. Proc Fenno Scand Assoc Dermatol 1965; 36–37.

56. Lubach D. Erbliche onychogryphosis. Hautarzt 1982; 33: 331.

57. Leachman SA, Kaspar RL, Fleckman P, et al. Clinical and pathological features of pachyonychia congenita. J Invest Dermatol Symp Proc 2005; 10: 3–17.

58. Baran R, Bureau H. Congenital malalignment of the big toenail as a cause of ingrowing toenail in infancy: pathology and treatment (a study of thirty cases). Clin Exp Dermatol 1983; 8: 619–623.

59. Harper KJ, Beer WE. Congenital malalignment of the great toenails – an inherited condition. Clin Exp Dermatol 1986; 11: 514–516.

60. Cohen JL, Scher RK, Pappert AS. Congenital malalignment of the great toenails. Pediatr Dermatol 1991; 8: 40–42.

61. Dawson TAJ. Great toe-nail dystrophy. Br J Dermatol 1989; 20: 139.

62. Baran R. Significance and management of congenital malalignment of the big toenail. Cutis 1996; 58: 181–184.

63. Hammerton MD, Shrank AB. Congenital hypertrophy of the lateral nailfolds of the hallux. Pediatr Dermatol 1988; 5: 243–245.

64. Honig PJ, Spitzer A, Bernstein R, Leyden JJ. Congenital ingrown toenails. Clin Pediatr 1982; 21: 424–426.

65. Bailie FB, Evans DM. Ingrowing toenails in infancy. Br Med J 1978; 2: 737–738.

66. Ito T, Ito N, Saathoff M, et al. Immunology of the human nail apparatus: The nail matrix is a site of relative immune privilege. J Invest Dermatol 2005; 125: 1139–1148.

67. Raval DS, Barton LL, Hansen RC, et al. Congenital cutaneous candidiasis: case report and review. Pediatr Dermatol 1995; 12: 355–358.

68. Sinniah D, Sandiford BR, Dugdale AE. Subungual infection in the newborn: an institutional outbreak of unknown etiology, possibly due to Veillonella. Clin Pediatr 1972; 11: 690–692.

69. De Berker D, Lever LR, Windebank K. Nail features in Langerhans cell histiocytosis. Br J Dermatol 1994; 130: 523–527.

70. Russo F, Collantes C, Guerrero J. Severe paronychia due to zidovudine-induced neutropenia in a neonate. J Am Acad Dermatol 1999; 40: 322–324.

71. Clegg HW, Prose NS, Greenberg DN. Nail dystrophy in congenital cutaneous candidiasis. Pediatr Dermatol. 2003; 20: 342–344.

72. Sardana K, Garg VK, Manchanda V, Rajpal M. Congenital candidal onychomycosis: effective cure with ciclopirox olamine 8% nail lacquer. Br J Dermatol 2006; 154: 573–575.

73. Jewell EW. Trichophyton rubrum onychomycosis in a 4-month-old infant. Cutis 1970; 6: 1121–1122.

74. Paradisis M, Van Asperen P. Yellow nail syndrome in infancy. J Paediatr Child Health 1997; 33: 454–457.

75. Zaun H. Leukonychias. Semin Dermatol 1991; 10: 17–20.

76. Stevens KR, Leis PF, Peters S, et al. Congenital leukonychia. J Am Acad Dermatol 1998; 39: 509–512.

77. Arbegast KD, Lamberty LF, Koh JK, et al. congenital candidiasis limited to the nail plates. Pediatr Dermatol 1990; 7: 310–312.

78. Baran R, Tosti A, Piraccini BM. Uncommon clinical patterns of fusarium nail infection: report of 3 cases. Br J Dermatol 1997; 136: 424–427.

79. Shelly WB, Humphrey GB. Transverse leukonychia (Mees' lines) due to daunorubicin chemotherapy. Pediatr Dermatol 1997; 14: 144–145.

80. Goettmann-Bonvallot S, André J, Belaich S. Longitudinal melanonychia in children: A clinical and histopathologic

study of 40 cases. J Am Acad Dermatol 1999; 41: 17–22.

81. Silverman RA. Nail and appendageal abnormalities. In: Schachner LA, Hansen RD, eds. Pediatric dermatology, 2nd edn. New York: Churchill Livingstone, 1994; 635–636.

82. Tosti A, Baran R, Piraccini BM, et al. Nail matrix nevi: A clinical and histopathologic study of twenty-two patients. J Am Acad Dermatol 1996; 34: 765–771.

83. Léauté-Labreze C, Bioulac-Sage P, Taîeb A. Longitudinal melanonychia in children: a study of eight cases. Arch Dermatol 1996; 132: 167–169.

84. Tosti A, Baran R, Morelli R, et al. Progressive fading of a longitudinal melanonychia due to a nail matrix melanocytic nevus in a child. Arch Dermatol 1994; 130: 1076–1077.

85. Antonovich DD, Grin C, Grant-Kels JM. Childhood subungual melanoma in situ in diffuse sail melanosis beginning as expanding longitudinal melanonychia. Pediatr Dermatol 2005; 22: 210–212.

Index

Page numbers followed by *f, t* or *b* indicate Figures, Tables and Boxes.

erythematous lesions in 280
zinc abnormalities in 240
Cystic hygroma 108, 348*f*, 505, 505*f*. *See also*
Lymphangiomas
Cysts
arachnoid 360
branchial 115, 115*f*
bronchogenic 116
dental lamina 85
dermoid 36*b*, 118–19, 118*f*, 119*f*, 362
epidermal inclusion 85
epidermoid 118
eruption 504–5, 504*f*, 504*t*
foreskin 85–6
gingival (alveolar) 85
median raphe 116, 116*f*
of omphalomesenteric duct 127
oral mucosal 85
palatal 85
perineal median raphe 85–6
preauricular 113, 114, 114*t*
renal 479
thyroglossal 115–16
urachal 126, 127*f*
urethral retention 512
Cytokines
in atopic dermatitis 232
in neonates 27
Cytomegalic inclusion disease 331*f*
Cytomegalovirus (CMV) infection 81, 141
cutaneous findings 201
dermal erythropoiesis with 331
diagnosis of 195*t*, 201
etiology/pathogenesis 201
extracutaneous findings 201
treatment 201

D

Dandy-Walker malformation 355, 360, 415
Darier-White disease 288*t*
Darier's sign 80, 147, 269, 407, 408, 431, 438, 461,
468, 468*f*
Darkfield examination 80, 80*b*
for congenital syphilis 138
for treponemal antigen 80
De Barsy syndrome 482*t*, 483
Deep vein thrombosis 353
Deerfly bites 224*t*
DEET (*N,N,*-diethyl-*m*-toluamide) 64
Dellman syndrome 453
Demarcation lines, pigmentary 412
Demodicidosis 222, 222*t*
Depigmentation. *see* Albinism; Hypopigmentary
disorders
Dermablend 384
Dermabrasion, for epidermal nevus 438
Dermal hypoplasia 7
focal 100, 122, 138*t*
Dermal immune system (DIS) 26
Dermal melanosis (Mongolian spots) 346*f*. *See also*
Mongolian spots
Dermal microvascular unit (DMU) 26
Dermal ridge patterns, absent 138*t*, 153
Dermal webbing 8
Dermal-epidermal junction (DEJ)
in fetal development 8–9, 9*f*
in newborn skin 22, 22*f*
in premature infants 59
Dermatan sulfate 23

Dermatitis. *See also* Atopic dermatitis; Contact
dermatitis; Irritant diaper dermatitis;
Seborrheic dermatitis
'ammoniacal' 60
'baby-wipe' 63
Candida diaper 214–15, 215*f*, 248*t*
described 241
nickel 238
perianal/perineal streptococcal 248*t*, 258, 258*f*
zinc deficiency 260, 260*f*
Dermatofibrosarcoma protuberans (DFSP) 362, 464–
5, 465*f*
Dermatoglyphics 12
Dermatographism 467, 468
Dermatomal configuration 40*b*
Dermatophyte test medium (DTM) 74
Dermatophytosis
diagnosis of 220
diaper 248*t*
onychomycosis 220
tinea capitis 219–20
tinea corporis 219, 220
tinea faciei 219, 220
Trichophyton spp. 219
Dermatosis
acute febrile neutrophilic 320–21, 320*f*
chronic 137*t*
chronic bullous dermatosis of childhood
(CBDC) 149, 149*f*
congenital erosive and vesicular 137*t*, 150
erosive pustular dermatosis of the scalp 135*t*,
145
Dermis
anatomy of 20f
in embryonic dermal development 6–7
in fetal skin development 7–8
in newborn skin 22–23
specialized components of 8
Dermographism 147, 316, 318, 408
Dermoid cysts 36*b*, 118–19, 118*f*, 119*f*, 362
Dermopathy, restrictive 7, 137*t*, 152, 305, 305*f*
Dermoscopy 416–17
Desmoglein 3 3
Desmoid fibromatoses 425–6, 426*f*
Desquamation
of boric acid poisoning 268
in collodion baby 285*f*
neonatal 45, 61, 93, 95*f*, 96
of SSSS 269
Developmental abnormalities
accessory tragi 113, 114, 114*f*
adnexal polyp 126, 127*f*
amnion rupture malformation sequence 127–8,
128*f*
aplasia cutis 122–5, 122*f*, 124*f*, 125*f*
branchial cysts 115
bronchogenic cysts 116
cervical tabs 114–15
cranial dysraphism 116
cutaneous dimples 126
median raphe cysts 116
midline cervical clefts 116
neural tube dysraphism 116
preauricular pits and sinuses 113–14, 114*f*
supernumary digits 115, 115*f*
supernumary mammary tissue 113
supra umbilical cleft 116
of umbilicus 126–7, 127*f*
Developmental venous anomalies (DVAs) 347

Diabetes
gestational 33, 113
insipidus 463
Diagnostic procedures. *See also specific disorders*
bacterial cultures
Darier's sign 80
darkfield examination 80, 80*b*
direct fluorescent antibody (DFA) 74–5
EMLA in 78–9, 78*f*, 78*t*
fluorescence in situ hybridization 73, 81
for herpesvirus infection 74–5
immunofluorescence 73, 77–8
microscopic hair examination 76, 76*t*
Nikolsky sign 79–80, 268
polymerase chain reaction 73, 75, 80–81, 140
postoperative wound care 73, 79
potassium hydroxide preparation 73–4, 73*b*, 74*f*
prenatal 81
for scabies 73, 76*b*, 76*f*
skin biopsy 73, 77, 77*b*
Tzanck preparation 73, 74, 75*b*, 75*f*, 76*t*
viral culture 75
Wood's light exam 80
Diaper care products 245–6
Diaper dermatitis 60, 143, 389
candidal 214–15, 215*f*, 256–7, 256*f*, 268
with psoriasiform id 248*t*, 255, 255*f*
causes 245*b*
cutaneous findings in 246
differential diagnosis 251
etiology/pathogenesis of 250–51
incidence of 245
irritant (IDD) 50, 63, 229, 245, 246, 246*f*
management of 251
in premature infant 50
tinea 220, 220*f*
treatment and care 251
Diaper dermatophytosis 248*t*, 258, 259*f*
Diaper erosions 22, 143
Diapering: care of the diaper area in the
newborn 245–46
Diazoxide
hypertrichosis induced by 528
maculopapular eruption caused by 315*f*
Differentiation 5t
Diffuse cutaneous mastocytosis 167, 468
DiGeorge anomaly 276, 278*t*
Digital fibromatoses, infantile 427, 427*f*
Digits, supernumary 109, 109*f*, 115, 115*f*
Dilantin, effect on nails of 12
Dilate cardiopathy 290*t*
Dimples, cutaneous 117, 126
and amniocentesis 99, 99*f*
genetic disorders associated with 126, 126*b*
location of 126, 126*b*
lumbosacral 121, 121*f*
Diphenhydramine, hazards of percutaneous
absorption 60*t*
Diplegia, spastic 365
Direct fluorescent antibody (DFA) test 73
for herpes virus infection 74–75
for treponemal antigen 138
Disseminated intravascular coagulation (DIC)
due to congenital hypercoagulability 153*f*
purpura fulminans in 153
Distichiasis 531
DNA
and congenital skin disorders 13, 73
and CVS 99

PPK *see* Palmoplantar keratoderma
Prader-Willi syndrome 376
Preauricular pits and sinuses 113–14, 114*b*, 114*f*
Pregnancy, and parvovirus B19 205
Preimplantation genetic diagnosis (PGD) 81
Premature infant skin
 affect of light on 51
 anetoderma of 52, 100–101, 100*f*, 108
 care of 53–4
 characteristics of 19, 43
 diseases of 52–53
 and a fluid environment 59
 hemangiomas of 52–53
 increased permeability of 50
 and infection 50–51
 mechanical injury to 50
 neurocutaneous development in 52
 permeability of 21
 scarring of 52
 and thermal homeostasis 51 52
Premature infants
 consequences of skin immaturity for 43
 hemangiomas in 34
 major complications of 48
 skin care recommended for 69*b*
prenatal counseling 13
Prenatal diagnosis, DNA-based 81
Preservatives 60, 62
Presumptive epidermis 2
Preterm infants. *See also* Premature infants
 cutaneous water losses in 46
 permeability barrier in 45–46
 topical medications for 50
Prickly heat 86, 142
Prilocaine, hazards of percutaneous absorption 60*t*
Primary cutaneous aspergillosis (PCA) 139, 218, 218*f*
Probiotics 235
Procainamide, drug eruption caused by 315*f*
Profilaggrin 21
Proflavine hemisulfate 64
Progressive osseous heteroplasia (POH) 432–3, 434
Progressive symmetric erythrokeratoderma 300
Proprionobacteria, in premature infant skin 51
Propylene glycol, cautious use of 61*t*
Protein C concentrate 332–3
Protein S concentrate 333
Proteinosis, lipoid 473–4
Proteins C and S deficiency 331–3, 332*f*
Proteoglycans (PGs) 23
Proteus spp. 175
Proteus syndrome 7, 344*t*, 355, 437, 441, 487–8, 488*f*, 541
 clinical findings 487–8
 diagnostic criteria 488*b*
 differential diagnosis 488
 etiology/pathogenesis 488
 treatment and care 488
Prothrombin complex concentrate 332
'Prune-belly' syndrome 483, 483*f*
Pruritis. *See also* Urticaria
 of atopic dermatitis 229, 230, 232*b*, 234, 267
 in diffuse cutaneous mastocytosis 467
 in eosinophilic pustular folliculitis 144
 in erythema gyratum perstans 311
 in mastocytosis 467
 and moisturizers 62
 of scabies 220–21
 in seborrheic dermatitis 237
 in Sjögren-Larsson syndrome 296

Pseudo-Darier's sign 80
Pseudoanuria 63
Pseudoarthrosis, congenital 479
Pseudoclefts, of lip 355
Pseudohyphae 74*f*, 90
Pseudohypoparathyroidism (HP) 433, 448
Pseudomonas aeruginosa 62, 135, 138, 179, 180*f*
Pseudomonas infection infection 47, 80, 135, 138, 175
 diagnosis of 134*t*, 136*t*
 ecthyma gangrenosum 179–80, 180*f*
Pseudopseudohypoparathyroidism (PPHP) 433
Pseudosyndactyly 164
Pseudotail 121, 121*f*
Pseudothalidomide syndrome 355
Psoriasis 41*b*, 216, 237–8, 254*f*, 389
 candidal diaper dermatitis with psoriasiform id 248*t*, 255, 255*f*
 candidiasis with psoriasiform id 238
 characteristics of 237
 compared with atopic dermatitis 233
 compared with SD 237
 cutaneous findings in 237, 247*f*, 254
 diagnosis of 135*t*, 237, 247*t*
 differential diagnosis 237–8, 254, 267–8
 etiology/pathogenesis of 237, 254
 evaluation of 275*t*
 extracutaneous findings 254
 in HIV-infected patients 203
 incidence of 237
 linear 438
 prognosis/treatment 238, 254, 268, 275*t*
 pustular 75*t*, 135*t*, 147, 147*f*, 268
Ptychotropism 301
Pulse oximetry, complications of 107
Punch biopsy 77
 technique 77*b*
Purpura
 Henoch-Schönlein 325
 macular 462*f*
 in newborn 330, 330*b*
 in NLE 314
Purpura fulminans (PF) 180–81, 180*f*
 course/management/treatment/prognosis 181
 cutaneous findings 180
 diagnosis of 138*t*, 181
 differential diagnosis 181
 etiology/pathogenesis 181
 extracutaneous findings 180–81
 neonatal 138*t*, 153, 331–3, 332*f*
Purpuric EMLA-induced eruption 78–9, 78*f*
Purpuric phototherapy-induced eruption 333
Pustules
 acropustulosis of infancy 144, 144*f*
 in atopic dermatitis 133
 of *Candida* diaper dermatitis 215, 215*f*
 conditions presenting 131, 131*b*
 of congenital candidiasis 213, 214*f*
 described 37*b*
 of eosinophilic pustular folliculitis 144, 145*f*
 of erythema toxicum neonatorum 87, 88*f*, 141, 141*f*, 142
 infantile acne 90, 91
 in Langerhans' cell histiocytosis 462*f*
 of miliaria 142
 neonatal acne 90, 90*f*
 of PCA 218
 scabies 221, 221*f*
 in tinea infection 219, 220

 transient neonatal pustular melanosis 88, 89, 89*f*, 142, 142*f*
Pustulosis
 and erythroderma 268
 neonatal cephalic (neonatal acne) 90, 90*f*, 135*t*, 143*f*, 217
 staphylococcal 174*f*, 269
Pyloric atresia, EB with (PA-JEB) 9*f*, 22, 33, 159*t*, 161, 162
Pyoderma gangrenosum (PG) 263, 511–12
 clinical findings in 150–51, 151*f*
 diagnosis of 137*t*, 250*t*
Pyodermas 37*b*
Pyogenic granuloma 91, 368
Pyramidal perianal protrusion 249*t*, 511, 511*f*

R

'Raccoon eyes' 313, 313*f*
'Raccoon facies' 59
Racquet nails 538
Radiant warmers 50, 63, 67, 67*f*, 68, 68*f*, 167
Radiologic examination
 for aplasia cutis 125
 for Farber disease 471
 in NOMID 319
 of pseudotail 121
Ranulas 85
 congenital 503
Rapp-Hodgkin syndrome 491, 518, 522
Reaction patterns, in newborns 43
Recessive dystrophic EB (RDEB) 159, 159*t*, 164–5, 165*f*, 169
Red scaly baby, evaluation of 274, 274*b*. *See also* Erythrodermas
red-baby syndrome 315–16
Refsum disease 288*t*
Renal disease
 nail-patella syndrome in 540
 nodular calcification associated with 431
Rendu-Osler-Weber disease 349–50
Respiratory distress syndrome 50
Restrictive dermopathy 7, 137*t*, 152
Reticulate configuration 42*b*
Retiform configuration 42*b*
Retinoids, for harlequin ichthyosis 292
Retinopathy
 pigmentary 527
 of prematurity 51
Rh incompatibility, dermal erythropoiesis in 331*f*
Rhabdomyosarcomas 36*b*, 362, 466, 466*f*
Rhizopus infection 41*b*, 51, 219*f*
Richner-Hanhart syndrome 290*t*, 304
Riga-Fede disease 497, 506, 507*f*
Riley-Day syndrome 496–7, 497*b*
Riley-Smith syndrome 355, 411
Roberts syndrome 355
Rothmund-Thomson syndrome 346, 409, 489–90, 523
Rubella 195*t*, 202
 congenital 330, 330*f*, 513
 dermal erythropoiesis in 331
Rubenstein Taybi syndrome 434, 528
Rubor, from excessive hemoglobin 94
Ruvalcaba-Myhre-Smith syndrome 355, 411

S

Sabin-Feldman dye test 223
Sabinas brittle hair syndrome 519
Sacral medial telangiectatic vascular nevi 343

563

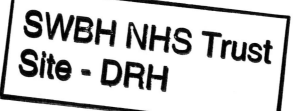